Life stage group	Choline (mg/d)	Calcium (mg/d)	Phosphorus (mg/d)	Magnesium (mg/d)	Iron (mg/d)	Zinc (mg/d)	Selenium (µg/d)	Iodine (µg/d)	Copper (µg/d)	Manganese (mg/d)	Fluoride (mg/d)	Chromium (µg/d)	Molybdenum (µg/d)
Infants													
0-6 mo	125*	210*	100*	30*	0.27*	2*	15*	110*	200*	0.003*	0.01*	0.2*	2*
7-12 mo	150*	270*	275*	75*	11	3	20*	130*	220*	0.6*	0.5*	5.5*	3*
Children													
1-3 y	200*	500*	460	80	7	3	20	90	340	1.2*	0.7*	11*	17
4-8 y	250*	800*	500	130	10	5	30	90	440	1.5*	1*	15*	22
Males													
9-13 y	375*	1,300*	1,250	240	8	8	40	120	700	1.9*	2*	25*	34
14-18 y	550*	1,300*	1,250	410	11	11	55	150	890	2.2*	3*	35*	43
19-30 y	550*	1,000*	700	400	8	11	55	150	900	2.3*	4*	35*	45
31-50 y	550*	1,000*	700	420	8	11	55	150	900	2.3*	4*	35*	45
51-70 y	550*	1,200*	700	420	8	11	55	150	900	2.3*	4*	30*	45
>70 y	550*	1,200*	700	420	8	11	55	150	900	2.3*	4*	30*	45
Females													
9-13 y	375*	1,300*	1,250	240	8	8	40	120	700	1.6*	2*	21*	34
14-18 y	400*	1,300*	1,250	360	15	9	55	150	890	1.6*	3*	24*	43
19-30 y	425*	1,000*	700	310	18	8	55	150	900	1.8*	3*	25*	45
31-50 y	425*	1,000*	700	320	18	8	55	150	900	1.8*	3*	25*	45
51-70 y	425*	1,200*	700	320	8	8	55	150	900	1.8*	3*	20*	45
>70 y	425*	1,200*	700	320	8	8	55	150	900	1.8*	3*	20*	45
Pregnancy													
≤18 y	450*	1,300*	1,250	400	27	13	60	220	1,000	2.0*	3*	29*	50
19-30 y	450*	1,000*	700	350	27	11	60	220	1,000	2.0*	3*	30*	50
31-50 y	450*	1,000*	700	360	27	11	60	220	1,000	2.0*	3*	30*	50
Lactation													
≤18 y	550*	1,300*	1,250	360	10	14	70	290	1,300	2.6*	3*	44*	50
19-30 y	550*	1,000*	700	310	9	12	70	290	1,300	2.6*	3*	45*	50
31-50 y	550*	1,000*	700	320	9	12	70	290	1,300	2.6*	3*	45*	50

Sources: Data compiled from *Dietary Reference Intakes for Calcium, Phosphorus, Magnesium, Vitamin D, and Fluoride.* Washington, DC: National Academy Press; 1997. *Dietary Reference Intakes for Thiamin, Riboflavin, Niacin, Vitamin B$_6$, Folate, Vitamin B$_{12}$, Pantothenic Acid, Biotin, and Choline.* Washington, DC: National Academy Press; 1998. *Dietary Reference Intakes for Vitamin C, Vitamin E, Selenium, and Carotenoids.* Washington, DC: National Academy Press; 2000. *Dietary Reference Intakes for Vitamin A, Vitamin K, Arsenic, Boron, Chromium, Copper, Iron, Manganese, Molybdenum, Nickel, Silicon, Vanadium, and Zinc.* Washington, DC: National Academy Press; 2001. These reports may be accessed via http://nap.edu.

Nutrition

Paul Insel
Stanford University

R. Elaine Turner
University of Florida

Don Ross
California Institute of Human Nutrition

American Dietetic Association

JONES AND BARTLETT PUBLISHERS

Sudbury, Massachusetts

BOSTON   TORONTO   LONDON   SINGAPORE

World Headquarters
Jones and Bartlett Publishers
40 Tall Pine Drive
Sudbury, MA 01776
978-443-5000
info@jbpub.com
www.jbpub.com

Jones and Bartlett Publishers Canada
2406 Nikanna Road
Mississauga, ON L5C 2W6
CANADA

Jones and Bartlett Publishers International
Barb House, Barb Mews
London W6 7PA
UK

Production Credits

Chief Executive Officer: Clayton Jones
Chief Operating Officer: Don W. Jones, Jr.
V.P., Managing Editor: Judith H. Hauck
V.P., Design and Production: Anne Spencer
V.P., Manufacturing and Inventory Control: Therese Bräuer
Sponsoring Editor: Suzanne Jeans
Senior Production Editor: Lianne Ames
Developmental Editor: Ohlinger Publishing Services
Art Development: Judith H. Hauck
Associate Editor: Amy Austin
Editorial/Production Assistant: Amanda Green
Interactive Technology Project Editor: Nicole Healy
Web Product Manager: Adam Alboyadjian
Web Site Designer: Kristin Ohlin
Design and Composition: Studio Montage
Copyediting: Joan Flaherty
Editorial Production Service: Ohlinger Publishing Services
Illustration: Imagineering Scientific and Technical Artwork, Studio Montage
Cover Design: Anne Spencer
Cover Photo: © Minori Kawana/Photonica
Printing and Binding: Courier Companies
Cover Printing: John Pow Company

Dedication

To Michelle whose unwavering warmth, support and patience sustained me through an arduous two years of this creative challenge.

To Allen, Mitchell, and Teddy for their love, patience, and understanding.

To Donna and Mackinnon whose inspiration and support helped bring this allconsuming task to fruition.

ISBN 0-7637-1985-4
This text (ISBN 0-7637-1985-4 © 2002) represents an update of the original © 2001 edition (ISBN 0-7637-0893-3).

Library of Congress Cataloging-in-Publication Data

Insel, Paul
    Nutrition / Paul Insel, R. Elaine Turner, Don Ross.
       p. cm.
    Includes bibliographical references and index.
    ISBN 0-7637-0893-3
       1. Nutrition I. Turner, R. Elaine II.Ross, Don. III. Title
QP141.I63 2001
612.3'9–dc21
                   00-052008

Printed in the United States of America
04 03 02   10 9 8 7 6 5 4 3

The material in this book has been favorably reviewed by the American Dietetic Association.

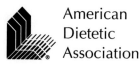 **American Dietetic Association**

216 W. Jackson Blvd. Chicago, IL 60606 (800) 877-1600

www.eatright.org

With nearly 70,000 members, the American Dietetic Association is the nation's largest organization of food and nutrition professionals.

ADA was founded in Cleveland, Ohio, in 1917 by a visionary group of women, led by ADA's first president, Lulu C. Graves, and co-founder Lenna F. Cooper, who were dedicated to helping the government conserve food and improve the American public's health and nutrition during World War I.

Members

Approximately 75 percent of ADA's members are registered dietitians (RDs) and four percent are dietetic technicians, registered (DTRs). Other ADA members include clinical and community dietetics professionals, consultants, food service managers, educators, researchers, dietetic technicians and students.

ADA members represent a wide range of practice areas and special interests, including: public health; sports nutrition; medical nutrition therapy; nutrition counseling for weight control, cholesterol reduction, diabetes, heart and kidney disease and many other health concerns; food service management in business, hospitals, restaurants, long-term care facilities, and education systems; education of other health-care professionals; and scientific research. Members can also join 28 special interest or dietetic practice groups.

What is a registered dietitian?

A registered dietitian is a food and nutrition expert who has met the minimum academic and professional requirements to qualify for the credential "RD." In addition to RD credentialing, many states have laws that regulate the licensure or credentialing of dietitians and nutrition practitioners. Frequently these state requirements are met through the same education and training required to become an RD.

Registered dietitians must:

- Complete at least a bachelor's degree and course work approved by ADA's Commission on Accreditation for Dietetics Education.
- Complete an accredited and supervised experiential practice program at a health-care facility, community agency or foodservice corporation.
- Pass a national examination administered by the Commission on Dietetic Registration.
- And complete continuing professional educational requirements to maintain registration.

What is a dietetic technician, registered?

Dietetic technicians, registered (DTRs), often working in partnership with registered dietitians, screen, evaluate and educate patients; provide guidance in prevention of diseases such as diabetes and obesity; and monitor the progress of a patient or client. DTRs provide expert assistance in hospices, home health-care programs, day-care centers, foodservice operations, government and community programs such as Meals on Wheels.

Dietetic technicians, registered must:

- Complete at least a two-year associate's degree in an approved dietetics technology program from an accredited U.S. college or university
- Complete a minimum of 450 hours of supervised practice experience in community programs, health care and food service facilities
- Pass a nationwide examination and continuing education courses throughout their careers.

Commission on Dietetic Registration

The Commission on Dietetic Registration, the credentialing agency for ADA, awards credentials at entry, fellow and specialty levels to individuals who have met its standards for competency to practice in the profession, including successful completion of its national certification examination and recertification by continuing professional education and/or examination.

Brief Contents

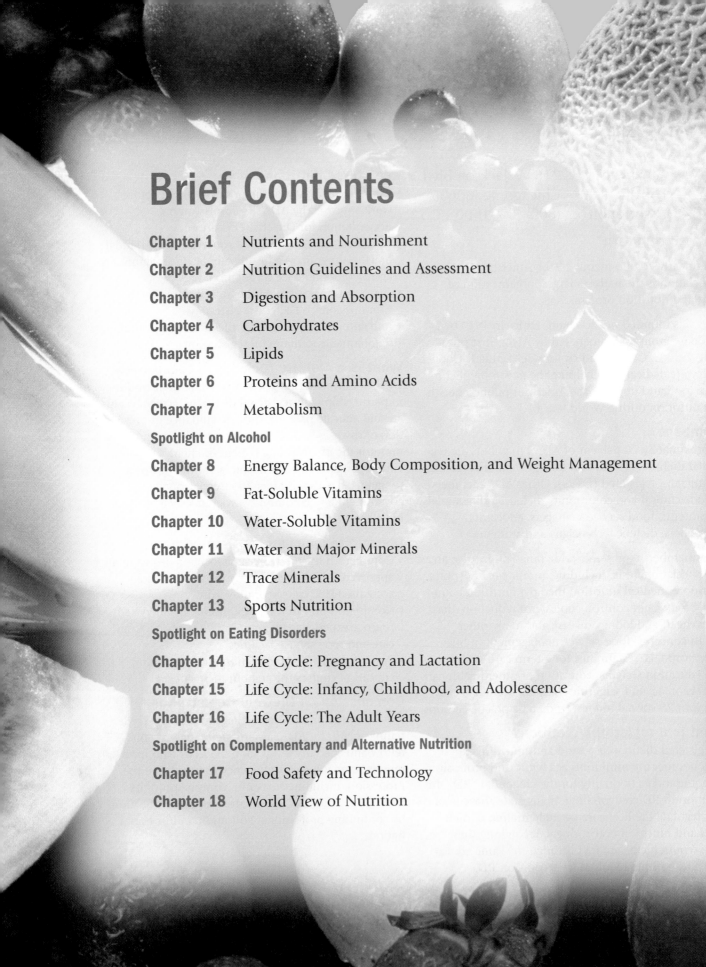

Table of Contents

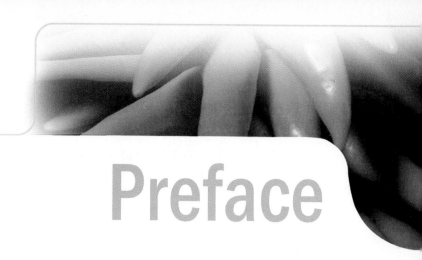

Preface

*P*eople's food preferences differ. They overeat. They undereat. They shop at health food stores. They eat mostly at fast-food restaurants. They don't eat eggs. But they eat fish. They eat only "organic" foods.

Perhaps the most significant development in the field of nutrition is the recognition that behavior and personal decision making play important roles in the way people eat. Most of us know the difference between healthful and unhealthful diets, but we often ignore what we know. Many people mistakenly believe that good nutrition is incompatible with pleasurable eating. A Harris poll suggests that two in three Americans think they'd be healthier if they changed their diets, but they continue to eat the way they always have because they enjoy it and believe they lack the willpower to change. Willpower, however, is not usually the issue. Instead, many people lack the basic skills and understanding to change their behaviors and make good and healthful choices.

Healthful Choices

Learning nutrition can be fun and exciting, *and* understandable. Our new book, *Nutrition*, will guide students on a fascinating journey beginning, perhaps, with curiosity and, we hope, ending with a solid knowledge base and a healthy dose of skepticism for the endless ads and infomercials promoting "new" diets and food products. We want students to learn enough about their nutritional and health status to use this new knowledge in their everyday lives. Our mission is to give students the tools to interpret more logically the nutrition information provided by the evening news, on food labels, in popular magazines, and by government agencies. Our goal is to help them become sophisticated consumers of both nutrients and nutrition information. Through this course they will come to understand that knowledge of nutrition allows them to personalize information, rather than follow every guideline issued for an entire population.

Nutrition is unique in its behavioral approach. It challenges students to act, not just memorize the material.

Familiar experiences and choices draw students into each chapter and analogies illuminate difficult concepts.

In addition, we address important questions that students often raise concerning ethnic diets, eating disorders, nutrient supplements, phytochemicals, vegetarianism, diets for athletes, food safety, and fad diets. We spotlight alcohol, eating disorders, and alternative nutrition. Throughout the book, the relationship of diet and health is incorporated into appropriate chapters (e.g., lipids and cardiovascular disease, carbohydrates and diabetes).

Nutrition research shows that people often respond idiosyncratically to food. Some of us, for example, find that we can liberally salt our food with no effect on our blood pressure. Others, who are salt sensitive, find that even a small amount of salt sends their systolic blood pressure soaring. *Nutrition* brings up-to-date nutritional research into your class. It features the latest standards, such as the *Dietary Reference Intakes* and *Dietary Guidelines for Americans* published in 2000. In addition, the book's web site, **nutrition.jbpub.com**, offers access to the constantly emerging developments in nutrition.

Accessible Science

Nutrition is based on the latest in learning theory and balances the behavioral aspects of nutrition with an accessible approach to scientific concepts. This introduction to the field allows students to master both areas so that they succeed in subsequent nutrition courses. Scientifically, nothing is left out. You will find the book to be a comprehensive resource that communicates graphically in a personal, interesting way.

We present chemistry in an engaging, non-intimidating way with an appealing, stepwise, parallel development of text and annotated illustrations. Understanding molecular structure, shape, and reactivity is central to understanding nutritional chemistry, so each type of nutrient molecule in this book has a distinct color and shape. Icons of an amino acid, a protein, a triglyceride, and a glucose molecule represent "characters" in a chemical event, instantly recognizable when they appear in later chapters.

This textbook is unique in the field of nutrition and leads the way in depicting important biological and physiological phenomena, such as transport across cell membranes, emulsification, glucose regulation, digestion and absorption, and fetal development. Extensive graphic presentations make nutrition and physiological principles come alive. Illustrations depict the fine details of important processes in the part of the cell or tissue where the processes occur.

In addition to these strengths, the contents of this book have been favorably reviewed by the American Dietetic Association, the nation's largest organization of food and nutrition professionals with nearly 70,000 members.

The Pedagogy

Nutrition focuses on teaching behavioral change, personal decision making, and up-to-date scientific concepts in a number of novel ways. The interactive approach that addresses different learning styles makes it the ideal text to ensure a high likelihood of success by students. Beginning with Chapter 1, the material engages students in considering their own behavior in light of the knowledge they are gaining. The pedagogical aids that appear in most chapters include:

Think About It questions at the beginning of each chapter present realistic nutrition-related situations and ask the students to consider how they would behave in such circumstances.

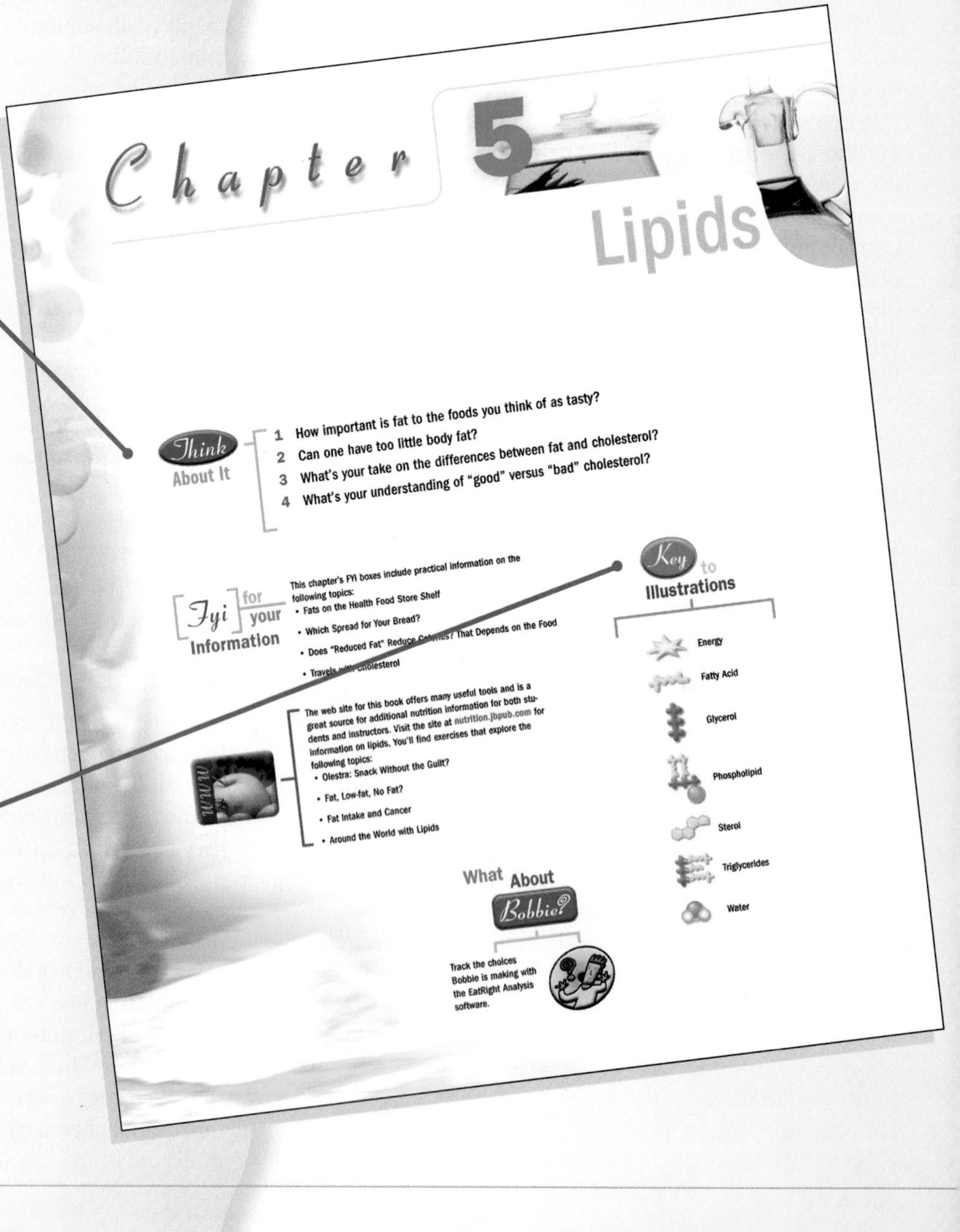

The **Key to Illustrations** at the beginning of each chapter identifies the icons students will encounter throughout the book. These *chemical icons* identify molecular components of nutrient molecules, making their construction and deconstruction visually and conceptually accessible.

Chapter 5 Lipids

Think About It

1 How important is fat to the foods you think of as tasty?
2 Can one have too little body fat?
3 What's your take on the differences between fat and cholesterol?
4 What's your understanding of "good" versus "bad" cholesterol?

Fyi for your Information

This chapter's FYI boxes include practical information on the following topics:
• Fats on the Health Food Store Shelf
• Which Spread for Your Bread?
• Does "Reduced Fat" Reduce Calories? That Depends on the Food
• Travels with Cholesterol

The web site for this book offers many useful tools and is a great source for additional nutrition information for both students and instructors. Visit the site at nutrition.jbpub.com for information on lipids. You'll find exercises that explore the following topics:
• Olestra: Snack Without the Guilt?
• Fat, Low-fat, No Fat?
• Fat Intake and Cancer
• Around the World with Lipids

Key to Illustrations

Energy
Fatty Acid
Glycerol
Phospholipid
Sterol
Triglycerides
Water

What About Bobbie?

Track the choices Bobbie is making with the EatRight Analysis software.

Key terms are in boldface type the first time they are mentioned. Their definitions also appear in the margins near the relevant textual discussion, making it easy for students to review material and terms.

---

718 *Chapter 18* WORLD VIEW OF NUTRITION

Food and Agriculture Organization (FAO) The largest autonomous UN agency; the FAO works to alleviate poverty and hunger by promoting agricultural development, improved nutrition, and the pursuit of food security

Quick Bites

Where were you born?

Your survival was greatly influenced by the location of your birth. Angola has the highest infant mortality rate (195 deaths per 1,000 live births), according to estimates for 2000. Other countries with high infant mortality rates include Sierra Leone (148 per 1,000), Afghanistan (149 per 1,000), and Liberia (134 per 1,000). At the other end of the spectrum is Finland (4 per 1,000). Canada (5 per 1,000) does better than the United States (7 per 1,000).

Hunger in the developing world is chronic. "It is debilitating. It blights the lives of all who are affected and undermines national economies and development processes where it is found on a large scale," says the **Food and Agriculture Organization** of the United Nations.[20] Although food shortages severe enough to cause endemic starvation or famine have lessened significantly, natural disasters, epidemics, economic or political upheaval, or war can quickly precipitate famine.[21]

Why Hunger?

Why, in a world of plenty, does hunger still exist? The causes are simple, but the solutions are tremendously complex; they require economic, political, and social change, as well as improvements in nutrition, food production, and environmental safeguards. As you study the critical nutrient deficiencies in the developing world, you will see that poverty, infection, poor sanitation, and social upheaval interact with nutrient shortages to bring about the deficiencies.

Social and Economic Factors

Poverty, overpopulation, and the migration to overcrowded cities are closely interrelated causes of hunger (**Figure 18.6**). Each situation worsens the effects of the others as they steadily drive a population toward malnutrition.

Poverty

Poverty is the most important underlying reason for chronic hunger. It limits access to food, obviously. It limits purchase of farming supplies to grow food, boats and equipment to fish, and storage equipment to prevent spoilage. It limits access to medical care. It compromises efforts at sanitation. It discourages education and the chance for personal advancement. For nations, poverty means paralyzed economic development and too few jobs; inadequate investments in infrastructure and basic housing; and too few resources to train doctors, nutritionists, nurses, and other health-care workers.

Fyi
FOR YOUR INFORMATION
AIDS and Malnutrition

Like other infections, HIV interacts with malnutrition in a vicious, devastating cycle. Left untreated, HIV infection progresses to the acquired immunodeficiency syndrome (AIDS). The virus attacks by destroying its victim's immune system. Unable to fight infections and malignancies, disease quickly depletes marginal nutrient stores, speeding the way to severe malnutrition and death. But malnutrition and HIV interact on several other levels, as well:

• Low vitamin A levels in pregnant women increase the rate of HIV transmission to their unborn babies.[1]

• HIV is transmitted to infants in breast milk; but in impoverished regions, substitutions for breast milk typically increase infantile diarrhea, malnutrition, and death.[2]

• AIDS leaves mothers too weak to feed and care for their children. Eventually AIDS turns children into orphans.

• AIDS disables parents so they cannot work to support and feed their families.

• Reduced levels of micronutrients in an HIV-infected person are associated with faster progression of HIV disease and AIDS.[3]

• Weight loss and muscle wasting in an infected person are associated with faster progression of HIV disease and AIDS.[4]

• Infections that accompany AIDS cause fever and diarrhea, worsening malnutrition. Nausea and loss of appetite also contribute to malnutrition.

• Severe protein-energy malnutrition (PEM) is characteristic of untreated AIDS, and frequently the ultimate cause of death.

Quick Bites are sprinkled throughout the book. They offer fun facts about nutrition-related topics such as exotic foods, social customs, origins of phrases, folk remedies, medical history, and so on.

For Your Information offer more in-depth treatment of controversial and timely topics, such as unfounded claims about the effects of sugar, whether athletes need more protein, and megadoses of vitamins.

Key Concepts summarize previous text and highlight important information.

Label to Table helps students apply their new decision-making skills at the supermarket. It walks students through the various types of information that appear on food labels, including government-mandated terminology, misleading advertising phrases, and amounts of ingredients.

---

172   Chapter 5   LIPIDS

13. Do not eat charred food. For meat and fish eaters, avoid burning meat juices. Consume the following only occasionally: meat and fish grilled (broiled) in a direct flame; cured or smoked meats.

14. For those who follow these recommendations, dietary supplements are probably unnecessary, and possibly unhelpful, for reducing cancer risk.

Key Concepts: *Excessive fat intake has been linked to obesity, heart disease, and cancer. There is a major public heath effort to reduce intake of fat, saturated fat, and cholesterol. Cholesterol-lowering diets have changed over the years, with somewhat less emphasis on reducing dietary cholesterol, and more on reducing fats and saturated fats, and increasing fruits, vegetables, and whole grains. The evidence linking dietary fats with cancer is less clear, but many other dietary factors are important in reducing risk.*

Label [to] Table

The Nutrition Facts panel shown here highlights all of the lipid-related information you can find on a food label. Look to the top of the label where it states that this product contains 35 Calories from Fat. Do you know how you can estimate this number from another part of the label? Recall (or look to the bottom of the label) that each gram of fat contains 9 kilocalories. If this food item has 4 grams of fat, then it should make sense that there are approximately 36 kilocalories provided by fat. In this case, because the manufacturer listed only 35 you can assume that the 4 grams fat on the label is rounded up from the actual total fat content of 3.9 grams (3.9 grams of fat × 9 kilocalories per gram = 35 kilocalories of fat).

Total Fat is the second thing you'll see along with saturated fat. Recall that fats are classified into 3 types: saturated, monounsaturated, and polyunsaturated. Manufacturers are required to list only saturated fat on the label but they can voluntarily list the others. Using this food label, you can estimate the amount of unsaturated fat by simply looking at the highlighted sections. There are 4 total grams of fat and 2.5 of them are saturated. That means the remaining 1.5 grams are either polyunsaturated or monounsaturated. Without even knowing what food item this label represents, you can decipher that it contains more saturated fat than unsaturated fat (2.5g vs. 1.5g). This is typical of a food that contains fat from an animal source or tropical oil.

Do you see the 6% to the right of "Total Fat"? This does not mean that the food item contains 6% of its calories from fat. In fact, this food item contains 23% of its calories from fat (35 fat kcal / 154 total kilocalories = .23, or 23% fat). The 6% refers to the Daily Values found below. You can see that a person who consumes 2,000 kcalories per day could consume up to 65 grams of fat per day. This product contributes just 4 grams per serving, which is 6% of that amount (4 / 65 = .06, or 6%). Note that the % Daily Value for saturated fat is 12% which means that just a few servings of this food can contribute quite a bit of saturated fat to your diet. Cholesterol is also highlighted on this label (20 mg) along with its Daily Value contribution (7%).

Nutrition Facts

Serving Size: 1 cup (248g)
Servings Per Container: 4

Amount Per Serving

Calories 154   Calories from fat 35

	% Daily Value*
Total Fat 4g	6%
Saturated Fat 2.5g	12%
Cholesterol 20mg	7%
Sodium 170mg	7%
Total Carbohydrate 19g	6%
Dietary Fiber 0g	0%
Sugars 14g	
Protein 11g	

Vitamin A 4%	•	Vitamin C 6%
Calcium 40%	•	Iron 0%

* Percent Daily Values are based on a 2,000 calorie diet. Your daily values may be higher or lower depending on your calorie needs:

		Calories:	2,000	2,500
Total Fat	Less Than		65g	80g
Sat Fat	Less Than		20g	25g
Cholesterol	Less Than		300mg	300mg
Sodium	Less Than		2,400mg	2,400mg
Total Carbohydrate			300g	375g
Dietary Fiber			25g	30g

Calories per gram:
Fat 9 • Carbohydrate 4 • Protein 4

The **Learning Portfolio** at the end of each chapter collects, in one place, all aspects of nutrition information students need to solidify their understanding of the material. The various formats will appeal to students according to their individual learning and studying styles.

Key Terms lists all new vocabulary alphabetically with the page number of the first appearance. This arrangement allows students to review any term they do not recall and turn immediately to the definition and discussion of it in the chapter. This approach promotes the acquisition of knowledge, not simply memorization.

Study Points is a bulleted list that summarizes the content of each chapter with a synopsis of each major topic. The points are in the order in which they appear in the chapter, so related concepts flow together.

---

174 Chapter 5 LIPIDS

LEARNING *Portfolio*

c h a p t e r 5

Key Terms

	page
adipocyte	144
adipose tissue	144
alpha-linolenic acid [Al-fah-lin-oh-LEN-ik]	
atherosclerosis [ath-e-roh-scle-ROH-sis]	142
bioavailability	151
cardiovascular disease (CVD)	144
chain length	167
cholesterol [ko-LES-te-rol]	136
choline	151
chylomicron [kye-lo-MY-kron]	149
cis fatty acids	155
conjugated linoleic acid	140
depot fat	140
desaturation	144
diglyceride	140
eicosanoids	143
elongation	140
enterocytes	140
essential fatty acids	155
ester	140
esterification [e-ster-ih-fih-KAY-shun]	143
fat substitutes	143
fatty acid	163
glycerol [GLISS-er-ol]	136
high-density lipoprotein (HDL)	142
hydrogenation [high-dro-jen-AY-shun]	159
hydrophobic	140
hypercholesterolemia	136
lipophilic	167
hydrophilic [high-dro-FILL-ik]	136
	136

	page
intermediate-density lipoprotein (IDL)	159
lanugo [lah-NEW-go]	144
lecithin	149
linoleic acid [lin-oh-LAY-ik]	142
lipophobic	136
lipoprotein	165
lipoprotein lipase (LPL)	158
low-density lipoprotein (LDL)	
lycopene	159
micelles	144
monoglyceride	154
monounsaturated fatty acid	143
nonessential fatty acid	138
obesity	140
olestra	166
omega-3 fatty acid	163
omega-6 fatty acid	140
omega-9 fatty acid	140
oxidation	140
phosphate group	147
phospholipid	148
phytosterols	136
polyunsaturated fatty acid	153
saturated fatty acid	138
squalene	138
steatorrhea	153
sterols	155
subcutaneous fat	136
trans fatty acids	144
unsaturated fatty acid	140
very-low-density lipoprotein (VLDL)	158
visceral fat	144

Study Points

- Lipids are a group of compounds that are soluble in organic solvents but not in water. Fats and oils are part of the lipids group.
- There are three main classes of lipids: triglycerides, phospholipids, and sterols.
- Fatty acids-long carbon chains with methyl and carboxyl groups on the ends-are components of both triglycerides and phospholipids, and are often attached to cholesterol.
- Saturated fatty acids have no double bonds between carbons in the chain, monounsaturated fatty acids have one double bond, and polyunsaturated fatty acids have more than one double bond.
- Two polyunsaturated fatty acids, linoleic acid and alpha-linolenic acid, are essential; they must be supplied in the diet. Phospholipids and sterols are made in the body and do not have to be supplied in the diet.
- Essential fatty acids are elongated and desaturated in the process of making "local hormones" called eicosanoids. These compounds regulate many body functions.
- Triglycerides are food fats and storage fats. They are composed of glycerol and three fatty acids.
- In the body, triglycerides are an important source of energy. Stored fat provides an energy reserve.
- Phospholipids are made of glycerol, two fatty acids, and a phosphate group with a nitrogen-containing component.
- Phospholipids are components of cell membranes and lipoproteins. Their unique affinity for both fat and water allows them to be effective emulsifiers in foods and in the body.
- Cholesterol is found in cell membranes and is used to synthesize vitamin D, bile acids, and steroid hormones. High levels of blood cholesterol are associated with heart disease risk.
- Most sources recommend that Americans consume no more than 30 percent of calories as fat, no more than 10 percent of calories as saturated fat, and no more than 300 milligrams of cholesterol each day.
- Diets high in fat and saturated fat tend to increase blood levels of LDL cholesterol and increase risk for heart disease.
- Excess fat in the diet is linked to obesity and some types of cancer.

The **Learning Portfolio** (continued)

Study Questions encourage students to probe deeper into the chapter content, making connections and gaining new insights. Although these questions can be used for pop quizzes, they will also help students to review, especially students who study by writing out material. They can check their work by looking at the **Study Questions with Answers** feature, which appears at the end of the appendices.

What About Bobbie? tracks the eating habits and health-related decisions of a typical college student so that students can apply the material they have learned in the chapter to a typical situation. Following the individual case of Bobbie takes students from the general concepts to the specific application of new information. As a complement to this textual feature, the EatRight Analysis CD allows students to track the various choices Bobbie makes, as well as their own food choices.

Try This! activities are for curious students who like to experiment. These suggestions for hands-on activities encourage students to put theory into practice. It will especially help students whose major learning style is experiential.

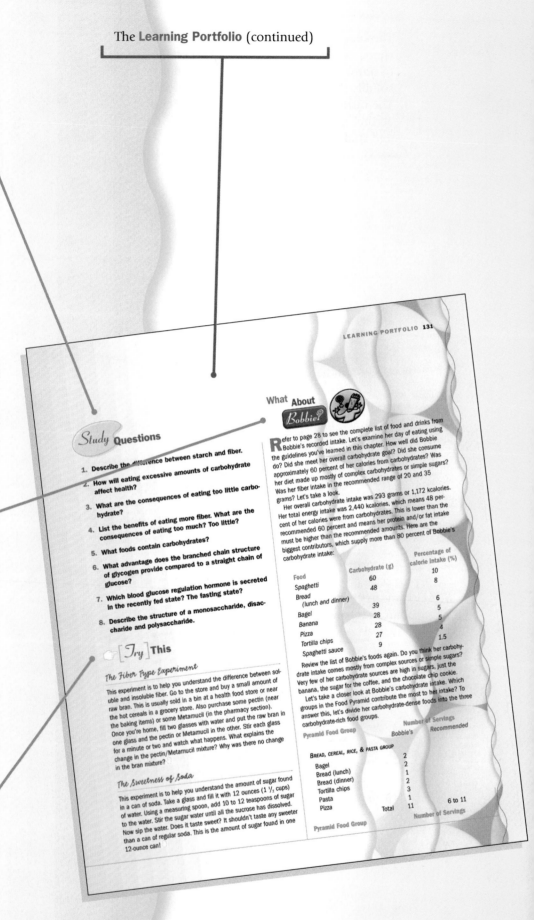

The Integrated Learning and Teaching Package

Integrating the text and ancillaries is crucial to deriving their full benefit. Based on feedback from instructors and students, Jones and Bartlett Publishers offers the following supplements.

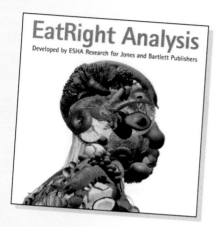

The **EatRight Analysis CD** is an important component of the behavioral change and personal decision-making focus. EatRight Analysis, developed by ESHA Research and tailored by the authors, enables students to analyze their diets by calculating their nutrient intake and comparing it to recommended intake levels.

The **web site** for *Nutrition*, **nutrition.jbpub.com**, offers students and instructors an unprecedented degree of integration between their text and the on-line world through many useful study tools, activities, and supplementary health information.

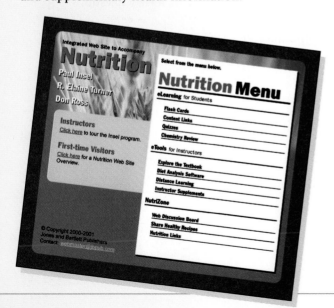

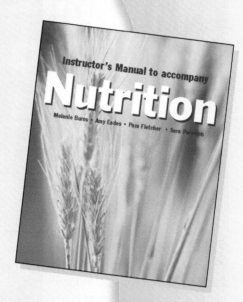

The **Instructor's Manual** is a comprehensive teaching resource available to adopters of the book. It includes chapter outlines, strategies for teaching difficult concepts, and a testbank.

The **Instructor's ToolKit CD-ROM** features an Image Bank of art that can be imported into tests or projected for class. It also includes:

- PowerPoint Lecture Presentation Slides
- Instructor's Guide
- Computerized TestBank

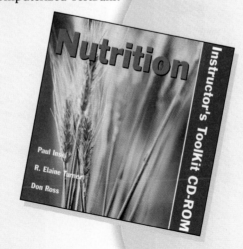

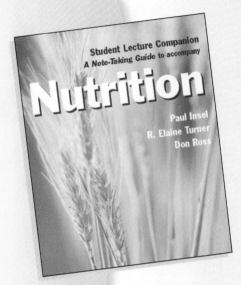

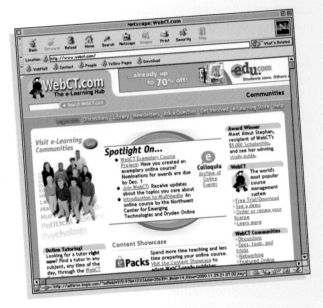

The **Student Lecture Companion for Nutrition** provides a visual guide that follows *Nutrition's* chapter topics and contains a print version of the PowerPoint slides included in the Instructor's ToolKit. Students can concentrate better during lectures and take notes without having to copy down the text from the slides.

WebCT is a customizable, web-based teaching and learning environment that offers distance learning tools for you and your students. Pre-loaded and fully customizable, the WebCT e-Pack offers:

- PowerPoint presentations, lecture outlines, and course syllabus
- Electronic posting and submission of assignments
- TestBank to create and administer online tests or quizzes
- Course management tools such as student rosters and immediate grade tracking and posting
- Student review tools such as review questions, web links, and flashcards
- Communications tools such as discussion boards, chat rooms, and e-mail

CyberClass is a Web-based customizable teaching and learning environment that offers on-line course-management tools for instructors (e.g., on-line quizzes) and learning tools for students (e.g., on-line flashcards). You can put your course on-line in less than an hour! Visit **www.jbcyberclass.com**, for more information.

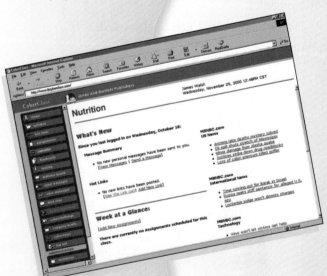

About the Authors

The *Nutrition* author team represents a culmination of years of teaching and research in psychology and nutrition science. The combined experience of the authors yields a balanced presentation of both the science of nutrition and the components of behavioral change.

Dr. Paul Insel is Clinical Associate Professor of Psychiatry and Behavioral Sciences at Stanford University (Stanford, California). In addition to being the principal investigator on several nutrition projects for the National Institutes of Health (NIH), he is the senior author of the seminal text in health education and has co-authored several best-selling nutrition books.

Dr. R. Elaine Turner is a Registered Dietitian and Assistant Professor in the Food Science and Human Nutrition Department at the University of Florida (Gainesville, Florida). Dr. Turner has been teaching courses in introductory and life-cycle nutrition for nearly 15 years. Her interests include nutrition labeling and dietary supplement regulations, computer applications in nutrition and education, maternal and infant nutrition, and consumer issues. Dr. Turner was named Undergraduate Teacher of the Year, 2000-2001, for the College of Agricultural and Life Sciences.

Don Ross is co-director of the California Institute of Human Nutrition (Redwood City, California). For 15 years he has created educational materials about health and nutrition for consumers, professionals, and college students. He has special expertise in communicating complicated physiological processes with easily understood graphical presentations. The National Institutes of Health selected his Travels with Cholesterol for distribution to consumers. His multidisciplinary focus brings together the fields of psychology, nutrition, biochemistry, and medicine.

Contributors

The following people contributed to this project:

Janine T. Baer, PhD, RD
University of Dayton
Chapter 13 Sports Nutrition
Chapter 14 Life Cycle: Pregnancy and Lactation

Toni Bloom, MS, RD, CDE
Past President of Nutrition Entrepreneurs DPG
Pedagogy

Boyce W. Burge, PhD
Chapter 17 Food Safety and Technology

Eileen G. Ford, MS, RD
Drexel University
Chapter 15 Life Cycle: Infancy, Childhood, and Adolescence

Ellen B. Fung, PhD, RD
University of Pennsylvania
Chapter 12 Trace Minerals

Sujatha Ganapathy, MS
University of Massachusetts
Chapter 8 Energy Balance, Body Composition, and Weight Management

Michael I. Goran, PhD
University of Southern California
Chapter 8 Energy Balance, Body Composition, and Weight Management

Nancy J. Gustafson, MS, RD, FADA
Chapter 4 Carbohydrates
Chapter 6 Proteins and Amino Acids

Rita H. Herskovitz, MS
University of Pennsylvania
Chapter 12 Trace Minerals

Jocie Iszler, MS, RD
Chapter 17 Food Safety and Technology

Nancy I. Kemp, MD
University of California, San Francisco
Chapter 11 Water and Major Minerals

Sarah Harding Laidlaw, MS, RD, MPA
Chapter 16 Life Cycle: The Adult Years

Rick D. Mattes, MPH, PhD, RD
Purdue University
Chapter 1 Food Choices

Lois McBean, MS, RD
National Dairy Council
Chapter 4 Lactose intolerance

Virginia L. Mermel, PhD, CNS
California Polytechnic State University
Chapter 3 Digestion and Absorption
Spotlight on Eating Disorders

Maye Musk, MS, RD
Chapter 18 World View of Nutrition

Joyce D. Nash, PhD
Chapter 8 Energy Balance, Body Composition,
and Weight Management

Barbara Quinn, MS, RD
Chapter 13 Sports Nutrition

Rachel Stern, MS, RD, CNS
Chapter 5 Lipids
Spotlight on Alcohol
Chapter 18 World View of Nutrition

Lisa Stollman, MA, RD, CDE, CDN
Chapter 3 Digestion and Absorption

Barbara Sutherland, PhD
University of California, Davis
Chapter 7 Metabolism

Scott Turner, BA, PhD
University of California, Berkeley
Chapter 11 Water and Major Minerals

Debra M. Vinci, PhD, RD, CD
Appalachian State University
Chapter 13 Sports Nutrition

Stella L. Volpe, PhD, RD, FACSM
University of Massachusetts
Chapter 8 Energy Balance, Body Composition,
and Weight Management

Paula Kurtzweil Walter, MS, RD
Federal Trade Commission
Chapter 17 Food Safety and Technology

The authors would also like to acknowledge the valuable
contributions from the following graduate students:

Ryan DeLee, *Stanford University*
Leigh Fish, *University of Florida*
Jacinda Mawson, *Stanford University*
Raj Rathod, *Stanford University*
David Zapol, *Stanford University*

Reviewers

Focus Group

Katie Brown, BS, MS
Central Missouri State University

Christine Goodner, MS, RD
Winthrop University

Nancy Gordon Harris, MS, RD, LDN
East Carolina State University

Mary K. Head, PhD, RD, LD
University of West Virginia

Mary Murimi, PhD
Louisiana Technical University

Barbara A. Stettler, MEd
Bluffton College

Anna Sumabat Turner, MEd
Bob Jones University

Reviewers

Nancy K. Amy, PhD
University of California-Berkeley

Susan I. Barr, PhD, RDN
University of British Columbia

Richard C. Baybutt PhD
Kansas State University

Beverly A. Benes, PhD, RD
University of Nebraska-Lincoln

Melanie Tracy Burns, PhD, RD
Eastern Illinois University

N. Joanne Caid, PhD
College of Agricultural Sciences and Technology

Holly A. Dieken, PhD, MS, BS, RD
University of Tennessee-Chattanooga

Christine Goodner, MS, RD
Winthrop University

Margaret Gunther, PhD
Palomar Community College

Shelley R. Hancock, MS, RD, LD
University of Alabama

Nancy Gordon Harris, MS, RD, LDN
East Carolina University

Mary K. Head, PhD, RD, LD
West Virginia University

Deloy G. Hendricks, PhD, CNS
Utah State University

Michael Jenkins
Kent State University

Zaheer Ali Kirmani, PhD, RD, LD
Sam Houston State University

Samantha R. Logan, DrPH, RD
University of Massachusetts

Michael P. Maina, PhD
Valdosta State University

Patricia Z. Marincic, PhD, RD, LD, CLE
College of Saint Benedict/Saint John's University

Melissa J. Martilotta, MS, RD
Pennsylvania State University

Jennifer McLean, MSPH
Corning Community College

Mark S. Meskin, PhD, RD
California State Polytechnic University-Pomona

Stella Miller, BA, MA
Mount San Antonio College

Marilyn Mook, BS, MS
Michigan State University

Mary W. Murimi, PhD
Louisiana Technical University

Katherine O. Musgrave, MS, RD, CAS
University of Maine-Orono

J. Dirk Nelson, PhD
Missouri Southern State College

Anne O'Donnell, MS, MPH, RD
Santa Rosa Junior College

Rebecca S. Pobocik, PhD, RD
Bowling Green State University

Brian Luke Seaward, PhD
University of Colorado-Boulder

Melissa Shock, PhD, RD
University of Central Arkansas

Christine Stapell, MS, RD, LDN
Tallahassee Community College

Bernice Gales Spurlock, PhD
Hinds Community College

Susan T. Saylor, RD, EdD
Shelton State University

Mohammad R. Shayesteh, PhD, RD, LD
Youngstown State University

LuAnn Soliah, PhD, RD
Baylor University

Beth Stewart, PhD, RD
University of Arizona

Shahla M. Wunderlich, PhD
Montclair State University

Janelle Walter, PhD
Baylor University

Erika M. Zablah
Louisiana State University-Baton Rouge

Acknowledgments

We are most grateful to Dr. Nancy Amy (University of California, Berkeley) and Dr. Sally Lederman (Columbia University) whose special nutrition expertise helped us strive for accuracy and precision. We would also like to thank the following people for their hard work and dedication. They have helped make this book a reality. Thank you to Monica Ohlinger and Joanne Vickers of Ohlinger Publishing Services for their help and patience during both the developmental editing phase and production phase of this manuscript. Thanks also to Judy Hauck of Jones and Bartlett Publishers for her thoughtful art development; to Joan Flaherty for a thorough and careful copyedit; to Donna Williams of Imagineering Scientific and Technical Artworks for carefully and speedily managing the process of getting artwork rendered; to Lianne Ames of Jones and Bartlett Publishers for shepherding the manuscript through to completion; and to MaryJo Gordon, Seann Dwyer and Elaine Coder of Studio Montage and John May of Graphic World for making this book look so great! We would also like to thank Suzanne Jeans and Paul Shepardson of Jones and Bartlett Publishers for giving us help and direction when we needed it.

Thanks also go to Ken Sammonds of the University of Massachusetts, Amherst and his students Marcie Lockenwitz, Krista Farrington, Sarah Lynch, Saima Dizdarevic, Danielle Blanchard, Carrieann Barnes, Kathryn Barron, E. Brooke Eaton, Corinne Arnold, Molly Lyon, Christina Bowman, Marc E. Hitchcock, Candice Shea, Jillian Grothusen, Tondy Lee Baumgartner, Michelle Croswell, Jacqueline L. Jones, Lucia M. MacMillan, Yukiko Hatanaka, Andrea B. Desjardins, Donna M. Pirog, Jessenatha Kimler, Jenny Allen, Angela Blomquist, and Briana Reardon, for class testing our manuscript in the fall of 2000. Thanks also to his honors class who have spent time in careful review of each chapter. Thanks to Kelly Anne Sullivan, Laura Dignard, Rebecca Odabasnian, Margaret M. Eng, and Erica Stengel.

Thanks also go to W. Scott Smith, Adam Alboyadjian, Nichole Healy, Kristin Ohlin and Tara Whorf for spending countless hours on the nutrition media package.

Finally the authors would also like to thank Kim Hyatt of Weber State University for reviewing web sites; Pam Fletcher and Sara Perovich of TVI Community College—Albuquerque for creating the Test Bank; Melanie Burns of Eastern Illinois University for creating the Lecture Outlines and PowerPoint Presentations; Amy Eades of Eastern Illinois University for sharing and creating the Classroom Activities; Wendy Schiff of St. Louis Community College-Meramec Campus for creating Cyberclass Flashcards and Practice Tests; and Amy Austin of Jones and Bartlett Publishers for coordinating the supplemental material that accompanies this book.

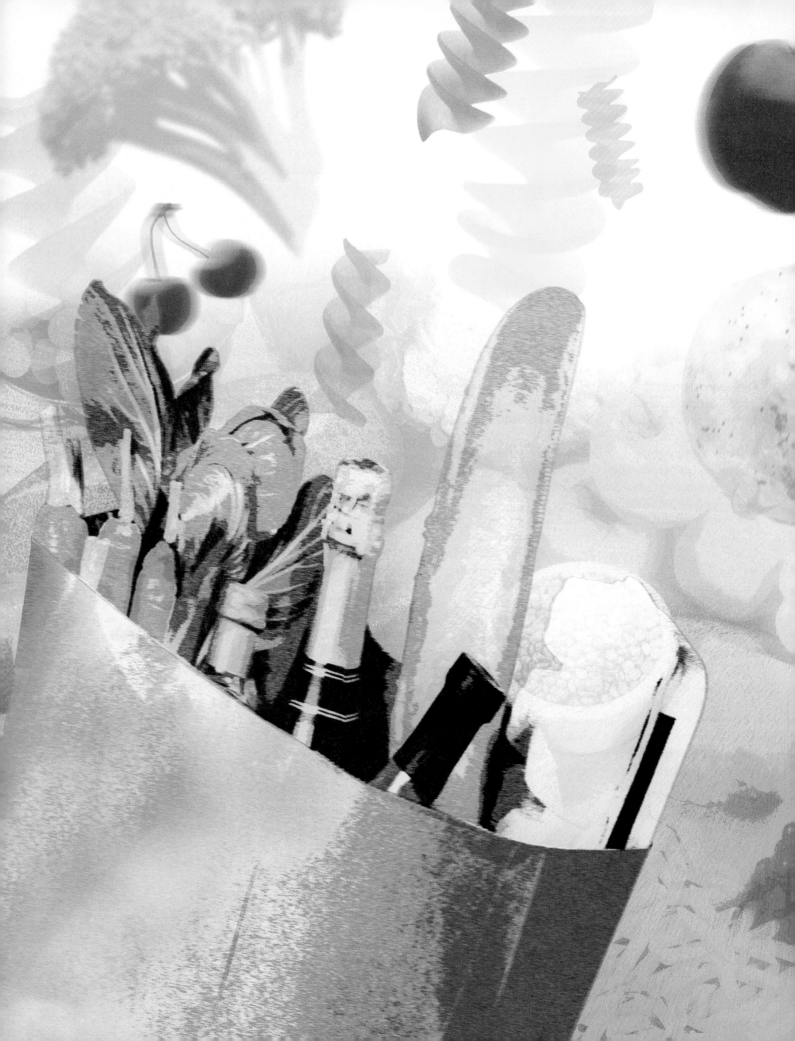

Chapter 1

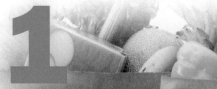

Nutrients and Nourishment

Think About It

1 How many different foods have you eaten in the last 24 hours? The last week?

2 Do you have a preference for sweets? Chocolate? Ice cream? If so, where do you think it comes from?

3 What do you think is driving the popularity of vitamins and other supplements?

4 Where do you get the majority of your information about nutrition?

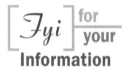

Fyi for your Information

This chapter's FYI boxes include practical information on the following topics:

• Phytochemicals: Why You should Eat More Fruits, Vegetables, Whole Grains, and Legumes!

• Do You Speak Metric?

• Evaluating Information on the Internet

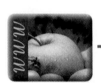

The web site for this book offers many useful tools and is a great source for additional nutrition information for both students and instructors. Visit the site at nutrition.jbpub.com for information on nutrients and nourishment. You'll find exercises that explore the following topics:

• The French Diet (*bon appetit!*)

• Why Are the Jains Vegetarians?

• Taste and Smell Disorders

What About Bobbie?

Track the choices Bobbie is making with the EatRight Analysis software.

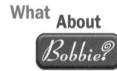

Key to Illustrations

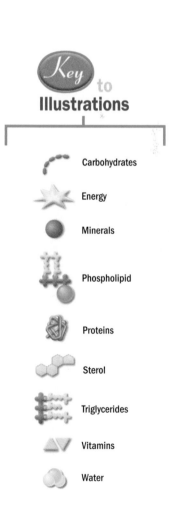

Carbohydrates

Energy

Minerals

Phospholipid

Proteins

Sterol

Triglycerides

Vitamins

Water

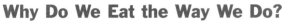

A college freshman expresses astonishment when her roommate chooses to serve pickled herring to their guests at a dinner party. A parent punishes a misbehaving child by withholding dessert. A professor recently recruited from a Chinese university feels dissatisfied unless he eats a bowl of rice daily. A policeman when asked to explain why hot dogs are his favorite food says it has something to do with going to baseball games with his father. A group of students go out for pizza every Tuesday night. What do these people have in common? They are all using food for something other than its nutrient value. Food has many symbolic meanings. Can you think of a holiday that is *not* celebrated with food? For most of us, food is more than a collection of nutrients and many factors affect what we choose to eat. Many of the foods people choose are nourishing and contribute to good health. The same, of course, may be true of the foods we reject.

The science of nutrition helps us improve our food choices by identifying the amounts of nutrients we need, the best food sources of those nutrients, and the other components in foods that may be helpful or harmful. Learning about nutrition will help us make better choices and not only improve our health, but reduce our risk of disease and increase our longevity. Keep in mind, though, that no matter how much you know about nutrition, you are still likely to choose some foods simply for their taste or because they make you feel good.

neophobia A dislike for anything new or unfamiliar.

Why Do We Eat the Way We Do?

Do you "eat to live" or "live to eat"? For most of us, the first is certainly true—you *must* eat to live. But there may be times that your *enjoyment* of food is more important to you than the nourishment you get from it. Such factors as age, sex, genetic makeup, occupation, lifestyle, family, and cultural background affect our daily food choices. We use food to project a desired image, bond relationships, express friendship, show creativity, and demonstrate feelings through gifts. We cope with anxiety or stress by eating or not eating; we reward ourselves with food for a good grade or a job well done, or in extreme cases, punish failures by denying ourselves the benefit and comfort of eating.

Food preferences begin early in life and then change as we interact with parents, friends, and peers. Additional exposure to different peoples, places, and situations often—but not always—causes us to expand or change our preferences. Taste and texture are the two most important things that influence our food choices; next are cost and convenience.[1] What we eat reveals much about who we are.

Age is a factor in food preferences. Young children prefer sweet or familiar foods; babies and toddlers are generally willing to try new things (see **Figure 1.1**); preschoolers typically go through a period of food **neophobia** (a dislike for anything new or unfamiliar); school-age children tend to accept a wider array of foods; and teenagers are

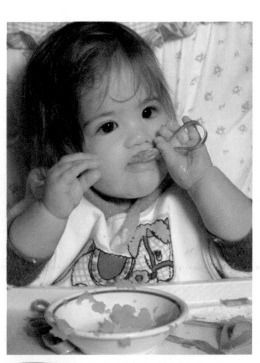

Figure 1.1 Babies and toddlers are generally willing to try new things.

think
out It
1

strongly influenced by the preferences and habits of their peers. If you track the kinds of foods you have eaten in the past year, you might be surprised to discover how few basic foods are in your diet. By the time we reach adulthood, we have formed a core group of foods we prefer. Of this group, only about 100 basic items account for 75 percent of our food intake.

Like many aspects of human behavior, food choices can be described in terms of both inborn (biological) factors and environmental influences; and as with other behaviors, the lines between nature and nurture are often blurred. However, we can look at food preferences in terms of the sensory properties of foods, cognitive factors that influence our choices, and long-term influences like culture. Exploring each of these areas may help you understand why you prefer certain foods.

Sensory Influences: Taste, Texture, and Smell

A very important determinant of food choice is what appeals to our senses. People often refer to **flavor** as a collective experience that describes both taste and smell. Texture is also part of the picture. You may prefer foods that have a crisp, chewy, or smooth texture. You may reject foods that feel grainy, slimy, or rubbery. Other sensory characteristics that affect food choice are color, moisture, and temperature.

Studies of taste physiology show that there are more tastes than the classic four of sweet, sour, bitter, and salty (see **Figure 1.2**). One of these additional taste sensations is **umami**, which is a Japanese term that describes the taste produced by glutamate.[2] Glutamate is an amino acid (a building block of protein) that is found in monosodium glutamate (MSG). It gives food a distinctive meaty or savory taste (see Chapter 3 for more information about taste and smell).

Key Concepts *Many factors influence our decisions about what to eat and when to eat. The four main factors are taste, texture, cost, and convenience.*

Cognitive Influences

Along with our experiences, our thoughts and feelings about food influence decisions about what to eat and when. We can call these factors *cognitive* influences because they affect how we think and the decisions we make.

flavor The collective experience that describes both taste and smell.

umami [ooh-MA-mee] A Japanese term that describes a delicious meaty or savory sensation. Chemically, this taste detects the presence of glutamate.

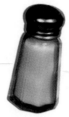

Quick Bites

Sweetness and Salt

Salt can do more than just make your food taste salty. Researchers at the Monell Chemical Senses Center demonstrated that salt also suppresses the bitter flavors in foods. When combined with chocolate, in a chocolate-covered pretzel for example, salt blocks some of the bitter flavor, making the chocolate taste sweeter. This phenomenon might explain why people in many cultures salt their fruit.

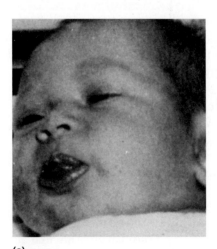
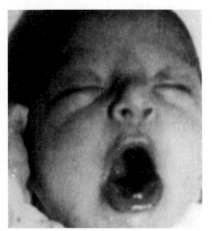

(a)   (b)

Figure 1.2 **The taste reflex of newborns.** (a) Response to sugar. (b) Response to bitter.

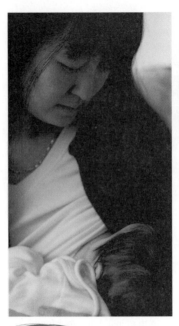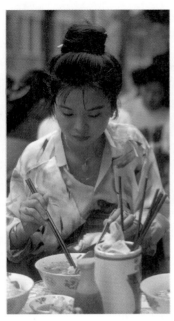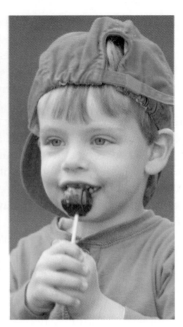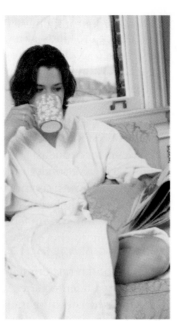

Figure 1.3 How you were nurtured as a child can shape your eating and cooking habits.

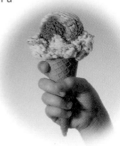

Day-to-Day Influences on Food Choices: Habits

Your eating and cooking habits are likely to reflect what you learned from your parents (see **Figure 1.3**). We typically learn to eat three meals a day, at about the same time each day. Quite often we eat the same foods, particularly for breakfast (e.g., cereal and milk) and lunch (e.g., sandwiches). This routine makes life convenient and we don't have to think much about when or what to eat. But we don't have to follow this routine! How would you feel about eating mashed potatoes for breakfast and cereal for dinner? Some people might get a stomachache just thinking about it, while others may enjoy the prospect of doing things differently. Look at your eating habits and see how often you make the same choices, every single day.

Comfort / Discomfort Foods

Our desire for particular foods is often based on behavioral motives of which we are unaware. For some people, food becomes an emotional security blanket. Consuming our favorite foods can make us feel better, relieve stress, and allay anxiety. Starting with the first days of life, food and affection are intertwined. Infants experience both physical and psychological satisfaction when eating. As we grow older, this experience is continually reinforced. For example, chicken soup and hot tea with honey are favorites when we feel under the weather because Mom and Dad fixed them especially for us. If we were rewarded for good behavior with a particular food (e.g., ice cream, candy, cookies), we tend to have positive feelings about that food that persist for a lifetime. Thus foods that we associate with positive childhood experiences often continue to generate secure and supportive feelings.

On the other hand, children who have negative associations with certain foods are unlikely to choose those foods as adults. Maybe there is a food that you avoid because you *know* it will make you sick. Chances are that at some point in your childhood, you got sick soon after eating that food, and consequently the two events are linked forever. Repeated power struggles with your parents over a helping of broccoli or zucchini may have turned you away from eating these vegetables. Fortunately, these behaviors can be reversed. Psychologists have shown us that negative associations are easier to extinguish than positive ones. Thus time and the knowledge that vegetables are beneficial may help us overcome negative associations.

Food Cravings

Chocolates for breakfast? Only if you are one of those people who can't survive more than one waking hour without a chocolate rush. Is the intense desire or craving for a particular food psychological or physiological? It's likely to be both and these factors may interact to increase the intensity of the desire. Add ice cream to chocolate and you have the top two candidates on the food craver's agenda. The use of chocolate and ice cream as rewards in early childhood often sets the stage for later cravings. Frequently just the thought of this pleasurable experience can achieve the change in behavior a parent or caretaker desires. The most popular theory to explain this phenomenon relates to an opiate called **beta-endorphin**. The brain releases this chemical "pleasure trigger" whenever foods like chocolate and ice cream are eaten.

Some people offer a nutritional explanation for food cravings: The body is sensing a nutrient deficit and influencing desire for a food rich in that nutrient. One example is the practice of eating nonfood items such as dirt, clay, and laundry starch. The craving for and consumption of such substances is called **pica** and is often associated with pregnancy. It has been suggested that iron deficiency drives the pregnant woman's craving so she seeks iron in any form possible, including dirt. Although this is a plausible explanation, current research has not found such a link. Rather, family traditions and cultural acceptance of pica have made it an expected behavior in some groups.[3]

Advertising and Promotion

It is not surprising that some of the most popular food products sold are high-fat and high-sugar baked goods and alcoholic beverages. Aggressive and sometimes deceptive advertising programs can influence people to buy foods of poor nutritional quality. On the other hand, we are seeing more innovative and aggressive advertising from the commodity boards who promote milk, meat, cranberries, and other more nutrient-dense products.

When the nutritional merits of food products are emphasized accurately, advertising like that in **Figure 1.4** can be helpful, especially to consumers whose diets require monitoring. In the mid-1980s, Kellogg's launched a print and television ad campaign for All-Bran cereal to suggest that a high-fiber diet would reduce the risk of cancer. Not only did sales of All-Bran increase dramatically in the months that followed, but the sales of all high-fiber cereals increased.[4] When the oat bran craze first hit in the late 1980s, sales of oat bran products by Quaker Oats Company increased 700 percent in one year.

Social Factors

Social factors exert a powerful influence on food choice. By observing their parents, infants and children learn which foods and combinations of foods are appropriate to consume and under what circumstances. Perhaps even more influential, though, are the messages gleaned from their peers.[5] Although food neophobia is common among children, it can often be over-

Think about It **2**

beta-endorphin A type of opiate that produces a sensation of pleasure.

pica The craving for and consumption of nonfood items like dirt, clay, or laundry starch.

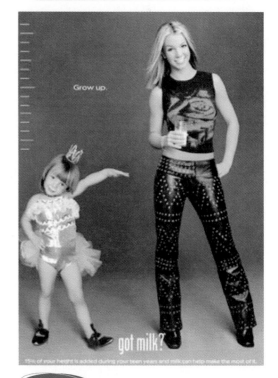

Grow up.

got milk?

Figure 1.4 **Healthy advertising.** Got milk? is an example of a successful healthy advertising campaign.

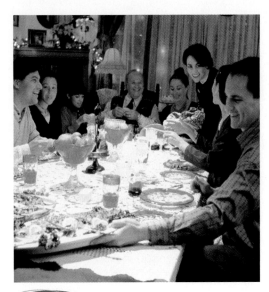

Figure 1.5 **Social facilitation.**

social facilitation Encouragement of the interactions between people.

come by allowing them to observe another child enjoying a food they have yet to sample. With age and increased social contact, children and teens are likely to adopt more and more of their peers' preferences for foods and for specific preparation and serving methods of those foods: "Mark eats his sandwiches in triangles; that's the way I want mine!"

As **Figure 1.5** illustrates, eating is also a social event that brings together different people for a variety of purposes (e.g., religious or cultural celebrations, business meetings, and family dinners). By virtue of a phenomenon termed **social facilitation,** food intake increases because of the social climate surrounding its consumption.[6]

However, social pressures can also restrict our food intake and selection. This is true, for example, in situations where one is attempting to make a certain impression on a dining partner(s). A person might choose foods on the basis of appropriateness and according to the guest's food preferences, rather than one's own, or perhaps out of courtesy to the host.

Nutrition and Health Beliefs

Information about food and nutrition is abundant, as **Figure 1.6** shows. Why do some people ignore health information and indulge themselves with foods that may lead to health problems, while others take the same information and commit themselves to a healthful diet?[7] To examine these questions, we need to consider the health beliefs of consumers, their perceptions of susceptibility to disease and whether they can take action to prevent or delay its onset.[8] For instance, if people feel vulnerable to disease and believe that dietary changes will lead to positive results, they are more likely to heed information about the links between dietary choices, dietary fat, and risks for diseases such as heart disease and cancer. Information about nutrient content on food labels along with health claims that describe links between food components and diseases further aid consumers who are trying to make positive choices.

Key Concepts *Habits, experiences, social factors, advertising, and knowledge of relationships between food and health all influence our food decisions.*

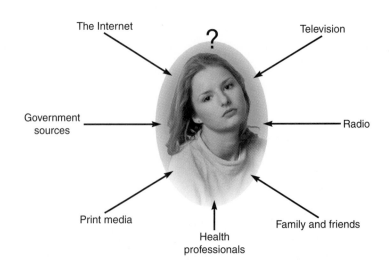

Figure 1.6 We endure a constant bombardment of food messages.

Cultural Influences

One of the strongest influences on food preferences is tradition or cultural background. In all societies, no matter how simple or complex, eating is the primary way of initiating and maintaining human relationships. People around us influence our food choices, and we prefer the foods we grew up eating. Sometimes these culturally acquired preferences can seem quite peculiar to those of a different culture. The college student who serves pickled herring to her friends may have learned to enjoy it from her Jewish parents, who introduced it to her as a child in comforting surroundings. Likewise, it is not uncommon for people of Mexican heritage to enjoy eating hot peppers, which were introduced to them early in life in highly gregarious social settings.

To a large extent, culture defines attitudes. "One man's food is another man's poison." Look at **Figure 1.7**. How does the photo make you feel? Insects, maggots, and entrails are delicacies to some, while just the thought of ingesting them is enough to make others retch. So powerful are cultural forces that if you were permitted only a single question to establish someone's food preferences, a good choice would be "To what ethnic group do you belong?"[9]

Knowledge, beliefs, customs, and habits all are defining elements of human culture.[10] Although there are genetic characteristics that tie people of one ethnic group together, culture is a learned behavior and, consequently, can be modified through education, experience, and sociopolitical forces.[11]

Cultural Beliefs and Traditions

In many cultures, food has symbolic meanings related to family traditions, social status, and health.[12] The latter is reflected by the many and varied food-based folk remedies one encounters. Some have gained wide acceptance, such as the use of spices and herb teas for purposes ranging from allaying anxiety to preventing cancer and heart disease.[13] Traditional medical practices in many cultures follow the belief that nature is composed of two opposing forces (e.g., yin and yang in traditional Chinese medicine). This idea of balance and the terms describing illness and foods as either "hot" or "cold" are found in other Asian cultures, including India and the Philippines, and in Latin American cultures. It is typically believed that good health reflects a balance of these two forces. Excesses in either direction causes illness which, therefore must be treated by giving foods of the opposite force.

As cultural distinctions blur, so do many of the unique expectations about the ability of certain foods to prevent disease, restore health among those with various afflictions, or enhance longevity. They are still apparent, however, in older, less assimilated groups. Food habits are among the last to change when an immigrant adapts to a new culture.[14]

Religion

Food is an important part of religious rites, symbols, and customs as well as of daily activities that are intended to promote an orderly relationship with supernatural forces. Some religious rules apply to everyday eating, whereas others are concerned with special celebrations.

Christianity, Judaism, Hinduism, Buddhism, and Islam all have distinct dietary laws, but within each religion different interpretations of these laws give rise to variations in dietary practices. For example, Jewish dietary laws

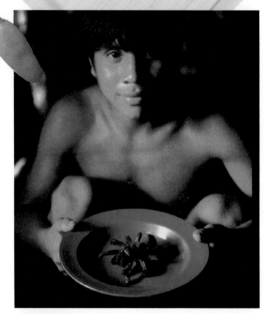

Figure 1.7 **Cultural influences.** What would you do if you were visiting this country? Would you be willing to try this delicacy?

Quick Bites

Nerve Poison for Dinner?

The puffer fish is a delicacy in Japan. Danger is part of its appeal; eating a puffer fish can be life-threatening! The puffer fish contains a poison called tetrodotoxin (TTX), which blocks the transmission of nerve signals and can lead to death. Chefs who prepare the puffer fish must have special training and licenses to prepare the fish properly, so diners feel nothing more than a slight numbing feeling.

specify the foods that are "fit and proper," or *kosher*, to eat. To be kosher, meat must come from clean animals that chew their cud and have cloven hooves. Fish must have fins and scales. Pork, crustaceans and shellfish, and birds of prey are not acceptable. The Orthodox laws of Judaism prohibit eating meat and milk in the same meal or even preparing or serving them with the same dishes and utensils. Islam identifies acceptable foods as *halal*, and has rules for slaughtering animals similar to those of Judaism. Islamic faith prohibits the consumption of pork, flesh of clawed animals, alcohol, and other intoxicating drugs. Intoxicating beverages are also prohibited in Buddhism.[15] The Church of Jesus Christ of Latter Day Saints disapproves of alcoholic and caffeine-containing beverages, but these are not problematic among other Christian traditions such as those of the Greek Orthodox Church. Most Hindus are vegetarians and do not eat eggs. The Jain religion (in India) forbids eating meat or animal products (milk, eggs, etc.) and anything grown in darkness (e.g., potato or garlic).

Religious rules may also define eating frequency and periodicity. During the holy month of Ramadan, Muslims fast from dawn to sunset. They consume two meals per day, one before the sunrise and one after sunset.[16] Religious laws (e.g., the traditional Catholic and Greek Orthodox practice of abstaining from eating meat on Fridays during Lent) also define the types of foods eaten on specific occasions.[17]

Cultural Cuisine

A culture and the foods its people choose to eat are reciprocally linked. Each contributes to the identity of the other and both help to define a person's values, preferences, and practices. Consequently, neither is abandoned easily or quickly, even in the face of changing world events. Nevertheless, the question arises: What impact will the population's increasing mobility have on food choice? Cultural interactions and exposure to various cuisines will undoubtedly increase. Will this ultimately lead to a heightened appreciation and preservation of different culinary practices or the synthesis of a single new hybrid cuisine?

Key Concepts *The cultural environments in which people grow up have a major influence on what foods they prefer, what foods they consider edible, and what foods they eat in combination and at what time of day. Many factors work to define a group's culture: economics, geographic location, traditions, and religious beliefs. As people from other cultures immigrate to new lands, they will adopt new behaviors consistent with their new homes. However, food habits are among the last to change.*

The American Diet

What then is a typical *American* diet? As a country influenced by the practices of both Native Americans and immigrants, there is no easy, single answer to this question. The U.S. diet is as diverse as Americans themselves. To many around the world, the American diet is hamburgers, french fries, and cola drinks! Our fondness for fast food and the marketability of such restaurants overseas make these a cultural symbol to many. And, many of the stereotypes are true. The most commonly consumed grain in the United States is white bread, the favorite meat is beef, and the most frequently eaten vegetable is the potato, usually as french fries. Despite the variety available to us, the American diet is still heavy on meat and potatoes and light on fruits and whole grains. We also are eating more cereals, snack foods, soft drinks, and non-citrus juices than ever before.[18]

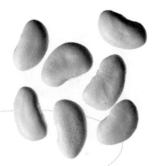

Quick Bites

The Lima Bean

The lima bean has been in cultivation in Peru since 6000 B.C.E. Not so coincidentally, Peru's capital is Lima.

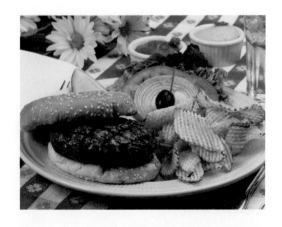

So, how healthful is the "American" diet? Although we are bombarded with information about health and nutrition, this doesn't necessarily translate into better food choices. People are not "natural nutritionists"; that is, they don't know instinctively which foods to choose for good health. The majority of the population has never taken a course in nutrition. They will probably never take the time to become well-informed consumers—not just of food, but of information about food and nutrition. So it is probably not surprising when national surveys indicate that although Americans *know* that nutrition and food choices are important determinants of health, few have made the recommended changes (e.g., eating less fat, sugar, and salt and more fruits and vegetables).

Consider some of the following facts from the United States Department of Agriculture's (USDA) 10th nationwide food consumption survey:[19]

- Americans agree (more than 90 percent of adults surveyed) that it is important to maintain a healthy weight. However, almost 40 percent admit they eat too many calories. And more than 50 percent of adults are overweight.

- Thirty minutes of moderate physical activity is recommended daily, but 28 percent of men and 44 percent of women say they rarely or never exercise vigorously.

- Two-thirds of adults think it is "very important" to choose a diet rich in vegetables and fruits; yet consumption of such foods has increased only slightly since the late 1970s.

- On the other hand, less than one-third of adults think it is very important to choose a diet with plenty of breads, cereals, rice, and pasta. Even so, consumption of those foods has increased by more than 40 percent since the late 1970s.

- Eighty-five percent of adults think it is important to use sugars only in moderation, yet Americans consume an average of 20 teaspoons of added sugars per day—accounting for 16 percent of calories.

- About two-thirds of adults eat more than the recommended intake level for fat, but only 50 percent think they eat too much. About 60 percent eat more saturated fat than is recommended, but only about one-third think they eat too much.

We are getting at least some of the message, but either not understanding how to implement it or choosing not to heed it. It's important to remember that health messages must compete with those conveyed by product labels, pricing, celebrity spokespeople, and societal conventions.

You are in a position to gather more information than the average consumer. By taking this course in nutrition, you will be getting the full story: the nutrients we need for good health, the science behind the health messages, and the food choices it will take to implement them. Whether you use this information (see **Figure 1.8**) is up to you; but at least you will be a well-informed consumer!

Key Concepts *What we think of as "American" cuisine is truly a melting pot of cultural contributions to foods and tastes. Although Americans receive and believe many messages about the role of diet in good health, these beliefs do not always translate into healthful food choices.*

Quick Bites

America's Favorite Vegetables

When Americans eat vegetables, they are most likely to eat potatoes (especially french fries), tomatoes (usually part of tomato sauce or ketchup), onions, and iceberg lettuce.

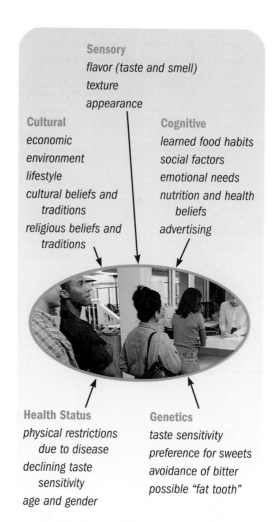

Sensory
flavor (taste and smell)
texture
appearance

Cultural
economic
environment
lifestyle
cultural beliefs and
*   traditions*
religious beliefs and
*   traditions*

Cognitive
learned food habits
social factors
emotional needs
nutrition and health
*   beliefs*
advertising

Health Status
physical restrictions
*   due to disease*
declining taste
*   sensitivity*
age and gender

Genetics
taste sensitivity
preference for sweets
avoidance of bitter
possible "fat tooth"

Figure 1.8   **Factors that affect food choices.** Selecting a food to eat often is done automatically, without thought. But in fact, your choices are complex events involving the interactions of a multitude of factors.

nutrient Any substance in food that the body can use to obtain energy, synthesize tissues, or regulate functions.

essential nutrient A substance that must be obtained in the diet because the body either cannot make it or cannot make adequate amounts of it.

antioxidant A substance that combines with or otherwise neutralizes a free radical, thus preventing oxidative damage to cells and tissues.

macronutrient A nutrient, such as carbohydrate, fat, or protein, that is needed in relatively large amounts in the diet.

micronutrient A nutrient, such as a vitamin or mineral, that is needed in relatively small amounts in the diet.

organic [or-GAN-ick] In chemistry, any compound that contains carbon, except carbon oxides (e.g., carbon dioxide) and sulfides and metal carbonates (e.g., potassium carbonate). The term sometimes is used to denote crops that are grown without synthetic fertilizers or chemicals.

inorganic Any substance that does not contain carbon, excepting certain simple carbon compounds such as carbon dioxide and monoxide. Common examples include table salt (sodium chloride) and baking soda (sodium bicarbonate).

Introducing the Nutrients

Although we give food meaning through our culture and experience and make dietary decisions based on a whole host of factors, ultimately the reason for eating is to obtain nourishment—nutrition.

Just like your body, food is a mixture of chemicals, some of which are essential for normal body function. These essential chemicals are called **nutrients.** You need nutrients for normal growth and development, for maintaining cells and tissues, for fuel to do physical and metabolic work, and for regulating the hundreds of thousands of body processes that go on inside you every second of every day. Further, food must provide these nutrients; the body either cannot make or cannot make adequate amounts of the **essential nutrients.** There are six classes of nutrients in food: *carbohydrates, lipids* (fats and oils), *proteins, vitamins, minerals,* and *water* (see **Figure 1.9**). The minimum diet for human growth, development, and maintenance must supply about 45 essential nutrients.

Definition of Nutrients

In studying nutrition, we focus on the functions of nutrients in the body so that we can see why they are important in the diet. However, to define a nutrient in technical terms, we focus on what happens in its absence. A nutrient is a chemical whose absence from the diet for a long enough time results in a specific change in health; we say that a person has a deficiency of that nutrient. A lack of vitamin C, for example, will eventually lead to scurvy. A diet with too little iron will result in iron-deficiency anemia. To complete the definition of a nutrient, it also must be true that putting the essential chemical back in the diet will reverse the change in health, if done before permanent damage occurs. If taken early enough, supplements of vitamin A can reverse the effects of deficiency on the eyes. If not, prolonged vitamin A deficiency can cause permanent blindness.

Nutrients are not the only chemicals in food. Other substances add flavor and color, some contribute to texture, and others, like caffeine, have physiological effects on the body. Some substances in food, like fiber, have important health benefits (as you will discover in Chapter 4), but do not fit the classical definition of a nutrient. One of the newest areas of research in nutrition is the area of phytochemicals. Although these "plant chemicals"

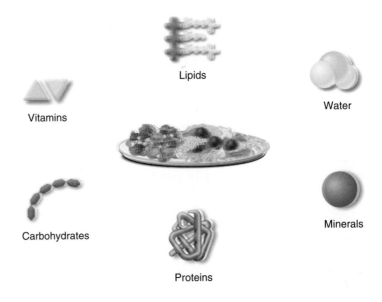

Figure 1.9 **The six classes of nutrients.** Water is our most important nutrient and we cannot survive long without it. Because our bodies need large quantities of carbohydrate, protein, and fat, they are called macronutrients. Our bodies need comparatively small amounts of vitamins and minerals, so they are called micronutrients.

Lipids

Water

Vitamins

Minerals

Carbohydrates

Proteins

are not nutrients, they have important health functions, such as **antioxidant** activity, which may reduce risk for heart disease or cancer.

The six classes of nutrients serve three general functions: provide fuel or energy, regulate body processes, and contribute to body structures (see **Figure 1.10**). While virtually all nutrients can be said to regulate body processes and many contribute to body structures, only the nutrients protein, carbohydrate, and fat are sources of energy. Because the body needs large quantities of carbohydrate, protein, and fat, these are called **macronutrients**; the vitamins and minerals are **micronutrients** because the amounts the body needs are comparatively small.

In addition to their functions, there are several other key differences among the classes of nutrients. First, the chemical composition of nutrients varies widely. One way to divide the nutrient groups is based on whether the compounds contain the element carbon. Substances that contain carbon are **organic** substances; those that do not are **inorganic**. Carbohydrates, lipids, proteins, and vitamins are all organic; minerals and water are not. Structurally, nutrients can be very simple—minerals are single elements (sodium, for example), although we often consume them as larger compounds (sodium chloride, or table salt). Water is also very simple in structure. The organic nutrients have more complex structures—the carbohydrates, lipids, and proteins we eat are made of smaller building blocks—while the vitamins are elaborately structured compounds.

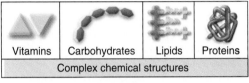

Organic – contains carbon ●

Simple chemical structures

Inorganic – no carbon

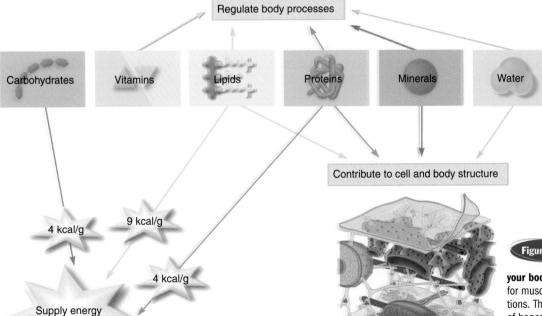

Figure 1.10 **Nutrients have three general functions in your body.** Nutrients are an energy source for muscle contractions and cellular functions. They are important to the structure of bones, muscles and all cells. Some nutrients help regulate bodily processes such as blood pressure, energy production, and temperature regulation.

carbohydrate A large group of compounds, including sugars, starches, and dietary fibers, that usually have the general chemical formula $(CH_2O)n$ where n represents the number of CH_2O units in the molecule. Carbohydrates are the primary source of energy for all body functions.

circulation Movement of substances through the vessels of the cardiovascular or lymphatic system.

lipids A group of fat-soluble compounds that includes triglycerides, sterols, and phospholipids.

hormone A chemical messenger that is secreted into the blood by one tissue and acts on cells in another part of the body.

protein Large, complex compounds consisting of many amino acids connected in varying sequences and forming unique shapes.

vitamin An organic compound necessary for promotion of reproduction, growth, and maintenance of the body. Vitamins are required in minuscule amounts.

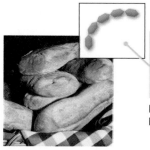

Whenever you see this icon, we'll be talking about **carbohydrates**

Provide:
Energy (4 kcal/g)

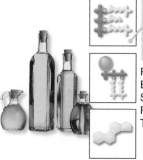

Whenever you see one of these 3 icons, we'll be talking about **lipids**

Provide:
Energy (9 kcal/g)
Structure
Regulation (hormones)
Transport

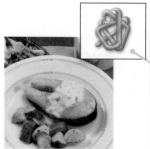

Whenever you see this icon, we'll be talking about **proteins**

Provide:
Energy (4 kcal/g)
Structure
Regulation

It is rare for a food to contain just one nutrient. Meat is not just protein any more than bread is solely carbohydrate. Foods contain mixtures of nutrients, although in most cases, protein, fat, or carbohydrate dominates. So while bread is certainly rich in carbohydrates, it also contains some protein, a little fat, and many vitamins and minerals. If it's whole-grain bread you're eating, you also get fiber, not technically a nutrient, but an important compound for good health nonetheless.

Key Concepts *Nutrients are the essential chemicals in food that the body needs for normal functioning and good health and that must come from the diet because they either cannot be made in the body or cannot be made in sufficient quantities. Six classes of nutrients—carbohydrates, proteins, lipids, vitamins, minerals, and water—can be described by their composition or by their function in the body.*

Carbohydrates

The word **carbohydrate,** or literally "hydrate of carbon," tells you exactly what this nutrient is made of, if you think "water" when you hear the word *hydrate.* Carbohydrates are made of carbon, hydrogen, and oxygen, and are a major source of fuel for the body. Dietary carbohydrates are the starches and sugars found in grains, vegetables, legumes (dry beans and peas), and fruits. We also get carbohydrates from dairy products, but practically none from meats. Your body converts most dietary carbohydrates to glucose, a simple sugar compound. It is glucose that we find in **circulation,** providing a source of energy for cells and tissues.[20]

Lipids

The term **lipids** refer to substances we know as fats and oils, but also to fat-like substances in foods such as cholesterol and phospholipids. Lipids are organic compounds and, like carbohydrates, contain carbon, hydrogen, and oxygen. Fats or, more correctly, triglycerides are another major fuel source for the body. In addition, triglycerides, cholesterol, and phospholipids have other important functions: providing structure for body cells, carrying the fat-soluble vitamins (A, D, E, and K), and providing the starting material (cholesterol) for making many **hormones.** Dietary lipids are provided by the fats and oils we add to foods or cook with, the naturally occurring fats in meats and dairy products, and less obvious sources in plants such as coconut, olives, and avocado.

Proteins

Proteins are organic compounds made of smaller building blocks called amino acids. The composition of amino acids is different from carbohydrates and lipids. In addition to carbon, hydrogen, and oxygen, amino acids contain nitrogen. Some amino acids also contain the mineral sulfur. The amino acids that we get from dietary protein combine with the amino acids made in the body to make hundreds of different body proteins. Body proteins help build and maintain body structures and regulate body processes. Protein can also be used for energy.

Proteins are found in a variety of foods, but meats and dairy products are among the most concentrated sources. Grains, legumes, and vegetables all contribute protein to the diet, while fruits contribute negligible amounts.[21]

Vitamins

Vitamins are organic compounds that contain carbon, hydrogen, and perhaps nitrogen, oxygen, phosphorus, sulfur, or other elements. Vitamins regulate body processes such as energy production, blood clotting, and calcium balance. Vitamins help to keep organs and tissues functioning and healthy. Because the functions of vitamins are so diverse, a lack of a particular vitamin can have widespread effects. While the body does not break down vitamins to yield energy, vitamins have vital roles in the extraction of energy from carbohydrate, fat, and protein.

Vitamins are usually divided into two groups: fat-soluble and water-soluble. The four fat-soluble vitamins—A, D, E, and K—have very diverse roles. What they have in common, is the way they are absorbed and transported in the body, and the fact that they are more likely to be stored in larger quantities than the water-soluble vitamins. The water-soluble vitamins include vitamin C and eight B vitamins: thiamin (B_1), riboflavin (B_2), niacin (B_3), pyridoxine (B_6), cobalamin (B_{12}), folate, pantothenic acid, and biotin. Most of the B vitamins are involved in some way with the pathways for energy metabolism.

Vitamins are found in a wide variety of foods, not just fruits and vegetables—although these are important sources—but also meats, grains, legumes, dairy products, and even fats. Choosing a well-balanced diet usually makes vitamin supplements unnecessary. In fact, when taken in large doses, vitamin supplements can be harmful, especially vitamins A and D, pyridoxine, and niacin.

Think
About It
3

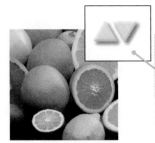

Whenever you see these icons, we'll be talking about **vitamins**

Provide:
Regulation

Minerals

Structurally, **minerals** are simple, inorganic substances. At least 16 minerals are essential to health; among them are sodium, chloride, potassium, calcium, phosphorus, magnesium, and sulfur.[22] Because the body needs these minerals in relatively large quantities compared to other minerals, they are often called **macrominerals.** The body needs the remaining minerals only in small amounts. These **microminerals,** or **trace minerals,** include iron, zinc, copper, manganese, molybdenum, selenium, iodine, and fluoride. Like vitamins, the functions of minerals are diverse. Minerals can be found in structural roles (e.g., calcium, phosphorus, and fluoride in bones and teeth) as well as regulatory roles (e.g., control of fluid balance and regulation of muscle contraction).

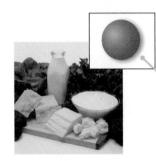

Whenever you see this icon, we'll be talking about **minerals**

Provide:
Structure
Regulation

Food sources of minerals are just as diverse. Although we often associate minerals with animal foods such as meats and milk, plant foods are important sources as well. Deficiencies of minerals, except iron and perhaps calcium, are uncommon. A balanced diet provides enough minerals for most people. However, individuals with iron-deficiency anemia may need iron supplements, and others may need calcium supplements if they cannot or will not drink milk or eat dairy products. As is true for vitamins, excessive intake of some minerals as supplements can be toxic.

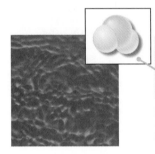

Whenever you see this icon, we'll be talking about **water**

Provides:
Regulation
Structure

Water

Next to the mineral elements, water is chemically the simplest nutrient. Water is also the most important nutrient! We can survive far longer without any of the other nutrients in the diet, indeed without food at all, than we can without water. Water has many roles in the body, including temperature control, lubrication of joints, and transportation of nutrients and wastes.

Your body is nearly 60 percent water, so maintaining adequate hydration means regular fluid intake is very important. Water is found not only in beverages, but also in most food products. Fruits and vegetables in particular

mineral An inorganic compound needed for growth and for regulation of body processes.

macromineral Major minerals are required in the diet and present in the body in large amounts compared to trace minerals.

micromineral Microminerals are present in the body and required in the diet in relatively small amounts compared to major minerals. Also known as trace minerals.

trace mineral Trace minerals are present in the body and required in the diet in relatively small amounts compared to major minerals. Also known as microminerals.

energy The capacity to do work. The energy in food is chemical energy, which the body converts to mechanical, electrical, or heat energy.

kilocalorie (kcal) [KILL-oh-kal-oh-ree] A unit used to measure energy. Food energy is measured in kilocalories (1000 calories = 1 kilocalorie).

calorie The general term for energy in food and used synonymously with the term *energy*. Often used instead of *kilocalorie* on food labels, in diet books, and in other sources of nutrition information.

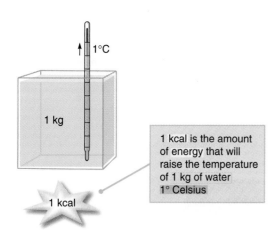

1 kcal is the amount of energy that will raise the temperature of 1 kg of water 1° Celsius

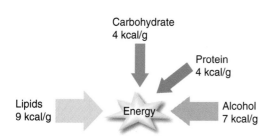

Energy potential in food

Figure 1.11 **Energy potential in food.** Your body can burn carbohydrate, fat, protein, and alcohol to extract energy (calories) for fuel.

are high in water content. Through many chemical reactions, the body makes some of its own water, but this is only a fraction of the amount needed for normal function.

Key Concepts *The body needs larger amounts of carbohydrates, lipids, and proteins (macronutrients) than vitamins and minerals (micronutrients). Carbohydrates, lipids, and proteins provide energy; proteins, lipids, minerals, and water add to body structure; and proteins, vitamins, minerals, and some fatty acids regulate body processes.*

Nutrients and Energy

One of the main reasons we eat food, and the nutrients it contains, is for **energy.** Every cellular reaction, every muscle movement, every nerve impulse requires energy. Three of the nutrient classes—carbohydrates, lipids (triglycerides only), and proteins—are energy sources. When we speak of the energy in foods, we are really talking about the *potential* energy that foods contain. Energy itself is not a food component.

Different scientific disciplines use different measures of energy. In nutrition, we discuss the potential energy in food, or the body's use of energy, in units of heat called **kilocalories** (1,000 calories). One kilocalorie (or kcal) is the amount of energy (heat) it would take to raise the temperature of 1 kilogram (kg) of water by 1° Celsius. For many, this may be an abstract concept. It is unlikely that you would ever want to burn sticks of butter or sugar cubes to boil water on your next camping trip! As you learn more about nutrition, you will discover the amount of energy you likely need to fuel your daily activities. And you will also learn about the amounts of potential energy in various foods.

Energy in Foods

Energy is available from foods because foods contain carbohydrate, fat, and protein. These nutrients can be broken down completely (metabolized) to yield energy in a form that cells can use. When completely metabolized in the body, carbohydrate and protein yield 4 kcal of energy for every gram (g) consumed; fat yields 9 kcal/g; and alcohol contributes 7 kcal/g (see **Figure 1.11**). Therefore, the energy available from a given food or from a total diet is reflected by the amount of each of these substances consumed. Because fat is a concentrated source of energy, adding or removing fat from the diet can have a big effect on available calories.

When is a kcalorie a calorie?

Many people inappropriately use the terms *calorie* and *kilocalorie* interchangeably. To clear up this confusing situation, you should use the term *calorie* as a general term for energy and *kilocalorie* as a specific measurement or unit of that energy. Using *calories* is like referring to gas for a car and *kilocalories* is like referring to gallons of fuel. When in doubt, substitute the word *energy* for calories. The following sentence illustrates the use of *kilocalorie* and *calorie*: Because fat contains 9 *kilocalories* per gram, more than double that of protein or carbohydrate, foods high in fat are rich in *calories* (energy).

You'll find that food labels, diet books, and other sources of nutrition information use the term **calorie,** not kilocalorie. Technically, the potential energy in foods is best measured in kilocalories; however, the term *calorie* has become familiar and commonplace.

How can we calculate the energy available from foods?

To calculate the energy available from food, multiply the number of grams of fat, carbohydrate, and/or protein by 9, 4, and 4, respectively; then add the results. For example, if we assume that one bagel plus one and a half ounces of cream cheese contains 39 grams of carbohydrate, 10 grams of protein, and 16 grams of fat, we can determine the available energy from each component.

To calculate the *percentage* of calories each of these components contributes to the total, divide the individual results by the total, and then multiply by 100. For example, to determine the percentage of calories from fat in the above example, divide the 144 fat kcal by the total of 340 kcal and then multiply by 100 (144 ÷ 340 × 100 = 42%).

Be Food Smart: Calculate the Percentages of Calories in Food

Current health recommendations suggest limiting fat intake to 30 percent of *total* energy intake. This means that during the course of the day, we should strive to eat less than 30 percent of our calories from fat. You can monitor this for yourself in two ways. If you like counting fat grams, you can first determine your suggested maximum fat intake. For example, if you need to eat 2000 kcal each day to maintain your current weight, 30 percent of those calories can come from fat. Therefore, your maximum fat intake should be about 67 grams. You can check food labels to see how many fat grams you typically eat.

Another way to monitor your fat intake is to know the percentage of calories that come from fat in various foods. If the proportion of fat in each food choice throughout the day exceeds 30 percent of calories, then the day's total of fat will be too high as well. Some foods contain nearly 0 percent of calories from fat (e.g., fruits and vegetables) while others are nearly 100 percent fat calories (e.g., margarine, salad dressing). Being aware that a snack like the bagel and cream cheese provides 42 percent of its calories from fat can help you select lower-fat foods at other times of the day.

Food Choices Provide Essential Nutrients

Food choices can provide more than an adequate diet. The balance of energy sources can affect our risk of chronic disease. For example, high-fat diets have been linked to heart disease and cancer. Excess calories contribute to obesity, which also increases disease risk. Other nutrients, such as the minerals sodium, chloride, calcium, and magnesium, affect blood pressure, while lack of the vitamin folate prior to conception and in early pregnancy can cause serious birth defects. Non-nutrient components in the diet (e.g., **phytochemicals**) may have antioxidant or immune-enhancing properties that also keep us healthy. The choices we make can reduce our disease risk, as well as provide energy and essential nutrients.

Key Concepts All cells and tissues need energy to keep the body functioning. Energy in foods and in the body is measured in kilocalories. The carbohydrates, lipids, and proteins in food are potential sources of energy, meaning that the body can extract energy from them. Lipids, specifically the triglycerides in fats, are the most concentrated source of energy, with 9 kcal/g. Carbohydrates and proteins can yield 4 kcal/g, while alcohol can yield 7 kcal/g.

CALCULATING THE ENERGY
AVAILABLE FROM FOODS

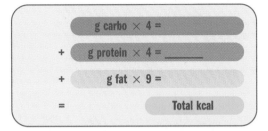

Example:
275 g carbohydrate × 4 kcal/g   =   1,100 kcal

75 g protein × 4 kcal/g = 300 kcal

67 g fat × 9 kcal/g = 600 kcal (rounded
from 603 kcal)

Total = 2000 kcal

CALCULATING THE PERCENTAGE OF
KILOCALORIES FROM NUTRIENTS

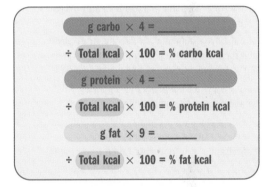

Example:
275 g carbohydrate × 4 = 1,100 kcal
÷ 2,000 kcal × 100 = 55% carbohydrates
kcal

75 g protein × 4 = 300 kcal
÷ 2,000 kcal × 100 = 15% protein kcal

67 g fat × 9 = 600 kcal (rounded
from 603kcal)

÷ 2,000 kcal × 100 = 30% fat kcal

phytochemicals Substances in plants that may possess health-protective effects, even though they are not essential for life.

Applying the Scientific Process to Nutrition

Whether it's identifying essential nutrients, establishing recommended intake levels, or exploring the effects of vitamins on cancer risk, scientific studies are the cornerstone of nutrition. Although the application of nutrition information may require some artistry to choose a pleasing array of foods, the fundamentals of nutrition are developed through the scientific process of observation and inquiry.

The scientific process enables researchers to test the validity of **hypotheses** that arise from observations of natural phenomena. For example, as **Figure 1.12** illustrates, it was well known in the 18th century that sailors on long voyages would likely develop scurvy. We now know that scurvy

hypothesis A scientist's "educated guess" to explain a phenomenon.

[Fyi] Phytochemicals: Why You Should Eat More Fruits, Vegetables, Whole Grains, and Legumes! Boyce Burge, Ph.D.

FOR YOUR INFORMATION

It seems you can't pick up a health magazine these days without seeing an article about phytochemicals. While the word phytochemical itself may sound futuristic, its meaning is simple: "plant chemical." The benefits of many phytochemicals are legendary! But what do we really mean when we talk about phytochemicals, and why is there so much interest in these compounds?

A vitamin is a food substance essential for health. Phytochemicals, in contrast, are substances in plants that may possess health-protective effects, even though they are not essential for life. Phytochemicals are complex chemicals that vary from plant to plant. They include thousands of compounds, pigments,

and natural antioxidants, many of which have been associated with protection from heart disease, hypertension, cancer, and diabetes.

Plants contain phytochemicals because these substances are of benefit to the plant itself. To illustrate their abundance, note that an orange has at least 170 distinct phytochemicals. Singly and together, these compounds help plants resist the attacks of bacteria and fungi, the ravages of free radicals, and high levels of ultraviolet light from the sun. When we eat these plants, the phytochemicals end up in our tissues and provide many of the same protections that plants enjoy.

Because we humans and our primate ancestors have been eating a wide variety of plants for millions of years, we have entered into a symbiosis of sorts with the plant world, and our bodies now "expect" a certain level and variety of phytochemicals for optimal health. Also, perhaps through natural selection, we humans have come to prefer the plants that have the greatest health benefits for us.

Unfortunately, this natural affinity for fresh fruits, vegetables, and grains has been corrupted by a recent emphasis on the processed, calorie-dense foods that are too common in the modern diet. Burgers, fries, chips, and pizza taste good, yet often crowd more healthful fruits, vegetables, and whole grains out of the diet.

Phytochemicals are part of the reason why the U.S. Department of Agriculture Food

Guide Pyramid recommends five servings per day of fruits and vegetables. Of course, fruits and vegetables are also naturally low in fat and calories and tend to be rich in fiber, potassium, and vitamins. In addition, studies show that populations who consume more fruits and vegetables tend to have lower rates of common chronic diseases.

What are some of the benefits of phytochemicals? One study of 2,400 Greek women found that those who ate the most vegetables (roughly five servings per day) had a 46 percent lower risk of breast cancer than the women who ate the fewest. In another study, Chinese who regularly consumed soybeans and/or tofu were found to have a 50 percent lower risk of cancers of the stomach, colon, breast, and lung, compared to those who rarely consumed soy products. The foods and herbs with the highest anticancer activity include garlic, soybeans, cabbage, ginger, and licorice, as well as the family of vegetables that includes celery, carrots, and parsley.

How do phytochemicals work to prevent cancer? Two of the major phytochemical mechanisms of cancer prevention are modification of hormone effects and neutralization of free radicals. A number of phytochemicals, including those from soybeans and from the cab-

results from a deficiency of vitamin C. Scurvy had been reported since ancient times, and its common symptoms—pinpoint skin hemorrhages (petechiae), swollen and bleeding gums, joint pain, fatigue and lethargy, and psychologic changes such as depression and hysteria—were well known. Indigenous populations discovered plant foods that would cure this illness; among Native Americans these included cranberries in the Northeast and many tree extracts in other parts of the country. From observations such as this come questions that lead to hypotheses, or "educated guesses," about which factors might be responsible for the observed phenomenon. Scientists then test hypotheses using appropriate research designs. Poorly designed research produces useless results or false conclusions.

bage family, are able to modify estrogen metabolism or block the effect of estrogen on cell growth. Since levels of estrogen and other hormones are in turn closely linked to the development of breast, ovarian, and prostate tumors, it is apparent how phytochemicals might inhibit development of such cancers.

Free radicals (active oxidants) are continually produced in our cells and over time can result in damage to DNA and other important cell structures. Eventually, this damage can promote both cancer and cell aging. A great variety of plant chemicals, such as the phenolic compounds and pigments in grapes and red wine, are able to neutralize or reduce concentrations of free radicals, thus protecting us against the development of both cancer and atherosclerosis.

While the phytochemicals in citrus help protect against cancer, they have additional benefits. Pink grapefruit, for instance, con-

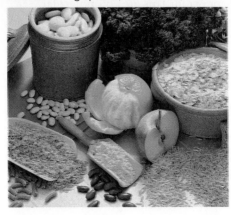

tains high levels of beta-carotene and a variety of other carotenoids with significant antioxidant activity. These compounds are associated with a lower incidence of age-related macular degeneration, the leading cause of age-related blindness. The phytochemicals in whole grains are generally similar to those found in fruits and vegetables and are important in prevention of both cancer and heart disease. One class of grain phytochemicals, the terpenoids, produces a significant reduction in total and LDL cholesterol levels, thus reducing the risk of heart disease. Before you reach for your next slice of bread, it is worth remembering that refined wheat, the source of white flour, has lost more than 99 percent of its phytochemical content, and only four vitamins and one mineral are added back when refined grains are enriched.

Since phytochemicals are so beneficial, why can't we just purify the important ones and add them to our diet as supplements, the way we add back to white flour the vitamins that are removed during processing? The short answer is that we don't know enough about how phytochemicals function. There are thousands of them, and many appear to act synergistically, both as antioxidants and as modifiers of hormonal influences. It is not surprising, then, that when a single pure phytochemical, such as beta-carotene, is given as a long-term supplement, only minor benefits are seen. In fact, some studies have shown no health benefits

from such purified supplements. Yet there is no doubt that consumption of plant foods containing multiple antioxidants is strongly associated with health benefits. The weight of evidence and experience strongly favors finding a place for a minimum of five servings of fruits and vegetables, and an emphasis on whole grains for the six to eleven servings recommended each day. Choosing legumes and soy products at least some of the time as alternatives to meat will introduce even more phytochemicals to the diet.

Changing your diet to include more plants and fewer empty calories needn't be painful if you use your imagination. Sometimes you can have your pizza and eat it too. The next time you indulge, ask for a pizza with minimum cheese and maximum vegetables. The combination of lycopene from tomato sauce, quercetin from onions, glucarates from green peppers, and carotenoids from basil and spinach can turn a potential nutritional train wreck into a phytochemical cornucopia.

Dr. Burge received his doctorate in microbiology from Harvard University. He has been a faculty member at MIT and a researcher in cancer and infectious disease.

Note: For more information on the possible benefits of various phytochemicals, see Appendix D.
Source: Healthline, November 1998.

epidemiology The science of determining the incidence and distribution of diseases in different populations.

correlation A connection, a co-occurrence more frequent than can be explained by chance or coincidence, but without a proven cause.

case control study An investigation that uses a group of people with a particular condition, in contrast to a randomized population. These cases are compared to a control group of people who do not have the condition.

experiment A test to examine the validity of a hypothesis.

Epidemiological Studies

An epidemiological study compares disease rates among population groups and can identify conditions related to diseases such as diet or smoking habits. This enables researchers to identify associations with the disease being studied. The observation that scurvy (see **Figure 1.12**) developed during prolonged time at sea is an example of one aspect of **epidemiology.** Based on observations, diseases that we now know as nutrient deficiencies, such as beriberi (thiamin deficiency) or pellagra (niacin deficiency), previously were thought to be caused by infectious agents. Further observation of factors, such as potential for spreading disease through close contact or differences in eating habits, often ruled out infectious causes. Another example is the association between dietary intakes of soy and breast cancer rates. While Japanese women have high dietary intakes of soy and low breast cancer rates, American women have comparatively low dietary intakes of soy and high breast cancer rates.

Epidemiological studies provide information about relationships but do not clarify cause and effect. The results of these studies show **correlations—** relationships between two factors. For example, with soy and breast cancer, epidemiological studies show only that populations with higher soy intake (Japanese women) have lower breast cancer rates; they do not establish that soy intake prevents breast cancer. However, epidemiological studies provide clues and insights that lead to animal and human studies that can further clarify diet and disease relationships.

Animal Studies

Animal studies can provide preliminary data that lead to human studies, or can be used to study hypotheses that cannot be tested on humans. It was shown in the 1890s that feeding polished (refined) rice to chickens led to a disease similar to beriberi, while a diet of rice with the hull intact did not. Although animal studies give scientists important information that furthers nutrition knowledge, it's important to keep in mind that results of animal studies cannot be transferred directly to humans. Following animal studies with cell culture studies or human clinical studies is important for determining specific effects in humans.

Cell Culture Studies

Another way to study nutrition is to isolate specific types of cells and grow them in culture. Scientists can then use these cells to study the effects of nutrients or other components on metabolic processes in the cell. An important area of nutrition research is the effect of specific nutrients and other chemical compounds on gene expression. This area of molecular biology will help us to explain individual differences in chronic disease risk factors and may lead to designing diets based on an individual's genetic profile, rather than guidelines for the population in general.

Human Studies

The **case control study** and clinical trials are the two primary types of **experiments** used to research hypotheses in humans. Case control studies are small-scale epidemiological studies in which one group of individuals who have a condition (e.g., breast cancer) are compared to a similar group of individuals who do not have the condition. Researchers then identify factors other than the disease in question, such as fruit and vegetable intake, that differ between the two groups. These factors provide researchers

1. Observation
Sailors on long voyages all became ill with scurvy

2. Hypothesis
Lack of certain foods causes scurvy

3. Experimentation:
Experiment to test hypothesis
Predicts that some dietary element will cure scurvy

Key
| Controlled variables |
| Experimental variables |
| Results |
| Conclusions |

James Lind: A Treatise of the Scurvy in Three Parts. Containing an inquiry into the Nature, Causes and Cure of that Disease, together with a Critical and Chronological View of what has been published on the subject. A. Millar, London, 1753.

On the 20th May, 1747, I took twelve patients in the scurvy on board the Salisbury at sea. Their cases were as similar as I could have them. They all in general had putrid gums, the spots and lassitude, with weakness of their knees. They lay together in one place, being a proper apartment for the sick in the fore-hold; and had one diet in common to all, viz., water gruel sweetened with sugar in the morning; fresh mutton broth often times for dinner; at other times puddings, boiled biscuit with sugar etc.; and for supper barley, raisins, rice and currants, sago and wine, or the like. Two of these were ordered each a quart of cyder a day. Two others took twenty five gutts of elixir vitriol three times a day upon an empty stomach, using a gargle strongly acidulated with it for their mouths. Two others took two spoonfuls of vinegar three times a day upon an empty stomach, having their gruels and their other food well acidulated with it, as also the gargle for the mouth. Two of the worst patients, with the tendons in the ham rigid (a symptom none the rest had) were put under a course of sea water. Of this they drank half a pint every day and sometimes more or less as it operated by way of gentle physic. Two others had each two oranges and one lemon given them every day. These they eat with greediness at different times upon an empty stomach. They continued but six days under this course, having consumed the quantity that could be spared. The two remaining patients took the bigness of a nutmeg three times a day of an electuary recommended by an hospital surgeon made of garlic, mustard seed, rad. raphan., balsam of Peru and gum myrrh, using for common drink narley water well acidulated with tamarinds, by a decoction of wich, with the addition of cremor tartar, they were gently purged three or four times during the course.

The consequence was that the most sudden and visible good effects were perceived from the use of the oranges and lemons; one of those who had taken them being at the end of six days fit four duty. The spots were not indeed at that time quite off his body, nor his gums sound; but without any other medicine than a gargarism or elixir of vitriol he became quite healthy before we came into Plymouth, which was on the 16th June. The other was the best recovered of any in his condition, and being now deemed pretty well was appointed nurse to the rest of the sick …

As I shall have occasion elsewhere to take notice of the effects of other medicines in this disease, I shall here only observe that the result of all my experiments was that oranges and lemons were the most effectual remedies for this distemper at sea. I am apt to think oranges preferable to lemons…

4. Publication

5. More experiments

6. Theory

Figure 1.12 **The first clinical trial.** In 1758, physician James Lind reported the careful process of his clinical trial among British sailors afflicted with scurvy.

with clues about the cause, progression, and prevention of the disease. It is important that the two groups are matched as closely as possible for major characteristics such as age, gender, and race.

Clinical trials are controlled studies where some type of intervention—a nutrient supplement, controlled diet, or exercise program is used to determine its impact on certain health parameters. Studies include an **experimental group** (the subjects who are given the intervention) and a **control group** (similar subjects who are not treated). Scientists measure aspects of health or disease in each group and compare the results.

Lind's experiments with sailors aboard the *Salisbury* in 1747 are considered to be the first dietary clinical trial. His observation that oranges and lemons were the only dietary elements that seemed to cure scurvy was an important finding. However, it took more than 40 years for the British Navy to begin routinely giving all sailors citrus juice or fruit—a practice that led to the nickname "limey" when referring to British sailors. It took nearly 200 years (until the 1930s) for scientists to isolate the compound we call vitamin C and show that it had antiscurvy activity.[23] The chemical name for vitamin C, ascorbic acid, comes from its role as an "antiscorbutic" (antiscurvy) compound.

There are several important elements in a modern clinical trial: random assignment to groups, use of placebos, and blinding of subjects and researchers. Subjects are assigned randomly—as by the flip of a coin—to the experimental group or the control group. This reduces the risk of introducing bias into either group. The experimental group receives the treatment or specific protocol (e.g., consuming a certain nutrient at a specific level). The control group does not receive the treatment but often does receive a **placebo.** A placebo is an imitation treatment that looks the same as the experimental treatment but has no effect (such as a sugar pill). The placebo is also important for reducing bias because subjects do not know if they are receiving the intervention and would be less inclined to alter their responses or reported symptoms based on what they think should happen.

When the members of neither the experimental nor the control groups know what treatment they are receiving, we say the subjects are "blinded" to the treatment. If a clinical trial is designed so neither the subjects nor the researchers collecting data are aware of the subjects' group assignments (treatment or placebo), the study is called **double blind.** This reduces the possibility that researchers will see the results they want to see even if these results do not occur. In this case, another member of the research team holds the code for subject assignments and does not participate in the data collection. Double-blind, placebo-controlled clinical trials are considered the "gold standard" of nutrition studies. These studies can show clear cause-and-effect relationships, but often require large numbers of subjects, and are expensive and time-consuming to conduct.

More on the Placebo Effect

The **placebo effect** exerts a powerful influence. At least one-third of participants show improvement after receiving a placebo regardless of the illness.[24] Thus, it is critical to make allowances for the placebo effect in research studies. For example, a double-blind study tested the effectiveness of a medication in reducing binge eating among people with bulimia.[25] After a baseline number of binge-eating episodes was determined, 22 women with bulimia were given the medication or a placebo. After a period of time, the number of binge-eating episodes was reassessed. The study found a 78 per-

clinical trials Studies that collect large amounts of data to evaluate the effectiveness of a treatment.

experimental group A set of people being studied to evaluate the effect of an event, substance, or technique.

control group A set of people used as a standard of comparison to the experimental group. The people in the control group have similar characteristics to those in the experimental group and are selected at random.

placebo An inactive substance that is outwardly indistinguishable from the active substance whose effects are being studied.

double-blind study A research study set up so that neither the subjects nor the investigators know which study group is receiving the placebo and which is receiving the active substance.

placebo effect A physical or emotional change that is not due to properties of an administered substance. The change reflects participants' expectations.

cent reduction in binge-eating episodes among those taking the medication, and a 70 percent reduction in the control group. This showed that the *expectation* that the medication would be effective was nearly as effective as the medication itself.

Peer Review of Experimental Results

Once an experiment is complete, scientists publish the results in a scientific journal to communicate new information to other scientists. Generally before articles are published in scientific journals, other scientists who have expert knowledge of the subject critically review them. **Peer review** ensures that only high-quality research findings are published. This is an important step because the federal government, nonprofit foundations, drug companies, and others fund most scientific research in this country. Ideally, all scientists are fair in evaluating the results of their research and are not influenced by the funding agency. Peer review ensures this objectivity. Unfortunately, peer-reviewed journals such as the *American Journal of Clinical Nutrition* and the *Journal of The American Dietetic Association* are not the main sources of information presented in the popular media.

Key Concepts *The scientific method is used to expand our nutrition knowledge. Hypotheses are formed from observations, and are then tested by experiments. Epidemiological studies observe patterns in populations. Animal and cell culture studies can test effects of various treatments. For human studies, placebo-controlled, double-blind clinical trials are the best research tool for determining cause-and-effect relationships.*

From Research Study to Headline

What about the nutrition and health headlines we see in the newspapers, hear on TV, or read about on the Internet daily? Consumers are often confused by what they see as the "wishy-washyness" of scientists—e.g., coffee is good, then coffee is bad. Margarine is better than butter...no wait, maybe butter is better after all. These contradictions, despite the confusion they cause, show us that nutrition is truly a science: dynamic, changing, and growing with each new finding.

Each time research findings are summarized and reported some degree of opinion is introduced into the report. A large-scale clinical trial or a long-term observational report produces mountains of data. Researchers must decide, using their experience and judgment, which data analysis methods to use and which results to summarize for peer-reviewed publication. The journalist who regularly scans scientific journals for potential headlines decides which studies will get media attention and will summarize study results in nontechnical terms. A news article becomes a 30-second sound bite that is usually far removed from the original data. In some cases, the study may be distorted, with its results misstated or overstated.

peer review An appraisal of research against accepted standards by professionals in the field.

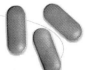

Quick Bites

Swallowing Your Beliefs

Patients' expectations also play an important role in their responses to a placebo. In one study, subjects swallowed a pill that contained only a magnet to measure their stomach contractions. Their stomach contractions increased, decreased, or did not change according to what they had been told would happen.

Think About It 4

SCIENTISTS DISPUTE CLAIMS OF GINKGO BILOBA EFFECTIVENESS

here have been over four hundred scientific udies conducted on proprietary stand

Schwabe Co. of Karlsruhe, Germa producer of the proprietary extra EGb 761. Ginkgo extract is a goo exa mu deli scie the for

Researchers Link Caffeine and Cancer

Some Say Ginkgo Biloba Improves Memory

cer and Vitamin E Link Disputed

Vitamin E Reduces Risk of Cancer

causing a multitude of other offenses human health, free radicals are the main

hardening of the arteries. Briefly, here's how it works: Excess free radicals in the bloodstream oxidize particles of LDL. Immune system cells in the oxidized LDLs as toxic to

The walls recognize the risk of oxidized LDLs as toxic to the body and gobble them up. This vitamin has been shown to be

Vitamin E reduces the risk of LDL cholesterol being oxidized and therefore attaching to the cell wall. Because it is fat

logical cells called foam cells. The foam cells attach readily t the vessel wall and start the

[*Fyi*] Do You Speak Metric?

FOR YOUR INFORMATION

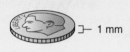

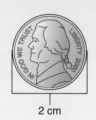

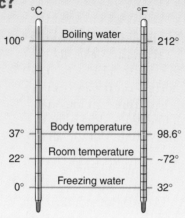

Although the metric system isn't really a language like English or Spanish, in some sense it is the language of science. Nutritionists must be fluent in metrics. Pick up any nutrition journal and you will find units of measurement expressed in terms *like kilograms* and *liters*.

The metric system is a decimal-based system of measurement units. Like our monetary system, units are related by factors of 10. There are 10 pennies in a dime and 10 dimes equal one dollar. Calculations involve the simple process of moving the decimal point to the right or to the left.

There are only seven basic units in the metric system. The most common units are the meter (m) to measure length, the kilogram (kg) for mass, the liter (L) for volume, and degree Celsius (°C) for temperature. The metric system avoids confusing dual use of terms, such as our current use of ounces to measure both weight and volume.

One strategy for learning metric is to find common or familiar associations. For example, when using degrees Celsius you should equate 20 degrees Celsius (20°C) with room temperature, 37 degrees Celsius (37°C) with body temperature, and 0 and

100 degrees Celsius with the freezing and boiling points of water, respectively. A millimeter (1 mm) is about the thickness of a dime and two centimeters (2 cm) is about the diameter of a nickel. Most people already recognize 1-L and 2-L soft-drink bottles. When you pick up a 2-lb bag of sugar, you are holding a little less than 1 kilogram. A fluid ounce can be tricky because it's a measure of liquid volume not weight. A 1-L bottle equals 33.8 fluid ounces.

The United States is the only industrial country in the world not officially using the metric system. Because of its many advantages (e.g., easy conversion between units of the same quantity), the metric system has become the internationally accepted system of measurement.

Many members of the international scientific community use the International System of Units (SI). The SI is the modern metric system and has adopted the joule rather than the calorie to measure food energy. Although we think of the calorie as a measure of energy, it is more accurately a measure of heat. Joules are a measure of work, not heat, and the amount of energy in foods is expressed best in kilojoules (kjoules). Each kcal is equivalent to approximately 4.2 (4.184) kjoules. For example, a 100 kcal glass of juice provides about 420 kjoules.

In most cases, familiarity with the following metric units will be sufficient in your study of nutrition.

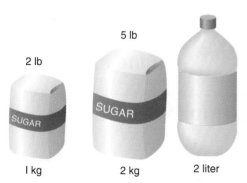

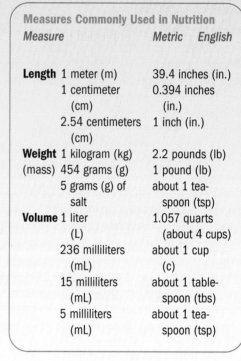

Measures Commonly Used in Nutrition

Measure		Metric	English
Length	1 meter (m)	39.4 inches (in.)
	1 centimeter (cm)	0.394 inches (in.)
	2.54 centimeters (cm)	1 inch (in.)
Weight (mass)	1 kilogram (kg)	2.2 pounds (lb)
	454 grams (g)	1 pound (lb)
	5 grams (g) of salt	about 1 teaspoon (tsp)
Volume	1 liter (L)	1.057 quarts (about 4 cups)
	236 milliliters (mL)	about 1 cup (c)
	15 milliliters (mL)	about 1 tablespoon (tbs)
	5 milliliters (mL)	about 1 teaspoon (tsp)

1 gram = 1000 milligrams

1 milligram = 1000 micrograms (μg or mcg)

The Celsius (C) temperature scale should be used instead of the Farenheit (F) scale. The following are familiar points:

	°C	°F
Temperature at which water freezes	*0*	*32*
Temperature at which water boils	*100*	*212*
Normal body temperature	*37*	*98.6*
Comfortable room temperature	*20–25*	*68–77*

Sorting Facts and Fallacies in the Media

People tend to believe what they hear repeatedly. Even when it has no basis in fact, a claim can seem credible if heard often enough. For example, do you believe that sugar makes kids hyperactive? There is no *scientific* evidence to support this claim! The public is surrounded by messages from various media: TV, radio, newspapers, magazines, books, and the Internet. The media makes money attracting viewers, listeners, and readers, which translates into higher ratings or sales and subsequently high advertising rates. To increase viewers or listeners, media may sensationalize and over-simplify nutrition-related topics. This is particularly true of stories related to obesity, cancer, vitamins and minerals, and food safety. Although news stories may be based on reports in the scientific literature, the media may present a distorted representation of the facts through omission of details.

As you learn about nutrition, you will undoubtedly be more aware not only of your eating and shopping habits but of nutrition-related information in the media. As you see and hear reports, stop to think carefully about what you are hearing. You may want to find the scientific article and see for yourself: Headlines often overstate the findings of a study. At first, reading journal articles will be difficult, but with experience (and growing nutrition knowledge) you will understand more of the information presented. Talk to your instructor for ideas about journal articles that might help you evaluate headlines you are seeing. Two other things to keep in mind: One study does not provide all the answers to our nutrition questions; and if it sounds too good to be true, it probably is!

Your study of nutrition is just beginning. As you learn about the essential nutrients, their functions and food sources, be alert to your food choices and the factors that influence them. When the discussion turns to the role of diet in health, think about your preconceived ideas, and evaluate your beliefs in the light of current scientific evidence. Keep an open mind, but also think critically. Most of all, remember that food is more than the nutrients it provides; it is part of the way we enjoy and celebrate life!

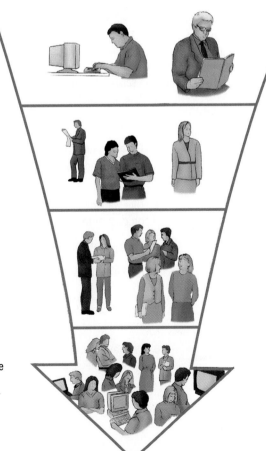

As scientific information is made accessible to more and more people, less detail is provided and more opinion and sensationalism are introduced.

Primary source: Professional journals in print and on the Internet.

Secondary source: Scientific magazines with articles based on primary source material written by specialists.

Generalist magazines and newspapers' science pages. Articles written by science writers.

Mass Media: Nightly news bites, "instant books", unattributed Internet sites.

Figure 1.13 **Sifting facts and fallacies.** Each time research findings are summarized and reported some degree of opinion is introduced. Researchers use their experience and judgment when analyzing data and summarizing results for peer-reviewed publication. Journalists usually select and summarize study results that generate the greatest media attention. A 30-second sound bite contains little information and is often a far cry from the original data. The best consumer information, whether in print, television, radio, or the Internet, attributes the sources for their facts.

[*Fyi*] Evaluating Information on the Internet

In many ways, "surfing" the Web has made life easier. You can buy a car, check stock prices, search out sources for a research paper, chat with like-minded people, and stay up to date on news or sports scores. Hundreds of Web sites are devoted to nutrition and health topics, and you may be asked to visit such sites as part of your course requirements. So, how do you evaluate the quality of information on the Web? Can you trust what you see?

First, it's important to remember that there are no rules for posting on the Internet. Anyone who has the equipment can set up a Web site and post any content he or she likes. Although the Health on the Net Foundation has set up a Code of Conduct for medical and health Web sites, following its eight principles is completely voluntary.[1]

Second, consider the source, if you can tell what it is! Many Web sites do not specify where the content came from, who is responsible for it, or how often it is updated. If the site lists the authors, what are their credentials? Who sponsors the site itself? Educational institutions (.edu), government agencies (.gov), and organizations (.org) generally have more credibility than commercial (.com) sites where selling rather than educating may be the motive.[2] Identifying the purpose for a site can give you more clues about the validity of its content.

Third, when you see claims for nutrients, dietary supplements, or other products, and results of studies or other information, keep in mind the scientific method and the basics of sound science. Who did the study? What type of study was it? How many subjects? Was it double-blind? Were the results published in a peer-reviewed journal? Think critically about the content, look at other sources, and ask questions of experts before you accept information as truth. Remember that just like books, magazines, and newspapers, just because it is in print or online, doesn't mean it's true.

Finally, be on the lookout for "junk science"—sloppy methods, interpretations, and claims that lead to public misinformation. The Food and Nutrition Science Alliance (FANSA) is a coalition of four professional societies: The American Dietetic Association (ADA), the American Society for Clinical Nutrition (ASCN), the American Society for Nutritional Sciences (ASNS), and the Institute of Food Technologists (IFT). FANSA has developed the "10 Red Flags of Junk Science" to help consumers identify potential misinformation. Use these red flags to evaluate Web sites.

Use the Internet. It's fun and can be educational. Don't forget about the library, though; many scientific journals are not available online. Treat claims as "guilty until proven innocent"—in other words, don't accept what you read at face value until you have evaluated the science behind it. If it sounds too good to be true, it probably is!

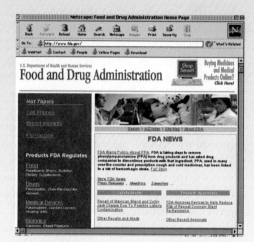

The 10 Red Flags of Junk Science

1. Recommendations that promise a quick fix

2. Dire warnings of danger from a single product or regimen

3. Claims that sound too good to be true

4. Simplistic conclusions drawn from a single study

5. Recommendations based on a single study

6. Dramatic statements that are refuted by reputable scientific organizations

7. Lists of "good" and "bad" foods

8. Recommendations made to help sell a product

9. Recommendations based on studies published without peer review

10. Recommendations from studies that ignore differences among individuals or groups

Source: ADA Serves Up 10 Red Flags to Spot Junk Science. http:www.eatright.org/pr/press021996a.html, accessed 9/16/00.

Note: *The Journal of The American Dietetic Association* has a list of several reliable Internet resources for dietetics professionals.

Evaluating Information on the Internet Box References

[1] http://www.hon.ch/HONcode/Conduct.html

[2] The wheat from the chaff: sorting out nutrition information on the Internet. *J Am Diet Assoc.* 1998;98:1270-1272.

LEARNING *Portfolio* chap

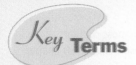 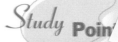 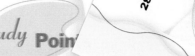

Key Terms

Study Points

➤ Most people have reasons ... than nutrient value.

➤ Taste and texture are the two most import... that influence food choices.

➤ In all cultures, eating is the primary way of maintaining social relationships.

➤ Although Americans know about healthful food choices, their eating habits do not always reflect this knowledge.

➤ Food is a mixture of chemicals. Essential chemicals in food are called nutrients.

➤ Carbohydrates, lipids, proteins, vitamins, minerals, and water are the six classes of nutrients found in food.

➤ Nutrients have three general functions in the body: energy source, structural component, and regulator of metabolic processes.

➤ Vitamins regulate body processes such as energy metabolism, blood clotting, and calcium balance.

➤ Minerals contribute to body structures and to regulating processes such as fluid balance.

➤ Water is the most important nutrient in the body. We can survive much longer without the other nutrients than we can without water.

➤ Energy in foods and the body is measured in kilocalories. Carbohydrates, fats, and proteins are sources of energy.

➤ Carbohydrate and protein have a potential energy value of 4 kcal/g and fat provides 9 kcal/g.

➤ Scientific studies are the cornerstone of nutrition. The scientific method uses observation and inquiry to test hypotheses.

➤ Double-blind, placebo-controlled clinical trials are considered the "gold standard" of nutrition studies.

➤ Research designs used to test hypotheses include epidemiological, animal, cell culture, and human studies.

➤ Information in the public media is not always an accurate or complete representation of the current state of the science on a particular topic.

Questions

1. List the six classes of nutrients.

2. What are the three main factors that influence our food choices?

3. How do our health beliefs affect our food choices?

4. How many kcalories are in 1 gram of carbohydrate, of protein, and of fat?

5. List the 13 vitamins.

6. What determines whether a mineral is a macromineral or a micro (trace) mineral?

7. What is an epidemiological study?

8. What's the difference between an experimental and a control group?

9. What's a placebo?

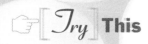 **This**

Try a New Cuisine Challenge

The purpose of this exercise is to expand your culinary taste buds and try a new cuisine. Take your local phone book and see how many ethnic restaurants are near campus. Choose a cuisine you are not that familiar with and take some friends along for dinner so you can order and share several dishes. While you're there, don't be afraid to ask questions about the menu, so you can gain a better understanding of the foods, preparation techniques, spices, and even the cultural meaning attached to some of the dishes.

Food Label Puzzle

The purpose of this exercise is to put the individual pieces of the food label together to determine how many kilocalories are in a serving. Take all the foods in your dorm room or apartment that have complete food labels and ask a friend to black out the value for Calories on each. Remember that the familiar term "Calories" on a food table is really referring to kilocalories. Your job is to determine how many kilocalories are in a serving of each of these foods. You can do this by putting together the individual pieces (carbohydrate, protein, and fat). If you need help, review this chapter and pay close attention to the section on the caloric nutrients. How many kilocalories does each have per gram? You may find that your calculations don't match the numbers on the label. Within labeling guidelines, food manufacturers can round values.

What About 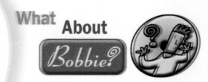 Bobbie?

The "What about Bobbie" feature appears in most chapters. Bobbie is a college student whom you'll follow chapter by chapter to learn the strengths and weaknesses of her diet. Look for this feature to see how the information you learn in each chapter can be applied to real life.

Bobbie is a 20-year-old college sophomore. She lives in the dorm and has one roommate. She has the standard meal plan with her university, so she eats most of her meals in the cafeteria. Sometimes she'll get a snack from the local coffee shop or a dorm vending machine. Her schedule is fairly typical with classes spread out in both the morning and afternoon. Occasionally at night, she and her friends will order pizza or go out for ice cream.

Bobbie weighs 155 pounds and is 5'4". She gained 10 pounds her freshman year in college and would like to lose it because she feels that her ideal weight is more like 145 pounds. She exercises infrequently but likes to walk with her friends and take an occasional aerobics class. Here is a typical day of eating for Bobbie:

Sample one-day menu from Bobbie's diet

7:45 A.M.
1 raisin bagel
   3 tablespoons light cream cheese
10 ounces regular coffee
   2 packets of sugar
   2 tablespoons of 2% fat milk

10:15 A.M.
1 banana

12:15 P.M.
Turkey and cheese sandwich
   2 slices sourdough bread
   2 ounces sliced turkey lunch meat
   2 teaspoons regular mayonnaise
   2 teaspoons mustard
   2 slices tomato
   2 slices dill pickle
   shredded lettuce
Salad from cafeteria salad bar
   2 cups shredded iceberg lettuce
   2 tablespoons each: shredded carrot chopped egg croutons

kidney beans
Italian dressing
12-ounce diet soda
1 small chocolate chip cookie

3:30 P.M.
16 ounces water
1.5 ounces regular tortilla chips
½ cup salsa

6:00 P.M.
Spaghetti with meatballs
   1.5 cups pasta
   3 ounce ground beef meatballs
   3 ounces spaghetti sauce with mushrooms
   2 tablespoons parmesan cheese
1 piece garlic bread
½ cup green beans
   1 teaspoon butter
12-ounce diet soda

10:15 P.M.
1 slice cheese pizza

References

1 Lernmer CM, Mattes R. Cognitive influences on food intake. *Healthline.* June 1999; 18:6–7.

2 Yamaguchi S, Ninomiya K. Umami and food palatability. *J Nutr.* 2000; 30:921S–926S.

3 Lacey EP. Broadening the perspective of pica: Literature review. *Public Health Reports.* 1990;105(1):29–35.

4 Levy AS, Stokes, RC. Effects of a health promotion advertising campaign on sales of ready-to-eat cereals. *Public Health Reports.* 1987;102(4):398–403.

5 Birch LL. Development of food preferences. *Ann Rev Nutr.* 1999; 19:41–62.

6 De Castro JM, Brewer ME. The amount eaten in meals by humans is a power function of the number of people present. *Physiol Behav.* 1991;51:121–125.

7 Lernmer CM, Mattes R, op. cit.

8 Cockerham WC. *Medical Sociology.* Englewood Cliffs, NJ: Prentice-Hall; 1978.

9 Rozin P. Human food selection: why do we know so little and what can we do about it? *Int J Obes.* 1980;4:333–337.

10 Kittler GO, Sucher K. *Food and Culture in America: A Nutrition Handbook.* Belmont, CA: Wadsworth; 1998.

11 Fieldhouse P. *Food and Nutrition: Customs and Culture.* UK: Chapman and Hall; 1996.

12 Zeman FJ, Ney DM. Cultural factors in nutrition care. In: Davis KM, ed. *Applications in Medical Nutrition Therapy.* Englewood Cliffs, NJ: Prentice-Hall; 1996:125–138.

13 Sloan AE. America's appetite '96: the top 10 trends to watch and work on. *Food Technology.* 1996;50:55–71.

14 Kittler GP, Sucher K, Op. cit.

15 Zeman FJ, Ney DM, *loc. cit.*; and Fieldhouse P. *Food and Nutrition: Customs and Culture.* UK: Chapman and Hall; 1996; and Kittler GP, Sucher K, Op. cit.

16 Chiva M. Cultural aspects of meals and meal frequency. Brit J Nutr. 1997;77:S21–28; and Zeman FJ, Ney DM, Loc. cit.

17 Fieldhouse P, Op. cit.

18 USDA. Results from the 1994–96 Continuing Survey of Food Intakes by Individuals. http://www.barc.usda.gov/bhnrc/food-survey/96result.html. Accessed 9/16/00.

19 Ibid.

20 Goran MI. Variation in total energy expenditure in humans. *Obes Res.* 1995;3(1 suppl):59–66.

21 Fuller MF, Garlich PJ. Human amino acid requirements: can the controversy be resolved? *Ann Rev Nutr.* 1994;14:217–241.

22 National Research Council Subcommittee on the Tenth Edition of the RDAs. Recommended Dietary Allowances. 10th ed., Washington, DC: National Academy Press; 1989.

23 Levine M, Rumsey S, Wang Y, Park J, Kwon O, Xu W, Amano N. Vitamin C. In: Ziegler EE, LJ Flier, eds. *Present Knowledge in Nutrition.* 7th ed. Washington DC: ILSI Press; 1996.

24 Turner JA. Placebo effects on pain. *Healthline.* April 1995.

25 Alger SA, Schwalberg MD, Bigaouette JM, Michalek AV, Howard LJ. Effect of a tricyclic antidepressant and opiate antagonist on binge-eating behavior in normal weight, bulimic, and obese binge-eating subjects. *Am J Clin Nutr.* 1991;53:865–871.

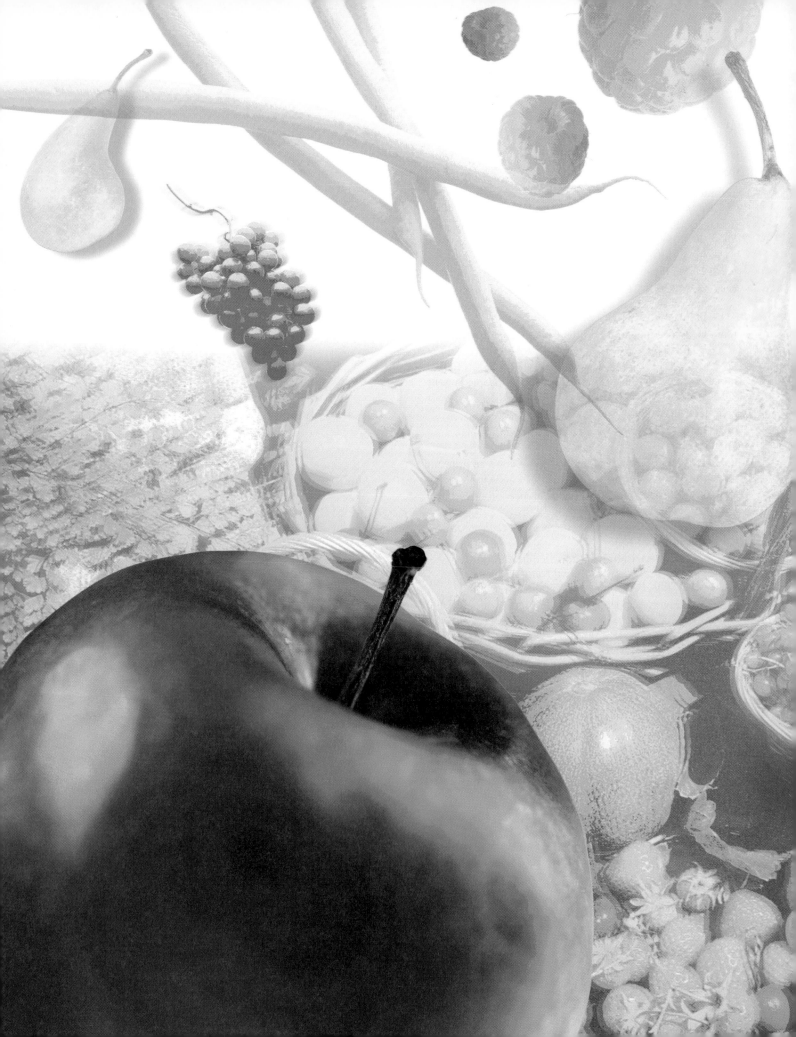

Chapter 2

Nutrition Guidelines and Assessment

 Think About It

1 Do you and your friends discuss food and diet?

2 Have you ever taken a very large dose of a vitamin or mineral? If so, why? How did you determine if it was safe?

3 Do you eat the same foods most days, or do you like variety?

4 What is your favorite drink?

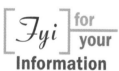 **Fyi for your Information**

This chapter's FYI boxes include practical information on the following topics:

• Are All Food Pyramids Created Equal?

• Food Guide Pyramid: Foods, Serving Sizes, and Tips

• Definitions for Descriptors on Food Labels

 www

The web site for this book offers many useful tools and is a great source for additional nutrition information for both students and instructors. Visit the site at nutrition.jbpub.com for information on nutrition guidelines and assessment. You'll find exercises that explore the following topics:

• Pros and Cons of Food Labeling

• Examining the New DRIs

• Assessing a Diet Assessor

• The Healthy Eating Index

Key to Illustrations

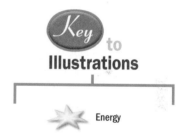 Energy

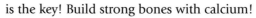

*S*o, you want to be healthier—
that may be the reason you
are taking this course! If so,
you already know one of the important elements of being healthy: a
well-planned diet. Many people
have come to realize that the foods
we choose have major impacts on
our health, but it's sometimes hard
to know exactly what choices to
make. This is especially true because
we are bombarded by headlines and
advertisements: Eat less fat! Get
more fiber in your diet! Moderation
is the key! Build strong bones with calcium!

To many Americans, nutrition is simply a lot of hearsay...or maybe the
latest slogan coined from last week's news headline. Conversations about
nutrition start off with *"They* say you should..." or "Now *they* think that... ."
Have you ever wondered who "they" are and why "they" are telling you
what to eat or what not to eat?

It's no secret that a healthy population is a more productive population,
so many of our nutrition guidelines come from the federal government's
efforts to improve our overall health. Thus the government is one "they."
Many important elements of nutrition policy stem from the recognition of
undernutrition in some segments of the population. The government
requires food manufacturers to add nutrients to certain foods to prevent
widespread deficiencies: iodide in salt, vitamin D in milk, and thiamin,
riboflavin, niacin, iron, and folic acid in enriched grains. Dietary standards
such as the Dietary Reference Intakes make it easier to define adequate diets
for large groups of people.

Overnutrition has led to changes in public policy as well. Links between
diet and high blood pressure, cancer, and heart disease have led to dietary
guidelines that suggest reductions in sodium and saturated fat. The public's
need to know where these and other substances are found in the food supply has led to increased nutrition information on food labels. Also, public
education efforts have resulted in development of teaching tools such as
the Food Guide Pyramid.

New information about diet and health will continue to drive public
policy. This chapter explores current dietary standards, guidelines, and
planning tools, as well as the measurements that evaluate nutritional
health. While you're reading, think about your diet and how it measures
up to current guidelines and standards.

Quick Bites

Early "Laws of Health"

*S*ome consider Galen the best known physician
who ever lived. During the second century,
Galen expounded his "laws of health": eat proper
foods, drink the right beverages, exercise, breathe
fresh air, get enough sleep, have a daily bowel
movement, and control one's emotions.

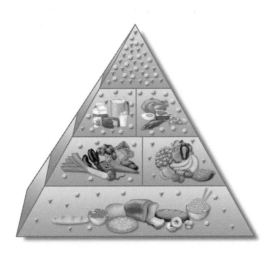

Linking Nutrients, Foods, and Health

It is universally accepted that what you eat affects your health. Nutrition
science has made many advances in identifying the essential nutrients and
the foods in which they are found. Eating foods with all the essential nutrients prevents nutritional deficiencies such as scurvy (vitamin C deficiency)
or pellagra (deficiency of the B vitamin niacin). Nutritional deficiencies due
to dietary inadequacies are relatively rare in the United States. More often,

Americans suffer from chronic diseases such as heart disease, cancer, hypertension, and diabetes—all linked to overconsumption and lifestyle choices. The focus of current research, therefore, is on identifying these links more specifically. Your future health depends on today's lifestyle choices, including your food choices.

Moderation, Variety, and Balance: Words to the Wise

Our cultural mindset leads us to expect immediate solutions to long-term problems. It would be nice if we could keep the consequences of overconsumption at bay just by taking a pill, drinking a beverage, or getting a shot. But no such magic food, nutrient, or other substance exists. Instead, you have to rely on a healthful diet, exercise, and lifestyle choices to reduce your risk of chronic disease. Even into the new millennium, we will need to follow the same advice we have been hearing for decades—healthful eating requires moderation, variety, and balance.

Moderation

Not too much or too little of anything—that's what moderation means. Moderation does *not* mean that you have to eliminate high-fat foods from your diet, but rather that you can include small amounts of them on occasion. Moderation also means not taking anything to extremes. Maybe you have heard about the positive effects of vitamin E, but that doesn't mean huge doses of this essential nutrient are appropriate for you. It is important to remember that substances that are healthful in small amounts can sometimes be dangerous in large quantities. For example, the body needs zinc for hundreds of chemical reactions including those that support normal growth, development, and immune function. Too much zinc, however, can cause deficiency of another essential mineral, copper, and can impair immune function.

Variety

How many *different* foods do you eat on a daily basis? 10? 15? Would it surprise you that the first of Japan's dietary guidelines (see **Figure 2.1**) suggests 30 different foods each day?[1] Now that's variety! Variety means lots of different foods in the diet: food from groups such as fruits, vegetables, grains; and also different foods within each group. Eating two bananas and three carrots each and every day may meet the minimum number of recommended daily servings for fruits and vegetables, but it doesn't add much variety. Variety is important for a number of reasons. It tends to balance the potential positive and negative interactions among food components, and it also balances the overall availability of nutrients to the body by providing nutrients in different forms from different food sources. Variety can add interest and even mystery to your meals while preventing boredom with your diet. Perhaps most important, variety helps ensure that you get all the nutrients you need. Studies have associated varied diets with increased intake of vitamin C and reduced intakes of sodium, sugar, and saturated fat.[2]

Balance

Healthful food choices require a balance of food groups, energy sources (carbohydrates, protein, and fat), and other nutrients. Balance means variety and moderation in your choice of food. Balance also means matching the amount of energy (calories) coming into the body via foods with the amount of energy you expend in daily activities and exercise.

Quick Bites

How Much Do Doctors and Dentists Know About Nutrition?

Although nutrition is a growing concern for the food industry and the general public, medical and dental schools in the United States seem to be moving in the opposite direction. Currently, only 23 percent of medical and dental schools require that students take a nutrition course. In 1981, 37 percent of these schools required a nutrition course.

1. Obtain well-balanced nutrition with a variety of foods; eat 30 foodstuffs a day; take staple food, main dish and side dish together.

2. Take energy corresponding to daily activity.

3. Consider the amount and the quality of the fats and oils you eat: avoid too much; eat more vegetable oils than animal fat.

4. Avoid too much salt, not more than 10 grams a day.

5. Happy eating makes for happy family life; sit down and eat together and talk; treasure family taste and home cooking.

Figure 2.1 Japan's dietary guidelines.

U.S. Department of Agriculture (USDA) The government agency that monitors the production of eggs, poultry, and meat for adherence to standards of quality and wholesomeness. The USDA also provides public nutrition education, performs nutrition research, and administers the WIC program.

U.S. Department of Health and Human Services (DHHS) The principal federal agency responsible for protecting the health of all Americans and providing essential human services. The agency is especially concerned with those Americans who are least able to help themselves.

Dietary Guidelines The *Dietary Guidelines for Americans* are general goals relating to nutrient intake and diet composition developed by the U.S. Department of Agriculture (USDA) and the Department of Health and Human Services (DHHS). They are intended to reduce the number of Americans who develop chronic diseases such as hypertension, diabetes, cardiovascular disease, obesity, and alcoholism.

There is no magic diet, food, or supplement. Instead, your overall, long-term food choices can bring you the benefits of a healthful diet. Let's have a look at some general guidance for making those food choices.

Dietary Guidelines for Americans

A Brief History of the Guidelines

In 1980 the **U.S. Departments of Agriculture (USDA)** and **Health and Human Services (DHHS)** jointly released the first edition of the *Dietary Guidelines for Americans*. Revised guidelines have been released every five years following extensive review of scientific information about links between diet and chronic disease. The purpose of the **Dietary Guidelines** is to provide sound advice for building healthful diets, specifically targeting dietary factors related to heart disease and cancer, the two leading causes of death in the United States. The most recent edition of the *Dietary Guidelines* was released in 2000 (see **Figure 2.2**).

Focus of the Guidelines

The *Dietary Guidelines* promote food and lifestyle choices that reduce risk for chronic disease through three basic messages:

1. **Aim for Fitness.** Weight control is important for improving health and reducing chronic disease risk. Obesity has been linked to an increased risk of heart disease, many types of cancer, stroke, hypertension, and diabetes. Exercise is an important factor in weight control and overall fitness. The guidelines suggest getting at least 30 minutes of physical activity daily.

2. **Build a Healthy Base.** Grains (especially whole grains), fruits, and vegetables should be the foundation of a healthful diet. These foods are rich in carbohydrates, fiber, and many vitamins, minerals, and phytochemicals. Choosing a variety of grains, fruits, and vegetables helps ensure you get all the nutrients you need. In addition, most plant foods are naturally low in fat and saturated fat. The Food Guide Pyramid (discussed in the next section) promotes a pattern of eating that emphasizes plant foods. Safe handling and preparation of all foods is a key to avoiding foodborne illness. For more information on food safety, see Chapter 17.

3. **Choose Sensibly.** Limiting the amount of fat, sugar, salt, and alcohol in the diet is sensible. Reducing saturated fat, cholesterol, and total fat intake can reduce the risk of heart disease and cancer. Also, excess fat intake can contribute to weight gain and obesity. Sugars and many processed foods that contain added sugar are sources of energy but have little other nutritional value. Excessive sugar intake accompanied by poor dental hygiene can contribute to tooth decay, and excess calories from sugar may be a factor in obesity. Excess salt (sodium) intake can contribute to high blood pressure in some people. And although studies have shown that a moderate intake of alcohol may have some health benefits, excess alcohol intake contributes to several of the leading causes of death, including accidents, suicide, homicide, and chronic liver disease.

Use of the Guidelines in Diet Planning

The *Dietary Guidelines for Americans* are just that: guidelines. They don't identify specific foods to consume or avoid, but instead give

Figure 2.2 **Dietary Guidelines for Americans.** These guidelines from two federal departments help define how to apply the principles of moderation, balance and variety.
Source: USDA, USDHHS. *Dietary Guidelines for Americans.* Home and Garden Bulletin No. 232, 5th edition, 2000.

Aim for fitness

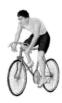

Aim for a healthy weight   Be physically active each day

Build a healthy base

Let the Pyramid guide your food choices

Choose a variety of grains daily, especially whole grains

Choose a variety of fruits and vegetables daily

Keep food safe to eat

Choose sensibly

Choose a diet that is low in saturated fat and cholesterol and moderate in total fat

Choose beverages and foods to moderate your intake of sugars

Choose and prepare foods with less salt

If you drink alcoholic beverages, do so in moderation

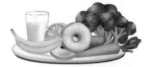

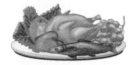

advice about the overall composition of the diet. To be consistent with the *Dietary Guidelines,* consider your overall intake. Choosing more fruits, vegetables, and grains will add variety to your diet and also lower your intake of saturated fat, fat, and cholesterol. Eating fewer high-fat toppings and fried foods will help you to balance intake and expenditure of energy. Then there are the extra things to use in moderation—sugar, salt, and alcohol. Choose water more often as a beverage than soft drinks; use less salt in your cooking and at the table; and if you choose to drink at all, be cautious with alcohol.

Sometimes, the lack of specificity of the *Dietary Guidelines* causes frustration. Many people like detailed information—how *many* fruits and vegetables? *Which* fat sources to minimize? What does "moderation" mean? The development of the Food Guide Pyramid as a diet-planning tool has helped resolve many of these questions.

Key Concepts *The Dietary Guidelines for Americans are a set of statements based on current science that "guide" us toward more healthful choices. The Guidelines embody the basic principles of balance, variety, and moderation.*

The Food Guide Pyramid

Food groups have long been used in nutrition education to illustrate the proper combination of foods in a healthful diet. Even young children can sort food into groups and fill a plate with foods from each group. Certainly different fruits represent similar parts of plants, but from a nutritional perspective, they have much more in common than that, such as the balance of macronutrients and the similarities in micronutrient composition. However, it is also important to understand that foods in one group may have significantly different vitamin and mineral profiles. Some fruits (e.g., citrus, strawberries, and kiwi) are rich in vitamin C and others (e.g., apples and bananas) have very little. Here again, we can see the importance of variety, of not simply including different food groups, but also choosing a variety of foods *within* each group.

A Brief History of Food Group Plans

The food group concept is quite an old one. The USDA published the first guide to food groups in 1916.[3] This guide used five food groups and indicated the percentage of the daily energy (calorie) intake that should come from each:

Food Group 1916	Recommended Percentage of Energy
Meats and other protein-rich food	*20% (10% from milk, 10% other)*
Cereals and other starchy food	*20%*
Vegetables and fruit	*30%*
Fatty foods	*20%*
Sugars	*10%*

Instead of focusing on limiting fat and sugar, this guide stressed the importance of using fat and sugar in order to consume enough energy to support daily activity. Because people performed more manual labor in those days, many people were simply not getting enough calories! More recent versions of food group plans, including the "Basic Four" that was popular from the 1950s through the 1970s, focus on fruits, vegetables, grains, dairy products, and meats and their substitutes. That Basic Four food plan (dairy, meats, fruits and vegetables, and grains) was usually depicted graphically as either a circle or a square with each group having an equal share. The implication

food group A category of similar foods, such as fruits.

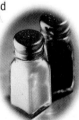

Food Guide Pyramid A graphic representation of the number of servings from the five major food groups needed daily to form a healthful diet. A sixth group consists of fats, oils, and sweets—all of which should be consumed sparingly.

was that people should consume equal amounts of food from each group. Nutrition science now tells us that those proportions would tend to lead to a diet too high in fat and protein and not high enough in carbohydrates and fiber. Consequently, toward the end of the 1980s, the USDA began work on a new graphic image for the food groups.

Development of the Food Guide Pyramid

The USDA introduced the **Food Guide Pyramid** (see **Figure 2.3**) in 1992 to provide a visual representation of a healthful diet—to illustrate the *Dietary Guidelines for Americans* in terms of food groups and recommended numbers of daily servings. The Pyramid shows that the foundation of a healthful diet (the bottom and largest section) is the group of bread, cereal, rice, and pasta. Foods in this group are sources of complex carbohydrates and provide important vitamins, minerals, and fiber. Working our way up the Pyramid, we come to the vegetable group and the fruit group. Unlike the Basic Four, the Pyramid separates fruits and vegetables because of differences in nutrient composition. Vegetables provide vitamins such as vitamins A, C, and folate, the minerals iron and magnesium, and carbohydrates including fiber. Fruits are rarely good sources of minerals other than potassium, but many are good sources of vitamins A and C. Taken together, these three groups at the bottom of the pyramid illustrate that plant foods should make up the bulk of the diet.

Next up are dairy foods, along with meat and meat alternatives (e.g., nuts, eggs, legumes). They are important components of the diet, but we

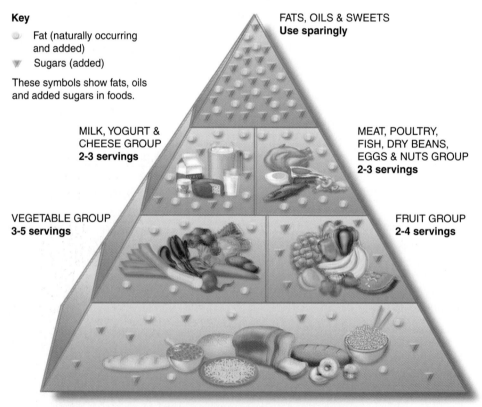

Key

⬤ Fat (naturally occurring and added)

▽ Sugars (added)

These symbols show fats, oils and added sugars in foods.

FATS, OILS & SWEETS
Use sparingly

MILK, YOGURT & CHEESE GROUP
2-3 servings

MEAT, POULTRY, FISH, DRY BEANS, EGGS & NUTS GROUP
2-3 servings

VEGETABLE GROUP
3-5 servings

FRUIT GROUP
2-4 servings

BREAD, CEREAL, RICE & PASTA GROUP
6-11 servings

Figure 2.3 **Food Guide Pyramid.** The USDA's Food Guide Pyramid is a research-based guidance system that help consumers put the Dietary Guidelines into action. The pyramid shows how many servings to eat from each food group every day.
Source: U.S. Department of Agriculture. *The Food Guide Pyramid.* Home and Garden Bulletin No. 252, August 1992, revised October, 1996.

don't need as many servings to obtain the important nutrients from these groups. Dairy products provide protein, vitamins (especially riboflavin and vitamins A and D), and minerals (calcium and phosphorus, in particular). Meats and their substitutes are also good sources of protein, some of the B vitamins, iron, and zinc. The pinnacle of the Pyramid (the smallest section) contains fats and sweets. These are the dietary "extras"—oil for cooking, butter or sour cream on potatoes, sugar in tea or coffee, soft drinks, and the like.

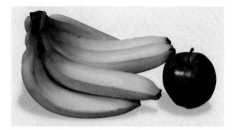

2–4 servings of fruit

The Pyramid's Relationship to the Dietary Guidelines for Americans

The Food Guide Pyramid illustrates the *Dietary Guidelines* in a number of ways. First, the large base of the Pyramid reinforces the advice to choose a variety of grains, vegetables, and fruits each day. Just as the *Guidelines* instruct us to eat less saturated fat, cholesterol, and total fat, the Pyramid shows us that we should eat fewer daily servings of dairy products, meats and alternatives, and few added fats. In addition, the ○ symbols scattered throughout the food groups show where one is likely to encounter fats in foods. You can see that the lower Pyramid groups have less fat, while the top of the Pyramid is more concentrated in fat sources. The ▼ symbol represents added sugars. The highest concentration of sugars is at the top of the Pyramid, in the smallest section, which is in line with the guideline that you should limit your sugar intake.

Using the Pyramid in Diet Planning

The first step in using the Food Guide Pyramid for diet planning is to be familiar with the types of food in each group, the number of recommended servings, and the appropriate serving sizes. The "Food Guide Pyramid: Foods, Serving Sizes, and Tips" feature shows examples of foods and serving sizes for each of the groups. Let's take fruits, for example. According to the Pyramid, our daily diets should include 2 to 4 servings of fruits. Suppose you have a 6-fluid ounce glass of orange juice for breakfast and a banana on your cereal. Add an apple for an afternoon snack, and you have already had three servings. Now let's try the grain group. A bowl (approximately 1 cup) of cereal and a slice of toast for breakfast would be two servings. A sandwich with two slices of bread for lunch adds two more servings. Dinner might include a cup of pasta and two slices of garlic bread. So far, that's 8 servings, which is right in the target zone of 6 to 11 servings per day. So, you see, it's not hard to meet the Pyramid recommendations. **Table 2.1** shows sample calorie intake levels and the associated numbers of servings. This table will give you an idea of how the number of Pyramid servings should vary with different energy needs.

Sometimes it is difficult to figure out how to account for foods that are mixtures of different groups—lasagna, casseroles, or pizza, for example. Try separating such foods into their components (e.g., pizza contains crust, tomato sauce, cheese, and toppings) to estimate the number of servings. You should be able to come up with a reasonable approximation. All in all, the Pyramid is an easy-to-use guideline that can help you select a variety of foods.

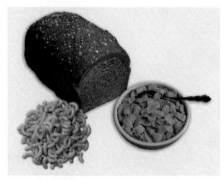

6–11 servings of bread, rice and cereal

Table 2.1 Suggested Numbers of Servings for Three Levels of Energy Intake

Food Group	Energy Intake Level		
	Low (about 1500 kcal)[a]	Moderate (about 2200 kcal)[b]	High (about 2800 kcal)[c]
	SERVINGS		
Bread/cereals/rice/pasta	6	9	11
Vegetable	3	4	5
Fruit	2	3	4
Milk/yogurt/cheese	2	2–3	3
Meat/fish/beans/eggs	2	2–3	3
Equivalent amount of meat	(5 ounces)	(6 ounces)	(7 ounces)
Fats/sugars[d]	use sparingly	use sparingly	use sparingly

[a] 1500 kcal is about right for many sedentary women and some older adults.
[b] 2200 kcal is about right for most children, teenage girls, active women, and many sedentary men.
[c] 2800 kcal is about right for teenage boys, many active men, and some very active women.
[d] Although fats and sugars are part of a normal diet, they should be used sparingly, so the Food Guide Pyramid has no recommended number of servings for this group.

Note: Your calorie needs may be higher or lower than those shown. Women need more calories when they are pregnant or breastfeeding.

Source: Adapted from: USDA. *The Food Guide Pyramid.* Home and Garden Bulletin No. 252, August 1992, revised October, 1996.

Exchange Lists for Meal Planning A list of foods that in specified portions provide equivalent amounts of carbohydrate, fat, protein, and energy. Any food in an exchange list can be substituted, for any other without markedly affecting nutrient intake.

Key Concepts *The Food Guide Pyramid is a visual representation of the Dietary Guidelines for Americans. This graphic tool shows the appropriate balance of food groups in a healthful diet: more grains, vegetables, and fruits, and less dairy, meat, and added fats and sugars.*

Exchange Lists

Another tool for diet planning that uses food groupings is called the **Exchange Lists for Meal Planning.** Like the Food Guide Pyramid and other food group plans, the exchange lists divide foods into groups. Diets can be planned by choosing a certain number of servings, or exchanges, from each group each day. The original purpose of the exchange lists was to help people with diabetes plan diets that would provide consistent levels of energy and carbohydrates—both essential for dietary control of diabetes. For this reason, the foods are organized into groups or lists not

---

[Fyi] Are All Food Pyramids Created Equal?
Alyson Escobar, M.S., R.D., Center for Nutrition Policy and Promotion
FOR YOUR INFORMATION

At the moment several dietary pyramids are competing for the public's attention: the USDA Food Guide Pyramid, the Mediterranean Pyramid, the Asian Pyramid, and the Latin American Pyramid, among others. What do these pyramids, all with seemingly different messages, mean for the American consumer?

The Mediterranean, Asian, and Latin American Diet Pyramids were produced by Oldways Preservation and Exchange Trust of Cambridge, Massachusetts. Oldways, a non-profit company, developed these diet pyramids to illustrate traditional food patterns that epidemiological studies have associated with good health.

The USDA Food Guide Pyramid and the Oldways pyramids have much in common. All illustrate eating patterns consistent with current nutritional recommendations and each can be used to plan diets consisting of different foods. Common emphases of all three pyramids include eating plenty of grain products and vegetables and fruits.

Physical activity, moderate consumption of alcoholic beverages, and enjoyment of meals are healthy lifestyle factors suggested by the Oldways Pyramids and the *Dietary Guidelines for Americans.*

The USDA Food Guide Pyramid is based on American eating patterns. Flexibility in food choices is an important objective of the USDA Pyramid. Thus, a person can easily

choose to eat "Mediterranean," "Asian," or "Latin American" style within the framework of the USDA Food Pyramid.

In fact, several other pyramids have been developed. The Puerto Rican Pyramid, the Vegetarian Pyramid, and the Soul Food Pyramid all use the USDA Food Guide Pyramid framework but emphasize a different range of foods. These pyramids, used in conjunction with the guidance of the USDA, can help the public choose foods that fit a specific ethnic or cultural diet.

The Oldways pyramids illustrate proportions rather than specific types and amounts of food. They don't recommend serving sizes and numbers of servings of foods. Neither do they specify levels of total fat and saturated fat.

Because they represent cultural eating patterns, the Oldways pyramids include a more limited range of foods than the USDA Food

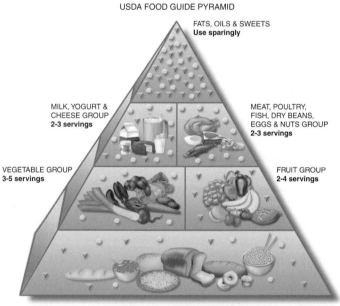

USDA FOOD GUIDE PYRAMID

FATS, OILS & SWEETS
Use sparingly

MILK, YOGURT & CHEESE GROUP
2-3 servings

MEAT, POULTRY, FISH, DRY BEANS, EGGS & NUTS GROUP
2-3 servings

VEGETABLE GROUP
3-5 servings

FRUIT GROUP
2-4 servings

BREAD, CEREAL, RICE & PASTA GROUP
6-11 servings

Guide Pyramid. A major difference between the Mediterranean and Asian diet pyramids and the USDA Food Guide Pyramid is their distinction between plant and animal proteins. The Oldways pyramids group plant-based proteins—legumes, soybeans, nuts, and seeds—separately from animal proteins found in meat, poultry, eggs, and dairy products.

Red meat is included only occasionally in both the Mediterranean and Asian pyramids

only by the type of food (e.g., fruits or vegetables) but also to contain relatively equal amounts of macronutrients (carbohydrate, protein, and fat). The portions are defined so that each "exchange" has a similar composition. For example, 1 fruit exchange is ½ cup of orange juice, or 12 grapes, or 1 medium apple, or ½ cup of applesauce. All of these exchanges have approximately 60 kilocalories, 15 grams of carbohydrate, 0 grams of protein, and 0 grams of fat. In the exchange list groupings, starchy vegetables such as potatoes, corn, and peas are grouped with breads and cereals instead of with other vegetables because their balance of macronutrients is more similar to that of bread or pasta than to that of carrots or tomatoes. A diet plan based on the exchange lists would specify the number of exchanges to be consumed from each group at each meal, and then the person could pick anything from the lists to fit that plan.

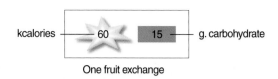

kcalories — 60 ⎯ 15 — g. carbohydrate

One fruit exchange

One fruit exchange

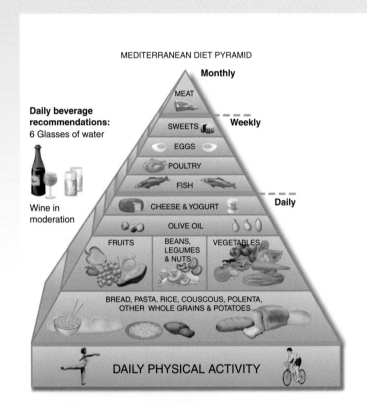

© 2000 Oldways Preservation & Exchange Trust

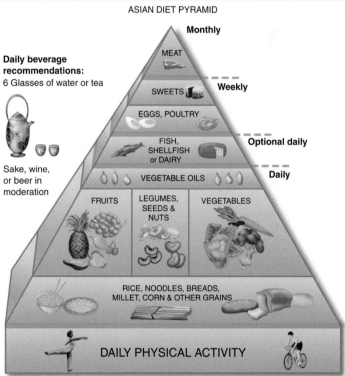

© 2000 Oldways Preservation & Exchange Trust

(a few times a month or less), while poultry and eggs appear slightly more often. The Asian Diet Pyramid contains limited dairy products, considering them optional and to be eaten in their low-fat forms only. Another important distinction among the pyramids concerns fat. Fat in the Oldways pyramids comes largely from vegetable oils high in monounsaturated fats, such as olive oil in the Mediterranean Pyramid and peanut oil in the Asian.

Neither the USDA Food Guide Pyramid nor the Oldways pyramids can convey all that consumers need to know to make food choices for a healthful diet. The USDA Food Guide Pyramid is accompanied by additional information such as the number of servings from each food group appropriate for people of different ages, sexes, and calorie needs.

Source: Adapted from "Are All Food Pyramids Created Equal?" Nutrition Insights, No. 2, USDA, April 1997.

For more information, contact the Center for Nutrition Policy and Promotion, Office of Public Information at (202) 418-2312, or Oldways Preservation & Exchange Trust, 25 First Street, Cambridge, MA 02141 at (617) 621-3000; fax (617) 621-1230. To receive the handbook *Reaching Consumers with Meaningful Health Messages: A Handbook for Nutrition and Food Communicators* contact the International Food Information Council, 1100 Connecticut Avenue, NW, Suite 430, Washington, DC 20036.

Fyi Food Guide Pyramid: Foods, Serving Sizes, and Tips

FOR YOUR INFORMATION

Breads, Cereals, Rice, and Pasta
(6–11 servings daily)

	Serving Size
Bread	1 slice
English muffin	½ muffin
Bagel	½ small bagel
Hamburger bun	½ bun
Cereal, flake type	1 ounce (approx. 1 cup)
Cereal, granola type	1 ounce (approx. ⅓ cup)
Cereal, cooked	½ cup
Rice, cooked	½ cup
Noodles, cooked	½ cup

Choose grains made with little fat or sugar. Go easy on high-fat and sugary toppings. Choose whole-grain products to increase fiber intake.

Vegetables
(3–5 servings daily)

	Serving Size
Raw spinach, lettuce, kale, other leafy greens.	1 cup
Cooked carrots, green beans, corn, other vegetables	½ cup
Baked potato	1 medium
Raw carrots, tomato, cucumber	½ cup
French fries	10 pieces

Choose a variety of vegetables to obtain different nutrients. Include dark green leafy vegetables several times each week. Limit fried vegetables and high-fat sauces or toppings to keep fat content low.

Fruits
(2–4 servings daily)

	Serving Size
Apple, orange, banana	1 medium
Grapes	12
Canned fruit or diced raw fruit	½ cup
Fruit juice	¾ cup
Avocado	½ whole

Variety is important here, too. Whole fruits contain more fiber than canned fruits, fruit sauces, or juice. When choosing a juice, look for "100% juice" on the label.

Milk, Yogurt, and Cheese
(2–3 servings daily)

	Serving Size
Milk	1 cup
Cottage cheese	2 cups
Yogurt	8 ounces
Natural cheeses (cheddar, Swiss, provolone, etc.)	1 ½ ounces
Processed cheeses	2 ounces
Ricotta cheese	½ cup

For the lowest fat intake, choose skim milk and nonfat yogurt. Look for part-skim or reduced-fat cheeses. Ice cream, ice milk, and frozen yogurt tend to have more fat and sugar and less calcium than other dairy foods.

Meat, Poultry, Fish, Dry Beans, Eggs and Nuts
(2–3 servings daily)

	Serving Size
Cooked lean meat, poultry, fish	3 ounces
Cooked ground meat	3 ounces
Bologna or other luncheon meat	2 slices (1 oz)

The following are equivalent to 1 ounce of meat (about 1/3 serving): 1 egg; 1/2 cup cooked dry beans and peas; 2 tablespoons peanut butter; 1/3 cup of nuts.

Choose lean meats, skinless poultry, fish, and beans and peas most often. Use lower-fat cooking methods like broiling, grilling, and roasting instead of frying. Egg yolks, liver, and shellfish are higher in cholesterol than other foods in this group. Nuts, seeds, nut butters, and luncheon meats are higher in fat than other choices, so eat them less often.

Fats, Oils, and Sweets

	Serving Size
Butter or margarine	Use sparingly
Cooking oil	Use sparingly
Mayonnaise	Use sparingly
Salad dressing (regular)	Use sparingly
Sour cream	Use sparingly
Cream cheese	Use sparingly
Sugar, jam, or jelly	Use sparingly
Honey, syrup	Use sparingly
Soft drink	Use sparingly
Fruit drink	Use sparingly
Chocolate bar	Use sparingly
Sherbet	Use sparingly
Gelatin dessert	Use sparingly

Although fats, oils, and sweets are not a food group, they contribute flavor, texture, and variety to our diet. In a 2,000-kilocalorie diet, no more than 65 grams of fat per day should be eaten on average. For the same 2,000-kilocalorie level, try to keep added sugars to a maximum 10 teaspoons each day.

Source: USDA. *The Food Guide Pyramid.* Home and Garden Bulletin No. 252, August 1992, revised October, 1996.

Figure 2.4 shows the amounts of carbohydrate, protein, fat, and calories in one exchange from each group, along with a sample serving size. For a complete set of exchange lists, see the appendix or go to www.jbpub.com/nutrition.

Using the Exchange Lists in Diet Planning

Many weight control programs use the exchange lists. Planning a diet using the exchange lists is done in much the same manner as using the Food Guide Pyramid. The first step is to become very familiar with the components of each group, the variations in fat content for the dairy and meat lists, and how other foods may be included. Then, an individual diet plan can be used to select meals and snacks throughout the day. For example, a 1,500-kilocalorie weight-reduction diet plan might have the following meal pattern:

Breakfast: 2 starch, 1 fruit, 1 milk, 1 fat

Lunch: 3 meat, 2 starch, 1 fruit, 1 vegetable, 1 fat

Snack: 1 milk, 1 starch, 1 fat

Dinner: 2 meat, 1 starch, 2 vegetable, 2 fat

Snack: 2 starch, 1 fruit

Using this pattern and a complete set of exchange lists, you could then plan out a day or a week of menus. Here's a sample for a day:

Breakfast: ½ cup orange juice, ¾ cup corn flakes, 1 cup 2% milk, 1 slice toast, 1 tsp margarine

Lunch: 3 oz cooked hamburger on bun, 1 tsp mayonnaise, ½ cup baby carrots, 1 medium apple

Snack: ¾ cup low-fat yogurt, ½ bagel with 1 Tbsp cream cheese

Dinner: 2 oz cooked pork chop, ½ cup rice with 1 tsp margarine, ½ cup yellow squash and ½ cup zucchini stir-fried in 1 tsp vegetable oil

Snack: 1 toasted English muffin, 1 medium pear

Key Concepts *The exchange lists are a diet planning tool that uses the idea of food groups, but defines groups specifically in terms of macronutrient (carbohydrate, fat, and protein) content. Individual diet plans can be developed for people who need to control energy or carbohydrate intake, such as for weight control or management of diabetes mellitus.*

Recommendations for Nutrient Intake: The RDAs and DRIs

So far, the tools we have described (*Dietary Guidelines for Americans,* Food Guide Pyramid, and exchange lists) deal with whole foods and food groups, which tend to be more understandable to the average consumer than are individual nutrient values. Sometimes, though, we need more specific information about our nutritional needs—a healthful diet is healthful because of the balance of *nutrients* it

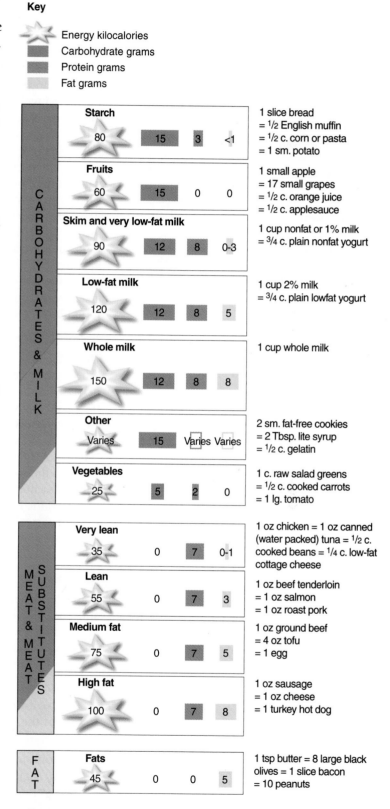

Key

- Energy kilocalories
- Carbohydrate grams
- Protein grams
- Fat grams

CARBOHYDRATES & MILK

Starch				
80	15	3	<1	1 slice bread = ½ English muffin = ½ c. corn or pasta = 1 sm. potato

Fruits				
60	15	0	0	1 small apple = 17 small grapes = ½ c. orange juice = ½ c. applesauce

Skim and very low-fat milk				
90	12	8	0-3	1 cup nonfat or 1% milk = ¾ c. plain nonfat yogurt

Low-fat milk				
120	12	8	5	1 cup 2% milk = ¾ c. plain lowfat yogurt

Whole milk				
150	12	8	8	1 cup whole milk

Other				
Varies	15	Varies	Varies	2 sm. fat-free cookies = 2 Tbsp. lite syrup = ½ c. gelatin

Vegetables				
25	5	2	0	1 c. raw salad greens = ½ c. cooked carrots = 1 lg. tomato

MEAT & MEAT SUBSTITUTES

Very lean				
35	0	7	0-1	1 oz chicken = 1 oz canned (water packed) tuna = ½ c. cooked beans = ¼ c. low-fat cottage cheese

Lean				
55	0	7	3	1 oz beef tenderloin = 1 oz salmon = 1 oz roast pork

Medium fat				
75	0	7	5	1 oz ground beef = 4 oz tofu = 1 egg

High fat				
100	0	7	8	1 oz sausage = 1 oz cheese = 1 turkey hot dog

FAT

Fats				
45	0	0	5	1 tsp butter = 8 large black olives = 1 slice bacon = 10 peanuts

Figure 2.4 **Exchange Lists for Meal Planning.** This is a widely-used system for meal planning for people with diabetes. It is also helpful for people interested in healthy eating and weight control. See Appendix B for the complete exchange lists.

Recommended Dietary Allowances (RDA) The nutrient intake that meets the nutrient needs of almost all (97 to 98 percent) individuals.

Food and Nutrition Board (FNB) A board within the Institute of Medicine in the National Academy of Sciences. Responsible for assembling the group of nutrition scientists who review available scientific data to determine appropriate intake levels of the known essential nutrients for the RDA values.

Dietary Reference Intakes (DRI) A generic term used to refer to the following types of values: Estimated Average Requirement (EAR), Recommended Dietary Allowance (RDA), Adequate Intake (AI), and Tolerable Upper Intake Level (UL).

requirement The lowest continuing intake level of a nutrient that prevents deficiency in an individual.

Estimated Average Requirement (EAR) The intake value that meets the estimated nutrient needs of 50 percent of individuals in a specific life-stage and gender group.

contains. In order to determine how well our food choices reflect our needs for specific nutrients, we need some sense of how much of each nutrient we require daily. This is the purpose of dietary standards—to define healthful diets in terms of specific amounts of the nutrients.

Meaning of Dietary Standards

Dietary standards are sets of recommended intake values for nutrients. It's a way to tell us how much of each nutrient we should have in our diets. In the United States, we have been using a set of recommended intake values called the **Recommended Dietary Allowances,** or RDAs.

Consider the following scenario. You are running a North Polar research center staffed by 60 people. You must provide all of their food because they will not have other sources. You must keep the group adequately nourished; you certainly don't want anyone to become ill as a result of a nutritional deficiency. How would you start planning? How could you be sure to provide adequate amounts of the essential nutrients? Your most important tool would be a set of dietary standards! Essentially the same scenario faces people who plan and provide food for groups of people in more routine circumstances—the military, prisons, and even schools. To assess nutritional adequacy, diet planners can compare the nutrient composition of their food plans to RDA values.

A Brief History of RDAs

The RDAs were first published in 1941. The date is significant because at that time there was a pressing need to ensure that American military troops were being fed adequately. By the 1940s, nutrition science had advanced to the point that many essential nutrients had been isolated from foods. This advance allowed scientists to measure the amounts of these nutrients in foods and to recommend daily intake levels. The **Food and Nutrition Board** of the National Academy of Sciences assembled a group of nutrition scientists, who reviewed the scientific data to determine appropriate intake levels of the known essential nutrients. These levels then became the first RDA values. Since that time, the Food and Nutrition Board has periodically appointed committees to review the RDAs, which has resulted in ten editions of RDAs through 1989. The RDA values are currently being revised as part of a more comprehensive set of dietary standards called the **Dietary Reference Intakes (DRIs).**

RDAs in Transition: Dietary Reference Intakes

Since the inception of the RDAs, we have learned more about the relationships between diet and chronic disease, and the incidence of nutrient-deficiency diseases has dramatically declined. New dietary standards reflect not just dietary adequacy but optimal nutrition. The Food and Nutrition Board's objectives for the development of Dietary Reference Intakes are to:

1. establish a set of reference values that would replace the RDAs,
2. have a single set of values for the United States and Canada (for the first time),
3. document clearly the derivation of the reference values,
4. promote optimal nutrient use and biologic-physical well-being,
5. use evidence concerning the prevention of disease and developmental disorders in addition to more traditional evidence of sufficient nutrient intake,
6. examine data about selected food components that have not been considered essential nutrients, and
7. recommend research based on the knowledge gaps identified.[4]

Similar to the RDAs, the DRIs are reference values for nutrient intakes to be used in assessing and planning diets for healthy people (see **Figure 2.5**). The Dietary Reference Intakes consist of four types of values: Estimated Average Requirement (EAR), Recommended Dietary Allowance (RDA), Adequate Intake (AI), and Tolerable Upper Intake Level (UL). Underlying each of these values is the definition of a **requirement** as the "lowest continuing intake level of a nutrient that, for a specific indicator of adequacy, will maintain a defined level of nutriture in an individual."[5]

Estimated Average Requirement The **Estimated Average Requirement (EAR)** reflects the nutrient intake level estimated to meet the needs of 50 percent of the people in a life-stage and gender group. For each nutrient, this requirement is defined using a specific indicator of dietary adequacy. This indicator could be the level of the nutrient or one of its break-down products in the blood, or the amount of an enzyme associated with that nutrient.[6] For example, the indicators for thiamin adequacy in adults are urinary thiamin excretion and the activity of a thiamin-requiring enzyme in red blood cells. The EAR is used to set the RDA, and it can also be used to assess dietary adequacy or plan diets for groups of people.

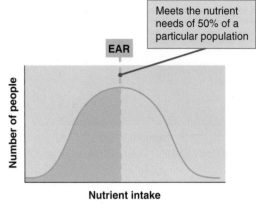

ESTIMATED AVERAGE REQUIREMENT

THE DRIs: DIETARY REFERENCE INTAKES

All DRI values refer to intakes averaged over time

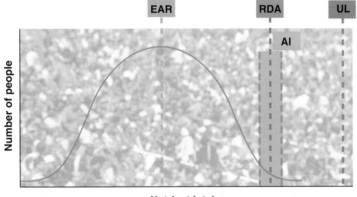

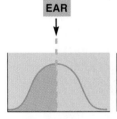

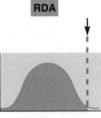

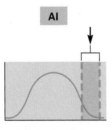

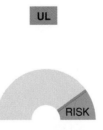

The **Estimated Average Requirement** is the nutrient intake level estimated to meet the need of 50% of the individuals in a life stage and gender group

The **Recommended Dietary Allowance** is the nutrient intake level that is sufficient to meet the need of 97-98% of the individuals in a life stage and gender group. The RDA is calculated from the EAR

Adequate Intake is based upon expert estimates of nutrient intake by a defined group of healthy people. These estimates are used when there is insufficient scientific evidence to establish an EAR. AI is not equivalent to RDA

Tolerable Upper Intake Level is the maximum level of daily nutrient intake that poses little risk of adverse health effects to almost all of the individuals in a defined group. In most cases, supplements must be consumed to reach a UL

Figure 2.5 **Dietary reference intakes.** The Dietary Reference Intakes are a set of dietary standards that include Estimated Average Requirement (EAR), Recommended Dietary Allowance (RDA), Adequate Intake (AI) and Tolerable Upper Level (UL).

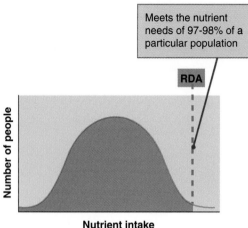

Meets the nutrient needs of 97-98% of a particular population

RDA

Number of people

Nutrient intake

RECOMMENDED DIETARY ALLOWANCE

Recommended Dietary Allowance The Recommended Dietary Allowance (RDA) is the daily intake level that meets the needs of most people (97 to 98 percent) in a life-stage and gender group. In the DRI values, the RDA will always be set at two standard deviations above the EAR. For a particular nutrient, this definition of RDA requires that first an Estimated Average Requirement (EAR) be set. In the past, RDAs were established for nutrients even when data did not provide enough information to estimate requirements. These RDAs were usually based on observed levels of intake that appeared to be adequate for health or growth. In the DRI framework, a nutrient for which an EAR cannot be set, cannot have an RDA value. For adults, calcium, fluoride, vitamin D, pantothenic acid, biotin, and choline do not have EAR or RDA values.

People can use the RDA value as a target or goal for dietary intake, but assessing actual intake as a percentage of the RDA is problematic. The RDAs do not define an *individual's* nutrient requirements. Your nutrient needs may be much lower than average, and therefore the RDA would be much more than you need. An analysis of your diet might show, for example, that you consume 45 percent of the RDA for a certain vitamin, but that might be adequate for your needs. Only specific laboratory or other tests can determine a person's true nutrient requirements and actual nutritional status.

Adequate Intake If not enough scientific data are available to set an EAR level, a value called an **Adequate Intake (AI)** is determined instead. AI values are determined in part by observing healthy groups of people and estimating their dietary intake. All the current DRI values for infants are AI levels because there have been too few scientific studies to determine specific requirements in infants. Instead, AI values for infants are usually based on nutrient levels in human breast milk, a complete food for newborns and young infants. Values for older infants and children are extrapolated

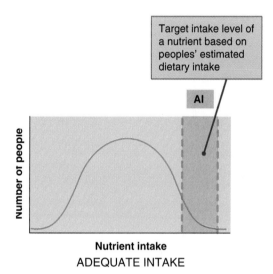

Target intake level of a nutrient based on peoples' estimated dietary intake

AI

Number of people

Nutrient intake

ADEQUATE INTAKE

Adequate Intake (AI) The nutrient intake that appears to sustain a defined nutritional state or some other indicator of health (e.g., growth rate or normal circulating nutrient values) in a specific population or subgroup. AI is used when there is insufficient scientific evidence to establish an EAR.

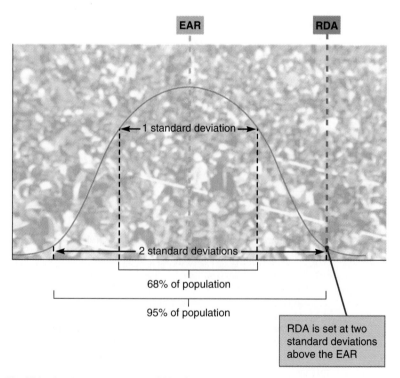

EAR   RDA

1 standard deviation

2 standard deviations

68% of population

95% of population

RDA is set at two standard deviations above the EAR

The RDA takes into account about 98% of the population.

from human milk and from data on adults. For older life-stage groups, AI values have been set for calcium, vitamin D, fluoride, pantothenic acid, biotin, and choline. For some of these nutrients, RDA values existed in the previous edition (1989) even though there were not enough data to estimate requirements.[7] In the new DRI values, AI levels reflect this lack of knowledge and the need for more scientific research. AI values can be considered target intake levels for individuals.

Tolerable Upper Intake Level Finally, values are being developed to define the **Tolerable Upper Intake Level (UL),** that is, the point at which higher intake of a nutrient could be harmful. The ULs are being developed partly in response to the growing interest in dietary supplements that contain large amounts of essential nutrients. In most cases, the UL applies to nutrient intake from supplements alone. The UL is *not* to be used as a target for intake.

The establishment of DRI values is an ongoing process that the Food and Nutrition Board is releasing in seven reports. The first report was released in 1997 and covered calcium, phosphorus, magnesium, vitamin D, and fluoride—the nutrients related to bone health. Since then reports have been released every year or so. Some of the key differences between the new DRIs and 1989 RDAs are summarized below[8]:

- Change in age categories
- For calcium, change from RDA to AI, with higher levels for children, teens, and adults
- Lower RDAs for phosphorus, vitamin A and zinc
- For vitamin D, change from RDA to AI, with higher levels for older adults
- Higher RDA for folate, with the recommendation that women of child-bearing age obtain, in addition to food folate, 400 µg per day of folic acid from fortified foods or supplements
- Recommendation that older adults use fortified foods or supplements to obtain adequate amounts of vitamin B_{12}
- AI values for choline, chromium, and manganese and RDA values for copper and molybdenum
- Slightly higher RDA for vitamin C for adults, changed from 60 mg to 75 mg per day for women and to 90 mg per day for men
- Slightly higher RDA for vitamin E for adults, changed from 8 mg per day for women and 10 mg for men to 15 mg per day for adults in general
- Slightly lower RDA for selenium for men, changed from 55 µg per day for women and 70 µg per day for men to 55 µg for all adults

Use of Dietary Standards

The most appropriate use of DRIs is as a tool for planning and evaluating diets for large groups of people. Remember the North Pole scenario at the beginning of this section? If you had planned menus and evaluated the nutrient composition of all those foods and if the nutrient levels of those daily menus averaged or exceeded the RDA/AI levels, you could be confident that your group would be adequately nourished. If you had a very large group—thousands of soldiers for instance—the EAR would be a more appropriate guide.

Tolerable Upper Intake Level (UL) Tolerable Upper Intake Level is the maximum level of daily nutrient intake that is unlikely to pose health risks to almost all of the individuals in the group for whom it is designed.

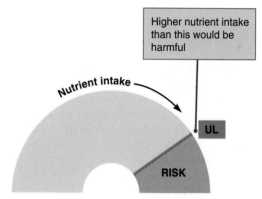

TOLERABLE UPPER INTAKE LEVEL

food label Labels required by law on virtually all packaged foods with five requirements: (1) a statement of identity; (2) the net contents (by weight, volume, or measure) of the package; (3) the name and address of the manufacturer, packer, or distributor; (4) a list of ingredients; and (5) nutrition information.

Food and Drug Administration (FDA) The federal agency responsible for assuring that foods sold in the United States (except for eggs, poultry, and meat, which are monitored by the USDA) are safe, wholesome, and labeled properly. The FDA sets standards for the composition of some foods, inspects food plants, and monitors imported foods. The FDA is part of the Public Health Services, a component of the Department of Health and Human Services (DHHS).

Nutrition Labeling and Education Act (NLEA) An amendment to the Food, Drug and Cosmetic Act of 1938. The NLEA made major changes to the content and scope of the nutrition label and to other elements of food labels. Final regulations were published in 1993, and went into effect in 1994.

statement of identity requirement Mandate that commercial food products display prominently the common or usual name of the product or identify the food with an "appropriately descriptive term."

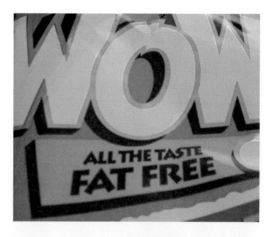

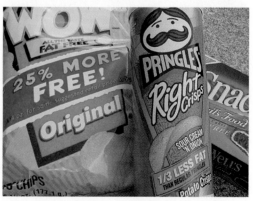

Dietary standards are also used to make decisions about nutrition policy. The Special Supplemental Food Program for Women, Infants, and Children (WIC), for example, takes into account the RDAs as it provides food. The goal of this federally funded supplemental feeding program is to improve the nutrient intake of low-income pregnant and breastfeeding women, their infants, and young children. The guidelines for school lunch and breakfast programs are also based on RDA values.

Often, we use dietary standards as comparison values for individual diets, an activity you may be pursuing in class. It can be interesting to see what percentage of the RDA or AI you routinely consume for a nutrient. However, an intake that is less than the RDA/AI doesn't necessarily mean deficiency; your individual requirement for a nutrient may be less than the RDA value. You can use the RDA/AI values as targets for dietary intake, while avoiding nutrient intake that exceeds the UL.

Future of the DRIs

Development of DRI values is an ongoing process of review and revision. As new values become available and replace the 1989 RDAs, nutrition professionals in all settings will be working to adapt existing educational materials, revise nutrient analysis programs, reevaluate menus and food plans, and change educational strategies. The first order of business is to understand the science behind the DRIs, and the methods used to set each of the values, and then to translate this information into dietary applications.

Key Concepts *Dietary standards are levels of nutrient intake recommended for healthy people. These standards help set nutrition policy as well as guide the planning and evaluation of diets for groups and individuals. The RDAs are being reevaluated and expanded into the Dietary Reference Intakes (DRIs), which focus instead on optimal health and lowering the risks of chronic disease.*

Food Labels

Now that you understand diet planning tools and dietary standards, let's focus on your use of these tools—for example, when making decisions at the grocery store. One of the most useful tools in planning a healthful diet is the **food label**.

A Brief History of Food Labeling

Specific federal regulations control what can and cannot appear on a food label, and what must appear on it. The **Food and Drug Administration** is responsible for assuring that foods sold in the United States are safe, wholesome, and labeled properly. The FDA's jurisdiction does not include meat, meat products, poultry or poultry products; the USDA regulates these foods.

In 1973 the FDA developed regulations pertaining to nutrition information on food labels. Initially, few foods had nutrition labels. But as consumer interest in nutrition grew in the 1980s, so did the food industry's response in providing nutrition labels, even when not required by the regulations. By 1990, approximately 60 percent of packaged foods carried nutrition labeling, often voluntarily.

As information about the role of diet in chronic disease grew, so did the demand for nutrition labels on all food products. As a result, in 1990 Congress passed the **Nutrition Labeling and Education Act (NLEA)**. Following development of the necessary regulations, new "Nutrition Facts" labels began appearing on food packages in 1994.

Components of the Food Label

Ingredients and Other Basic Information

Our current food label has been shaped by many sets of regulations. Today nutritional labeling is required on virtually all packaged foods. As **Figure 2.6** shows, food labels have five mandatory components:

1. a statement of identity
2. the net contents of the package
3. the name and address of the manufacturer, packer, or distributor
4. a list of ingredients
5. nutrition information

The **statement of identity** requirement means that the product must display prominently the common or usual name of the product, or identify the food with an "appropriately descriptive term." For example, it would be misleading to label a fruit beverage containing only 10 percent fruit juice as a "juice." The statement of net package contents must reflect accurately the quantity in terms of weight, volume, measure, or numerical count. Information about the manufacturer, packer, or distributor gives consumers a place to contact in case they have questions about the product. Ingredients must be listed by common or usual name, in descending order by weight, so the first ingredient listed is the predominant ingredient in that food product. Let's compare two cereals:

Cereal A ingredients: *Milled corn, sugar, salt, malt flavoring, high-fructose corn syrup*

Cereal B ingredients: *Sugar, yellow corn flour, rice flour, wheat flour, whole oat flour, partially hydrogenated vegetable oil (contains one or more of the following oils: canola, soybean, cottonseed), salt, cocoa, artificial flavor, corn syrup*

In Cereal B, the first ingredient listed is sugar, which means this cereal contains more sugar by weight than any other ingredient. Cereal A's primary ingredient is milled corn. If we were to read the nutrition information, we would find that a 1 cup serving of Cereal A contains 2 grams of sugars, while a similar amount of Cereal B contains 12 grams of sugars. Quite a difference!

As you have probably noticed, the presence of the artificial sweeteners saccharin or aspartame in an ingredient list is accompanied by a warning statement. Also, preservatives that are added to foods must be listed, along with an explanation of their functions. Accurate and complete ingredient information is vital for people with food allergies who must avoid certain food components.

Nutrition Facts Panel

The Nutrition Facts panel contains the most important label information for the health-conscious consumer. The Food Marketing Institute's 1997 survey "Shopping for Health" indicates that 54 percent of consumers check the food label before buying a product for the first time. The top three numbers they look for

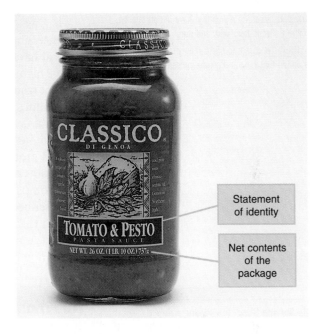

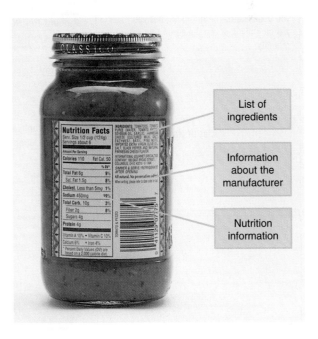

Figure 2.6 **The Five Mandatory requirements for food labels.**

Nutrition Facts A portion of the food label that states the content of selected nutrients in a food in a standard way prescribed by the Food and Drug Administration. By law Nutrition Facts must appear on nearly all processed food products in the United States.

Daily Values (DVs) A single set of nutrient intake standards developed by the Food and Drug Administration to represent the needs of the "typical" consumer. Used as standards for expressing nutrient content on food labels, DVs are based on two types of standards: Daily Reference Values (DRVs) and Reference Daily Intakes (RDIs).

enriched Refers to grains that have added thiamin, riboflavin, niacin, folic acid, and iron.

fortified Foods are fortified when vitamins or minerals are added that weren't originally present.

are total fat, calories, and sodium. The Nutrition Facts panel not only is a source of information about the nutritional value of a food product; it can also be used to compare similar products. Let's take a closer look at the elements of the Nutrition Facts panel (see **Figure 2.7**). It was designed so that the nutrition information would be easy to find on the label. The heading **Nutrition Facts** stands out clearly. Just under the heading is information about the serving size and number of servings per container. It is important to note the serving size because all of the following nutrient information is based on that amount of the food, and the listed serving size may be different from what you usually eat. An 8-ounce bag of potato chips may be a "small" snack to a hungry college student, but the manufacturer states the bag really contains 8 servings! Serving sizes are standardized based on reference amounts developed by the FDA. Similar products (cereals, for instance) will have similar serving sizes (1 ounce).

The next part of the label shows the calories per serving and the calories that come from fat. This information reveals at a glance whether a food product is high or low in fat. If most of the calories in a product come from fat, it is a high-fat food. Following this is a list of the amounts of total fat, saturated fat, cholesterol, sodium, total carbohydrate, dietary fiber, sugars, and protein in one serving. This information is given both in quantity (grams or milligrams per serving) and as a percentage of the **Daily Value**— a comparison standard specifically for food products (this standard is described below). Listed next are percentages of Daily Values for vitamins A and C, calcium, and iron, which are the only micronutrients that must appear on all standard labels. Manufacturers may choose to include information about other nutrients in the Nutrition Facts, such as potassium,

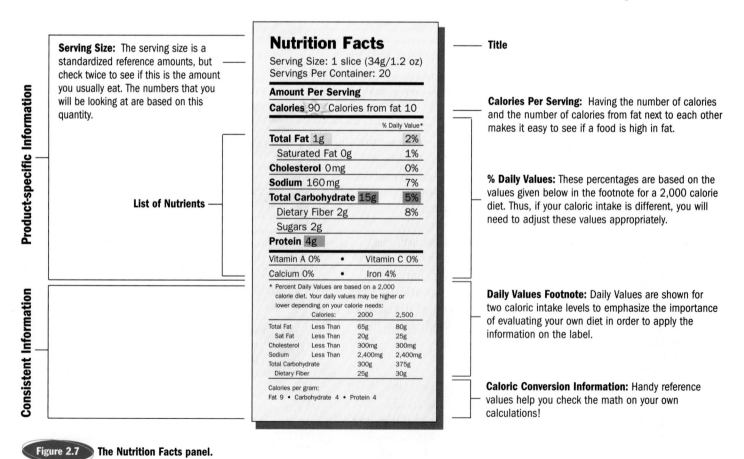

Figure 2.7 The Nutrition Facts panel.

polyunsaturated fat, additional vitamins, or other minerals. However, if they make a claim about an optional component (e.g., "good source of soluble fiber") or if the food is **enriched** or **fortified**, the manufacturer must include specific nutrition information. They must include this information even when government regulations require enrichment or fortification, such as the fortification of milk with vitamin D to increase absorption of calcium and phosphorus and the fortification of grain products with folic acid to reduce risk of birth defects. Food products that come in small packages (e.g., gum, candy, and tuna) or that have little nutritional value (e.g., diet soft drinks) can have abbreviated versions of the Nutrition Facts on the label, as **Figure 2.8** shows.

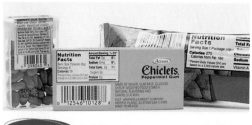

Figure 2.8 Nutrition Facts on small packages.

Daily Values

Let's come back to the Daily Values part of the label. The Daily Values (DV) are a set of dietary standards used to compare the amount of a nutrient (or other component) in a serving of food to the amount recommended for daily consumption. This information lets consumers see at a glance how a food fits into their diets. Let's say you rely on your breakfast cereal as a major source of dietary fiber. Comparing two packages, as in **Figure 2.9,** you find that a serving of corn-flake cereal has 4 percent of the DV for dietary fiber, but choosing a wheat-bran cereal will give you 52

Figure 2.9 These cereal labels come from different types of breakfast cereal: corn-flakes cereal (left) and bran-flakes cereal (right). What might influence your decision to buy one over the other?

Nutrition Facts

Serving Size:		1 Cup (28g/1.0 oz.)	
Servings Per Container:		About 18	

Amount Per Serving	Cereal	with ½ cup Skim Milk	
Calories	100	140	
Fat Calories	0	0	

	% Daily Value		
Total Fat 0g	0%	0%	
Saturated Fat 0g	0%	0%	
Cholesterol 0mg	0%	0%	
Sodium 300mg	13%	15%	
Potassium 25mg	1%	7%	
Total Carbohydrate 24g	8%	10%	
Dietary Fiber 1g	4%	4%	
Sugars 2g			
Other Carbohydrates 21g			
Protein 2g			
Vitamin A	15%	20%	
Vitamin C	25%	25%	
Calcium	0%	15%	
Iron	45%	45%	
Vitamin D	10%	25%	
Thiamin	25%	30%	
Riboflavin	25%	35%	
Niacin	25%	25%	
Vitamin B₆	25%	25%	
Folate	25%	25%	
Vitamin B₁₂	25%	35%	

Nutrition Facts

Serving Size:		3/4 Cup (30g)	
Servings Per Container:		About 15	

Amount Per Serving	Cereal	with ½ cup Skim Milk	
Calories	100	140	
Calories from Fat	5	5	

	% Daily Value		
Total Fat 0.5g	1%	1%	
Saturated Fat 0g	0%	0%	
Cholesterol 0mg	0%	0%	
Sodium 210mg	9%	12%	
Potassium 200mg	6%	11%	
Total Carbohydrate 24g	8%	10%	
Dietary Fiber 5g	20%	20%	
Sugars 5g			
Other Carbohydrates 14g			
Protein 3g			
Vitamin A	15%	20%	
Vitamin C	0%	2%	
Calcium	0%	15%	
Iron	45%	45%	
Vitamin D	10%	25%	
Thiamin	25%	30%	
Riboflavin	25%	35%	
Niacin	25%	25%	
Vitamin B₆	25%	25%	
Folic Acid	25%	25%	
Vitamin B₁₂	25%	35%	

percent. You don't have to know anything about grams to see which has more fiber!

The comparison standards used to determine the percentage of the Daily Values (%DV) on a food label actually consist of two sets of values: Reference Daily Intakes (RDIs) and Daily Reference Values (DRVs) (see **Table 2.2**). These comparison standards reflect values for a diet of approximately 2000 kilocalories per day. Your usual intake may be higher or lower, so you may want to make mental adjustments in the %DV to suit your diet.

Reference Daily Intakes Reference Daily Intakes (RDIs) provide comparison values for nutrients with RDA values, like protein, vitamins, and most minerals. **Table 2.3** shows the individual RDI values. Manufacturers determine the %DV for vitamin C in a food product, for example, by dividing the amount of vitamin C in the food (e.g., 30 mg) by the RDI (60 mg). In

Table 2.2 Summary of Dietary Standards

Food Labeling

Abbreviation	Term	Definition
DV	Daily Value	Recommended daily consumption level for a food component based on a 2,000 kcalorie diet
RDI	Reference Daily Intakes	Values for protein, vitamins, and most minerals
DRV	Daily Reference Values	Values for carbohydrate, fat, saturated fat, protein, cholesterol, sodium, potassium, and dietary fiber

Nutrient Standards

Abbreviation	Term	Definition
DRI	Dietary Reference Intakes	Term applied to the collection of EAR, RDA, AI, and UL values
EAR	Estimated Average Requirement	Intake level required to meet the need of 50% of the individuals in a life-stage and gender group
RDA	Recommended Dietary Allowance	Intake level meet the need of 97 to 98% of the individuals in a specific life-stage and gender group
AI	Adequate Intake	Based on estimates of nutrient intake by a defined group of healthy people, and used when there is insufficient scientific evidence to establish an EAR and RDA; not equivalent to RDA
UL	Tolerable Upper Intake Level	Maximum level of daily nutrient intake that poses little health risk to almost all of the individuals in a defined group; generally, supplements must be consumed to reach these high levels of intake

Table 2.3 Reference Daily Intakes for People Older Than 4 Years

Food Component	RDI
Protein	50 g
Vitamin A	1000 RE[a]
Vitamin D	400 IU[b]
Vitamin E	30 IU
Vitamin K	80 µg[c]
Vitamin C	60 mg[d]
Folate	400 µg
Thiamin	1.5 mg
Riboflavin	1.7 mg
Niacin	20 mg
Vitamin B_6	2 mg
Vitamin B_{12}	6 µg
Biotin	0.3 mg
Pantothenic acid	10 mg
Calcium	1000 mg
Phosphorus	1000 mg
Iodide	150 µg
Iron	18 mg
Magnesium	400 mg
Copper	2 mg
Zinc	15 mg
Chloride	3400 mg
Manganese	2 mg
Selenium	70 µg
Chromium	120 µg
Molybdenum	75 µg

[a] RE = retinol equivalents
[b] IU = international units
[c] µg = micrograms
[d] mg = milligrams

Note: RDI values were developed based on older RDAs and do not reflect new DRI values.

Source: FDA from www.fda.gov

this example, the %DV is 50 percent, which means that one serving of this food product provides half the daily recommendation for vitamin C.

Daily Reference Values Daily Reference Values (DRVs) are for nutrients and other food components (like fiber and cholesterol) for which RDA values do not exist (see **Table 2.4**). There is also a DRV for protein. The DRVs are based on current recommended intake levels for these substances. For example, no more than 30 percent of our kilocalories should come from fat. Using the 2,000 kilocalorie per day standard, this comes to

2,000 kilocalories X .30 = 600 kilocalories from fat

600 kilocalories ÷ 9 kilocalories per gram ≈ 67 grams of fat

This is rounded down to 65 grams, which becomes the DRV for fat. So, if a 1-ounce serving of cheese contains 9 grams of fat, it would have 14 percent of the Daily Value (9 ÷ 65 = 0.14, or 14 percent). To take this one step farther, 7 ounces of this cheese (about 7 1-inch cubes) would provide almost the total amount of fat recommended for one day!

For people whose typical energy intake exceeds 2,000 kcal (e.g., most adult males reading this textbook), DRV levels have been set for a 2,500 kilocalorie diet. You can see these numbers in Table 2.4 and on the Nutrition Facts panel.

Descriptive Terms

Under the provisions of the NLEA and the resulting FDA regulations, food manufacturers are allowed to use a variety of descriptive terms on labels. The guidelines for terms like *low fat* and *high fiber* are clear. The feature "Definition for Descriptors on Food Labels" shows a list of allowable adjectives. The FDA has made an effort to make the terms meaningful, and the regulations have reduced the number of potentially misleading label statements. Companies can no longer take liberties with label statements, such as printing "cholesterol free" on a can of vegetable shortening—a food that is 100 percent fat and high in saturated fatty acids (this type of fat raises blood cholesterol levels in the body). This type of statement misleads consumers who associate "cholesterol free" with "heart healthy." Under the NLEA regulations, descriptors related to cholesterol can be used only when the product is also low in saturated fat (less than 2 grams per serving).

Health Claims

With the passage of the NLEA, manufacturers also were allowed to add health claims to food labels. Before the NLEA, products making such claims were considered drugs, not foods. A **health claim** is a statement that links one or more dietary components (e.g., calcium) to reduced risk of disease (e.g., osteoporosis). A health claim must be supported by scientifically valid evidence for it to be approved for use on a food label. In addition, there are specific criteria for the use of claims. For example, a high-fiber food that is also high in fat is not eligible for a health claim. So far, FDA has approved 12 health claims:

- Calcium and osteoporosis: adequate calcium may reduce the risk of osteoporosis.
- Sodium and hypertension (high blood pressure): low-sodium diets may help lower blood pressure.
- Dietary fat and cancer: high-fat diets increase risk for some types of cancer.
- Dietary saturated fat and cholesterol and risk of coronary heart disease (CHD): diets high in saturated fat and cholesterol increase risk for heart disease.

Table 2.4 Daily Reference Values on Food Labels

	2,000 kcal intake	2,500 kcal intake
Fat	< 65 g	< 80 g
Saturated fat	< 20 g	< 25 g
Protein	50 g	65 g
Cholesterol	< 300 mg	< 300 mg
Carbohydrate	300 g	375 g
Fiber	25 g	30 g
Sodium	< 2,400 mg	< 2,400 mg

Source: FDA from www.fda.gov

Reference Daily Intakes (RDIs) A set of nutrient standards used to calculate the % Daily Values on nutrition labels.

Daily Reference Values (DRVs) Standards set for the intake of carbohydrate, fat, saturated fat, cholesterol, sodium, potassium, and dietary fiber. They are used to calculate the %DVs on nutrition labels.

Health Claim Any statement that associates a substance in food to a disease or health-related condition. The FDA monitors health claims.

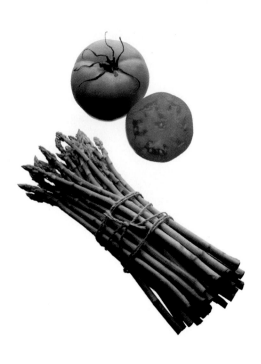

- Fiber-containing grain products, fruits, and vegetables and cancer: diets low in fat and rich in high-fiber foods may reduce the risk of certain cancers.

- Fruits, vegetables, and grain products that contain fiber, particularly soluble fiber, and risk of CHD: diets low in fat and rich in soluble fiber sources may reduce risk of heart disease.

- Fruits and vegetables and cancer: diets low in fat and rich in fruits and vegetables may reduce the risk of certain cancers.

- Folate and neural tube defects: adequate folate status prior to and early in pregnancy may reduce the risk of neural tube defects (a birth defect).

- Dietary sugar alcohols and dental caries (cavities): foods sweetened with sugar alcohols do not promote tooth decay.

- Dietary soluble fiber, such as that found in whole oats and psyllium seed husk, and CHD: diets low in fat and rich in these types of fiber can help reduce the risk of heart disease.

- Soy protein and CHD: foods rich in soy protein as part of a low-fat diet may help reduce the risk of heart disease.

- Whole-grain foods and CHD or cancer: diets high in whole-grain foods and other plant foods and low in total fat, saturated fat, and cholesterol may help reduce the risk of heart disease and certain cancers.

Fyi Definitions for Descriptors on Food Labels

FOR YOUR INFORMATION

Free: Food contains no amount (or trivial or "physiologically inconsequential" amounts). May be used with one or more of the following: fat, saturated fat, cholesterol, sodium, sugar, and calorie. Synonyms include *without, no,* and *zero.*

Fat-free: *less than 0.5 g of fat per serving*

Saturated fat free: *less than 0.5 g of saturated fat per serving, and no more than 0.5 g of trans fatty acids per serving*

Cholesterol-free: *less than 2 mg of cholesterol and 2 grams or less of saturated fat per serving*

Sodium-free: *less than 5 mg of sodium per serving*

Sugar-free: *less than 0.5 g of sugar per serving*

Calorie-free: *fewer than 5 calories per serving*

Low: Food can be eaten frequently without exceeding dietary guidelines for one or more of these components: fat, saturated fat, cholesterol, sodium, and calories. Synonyms include *little, few,* and *low source of.*

Low-fat: *3 g or less per serving*

Low-saturated fat: *1 g or less per serving*

Low-cholesterol: *20 mg or less and 2 g or less of saturated fat per serving*

Low-sodium: *140 mg or less per serving*

Very low sodium: *35 mg or less per serving*

Low calories: *40 calories or less per serving*

High: Food contains 20 percent or more of the Daily Value for a particular nutrient in a serving.

Good source: Food contains 10 to 19 percent of the Daily Value for a particular nutrient in one serving.

Lean and extra lean: Describes the fat content of meat, poultry, seafood, and game meat.

Lean: *less than 10 g fat, 4.5 g or less saturated fat, and less than 95 mg of cholesterol per serving and per 100 g*

Extra lean: *less than 5 g fat, less than 2 g saturated fat, and less than 95 mg of cholesterol per serving and per 100 g*

Reduced: Nutritionally altered product containing at least 25 percent less of a nutrient or of calories than the regular or reference product. (*Note:* A "reduced" claim can't be used if the reference product already meets the requirement for "low.")

Less: Food, whether altered or not, contains 25 percent less of a nutrient or of calories than the reference food. *Fewer* is an acceptable synonym.

A new health claim may be proposed at any time, so this list will expand. In fact, in September, 2000, FDA tentatively authorized a health claim for plant sterol or stanol esters and CHD. These compounds, which are being added to some margarines, have been shown to reduce blood cholesterol levels. In the NLEA and the FDA regulations that followed, health claims were intended to cover both foods and dietary supplements. However, the regulatory requirements for **dietary supplements** changed following the passage of the **Dietary Supplement Health and Education Act (DSHEA)** in 1994. Dietary supplements are products taken by mouth that contain so-called dietary ingredients and may include vitamins, minerals, herbs, or amino acids, as well as other substances such as enzymes, organ tissues, metabolites, extracts, or concentrates. Requirements related to specific health claims are the same for foods and for supplements; however, only a few of the health claims approved for foods are appropriate for dietary supplements:

- calcium and osteoporosis
- folate and neural tube defects
- soluble fiber from whole oats or psyllium seed husk and coronary heart disease
- soy protein and coronary heart disease

However, dietary supplement labels also may contain claims about potential effects on body structures or functions. So long as the product does not claim to diagnose, cure, mitigate, treat, or prevent a disease,

dietary supplements Any product taken by mouth that contains a so-called dietary ingredient, which may include vitamins, minerals, herbs, or amino acids, as well as other substances such as enzymes, organ tissues, metabolites, extracts, or concentrates.

Dietary Supplement Health and Education Act (DSHEA) Legislation that regulates dietary supplements.

Light: this descriptor can have two meanings:
1. a nutritionally altered product contains one-third fewer calories or half the fat of the reference food. If the reference food derives 50 percent or more of its calories from fat, the reduction must be 50 percent of the fat.
2. the sodium content of a low-calorie, low-fat food has been reduced by 50 percent. Also, *light in sodium* may be used on a food in which the sodium content has been reduced by at least 50 percent.

Note: The term *light* can still be used to describe such properties as texture and color as long as the label clearly explains its meaning (e.g., *light brown sugar* or *light and fluffy*).

More: A serving of food, whether altered or not, contains a nutrient that is at least 10 percent of the Daily Value more than the reference food. This also applies to *fortified*, *enriched*, and *added* claims, but in those cases, the food must be altered.

Healthy: A *healthy* food must be low in fat and saturated fat and contain limited amounts of cholesterol (< 60 mg) and sodium (< 360 mg for individual foods and < 480 mg for meal-type products). In addition, a single item food must provide at least 10 percent or more of one of the following: vitamins A or C, iron, calcium, protein, or fiber. A meal-type product, such as a frozen entree or dinner, must provide 10 percent of two or more of these vitamins or minerals or, protein, or fiber, in addition to meeting the other criteria. Additional regulations allow the term "healthy" to be applied to raw, canned, or frozen fruits and vegetables and enriched grains even if the 10 percent nutrient content rule is not met. However, frozen or canned fruits or vegetables cannot contain ingredients that would change the nutrient profile.

Fresh: Food is raw, has never been frozen or heated, and contains no preservatives. *Fresh frozen*, *frozen fresh*, and *freshly frozen* can be used for foods that are quickly frozen while still fresh. Blanched foods also can be called fresh.

Percent fat free: Food must be a low-fat or a fat-free product. In addition, the claim must reflect accurately the amount of non-fat ingredients in 100 g of food.

Implied claims: These are prohibited when they wrongfully imply that a food contains or does not contain a meaningful level of a nutrient. For example, a product claiming to be made with an ingredient known to be a source of fiber (such as "made with oat bran") is not allowed unless the product contains enough of that ingredient (e.g., oat bran) to meet the definition for "good source" of fiber. As another example, a claim that a product contains "no tropical oils" is allowed, but only on foods that are "low" in saturated fat, because consumers have come to equate tropical oils with high levels of saturated fat.

Source: FDA from www.fda.gov

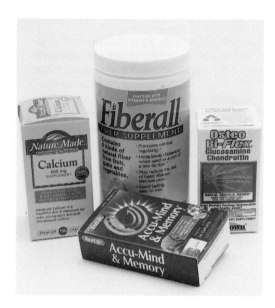

a manufacturer can claim that a product "helps promote urinary tract health" or is an "energizer" if *some* evidence can be provided to support the claim. Many scientists are concerned about the lack of a consistent scientific standard for both health claims and structure/function claims.

Using Labels to Make Healthful Food Choices

The best way to start using food label information to make food choices is by looking at some examples. Let's say that one of your goals is to add more iron to your diet. Compare the cereal labels in **Figure 2.9**. Which cereal contains a higher percentage of the Daily Value for iron? How do they compare in terms of sugar content? Vitamins and other minerals?

Maybe it's a frozen entrée you're after. Look at the two examples in **Figure 2.10**. Which is the best choice nutritionally? Are you sure? Sometimes the answer is not clear-cut. Product A is higher in sodium, while Product B has more saturated fat. It would be important to know about the rest of your dietary intake before making a decision. Do you already have quite a bit of sodium in your diet, or are you likely to add salt at the table? Maybe you never salt your food, so a bit extra in your entrée is OK. If you know that your saturated fat intake is already a bit high, however, Product A might be a better choice. To make the best choice, you should know which substances are most important in terms of your own health risks. The label is there to help you make these types of food decisions.

Key Concepts *Making food choices at the grocery store is your opportunity to implement the Dietary Guidelines and your Pyramid-planned diet. The Nutrition Facts panel contains not only the specific amounts of nutrients shown in grams or milligrams, but also comparisons between the amounts of nutrients in a food and the recommended intake values. These comparisons are reported as %DV (Daily Values). The %DV information can be used to compare two products or to see how individual foods contribute to the total diet.*

Label [to] **Table**   Nutrition Labels: Do They Help Us Choose a Healthful Diet?

The Nutrition Labeling and Education Act of 1990 (NLEA) changed food labeling and brought us the Nutrition Facts panel we see on food labels today. One of the NLEA's primary objectives was to help consumers select foods for a healthful diet. Labels were designed to be educational rather than merely informational. Thus, rather than just listing the amounts (e.g., grams and milligrams) of a product's nutrients, Daily Values were developed to make comparisons possible; terms such as *reduced, light, low,* and *free* were defined; and health claims for certain diet-disease relationships were developed. These were dramatic changes from the informational labels of the 1970s and 1980s. But did they work? Does the additional information and the new format encourage more healthful purchases? Policy makers had high hopes for the effect of changes to nutrition labels. Zarkin and colleagues predicted four scenarios for behavior change resulting from implementation of the NLEA.[1] Taking those changes over a 20-year period, the number of potential life-years gained ranged from 40,000 to 1.2 million. The potential dollar value of such effects is staggering, ranging from $3 billion to more than $100 billion!

A study of adults found that nutrition labels *are* useful for people who want to lower the fat content of their diets—an important health goal for most Americans.[2] In this study, adults in Washington state were surveyed by telephone about their use of nutrition labels, their dietary habits as they relate to fat, fruit, and vegetable intake, their health behaviors, and their demographic characteristics. Women were more likely than men to read nutrition labels and to look at information on serving size, calories, and grams of fat; men were more likely to look at cholesterol information. People younger than 35 were more likely to consider serving size, calories from fat, and grams of fat, while those 35 and older read cholesterol information more frequently. Label use was associated with a lower intake of fat, but there was no relation between label use and fruit and vegetable intake. Regular reading of nutrition labels was associated with a reduction in fat intake of at least 5 percent. Although this is lower than the 13 percent used by Zarkin and colleagues in predicting potential outcomes, this level of fat intake reduction

Nutrition Facts

Serving Size: 1 Entree (240g)
Servings Per Container: 1

Amount Per Serving

Calories 400   Calories from fat 150

	% Daily Value*
Total Fat 16g	25%
Saturated Fat 3.5 g	18%
Cholesterol 10mg	3%
Sodium 780mg	33%
Total Carbohydrate 56g	19%
Dietary Fiber 2g	8%
Sugars 2g	
Protein 8g	

Vitamin A 2%	•	Vitamin C 4%
Calcium 6%	•	Iron 4%

Nutrition Facts

Serving Size: 1 package (269g)

Amount Per Serving

Calories 400   Calories from fat 140

	% Daily Value*
Total Fat 16g	24%
Saturated Fat 8 g	40%
Cholesterol 40mg	14%
Sodium 690mg	29%
Total Carbohydrate 48g	16%
Dietary Fiber 2g	9%
Sugars 5g	
Protein 15g	

Vitamin A 10%	•	Vitamin C 8%
Calcium 20%	•	Iron 15%

Figure 2.10 Labels may look similar, but appearances can be deceptive.

Nutrition Assessment: Determining Nutritional Health

In a nutritional sense what does it mean to be healthy? In this chapter we have focused on food choices and the tools available to make better choices. Nutritional health is quite simply obtaining all the nutrients in amounts needed to support body processes. We can measure nutritional health in a number of ways. Taken together, such measurements can give you much insight into your current and long-term well-being. The process of measuring nutritional health is usually termed **nutrition assessment.**

nutrition assessment Measurement of the nutritional health of the body. It can include anthropometric measurements, biochemical tests, clinical observations, and dietary intake, as well as medical histories and socioeconomic factors.

would still have significant health benefits for the population as a whole.

In another survey of adults, people who ate diets lower in fat and higher in fruits, vegetables, and fiber, were more likely to use labels in making food purchase decisions. Further, people with high blood cholesterol or hypertension focused their attention on key aspects of the labels—saturated fat and cholesterol and sodium, respectively.[3]

It appears that most label readers still focus on the numbers of grams, calories, or milligrams rather than the %DV. Neuhouser and colleagues found that while 80 percent of the subjects read nutritional labels, only 39 percent of those label readers used the %DV for fat. It is possible that this information is not well understood by consumers and that the

"E" in NLEA (Education) has not been extensive enough to facilitate full use of the information provided. Other surveys indicate that consumers are not clear on the definition of other terms such as *low fat* or *cholesterol free*.[4] While these terms are strictly defined in the regulations, the average shopper is not aware of the definitions. Other surveys indicate that interest in labels is waning and that the %DV is not interpreted correctly.[5]

If we are to realize savings in health-care costs, it will be up to registered dietitians, health-care providers, and public information systems to continue to educate consumers about how to use the valuable information provided on food labels. Without adequate education, more health claims or label statements will just be part of consumers'

information overload, rather than a pathway to healthful dietary choices.

1 Zarkin GA, Dean N, Mauskopf JA, Williams R. Potential health benefits of nutrition label changes. *Am J Public Health.* 1993;83:717–724.

2 Neuhouser ML, Kristal AR, Patterson RE. Use of food nutrition labels is associated with lower fat intake. *J Am Diet Assoc.* 1999;99:45–53.

3 Kreuter MW, Brennan LK, Schaff DP, Lukwago SN. Do nutrition label readers eat healthier diets? Behavioral correlates of adults' use of food labels. *Am J Prev Med.* 1997;13:277–283.

4 Resnick ML. *Proceedings of the Human Factors and Ergonomics Society 41st Annual Meeting.* 1997;395–399.

5 Sloan AE. Lessons from labels. *Food Technology.* 1998;52:24.

Nutrition assessment serves a variety of purposes. It may help evaluate nutrition-related risks that may jeopardize a person's current or future health. Nutrition assessment is a routine part of the nutritional care of hospitalized patients. In this setting, nutrition assessment can not only identify risks, but also measure the effectiveness of treatment. In public health, nutrition assessment helps identify people in need of nutrition-related interventions, and also to monitor the effectiveness of intervention programs. Sometimes, assessments determine the nutritional health of an entire population—to identify health risks common in a population group so specific policy measures can be developed to combat them.

The Continuum of Nutritional Status

| Undernutrition | Good Nutrition | Overnutrition |

We can view nutritional status as a continuum of conditions, with the extremes being undernutrition and overnutrition. Chronic undernutrition results in the development of nutritional deficiency diseases, as well as conditions of energy and protein malnutrition such as **marasmus** and **kwashiorkor,** and can lead to death. **Undernutrition** differs from starvation in that *some* food is being consumed, but the intake is not nutritionally adequate. Although chronic undernutrition and associated deficiency diseases were common in the United States in the 1800s and early 1900s, today they are rare. Undernutrition now is most often associated with extreme poverty, alcoholism, illness, or some eating disorders.

Overnutrition is the chronic consumption of more than is necessary for good health. Specifically, overnutrition is the regular consumption of excess calories, fats, saturated fats, or cholesterol—all of which increase risk for chronic disease. Today, nutrition-related chronic diseases such as coronary heart disease, cancer, stroke, and diabetes are among the 10 leading causes of death in the United States. All of these problems have been linked to dietary excess. (Remember that epidemiological (population) studies can show associations between various factors and diseases, but these correlations do not necessarily indicate cause and effect.)

Between these two extremes lies a region of good health. In 1988, the U.S. Surgeon General wrote: "for the two out of three adult Americans who do not smoke and do not drink excessively, one personal choice seems to influence long-term health prospects more than any other: what we eat."[9] Good food and lifestyle choices, a balanced diet, and regular exercise help to reduce the risk of chronic disease and delay its onset, keeping us in a region of good health for more of our lifetime.

Nutrition Assessment of Individuals

In health-care settings, a registered dietitian or physician may do an individual nutrition assessment of a patient or client. Depending on the purpose of the nutrition assessment, the measures may be very comprehensive and detailed. A dietitian can then use this information to plan individualized nutrition counseling. Nutrition assessment measures are often repeated in order to assess the effectiveness of nutrition counseling or a change in diet.

Nutrition Assessment of Populations

Population-based nutrition assessment is done in conjunction with programs to monitor the status of nutrition in the United States or as part of

marasmus A type of malnutrition resulting from chronic protein-energy undernutrition characterized by wasting of muscle and other body tissue.

kwashiorkor A type of malnutrition that occurs primarily in young children who have an infectious disease and whose diets supply marginal amounts of energy and very little protein. Common symptoms include poor growth, edema, apathy, weakness, and susceptibility to infections.

undernutrition Poor health resulting from the depletion of nutrients due to inadequate nutrient intake over time. It is now most often associated with poverty, alcoholism, and some types of eating disorders.

overnutrition The long-term consumption of an excess of nutrients. The most common type of overnutrition in the United States is due to the regular consumption of excess calories, fats, saturated fats, and cholesterol.

large-scale epidemiological studies. Typically, nutrition assessment of populations is not as comprehensive as an assessment of an individual. One of the largest ongoing nationwide surveys of dietary intake and health status is the National Health and Nutrition Examination Survey (NHANES). To date, four of these surveys have been completed, and they have told us a great deal about the nutritional status of our population. Another tool for monitoring the dietary intake of Americans is the Continuing Survey of Food Intake by Individuals (CSFII). Some of the results of the 10th edition of this survey (1994–1996) were highlighted in Chapter 1.

Nutrition Assessment Methods

Just as there is not one measure of physical fitness, there is not just one indicator of nutritional health. Nutrients play many roles in the body, so measures of nutritional status must look at many factors. Often these factors are termed the **ABCDs of nutrition assessment**: <u>A</u>nthropometric measurements, <u>B</u>iochemical tests, <u>C</u>linical observations, and <u>D</u>ietary intake (see **Table 2.5**).

Anthropometric Measurements

Anthropometric measurements are physical measurements of the body, such as height and weight, head circumference, girth measurement, or skinfold measurements.

Height and Weight

To provide useful information, height and weight must be measured accurately. For infants and young children, measurement of height is really measurement of recumbent length (that is, when they are lying down). Careful measurement of length at each checkup gives a clear indication of a child's growth rate. Standard growth charts show how the child's growth compares to that of others of the same age and sex. For children 2 to 20 years old, charts illustrating growth are based on standing height, or stature.

The standing height of older children and adults can be determined with a tape measure fixed to a wall and a sliding right-angle headboard for reading the measurement. Aging adults lose some height due to bone loss and curvature, so it is important to measure height and not simply rely on remembered values. Because many calculations/standards use metric measures, it's important to be familiar with standard conversion factors.

ABCDs of nutrition assessment Nutrition assessment components: <u>A</u>nthropometric measurements, <u>B</u>iochemical tests, <u>C</u>linical observations, and <u>D</u>ietary intake.

anthropometric measurement Measurement of the physical characteristics of the body, such as height, weight, head circumference, girth, and skinfold measurements. Anthropometric measurements are particularly useful in evaluating the growth of infants, children, and adolescents, and in determining body composition.

To convert inches to centimeters, multiply the number of inches by 2.54

inches X 2.54 = centimeters

To convert pounds to kilograms, divide the number of pounds by 2.2

pounds ÷ 2.2 = kilograms

Table 2.5 The ABCDs of Nutrition Assessment

Assessment Method	Why it's done
Anthropometric measures	measures growth in children; shows changes in weight that can reflect diseases (i.e. cancer or thyroid problems); monitors progress in fat loss
Biochemical tests	measures blood and/or urine, and/or feces for nutrients or metabolites that indicate infection or disease
Clinical observations	assesses change in skin color and health, hair texture, fingernail shape, etc.
Dietary intake	evaluate diet for nutrient (i.e. fat, calcium, protein) or food (i.e. number of fruits and vegetables) intake

Weight is a critical measure in nutrition assessment. It is used to assess children's growth, predict energy expenditure and protein needs, and determine body composition. Weight should be measured using a calibrated scale. For assessments that need a high degree of precision, subtract the weight of the clothing.

For the anthropometric assessment of infants and young children, a third measurement is common: head circumference. This is measured using a flexible tape measure, put snugly around the head. Head circumference measures are another useful indicator of normal growth and development, especially during rapid growth from birth to age three.

Skinfolds

skinfold measurement A method to estimate body fat by measuring with calipers the thickness of a fold of skin and subcutaneous fat.

Skinfold measurements serve a variety of purposes. Because a significant amount of the body's fat stores are right beneath the skin (subcutaneous fat), the sizes of skinfolds at various sites around the body can give a good indication of body fatness. This information may be used to evaluate the physical fitness of an athlete or predict the risk of obesity-related disorders. Skinfold measurements are also useful in cases of illness; the maintenance of fat stores in a patient's body may be a valuable indicator of dietary adequacy. Skinfold measurements are done with special calipers (see **Figure 2.11**). For reliable measurements, training in the use of calipers is essential. Skinfold measurements can be used to estimate the percentage of body fat, or can be compared to percentile tables for specific sex and age categories.

Biochemical Tests

Because of their relation to growth and body composition, anthropometric measurements give a broad picture of nutritional health—if the diet contains enough calories and protein to maintain normal patterns of growth, normal body composition, and normal levels of lean body mass. However,

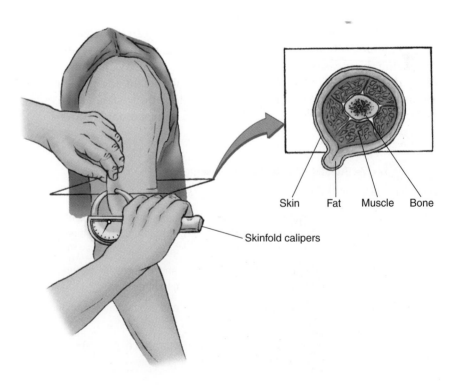

Figure 2.11 **Skinfold measurements.** A significant amount of the body's fat stores lie just beneath the skin, so when done correctly skinfold measurements can provide an indication of body fatness. An inexperienced or careless measurer, however, can easily make large errors. Skinfold measurements usually work better for monitoring malnutrition, rather than for identifying overweight and obesity. They also are widely used in large population studies.

Skin   Fat   Muscle   Bone

Skinfold calipers

anthropometric measures do not give specific information about *nutrients*. For that information, a variety of biochemical tests are useful.

Biochemical assessment measures a nutrient or metabolite (a related compound) in one or more body fluids such as blood and urine, or in feces. For example, the concentration of albumin (an important transport protein) in the blood can be an indicator of the body's protein status. If little protein is eaten, the body produces smaller amounts of body proteins such as albumin.

Functional measures are biochemical measurements of a nutrient metabolite, a storage or transport compound, an enzyme that depends on a vitamin or mineral, or another indicator of the body's functioning in relation to a particular nutrient. Functional measures usually are a better indicator of nutritional status than directly measuring blood levels of nutrients such as vitamin A or calcium. The levels of nutrients excreted in the urine or feces also provide valuable information.

Clinical Observations

Clinical observations—the characteristics of health that can be seen in physical exams—help complete the picture of nutritional health. While often nonspecific, clinical signs are clues to nutrient deficiency or excess that can be confirmed or ruled out by further testing. A clinical nutrition examination would observe the hair, nails, skin, eyes, lips, mouth, bones, muscles, and joints.[10] Specific findings, such as cracking at the corners of the mouth (suggestive of riboflavin, B_6 or niacin deficiency) or petechiae (small, pinpoint hemorrhages on the skin indicative of vitamin C deficiency) need to be followed by other assessments.

Dietary Intake

A picture of nutritional health would not be complete without information about dietary intake. Dietary information may confirm the lack or excess of a dietary component suggested by anthropometric, biochemical, or clinical evaluations.

There are a number of ways to collect dietary intake data. Each has strengths and weaknesses. It is important to match the method to the type and quantity of data needed. Remember, too, that the quality of information obtained about people's diets often relies heavily on people's memories, as well as their honesty in sharing those recollections. How well do you remember *everything* you ate yesterday?

Diet History

The most comprehensive form of dietary intake data collection is the **diet history.** In this method, a skilled interviewer finds out not only what the client has been eating in the recent past but also the client's long-term habits of food consumption. The interviewer's questions may also address other risk factors for nutrition-related problems, such as economic issues.

Food Record

Food records, or diaries, provide detailed information about day-to-day eating habits. Typically, a person records all foods and beverages consumed during a defined period, usually three to seven consecutive days. Because food records are recorded concurrently with intake, they are less prone to inaccuracy from lapses in memory. Because the data are completely self-reported, however, food records may not be accurate if the person fails to record all items. To make food records more precise, the items in a meal

biochemical assessment Assessment by measuring a nutrient or its metabolite in one or more body fluids such as blood and urine, and in feces. Also called laboratory assessment.

clinical observation Assessment by evaluating the characteristics of well-being that can be seen in a physical exam. Nonspecific, clinical observations can provide clues to nutrient deficiency or excess that can be confirmed or ruled out by biochemical testing.

diet history Record of food intake and eating behaviors that includes recent and long-term habits of food consumption. Done by a skilled interviewer, the diet history is the most comprehensive form of dietary intake data collection.

food record Detailed information about day-to-day eating habits which typically includes all foods and beverages consumed for a defined period, usually three to seven consecutive days.

Quick Bites

Nutrition and Nails

Do your nails have white marks or ridges? Contrary to popular belief, that does not necessarily mean you have a vitamin deficiency. Usually a slight injury to the nail causes white marks or ridges.

weighed food record A detailed food record obtained by weighing foods before eating, and then weighing leftovers to determine the exact amount consumed.

food frequency questionnaire (FFQ) A questionnaire for nutrition assessment that asks how often the subject consumes specific foods or groups of foods, rather than what specific foods the subject consumes daily. Also called food frequency checklist.

twenty-four-hour dietary recall A form of dietary intake data collection. The interviewer takes the client through a recent 24-hour period (usually midnight to midnight) to determine what foods and beverages the client consumed.

can be weighed before consumption. Remaining portions are weighed at the end of the meal to determine exactly how much was eaten. **Weighed food records** are much more time-consuming to complete.

Food Frequency Questionnaire

A **food frequency questionnaire (FFQ)** asks how often the subject consumes specific foods or groups of foods, rather than what specific foods the subject consumes daily. A food frequency questionnaire may ask, for example, "How often do you drink a cup of milk?" with response options of daily, weekly, monthly, and so on (see **Figure 2.12**). This information is used to estimate that person's average daily intake.

Although food frequency questionnaires do not require a trained interviewer and can be completed relatively quickly, there are disadvantages to this method of data collection. One problem is that it is often difficult to translate a person's response to how often they drink milk, or how many cups of milk they drink per week, into specific nutrient values without more detailed information. More important, food frequency questionnaires require a person to average, over a long period, foods that may be consumed erratically in portions that are sometimes large and sometimes small.

Twenty-Four-Hour Recall

The **twenty-four-hour recall** is the simplest form of dietary intake data collection. In a twenty-four-hour recall, the interviewer takes the client through a recent 24-hour period (usually midnight to midnight) to determine what foods and beverages the client consumed. To get a complete, accurate picture of the subject's diet, the interviewer must ask probing questions like, "Did you put anything on your toast?" but not leading questions like, "Did you put butter and jelly on your toast?" Comprehensive population surveys frequently use twenty-four-hour recalls as the main method of data collection. While a single twenty-four-hour recall is not very useful for describing the nutrient content of an individual's overall diet (there's too

Food Item	Average Use During Past Year					
	<1 serving per month	1–3 servings per month	1–4 servings per week	5–7 servings per week	2–4 servings per day	5+ servings per day
coffee					√	
dark bread	√					
ice cream				√		

Food Item	Your Serving Size				How Often?				
	Medium Serving	S	M	L	Day	Week	Month	Year	Never
coffee	(1 cup)			√	2				
dark bread	(1 slice)								√
ice cream	(1/2 cup)		√			3			

Figure 2.12 **Examples of food frequency questionnaire formats.**
Source: Adapted from Lee RD, Nieman DC. *Nutritional Assessment*, 2nd ed. St. Louis: mosby, 1996.

much day-to-day variation), in large-scale studies it gives a reasonably accurate picture of the average nutrient intake of a population. Multiple diet recalls also are useful for estimating nutrient intake of individuals.

Methods of Evaluating Dietary Intake Data

Once the data are collected, the next step is to determine the nutrient content of the diet and evaluate that information in terms of dietary standards or other reference points. This is commonly done using nutrient analysis software. Computer programs remove the tedium of looking up foods in tables of nutrient composition; large databases allow for simple access to food composition, and the computer does the math automatically.

Comparison to Dietary Standards

It is possible to compare a person's nutrient intake to dietary standards such as the RDA or AI values. Although this will give a qualitative idea of dietary adequacy, it cannot be considered a definitive evaluation of a person's diet because we don't know that individual's specific nutrient requirements. Comparisons of individual diets to RDA or AI values should be interpreted with caution.

Comparison to Food Guide Pyramid

Another type of dietary analysis compares a person's food intake to the Food Guide Pyramid. This involves categorizing foods into the various groups and determining the number of servings the subject has eaten. Evaluators often have trouble making these comparisons because many common foods (e.g., pizza, sandwiches, casseroles) contain servings or partial servings from multiple food groups.

Comparison to Dietary Guidelines for Americans

For a general picture of the subject's dietary habits, the evaluator can compare the person's diet to the *Dietary Guidelines for Americans*. While these evaluations usually are not specific, they give a general idea of whether the subject's diet is high or low in saturated fat, or whether the subject is eating enough fruits and vegetables.

Outcomes of Nutrition Assessment

When taken together, anthropometric measures, biochemical tests, clinical exams, and dietary evaluation, along with the individual's family history, socioeconomic situation, and other factors give a complete picture of nutritional health. A client's assessment may lead to a recommendation for a diet change to reduce weight or blood cholesterol, the addition of a vitamin or mineral supplement to treat a deficiency, the identification of abnormal growth due to inadequate infant feeding, or simply the affirmation that dietary intake is adequate for current nutrition needs.

Key Concepts *Nutrition assessment involves the collection of various types of data— anthropometric measurements, biochemical tests, clinical observations, and dietary intake—for a complete picture of one's nutritional health. Such data are compared to established standards to diagnose nutritional deficiencies, identify dietary inadequacies, or evaluate progress as a result of dietary changes.*

LEARNING *Portfolio* chapter 2

Key Terms

	page		page
ABCDs of nutrition assessment	57	food label	46
Adequate Intake (AI)	44	food record	59
anthropometric measurement	57	fortified	48
biochemical assessment	59	health claim	55
clinical observation	59	kwashiorkor	56
Daily Reference Values (DRVs)	51	marasmus	56
Daily Values (DVs)	48	nutrition assessment	55
diet history	59	Nutrition Facts	48
Dietary Guidelines	34	Nutrition Labeling and Education Act (NLEA)	46
Dietary Reference Intakes (DRI)	42	overnutrition	56
dietary supplements	53	Recommended Dietary Allowances (RDA)	42
Dietary Supplement Health and Education Act (DSHEA)	53	Reference Daily Intakes (RDIs)	51
enriched	48	requirement	42
Estimated Average Requirement (EAR)	42	skinfold measurement	58
Exchange Lists for Menu Planning	38	statement of identity requirement	46
Food and Drug Administration (FDA)	46	twenty-four-hour dietary recall	60
Food and Nutrition Board (FNB)	42	undernutrition	56
food frequency questionnaire (FFQ)	60	Tolerable Upper Intake Level (UL)	45
food group	35	U.S. Department of Agriculture (USDA)	34
Food Guide Pyramid	36	U.S. Department of Health and Human Services (DHHS)	34
		weighed food record	60

Study Points

➤ Moderation, balance, and variety are general guiding principles for healthful diets.

➤ The *Dietary Guidelines for Americans* give consumers advice regarding general components of the diet.

➤ The Food Guide Pyramid is a graphic representation of a food group plan that supports the principles of the *Dietary Guidelines for Americans.*

➤ Each food group in the Food Guide Pyramid has a recommended number of daily servings. Choose a variety of foods from each group to obtain all the nutrients.

➤ The exchange lists are a diet planning tool most often used for diabetic or weight-control diets.

➤ Servings for each food in the exchange lists are grouped so that equal amounts of carbohydrate, fat, and protein are provided by each choice.

➤ Dietary standards are values for individual nutrients that reflect recommended intake levels. These values are used for planning and evaluating diets for groups and individuals.

➤ The Dietary Reference Intakes are the current dietary standards in the United States. The DRIs consist of four sets of values: EAR, RDA, AI, and UL.

➤ Nutrition information on food labels can be used to select a more healthful diet.

➤ Label information provides not only the amounts (in grams or milligrams) of the nutrients present, but gives a percentage of Daily Values to compare the amount in the food and the amount recommended for consumption each day.

➤ Nutrition information, label statements, and health claims are defined by the regulations developed based on the Nutritional Labeling and Education Act of 1990.

➤ Nutrition assessment is a process of determining the overall health of a person as related to nutrition.

➤ Nutrition assessment involves four major factors: anthropometric measurements, biochemical tests, clinical observations, and dietary intake.

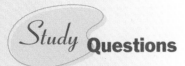 **Questions**

1. **List the four Dietary Reference Intake categories. How do they differ?**

2. **What is the recommended number of servings for each of the food groups in the Food Guide Pyramid?**

3. **Describe how the exchange system works and why diabetics might use it.**

4. **Which food components must be listed on food labels?**

5. **What is the purpose of the "% Daily Value" listed next to most nutrients on a food label?**

6. **Many labels show Daily Values for two calorie levels at the bottom of the Nutrition Facts panel. What are these two calorie levels? Which is used as the basis for "% Daily Values" on all food labels?**

☞ [*Try*] **This**

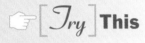

Keep a detailed food diary for three days. Make sure to include things you drink along with the amounts (cups, ounces, tablespoons, etc.) of each food or beverage. Using the serving sizes described in this chapter, translate each food in your three-day diary into the correct number of Food Guide Pyramid serving sizes. Remember that one of your portions may equal several servings as defined in the pyramid. Add up the number of servings you ate each day from each pyramid group; compare the total to the recommended number of servings. How did you do? From which groups did you tend to eat more than is recommended? Were there any groups for which you did not meet the recommendations? Was there a day-to-day variation in the number of servings you ate of each group? Use the results of this activity to plan ways to improve your diet. ✍

Grocery Store Scavenger Hunt

On your next trip to the grocery store, find a food item that has any number other than a "0" listed for the two vitamins and two minerals required to be listed on the food label %DV. It doesn't matter if you choose a cereal, soup, cracker, or snack item; it just has to have numbers other than "0" for all four items. Once you're home, review the Reference Daily Intakes (RDIs) and calculate the number of milligrams of calcium, iron, and vitamin C found in each serving of your food. Next, take a look at vitamin A, how many International Units (IUs) does each serving of your product have? If you can calculate this, you should have a better understanding of % Daily Values. ✍

References

1 Truswell AS. Dietary Goals and Guidelines: National and International Perspectives. In: Shils ME, Olson JA, Shike M, Ross AC, eds. *Modern Nutrition in Health and Disease.* 9th ed. Baltimore, MD: Williams & Wilkins, 1998.

2 Drewnowski, A, Henderson, SA, Drisscoll, A, Rolls, BJ. The Dietary Variety Score: Assessing diet quality in healthy young and older adults. *J Am Diet Assoc.* 1997;97:266–271.

3 Welsh S, Davus C, Shaw A. A brief history of food guides in the United States. *Nutr Today.* 1992;Nov/Dec:6–11.

4 Institute of Medicine, Food and Nutrition Board. *Dietary Reference Intakes for Calcium, Phosphorus, Magnesium, Vitamin D, and Fluoride.* Washington, DC: National Academy Press; 1997.

5 Ibid.

6 Yates, AA, Schlicker, SA, Suitor, CW. Dietary Reference Intakes: The new basis for recommendations for calcium and related nutrients, B vitamins and choline. *J Am Diet Assoc.* 1998;98:699–706.

7 National Academy of Sciences. *Recommended Dietary Allowances.* 10th ed. Washington, DC: National Academy Press; 1989.

8 Institute of Medicine, Food and Nutrition Board. Op cit., and Institute of Medicine, Food and Nutrition Board. *Dietary Reference Intakes for Thiamin, Riboflavin, Niacin, Vitamin B_6, Folate, Vitamin B_{12}, Pantothenic Acid, Biotin, and Choline.* Washington, DC: National Academy Press; 1998 and Institute of Medicine, Food and Nutrition Board. *Dietary Reference Intakes for Vitamin C, Vitamin E, Selenium, and Carotenoids.* Washington, DC: National Academy Press; 2000.

9 US Department of Health and Human Services. *The Surgeon General's Report on Nutrition and Health.* Washington DC: US Government Printing Office; 1988.

10 Lee RD, Nieman DC. *Nutritional Assessment.* 2nd ed. St. Louis, MO: Mosby Year-Book; 1996.

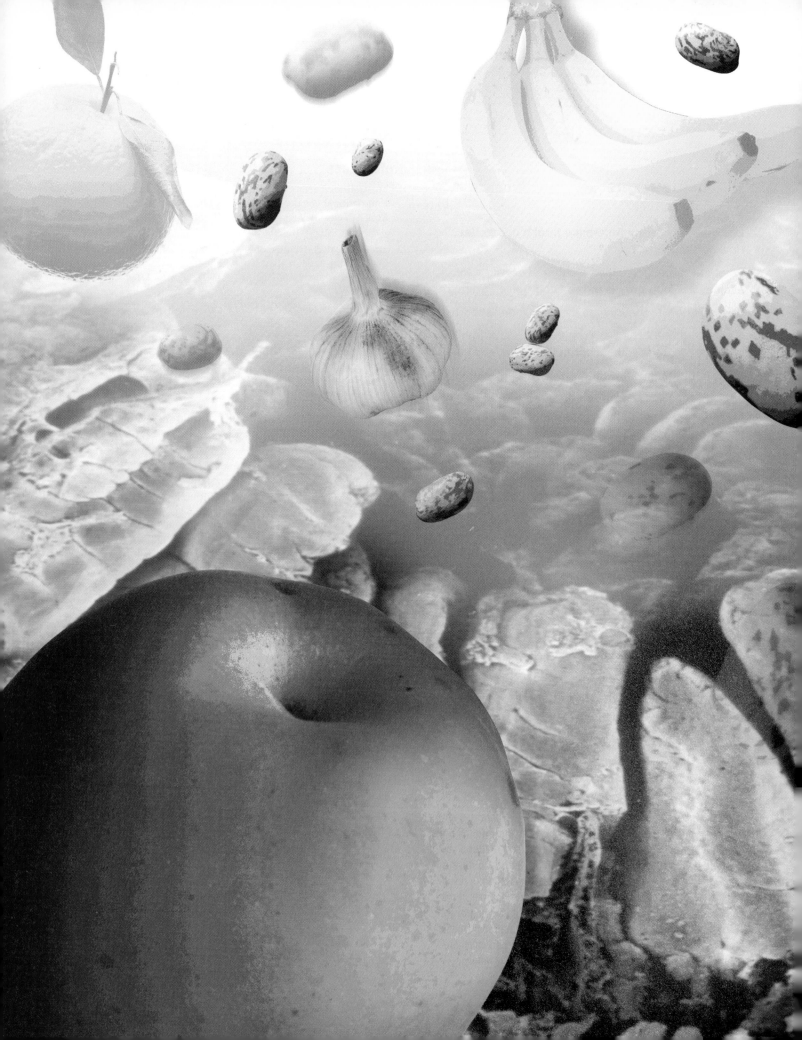

Chapter 3

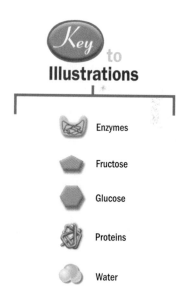

Digestion and Absorption

Think About It

1 Your friend warns you that eating some foods together is not healthful. Is this likely to change your eating behavior?

2 How good are you at identifying tastes?

3 Have you ever noticed that food sometimes tastes sweeter after chewing it for a while?

4 You feel particularly happy and you find a meal prepared by your friend tastes especially good. Any connection?

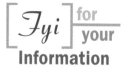

Fyi for your Information

This chapter's FYI boxes include practical information on the following topics:

• Bugs in Your Gut? Health Effects of Intestinal Bacteria

• Lactose Intolerance

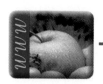

The web site for this book offers many useful tools and is a great source for additional nutrition information for both students and instructors. Visit the site at **nutrition.jbpub.com** for information on digestion and absorption. You'll find exercises that explore the following topics:

• Gastrointestinal Disorders

• Have You Heard about GERD?

• Gallbladder Health

• Lactose Intolerance

Key to Illustrations

Enzymes

Fructose

Glucose

Proteins

Water

What About Bobbie?

Track the choices Bobbie is making with the EatRight Analysis software.

The aroma from a roasting turkey floats past your nose. You haven't eaten for six or seven hours. Your mouth waters, anticipating a delicious experience. Your digestive juices are turned on! Is this virtual reality? Not at all! Before you eat a morsel of food, fleeting thoughts from your brain signal your body to prepare for the coming feast.

The body's machinery to process food and turn it into nutrients is not only efficient but elegant. The action unfolds in the digestive tract in two stages: **digestion**—the breaking apart of foods into smaller and smaller units—and **absorption**—the movement of those small units from the gut into the bloodstream or lymphatic system for circulation. Remarkably, your digestive system is designed to digest carbohydrates, proteins, and fats simultaneously, all the while preparing other substances—vitamins, minerals, and cholesterol, for example—for absorption. And the best part is that it doesn't need any help! You may see promotions for enzyme supplements or read diet books that recommend consuming food or nutrient groups separately. There is no scientific basis for most of these claims. Unless you have a specific medical condition, your digestive system is ready, willing, and able to digest and absorb the foods you eat, in whatever combination you eat them.

But go back to the aroma of that roast turkey for a moment. Before digestion and absorption, our senses of taste and smell attract us to the foods we are likely to consume.

Taste and Smell: The Beginnings of Our Food Experience

As you learned in Chapter 1, you probably wouldn't eat a food if it didn't appeal in some way to your senses. Smell and taste belong to our chemical sensing system, or the **chemosenses.** The complicated processes of smelling and tasting begin when tiny molecules released by the substances around us bind to receptors on special cells in the nose, mouth, or throat. These special sensory cells transmit messages through nerves to the brain, where specific smells or tastes are identified.

The Chemosenses

Olfactory (smell) **cells** are stimulated by the odors around us, such as the fragrance of a gardenia or the smell of bread baking. These nerve cells are found in a small patch of tissue high inside the nose, and they connect directly to the brain.

Gustatory (taste) **cells** react to food and beverages. These surface cells in the mouth send taste information along their nerve fibers. The taste cells are clustered in the taste buds of the mouth and throat, as **Figure 3.1** shows. Many of the visible small bumps on the tongue contain taste buds.

A third chemosensory mechanism, the **common chemical sense,** contributes to our senses of smell and taste. In this system, thousands of nerve

digestion The process of transforming the foods we eat into units for absorption.

absorption The movement of substances into or across tissues; in particular, the passage of nutrients and other substances into the walls of the gastrointestinal tract and then into the bloodstream.

chemosenses [key-mo-SEN-sez] The chemical sensing system in the body, including taste and smell.

olfactory cells Nerve cells in a small patch of tissue high in the nose connected directly to the brain to transmit messages about specific smells.

gustatory cells Surface cells in the throat and on the taste buds in the mouth that transmit taste information.

common chemical sense A chemosensory mechanism that contributes to our senses of smell and taste. It comprises thousands of nerve endings, especially on the moist surfaces of the eyes, nose, mouth, and throat.

essential fatty acid Fatty acids that the body needs but cannot synthesize and must be obtained from diet.

cephalic phase responses The responses of the parasympathetic nervous system to the sight, smell, thought, taste, and sound of food.

Quick Bites

How Many Taste Buds Do You Have?

We have almost 10,000 taste buds in our mouths, including those on the roofs of our mouths. In general, females have more taste buds than males.

Think About It
1

Think About It
2

endings—especially on the moist surfaces of the eyes, nose, mouth, and throat—give rise to sensations like the sting of ammonia, the coolness of menthol, and the irritation of chili peppers.

In the mouth, along with texture, temperature, and the sensations from the common chemical sense, tastes combine with odors to produce a perception of flavor. It is flavor that lets us know whether we are eating a pear or an apple. You recognize flavors mainly through the sense of smell. If you hold your nose while eating chocolate, for example, you will have trouble identifying it, even though you can distinguish the food's sweetness or bitterness. That's because the familiar flavor of chocolate is sensed largely by odor, as is the well-known flavor of coffee.

Many nutritionists have suggested that fat has no taste and that its appeal is due solely to its texture. However, this may not be the case. Animal studies have found a taste receptor for fat, and **essential fatty acids** (fatty acids that must be obtained from the diet) elicit the strongest taste response.[1]

The sight, smell, thought, taste, and in some cases, even the sound of food can trigger a set of physiologic responses known as the **cephalic phase responses.**[2] These responses (see **Figure 3.2**) involve more than just the digestive tract, and follow rapidly on the heels of sensory stimulation. In the digestive tract, salivary and gastric secretions flow, preparing for the consumption of food. If no food is consumed, the response diminishes; but eating continues the stimulation of the salivary and gastric cells.

Figure 3.1 **Taste buds.** Although different regions of the tongue have slight differences in sensitivity, all taste buds can detect the qualities of taste—salty, bitter, sweet, sour, and possibly umami. The photomicron shows a taste cell.
Source: Micrograph courtesy of Dr. Gene Shih and Dr. R.G. Kessel, all rights reserved.

Figure 3.2 **The cephalic (preabsorptive) phase responses.** In response to sensory stimulation, your body primes its resources to better absorb and use anticipated nutrients.

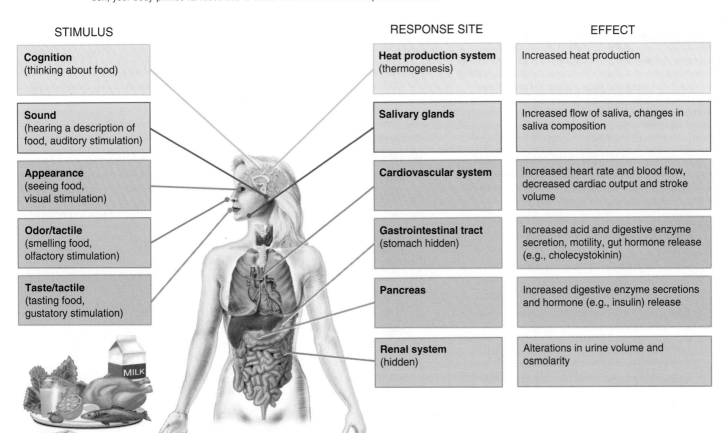

STIMULUS	RESPONSE SITE	EFFECT
Cognition (thinking about food)	**Heat production system** (thermogenesis)	Increased heat production
Sound (hearing a description of food, auditory stimulation)	**Salivary glands**	Increased flow of saliva, changes in saliva composition
Appearance (seeing food, visual stimulation)	**Cardiovascular system**	Increased heart rate and blood flow, decreased cardiac output and stroke volume
Odor/tactile (smelling food, olfactory stimulation)	**Gastrointestinal tract** (stomach hidden)	Increased acid and digestive enzyme secretion, motility, gut hormone release (e.g., cholecystokinin)
Taste/tactile (tasting food, gustatory stimulation)	**Pancreas**	Increased digestive enzyme secretions and hormone (e.g., insulin) release
	Renal system (hidden)	Alterations in urine volume and osmolarity

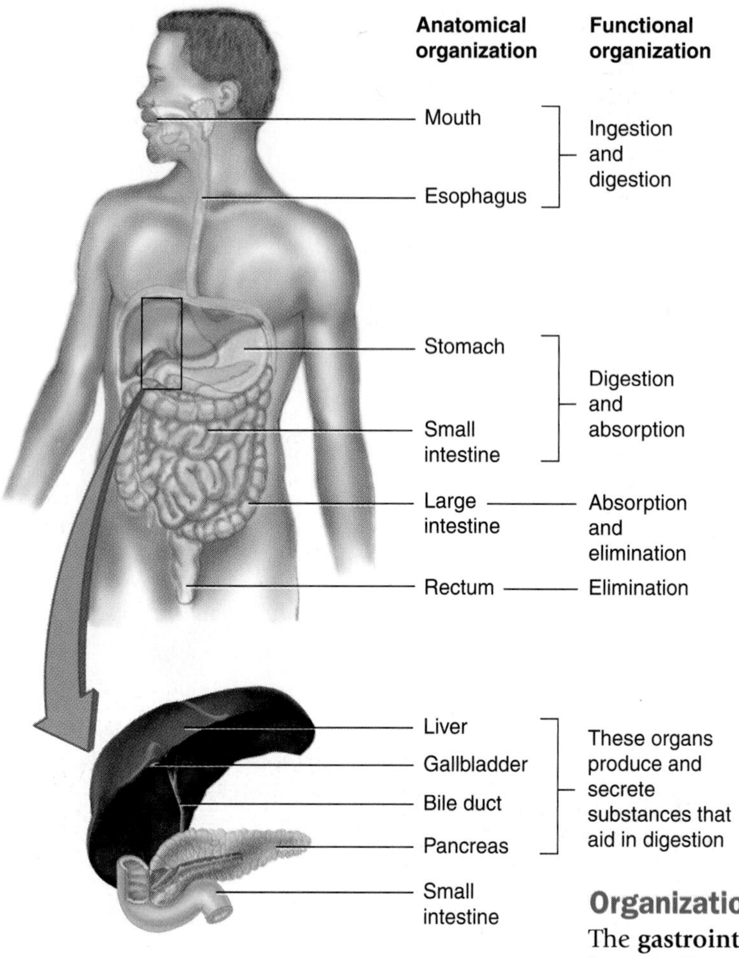

Anatomical organization

Functional organization

Mouth
— Ingestion and digestion
Esophagus

Stomach
— Digestion and absorption
Small intestine

Large intestine — Absorption and elimination

Rectum — Elimination

Liver
Gallbladder
Bile duct — These organs produce and secrete substances that aid in digestion
Pancreas

Small intestine

> **Figure 3.3** **Anatomic and functional organization of the GI tract.** Although digestion begins in the mouth, most digestion occurs in the stomach and small intestine. Absorption primarily takes place in the small and large intestines. For a detailed description of the GI tract and assisting organs, see Appendix E.

gastrointestinal (GI) tract [GAS-troh-in-TES-tin-al] The connected series of organs and structures used for digestion of food and absorption of nutrients; also called the alimentary canal or the digestive tract.

excretion The process of separating and eliminating waste products of metabolism and undigested food from the body.

mucosa [myu-KO-sa] The innermost layer of a cavity. The inner layer of the gastrointestinal tract, also called the intestinal wall. It is composed of epithelial cells and glands.

submucosa The layer of loose fibrous connective tissue under the mucous membrane.

circular muscle Layers of smooth muscle that surround organs, including the stomach and the small intestine.

longitudinal muscle Muscle fibers aligned lengthwise.

serosa A smooth membrane composed of a mesothelial layer and connective tissue. The intestines are covered in serosa.

Key Concepts *Taste and smell are the first interactions we have with food. The flavor of a particular food is really a combination of olfactory, gustatory, and other stimuli. Smell (olfactory) receptors receive stimuli through odor compounds. Taste (gustatory) receptors in the mouth sense flavors. Other nerve cells (the common chemical senses) are stimulated by other chemical factors. If one of these stimuli is missing, our sense of flavor is incomplete.*

The Gastrointestinal Tract

If, instead of teasing the body with mere sights and smells, we actually sit down to a meal and experience the full flavor and texture of foods, the real work of the digestive tract begins. In order for the food we eat to nourish our bodies, we need to digest it, (break it down into smaller units) absorb it, or move it from the gut into circulation; and finally transport it to the tissues and cells of the body. The digestive process starts in the mouth and continues as food journeys down the gastrointestinal, or GI, tract. At various points along the GI tract, nutrients are absorbed, meaning they move from the GI tract into circulatory systems so they can be transported throughout the body. If there are problems along the way, with either incomplete digestion or inadequate absorption, the cells will not receive the nutrients they need to grow, perform daily activities, fight infection, and maintain health. A closer look at the gastrointestinal tract will help you see just how amazing this organ system is.

Organization of the GI Tract

The **gastrointestinal (GI) tract,** also known as the alimentary canal, is a long, hollow tube that begins at the mouth and ends at the anus. The specific parts include the mouth, esophagus, stomach, small intestine, large intestine, and rectum. The GI tract works with the assisting organs—the salivary glands, liver, gallbladder, and pancreas—to turn food into small molecules that the body can absorb and use (see **Figure 3.3**). The GI tract has an amazing variety of functions, including

1. ingestion—the receipt and softening of food,
2. transport of ingested food,
3. secretion of digestive enzymes, acid, mucus, and bile,
4. absorption of end products of digestion,
5. movement of undigested material, and
6. elimination—the transport, storage and **excretion** of waste products.

A Closer Look at Gastrointestinal Structure

Although it's convenient to describe the GI tract as a hollow tube, its structure is really much more complex. As you can see in **Figure 3.4**, there are several layers to this tube:

- The innermost layer, called the **mucosa,** is a layer of epithelial (lining) cells and glands.
- Next, the **submucosa,** is a layer of loose fibrous connective tissue.
- Continuing outward are two layers of muscle fibers:
  - First is a layer of **circular muscle,** where muscle fibers go around the tube,
  - Next is a layer of **longitudinal muscle,** where fibers lie lengthwise along the tube.

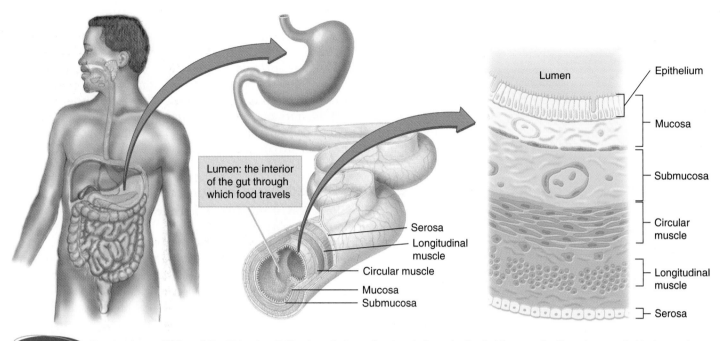

Lumen: the interior of the gut through which food travels

Serosa
Longitudinal muscle
Circular muscle
Mucosa
Submucosa

Lumen
Epithelium
Mucosa
Submucosa
Circular muscle
Longitudinal muscle
Serosa

Figure 3.4 **Structural organization of the GI tract wall.** Your intestinal tract is a long hollow tube lined with mucosal cells and surrounded by layers of muscle cells.

- Finally the outer surface, or **serosa,** provides a covering for the entire GI tract.

At several points along the tract, where one part connects with another (e.g., where the esophagus meets the stomach) the muscles are thicker and form **sphincters.** As you can see in **Figure 3.5,** by alternately contracting and relaxing, a sphincter acts as a valve controlling the movement of food material so that it goes only in one direction.

Key Concepts *The gastrointestinal tract consists of the mouth, esophagus, stomach, small intestine, large intestine, and rectum. The function of the GI tract is to ingest, digest, and absorb nutrients, and eliminate waste. The general structure of the GI tract consists of many layers, including an inner mucosal lining, a layer of connective tissue, layers of muscle fibers, and an outer covering layer. Sphincters are muscular valves along the GI tract that control movement from one part to the next.*

Overview of Digestion: Physical and Chemical Processes

The breakdown of food into smaller units and finally into absorbable nutrients involves both chemical and physical processes. First, there is the physical breaking of food into smaller pieces, such as happens when we chew. In addition, the muscular contractions of the GI tract continue to break food up and mix it with various secretions, while at the same time moving the mixture (called **chyme**) along the tract. Enzymes, along with other chemicals, help complete the breakdown process and promote absorption.

The Physical Movement and Breaking Up of Food

Distinct muscular actions of the GI tract take the food on its long journey. From mouth to anus, wavelike muscular contractions called **peristalsis** transport food and nutrients along the length of the GI tract. Peristaltic waves from the stomach muscles occur about three times per minute. In the small intestine, circular and longitudinal bands of muscle contract approximately every four to five seconds. The large intestine uses slow peristalsis to move the end products of digestion (feces).

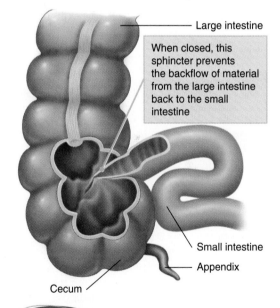

Large intestine

When closed, this sphincter prevents the backflow of material from the large intestine back to the small intestine

Small intestine
Appendix
Cecum

Figure 3.5 **Sphincters in action.** Movement from one section of the GI tract to the next is controlled by muscular valves called sphincters.

sphincter [SFINGK-ter] A circular band of muscle fibers that surround the entrance or exit of a hollow body structure (e.g., the stomach) and act as valves to control the flow of material.

chyme [KIME] A mass of partially digested food and digestive juices moving from the stomach into the duodenum.

peristalsis [Per-ih-STAHL-sis] The wavelike, rhythmic muscular contractions of the GI tract that propel its contents down the tract.

PERISTALSIS

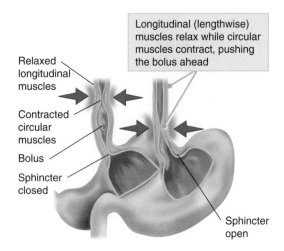

Relaxed longitudinal muscles

Longitudinal (lengthwise) muscles relax while circular muscles contract, pushing the bolus ahead

Contracted circular muscles

Bolus

Sphincter closed

Sphincter open

SEGMENTATION

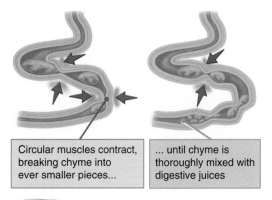

Circular muscles contract, breaking chyme into ever smaller pieces...

... until chyme is thoroughly mixed with digestive juices

Figure 3.6 **Peristalsis and segmentation.** Peristalsis and segmentation help break up, mix and move food through the GI tract.

segmentation Periodic muscle contractions at intervals along the GI tract that alternate forward and backward movement of the contents, thereby breaking apart chunks of the food mass and mixing in digestive juices.

enzyme [EN-zime] Large proteins in the body that accelerate the rate of chemical reactions but are not altered in the process.

catalyze To speed up a chemical reaction.

hydrolysis A reaction that breaks apart a compound through the addition of water.

lumen Cavity or hollow channel in any organ or structure of the body.

passive diffusion The movement of substances into or out of cells without the expenditure of energy or the involvement of transport proteins in the cell membrane. Also called simple diffusion.

Segmentation, a muscular movement that occurs in the small intestine, divides and mixes the chyme by alternating the forward and backward movement of the GI tract's contents. Segmentation also enhances absorption by bringing chyme into contact with the intestinal wall. In contrast, peristaltic contractions proceed in one direction for variable distances along the length of the intestine. Some even travel the entire distance from the beginning of the small intestine to the end. Peristaltic contractions of the small intestine often are continuations of contractions that began in the stomach. **Figure 3.6** shows peristalsis and segmentation.

The Chemical Breakdown of Food

Chemically, it is the action of enzymes that divide nutrients into compounds small enough for absorption.

Enzymes are protein compounds that **catalyze** or speed up chemical reactions but are not altered in the process. Most enzymes can catalyze only one or a few related reactions, a property called enzyme specificity. Enzymes act in part by bringing the reacting molecules close together. In digestion, these chemical reactions divide substances into smaller compounds by a process called **hydrolysis** (breaking apart by water), as **Figure 3.7** shows. Most of the digestive enzymes can be identified by names; they commonly end in *-ase* (amylase, lipase, etc.). For example, the enzyme needed to digest sucrose is sucr*ase*.

In addition to enzymes, other chemicals support the digestive process. These include acid in the stomach, a neutralizing base in the small intestine, bile that prepares fat for digestion, and mucus secreted along the GI tract. This mucus does not break down food but lubricates it and protects the cells that line the GI tract from the strong digestive chemicals. Fluids containing various enzymes and other substances are added to the consumed food along the GI tract. In fact, the volume of fluid secreted into the GI tract is about 7,000 milliliters (about $6^2/_3$ quarts) per day.[3] **Figure 3.8** shows the average daily fluids in the GI tract.

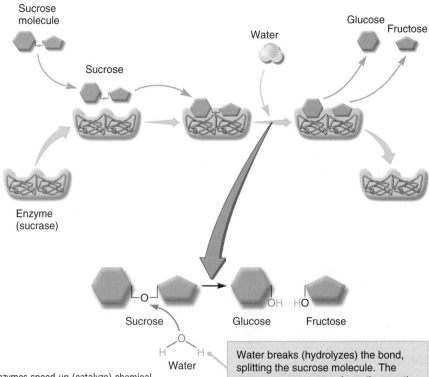

Sucrose molecule

Sucrose

Water

Glucose Fructose

Enzyme (sucrase)

Sucrose

Glucose Fructose

Water

Water breaks (hydrolyzes) the bond, splitting the sucrose molecule. The enzyme sucrase speeds up the reaction

Figure 3.7 **Water and enzymes in chemical reactions.** Enzymes speed up (catalyze) chemical reactions. When water breaks a chemical bond, the action is called hydrolysis.

Key Concepts *Digestion involves both physical and chemical activity. Physical activity includes chewing and the movement of muscles along the GI tract that divide food into smaller pieces and mix it with digestive secretions. Chemical digestion is the breaking of bonds in nutrients, such as carbohydrates or proteins, to produce smaller units. Enzymes—proteins that encourage chemical processes—catalyze these hydrolytic reactions.*

Overview of Absorption

Food is broken apart during digestion and moved from the GI tract into circulation and on to the cells. Many of the nutrients—vitamins, minerals, and water—do not need to be digested before they are absorbed. But the energy-yielding nutrients—carbohydrate, fat, and protein—are too large to be absorbed intact and must be digested first. At this point, we need to outline how nutrients are moved from the interior, or **lumen,** of the gut through the lining cells (mucosa) and into circulation.

The Four Roads to Nutrient Absorption

There are four processes by which nutrients are absorbed: passive diffusion, facilitated diffusion, active transport, and endocytosis (see **Figure 3.9**). Let's take a look at each one in turn.

Passive diffusion is movement of molecules without the expenditure of energy through the cell membrane, through either special watery channels or intermolecular gaps in the cell membrane. Molecules cross permeable cell membranes as a result of random movements that tend to equalize the concentration of substances on both sides of a membrane. **Concentration gradients** (e.g., a high outside concentration and a low inside concentration of molecules) drive passive diffusion. The larger the concentration of molecules on one side of the cell membrane, the faster those molecules move across the membrane to the area of lower concentration.

Since the cell membrane mainly consists of fat-soluble substances, it welcomes fats and other fat-soluble molecules. Oxygen, nitrogen, carbon dioxide, and alcohols are highly soluble in fat and readily dissolve in the cell membrane and diffuse across it. Large amounts of oxygen are delivered this way, passing easily into a cell's interior almost as if it had no membrane barrier at all. Although water crosses cell membranes easily, most water-soluble nutrients (carbohydrates, **amino acids,** vitamins, and minerals) cannot be absorbed via passive diffusion. They need help to cross into the intestinal cells. This help comes in the form of a carrier, and may also require energy.

In **facilitated diffusion,** special carriers help transport a substance (such as the simple sugar fructose) across the cell membrane. The facilitating carriers are proteins that reside in the cell membrane. The diffusing molecule becomes lightly bound to the carrier protein, which changes its shape to open a pathway for the diffusing molecules to move into the cell. Concentration gradients also help to drive facilitated diffusion, which is passive and can move substances only from a region of higher concentration to one of lower concentration.

Energy is required to **actively transport** substances in an unfavorable direction. Substances cannot diffuse "uphill" against an unfavorable gradient, whether the difference is one of concentration, electrical charge, or pressure. Substances that usually require active transport across some cell membranes include many minerals (sodium, potassium, calcium, iron,

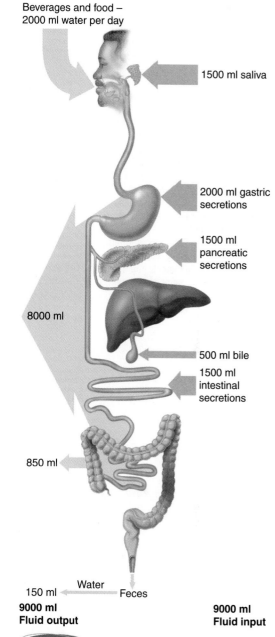

Beverages and food – 2000 ml water per day

1500 ml saliva

2000 ml gastric secretions

1500 ml pancreatic secretions

8000 ml

500 ml bile

1500 ml intestinal secretions

850 ml

150 ml — Water — Feces

9000 ml Fluid output

9000 ml Fluid input

Figure 3.8 **Average daily fluids in the GI tract.** Your GI tract performs a critical balancing act—accepting, secreting, absorbing, and excreting fluids every day.

concentration gradient A difference between the solute concentrations of two substances.

amino acid An organic compound that functions as one of the building blocks of protein.

facilitated diffusion A process by which carrier (transport) proteins in the cell membrane transport substances into or out of cells down a concentration gradient.

active transport The movement of substances into or out of cells against a concentration gradient. Active transport requires energy (ATP) and involves carrier (transport) proteins in the cell membrane.

Figure 3.9 **(a) Passive diffusion.** Using passive diffusion, some substances easily move in and out of cells, either through protein channels or directly through the cell membrane.
(b) Facilitated diffusion. Some substances need a little assistance to enter and exit cells. The transmembrane protein helps out by changing shape.
(c) Active transport. Some substances need a lot of assistance to enter cells. Similar to swimming upstream, energy is needed for the substance to penetrate against an unfavorable concentration gradient.
(d) Endocytosis. Cells can use their cell membranes to engulf a particle and bring it inside the cell. The engulfing portion of the membrane separates from the cell wall and encases the particle in a vesicle.

PASSIVE DIFFUSION

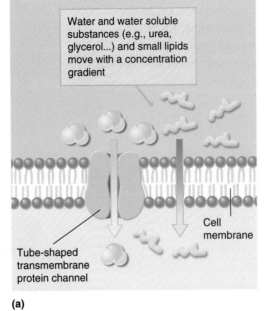

Water and water soluble substances (e.g., urea, glycerol...) and small lipids move with a concentration gradient

Cell membrane

Tube-shaped transmembrane protein channel

(a)

FACILITATED DIFFUSION

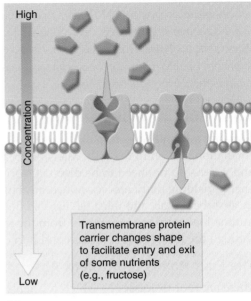

High

Concentration

Low

Transmembrane protein carrier changes shape to facilitate entry and exit of some nutrients (e.g., fructose)

(b)

ACTIVE TRANSPORT

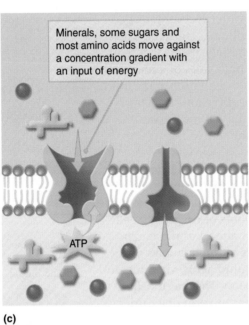

Minerals, some sugars and most amino acids move against a concentration gradient with an input of energy

ATP

(c)

ENDOCYTOSIS

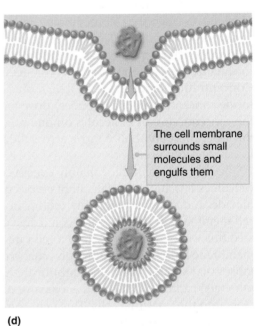

The cell membrane surrounds small molecules and engulfs them

(d)

endocytosis The uptake of material by a cell by the indentation and pinching off of its membrane to form a vesicle that carries material into the cell.

pinocytosis The process by which cells internalize fluids and macromolecules. To do so, the cell membrane invaginates and forms a pocket around the substance. From *pino*, "drinking," and *cyto*, "cell."

phagocytosis The process by which cells engulf large particles and small microorganisms. Receptors on the surface of cells bind these particles and organisms to bring them into large vesicles in the cytoplasm. From *phago*, "eating," and *cyto*, "cell."

chloride, and iodide), several sugars (glucose and galactose), and most amino acids (simple components of protein). These substances can move from the intestine even though their concentration in the intestinal lumen is lower than their concentration in the absorptive cell.

Most substances either diffuse or are actively transported across cell membranes, but some are engulfed and ingested in a process known as **endocytosis**. This occurs, for example, when a newborn infant absorbs antibodies from breast milk.[4] In endocytosis, a portion of the cell membrane forms a sac around the substance to be absorbed, pulling it into the interior of the cell. When cells ingest small molecules and fluids the process is known as **pinocytosis**. A similar ingestion process, **phagocytosis**, is used by specialized cells to absorb large particles.

Key Concepts *Absorption through the GI cell membranes occurs by one of four basic processes. Passive diffusion occurs when nutrients permeate the intestinal wall without a carrier or energy expenditure (e.g., water). Facilitated diffusion occurs when a carrier brings substances into the absorptive intestinal cell without expending energy (e.g., fructose). Active transport requires energy to transport a substance across a cell membrane in an unfavorable direction (e.g., glucose and galactose). Endocytosis (phagocytosis or pinocytosis) occurs when the absorptive cell's membrane engulfs particles or fluids (e.g., absorption of antibodies from breast milk).*

Assisting Organs

The salivary glands, liver, gallbladder, and pancreas all have critical roles in the digestive process. The GI tract works in concert with these organs, which assist digestion by providing fluid, acid neutralizers, enzymes, and **emulsifiers.**

Salivary Glands

Three pairs of **salivary glands** (parotid, sublingual, and submandibular) located in or near the mouth secrete saliva into the oral cavity (see **Figure 3.10**). Saliva moistens food, lubricating it for easy swallowing. Saliva also contains enzymes that begin the process of chemical digestion. We secrete approximately 1,500 milliliters (about 1.5 quarts) of saliva each day. The mere sight, smell, or thought of food can start the flow of saliva.

Liver

The **liver** produces and secretes 600 to 1,000 milliliters of bile daily. Bile is a yellow-green, pasty material that contains water, bile salts and acids, pigments, cholesterol, phospholipids (a type of fat molecule), and electrolytes (electrically charged minerals). Bile tastes bitter, and this is why the word *bile* has come to denote bitterness. Bile acts as an emulsifier by reducing large globs of fat to smaller globs. This process breaks no bonds in fat molecules; it increases the surface area of fat, allowing more contact between fat molecules and enzymes in the small intestine.

Bile is concentrated in your gallbladder and released to the small intestine on demand. After it has done its work, most bile salts are reabsorbed and returned to the liver for recycling. This recirculation is known as the **enterohepatic** (*entero* meaning intestines, *hepatic* referring to the liver) **circulation** of bile salts (see **Figure 3.11**).

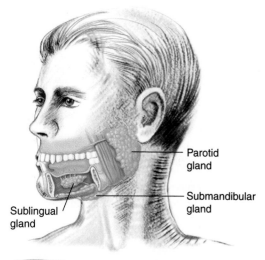

Figure 3.10 **The salivary glands.** The three pairs of salivary glands supply saliva which moistens and lubricates food. Saliva also contains salivary enzymes that begin the digestion of starch.

Labels: Parotid gland; Submandibular gland; Sublingual gland

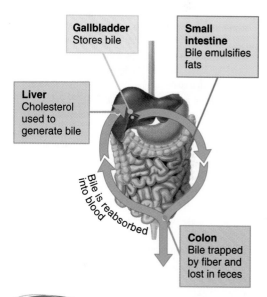

Gallbladder Stores bile

Small intestine Bile emulsifies fats

Liver Cholesterol used to generate bile

Bile is reabsorbed into blood

Colon Bile trapped by fiber and lost in feces

Figure 3.11 **Enterohepatic circulation.** During this recycling process, bile travels from the liver to the small intestine where it assists digestion. In the small intestine, bile is reclaimed and then sent back to the liver to be reused.

emulsifier An agent that blends fatty and watery liquids by promoting the breakup of fat into small particles and stabilizing their suspension in aqueous solution.

salivary glands Glands in the mouth that release saliva.

liver The largest glandular organ in the body, it produces and secretes bile, detoxifies harmful substances, and helps metabolize carbohydrates, lipids, proteins, and micronutrients.

bile An alkaline, yellow-green fluid that is produced in the liver and stored in the gallbladder. The primary constituents of bile are bile acids, phospholipids, cholesterol, and bicarbonate. Bile emulsifies dietary fats, aiding fat digestion and absorption.

enterohepatic circulation [EN-ter-oh-heh-PAT-ik] Recycling of certain compounds between the small intestine and the liver.

gallbladder A pear-shaped sac that stores and concentrates bile from the liver.

cholecystokinin (CCK) [ko-la-sis-toe-KY-nin] A hormone produced by cells in the small intestine that stimulates the release of digestive enzymes from the pancreas and bile from the gallbladder.

pancreas The pancreas secretes enzymes that affect the digestion and absorption of nutrients and releases hormones, such as insulin, which regulate metabolism as well as the disposition of the end products of food in the body.

amylase [AM-ih-lace] A salivary enzyme that catalyzes the hydrolysis of amylose, a starch. Also called ptyalin.

lingual lipase A fat-splitting enzyme secreted by cells at the base of the tongue.

bolus [BOH-lus] A chewed, moistened lump of food that is ready to be swallowed.

esophagus [ee-SOFF-uh-gus] The food pipe that extends from the pharynx to the stomach.

stomach The enlarged, muscular, sac-like portion of the digestive tract between the esophagus and the small intestine.

esophageal sphincter The opening between the esophagus and the stomach that relaxes and opens to allow the bolus to travel into the stomach, and then closes behind it. Also acts as a barrier to prevent the reflux of gastric contents.

hydrochloric acid An acid of chloride and hydrogen atoms made by the gastric glands and secreted into the stomach.

pH A measurement of the hydrogen ion concentration, or acidity, of a solution.

mucus A slippery substance secreted in the GI tract (and other body linings) that protects cells from irritants.

pepsinogen The inactive form of the enzyme pepsin.

pepsin A protein-digesting enzyme produced by the stomach.

gastric lipase An enzyme in the stomach that hydrolyzes certain triglycerides into fatty acids and glycerol.

triglycerides A fat composed of three fatty acid chains esterified to a glycerol molecule.

gastrin [GAS-trin] A polypeptide hormone released from the walls of the stomach mucosa and duodenum that stimulates gastric secretions and motility.

intrinsic factor A protein released from cells in the stomach wall that binds to and aids in absorption of vitamin B_{12}.

The liver also is a detoxification center that filters toxic substances and alters their chemical forms. These altered substances may be sent to the kidney for excretion or carried by bile to the small intestine and routed out of the body in feces.

Gallbladder

The primary function of the **gallbladder** is to store and concentrate bile from the liver. A small, muscular, pear-shaped sac nestled in a depression on the right underside of the liver, the gallbladder holds about a quarter of a cup of bile. The gallbladder is a storage stop for bile between the liver and the small intestine. It fills with viscous bile and thickens it, until a hormone released after eating signals the gallbladder to squirt out its colorful contents.

The gallbladder is normally relaxed and full between meals. When dietary fats enter the small intestine, they stimulate the production of **cholecystokinin (CCK),** a hormone, in the intestinal wall. Cholecystokinin causes the gallbladder to contract and the sphincter of Oddi, which is at the end of the common bile duct, to relax. Like a squeeze bulb, the gallbladder squirts bile into the duodenum (the upper part of the small intestine), about 500 milliliters each day. The common bile duct also carries digestive enzymes from the pancreas.

Pancreas

The **pancreas** secretes enzymes that affect the digestion and absorption of nutrients. During the course of a day, the pancreas secretes about 1,500 milliliters of fluid, which contains mostly water, bicarbonate, and digestive enzymes. The pancreas also releases hormones that are involved in other aspects of nutrient use by the body. For example, the pancreatic hormones insulin and glucagon regulate blood glucose levels. The combination of these two functions makes the pancreas one of the most important organs in the digestion and use of food.

Key Concepts *The salivary glands, liver, gallbladder, and pancreas all make important contributions to the digestive process. The salivary glands release saliva, which contains mucus and enzymes, into the mouth. The liver produces bile, which is stored in the gallbladder and released into the small intestine, where bile helps to prepare fats for digestion. The pancreas also secretes liquid containing bicarbonate and several types of enzymes into the small intestine.*

Putting It All Together: Digestion and Absorption

Up to this point, our discussion has centered on structures, mechanisms, and processes to give you a general idea of the workings of the GI tract. Now you're ready for a complete tour, a journey along the GI tract to see what happens and how digestion and absorption are accomplished. Detailed descriptions of specific enzymes and actions on individual nutrients are covered in later chapters.

Mouth

As soon as you put food in your mouth the digestive process begins. As you chew, you break down the food into smaller pieces, increasing the surface area available to enzymes. Saliva contains the enzyme salivary **amylase** (ptyalin), which breaks down starch into small sugar molecules. Food remains in the mouth only for a short time, so only about 5 percent of the starch is completely broken down. The next time you eat a cracker or a piece of bread, chew slowly and notice the change in the way it tastes. It gets sweeter. That's the salivary amylase breaking down the starch into sugar. Salivary amylase continues to work until the strong acid content of the stomach deactivates it. To start the process of fat digestion, the cells at the base of the tongue secrete another enzyme, **lingual lipase.** The overall impact of lingual lipase on fat digestion, though, is small.

Saliva and other fluids, including mucus, blend with the food to form a **bolus,** a chewed, moistened lump of food that is soft and easy to swallow. When you swallow, the bolus slides past the epiglottis, a valvelike flap of tissue that closes off your air passages so you don't choke. The bolus then moves rapidly through the **esophagus** to the stomach, where it will be digested further. **Figure 3.12** shows the process of swallowing.

Stomach

The bolus enters the **stomach** through the **esophageal sphincter,** commonly called the cardiac sphincter, which immediately closes to keep the bolus from sliding back into the esophagus. Quick and complete closure by the esophageal sphincter is essential to prevent the acidic stomach contents from backing up into the esophagus, causing pain and tissue damage. Heartburn is the movement of acid from the stomach back into the esophagus.

Nutrient Digestion in the Stomach

The stomach cells produce secretions that are collectively called gastric juice. Included in this mixture are water, hydrochloric acid, mucus, pepsinogen (the inactive form of the enzyme pepsin), the enzyme gastric lipase, the hormone gastrin, and intrinsic factor.

- **Hydrochloric acid** makes the stomach contents extremely acidic. See the pH scale in **Figure 3.13** (a **pH** of 2, compared to a neutral pH of 7). This acidic environment kills many pathogenic (disease-causing) bacteria that may have been ingested, and also aids in the digestion of protein. **Mucus** secreted by the stomach cells coats the stomach lining, protecting these cells from damage by the strong gastric juice.

  Hydrochloric acid works in protein digestion in two ways. First, it demolishes the functional, three-dimensional shape of proteins, unfolding and breaking proteins into linear chains; this increases their vulnerability to attacking enzymes. Second, it promotes the breakdown of proteins by converting the enzyme precursor **pepsinogen** to its active form, **pepsin.**

- Pepsin then begins breaking the links in protein chains, cutting dietary proteins into smaller and smaller pieces.

- Stomach cells also produce an enzyme called **gastric lipase.** It has a minor role in the digestion of lipids, specifically **triglycerides** with an abundance of short chain fatty acids.

- **Gastrin,** another component of gastric juice, is a hormone that stimulates gastric secretion and motility.

- **Intrinsic factor** is a substance necessary for the absorption of vitamin B_{12} that occurs further down the GI tract, near the end of the small intestine. In the absence of intrinsic factor, only about $1/50$ of ingested vitamin B_{12} is absorbed.

After you swallow something, salivary amylase continues to digest carbohydrates. After about an hour, acidic stomach secretions become well

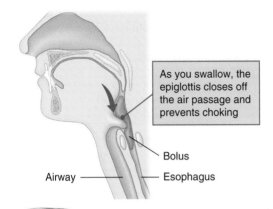

As you swallow, the epiglottis closes off the air passage and prevents choking

Bolus

Airway — Esophagus

Figure 3.12 **Swallowing.** Your epiglottis didn't completely do its job if you have ever choked and had a drink go "down the wrong pipe."

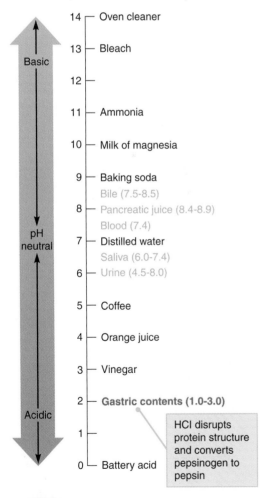

TYPICAL pHs OF COMMON SUBSTANCES

14	Oven cleaner
13	Bleach
12	
11	Ammonia
10	Milk of magnesia
9	Baking soda
	Bile (7.5-8.5)
8	Pancreatic juice (8.4-8.9)
	Blood (7.4)
7	Distilled water
	Saliva (6.0-7.4)
6	Urine (4.5-8.0)
5	Coffee
4	Orange juice
3	Vinegar
2	Gastric contents (1.0-3.0)
1	
0	Battery acid

Basic — pH neutral — Acidic

HCl disrupts protein structure and converts pepsinogen to pepsin

Figure 3.13 **The pH scale.** Because pancreatic juice has a pH around 8, it can neutralize the acidic chyme which leaves the stomach with a pH around 2.

pyloric sphincter [pie-LORE-ic] A circular muscle that forms the opening between the duodenum and the stomach. It regulates the passage of food into the small intestine.

mixed with the food. This increases the acidity of the food and effectively blocks further salivary amylase activity.

Do you sometimes feel your stomach churning? An important action of the stomach is to continue mixing food with GI secretions and produce the semiliquid chyme. To accomplish this, the stomach has an extra layer of diagonal muscles. These, along with the circular and longitudinal muscles, contract and relax to mix food completely. When the chyme is ready to leave the stomach, about 30 to 40 percent of carbohydrate, 10 to 20 percent of protein, and less than 10 percent of fat have been digested.[5] The stomach slowly releases the chyme through the **pyloric sphincter** and into the small intestine. The pyloric sphincter then closes to prevent the chyme from returning to the stomach (see **Figure 3.14**).

The stomach normally empties in one to four hours, depending on the types and amounts of food eaten. Carbohydrates speed through the stomach in the shortest time, followed by protein and fat. Thus, the higher the fat content of a meal, the longer it will take to leave the stomach.

Nutrient Absorption in the Stomach

Although a substantial fraction of digestion has been accomplished by the time chyme leaves the stomach, very little absorption has occurred. Only some lipid-soluble compounds and weak acids, such as alcohol and aspirin, are absorbed through the stomach. Chyme moves on to the small intestine, the digestive and absorptive workhorse of the gut.

Figure 3.14 **The stomach.** Stomach acid unfolds proteins as the stomach churns and mixes food.

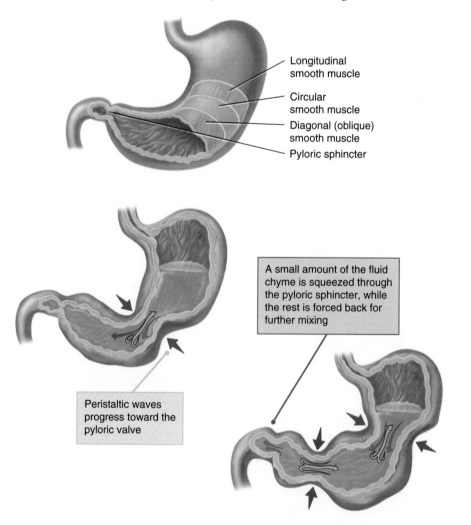

Longitudinal smooth muscle

Circular smooth muscle

Diagonal (oblique) smooth muscle

Pyloric sphincter

A small amount of the fluid chyme is squeezed through the pyloric sphincter, while the rest is forced back for further mixing

Peristaltic waves progress toward the pyloric valve

Small Intestine

The **small intestine** is where the digestion of protein, fat, and nearly all carbohydrate is completed and where most nutrients are absorbed. As you can see in **Figure 3.15,** the small intestine is a tube approximately 10 feet long, divided into three parts:

- **Duodenum** (the first 10 to 12 inches)
- **Jejunum** (about 4 feet)
- **Ileum** (about 5 feet)

Most digestion occurs in the duodenum, where the small intestine receives **digestive secretions** from the pancreas, gallbladder, and its own glands. The remainder of the small intestine primarily absorbs previously digested nutrients.

small intestine The tube (approximately 10 feet long) where the digestion of protein, fat and carbohydrate is completed, and where the majority of nutrients are absorbed. The small intestine is divided into three parts: the duodenum, the jejunum, and the ileum.

duodenum [doo-oh-DEE-num, or doo-AH-den-um] The portion of the small intestine closest to the stomach. The duodenum is 10 to 12 inches long and wider than the remainder of the small intestine.

jejunum [je-JOON-um] The middle section (about 4 ft) of the small intestine lying between the duodenum and ileum.

ileum [ILL-ee-um] The terminal segment (about 5 feet) of the small intestine, which opens into the large intestine.

digestive secretions Substances released at different places in the GI tract to speed the breakdown of ingested carbohydrates, fats, and proteins.

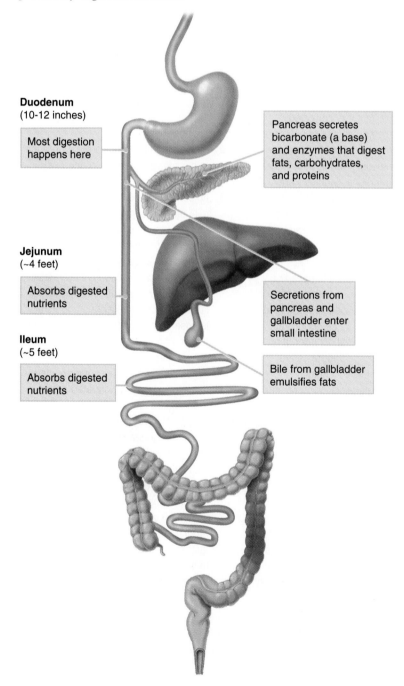

Duodenum
(10-12 inches)

Most digestion happens here

Pancreas secretes bicarbonate (a base) and enzymes that digest fats, carbohydrates, and proteins

Jejunum
(~4 feet)

Absorbs digested nutrients

Ileum
(~5 feet)

Absorbs digested nutrients

Secretions from pancreas and gallbladder enter small intestine

Bile from gallbladder emulsifies fats

Figure 3.15 **The small intestine.** The duodenum is mainly responsible for digesting food; the jejunum and ileum primarily deal with the absorption of food. In addition to the digestive juices from assisting organs, the duodenum secretes mucus, enzymes and hormones to aid digestion. All along the intestinal walls, nutrients are absorbed into blood and lymph. Undigested materials are passed on to the large intestine.

secretin [see-CREET-in] An intestinal hormone released during digestion that stimulates the pancreas to release water and bicarbonate.

Nutrient Digestion in the Small Intestine

In the duodenum, the acidic chyme from the stomach is neutralized by a base, bicarbonate, from the pancreas. The slow delivery of chyme through the pyloric sphincter (about 2 mL/min) allows chyme to be adequately neutralized. This is important because the enzymes of the small intestine need a more neutral environment to work effectively. The stimulus for release of bicarbonate from the pancreas is the hormone **secretin**. This hormone is released from intestinal cells in response to the appearance of chyme.

Fyi Lactose Intolerance

FOR YOUR INFORMATION

When drinking a milkshake is followed shortly by bloating, gas, abdominal pain, and diarrhea, it could be lactose intolerance—the incomplete digestion of the lactose in milk due to low levels of the intestinal enzyme lactase. Lactose is the primary carbohydrate in milk and other dairy foods. Nondairy foods—such as instant breakfast mixes, cake mixes, mayonnaise, luncheon meats, medications, and vitamin supplements—also contain small amounts of lactose. Lactase is necessary to digest lactose in the small intestine. If lactase is deficient, undigested lactose enters the large intestine, where it is fermented by colonic bacteria, producing short chain organic acids and gases (hydrogen, methane, carbon dioxide).

With the exception of a rare congenital disorder in which infants are born without lactase, infants have sufficiently high levels of lactase. However, lactase activity declines with weaning in many racial/ethnic groups. This normal, genetically controlled decrease in lactase activity, called lactose maldigestion, is prevalent among Asians, Native Americans, and African-Americans. However, among U.S. Caucasians, Northern and Central Europeans, lactose maldigestion is far less common because lactase activity tends to persist. Lactose maldigestion occurs in about 25 percent of the U.S. population and in 75 percent of the worldwide population.

In addition to primary lactose intolerance, lactose intolerance can be secondary to diseases or conditions (e.g., inflammatory bowel disease such as Crohn's disease or celiac disease, gastrointestinal surgery, and certain medications) which injure the intestinal

mucosa where lactase is expressed. Secondary lactose maldigestion is temporary and lactose digestion improves once the underlying causative factor is corrected.

Lactose intolerance is far less prevalent than commonly believed. Many factors unrelated to lactose, including strong beliefs, can contribute to this condition. Studies have demonstrated that among self-described lactose-intolerant individuals, one-third to one-half develop few or no gastrointestinal symptoms following intake of lactose under well-controlled, double-blind conditions.

Self-diagnosis of lactose intolerance is a bad idea because it could lead to unnecessary dietary restrictions, expense, nutritional shortcomings, and failure to detect or treat a more serious gastrointestinal disorder. If lactose maldigestion is suspected, tests are available to diagnose this condition.

People with real or perceived lactose intolerance may limit their consumption of dairy foods unnecessarily and jeopardize their intake of calcium and other essential nutrients. A low intake of calcium is associated with increased risk of osteoporosis (porous bones), hypertension, and colon cancer.

With the exception of the few individuals who are sensitive to very small amounts of lactose, avoiding all lactose is neither necessary nor recommended because some lactase is still being produced. Lactose maldigesters need to determine the amount of lactose they can comfortably consume at any one time. Here are some strategies for including milk and other dairy foods in your diet without developing symptoms:

1. Initially, consume small servings of lactose-containing foods such as milk (e.g., $\frac{1}{2}$ cup). Gradually increase the serving size until symptoms begin to appear, then back off.
2. Consume lactose with a meal or foods (e.g., milk with cereal) to improve tolerance.
3. Adjust the type of dairy food. Whole milk may be tolerated better than low-fat milk, and chocolate milk may be tolerated better than unflavored milk. Many cheeses (e.g., Cheddar, Swiss, Parmesan) contain considerably less lactose than does milk. Aged cheeses generally have negligible amounts of lactose. Yogurts with live, active cultures are another option; these bacteria will digest lactose. Sweet acidophilus milk, yogurt milk, and other nonfermented dairy foods may be tolerated better than regular milk by lactose maldigesters. However, factors such as the strain of bacteria used, may influence tolerance to these dairy foods.
4. Lactose-hydrolyzed dairy foods and/or commercial enzyme preparations (e.g., lactase capsules, chewable tablets, solutions) are another option. Lactose-reduced (70 percent less lactose) and lactose-free (99.9 percent less lactose) milks are available, although at a higher cost than regular milk.

Lactose maldigestion need not be an impediment to meeting the needs for calcium and other essential nutrients provided by milk and other dairy foods.

Pancreatic juice contains a variety of digestive enzymes that help to digest fats, carbohydrates, and proteins. Secretions from the intestinal wall cells add enzymes to complete carbohydrate digestion.

The presence of fat in the duodenum stimulates the release of stored bile by the gallbladder. The specific signal comes from the intestinal hormone cholecystokinin. Lipids ordinarily do not mix with water, but bile acts as an emulsifier, keeping lipid molecules mixed with the watery chyme and digestive secretions. Without the action of bile, lipids might not come into contact with pancreatic lipase, and digestion would be incomplete.

Distribution of lactose intolerance worldwide.

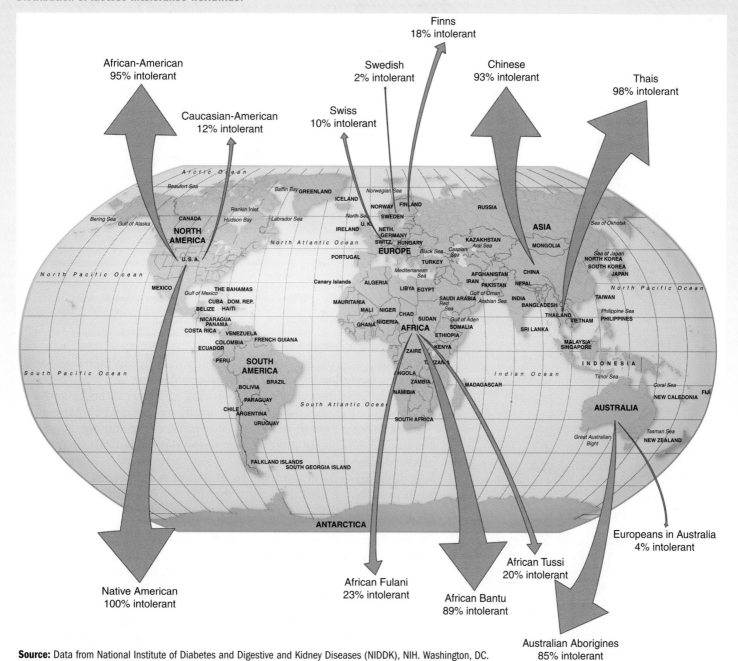

Source: Data from National Institute of Diabetes and Digestive and Kidney Diseases (NIDDK), NIH. Washington, DC.

villi Small fingerlike projections that blanket the folds in the lining of the small intestine. Singular is villus.

microvilli Minute, hairlike projections that extend from the surface of absorptive cells facing the intestinal lumen.

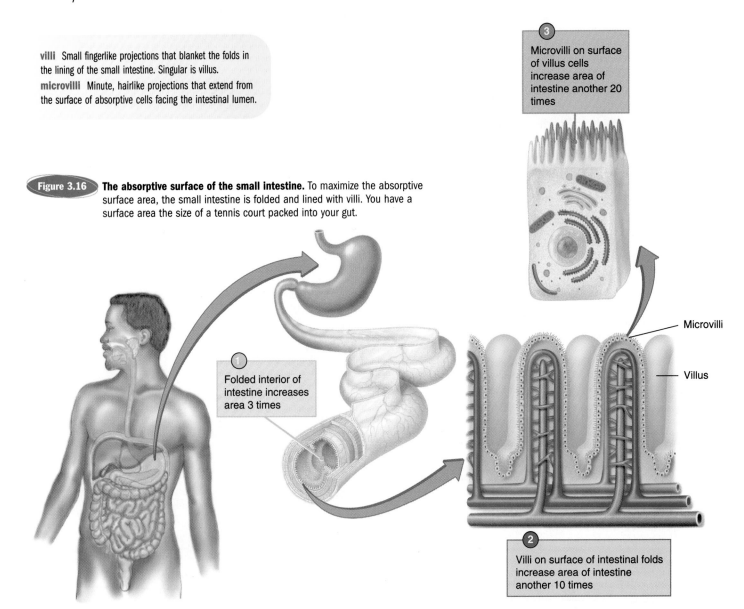

Figure 3.16 **The absorptive surface of the small intestine.** To maximize the absorptive surface area, the small intestine is folded and lined with villi. You have a surface area the size of a tennis court packed into your gut.

3 Microvilli on surface of villus cells increase area of intestine another 20 times

1 Folded interior of intestine increases area 3 times

2 Villi on surface of intestinal folds increase area of intestine another 10 times

Microvilli

Villus

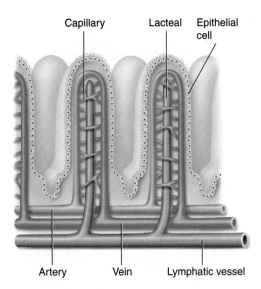

Capillary   Lacteal   Epithelial cell

Artery   Vein   Lymphatic vessel

Anatomy of the villi.

With the pancreatic and intestinal enzymes working together, digestion progresses nicely, leaving smaller protein, carbohydrate, and lipid compounds ready for absorption. Other nutrients, such as vitamins, minerals, and cholesterol, are not digested and generally are absorbed unchanged.

Just as the small intestine accomplishes much of the nutrient digestion, it is also responsible for most nutrient absorption. Its structure makes the process of absorption efficient and complete. In most cases, more than 90 percent of ingested carbohydrate, fat, and protein is absorbed. To see how this is possible, we need to examine the structure of the small intestine.

Absorptive Structures of the Small Intestine

The small intestine packs a gigantic surface area into a small space. As you can see in **Figure 3.16**, the interior surface of the small intestine is wrinkled into folds, tripling the absorptive surface area. These folds are carpeted with fingerlike projections called **villi** that expand the absorptive area another tenfold. Each cell lining the surface of each villus is covered with a "brush border" that contains as many as 1,000 hairlike projections called **microvilli**. The microvilli increase the surface area another 20 times. Taken together, the folds plus the villi and microvilli yield a 600-fold increase in surface area. In fact, your 10-foot (3-meter) long intestine has an absorptive surface area of more than 300 square yards (250 or more square meters)—equivalent to the surface of a tennis court!

Nutrient Absorption in the Small Intestine

As nutrients journey through the small intestine, they are trapped in the folds and projections of the intestinal wall and absorbed through the microvilli into the lining cells. Depending on your diet, each day your small intestine absorbs several hundred grams of carbohydrate, 60 or more grams of fat, 50 to 100 grams of amino acids, 50 to 100 grams of vitamins and minerals, and 7 to 8 liters of water. But the total absorptive capacity of the healthy small intestine is far greater. It actually has the capacity to absorb as much as several kilograms of carbohydrate, 500 grams of fat, 500 to 700 grams of amino acids, and 20 or more liters of water per day.[6] Approximately 85 percent of the water absorption by the gut occurs in the jejunum.[7]

Nutrients absorbed through the intestinal lining pass into the interior of the villi. Each villus contains blood vessels (veins, arteries, and capillaries) and a **lymph** vessel (known as a lacteal) that transport nutrients to other parts of your body. Water-soluble nutrients are absorbed directly into the bloodstream. Fat-soluble lipid compounds are absorbed into the lymph rather than directly into the blood.

Absorption takes place along the entire length of the small intestine. Most minerals, with the exception of the electrolytes sodium, chloride, and potassium, are absorbed in the duodenum and upper part of the jejunum. Carbohydrates, amino acids, and water-soluble vitamins are absorbed along the jejunum and upper ileum, while lipids and fat-soluble vitamins are absorbed primarily in the jejunum. At the very end of the small intestine, the terminal ileum is the site of vitamin B_{12} absorption. If there is damage to the lower small intestine, or surgical removal of this section in the treatment of cancer and other diseases, malabsorption of fat-soluble vitamins and vitamin B_{12} is likely.

The small intestine suffers constant wear and tear as it propels and digests the chyme. The intestinal lining is renewed continually as the mucosal cells are replaced every two to five days. As the chyme completes its three- to ten-hour journey through the small intestine, it passes through the **ileocecal valve,** the connection to the large intestine.

The Large Intestine

The chyme's next stop is the **large intestine.** As **Figure 3.17** shows, this tube is about five feet long and includes the cecum, **colon,** rectum, and anal canal. As chyme fills the cecum, a local reflex signals the ileocecal valve to close, preventing material from reentering the ileum of the small intestine.

Digestion in the Large Intestine

The peristaltic movements of the large intestine are sluggish compared to those of the small intestine. Normally 18 to 24 hours are required for material to traverse its length. During that time, the colon's large population of bacteria digest small amounts of fiber, providing a negligible number of calories daily. Of more significance are the other substances formed by this bacterial activity, including vitamin K, vitamin B_{12}, thiamin, riboflavin, biotin, and various gases that contribute to flatulence.[8] Other than bacterial action, no further digestion occurs in the large intestine.

lymph Fluid that travels through the lymphatic system, made up of fluid drained from between cells and large fat particles.

lacteal A small lymphatic vessel in the interior of each intestinal villus that picks up chylomicrons and fat-soluble vitamins from intestinal cells.

ileocecal valve The sphincter at the junction of the small and large intestines.

large intestine The tube (about 5 feet) extending from the ileum of the small intestine to the anus. The large intestine includes the appendix, cecum, colon, rectum, and anal canal.

colon The portion of the large intestine extending from the cecum to the rectum. It is made up of four parts—the ascending, transverse, descending, and sigmoid colons.

Quick Bites

Short Bowel Syndrome

*P*atients who suffer from short bowel syndrome commonly have difficulty absorbing fat-soluble vitamins. To enhance absorption, treatment includes taking a fat-soluble vitamin supplement that easily mingles with water. These patients may also need to take intramuscular shots of B_{12} because they are unable to absorb this water-soluble vitamin.

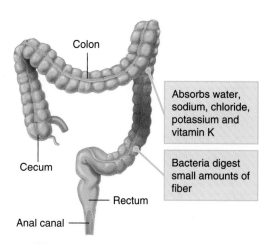

Colon

Absorbs water, sodium, chloride, potassium and vitamin K

Bacteria digest small amounts of fiber

Cecum

Rectum

Anal canal

Figure 3.17 **The large intestine.** In the large intestine, bacteria break down dietary fiber and other undigested carbohydrates, releasing acids and gas. The large intestine absorbs water and minerals, and forms feces for excretion.

The Clever Colon

Though it has been presumed that the colon has no digestive function, recent research shows that the human colon can be an important digestive site in patients who are missing significant sections of their intestines. These patients can actually absorb energy from starch and nonstarch polysaccharides in the colon.

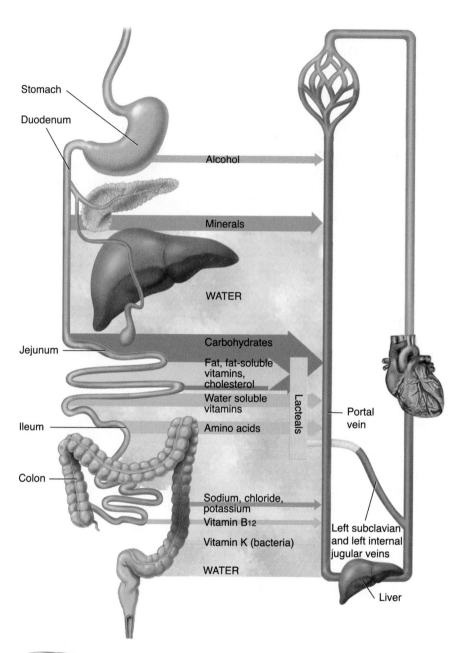

Figure 3.18 **Absorption of nutrients.**

Labels in figure: Stomach, Duodenum, Alcohol, Minerals, WATER, Jejunum, Carbohydrates, Fat, fat-soluble vitamins, cholesterol, Water soluble vitamins, Amino acids, Ileum, Lacteals, Portal vein, Colon, Sodium, chloride, potassium, Vitamin B12, Vitamin K (bacteria), WATER, Left subclavian and left internal jugular veins, Liver

Nutrient Absorption in the Large Intestine

Minimal nutrient absorption takes place in the large intestine, and is limited to water, sodium, chloride, potassium, and some of the vitamin K produced by bacteria. Although vitamin B_{12} is also produced by colonic bacteria, it is not absorbed. The colon dehydrates the watery chyme, removing and absorbing most of the fluid. Of the approximately 1,000 milliliters of material that enters the large intestine, only about 150 milliliters remains for excretion as feces. The semisolid feces, consisting of roughly 60 percent solid matter (food residues, which include dietary fiber, bacteria, and digestive secretions) and 40 percent water, then passes into the rectum. In the **rectum,** strong muscles hold back the waste until it is time to defecate. The rectal muscles then relax, and the anal sphincter opens to allow passage of the stool out the anal canal.[9] **Figure 3.18** illustrates nutrient absorption in the large intestine.

rectum The muscular final segment of the intestine, extending from the sigmoid colon to the anus.

Key Concepts *Digestion begins in the mouth with the action of salivary amylase. Food material next moves down the esophagus to the stomach where it mixes with gastric secretions. Protein digestion is begun through the action of pepsin, while salivary amylase action ceases due to the low pH level of the stomach. Some substances, such as alcohol, are absorbed directly from the stomach. The liquid material (chyme) next moves to the small intestine. Here, secretions from the gallbladder, pancreas, and intestinal lining cells complete the digestion of carbohydrates, proteins, and fats. The end products of digestion, along with vitamins, minerals, water, and other compounds, are absorbed through the intestinal wall and into circulation. Undigested material and some liquid move on to the large intestine where water and electrolytes are absorbed, leaving waste material to be excreted as feces.*

> **central nervous system (CNS)** Comprised of the brain and the spinal cord, the central nervous system transmits signals that control muscular actions and glandular secretions along the entire GI tract.
>
> **enteric nervous system** A network of nerves located in the gastrointestinal wall.
>
> **autonomic nervous system** The part of the central nervous system that regulates the automatic responses of the body; comprised of the sympathetic and parasympathetic systems.

Regulation of Gastrointestinal Activity

The processes of digestion and absorption are regulated by interaction of the nervous and hormonal systems. It would be wasteful to use energy for peristalsis or to secrete digestive enzymes when they were not needed. So, a system of signals is necessary to control GI movement and secretions. That's where nerve cells and hormones come in.

Nervous System

Nerves carry information back and forth between tissues and the brain. Chemicals called neurotransmitters send signals to either excite or suppress nerves, thereby stimulating or inhibiting activity in various parts of the body.

The **central nervous system** (CNS) regulates GI activity in two ways. The **enteric nervous system** is a local system of nerves in the gut wall that is stimulated both by the chemical composition of chyme and by the stretching of the GI lumen that results from food in the GI tract. This stimulation leads to nerve impulses that enhance the muscle and secretory activity along the tract. The enteric nervous system plays an essential role in the control of motility, blood flow, water and electrolyte transport, and acid secretion in the GI tract. A branch of the **autonomic nervous system** (the portion of the CNS that controls organ function) responds to the sight, smell, and thought of food. This branch of the CNS carries signals to and from the GI tract via the vagus nerve, and also enhances GI motility and secretion. In the past, treatments for some ulcers and other GI ailments included severing the vagus nerve, a measure that brought temporary, but not long-term relief.

Hormonal System

Hormones are also involved in GI regulation (see **Figure 3.19**). Hormones are chemical messengers that are produced at one location and travel in the bloodstream to affect another location in the body. Some GI hormones, however, are secreted by and active in the same tissue.

Gastrointestinal hormonal signals increase or decrease GI motility and secretions, and influence your appetite by sending signals

Figure 3.19 **Hormonal regulation of digestion.** In response to food moving through the digestive tract, hormones control the increase and decrease of digestive activities.

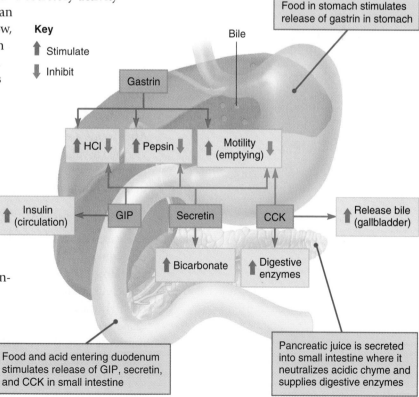

Key
- ↑ Stimulate
- ↓ Inhibit

Bile

Gastrin

↑ HCl ↓   ↑ Pepsin ↓   ↑ Motility (emptying) ↓

↑ Insulin (circulation)   GIP   Secretin   CCK   ↑ Release bile (gallbladder)

↑ Bicarbonate   ↑ Digestive enzymes

Food in stomach stimulates release of gastrin in stomach

Food and acid entering duodenum stimulates release of GIP, secretin, and CCK in small intestine

Pancreatic juice is secreted into small intestine where it neutralizes acidic chyme and supplies digestive enzymes

gastric inhibitory peptide (GIP) [GAS-trik in-HIB-ihtor-ee PEP-tide] A hormone released from the walls of the duodenum that slows the release of the stomach contents into the small intestine and also stimulates release of insulin from the pancreas.

vascular system A network of veins and arteries through which the blood carries nutrients.

to the central nervous system. Some GI hormones function as growth factors for the gastrointestinal mucosa and pancreas.

Four major hormones that regulate the GI function are gastrin, secretin, cholecystokinin, and gastric inhibitory peptide.

- Gastrin is released by cells in the stomach in response to distention of the stomach, nerve impulses from the vagus nerve, and the presence of chemicals such as alcohol and caffeine. Gastrin increases muscle movement in the stomach and enhances release of hydrochloric acid and pepsinogen to encourage digestion.

- Secretin is released by cells along the duodenal wall when acidic chyme begins to move into the duodenum. Secretin opposes the action of gastrin; it reduces gastric secretion and motility and stimulates the pancreas to release bicarbonate in order to neutralize chyme.

- Cholecystokinin (CCK) is released by cells along the small intestine as amino acids and fatty acids from digestion begin to enter the small intestine. CCK stimulates the pancreas to secrete enzymes, stimulates the gallbladder to contract and release bile, and slows gastric emptying.

- **Gastric inhibitory peptide (GIP)** is also released from the intestinal mucosal cells in response to fat and glucose in the small intestine. As its name implies, GIP inhibits gastric secretion, motility, and emptying. In addition, GIP stimulates the release of insulin, which is necessary for glucose utilization.

Taken together, nerve cells and hormones coordinate the movement and secretions of the GI tract so enzymes are released when and where they are needed and chyme moves at a rate that will optimize digestion and absorption.

Key Concepts *Both hormonal and nervous system signals regulate gastrointestinal activity. Nerve cells in both the enteric and autonomic nervous systems control muscle movement and secretory activity. Key hormones involved in regulation are gastrin, secretin, cholecystokinin, and gastric inhibitory peptide. The net effect of these regulators is to coordinate GI movement and secretion for optimal digestion and absorption of nutrients.*

Circulation of Nutrients

After foods are digested and nutrients are absorbed, they are transported via the vascular and lymphatic systems to specific destinations throughout the body. Let's take a closer look at how each of these circulatory systems delivers nutrients to the places they are needed.

Vascular System

The **vascular** or **blood circulatory system** is a network of veins and arteries through which the blood carries nutrients (see **Figure 3.20**). The heart is the pump that keeps the blood circulating through the body. From intestinal cells, water-soluble nutrients are absorbed directly into tiny capillary tributaries of the bloodstream where they travel to the liver before being dispersed throughout the body. Blood carries oxygen from the lungs and nutrients from the GI system to all body tissues. Once the destination cells have used the oxygen and nutrients, carbon dioxide and waste products are picked up by the blood and transported to the lungs and kidneys, respectively, for excretion.

Lymphatic System

Most fat-soluble nutrients are absorbed into the **lymphatic system,** a circulatory system that bypasses the liver before delivery to the bloodstream. The lymphatic system, which joins the bloodstream via two ducts in the neck, plays an important role in nutrition. Its vessels pick up and transport most end products of fat digestion. After a fatty meal, lymph can become as much as 1 to 2 percent fat. We'll discuss the specific process for absorption of lipids into the lymphatic system in Chapter 5.

The lymphatic system is a network of vessels that drain lymph, the clear fluid formed in the spaces between cells. Lymph moves through its system, eventually to empty into the bloodstream near the neck. Unlike nutrients absorbed directly into the vascular system, nutrients absorbed into the lymphatic system bypass the liver before entering the bloodstream.

Unlike the vascular system, the lymphatic system has no pumping organ. The major lymph vessels contain one-way valves and when filled with lymph, smooth muscles in the vessel walls contract and pump the lymph forward. The succession of valves allows each segment of the vessel to act

lymphatic system A system of small vessels, ducts, valves, and organized tissue (e.g., lymph nodes) through which lymph moves from its origin in the tissues toward the heart.

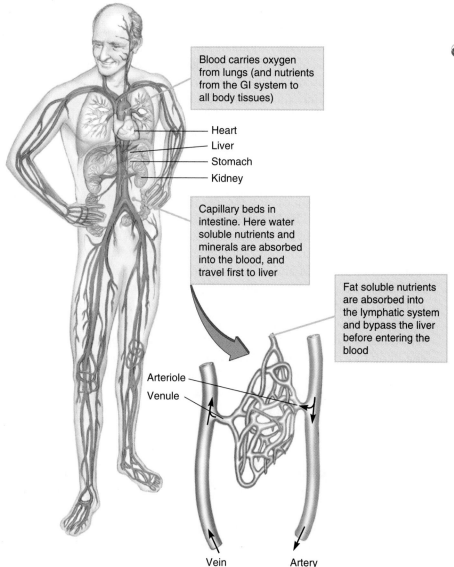

Blood carries oxygen from lungs (and nutrients from the GI system to all body tissues)

Heart
Liver
Stomach
Kidney

Capillary beds in intestine. Here water soluble nutrients and minerals are absorbed into the blood, and travel first to liver

Fat soluble nutrients are absorbed into the lymphatic system and bypass the liver before entering the blood

Arteriole
Venule

Vein   Artery

Figure 3.20 **Circulation.** Blood carries oxygen from the lungs and nutrients from the GI system to all body tissues. Intestinal cells absorb water-soluble nutrients and deliver them directly into tiny capillary tributaries of the bloodstream. From here, they travel to the liver before being dispersed throughout the body. Intestinal cells absorb fat-soluble nutrients and deliver most to the lymphatic system, a circulatory system that bypasses the liver before connecting to the bloodstream.

gastric acid A very strong acid, hydrochloric acid, secreted by glands in the stomach wall.

acrolein A pungent decomposition product of fats, generated from dehydrating the glycerol component of fats; responsible for the coughing attacks caused by the fumes released by burning fat. This toxic water-soluble liquid vaporizes easily and is highly flammable.

as an independent pump. Lymph also is moved along by skeletal muscle contractions that squeeze the vessels.

The lymphatic system also performs an important cleanup function. Proteins and large particulate matter in tissue spaces cannot be absorbed directly into the blood capillaries, but they easily enter the lymphatic system where they are carried away for removal. This removal process is essential—without it a person would die within 24 hours from buildup of fluid and materials around the cells.[10]

Key Concepts *Absorbed nutrients are carried by either the vascular or lymphatic system. Water-soluble nutrients are absorbed directly into the bloodstream, carried to the liver, and then distributed around the body. Fat-soluble vitamins and large lipid molecules are absorbed into the lymphatic vessels and carried by this system before entering the vascular system.*

Influences on Digestion and Absorption

Psychological Influences

The taste, smell, and presentation of foods can have a positive effect on digestion. Just the thought of food can trigger saliva production and peristalsis. Stressful emotions such as depression and fear can have the reverse effect (see **Figure 3.21**); they stimulate the brain to activate the autonomic nervous system. This results in decreased **gastric acid** secretion, reduced blood flow to the stomach, inhibition of peristalsis, and reduced propulsion of food.[11] The next time you sit down to a holiday meal, notice how you feel at the sight of your family's traditional foods as well as smells from your childhood. Happiness and positive memories add to the enjoyment of food, whereas sadness can bring on a poor appetite or upset stomach.

Think About It **4**

Chemical Influences

The type of protein you eat and the way it is prepared affects digestion. Plant proteins tend to be less digestible than animal proteins. Cooking food usually denatures protein (uncoils its three-dimensional structure), which increases digestibility. Cooking meat softens its connective tissue, making chewing easier and increasing the meat's accessibility to digestive enzymes. Food processing produces chemicals that may influence digestive secretions. For example, frying foods in fat at very high temperatures produces small amounts of **acrolein**,[12] which decreases the flow of digestive secretions; whereas meat extracts may stimulate digestion. The physical condition of a food sometimes causes problems with digestion. Cold foods may cause intestinal spasms in people who suffer from irritable bowel syndrome or Crohn's disease. Stomach contents can affect absorption. When food is consumed on an empty stomach, it has more contact with gastric secretions and will be absorbed faster than if it were consumed on a full stomach.

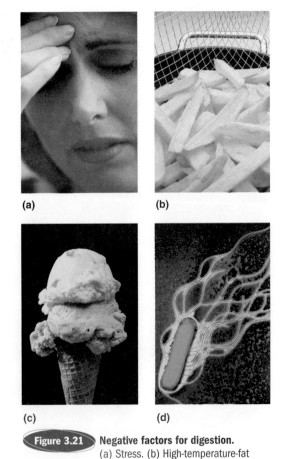

(a)

(b)

(c)

(d)

Figure 3.21 **Negative factors for digestion.** (a) Stress. (b) High-temperature-fat frying. (c) Cold foods. (d) Bacteria.

Bacterial Influences

In the healthy stomach, hydrochloric acid kills most bacteria. In conditions where there is a lower concentration of hydrochloric acid, more bacteria can survive and multiply; harmful bacteria can cause gastritis, an inflammation of the stomach lining, and peptic ulcer—a wound in the mucous membranes lining the stomach or duodenum. Bacteria that cause foodborne illness resist the germicidal effects of hydrochloric acid, so they survive to wreak havoc on the digestive process.

The large intestine has the largest population of helpful bacteria. Bacterial activity can form several vitamins and digest small amounts of cellulose, producing a small amount of energy. These bacteria also synthesize gases, such as hydrogen, ammonia, and methane, as well as acids and various substances that contribute to the odor of feces. If the digestion and absorption of food in the small intestine is incomplete, the debris enters the large intestine where bacterial action produces excessive gas, and possibly bloating and pain.

Key Concepts *Psychological, chemical, and bacterial factors can influence the processes of digestion and absorption. Emotions can influence GI motility and secretion. The temperature and form of food can also affect digestive secretions. Although stomach acid kills many types of bacteria, some are resistant to acid and cause foodborne illness. Helpful bacteria in the large intestine can cause bloating and gas if they receive and begin to digest food components that are normally digested in the small intestine.*

Quick Bites

Gastrointestinal Flora Abound

Your entire body has about 100 trillion cells, but this is only one-tenth the number of protective microorganisms normally living in your body. More than 500 bacterial species live in your GI tract.

Fyi Bugs in Your Gut? Health Effects of Intestinal Bacteria

FOR YOUR INFORMATION

Unseen and unnoticed, millions and millions of bacteria call your GI tract home. Although we often associate bacteria with illness, the right kinds of bacteria in the gut actually protect us from disease. The normal microflora of the gut, specifically strains of *lactobacilli* and *bifidobacteria*, have been linked to improved digestion, enhanced GI immune function, improved lactose tolerance, and even reduced risk of colon cancer. So how can we be good hosts to our intestinal guests, keeping them well-fed and happy? The answer may be in food products and dietary supplements known as probiotics and prebiotics.

Probiotics are foods (or supplements) that contain live microorganisms such as *Lactobacillus acidophilus*. Such lactic-acid-producing bacteria have been used for centuries to ferment milk into yogurt, cheeses, and other products. The bacteria convert lactose into lactic acid, which causes the milk to gel and imparts a tart flavor to the product. The resulting product has a much longer shelf-life than fresh milk and is associated with good health and longevity in many societies.

The term *prebiotic* describes an indigestible food product that stimulates the growth and/or activity of "good" gut bacteria. For example, it is thought that the composition of breast milk strongly favors the growth of *lactobacilli* and *bifidobacteria* in the newborn gut. Some scientists have found *bifidobacteria* to be the dominant species in breast-fed infants while the microflora of bottle-fed infants is more diverse. The reduced incidence of GI infections in breast-fed infants has been attributed to the dominance of *bifidobacteria*. Substances that may be effective prebiotics include fructooligosaccharides, galactooligosaccharides, and inulin.

So how does feeding your gut improve your health? Intestinal bacteria metabolize both indigestible and incompletely digested food material. Some bacteria may make potentially toxic byproducts that have been theorized as a cause of colon cancer. Other bacteria may produce more desirable byproducts, thus reducing risk. For example, acids produced by colon bacteria change the pH of the colon, and this may interfere with carcinogenesis. "Good" bacteria can digest the lactose that enters the colon of a person with lactose intolerance, reducing symptoms and discomfort. Successful colonization of helpful bacteria allows them to outnumber (and out-eat) disease-causing bacteria, thus reducing the likelihood of foodborne illness.

Fermented milk products such as yogurt or kefir are one way to keep your gut happy. Look for a seal recently adopted by the National Yogurt Association to identify products that contain a minimum of 100 million live lactic acid bacteria per gram of yogurt. Not all brands of yogurt contain live, active cultures. Supplemental probiotics must have sufficient numbers of live bacteria to be useful; currently, identification and standardization procedures are lacking. Prebiotics such as fructooligosaccharides are the subject of intense and promising research. Although results are preliminary, food and supplement sources of prebiotics may be another useful way to improve gut microflora and overall health.

constipation Infrequent and difficult bowel movements, followed by a sensation of incomplete evacuation.

diarrhea Watery stools due to reduced absorption of water.

Figure 3.22 **Common GI ailments.** Beans are familiar culprits in what is perhaps the most common GI ailment—gas. Rice is the only starch that does not cause gas.

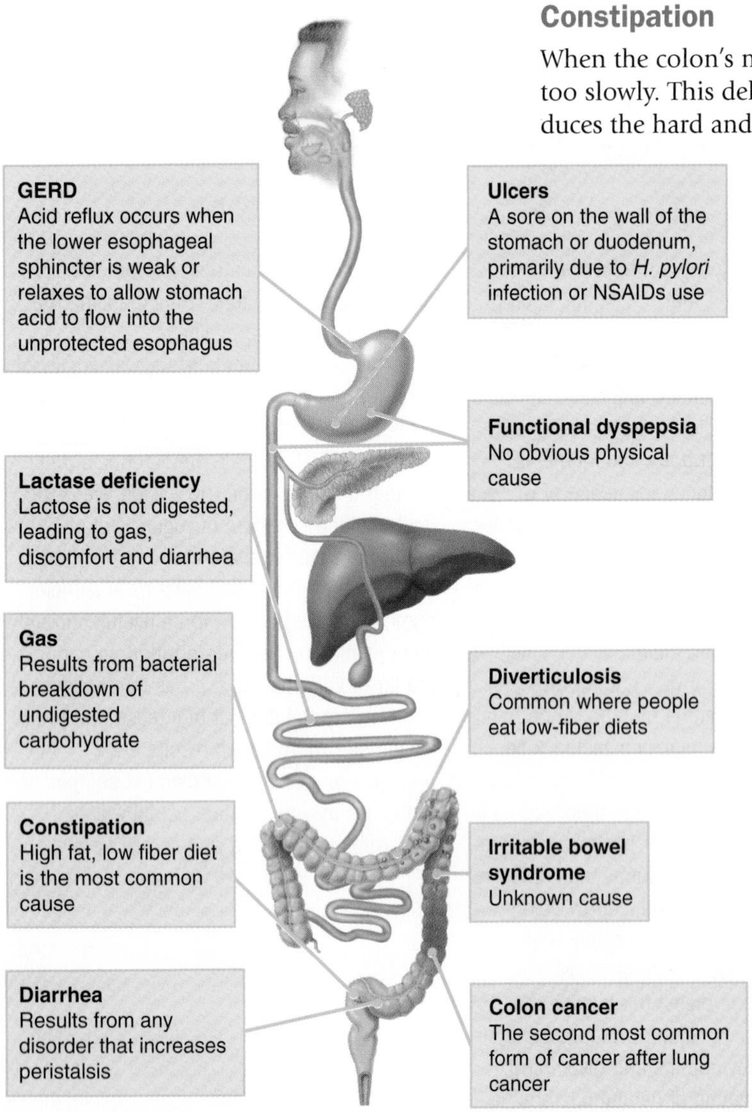

GERD
Acid reflux occurs when the lower esophageal sphincter is weak or relaxes to allow stomach acid to flow into the unprotected esophagus

Lactase deficiency
Lactose is not digested, leading to gas, discomfort and diarrhea

Gas
Results from bacterial breakdown of undigested carbohydrate

Constipation
High fat, low fiber diet is the most common cause

Diarrhea
Results from any disorder that increases peristalsis

Ulcers
A sore on the wall of the stomach or duodenum, primarily due to *H. pylori* infection or NSAIDs use

Functional dyspepsia
No obvious physical cause

Diverticulosis
Common where people eat low-fiber diets

Irritable bowel syndrome
Unknown cause

Colon cancer
The second most common form of cancer after lung cancer

Nutrition and GI Disorders

"I have butterflies in my stomach." "It was a gut-wrenching experience." Our language contains many references to the connection between emotional distress and the GI tract. Most of us have experienced intestinal cramping right before a big date or job interview, or a queasy stomach in response to something very disgusting. The brain, through numerous neurochemical connections with the gut, exerts a profound influence on GI function. Nearly all GI disorders are influenced to some degree by emotional state. On the other hand, a number of illnesses that were once attributed largely to emotional stress, such as peptic ulcer disease, have been shown to be caused primarily by infection and other physical causes. **Figure 3.22** shows some common ailments that affect the GI tract.

Although stress management may help and medical intervention can be required, we can prevent and manage most GI disorders with diet. For instance, adding fiber-rich foods (see **Table 3.1**) and water to the diet reduces intestinal pressure, decreases the time food byproducts remain in the colon, and promotes bowel regularity. You can avoid most problems and keep your GI tract operating at peak efficiency if you regularly eat a healthful diet, exercise, and maintain a healthy weight.

Constipation

When the colon's muscle contractions are slow or sluggish, the stool moves too slowly. This delay causes the colon to absorb too much water and produces the hard and dry stools of **constipation.**

A diet low in fiber and water and high in fats is the most common cause of constipation. Soluble fiber dissolves easily in water and takes on a soft, gel-like texture in the intestines. Insoluble fiber passes almost unchanged through the intestines. The bulk and soft texture of fiber help prevent hard, dry stools that are difficult to pass. People who eat plenty of high-fiber foods are not likely to become constipated.

Liquids like water and juice add fluid to the colon and bulk to stools, making bowel movements softer and easier to pass. Liquids that contain caffeine (e.g., coffee, tea, and many soft drinks) have a dehydrating effect.

Although treatment depends on the cause, severity, and duration, in most cases dietary changes help relieve symptoms and prevent constipation.

Diarrhea

Diarrhea—loose, watery stools that occur more than three times in one day—is caused by digestion products moving through the large intestine too rapidly for sufficient water to be reabsorbed.

Diarrhea is a symptom of many disorders that cause increased peristalsis. Culprits include stress, intestinal irritation or damage, and intolerance to gluten, fat, or lactose. Eating food contaminated with bacteria or viruses often causes diarrhea when the digestive tract speeds the offending food along the alimentary canal and out of the body.

Diarrhea can cause dehydration, which means the body lacks enough fluid to function properly.

Dehydration is particularly dangerous in children and the elderly, and it must be treated promptly to avoid serious health problems.

A diet of broth, tea, and toast and avoidance of lactose, caffeine, and sorbitol can reduce diarrhea until it subsides. As stools form, you can gradually introduce more foods. Pectin, a form of dietary fiber, may be helpful. Also, include foods high in potassium, if tolerated, to replace lost electrolytes. Fluid replacement is also important to avoid dehydration.

Diverticulosis

Like an inner tube that pokes through weak places in a tire, the colon develops small pouches that bulge outward through weak spots as people age. Known as diverticulosis, this condition afflicts about half of all Americans age 60 to 80, and almost everyone older than 80. Although it usually causes few problems, in 10 to 25 percent of these people the pouches become infected or inflamed—a condition called diverticulitis.

Diverticulosis and diverticulitis are common in developed or industrialized countries—particularly the United States, England, and Australia—where low-fiber diets are common. Diverticular disease is rare in countries of Asia and Africa, where people eat high-fiber, vegetable-based diets.

A low-fiber diet can make stools hard and difficult to pass. If the stool is too hard, muscles must strain to move it. This is the main cause of increased pressure in the colon, which causes weak spots to bulge outward.

Increasing the amount of fiber in the diet may reduce symptoms of diverticulosis and prevent complications such as diverticulitis. Fiber keeps stool soft and lowers pressure inside the colon so bowel contents can move through easily (**Table 3.2**).

Quick Bites

Halt! Who Goes There?

Be they friend or foe, antibiotics kill microorganisms in your GI tract, frequently causing diarrhea. About half of pharmaceutical drugs have gastrointestinal side effects.

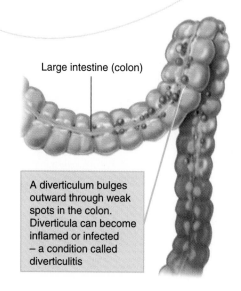

Large intestine (colon)

A diverticulum bulges outward through weak spots in the colon. Diverticula can become inflamed or infected – a condition called diverticulitis

Table 3.1 Dietary Fiber in Foods

Food Group	Serving Size	Fiber (g)
Legumes		
Kidney beans	$\frac{1}{2}$ cup	8
Lentils	$\frac{1}{2}$ cup	5
Split peas	$\frac{1}{2}$ cup	4.4
Fruit		
Stewed prunes	$\frac{1}{2}$ cup	4.5
Apple with skin	1 medium	3.1
Peach with skin	1 medium	2.3
Vegetables		
Broccoli	1 cup	4.6
Carrot, raw	1 medium	2.3
Tomato	1 medium	2.3
Grains		
Wheat-bran cereal	1 ounce	8
Bulgur wheat	$\frac{1}{2}$ cup, cooked	5.3
Whole-wheat bread	1 slice	2-3
Brown rice	$\frac{1}{2}$ cup, cooked	1.7
Spaghetti, enriched white	$\frac{1}{2}$ cup, cooked	1.1
White bread	1 slice	0.5
White rice	$\frac{1}{2}$ cup, cooked	0

Table 3.2 Benefits of Dietary Fiber

1. It has a positive impact on weight control because it delays gastric emptying and enhances a feeling of fullness.
2. It improves glucose tolerance by delaying the movement of carbohydrates into the small intestine.
3. It removes cholesterol by binding with bile in the intestine and causing it to be excreted.
4. It increases stool weight, thus promoting regularity.
5. It may protect against the development of colorectal cancer by decreasing colonic transit time.
6. It decreases pressure within the colon.

gastroesophageal reflux disease (GERD) Tissue damage to the esophagus due to the reflux of gastric contents.

Until recently, many doctors suggested avoiding foods with small seeds such as tomatoes or strawberries because they believed that particles could lodge in the diverticula and cause inflammation. However, this is now a controversial point and no evidence supports this recommendation.

If cramps, bloating, and constipation are problems, the doctor may prescribe a short course of pain medication. However, many medications cause either diarrhea or constipation, undesirable side effects for people with diverticulosis.

Gastroesophageal Reflux

Gastroesophageal reflux disease (GERD) occurs when the lower esophageal sphincter (LES) is weak or relaxes inappropriately allowing the stomach's contents to flow back into the esophagus. Unlike the stomach, the esophagus has no protective mucous lining, so acid can quickly damage it, causing pain. GERD has a variety of causes and many treatment strategies involve lifestyle and nutrition.

Doctors recommend avoiding foods and beverages that can weaken the LES, including chocolate, peppermint, fatty foods, coffee, and alcoholic beverages. Foods and beverages that can irritate a damaged esophageal lining, such as citrus fruits and juices, tomato products, and pepper, also should be avoided.

Decreasing both the portion size and the fat content of meals may help. High-fat meals remain in the stomach longer than low-fat meals. This creates back pressure on the lower esophageal sphincter. Eating meals at least two to three hours before bedtime may lessen reflux by allowing partial emptying and a decrease in stomach acidity. Elevating the head of the bed on six-inch blocks or sleeping on a specially designed wedge reduces heartburn by allowing gravity to minimize reflux of stomach contents into the esophagus.

In addition, cigarette smoking weakens the LES and being overweight often worsens symptoms. Stopping smoking is important and many overweight people find relief when they lose weight.

Label [to] **Table**

As you've learned in this chapter, fiber is one of the few things you do not digest fully. Instead, fiber moves through the GI tract and most of it leaves the body in feces. If it's not digested, then why all the fuss about eating more fiber? You'll learn later in this textbook (in the Carbohydrate chapter) that a healthy intake of fiber may lower your risk of cancer and heart disease and help with bowel regularity. So how do you know which foods have fiber? You have to check out the food label!

This Nutrition Facts panel is from the label on a loaf of whole-wheat bread. The highlighted sections show you that every slice of bread contains 3 grams of fiber. The 12% listed to the right of that refers to the Daily Values below. Look at the Daily Values at the bottom of the label, and note that there are two numbers listed for fiber. One (25 g) is for a person who consumes about 2,000 kilocalories per day and the other (30 g) is for a 2,500-kilocalorie level. It should be no surprise that if you are consuming more calories, you should also be consuming more fiber. The 12% Daily Value is calculated using the 2,000-kilocalorie fiber guideline as follows:

$$\frac{3 \text{ grams fiber per slice}}{25 \text{ grams Daily Value}} = .12, \text{ or } 12\%$$

This means if you make a sandwich with 2 slices of whole-wheat bread, you're getting 6 grams of fiber and almost $\frac{1}{4}$ (24% Daily Value) of your fiber needs per day. Not bad! Be careful though, many people inadvertently buy wheat bread thinking that it's as high in fiber as *whole-wheat* bread but it's not. Whole-wheat bread contains the whole (complete) grain but wheat bread often is stripped of its fiber. Check the label before you buy your next loaf

Irritable Bowel Syndrome

About 20 percent of people in western countries suffer from **irritable bowel syndrome (IBS)**, a poorly understood condition that causes abdominal pain, altered bowel habits (such as diarrhea or constipation), and cramps. Often IBS is just a mild annoyance, but for some people it can be disabling.

The cause of IBS remains a mystery, but emotional stress and specific foods clearly aggravate the symptoms in most sufferers.[13] Beans, chocolate, milk products, and large amounts of alcohol are frequent offenders. Fat in any form (animal or vegetable) is a strong stimulus of colonic contractions after a meal. Caffeine causes loose stools in many people, but it is more likely to affect those with IBS. Women with IBS may have more symptoms during their menstrual periods, suggesting that reproductive hormones can increase IBS symptoms.

The good news about IBS is that although its symptoms can be uncomfortable, it does not shorten life span or progress to a more serious illness. IBS can usually be controlled with diet and lifestyle modifications, and judicious use of medication if needed. Psychiatric treatment, biofeedback, and Transcendental Meditation (a deep relaxation technique) have all been reported to alleviate symptoms in some patients.[14]

Many researchers are convinced that IBS sufferers have abnormal patterns of intestinal motility, but studies show no consistent differences in the GI motion patterns of IBS patients compared with normal control subjects. Some researchers have postulated that IBS sufferers may be hypersensitive to GI stimuli but, again, research results are inconclusive. We are a long way from understanding what causes IBS, but it is likely that a number of physical and psychosocial factors combine to trigger this disorder.

irritable bowel syndrome (IBS) A disruptive state of intestinal motility with no known cause.

Colon Cancer

After lung cancer, colon cancer is the second most common form of cancer in the United States.[15] A diet high in animal fat and low in dietary fiber, which is the typical American diet today, has been linked to colon cancer.[16] Review of the relationships between diet and colon cancer suggests that

---

Nutrition Facts

Serving Size: 1 slice (43g)
Servings Per Container: 16

Calories 100
 Calories from Fat 15

Amount Per Serving	% Daily Value*
Total Fat 2g	**3%**
Saturated Fat 0g	**0%**
Polyunsaturated Fat 0g	
Monounsaturated Fat 0g	
Cholesterol 0mg	**0%**

Amount Per Serving	% Daily Value*
Sodium 230 mg	**9%**
Total Carbohydrate 18g	**6%**
Dietary Fibers 3g	**12%**
Sugars 2g	
Protein 5g	

Vitamin A 0% • Vitamin C 0% • Calcium 6% • Iron 6%

Thiamin 10% • Riboflavin 4% • Niacin 10% • Folate 10%

* Percent Daily Values are based on a 2,000 calorie diet. Your daily values may be higher or lower depending on your calorie needs:

		Calories:	2000	2,500
Total Fat		Less Than	65g	80g
Sat Fat		Less Than	20g	25g
Cholesterol		Less Than	300mg	300mg
Sodium		Less Than	2,400mg	2,400mg
Total Carbohydrate			300g	375g
Dietary Fiber			25g	30g

INGREDIENTS: STONE GROUND WHOLE WHEAT FLOUR, WATER, HIGH FRUCTOSE CORN SYRUP, WHEAT GLUTEN, WHEAT BRAN. CONTAINS 2% OR LESS OF EACH OF THE FOLLOWING: YEAST, SALT, PARTIALLY HYDROGENATED SOYBEAN OIL, HONEY, MOLASSES, RAISIN JUICE CONCENTRATE, DOUGH CONDITIONERS (MAY CONTAIN ONE OR MORE OF EACH OF THE FOLLOWING: MONO- AND DIGLYCERIDES, CALCIUM AND SODIUM STEAROYL LACTYLATES, CALCIUM PEROXIDE), WHEAT GERM, WHEY, CORNSTARCH, YEAST NUTRIENTS (MONOCALCIUM PHOSPHATE, CALCIUM SULFATE, AMMONIUM SULFATE).

flatus Lower intestinal gas that is expelled through the rectum.

diets high in vegetables and regular physical activity are the most significant factors in reducing colon cancer risk. Some scientists hypothesize that fiber (from vegetables) might bind to potential carcinogens and cause them to be excreted before they can cause harm, or that the enhanced movement of materials through the GI tract due to exercise or to a high-fiber diet reduces the time that carcinogens might have to come in contact with colon cells. Alternatively, the fermentation products of fiber produced by colonic bacteria, including acids that lower colon pH, might make carcinogens inactive.

Although these logical reasons point to a beneficial effect of fiber, some studies on animals and humans fail to show this benefit. A recent study of women does not support the protective effect of dietary fiber against colorectal cancer.[17]

Gas

Everyone has gas and eliminates it by burping or passing it through the rectum. Gas is made primarily of odorless vapors. The unpleasant odor of flatulence comes from bacteria in the large intestine that release small amounts of gases that contain sulfur. Although having gas is common, it can be uncomfortable and embarrassing.

Gas in the stomach is commonly caused by swallowing air. Everyone swallows small amounts of air when they eat and drink. However, eating or drinking rapidly, chewing gum, smoking, or wearing loose dentures can cause some people to take in more air. Burping, or belching, is the way most swallowed air leaves the stomach. The remaining gas moves into the small intestine where it is partially absorbed. A small amount travels into the large intestine for release through the rectum. (The stomach also releases carbon dioxide when stomach acid and bicarbonate mix, but most of this gas is absorbed into the bloodstream and does not enter the large intestine.)

Frequent passage of rectal gas may be annoying but it's seldom a symptom of serious disease. **Flatus** (lower intestinal gas) composition depends largely on dietary carbohydrate intake and the activity of the colon's bacterial population.

Most foods that contain carbohydrates can cause gas. By contrast, fats and proteins cause little gas. In the large intestine, bacteria partially break down undigested carbohydrate, producing hydrogen, carbon dioxide, and, in about one-third of people, methane. Eventually these gases exit through the rectum.

Foods that produce gas in one person may not cause gas in another. Some common bacteria in the large intestine can destroy the hydrogen that other bacteria produce. The balance of the two types of bacteria may explain why some people have more gas than others.

Sugars that commonly cause gas are (1) raffinose, found in large quantities in beans, (2) lactose, the natural sugar in milk, (3) fructose, a common sweetener in soft drinks and fruit drinks, (4) sorbitol, found naturally in fruits and used as an artificial sweetener, and (5) stachyose, found in dried beans, peas, and lentils.

Most starches, including potatoes, corn, noodles, and wheat, produce gas as they are broken down in the large intestine. Rice is the only starch that does not cause gas.

Soluble fiber, found in oat bran, beans, peas, and most fruits, is not broken down until it reaches the large intestine where digestion causes gas.

On the other hand, insoluble fiber, found in wheat bran and some vegetables, passes essentially unchanged through the intestines and produces little gas.

Ulcers

A gnawing, burning pain in the upper abdomen is the classic sign of a peptic **ulcer**, which also can cause nausea, vomiting, loss of appetite, and weight loss. A peptic ulcer is a sore that forms in the duodenum (the beginning of the small intestine) or the lining of the stomach.

It was once assumed that stress was a major factor in the development of peptic ulcer disease, particularly in people with "intense" personalities. Diet was also thought to be important, with spicy foods often cast as a major villain. But much to the amazement of most of the medical community, research over the last ten years has confirmed that the vast majority of ulcers are actually caused by infection with a bacterium, *Helicobacter pylori*. Use of nonsteroidal antiinflammatory drugs (NSAIDs), such as aspirin, ibuprofen, and naproxen sodium, is also a common cause of ulcers.

H. pylori causes 80 percent of stomach ulcers and more than 90 percent of duodenal ulcers. These bacteria weaken the protective mucous coating, allowing acid to penetrate to the sensitive lining beneath. Both the acid and the bacteria irritate the lining and cause a sore, or ulcer. *H. pylori* is able to survive in stomach acid because it secretes enzymes that neutralize the acid. This mechanism allows *H. pylori* to make its way to the "safe" area—the protective mucous lining. Once there, the bacterium's spiral shape helps it burrow through the mucous lining.[18]

Nonsteroidal anti-inflammatory drugs (NSAIDs) cause ulcers by interfering with the GI tract's ability to protect itself from acidic stomach juices. Normally the stomach and duodenum employ three defenses against digestive juices: mucus that coats the lining and shields it from stomach acid, the chemical bicarbonate that neutralizes acid, and blood circulation that aids in cell renewal and repair. NSAIDs hinder all these protective mechanisms, and with the defenses down, digestive juices can cause ulcers by damaging the sensitive lining of the stomach and duodenum. Fortunately, NSAID-induced ulcers usually heal once the person stops taking the medication.

If you had ulcers in the 1950s, you probably were told to quit your high-stress job and switch to a bland diet. Today, ulcer sufferers are usually treated with an antimicrobial regimen aimed at eradicating *H. pylori*. Although personality and life stress are no longer considered significant factors in the development of most ulcers, relapse after treatment is more common in people who are emotionally stressed or suffering from depression.

Functional Dyspepsia

Chronic pain in the upper abdomen not due to any obvious physical cause (such as inflammation of the esophagus, peptic ulcer, or gallstones) is referred to as **functional dyspepsia.** Like IBS, the cause of functional dyspepsia is unknown. Hypersensitivity to GI stimuli, abnormal GI motility, and psychosocial problems have all been postulated as causes of dyspepsia.[19] *H. pylori* may also be a factor in some cases of functional dyspepsia.

The treatment of functional dyspepsia includes drugs that speed up the transit of food through the upper part of the intestinal tract, agents that decrease stomach acid production, and antibiotics. Just as with IBS, stress

ulcer A craterlike lesion that occurs in the lining of the stomach or duodenum; also called a peptic ulcer to distinguish it from a skin ulcer.

functional dyspepsia Chronic pain in the upper abdomen not due to any obvious physical cause.

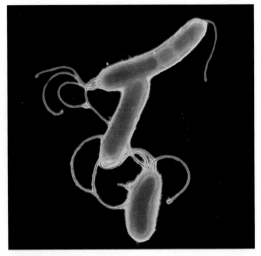

Helicobacter pylori.

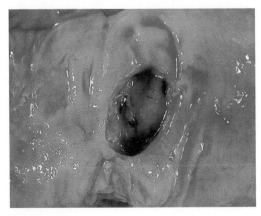

Stomach ulcer.

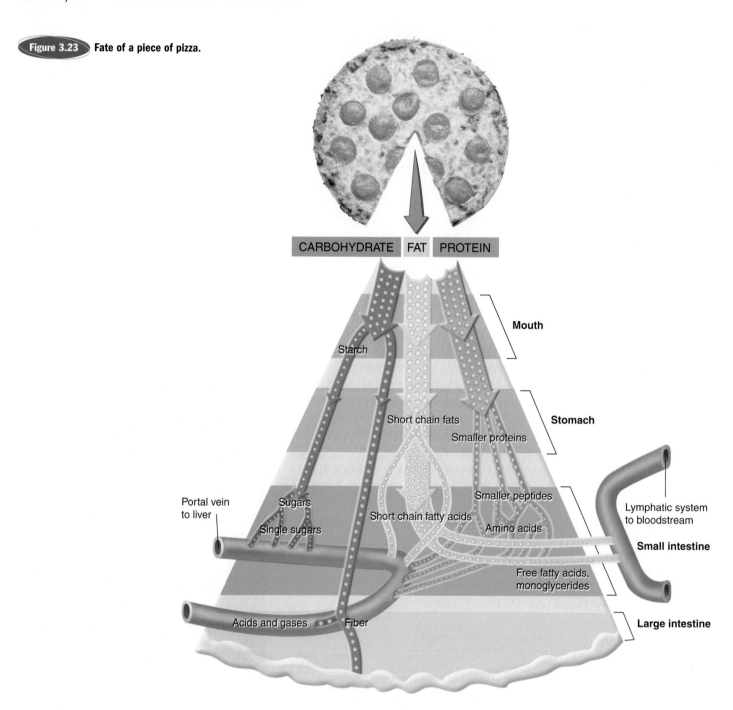

Figure 3.23 Fate of a piece of pizza.

CARBOHYDRATE · FAT · PROTEIN

Mouth

Starch

Stomach

Short chain fats

Smaller proteins

Smaller peptides

Portal vein to liver

Sugars

Short chain fatty acids

Amino acids

Single sugars

Lymphatic system to bloodstream

Small intestine

Free fatty acids, monoglycerides

Acids and gases   Fiber

Large intestine

reduction techniques such as meditation and biofeedback can often improve the symptoms of functional dyspepsia.

Key Concepts *GI disorders generally produce uncomfortable symptoms such as abdominal pain, gas, bloating, and change in elimination patterns. Some GI disorders, such as diarrhea, are generally symptoms of some other illness. Although medications are useful in reducing symptoms, many GI disorders are treatable with changes in diet, especially getting adequate fiber and fluids in the diet.*

As you have seen, the gastrointestinal tract is the key to turning food and its nutrients into nourishment for our bodies (see **Figure 3.23**). A healthy GI tract is an important factor in our overall health and well-being.

LEARNING *Portfolio* chapter 3

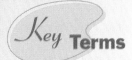

Key Terms

Study Points

- The GI tract is a tube that can be divided into regions: the mouth, esophagus, stomach, small intestine, large intestine, and rectum.

- Digestion and absorption of the nutrients in foods occur at various sites along the GI tract.

- Digestion involves both physical processes (e.g., chewing, peristalsis, and segmentation) and chemical processes (e.g., the hydrolytic action of enzymes).

- Absorption is the movement of molecules across the lining of the GI tract and into circulation.

- Four mechanisms are involved in nutrient absorption: passive diffusion, facilitated diffusion, active transport, and endocytosis.

- In the mouth, food is mixed with saliva for lubrication. Salivary amylase begins the digestion of starch.

- Secretions from the stomach lower the pH of stomach contents and begin the digestion of proteins.

- The pancreas and gallbladder secrete material into the small intestine to help with digestion.

- Most chemical digestion and nutrient absorption occur in the small intestine.

- Electrolytes and water are absorbed from the large intestine. Remaining material, waste, is excreted as feces.

- Both the nervous system and hormonal system regulate GI tract processes.

- Numerous factors affect GI tract functioning, including psychological, chemical, and bacterial factors.

- Problems that occur along the GI tract can affect digestion and absorption of nutrients. Dietary changes are important in the treatment of GI disorders.

Study Questions

1. The contents of which organ has the lowest pH? What organ produces an alkaline or basic solution to buffer this low pH?

2. What is the purpose of mucus in the GI tract? What would happen if it didn't line the stomach?

3. Where in the GI tract does the majority of nutrient digestion and absorption take place?

4. List the organs (in order) that make up the GI tract.

5. Name three "assisting" organs that are not part of the GI tract but are needed for proper digestion. What are their roles in digestion?

6. List the four major hormones involved in regulating digestion and absorption. What are their roles?

7. What is gastroesophageal reflux?

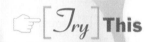 This

The Saltine Cracker Experiment

This experiment will help you understand the effect of salivary amylase. Remember, salivary amylase is the starch-digesting enzyme produced by the salivary glands. Chew two saltine crackers until a watery texture forms in your mouth. You have to fight the urge to swallow so you can pay attention to the taste of the crackers. Do you notice a change in the taste?

The crackers first taste salty and "starchy," but as amylase is secreted it begins to break the chains of starch into sugar. As it does this, the saltines begin to taste sweet like animal crackers!

What About *Bobbie?*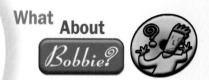

Because both fluid and fiber are important for a healthy gastrointestinal tract, let's check out Bobbie's intake of these. Refresh yourself with her day of eating by reviewing page 28. How do you think Bobbie did in terms of fiber? She did pretty well! At 24 grams of fiber, she's just right in the recommended range of 20 to 35 grams per day. Here are her best fiber sources:

Food	Fiber Grams
Spaghetti (pasta)	3.5
Tortilla chips	3
Banana	3
Salsa	2
Green beans	2

Are you surprised by the tortilla chips and the amount of fiber they add? Don't misinterpret this to mean that tortilla chips are a great source of fiber. There are two reasons why the chips rank so high. First, the other grain choices were not whole wheat and therefore don't contribute a lot of fiber. Second, her afternoon snack consisted of over 200 kilocalories of tortilla chips.

What could Bobbie have done differently if she wanted to reach the high end of the recommended range? Here are a few small changes that would add more fiber.

- By choosing a whole-wheat bagel, she'd add 4 grams of fiber.
- By having her sandwich on whole-wheat bread, she'd add at least 3 grams of fiber.
- By substituting the 2 tablespoons of croutons with 2 more tablespoons of kidney beans, she'd add 1.5 grams of fiber.
- If she ate another piece of fruit as a snack sometime during the day, it would add 1 to 3 grams of fiber.

Now let's look at Bobbie's fluid intake. Remember, when you increase your fiber it is critical to increase your fluid intake so you don't become constipated. Here's a list of Bobbie's drinks:

Breakfast—10 ounces coffee

Snack—none

Lunch—12 ounces diet soda

Snack—16 ounces water

Dinner—12 ounces diet soda

Snack—none

How do you think she did? Her total fluid intake is 50 ounces which, you'll learn in Chapter 11, is lower than the recommended intake of at least 64 ounces per day. Even more noteworthy is the fact that if 3 of her 4 beverages contained caffeine, a diuretic, she would have lost even more water. So although she drank some water in the afternoon, her overall intake of fluids is not enough to handle her fiber intake and keep her GI contents moving smoothly.

What suggestions do you have that will increase Bobbie's fluid intake? Any of the following would work:

- Carry a bottle of water to sip throughout the day.
- Wash down the morning banana snack with a cup or two of water.
- Consider decaffeinated coffee or decaffeinated soda.
- Drink more water with the tortilla chips in the afternoon.
- Add a fluid to dinner.
- Drink water with the piece of pizza at night.

References

1 Gilbertson TA, Fontenot DT, Liu L, et al. Fatty acid modulation of K+ channels in taste receptor cells: gustatory cues for dietary fat. *Am J Physiology.* 1997;272:4 (pt 1) C1203–10.

2 Mattes RD, Physiologic responses to sensory stimulation by food: nutritional implications. *J Am Diet Assoc.* 1997;97: 406–410.

3 Klein S, Cohn SM, Alpers DH. The alimentary tract in nutrition. In: Shils ME, Olson JA, Shike M, Ross AC, eds. *Modern Nutrition in Health and Disease.* 9th ed. Baltimore: Williams & Wilkins; 1998:605–629.

4 Caspary WF. Physiology and pathophysiology of intestinal absorption. *Am J Clin Nutr.* 1992;55:299S–307S; and Yamada T, Alper DH. *Textbook of Gastroenterology.* New York: JB Lippincott; 1995.

5 Guyton AC, Hall JE. *Textbook of Medical Physiology.* 9th ed. Philadelphia: WB Saunders Company; 1996.

6 Yamada T, Alper DH *Textbook of Gastroenterology.* Op. cit.

7 Klein S, Cohn SM, Alpers DH. The alimentary tract in nutrition. Op. cit., 605–629.

8 Guyton AC, Hall JE. Op. cit.

9 Yamada T, Alper DH. Op. cit.

10 Guyton AC, Hall JE. Op. cit.

11 Mahan LK, Escott-Stump S. *Krause's Food Nutrition and Diet Therapy.* 10th ed. Philadelphia: WB Saunders; 1999.

12 *Toxicological Profile for Acrolein.* Atlanta, GA: US Public Health Service, US Department of Health and Human Services, Agency for Toxic Substances and Disease Registry (ATSDR); 1989.

13 Clouse RE. Anxiety and gastrointestinal illness. *Psychiatr Clin North Am.* 1988;11:399–417; and Dancey CP, Taghavi M, Fox RJ. The relationship between daily stress and symptoms of irritable bowel: a time-series approach. *J Psychosom Res.* 1998;44:537–45; and Jarrett M, Heitkemper M, Cain KC, et al. The relationship between psychological distress and gastrointestinal symptoms in women with irritable bowel syndrome. *Nurs Res.* 1998;47:154–61.

14 Mine K, Kanazawa F, Hosoi M., et al. Treating nonulcer dyspepsia considering both functional disorders of the digestive system and psychiactric conditions. *Digest Dis & Sci.* 1998;43:124–7; and Lembo T, Munakata J, Merz H, et al., Evidence for the hypersensitivity of lumbar splanchnic afferants in irritable bowel syndrome. *Gastroenterol.* 1994;107:1686–1696.

15 Prevention of Colon Cancer. American Cancer Society; 1998.

16 Slattery ML, Boucher KM, Caan BJ, et al. Eating patterns and risk of colon cancer. *Am J Epidemiol.* 1998;148:4–16.

17 Fuchs CS, Giovannucci EL, Colditz GA, et al. Dietary fiber and the risk of colorectal cancer and adenoma in women. *N Engl J Med.* 1999; 340:169–176.

18 Helicobacter pylori in peptic ulcer disease. NIH Consensus Statement. 1994; 12:1–23.

19 Wiklund J, Butler-Wheelhouse P. Psychosocial factors and their role in symptomatic gastroesophageal reflux disease and functional dyspepsia. *Scand J Gastroenterol.* 1996;220(suppl): 94–100.

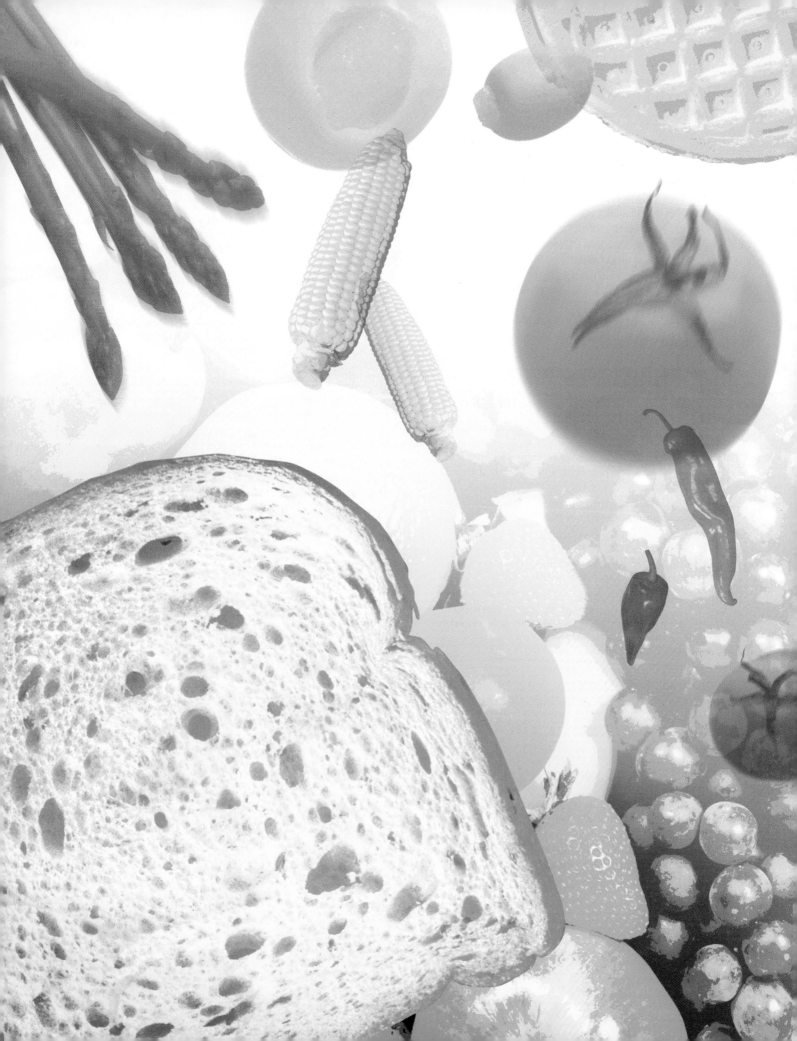

Chapter 4

Carbohydrates

Think About It

1   When you think of the word *carbohydrate,* what foods come to mind?

2   How does your dietary fiber intake stack up?

3   Many people choose honey instead of white sugar because they think it's more "natural." What do you think?

4   Do you prefer artificial sweeteners to sugar? Explain your preference.

Fyi for your Information

This chapter's FYI boxes include practical information on the following topics:

• Unfounded Claims Against Sugars

• The Glycemic Index of Foods: Useful or Useless?

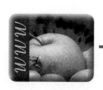

The web site for this book offers many useful tools and is a great source for additional nutrition information for both students and instructors. Visit the site at nutrition.jbpub.com for information on carbohydrates. You'll find exercises that explore the following topics:

• Aspartame: Your Friend or Foe?

• Are You in the Carbohydrate Zone?

• Constant Craving?

Key to Illustrations

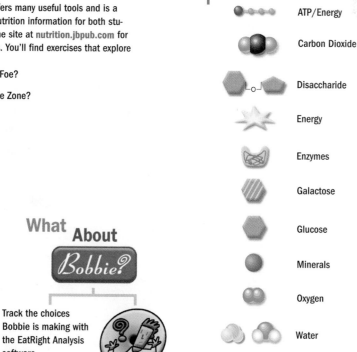

ATP/Energy	
Carbon Dioxide	
Disaccharide	
Energy	
Enzymes	
Galactose	
Glucose	
Minerals	
Oxygen	
Water	

What About Bobbie?

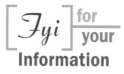

Track the choices Bobbie is making with the EatRight Analysis software.

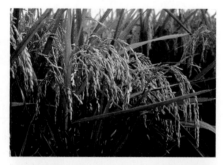

Sugar causes diabetes. Sugar causes hyperactivity. Sugar causes criminal behavior. Sugar rots your teeth. Starches make you fat. These and many other claims have been made about sugar and starch—dietary carbohydrates—over the years. But where do these claims come from? What is myth and what is fact? What links, if any, are there between carbohydrates in your diet and health? Are carbohydrates important in the diet?

Most of the world depends on carbohydrate-rich plant foods for daily sustenance. In some countries, 80 percent or more of daily calorie intake is carbohydrate. Rice provides the bulk of the diet in Southeast Asia, as does corn in South America, cassava in certain parts of Africa, and wheat in Europe and North America. Besides providing energy, foods rich in carbohydrates are also good sources of vitamins, minerals, dietary fiber, and phytochemicals that can help lower risk of chronic diseases. **Figure 4.1.** shows some carbohydrate-rich foods, which include whole grains, legumes, fruits, and vegetables.

Generous carbohydrate intake should provide the foundation for any healthful diet. Carbohydrates contain only 4 kilocalories per gram, compared with 9 kilocalories per gram for fat. Thus, a diet rich in carbohydrates provides fewer calories and a greater volume of food than the

Thin About **1**

Quick Bites

Is pasta a Chinese food?

Noodles were used in China as early as the first century; Marco Polo did not bring them to Italy until the 1300s.

Figure 4.1 Cassava, rice, wheat, and corn.

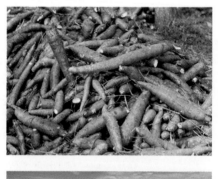
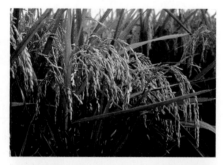
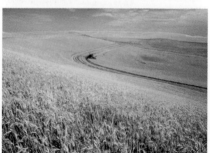
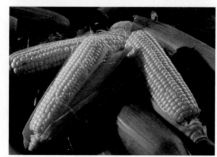

typical fat-laden American diet. As you explore the topic of carbohydrates, think about some of the claims you have heard for and against a high-carbohydrate intake.

What Are Carbohydrates?

Plants use carbon dioxide from the air, water from the soil, and energy from the sun to produce carbohydrates and oxygen through a process called photosynthesis.[1] (See **Figure 4.2**.) Carbohydrates are organic compounds that contain carbon (C), hydrogen (H), and oxygen (O) in the ratio of 1 carbon atom and 1 oxygen atom for every 2 hydrogen atoms (CH_2O). The sugar glucose, for example, contains 6 carbon atoms, 12 hydrogen atoms, and 6 oxygen atoms, giving this vital carbohydrate the chemical formula ($C_6H_{12}O_6$). Two or more sugar molecules can be assembled to form increasingly complex carbohydrates. The two main types of carbohydrates in food are simple carbohydrates (sugars) and complex carbohydrates (starches and dietary fiber).

Simple Sugars: Monosaccharides and Disaccharides

Simple carbohydrates are naturally present as simple sugars in fruits, milk, and other foods. Plant carbohydrates also can be refined to produce sugar products like table sugar and corn syrup. The two main types of sugars are monosaccharides and disaccharides. **Monosaccharides** consist of a single sugar molecule ("mono" meaning one and "saccharide" meaning sugar). **Disaccharides** consist of two sugar molecules chemically joined ("di" meaning two). Monosaccharides and disaccharides give various degrees of sweetness to foods.

> **simple carbohydrates** Sugars composed of a single sugar molecule (a monosaccharide) or two joined sugar molecules (a disaccharide).
>
> **monosaccharide** Any sugar that is not broken down during digestion and has the general formula (CH_2O)$_n$ where n = 3 to 7. For the common monosaccharides glucose, galactose, and fructose, n = 6.
>
> **disaccharide [dye-SACK-uh-ride]** Carbohydrates composed of two monosaccharide units linked by a glycosidic bond. They include sucrose (common table sugar), lactose (milk sugar), and maltose.

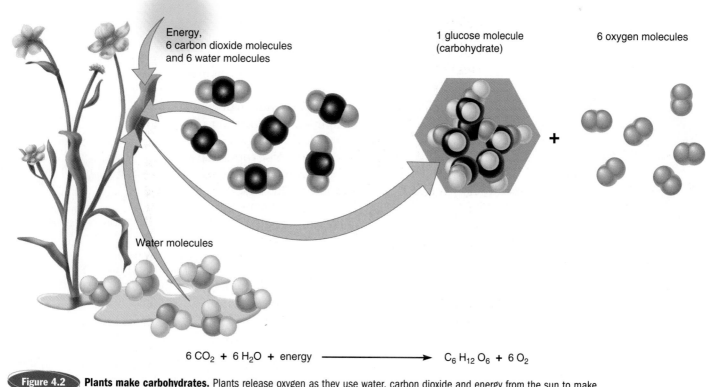

Energy,
6 carbon dioxide molecules
and 6 water molecules

1 glucose molecule
(carbohydrate)

6 oxygen molecules

Water molecules

$$6\ CO_2\ +\ 6\ H_2O\ +\ energy\ \longrightarrow\ C_6H_{12}O_6\ +\ 6\ O_2$$

Figure 4.2 **Plants make carbohydrates.** Plants release oxygen as they use water, carbon dioxide and energy from the sun to make carbohydrate (glucose) molecules.

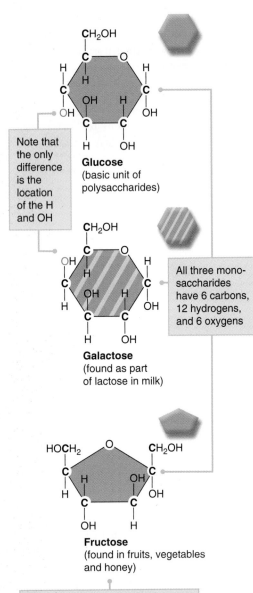

Note that the only difference is the location of the H and OH

Glucose
(basic unit of polysaccharides)

All three monosaccharides have 6 carbons, 12 hydrogens, and 6 oxygens

Galactose
(found as part of lactose in milk)

Fructose
(found in fruits, vegetables and honey)

Each of these molecules can exist in two forms – mirror images – called D or L optical isomers. The body can only use one of these forms, the D isomer

Figure 4.3 **The monosaccharides: glucose, galactose, and fructose.** Since glucose and galactose share similar 6-sided hexagonal structures, they can be difficult to tell apart. Fructose's 5-sided pentagon stands out.

Monosaccharides: The Single Sugars

The most common monosaccharides in the human diet are

- glucose
- galactose
- fructose

Glucose   **Galactose**   **Fructose**

All three monosaccharides have 6 carbons, and all have the chemical formula $C_6H_{12}O_6$ but each has a different arrangement of these atoms. The carbon and oxygen atoms of glucose and galactose can form a six-sided ring. The structures of glucose and galactose look almost identical except for the reversal of the OH and H groups on one of the carbon atoms. The carbons and oxygen of fructose form a five-sided ring. Look carefully at **Figure 4.3** to find all six carbons.

Glucose

The monosaccharide glucose is the most abundant simple carbohydrate unit in nature. (See **Figure 4.4**.) Also referred to as dextrose, **glucose** plays a key role in both foods and the body. Glucose imparts a mildly sweet flavor to food. It seldom exists as a monosaccharide in food but is usually joined to other sugars to form disaccharides, starch, or dietary fiber. Glucose makes up at least one of the two sugar molecules in every disaccharide.

In the body, glucose supplies energy to cells. The body closely regulates blood glucose (blood sugar) levels to ensure a constant fuel source for vital body functions. Glucose is virtually the only fuel used by the brain, except during prolonged starvation when the glucose supply is low.

Fructose

Also called levulose or fruit sugar, **fructose** tastes the sweetest of all the sugars—it is what commonly sweetens colas and other soft drinks. It occurs naturally in fruits and vegetables. Although the sugar in honey is about half fructose and half glucose, fructose is the primary source of the sweet taste. Food manufacturers use high-fructose corn syrup as an additive to sweeten many foods, including soft drinks, desserts, candies, jellies, and jams. Fructose currently provides about 5 percent of people's energy intake in the United States.[2]

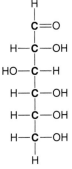

Glucose's linear representation shows all atoms and bonds

Simplified ring representation (omits ring carbons and lone hydrogens)

Figure 4.4 **Different ways to look at glucose.** Whether drawn as a linear form or a ring, the molecule is still glucose.

Galactose

Galactose rarely occurs as a monosaccharide in food. It usually is chemically bonded to glucose to form lactose, the primary sugar in milk. Galactose and glucose have almost but not quite identical atom arrangements. (See Figure 4.3.)

Other Monosaccharides and Derivative Sweeteners

Pentoses are single sugar molecules that contain five carbons. Although they are present in foods in only small quantities, they are essential components of nucleic acids, the genetic material of life. (See **Figure 4.5**.) The five-carbon sugar ribose is part of ribonucleic acid, or RNA. Another five-carbon sugar, deoxyribose, is a part of deoxyribonucleic acid, or DNA. Some pentoses also are components of indigestible gums and mucilages, which are classified as part of the dietary fiber component of foods.[3] Pentoses are synthesized in the body, and therefore are not needed in the diet.

Sugar alcohols are derivatives of monosaccharides. Like other sugars, they taste sweet and supply energy to the body. However, sugar alcohols are absorbed more slowly than sugars and the body processes them differently. Some fruits naturally contain minute amounts of sugar alcohols. Sugar alcohols such as sorbitol, manitol, lactitol, and xylitol also are used as nutritive sweeteners in foods.[4] For example, sorbitol, which is derived from glucose, sweetens sugarless gum, breath mints, and candy.

Disaccharides: The Double Sugars

Disaccharides consist of two monosaccharides chemically joined by a process called condensation. The following disaccharides (see **Figure 4.6.**) are important in human nutrition:

- sucrose (common table sugar)
- lactose (major sugar in milk)
- maltose (product of starch digestion)

glucose [GLOO-kose] A common monosaccharide containing six carbons that is present in the blood; also known as dextrose and blood sugar.

fructose [FROOK-tose] A common monosaccharide containing six carbons that is naturally present in honey and many fruits.

galactose [gah-LAK-tose] A monosaccharide containing six carbons that has a chemical structure similar to glucose.

pentose A sugar molecule containing five carbon atoms.

sugar alcohols Compounds formed from monosaccharides by replacing a hydrogen atom with a hydroxyl group (−OH).

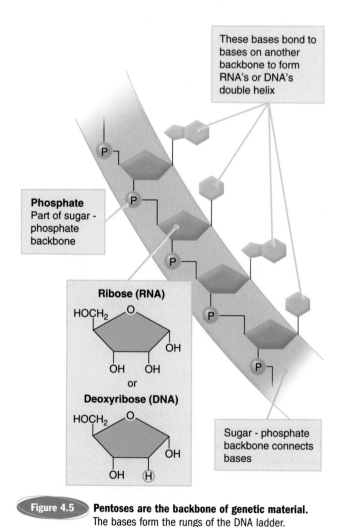

Figure 4.5 Pentoses are the backbone of genetic material.
The bases form the rungs of the DNA ladder.

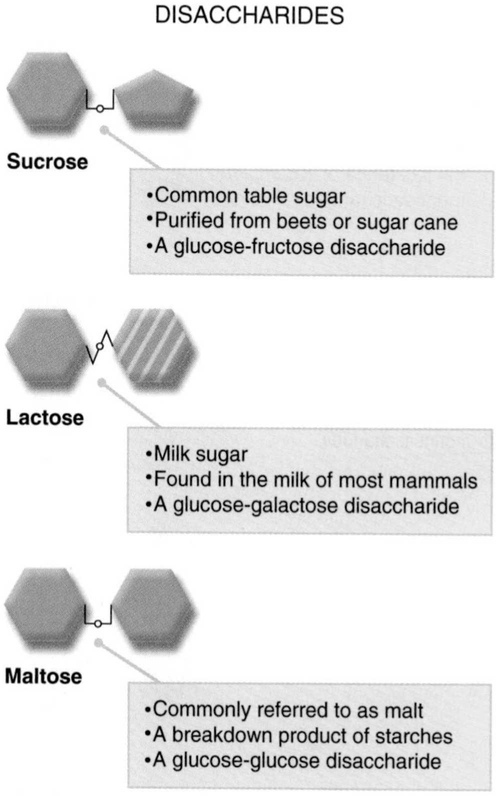

DISACCHARIDES

Sucrose
- Common table sugar
- Purified from beets or sugar cane
- A glucose-fructose disaccharide

Lactose
- Milk sugar
- Found in the milk of most mammals
- A glucose-galactose disaccharide

Maltose
- Commonly referred to as malt
- A breakdown product of starches
- A glucose-glucose disaccharide

Figure 4.6 The disaccharides: sucrose, lactose, and maltose.
The three monosaccharides pair up in different combinations to form the three disaccharides.

CONDENSATION

Glucose   Fructose

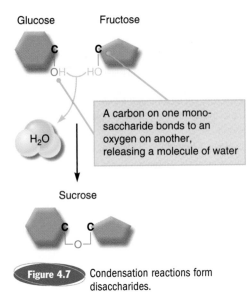

A carbon on one mono-saccharide bonds to an oxygen on another, releasing a molecule of water

Sucrose

Figure 4.7 Condensation reactions form disaccharides.

HYDROLYSIS

Maltose

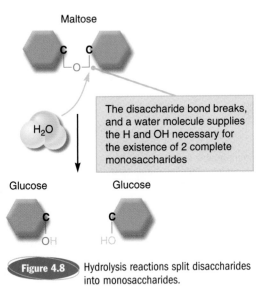

The disaccharide bond breaks, and a water molecule supplies the H and OH necessary for the existence of 2 complete monosaccharides

Glucose   Glucose

Figure 4.8 Hydrolysis reactions split disaccharides into monosaccharides.

Joining and Cleaving Sugar Molecules

Sugar molecules are joined or separated (cleaved) by the removal or addition of a molecule of water. A **condensation** reaction can chemically join two monosaccharides while removing an H from one sugar molecule and an OH from the other to form water (H_2O) (see **Figure 4.7**). A **hydrolysis** reaction can separate disaccharides into monosaccharides (see **Figure 4.8**). During hydrolysis, the addition of a molecule of water splits the bond between the two sugar molecules, providing the H and OH groups necessary for the sugars to exist as monosaccharides. Hydrolysis takes place during the digestion of carbohydrates.

Sucrose

Sucrose, most familiar to us as table sugar, is composed of one molecule of glucose and one molecule of fructose. Sucrose provides some of the natural sweetness of honey, maple syrup, fruits, and vegetables. Manufacturers use a refining process to extract sucrose from the juices of sugar cane or sugar beets. Full refining removes impurities; white sugar and powdered sugar are so highly refined they are virtually 100 percent sucrose. When a food label lists sugar as an ingredient, the term refers to sucrose.

Lactose

Lactose, or milk sugar, is composed of one molecule of glucose and one molecule of galactose. Lactose gives milk and other dairy products a slightly sweet taste. Human milk has a higher concentration (~7 g/100 mL) of lactose than cow's milk (~4.5 g/100 mL), so human milk tastes sweeter than cow's milk.

Maltose

Maltose is composed of two glucose molecules. Maltose seldom occurs naturally in foods, but forms whenever long molecules of starch break down. Human digestive enzymes in the mouth and small intestine break starch down into maltose. When you chew a slice of fresh bread, you may detect a slightly sweet taste as starch breaks down into maltose. Starch also breaks down into maltose in germinating seeds. Maltose is fermented in the production of beer.

Key Concepts: *Carbohydrates are composed of carbon, hydrogen, and oxygen and can be categorized as simple or complex. Simple carbohydrates include monosaccharides and disaccharides. The monosaccharides glucose, fructose, and galactose are single sugar molecules. The disaccharides sucrose, lactose, and maltose are double sugar molecules. A condensation reaction joins two monosaccharides to form a disaccharide.*

condensation In chemistry, a reaction in which a covalent bond is formed between two molecules by removal of a water molecule.

hydrolysis [High-DROL-ih-sis] A chemical reaction in which a compound is split into two products by the addition of water.

sucrose [SOO-crose] A disaccharide composed of glucose and fructose; also known as table sugar.

lactose [LAK-tose] A disaccharide composed of glucose and galactose; also called milk sugar.

maltose [MALL-tose] A disaccharide composed of two glucose molecules; sometimes called malt sugar. Maltose seldom occurs naturally in foods but is formed whenever long molecules of starch break down.

Complex Carbohydrates

Complex carbohydrates are chains of more than two sugar molecules. Short carbohydrate chains may have as few as three monosaccharide molecules, but long chains, the polysaccharides, can contain hundreds or even thousands.

Oligosaccharides

Oligosaccharides (*oligo* meaning "scant") are short carbohydrate chains of 3 to 10 sugar molecules. Dried beans, peas, and lentils contain the two most common oligosaccharides—raffinose and stachyose.[5] Raffinose is formed from three monosaccharide molecules—one galactose, one glucose, and one fructose. Stachyose is formed from four monosaccharide molecules—two galactose, one glucose, and one fructose. The body cannot break down raffinose or stachyose, but they are readily metabolized by intestinal bacteria and are responsible for the familiar gaseous effects of eating foods such as beans.

Human milk contains more than one hundred different oligosaccharides which vary with the duration of pregnancy, the duration of breastfeeding and the genetic makeup of the mother.[6] For breast-fed infants, oligosaccharides serve a function similar to dietary fiber in adults—making stools easier to pass. Some of these oligosaccharides also protect infants from disease-causing agents by binding to them in the intestine. Oligosaccharides in human milk may also be an important source of sialic acid, a compound essential for normal brain development.[7]

Polysaccharides

Polysaccharides (*poly* meaning "many") are long carbohydrate chains of monosaccharides. Some polysaccharides form straight chains, while others branch off in all directions. Such structural differences affect how the polysaccharide behaves in water and with heating. The way monosaccharides are linked may make them digestible (e.g., starch) or indigestible (e.g., dietary fiber).

Starch

Plants store energy as **starch** for use during growth and reproduction. Rich sources of starch include (1) grains such as wheat, rice, corn, oats, millet, and barley, (2) legumes such as peas, beans, and lentils, and (3) tubers

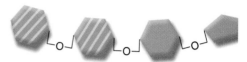

Stachyose

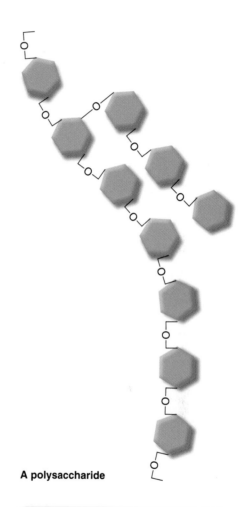

A polysaccharide

complex carbohydrate A chain of more than two monosaccharides. May be an oligosaccharide or a polysaccharide.

oligosaccharide A short carbohydrate chain composed of 3 to 10 sugar molecules.

polysaccharide Long carbohydrate chains composed of more than 10 sugar molecules. Polysaccharides can be straight or branched.

starch The major storage form of carbohydrate in plants; starch is composed of long chains of glucose molecules in a straight (amylose) or branching (amylopectin) arrangement.

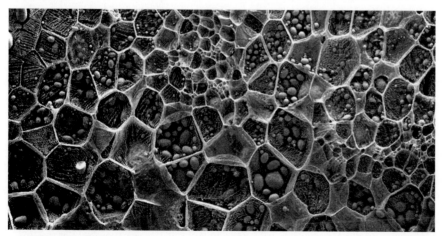

A scanning electron micrograph of a potato tuber cell shows the starch granules where energy is stored.

amylose [AM-uh-los] A straight-chain polysaccharide composed of glucose units.

amylopectin [am-ih-low-PEK-tin] A branched-chain polysaccharide composed of glucose units.

resistant starch A starch that is not digested.

glycogen [GLY-ko-jen] A very large, highly branched polysaccharide composed of multiple glucose units. Sometimes called animal starch, glycogen is the primary storage form of glucose in animals.

dietary fiber The indigestible parts of plants.

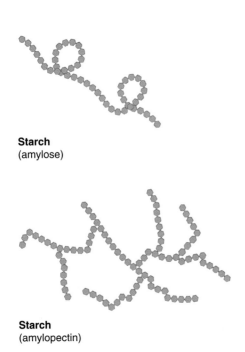

Starch
(amylose)

Starch
(amylopectin)

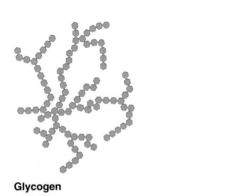

Glycogen

Figure 4.9 **Starch and glycogen.** Plants have two main types of starch—amylose which has long unbranched chains of glucose and amylopectin which has branched chains. Animals store glucose in highly branched chains called glycogen.

such as potatoes, yams, and cassava. Starch imparts a moist, gelatinous texture to food. For example, it makes the inside of a baked potato moist, thick, and almost sticky. The starch in flour absorbs moisture and thickens gravy.

Starch takes two main forms in plants: amylose and amylopectin. **Amylose** is made up of long, unbranched chains of glucose molecules, while **amylopectin** is made up of branched chains of glucose molecules. (See **Figure 4.9.**) Amylose and amylopectin typically occur in a ratio of about 1:4 in plants, although this proportion can vary.[8] Wheat flour contains a higher proportion of amylose, whereas cornstarch contains a higher proportion of amylopectin.

Our bodies treat amylose and amylopectin the same. However, the proportion of amylose to amylopectin in a food affects its functional properties. For example, food manufacturers often thicken gravies for frozen foods with cornstarch (rich in branched amylopectin) because it forms thicker, more stable gels than gravies thickened with wheat flour (rich in unbranched amylose).

Although the body easily digests most starches, a small portion of the starch in plants may remain enclosed in cell structures and escape digestion in the small intestine. Starch that is not digested is called **resistant starch.**[9] Some legumes, such as white beans, contain large amounts of resistant starch.[10]

Glycogen

Glycogen, also called animal starch, is the storage form of carbohydrate in living animals. (See **Figure 4.9.**) After slaughter, tissue enzymes break down most glycogen within 24 hours. While some organ meats, such as kidney, heart, and liver, contain small amounts of carbohydrate, meat from muscle contains none.[11] Since plant foods do not contain glycogen, it is a negligible carbohydrate source in our diets. Glycogen does, however, play an important role in our bodies as a readily mobilizable store of glucose.

Glycogen is composed of long, highly branched chains of glucose molecules. Its structure is similar to amylopectin, but glycogen is much more highly branched. Glycogen in our cells can be broken down rapidly into single glucose molecules as needed. Since enzymes can only attack the ends of glycogen chains, the highly branched structure of glycogen multiplies the number of sites available for enzyme activity.

Skeletal muscle and the liver are the two major sites of glycogen storage. In muscle cells, glycogen provides a reservoir of glucose for strenuous muscular activity. Liver cells also use glycogen to regulate blood glucose levels. If necessary, liver glycogen can provide as much as 100 to 150 milligrams of glucose per minute to the blood at a sustained rate for up to 12 hours.[12]

Normally, the body can store only about 200 to 500 grams of glycogen at a time.[13] Some athletes practice a carbohydrate-loading regimen by gradually tapering off rigorous training and emphasizing high-carbohydrate meals a few days to one week before competition. This can increase the amount of stored glycogen by about one and one-half times, providing a competitive edge for marathon running and other endurance events.[14] (See Chapter 13, "Sports Nutrition.")

Dietary Fiber

Dietary fiber provides structure to plant cell walls, and is also found inside plant cells. All types of plant foods contain fiber including fruits, vegetables, legumes, and whole grains. Dietary fibers resemble starches, but are impervious to human digestive enzymes, so they are not digested in the

GI tract.[15] Dietary fibers, often called nonstarch polysaccharides, include cellulose, hemicellulose, pectins, gums, and mucilages. Other types of dietary fiber, such as lignin, cutins, and waxes, are not polysaccharides. Food manufacturers add certain fibers to food products to thicken and stabilize them.

Cellulose **Cellulose** gives plant cell walls their strength and rigidity. It forms the woody fibers that support tall trees. It also forms the brittle shafts of hay and straw and the stringy threads in celery. Cellulose is made up of long, straight chains of glucose molecules. (See **Figure 4.10**.)

Hemicelluloses The **hemicelluloses** are a diverse group of polysaccharides that vary from plant to plant. They are mixed with cellulose in plant cell walls.[16] Hemicelluloses are composed of a variety of monosaccharides with many branching side chains. The outer bran layer on many cereal grains is rich in hemicelluloses, as are whole grain cereals and food products.

Pectins **Pectins** are gel-forming polysaccharides found in all plants, but especially in fruits. The pectin in fruits acts like a cement that gives body to fruits and helps them keep their shape. When fruit becomes overripe, pectin breaks down into monosaccharides and the fruit becomes mushy. Mixed with sugar and acid, pectin forms a gel that the food industry uses to add firmness to jellies, jams, sauces, and salad dressings.

Gums and Mucilages Like pectin, **gums** and **mucilages** are thick, gel-forming fibers that help hold plant cells together. The food industry uses plant gums such as gum arabic, guar gum, locust bean gum, and xanthan gum, and mucilages such as carrageenan, to thicken, stabilize, or add texture to foods such as salad dressings, puddings, pie fillings, candies, sauces, and even drinks.

cellulose [SELL-you-los] A straight-chain polysaccharide composed of hundreds of glucose units linked by beta bonds. It is indigestible by humans and a component of insoluble dietary fiber.

hemicellulose [hem-ih-SELL-you-los] A group of large polysaccharides in dietary fiber that are fermented more easily than cellulose.

pectin A type of soluble fiber found in fruits.

gum A dietary fiber, which contains galactose and other monosaccharides, found between plant cell walls.

mucilage A gelatinous soluble fiber containing galactose, mannose, and other monosaccharides.

Quick Bites

"An apple a day keeps the doctor away."

Most likely this adage persisted over time due to actual health benefits from apples. Apples have a high pectin content, a soluble fiber known to be an effective GI regulator.

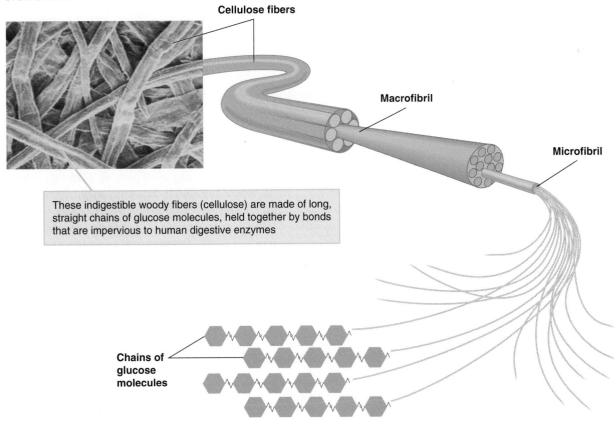

Cellulose fibers

Macrofibril

Microfibril

These indigestible woody fibers (cellulose) are made of long, straight chains of glucose molecules, held together by bonds that are impervious to human digestive enzymes

Chains of glucose molecules

Figure 4.10 **The structure of cellulose.** Cellulose forms the indigestible, fibrous component of plants and is part of grasses, trees, fruits, and vegetables.

| **Table 4.1** | Foods Rich in Soluble and Insoluble Dietary Fiber |

Rich in Soluble Fiber	Rich in Insoluble Fiber
Fruits	
Apples	Apples
Cranberries	Bananas
Grapefruit	Berries
Mango	Cherries
Oranges	Pears
Vegetables	
Asparagus	Broccoli
Broccoli	Green peppers
Brussels sprouts	Red cabbage
Carrots	Spinach
	Sprouts
Nuts and seeds	
Peanuts	Almonds
Pecans	Sesame seeds
Walnuts	Sunflower seeds
Legumes	
Most legumes	Most legumes
Grains	
Oat bran	Brown rice
Oatmeal	Whole-wheat breads
Psyllium	Wheat-bran cereals

Source: Adapted from Shils ME, Olson JA, Shike M, Ross AC, eds. *Modern Nutrition in Health and Disease.* 9th ed. Philadephia: Lippincott Williams & Wilkins, 1999.

lignin [LIG-nin] An insoluble fiber composed of multi-ring alcohol units.

soluble fiber Dietary fiber components that dissolve in or absorb water, including pectins, gums, mucilages, and some hemicelluloses.

insoluble fiber Dietary fiber components that do not dissolve in water, including cellulose, lignin, and some hemicelluloses.

pancreatic amylase Starch-digesting enzyme secreted by the pancreas.

alpha (α) bond A chemical bond linking two monosaccharides (glycosidic bond) that can be broken by human intestinal enzymes, releasing the individual monosaccharides.

beta (β) bond A chemical bond linking two monosaccharides (glycosidic bond) that cannot be broken by human intestinal enzymes.

Lignins Lignins are not actually carbohydrates, but these indigestible substances make up the woody parts of vegetables such as carrots and broccoli and the seeds of fruits such as strawberries.

Classification of Dietary Fiber: Soluble and Insoluble Researchers classify dietary fibers by their ability to dissolve in water.[17] Pectins, gums, mucilages, and some hemicelluloses dissolve in water and so are classified as **soluble fibers.** Cellulose, some hemicelluloses, and lignin don't dissolve in water, and are thus **insoluble fibers.**

Only plant foods contain dietary fiber. Foods rich in dietary fiber include whole-grain foods such as brown rice, rolled oats, and whole-wheat breads and cereals; legumes such as kidney beans, garbanzo beans (chickpeas), peas, and lentils; fruits; and vegetables. Oat bran, legumes, soybean fiber, and some fruits and vegetables are rich in soluble fiber; whereas wheat bran and most whole grains and cereals are rich in insoluble fiber (**Table 4.1**). Psyllium, derived from the husk of blonde psyllium seed, is a soluble fiber used in the laxative Metamucil. The soluble fiber from psyllium and oats has been shown to help lower blood cholesterol levels[18] (For more on this, see the later section on "Carbohydrates and Health.") and is being added to some breakfast cereals for this purpose.

Key Concepts: *Complex carbohydrates include starch, glycogen, and dietary fiber. Starch is composed of straight or branched chains of glucose molecules and is the storage form of energy in plants. Glycogen is composed of highly branched chains of glucose molecules and is the storage form of energy in animals. Dietary fibers include many different substances that cannot be digested by enzymes in the human intestinal tract and are found in plant foods such as whole grains, legumes, vegetables, and fruits.*

Carbohydrate Digestion and Absorption

Although glucose is a key building block of carbohydrates, you can't exactly find it on the menu at your favorite restaurant or campus hideout. You must first drink that chocolate milkshake, or eat the hamburger bun so your body can convert the food carbohydrate into glucose in the body. So, let's see what happens to carbohydrate foods you eat!

Digestion

Refer to **Figure 4.11** for an overview of the digestive process. Carbohydrate digestion begins in the mouth, where the starch-digesting enzyme salivary amylase hydrolyzes starch into shorter polysaccharides and maltose. Chewing stimulates saliva production and mixes salivary amylase with food. Disaccharides, unlike starch, are not digested in the mouth. Only about 5 percent of the starches in food are broken down by the time the food is swallowed.

When carbohydrate enters the stomach, the acidity of stomach juices eventually halts the action of salivary amylase by denaturing it, causing the enzyme (a protein) to lose its shape and function. This stops carbohydrate digestion, which will restart in the small intestine. Soluble dietary fibers provide a feeling of fullness and tend to delay digestive activity by slowing stomach emptying.

Most carbohydrate digestion takes place in the small intestine. As stomach contents enter the small intestine, the pancreas secretes pancreatic amylase through the pancreatic duct and into the small intestine. **Pancreatic amylase** continues the digestion of starch, breaking it into the disaccharide maltose.

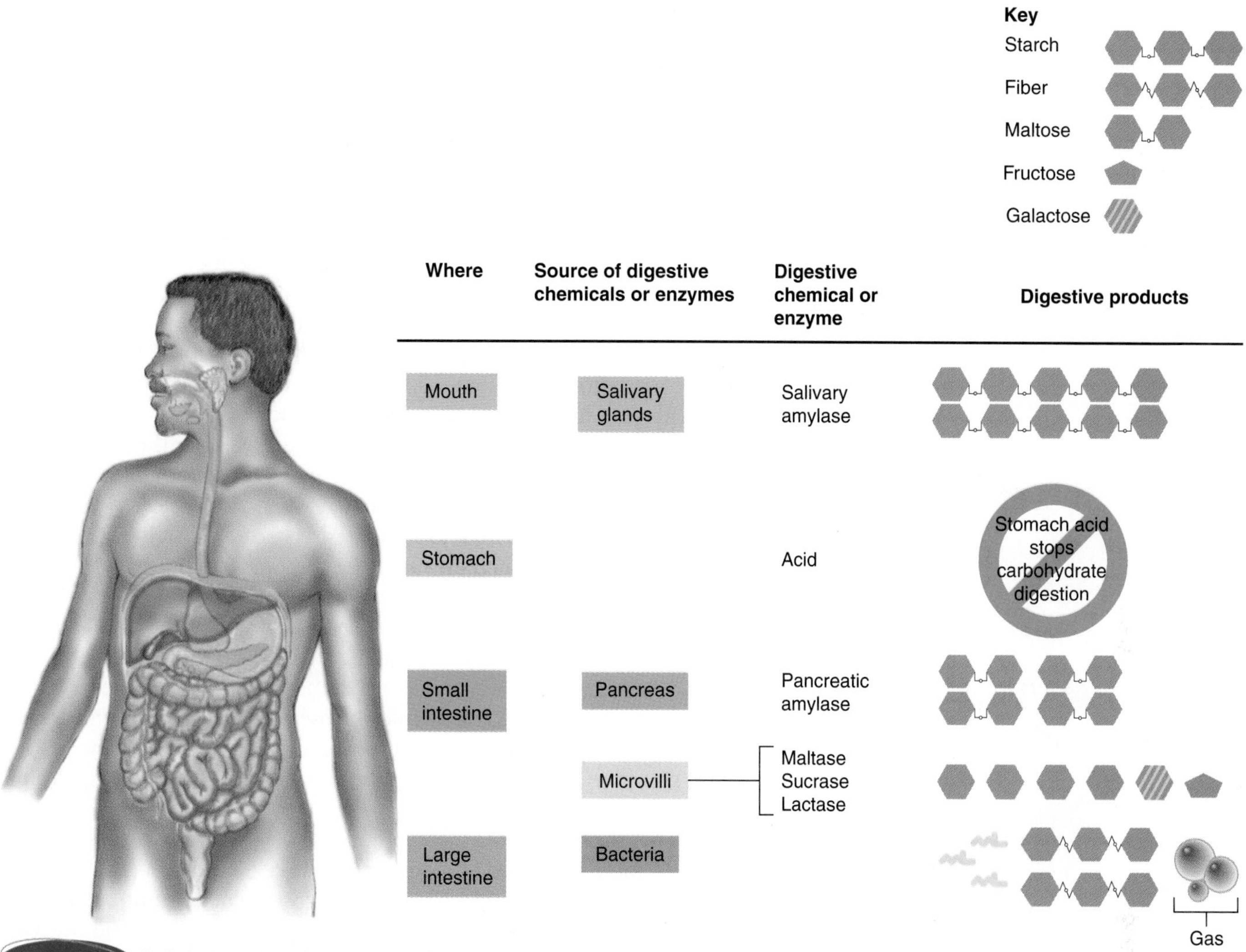

Key

Starch	
Fiber	
Maltose	
Fructose	
Galactose	

Where	Source of digestive chemicals or enzymes	Digestive chemical or enzyme	Digestive products
Mouth	Salivary glands	Salivary amylase	
Stomach		Acid	Stomach acid stops carbohydrate digestion
Small intestine	Pancreas	Pancreatic amylase	
	Microvilli	Maltase Sucrase Lactase	
Large intestine	Bacteria		Gas

Figure 4.11 **Carbohydrate digestion.** Most carbohydrate digestion takes place in the small intestine.

Meanwhile, enzymes attached to the brush border (microvilli) of the mucosal cells lining the intestinal tract go to work. (See Chapter 3 for a detailed explanation of the complex structure of the small intestine.) These digestive enzymes, called brush border disaccharidases, break disaccharides into monosaccharides for absorption. The enzyme maltase splits maltose into two glucose molecules. The enzyme sucrase splits sucrose into glucose and fructose. The enzyme lactase splits lactose into glucose and galactose.

The bonds that link glucose molecules in complex carbohydrates are called glycosidic bonds. The two forms of these bonds, **alpha bonds** and **beta bonds,** have important differences. (See **Figure 4.12.**) Human enzymes easily break alpha bonds, making glucose available from the polysaccharides starch and glycogen. Cellulose, which is an indigestible polysaccharide found in dietary fiber, contains long chains of glucose molecules linked by beta bonds, which the body's enzymes cannot break. Beta bonds also link the galactose and glucose molecules in the disaccharide lactose, but the enzyme lactase is specifically tailored to attack this small molecule. People with a sufficient supply of the enzyme lactase can break these bonds. But when lactase is lacking, the beta bonds remain unbroken and lactose remains undigested until bacteria in the colon can attack it. (See Chapter 3 for more on lactose maldigestion.)

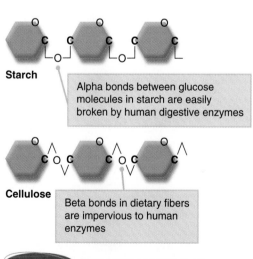

Starch

Alpha bonds between glucose molecules in starch are easily broken by human digestive enzymes

Cellulose

Beta bonds in dietary fibers are impervious to human enzymes

Figure 4.12 **Alpha bonds and beta bonds.** Human digestive enzymes easily can break the alpha bonds in starch, but they cannot break the beta bonds in cellulose.

Enzymes are highly specific; they speed up only specific reactions and work only on certain molecules. Humans lack the digestive enzymes to break down the oligosaccharides raffinose and stachyose. The commercial product Beano is an enzyme preparation. When taken right before eating beans or other gas-forming vegetables, Beano helps break oligosaccharides into monosaccharides so the body can absorb them.

Due to a lack of certain enzymes in the small intestine, or the presence of indigestible structures like dietary fiber or resistant starch, some carbohydrates move to the large intestine intact. In the large intestine, bacteria partially ferment (break down) these undigested carbohydrates, producing gas and a few short-chain fatty acids. These fatty acids are absorbed into the colon and are used for energy by the colon cells. In addition, these fatty acids may have other health effects such as reducing blood cholesterol levels,[19] and helping to protect against colon cancer.[20]

Soluble fiber dissolves easily in water, so during its journey through the GI tract it takes on a soft, gel-like texture. In the large intestine, soluble fiber that survives bacterial digestion softens the stool, and makes it easier to pass.[21] Insoluble fiber, which adds bulk to stools, resists bacterial activity so it passes essentially unchanged through the intestines and produces little gas.

Absorption

Monosaccharides are absorbed into the mucosal cells lining the small intestine by two mechanisms that you learned about in Chapter 3. Fructose is absorbed by facilitated diffusion, while glucose and galactose depend on an active transport mechanism. A sodium-potassium pump helps transport glucose and galactose across the intestinal cell's membrane. The carrier protein in the cell membrane is first loaded with sodium, and then either glucose or galactose can attach.[22] Fructose absorption is slower than that of glucose or galactose. In the villi, absorbed monosaccharides pass through the intestinal mucosal cells and enter the bloodstream. Glucose, galactose, and fructose molecules travel to the liver via the portal vein, where galactose and fructose are converted to glucose. The liver stores and releases glucose as needed to maintain constant blood glucose levels. **Figure 4.13** illustrates absorption in the small intestine.

Key

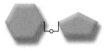

Lactose

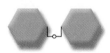

Sucrose

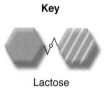

Maltose

Fructose

Galactose

Glucose

Enzyme

Na⁺

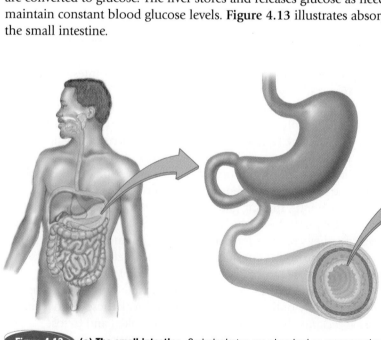

Figure 4.13 **(a) The small intestine.** Carbohydrates are absorbed as monosaccharides in the small intestine.

Key Concepts: *Carbohydrate digestion takes place primarily in the small intestine, where digestible carbohydrates are broken down and absorbed as monosaccharides. Bacteria in the large intestine partially ferment indigestible carbohydrates such as resistant starch and soluble fiber, producing gas and a few short-chain fatty acids that can be absorbed through the large intestine and used for energy. The liver converts absorbed monosaccharides into glucose.*

Carbohydrates in the Body

Through the processes of digestion and absorption, our varied diet of carbohydrates from vegetables, fruits, grains, and milk becomes glucose. Glucose has one major role—to supply energy for the body.

Normal Use of Glucose

Cells throughout the body depend on glucose for energy to drive chemical processes. Although most, but not all, cells can also burn fat for energy, the body needs some glucose to burn fat efficiently.

When we eat food, our bodies immediately use some glucose to maintain normal blood glucose levels. We store excess glucose as glycogen in liver and muscle tissue. Insulin and glucagon, two hormones produced by the pancreas, closely regulate blood glucose levels.

Absorbed monosaccharides enter capillaries, flow to liver where all are converted to glucose. Absorbed glucose travels to liver or remains in bloodstream to maintain constant blood glucose levels

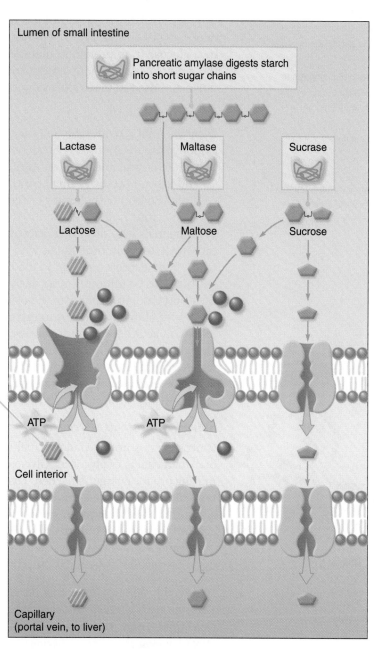

Lumen of small intestine

Pancreatic amylase digests starch into short sugar chains

Lactase

Maltase

Sucrase

Lactose

Maltose

Sucrose

ATP

ATP

Cell interior

Capillary (portal vein, to liver)

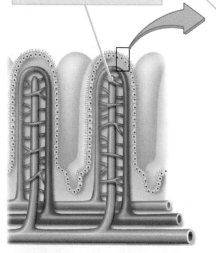

Figure 4.13 **(b) Absorption.**

ketone bodies Molecules formed when insufficient carbohydrate is available to completely metabolize fat. Formation of ketone bodies is promoted by a low glucose level and high acetyl CoA level within cells.

ketosis [kee-TOE-sis] Abnormally high concentration of ketone bodies in body tissues and fluids.

blood glucose level The amount of glucose in the blood at any given time.

insulin [IN-suh-lin] Produced by beta cells in the pancreas, this polypeptide hormone stimulates the uptake of blood glucose into muscle and adipose cells, the synthesis of glycogen in the liver, and various other processes.

glucagon [GLOO-kuh-gon] Produced by alpha cells in the pancreas, this polypeptide hormone promotes the breakdown of liver glycogen to glucose, thereby increasing blood glucose.

epinephrine A hormone released in response to stress or sudden danger, epinephrine raises blood glucose levels to ready the body for "fight or flight." Also called adrenaline.

glycemic index A measure of the effect of food on blood glucose levels.

diabetes mellitus A chronic disease in which uptake of blood glucose by body cells is impaired, resulting in high glucose levels in the blood and urine.

Glucose

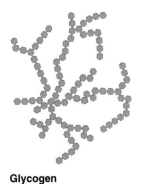

Glycogen

Using Glucose for Energy

Glucose is the primary fuel for most cells in the body and the preferred fuel for the brain, red blood cells, nervous system, fetus, and placenta. Even when fat is burned for energy, a small amount of glucose is needed to metabolize fat completely. To obtain energy from glucose, glucose from the blood must be taken up by cells. Once glucose enters cells, a series of metabolic reactions break it down into carbon dioxide and water, releasing energy in a form the body can use.[23]

Sparing Body Protein

In the absence of carbohydrate, both proteins and fats can be used for energy. Although most cells can break down fat for energy, brain cells and developing red blood cells require a constant supply of glucose.[24] (After an extended period of starvation, the brain adapts and is able to use ketones from fat breakdown for part of its energy needs.) If glycogen stores are depleted and glucose is not provided in the diet, the body must make its own glucose from protein to maintain blood levels and supply glucose to the brain. Dietary carbohydrate spares body proteins from being broken down and used to make glucose.

Preventing Ketosis

Even when fat provides the fuel for cells, cells require a small amount of carbohydrate to completely break down fat to release energy. When no carbohydrate is available, the liver cannot break down fat completely for energy, and instead produces small compounds called **ketone bodies.**[25] Most cells can use ketone bodies for energy.

When ketone bodies are produced faster than they are used, as happens in individuals who diet vigorously and consume only small amounts of carbohydrates or in individuals who cannot metabolize blood glucose normally, ketone levels build up in the blood, causing a condition known as **ketosis.** This condition is most likely to develop in starvation, diabetes mellitus, and chronic alcoholism. Ketosis can also develop when fluid intake is too low to allow the kidneys to excrete excess ketone bodies. Ketosis interferes with acid/base balance, causing the blood to become too acidic. Dehydration is a common consequence of ketosis because the body loses water excreting excess ketones in the urine. The body needs a minimum of 50 to 100 grams of carbohydrate per day to prevent ketosis.[26] (See Chapter 7 "Metabolism" for more details on ketosis.)

Storing Glucose as Glycogen

Glucose that is not needed as a fuel source is assembled into the long, branched chains of glycogen. Glycogen can be quickly disassembled, releasing glucose for energy as needed. Liver glycogen stores are used to maintain normal blood glucose levels and account for about one-third of body glycogen stores. Muscle glycogen stores are used to fuel muscle activity and account for about two-thirds of body glycogen stores.[27] The body can store only limited amounts of glycogen—usually enough to last from a few hours to one day, depending on activity level.[28]

Key Concepts: *Glucose circulates in the blood to provide immediate energy to cells. The body needs adequate carbohydrate intake to prevent the breakdown of body proteins for energy. The body needs some carbohydrate to completely break down fat and prevent the buildup of ketone bodies in the blood. The body stores excess glucose in the liver and muscle as glycogen.*

Regulating Blood Glucose Levels

The body closely regulates **blood glucose** (also known as blood sugar) to maintain an adequate supply of glucose for cells. If blood glucose levels drop too low, a person becomes shaky and weak. If blood glucose levels rise too high, a person becomes sluggish and confused, and may have difficulty breathing.

Two hormones produced by the pancreas tightly control blood glucose levels.[29] When blood glucose levels rise after a meal, special cells called beta cells in the pancreas release the hormone insulin into the blood. **Insulin** acts like a key, "unlocking" the cells of the body and allowing glucose to enter and fuel them. Insulin works on receptors on the surface of cells, increasing their affinity for glucose and increasing glucose uptake by cells. Insulin also stimulates liver and muscle cells to store glucose as glycogen. As glucose enters cells to deliver energy or be stored as glycogen, blood glucose levels return to normal. (See **Figure 4.14**.)

When an individual has not eaten in a while, and blood glucose levels begin to fall, alpha cells in the pancreas release another hormone called **glucagon.** Glucagon stimulates the breakdown of glycogen stores to release glucose into the bloodstream. Glucagon also stimulates gluconeogenesis, or the synthesis of glucose from protein. Another hormone, **epinephrine** (also called adrenaline), exerts effects similar to glucagon to ensure all body cells have adequate energy for emergencies. Released by the adrenal glands in response to sudden stress or danger, epinephrine is called the "fight-or-flight" hormone.

Different foods vary in their effect on blood glucose regulation. Foods rich in simple carbohydrates or starch but low in fat or fiber tend to be digested and absorbed rapidly. This rapid absorption causes a corresponding large and rapid rise in blood glucose levels.[30] The body reacts to this rise by pumping out extra insulin, which in turn can lower blood glucose levels too far before finally stabilizing. Other foods, especially foods rich in dietary fiber, resistant starch, or fat, cause a lesser blood glucose response with smaller swings in blood glucose levels.

The **glycemic index** measures the effect of a food on blood glucose levels. While foods with a high glycemic index cause a faster and higher rise in blood glucose, foods with a low glycemic index cause a slower rise in blood glucose. Although some experts disagree on the usefulness of the glycemic index for humans, diets that emphasize foods with a low glycemic index may offer important health benefits.[31]

High Blood Sugar: Diabetes Mellitus

Diabetes mellitus is a disease in which the body either does not produce enough insulin or does not properly use insulin, and thus, blood glucose levels are elevated. Diabetes mellitus is the seventh leading cause of death among Americans. While 16 million Americans have diabetes, only 10 million are aware they have it. About one in 20 people will develop diabetes sometime during their lives.[32] Although the causes of diabetes are not completely known, both genetics and environmental factors such as obesity and lack of exercise appear to be involved.

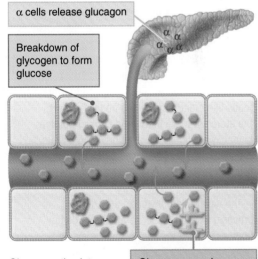

High blood glucose → Release of insulin from pancreas → Storage of glucose (glycogen) in liver and muscle cells

β cells release insulin

Insulin enters bloodstream, binds to cell receptors

Pancreas

Blood glucose

Glucose stored as glycogen in liver and muscle cells

Insulin stimulates:
• uptake of glucose
• storage as glycogen
• fat storage

(a)

Low blood glucose → Release of glucagon from pancreas → Breakdown of glycogen and protein – release of glucose into bloodstream

α cells release glucagon

Breakdown of glycogen to form glucose

Glucagon stimulates:
• breakdown of glycogen
• release of glucose
• synthesis of glucose from amino acids

Gluconeogenesis – the synthesis of glucose from amino acids

(b)

Figure 4.14 **Regulating blood glucose levels.** (a) In response to high blood glucose levels, the pancreas releases insulin which increases the uptake of glucose by cells. (b) If blood glucose is too low, the pancreas releases glucagon which stimulates the release of glucose into the bloodstream.

The glycemic index is a valuable and easy-to-use concept, claim some researchers.[1] It has no clinical benefit, according to others, and continued interest is like "flogging a dead horse."[2] So which is it?

How is the glycemic index measured?

The glycemic index classifies foods or meals based on their potential to raise blood glucose levels. It is expressed as a percentage of the response to a standard food or carbohydrate, usually white bread or pure glucose.[3]

Foods with a high glycemic index trigger a sharp rise in blood glucose followed by a dramatic fall, often to levels that are transiently below normal. The body more easily copes with low-glycemic-index foods, which trigger slower and more modest changes in blood glucose levels.

What factors affect the glycemic index of a food or meal?

The glycemic index of a food is not always easy to predict. Would you expect a high-sugar food such as ice cream to have a high glycemic index? Ice cream actually has a low index since the fat slows sugar absorption. On the other hand, wouldn't complex carbohydrate foods like bread or potatoes be low? In fact, the starch in white bread and cooked potatoes is readily absorbed, so each has a high value.[4] The glycemic index of some common foods is listed in **Table 1,** and lower glycemic index substitutions are given in **Table 2.**

The type of carbohydrate, the cooking process, and the presence of fat and dietary fiber all affect a food's glycemic index.[5] In a person's diet, it is the glycemic index of mixed meals, referred to as the glycemic load of a meal, rather than individual foods that counts.

Why do some researchers believe the glycemic index is useful?

Health benefits can be significant. Diets that emphasize low-glycemic-index foods decrease risk of developing type 2 diabetes[6] and improve blood sugar control in people who are already afflicted.[7] Such diets also reduce the risk of colon cancer[8] and may help reduce heart disease risk as well. They lower blood lipid levels[9] and improve insulin sensitivity,[10] two important factors in the development of heart disease.

Why do some researchers believe the glycemic index is useless?

Some researchers believe the glycemic index is a dead issue, calling it "much ado about (almost) nothing."[11] They believe it has little clinical usefulness and question the quality of the research that shows benefits. They point out that other dietary and behavioral changes, such as weight reduction, yield much stronger benefits.

They also believe the glycemic index is too complex for most people to use effectively. The American Diabetes Association seems to concur for people with diabetes and states that "from a clinical perspective first priority should be given to the total amount of carbohydrate consumed rather than the source of carbohydrate."[12]

We need more information about the glycemic index of specific foods. Processing affects the glycemic index of different foods differently and the glycemic index cannot always be predicted by starch, sugar, fiber, or fat content. In addition, predicting the glycemic effects of meals with mixed carbohydrate sources may be difficult, if not impossible.

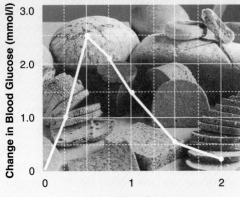

Time (hrs)
HIGH GLYCEMIC INDEX

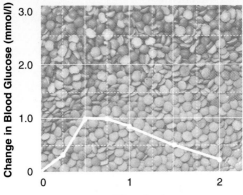

Time (hrs)
LOW GLYCEMIC INDEX

Are we really flogging a dead horse?

Although the glycemic index is a complex concept, this has not stopped researchers from advancing and applying it. Many researchers strongly believe that just as different types of fats affect blood lipid values differently, different types of carbohydrates affect blood glucose levels differently. Not only is the glycemic index horse not yet dead, it is still alive and kicking.

Table 1 **Glycemic Index of Some Foods Compared to Pure Glucose***

Food	Glycemic Index (%)*	Food	Glycemic Index (%)*
BAKERY PRODUCTS		*FRUITS*	
Angel food cake	67	Apples	36
Waffles	76	Bananas	53
		Pineapple	66
BREADS		*LEGUMES*	
White bread	70	Black-eyed peas	42
Wheat bread, whole-meal flour	69	Lentils	29
BREAKFAST CEREALS		*PASTA*	
All-Bran	42	Spaghetti	41
Corn flakes	84	Macaroni	45
Oatmeal	61	*VEGETABLES*	
CEREAL GRAINS		Carrots	71
Barley	25	Baked potatoes	85
Sweet corn	55	Green peas	48
White rice	56	*CANDY*	
Instant rice	91	Jelly beans	80
DAIRY FOODS		Life Savers	70
Ice cream	61		
Skim milk	32		

* Glycemic response to pure glucose is 100.

Source: Data compiled from Foster-Powell K, Miller JB. International table of glycemic index. *Am J Clin Nutr.* 1995; 62:8715-8935.

Table 2 **Sample Substitutions for High-Glycemic-Index Foods**

High-Glycemic-Index Food	Low-Glycemic-Index Alternative	High-Glycemic-Index Food	Low-Glycemic-Index Alternative
Bread, wheat	Oat bran, rye, or pumpernickel bread	Plain cookies and crackers	Cookies made with dried fruits and whole grains such as oats
Processed breakfast cereal	Unrefined cereal such as oats (either museli or oatmeal)	Cakes and muffins	Cakes and muffins made with fruit, oats, or whole grains
		Bananas	Apples
		Potatoes	Pasta or legumes

1 Miller JB, Colagiuri S, Foster-Powell K. The glycemic index is easy and works in practice. *Diabetes Care.* 1997;20:1628–1629.

2 Wolever TMS. The glycemic index: flogging a dead horse? *Diabetes Care.* 1997;20:452–456.

3 World Health Organization. *Carbohydrates in Human Nutrition: Report of a Joint FAO/WHO Expert Consultation, Rome,* 1997. FAO Food and Nutrition Paper 66, 1997.

4 Jenkins DJA, Jenkins AL. The glycemic index, fiber, and the dietary treatment of hypertriglyc-eridemia and diabetes. *J Am College Nutr.* 1987;6:11–17.

5 World Health Organization. Op. cit.

6 Salmeron J, Manson JE, Stampfer MJ, et al. Dietary fiber, glycemic load, and risk of non-insulin-dependent diabetes mellitus in women. *JAMA.* 1997; 277:472–477, and Salmeron J, Ascherio A, Rimm EB, et al. Dietary fiber, glycemic load, and risk of NIDDM in men. *Diabetes Care.* 1997;20:545–550.

7 Miller JB. Importance of glycemic index in diabetes. *Am J Clin Nutr.* 1994;59(suppl):747S–752S.

8 Slattery ML, Benson J, Berry TD, et al. *Cancer Epidemiological Biomarkers and Prevention,* 1997; 6:677–685., 1997.

9 Read NW, Eastwood MA. Gastrointestinal physiology and function. In: Schweizer TF, Edwards CA, eds. *Dietary Fibre. A Component of Food.* London: Springer-Verlag;1992:103–117.

10 Frost G, Leeds A, Trew G, et al. Insulin sensitivity in women at risk of coronary heart disease and the effect of a low glycemic diet. *Metabolism.* 1998;47:12545–1251.

11 Coulston AM, Reaven GM. Much ado about (almost) nothing. *Diabetes Care.* 1997;20:241–243.

12 Franz MJ, Horton ES, Bantle JP, et al.. Nutrition principles for the management of diabetes and related complications. (Technical Review). *Diabetes Care.* 1994;17:490–518.

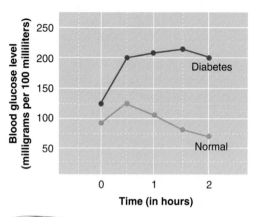

Figure 4.15 Glucose tolerance tests are used to detect diabetes.

Consequences of Diabetes

Hyperglycemia, or an abnormally high blood glucose level, is the hallmark of diabetes mellitus. (See **Figure 4.15.**) Even though blood glucose is overly abundant, it is unable to enter starving cells and fuel their needs. This is why diabetes is called the disease of "starvation in the midst of plenty." In an ironic twist of fate, these starving cells signal the liver to make more glucose, worsening the hyperglycemia. The kidneys are taxed beyond their capacities to reabsorb glucose and the excess spills into the urine where it can be detected by urine glucose tests.

Unable to use glucose, cells turn to other energy sources—fat and protein. But this leads to other problems. Excessive use of fat as an energy source, without available glucose in the cell, causes ketosis and acidosis, dangerously high acidity levels in the blood. Use of muscle proteins causes muscle wasting and weakness. Abnormalities in fat and protein metabolism often accompany hyperglycemia.[33]

Over time, abnormally high blood glucose levels increase risk of high blood pressure, heart disease, and kidney disease. High blood glucose levels enable sugars to react with and damage body proteins and tissues, especially in the eyes, kidneys, nerves, and blood vessels. Complications of this chronic disorder can contribute to a number of degenerative conditions including peripheral vascular disease, deterioration of the eye and eventual blindness, kidney disease, and progressive nerve damage. Diabetes is responsible for 50 percent of all amputations of the lower extremities and 25 percent of all kidney failure in adults.[34] Diabetes is also the leading cause of blindness in adults.[35] People with diabetes are two to four times more likely to develop heart disease than people without diabetes.

Forms of Diabetes

There are two main forms of diabetes:

- Type 1, previously known as insulin-dependent diabetes mellitus (IDDM) or juvenile-onset diabetes
- Type 2, previously known as non-insulin-dependent diabetes mellitus (NIDDM) or adult-onset diabetes

Type 2 diabetes is far more common, accounting for 90 to 95 percent of diabetes cases. Another type of diabetes, gestational diabetes, occurs during pregnancy (see Chapter 17 for more information on gestational diabetes).

Type 1 diabetes usually occurs in people under the age of 30 years and often develops suddenly. Symptoms include excessive thirst, frequent urination, nausea, and rapid weight loss.[36] As blood glucose levels rise, glucose spills into the urine, taking water with it and causing frequent urination and increased thirst. Although blood glucose levels are high, glucose cannot get into cells to be burned for energy, causing weight loss and feelings of hunger.

People with type 1 diabetes require lifelong, daily insulin injections balanced with a healthful diet and regular exercise to maintain blood glucose levels in the normal range. Since exercise lowers blood glucose levels, individuals must consider the timing of exercise in addition to food intake and insulin injections to avoid lowering blood glucose levels too far.

In **type 2 diabetes,** glucose has trouble entering body cells because either the pancreas cannot produce enough insulin or cells in the body become

hyperglycemia [HIGH-per-gly-SEE-me-uh]
Abnormally high concentration of glucose in the blood.

type 1 diabetes Type 1 diabetes occurs when the body's immune system attacks beta cells in the pancreas, causing them to lose the ability to make insulin.

type 2 diabetes Type 2 diabetes occurs when target cells (e.g., fat and muscle cells) lose the ability to respond normally to insulin.

resistant to the action of insulin. Although obesity is the cause of insulin resistance in most people with type 2 diabetes, genetic factors may play a role for some lean individuals with this type of diabetes. Type 2 diabetes usually develops in overweight people age 45 and older.

Diet and exercise are the primary management tools for type 2 diabetes, and weight loss often restores normal glucose metabolism.[37] Exercise increases the sensitivity of body cells to insulin, so the body needs less insulin to let glucose into cells. If diet and exercise fail to maintain blood glucose levels in the normal range, people with type 2 diabetes sometimes need medications to either increase insulin production or improve glucose uptake by cells. In some cases, insulin is needed to normalize blood glucose levels. (See **Figure 4.16**.)

Risk Factors for Diabetes

Some people are at higher risk than others of developing diabetes. **Table 4.2** lists the risk factors for type 1 and type 2 diabetes. Any person with a family history of diabetes has an increased risk. Diabetes also occurs more frequently in Native Americans, Hispanic Americans, and African Americans than in the general population.

Because it tends to run in families, the major risk factor for type 1 diabetes appears to be genetics. The risk of developing type 2 diabetes increases progressively as body fat increases, especially around the mid-section. Compared to a normal-weight person, an obese person can have 40 times the risk of type 2 diabetes.[38] Most, but not all, people diagnosed with type 2 diabetes are obese when the diagnosis is made.

Syndrome X is a relatively recent diagnosis characterized by hyperinsulinemia, hypertension, and insulin resistance. Within this syndrome is a complex interaction between hyperinsulinemia and dyslipidemia (altered blood lipid levels), hypertension, and glucose intolerance, all of which increase the risk of heart disease and type 2 diabetes.

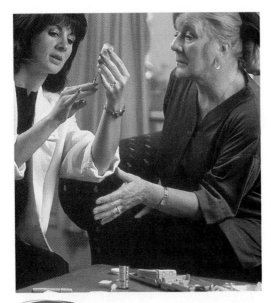

Figure 4.16 In some cases of diabetes, insulin is needed to normalize blood glucose levels.

Syndrome X A cluster of risk factors for heart disease associated with insulin resistance. These risk factors include hypertriglyceridemia (high blood lipid), low HDL cholesterol, hyperinsulinemia (high blood insulin), often hyperglycemia (high blood glucose), and hypertension (high blood pressure).

 Table 4.2 **Risk Factors for Type 1 and Type 2 Diabetes Mellitus**

Who is at greater risk for type 1 diabetes?

- Siblings of people with type 1 diabetes
- Children of parents with type 1 diabetes

Who is at greater risk for type 2 diabetes?

- People over age 45
- People with a family history of diabetes
- People who are overweight
- People who do not exercise regularly
- People with low HDL or high triglycerides
- Certain racial and ethnic groups (e.g., African Americans, Hispanic Americans, Asian and Pacific Islanders, and Native Americans)
- Women who had gestational diabetes, a form of diabetes that occurs in about 4 percent of pregnancies, or who have had a baby who weighed 9 pounds or more at birth

Source: American Diabetes Association. Position statement: Screening for type 2 diabetes, diabetes care. *Clinical Practice Recommendations*. 2000; 23 (1).

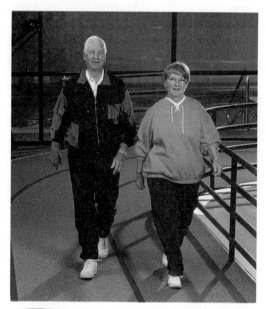

Figure 4.17 Exercise helps manage blood glucose levels.

Contrary to popular thought, high sugar or high carbohydrate intake does not by itself cause diabetes. In fact, current dietary recommendations for individuals with diabetes emphasize diets rich in complex carbohydrates (including fiber) and low in fat.[39] Although in the past, dietary treatment of diabetes eliminated simple sugars from the diet, current recommendations allow people with diabetes to include moderate amounts of simple sugars in their diet provided sugar intake does not contribute to excess energy intake and obesity.[40]

The best prevention for type 2 diabetes due to obesity or syndrome X is a healthful diet and regular exercise. Reducing excess body fat will improve glucose tolerance and reduce related risk factors for heart disease. Regular exercise will improve carbohydrate and lipid metabolism and increase insulin sensitivity. In addition, exercise improves capillary blood flow to the peripheral tissues, normalizing elevated blood pressure and reducing risk of heart disease. (See **Figure 4.17.**)

Low Blood Sugar: Hypoglycemia

Excess insulin results in low blood sugar, or **hypoglycemia.** Too much glucose enters cells, lowering blood glucose levels too far. When blood glucose levels drop too low, nervousness, irritability, hunger, headache, shakiness, rapid heartbeat, and weakness can develop. A further drop in blood glucose levels can cause coma and death.

A person with diabetes can develop hypoglycemia in response to an overdose of insulin or vigorous exercise. In nondiabetic people, two types of hypoglycemia occur. **Reactive hypoglycemia** occurs about one hour after eating carbohydrate-rich food. The body overreacts and produces too much insulin in response to food. Individuals can prevent reactive hypoglycemia by eating frequent, smaller meals to smooth out blood glucose responses to food. **Fasting hypoglycemia** occurs because the body produces too much insulin even when no food is eaten. Pancreatic tumors can cause fasting hypoglycemia.

Key Concepts: In healthy individuals, two hormones produced by the pancreas closely regulate blood glucose levels. Insulin allows glucose to enter cells and stimulates storage of glucose as glycogen, lowering blood glucose levels. Glucagon stimulates the release of glucose from glycogen and the formation of glucose from protein. Some individuals lack the ability to regulate blood glucose levels properly, resulting in diabetes (characterized by hyperglycemia) or hypoglycemia (low blood sugar). Individuals with type 1 diabetes cannot make insulin; individuals with type 2 diabetes are resistant to the action of insulin or make inadequate amounts.

Carbohydrates in the Diet

What foods supply our dietary carbohydrates? **Figure 4.18** shows many foods rich in carbohydrates. The food groups in the lower part of the Food Guide Pyramid are our main dietary sources of carbohydrates: grains and vegetables provide starches and fibers; fruits provide sugars and fibers. Additional sugar (mainly lactose) is found in dairy foods, while complex carbohydrates are also found in the legumes included in the meat and meat alternatives group. Sugars of all types are found at the tip of the Pyramid as sweeteners, beverages, jams, jellies, candy, and so forth.

hypoglycemia [HIGH-po-gly-SEE-mee-uh] Abnormally low concentration of glucose in the blood; any blood glucose value below 40 to 50 mg/dl of blood.

reactive hypoglycemia A type of hypoglycemia that occurs about one hour after eating carbohydrate-rich food. The body overreacts and produces too much insulin in response to food, rapidly decreasing blood glucose.

fasting hypoglycemia A type of hypoglycemia that occurs because the body produces too much insulin even when no food is eaten.

Quick Bites

Carbohydrate Companions

The word *companion* comes from the Latin word *companio,* meaning "one who shares bread."

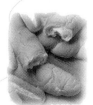

Recommendations for Carbohydrate Intake

The Surgeon General's Report on Nutrition and Health recommends that carbohydrate contribute about 55 to 60 percent of daily calories for individuals older than two years of age.[41] For the average American who eats about 2,000 kilocalories daily, a daily carbohydrate intake of 275 to 300 grams meets this recommendation. The Daily Value for carbohydrates is 300 grams, representing 60 percent of the calories in a 2,000-kilocalorie diet. The number of servings of food groups recommended for adults by the Food Guide Pyramid—6 to 11 servings of breads, cereals, rice, and pasta; 2 to 4 servings of fruits; 3 to 5 servings of vegetables; and 2 to 3 servings of milk— would provide this amount of carbohydrate. At a bare minimum, 50 to 100 grams of carbohydrate are required daily to prevent ketosis from incomplete fat metabolism.[42]

The *Dietary Guidelines for Americans* state general goals for consumption of sugars and complex carbohydrates.[43] One goal states "choose beverages and foods to moderate your intake of sugars." Other goals include "choose a variety of grains daily, especially whole grains" and "choose a variety of fruits and vegetables daily." These goals are reflected in the Food Guide Pyramid.

Other recommendations suggest that added sugars (excluding natural sugars in foods like fruits and milk) should provide no more than 10 percent of daily energy intake. For the typical adult consuming about 2,000 kilocalories daily, this amounts to about 50 grams or less of added sugar daily. Considering that a single can of soft drink contains 35 to 40 grams of sugar, it's not surprising that Americans generally consume more added sugar than recommended. Health experts also suggest we get about 10 to 13 grams of dietary fiber per 1,000 kilocalories, or about 20 to 35 grams of fiber daily for adults.[44] The Daily Value for fiber is 25 grams.

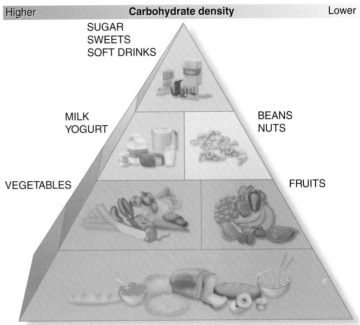

Key

Higher	Carbohydrate density	Lower

SUGAR
SWEETS
SOFT DRINKS

MILK
YOGURT

BEANS
NUTS

VEGETABLES

FRUITS

BREADS, CEREALS, RICE & PASTAS

Figure 4.18 **Carbohydrate sources from the Food Guide Pyramid.** Foods lower on the Food Guide Pyramid generally have a higher carbohydrate density. The sugars, sweets, and soft drinks in the top of the pyramid are rich in sugar (carbohydrate) but these should be consumed sparingly.
Source: US Department of Agriculture/ US Department of Health and Human Services.

Current Consumption

Adult Americans currently consume about 50 percent of their energy intake as carbohydrate.[45] Dietary fiber intake averages about 15 grams daily,[46] about half the recommended amount. Thus, Americans are not eating enough total carbohydrate or dietary fiber.

Natural sugars in milk, fruits, and grains make up about half of our sugar intake; refined sugars added to foods make up the other half. Consumption of sugars in the United States rose 15 percent between 1971 and 1991 and currently averages a little over 100 grams of sugar per person per day— equivalent to about one-half cup of sugar daily.[47] This value may be a little misleading, because it is based on food disappearance data (sugar that disappears from the food supply rather than sugar actually consumed) and includes sugar lost in processing or wasted, such as sugar poured out when the juice is drained from canned fruit. Actual sugar intake is lower and may be closer to the recommended maximum 10 percent of energy intake from added sugars.[48] However, the rapid increase in popularity of soft drinks, and

Think About It
2

Quick Bites

Liquid Candy

Soft drinks are the biggest source of refined sugars for Americans. Soft drinks provide 44 percent of the 34 teaspoons of sugar that 12- to 19-year-old boys consume every day. Girls of this age group average about 24 teaspoons of sugar each day, 40 percent from soft drinks.

germ The innermost part of a grain, located at the base of the kernel, that can grow into a new plant. The germ is rich in protein, oils, vitamins, and minerals.

endosperm The largest middle portion of a grain kernel, the endosperm is high in starch to provide food for the growing plant embryo.

bran The layers of protective coating around the grain kernel that are rich in dietary fiber and nutrients.

husk The inedible covering of grain. Also known as the chaff.

the addition of sugar in low-fat and fat-free foods probably means that our sugar intake remains higher than the recommended level.

Increasing Complex Carbohydrate Intake

The Food Guide Pyramid emphasizes grains, vegetables, and fruits as the foundation of a healthful diet.[49] While naturally low in fat, these foods are rich in complex carbohydrates, both starches and fibers. Legumes are rich in both protein and complex carbohydrate.

Whole kernels of grains consist of four parts: the germ, the endosperm, the bran, and the husk. (See **Figure 4.19**.) The **germ,** the innermost part at the base of the kernel, is the part that grows into a new plant. It is rich in protein, oils, vitamins, and minerals. The **endosperm** is the largest middle portion of the grain kernel. It is high in starch to provide food for the growing plant embryo. The **bran** is composed of layers of protective coating around the grain kernel and is rich in dietary fiber. The **husk** is an inedible covering.

When grains are refined, making white flour from wheat, for example, or making white rice from brown rice, the process removes the outer husk and bran layers and sometimes the inner germ of the grain kernel. Since the bran and germ portions of the grain contain much of the dietary fiber, vitamins, and minerals, the nutrient content of whole grains is far superior to that of refined grains. Although food manufacturers add iron, thiamin, riboflavin, and niacin back to white flour through enrichment, they usually do not add back dietary fiber and nutrients such as vitamin B_6, calcium, phosphorus, potassium, magnesium, and zinc, which are also lost in processing. Read labels carefully to choose foods that contain whole grains. Terms like *whole-wheat, whole-grain, rolled oats,* and *brown rice* indicate the entire grain kernel is included in the food.

To emphasize complex carbohydrates (including fiber) in your diet:

- Eat more breads, cereals, pasta, rice, fruits, vegetables, and legumes.

- Eat fruits and vegetables with the peel, if possible. The peel is high in fiber.

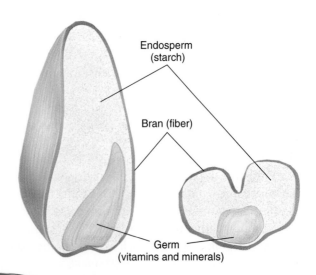

Endosperm (starch)

Bran (fiber)

Germ (vitamins and minerals)

Figure 4.19 Whole kernels of grains consist of four parts: germ, endosperm, bran, and husk (not shown in figure).

- Add fruits to muffins and pancakes.
- Add legumes like pinto, navy, kidney, and black beans and lentils to casseroles and mixed dishes as a meat substitute.
- Substitute whole-grain flour for all-purpose flour in recipes whenever possible.
- Use brown rice instead of white rice.
- Substitute oats for flour in crumb toppings.
- Choose high-fiber cereals.
- Choose whole fruits rather than fruit juices.

When increasing your fiber intake, do so gradually and drink plenty of fluids to allow your body to adjust. Add just a few grams a day; otherwise, abdominal cramps, gas, bloating, and diarrhea or constipation may result. Parents and caregivers should also emphasize foods rich in complex carbohydrate and dietary fiber for children older than two years, but must take care that these foods do not fill a child up before energy and nutrient needs are met. **Table 4.3** lists various foods that are high in simple and complex carbohydrates.

Although health food stores, pharmacies, and even grocery stores sell many types of fiber supplements, most experts agree that you should get your fiber from food rather than from a supplement. Foods rich in dietary fiber contain a variety of fibers as well as vitamins, minerals, and other phytochemicals that offer important health effects themselves.

Moderating Sugar Intake

Most of us enjoy the taste of sweet foods, and there's no reason that we should not. But for some individuals, habitually high sugar intake crowds out foods that are higher in complex carbohydrates, vitamins, and minerals.

To moderate sugars in your diet:

- Use less of all nutritive sugars, including white sugar, brown sugar, honey, and syrups.
- Limit use of soft drinks, high-sugar breakfast cereals, candy, ice cream, and sweet desserts.
- Use fresh or frozen fruits and fruits canned in natural juices or light syrup for dessert and to sweeten waffles, pancakes, muffins, and breads.

Read ingredient lists carefully. Food labels list the total grams of sugar in a food, which includes sugars naturally present in foods and sugars added to foods. Many terms for added sweeteners appear on food labels. Foods likely to be high in sugar list some form of sweetener as the first, second, or third ingredient on labels. **Table 4.4** lists the various forms of sugar used in foods.

Sugar substitutes such as artificial sweeteners can help many people lower sugar intake, but foods with artificial sweeteners may not provide less energy than similar products containing nutritive sweeteners. Rather than sugar, other energy-yielding nutrients, such as fat, are the primary source of the calories in these foods. Also, as artificial sweetener use in the United States has increased, so has sugar consumption, an interesting paradox!

Table 4.3 High-Carbohydrate Foods

High in Complex Carbohydrates	High in Simple Carbohydrates
Bagels	**Naturally present**
Tortillas	Fruits
Cereals	Fruit juices
Crackers	Skim milk
Rice cakes	Plain nonfat yogurt
Legumes	
Corn	**Added**
Potatoes	Angel food cake
Peas	Soft drinks
Squash	Sherbet
Popcorn	Syrups
	Sweetened nonfat yogurt
	Candy
	Jellies
	Jams
	Gelatin
	High-sugar breakfast cereals
	Cookies
	Frosting

Table 4.4 Forms of Sugar Used in Foods

Brown rice syrup	Invert sugar
Brown sugar	Lactose
Concentrated fruit juice sweetener	Levulose
	Maltose
Confectioners sugar	Mannitol
Corn syrup	Maple sugar
Dextrose	Molasses
Fructose	Natural sweeteners
Galactose	Raw sugar
Glucose	Sorbitol
Granulated sugar	Turbinado sugar
High-fructose corn syrup	White sugar
	Xylitol

Key Concepts: *Dietary guidelines recommend that carbohydrates provide 55 to 60 percent of energy intake, and that added sugars provide less than 10 percent of energy intake. Adults should aim for a fiber intake of 20 to 35 grams per day. Americans need to increase intake of complex carbohydrates and decrease intake of sugars to meet these recommendations. To increase complex carbohydrates (starches and fibers) in the diet, people should emphasize whole grains, legumes, fruits, and vegetables. To moderate sugar consumption, people should limit use of high-sugar foods such as high-sugar breakfast cereals, soft drinks, candies, jellies, jams, and some desserts.*

Nutritive Sweeteners

Nutritive sweeteners are digestible carbohydrates that provide energy. These include monosaccharides, disaccharides, and sugar alcohols from either natural or refined sources. White sugar, brown sugar, honey, maple syrup, glucose, fructose, xylitol, sorbitol, and mannitol are just some of the many nutritive sweeteners used in foods. **Figure 4.20** compares the sweetness of sweeteners. One slice of angel food cake, for example, contains about 5 teaspoons of sugar. Fruit-flavored yogurt contains about 7 teaspoons of sugar. Even two sticks of chewing gum contain about 1 teaspoon of sugar. Whether sweeteners come from natural sources or are refined, all are broken down in the small intestine and absorbed as monosaccharides. Since all the absorbed monosaccharides end up as glucose, the body cannot tell whether these monosaccharides came from honey or table sugar.

Sugar alcohols in sugarless chewing gums and candies are also nutritive sweeteners, but the body does not digest and absorb them fully, so they provide only 2 kilocalories per gram compared with the 4 kilocalories per gram that other sugars provide.

Natural Sweeteners Natural sweeteners such as honey and maple syrup contain monosaccharides and disaccharides that make them taste sweet. Honey contains a mix of fructose and glucose—the same two monosaccharides that make up sucrose. Bees make honey from the sucrose-containing nectar of flowering plants. Real maple syrup contains primarily sucrose and is made by boiling and concentrating the sap from sugar maple trees. Most maple-flavored syrups sold in grocery stores, however, are made from corn syrup with maple flavoring added.

Many fruits also contain sugars that impart a sweet taste. Usually the riper the fruit, the higher its sugar content—a ripe pear tastes sweeter than an unripe one.

Refined Sweeteners **Refined sweeteners** are monosaccharides and disaccharides that have been extracted from plant foods. White table sugar is sucrose extracted from either sugar beets or sugar cane. Molasses is a byproduct of the sugar-refining process. Most brown sugar is really white table sugar with some molasses added for coloring and flavor.

Manufacturers make high-fructose corn syrup by treating cornstarch with acid and enzymes to break the starch into glucose. Then different enzymes convert much of the glucose to fructose. High-fructose corn syrup tastes 1.5 times sweeter than table sugar and costs less to produce. An increase in high-fructose corn syrup in soft drinks and other processed foods accounts for much of the increased use of sweeteners in the United States since the 1970s.[50]

Sugar Alcohols The sugar alcohols sorbitol, xylitol, and mannitol occur naturally in foods and are additives in sugar-free products like gum and mints.

nutritive sweetener A substance that imparts sweetness to foods and can be absorbed and yield energy in the body.

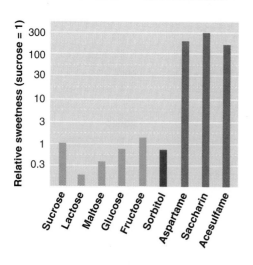

Key
Sugar alcohol
Refined sweeteners
Artificial sweeteners

Figure 4.20 **Comparing the sweetness of sweeteners.**

Although these sweeteners are not as sweet as sucrose, they do have the advantage of being less likely to cause tooth decay. When sugar alcohols are used as the sweetener, the product may be sugar (sucrose) free, but it is not calorie free. Check the label to be sure.

Artificial Sweeteners

Think About It 4

Gram for gram, most **artificial sweeteners** are many times sweeter than nutritive sweeteners. Thus, food manufacturers can use much less artificial sweetener to sweeten foods. Although some artificial sweeteners do provide energy, in the amounts used their energy contribution is minimal.

The most common artificial sweeteners in the United States are saccharin, aspartame, and acesulfame K. Cyclamates, banned in the United States in 1969 because of cancer concerns, are still used in Canada and many other countries. For people who want to decrease their intake of sugar and energy while still enjoying sweet foods, artificial sweeteners offer an alternative. Also, artificial sweeteners do not contribute to tooth decay.

Saccharin **Saccharin** tastes about 300 times sweeter than sucrose and has been used in foods since it was discovered in 1879. In the 1970s research indicated that very large doses of saccharin were associated with increased bladder cancer in laboratory animals. In 1977 the Food and Drug Administration (FDA) proposed banning saccharin from use in food. Widespread protests by consumer and industry groups, however, led Congress to impose a moratorium on the saccharin ban. This moratorium

Quick Bites

Why is honey dangerous for babies?
Honey should never be fed to infants younger than one year of age because it can contain spores of the bacterium *Clostridium botulinum*. Infants do not produce as much stomach acid as older children and adults, so these spores can germinate in an infant's GI tract and cause botulism, a deadly foodborne illness.

refined sweeteners Composed of monosaccharides and disaccharides that have been extracted and processed from other foods.

artificial sweetener Substances that impart sweetness to foods but supply little or no energy to the body; also called non-nutritive or alternative sweeteners.

saccharin [SAK-ah-ren] An artificial sweetener that tastes about 300 to 700 times sweeter than sucrose.

Label [to] **Table**

This label highlights all of the carbohydrate-related information you can find on a food label. Look at the center of the Nutrition Facts label and you'll see the Total Carbohydrates along with two of the carbohydrate "subgroups": Dietary Fiber and Sugars. Recall that carbohydrates are classified into simple carbohydrates and the two complex carbohydrates starch and fiber.

Using this food label you can determine all three of these components. There are 19 total grams of carbohydrate with 14 grams coming from sugars and 0 grams from fiber. This means the remaining 5 grams must be from starch, which is not required to be listed separately on the label. Without even knowing what food this label represents, you can decipher that it contains a high proportion of sugar (14 of the 19 grams) and is probably sweet. If this is a fruit juice, that level of sugar would be expected; but if this is cereal, you'd be getting a lot more sugar than complex carbohydrates, and probably not be making the best choice!

Do you see the 6% listed to the right of "Total Carbohydrates"? This doesn't mean

that the food item contains 6% of its calories from carbohydrate. Instead, it refers to the daily allotment (or Daily Value) of carbohydrates listed at the bottom of the label. You can see there that a person consuming 2,000 kcalories per day should consume 300 grams of carbohydrates each day. This product contributes 19 grams per serving, which is just 6% of the recommended 300 grams per day. Note that the % Daily Value for fiber is 0% because this food item lacks fiber.

The last highlighted section on this label, at the bottom of some Nutrition Facts labels, is the number of calories in a gram of carbohydrate. Recall that carbohydrates contain 4 kilocalories per gram. Armed with this information and the product's calorie information, can you calculate the percentage of calories that come from carbohydrate?

Here's how:

19 g carbohydrate $\times$ 4kcal per g = 76 carbohydrate kcal

76 carbohydrate kcal $\div$ 154 total kcal = .49 or 49% carbohydrate kcal

Nutrition Facts

Serving Size: 1 cup (248g)
Servings Per Container: 4

Amount Per Serving

Calories 154   Calories from fat 35

	% Daily Value*
Total Fat 4g	6%
Saturated Fat 2.5g	12%
Cholesterol 20mg	7%
Sodium 170mg	7%
Total Carbohydrate 19g	6%
Dietary Fiber 0g	0%
Sugars 14g	
Protein 11g	

Vitamin A 4%	•	Vitamin C 6%	
Calcium 40%	•	Iron 0%	

* Percent Daily Values are based on a 2,000 calorie diet. Your daily values may be higher or lower depending on your calorie needs:

		Calories:	2000	2,500
Total Fat	Less Than		65g	80g
Sat Fat	Less Than		20g	25g
Cholesterol	Less Than		300mg	300mg
Sodium	Less Than		2,400mg	2,400mg
Total Carbohydrate			300g	375g
Dietary Fiber			25g	30g

Calories per gram:
Fat 9 • Carbohydrate 4 • Protein 4

Quick Bites

The Discovery of Saccharin

A German student named Constantine Fahlberg discovered saccharin in 1879, while working with organic chemicals in the lab of Ira Remsen at Johns Hopkins University. One day, while eating some bread, he noticed a strong sweet flavor. He deduced that the flavor came from the compound on his hands, $C_6H_4CONHSO_2$. Fahlberg then patented saccharin by himself, without Remsen.

aspartame [AH-spar-tame] An artificial sweetener composed of two amino acids and methanol. It is 200 times sweeter than sucrose. Its trade name is NutraSweet.

has since been extended every few years, and products that contain saccharin are required to bear a warning label about saccharin and cancer risk in animals. In Canada, although saccharin is banned from food products, it can be purchased in pharmacies and carries a warning label.

Aspartame **Aspartame** is a combination of the two amino acids phenylalanine and aspartic acid. When digested and absorbed, it provides 4 kilocalories per gram. However, aspartame is so many times sweeter than sucrose, that the amount used to sweeten foods contributes virtually zero calories to the diet; and it does not promote tooth decay. The FDA approved aspartame for use in some foods in 1981 and for use in soft drinks in 1983. More than 90 countries allow aspartame in products such as beverages, gelatin desserts, gums, and fruit spreads. Because amino acids are damaged by heat, aspartame cannot be used in products that require cooking.

Several safety concerns have been raised regarding aspartame. Some groups believe aspartame could cause high blood levels of the amino acid phenylalanine. However, high-protein foods such as meats contain much more phenylalanine than foods sweetened with aspartame. Consuming

---

Fyi | Unfounded Claims Against Sugars

FOR YOUR INFORMATION

Sugar has become the vehicle for the diet zealots to create a new soapbox. Cut sugar to trim fat! Bust Sugar! Break the sugar habit! These battle cries falsely demonize sugar as a dietary villain. But what are the facts?

Sugar and Obesity

Many people believe that sugar is fattening and causes obesity. Sugar is a carbohydrate, and all carbohydrates provide 4 kilocalories per gram. High fat—not sugar—intakes are associated with a greater risk of obesity.[1] Fat is a more concentrated source of energy, and provides 9 kilocalories per gram. However, many foods high in sugar such as doughnuts and cookies are also high in fat. Excess energy intake from any source will cause obesity, but sugar by itself is no more likely to cause obesity than starch or protein. The increased availability of low-fat and fat-free foods has not reduced obesity rates in the United States; in fact, incidence of obesity is still climbing. Some speculate that consumers equate fat-free with calorie-free, and eat more of these foods, not realizing that fat-free foods often have a higher sugar content, which makes any calorie savings negligible.

Sugar and Heart Disease

Risk factors for heart disease include a genetic predisposition, smoking, high blood pressure, high blood cholesterol levels, diabetes, and obesity. Sugar by itself does not cause heart disease.[2] However, if intake of high-sugar foods contributes to obesity, then risk for heart disease increases. In addition, excessive intake of refined sugar can alter blood lipids in carbohydrate-sensitive people, increasing their risk for heart disease. However, a high fat intake is more likely to promote obesity than a high sugar intake. Thus, total fats, saturated fat, cholesterol, and obesity have a significantly more important relationship to heart disease than sugar.

Sugar and Behavior

Parents continue to talk about kids "bouncing off the walls" at birthday parties because of "all that sugar." So, what's going on? Most likely, the event (a party, trick-or-treating for Halloween, a carnival) is enhancing kids' normal levels of excitement and enthusiasm. From a brain-chemistry perspective, carbohydrates actually have a calming effect by increasing production of the sleep-inducing chemical serotonin! Well-controlled research studies have found no link between sugar

and hyperactivity, so blame the excitement of the party, but not the sugar for kids' "wild" behavior.[3]

In 1978 Dan White blamed his gunning down the mayor of San Francisco on his emotional state created by eating too many Hostess Twinkies, a legal strategy that became known as the Twinkie defense. But claims that sugar causes criminal behavior in adults are unfounded. Studies show no association between high sugar intake and adult behavior.[4]

1 Lichtenstein AH, Kennedy E, Barrier P, et al. Dietary fat consumption and health. *Nutr Rev.* 1998; 56:S3–S19.

2 World Health Organization (WHO). *Carbohydrates in Human Nutrition: Report of a Joint FAO/WHO Expert Consultation, Rome, 1997.* FAO Food and Nutrition Paper 66; 1997.

3 White JW, Wolraich M. Effect of sugar on behavior and mental performance. *Am J Clin Nutr.* 1995;62:S242–S249; and Wolraich ML, Lindgren SD, Stumbo PJ, et al. Effects of diets high in sucrose or aspartame on the behavior and cognitive performance of children. *N Engl J Med.* 1994;330:301–307,

4 White JW, Wolraich M. Ibid.

phenylalanine alone could raise blood or brain levels more than consuming phenylalanine mixed with other amino acids found in high-protein foods, but the amounts used in aspartame-sweetened products are low enough not to cause concern.

Although some people report headaches, dizziness, seizures, nausea, or allergic reactions with aspartame use, scientific studies have failed to confirm these effects. Most experts believe aspartame is safe for healthy people.[51] However, people with a genetic disease called **phenylketonuria (PKU)** cannot properly metabolize the amino acid phenylalanine, so they must carefully monitor their phenylalanine intake from all sources, including aspartame.

The FDA set a maximum allowable daily intake of aspartame of 50 milligrams per kilogram of body weight. This amount of aspartame equals the amount in 16 12-ounce diet soft drinks for adults and 8 diet soft drinks for children.

Acesulfame K Acesulfame K is about 200 times sweeter than table sugar and is marketed under the brand name Sunette. The FDA approved its use in the United States in 1988. Acesulfame K provides no energy because the body cannot digest it. Food manufacturers use acesulfame K in chewing gum, powdered beverage mixes, nondairy creamers, gelatins, and puddings. Heat does not destroy acesulfame K, so it can be used in cooking.

Sucralose Sucralose was approved for use in the United States in 1998, and has been used in Canada since 1992. Sucralose is made from sucrose, but the resulting compound is non-nutritive, and about 600 times sweeter than sugar. Sucralose has been approved for use in a wide variety of products including baked goods, beverages, gelatin desserts, frozen dairy desserts, and many others. It also can be used as a "table-top sweetener" and added directly to food by consumers.

Other Artificial Sweeteners Other artificial sweeteners such as alitame and D-tagatose are awaiting approval by the FDA for use in the United States.[52] **Alitame** is composed of two amino acids plus another nitrogen-containing compound and tastes 2,000 times sweeter than sucrose. **D-tagatose** is derived from lactose and has the same sweetness of sucrose with only one-half the energy.

Key Concepts: *Sweeteners add flavor to foods. Nutritive sweeteners provide energy, while artificial sweeteners provide little or no energy. The body cannot tell the difference between sugars derived from natural and refined sources.*

Carbohydrates and Health

Carbohydrates contribute both positively and negatively to health. Fiber helps to keep the gastrointestinal tract healthy and, along with other complex carbohydrates, may reduce the risk of heart disease and cancer. Excess sugar can contribute to poor nutrient intake and tooth decay.

Sugar and Nutrient Intake

Foods high in sugar are popular in American diets. These empty-calorie foods (e.g., candy, soft drinks, sweetened gelatin, and some desserts) provide most of their energy from sugar but contain little or no dietary fiber, vitamins, or minerals. Consider that one can of soft drink contains 10 to 12 teaspoons of sugar. Would you add that much sugar to a glass of iced tea?

phenylketonuria (PKU) An inherited disorder caused by a lack or deficiency of the enzyme that converts phenylalanine to tyrosine.

acesulfame K [ay-SUL-fame] An artificial sweetener that is 200 times sweeter than common table sugar (sucrose). Because it is not digested and absorbed by the body, acesulfame contributes no calories to the diet and yields no energy when consumed.

sucralose An artificial sweetener made from sucrose. Sucralose is non-nutritive and about 600 times sweeter than sugar.

alitame An artificial sweetener composed of two amino acids and a nitrogen compound. Alitame tastes 2,000 times sweeter than sucrose.

D-tagatose An artificial sweetener derived from lactose that has the same sweetness as sucrose with only half the calories.

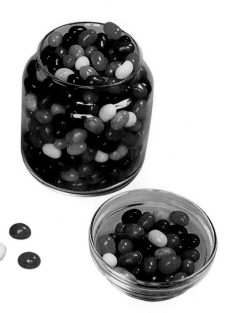

dental caries [KARE-ees] Destruction of the enamel surface of teeth caused by acids resulting from bacterial breakdown of sugars in the mouth.

People with high energy needs, such as active teenagers and young adults, can afford to get a bit more of their calories from high-sugar foods. People with low energy needs, such as some elderly or sedentary people or people trying to lose weight, cannot afford to get as many calories from high-sugar foods. Most people can include moderate amounts of sugar in their diet and still meet other nutrient needs.

Sugar and Dental Caries

High sugar intake contributes to **dental caries,** or cavities. (See **Figure 4.21.**) When bacteria in the mouth feed on sugars, they produce acids that eat away tooth enamel and dental structure, causing dental caries. Although these bacteria quickly metabolize sugars, they can feed on any carbohydrate, including starch.

The longer a carbohydrate remains in the mouth, the more likely it will promote dental caries. Foods that stick to the teeth, such as caramel, licorice, crackers, sugary cereals, and cookies, are more likely to cause dental caries than foods that are quickly washed out of the mouth. High sugar beverages such as soft drinks are more likely to cause dental caries when they are sipped slowly over an extended period of time. A baby should never be put to bed with a bottle, because the warm milk or juice may remain in the mouth all night, providing a ready source of carbohydrate for bacteria to break down.

Snacking on high-sugar foods throughout the day provides continuous carbohydrate and also promotes formation of dental caries. Good dental hygiene, adequate fluoride, and a well-balanced diet for strong tooth formation can all help prevent dental caries.[53]

Complex Carbohydrates and Obesity

A diet rich in complex carbohydrates promotes a healthy body weight and lowers the risk of obesity. These effects occur for several reasons.[54] Foods rich in complex carbohydrates are usually low in fat and energy. They are also more filling, offer a greater volume of food for fewer calories, and take longer to eat. Once eaten, foods high in dietary fiber take longer to leave the stomach and they attract water, giving a feeling of fullness. For example, three apple products with the same energy content have different complex carbohydrate contents: a large apple contains 5 grams of dietary fiber, $1/2$ cup applesauce contains 2 grams of fiber, and $3/4$ cup of apple juice contains 0.2 grams of fiber. For most of us, the whole apple would be more filling and satisfying than the applesauce or apple juice.

Complex Carbohydrates and Type 2 Diabetes

Populations with a high intake of complex carbohydrates have a low incidence of type 2 diabetes.[55] High intake of complex carbohydrates decreases the risk of becoming obese, and obesity greatly increases the risk for developing type 2 diabetes. High intake of soluble fiber also delays emptying of the stomach and smooths out blood glucose response, effects that are helpful for healthy people as well as people with type 2 diabetes. Current dietary recommendations for people with type 2 diabetes advise a high intake of complex carbohydrate, and dietary fiber.[56]

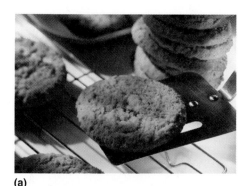

(a)

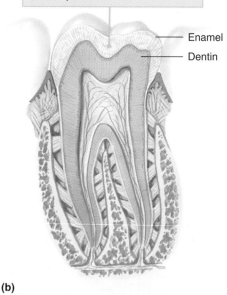

Bacteria feeding on sugar and other carbohydrates produce acids that eat away tooth enamel

— Enamel

— Dentin

(b)

Figure 4.21 **Dental caries.** Snacking on high-sugar foods promotes dental caries.

Complex Carbohydrates and Cancer

A diet rich in complex carbohydrates lowers risk of certain kinds of cancers.[57] Foods rich in complex carbohydrates, particularly fruits and vegetables, contain antioxidants that may protect against cell damage that can trigger cancer.

Do foods rich in dietary fiber protect against colon cancer? Some studies show this to be the case,[58] but the final answer is yet to be determined. High fiber intake may dilute cancer-causing agents in the gastrointestinal tract and speed their passage out of the body, decreasing their contact with mucosal cells. The short-chain fatty acids from fermentation of resistant starch and dietary fiber may also offer protection against colon cancer through several mechanisms.[59] However, a report from the large-scale Nurse's Health Study did not find a link between high intake of dietary fiber and reduced risk for colon cancer.[60] Further investigation is needed to resolve the relationship between dietary fiber and colon cancer.

Complex Carbohydrates and Cardiovascular Disease

High blood cholesterol levels increase risk for heart disease. Diets rich in soluble fiber can lower blood cholesterol levels by 20 percent or more.[61] Since every 1 percent decrease in blood cholesterol levels decreases risk of heart disease 2 percent, high fiber intake can decrease risk of heart disease by 40 percent or more.

Soluble fibers, such as oat bran, legumes, and psyllium, may lower serum cholesterol levels by binding bile acids in the gastrointestinal tract and preventing their reabsorption into the body. Bile acids are made from cholesterol in the liver and are secreted into the intestinal tract to aid with fat absorption. When dietary fiber prevents their reabsorption, more bile acids must be made in the liver from cholesterol, reducing blood cholesterol levels. The short-chain fatty acids produced from bacterial fermentation of fiber in the large intestine may also inhibit cholesterol synthesis.[62]

Studies also show an association between high intake of whole grains and low risk of heart disease.[63] Whole grains contain not only fiber but also antioxidants, which may protect against cellular damage that promotes heart disease.

Dietary Fiber and Gastrointestinal Disorders

A high intake of dietary fiber, particularly of insoluble types found in cereal grains, helps promote healthy gastrointestinal functioning. High fiber intake also helps in treating certain gastrointestinal disorders.[64]

Diets rich in insoluble fiber add bulk and increase water in the stool, softening the stool and making it easier to pass. Insoluble fiber also speeds passage of food through the intestinal tract, promoting regularity. If fluid intake is also ample, high fiber intake helps prevent and treat constipation, hemorrhoids (swelling of rectal veins), and diverticular disease (development of pouches on the intestinal wall).

Quick Bites

Fierce Fiber and Flatulence

The Jerusalem artichoke surpasses even dry beans in its capacity for facilitating flatulence. This artichoke contains large amounts of indigestible carbohydrate. After passing through the small intestine undigested, the fiber is attacked by gas-generating bacteria in the colon.

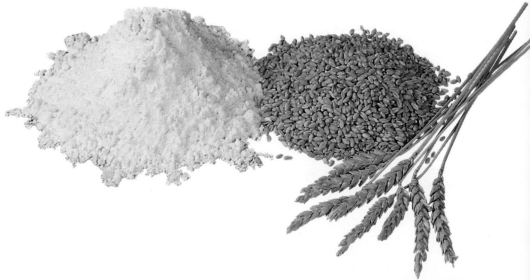

Negative Health Effects of Excess Dietary Fiber

Despite its health advantages, high fiber intake can cause problems, especially for people who drastically increase their fiber intake in a short period of time. When fiber intake increases, so should water intake to prevent the stool from becoming hard and impacted. A sudden increase in fiber intake also can cause increased intestinal gas and bloating. These problems can be prevented both by increasing fiber intake gradually over several weeks and by drinking plenty of fluids.

High fiber intake may also bind small amounts of minerals in the GI tract and prevent them from being absorbed. Fiber binds the minerals zinc, calcium, magnesium, and iron. For people who get enough of these minerals, however, the recommended amounts of dietary fiber do not significantly affect mineral status.[65]

If the diet contains high amounts of fiber, some people, such as young children and the elderly, may become full before meeting energy and nutrient needs. Because of a limited stomach capacity, they must be careful that fiber intake does not interfere with their ability to consume adequate energy and nutrients.

Key Concepts: *Diets high in starch and dietary fiber decrease risk of obesity, type 2 diabetes, cancer, cardiovascular disease, and gastrointestinal disorders. High sugar intake promotes dental caries and can contribute to nutrient deficiencies by replacing other more nutritious foods in the diet. High intake of complex carbohydrates offers many health benefits. Increase fiber intake gradually while drinking plenty of fluids; children and the elderly with small appetites should take care that energy needs are still met.*

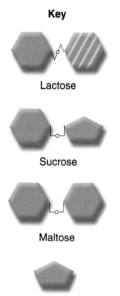

Key

Lactose

Sucrose

Maltose

Fructose

Galactose

Glucose

Enzyme

Na⁺

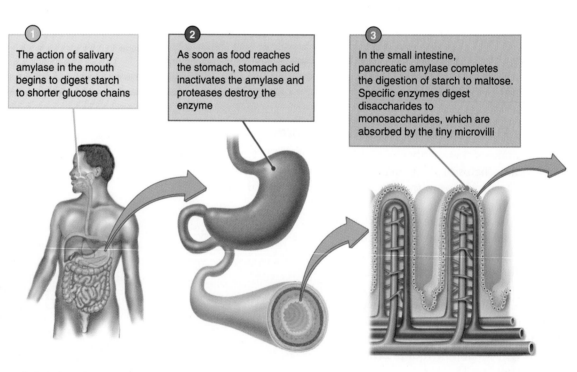

1. The action of salivary amylase in the mouth begins to digest starch to shorter glucose chains

2. As soon as food reaches the stomach, stomach acid inactivates the amylase and proteases destroy the enzyme

3. In the small intestine, pancreatic amylase completes the digestion of starch to maltose. Specific enzymes digest disaccharides to monosaccharides, which are absorbed by the tiny microvilli

Figure 4.22 **Summary figure.** Carbohydrate: From intake to utilization.

4 Intestinal cells absorb glucose and galactose through energy- and sodium-dependent active transport channels. Fructose uses facilitated diffusion to enter the cell. All three monosaccharides use facilitated diffusion to move out of the cell and into the bloodstream

5 Once in the bloodstream, the monosaccharides travel to the liver via the portal vein. The liver can convert fructose and galactose to glucose. The liver may form glucose into glycogen, burn it for energy, or release it to the bloodstream for use in other parts of the body

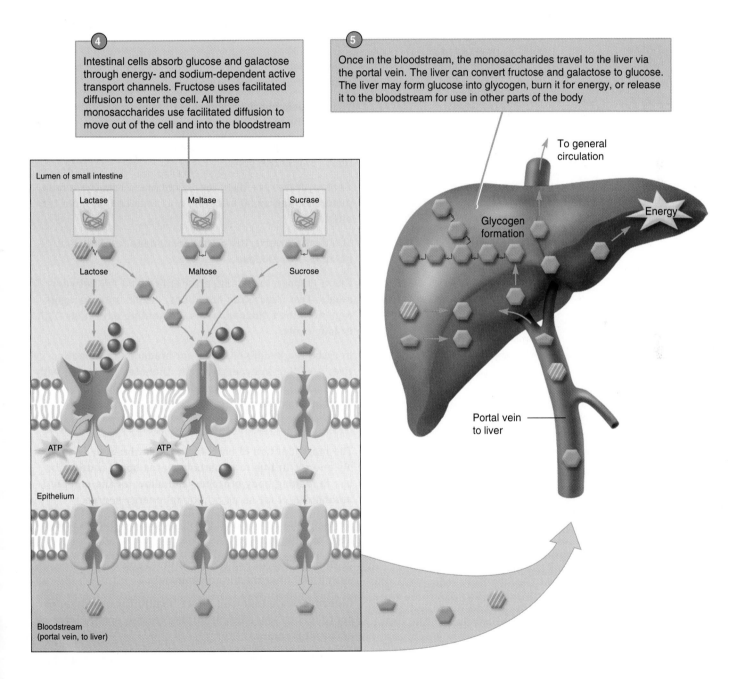

Lumen of small intestine

Lactase

Maltase

Sucrase

Lactose

Maltose

Sucrose

ATP

ATP

Epithelium

Bloodstream
(portal vein, to liver)

To general
circulation

Energy

Glycogen
formation

Portal vein
to liver

LEARNING *Portfolio* c h a p t e r 4

Key Terms

	page		page
acesulfame K [ay-SUL-fame]	125	hydrolysis [High-DROL-ih-sis]	104
alitame	125	hyperglycemia [HIGH-per-gly-SEE-me-uh]	116
alpha (α) bond	108	hypoglycemia [HIGH-po-gly-SEE-mee-uh]	118
amylopectin [am-ih-low-PEK-tin]	106	insoluble fiber	108
amylose [AM-uh-los]	106	insulin [IN-suh-lin]	112
artificial sweetener	123	ketone bodies	112
aspartame [AH-spar-tame]	124	ketosis [kee-TOE-sis]	112
beta (β) bond	108	lactose [LAK-tose]	104
blood glucose level	112	lignin [LIG-nin]	108
bran	120	maltose [MALL-tose]	104
cellulose [SELL-you-los]	107	monosaccharide	101
complex carbohydrate	105	mucilage	107
condensation	104	nutritive sweetener	122
D-tagatose	125	oligosaccharide	105
dental caries [KARE-ees]	126	pancreatic amylase	105
diabetes mellitus	112	pectin	107
dietary fiber	106	pentose	103
disaccharide [dye-SACK-uh-ride]	101	phenylketonuria (PKU)	125
endosperm	120	polysaccharide	105
epinephrine	112	reactive hypoglycemia	118
fasting hypoglycemia	118	refined sweeteners	123
fructose [FROOK-tose]	103	resistant starch	106
galactose [gah-LAK-tose]	103	saccharin [SAK-ah-ren]	123
germ	120	simple carbohydrates	101
glucagon [GLOO-kuh-gon]	112	soluble fiber	108
glucose [GLOO-kose]	103	starch	105
glycemic index	112	sucralose	125
glycogen [GLY-ko-jen]	106	sucrose [SOO-crose]	104
gum	107	sugar alcohols	103
hemicellulose [hem-ih-SELL-you-los]	107	Syndrome X	117
husk	120	type 1 diabetes	116
		type 2 diabetes	116

Study Points

➤ Carbohydrates include the simple sugars and complex carbohydrates.

➤ Monosaccharides are the building blocks of carbohydrates.

➤ Three monosaccharides are important in human nutrition: glucose, fructose, and galactose.

➤ The monosaccharides combine to make disaccharides: sucrose, lactose, and maltose.

➤ Starch, glycogen, and fiber are long chains (polysaccharides) of glucose units.

➤ Carbohydrates are digested by enzymes from the mouth, pancreas, and small intestine and absorbed as monosaccharides.

➤ The liver converts the monosaccharides fructose and galactose to glucose.

➤ Blood glucose levels rise after eating and fall between meals. Two pancreatic hormones, insulin and glucagon, regulate blood glucose levels, preventing extremely high or low levels.

➤ In diabetes, insulin either is not produced or is ineffective, resulting in hyperglycemia. Diabetes is treated with diet, exercise, and medication, including insulin injections in some cases.

➤ Hypoglycemia results when blood glucose falls too low.

➤ The main function of carbohydrates in the body is to supply energy. In this role, carbohydrates spare protein for use in making body proteins, and allow for the complete breakdown of fat as an additional energy source.

➤ Carbohydrates are found mainly in plant foods as starch, fiber, and sugar.

➤ In general, Americans consume more sugar and less starch and fiber than is recommended.

➤ Carbohydrate intake can affect health. Excess sugar can contribute to low nutrient intake, excess energy intake, and dental caries.

➤ Diets high in complex carbohydrates, including fiber, have been linked to reduced risk for GI disorders, heart disease, and cancer.

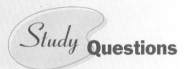

Study Questions

1. **Describe the difference between starch and fiber.**

2. **How will eating excessive amounts of carbohydrate affect health?**

3. **What are the consequences of eating too little carbohydrate?**

4. **List the benefits of eating more fiber. What are the consequences of eating too much? Too little?**

5. **What foods contain carbohydrates?**

6. **What advantage does the branched chain structure of glycogen provide compared to a straight chain of glucose?**

7. **Which blood glucose regulation hormone is secreted in the recently fed state? The fasting state?**

8. **Describe the structure of a monosaccharide, disaccharide and polysaccharide.**

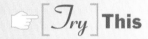 **This**

The Fiber Type Experiment

This experiment is to help you understand the difference between soluble and insoluble fiber. Go to the store and buy a small amount of raw bran. This is usually sold in a bin at a health food store or near the hot cereals in a grocery store. Also purchase some pectin (near the baking items) or some Metamucil (in the pharmacy section). Once you're home, fill two glasses with water and put the raw bran in one glass and the pectin or Metamucil in the other. Stir each glass for a minute or two and watch what happens. What explains the change in the pectin/Metamucil mixture? Why was there no change in the bran mixture?

The Sweetness of Soda

This experiment is to help you understand the amount of sugar found in a can of soda. Take a glass and fill it with 12 ounces (1 1/2 cups) of water. Using a measuring spoon, add 10 to 12 teaspoons of sugar to the water. Stir the sugar water until all the sucrose has dissolved. Now sip the water. Does it taste sweet? It shouldn't taste any sweeter than a can of regular soda. This is the amount of sugar found in one 12-ounce can!

What About Bobbie?

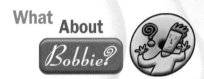

Refer to page 28 to see the complete list of food and drinks from Bobbie's recorded intake. Let's examine her day of eating using the guidelines you've learned in this chapter. How well did Bobbie do? Did she meet her overall carbohydrate goal? Did she consume approximately 60 percent of her calories from carbohydrates? Was her diet made up mostly of complex carbohydrates or simple sugars? Was her fiber intake in the recommended range of 20 and 35 grams? Let's take a look.

Her overall carbohydrate intake was 293 grams or 1,172 kcalories. Her total energy intake was 2,440 kcalories, which means 48 percent of her calories were from carbohydrates. This is lower than the recommended 60 percent and means her protein and/or fat intake must be higher than the recommended amounts. Here are the biggest contributors, which supply more than 80 percent of Bobbie's carbohydrate intake:

Food	Carbohydrate (g)	Percentage of calorie intake (%)
Spaghetti	*60*	*10*
Bread (lunch and dinner)	*48*	*8*
Bagel	*39*	*6*
Banana	*28*	*5*
Pizza	*28*	*5*
Tortilla chips	*27*	*4*
Spaghetti sauce	*9*	*1.5*

Review the list of Bobbie's foods again. Do you think her carbohydrate intake comes mostly from complex sources or simple sugars? Very few of her carbohydrate sources are high in sugars, just the banana, the sugar for the coffee, and the chocolate chip cookie.

Let's take a closer look at Bobbie's carbohydrate intake. Which groups in the Food Pyramid contribute the most to her intake? To answer this, let's divide her carbohydrate-dense foods into the three carbohydrate-rich food groups.

Pyramid Food Group	Number of Servings	
	Bobbie's	Recommended
BREAD, CEREAL, RICE, & PASTA GROUP		
Bagel	2	
Bread (lunch)	2	
Bread (dinner)	1	
Tortilla chips	2	
Pasta	3	
Pizza	1	
Total	11	6 to 11

What About *Bobbie?*

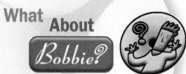

Pyramid Food Group	Number of Servings	
	Bobbie's	Recommended
FRUIT GROUP		
Banana	1	
Total	1	2 to 4
VEGETABLE GROUP		
Lettuce	2	
Carrot	$1/8$	
Spaghetti sauce	$1/2$	
Green beans	1	
Total	>3	3 to 5

So, now that you've reviewed Bobbie's food group totals, what can you conclude about her carbohydrate intake? Her total carbohydrate calories were lower than the recommended level, and her diet could use some improvement. Bobbie fulfills the recommendation from the bottom of the Pyramid but is very low in fruits and vegetables. This helps explain why her carbohydrate percentage (based on total calories) was only 48 percent. She needs to eat more foods from the fruit and vegetable groups.

References

1 Mathews CK, Van Holde KE. *Biochemistry.* 2nd ed. New York: Benjamin/Cummings; 1996.

2 Giboney M, Sigman-Grant M, Stanton JL, Keast DR. Consumption of sugars. *Am J Clin Nutr.* 1995;62(suppl):178S–194S.

3 Eastwood, M. *Principles of Human Nutrition.* New York: Chapman & Hall; 1997.

4 Finley JW, Leveille GA. Macronutrient substitutes. In: Ziegler EE, Filer LJ, eds. *Present Knowledge in Nutrition.* 7th ed. Washington DC: ILSI Press; 1996:581–595.

5 World Health Organization. (WHO) *Carbohydrates in Human Nutrition: Report of a Joint FAO/WHO Expert Consultation, Rome, 1997.* FAO Food and Nutrition Paper 66; 1997.

6 McVeagh P, Miller JB. Human milk oligosaccharides: only the breast. *J Pediatr Child Health.* 1977;33:281–286.

7 Ibid.

8 Eliasson, AC. *Carbohydrates in Food.* New York: Marcel Dekker; 1996.

9 World Health Organization. Op. cit.

10 Noah L, Guillon F, Bouchet B, et al. Digestion of carbohydrate from white beans (*Phaseolus vulgaris L.*) in healthy humans. *J Nutr.* 1998;128:977–985.

11 Conversion of muscle to meat, Meat Science at Texas A&M University, http://www.meat.tamu.edu/conversion.html, accessed 3/16/2000; and Meat Processing, Britannica.com, Encylclopaedia Britannica, 1999–2000., http://www.britannica.com/bcom/eb/article/6/0,5716,120856+6,00.html, accessed 3/16/2000.

12 Robyt JF. *Essentials of Carbohydrate Chemistry.* New York: Springer; 1998.

13 Flatt, JP. Use and storage of carbohydrates. *Am J Clin Nutr.* 1995;61(suppl):952S–959S.

14 Miller GD. Carbohydrates in ultra-endurance exercise and athletic performance. In: Wolinski I, Hickson JF, eds. *Nutrition in Exercise and Sport.* 2nd ed. Boca Raton, FL: CRC Press; 1994:49–64.

15 Morris ER. Fiber in foods. In: Kritchevsky D, Bonfield C., eds. *Dietary Fiber in Health and Disease.* St. Paul, MN: Eagan Press; 1995:37–45.

16 Ibid.

17 Ibid.

18 Olson BH, Anderson SM, Becker MP, et al. Psyllium-enriched cereals lower blood total cholesterol and LDL cholesterol, but not HDL cholesterol, in hypercholesterolemic adults: results of a meta-analysis. *J Nutr.* 1997;127:1973–1980.

19 Anderson JW. Short-chain fatty acids and lipid metabolism. In: Cummings JH, Rombeau JL, Sakata T, eds. *Physiological and Clinical Aspects of Short Chain Fatty Acids.* New York: Cambridge University Press; 1995:509–523.

20 Hylla S, Gostner A, Dusel G, et al. Effects of resistant starch on the colon in healthy volunteers: possible implications for cancer prevention. *Am J Clin Nutr.* 1998;67:136–142; and Scheppach W, Bartram HP, Richter F. Role of short-chain fatty acids in the prevention of colorectal cancer. *Eur J Cancer.* 1995;31A:1077–1080.

21 Morris ER. Fiber in foods. Loc. cit.

22 Groff JL, Gropper SS, eds. *Advanced Nutrition and Human Metabolism,* 3rd ed. Belmont CA: Wadsworth; 1999.

23 Berdanier CD. *Advanced Nutrition: Macronutrients.* Boca Raton, FL: CRC Press; 1995; and Stryer L. Biochemistry. 4th ed. New York: WH Freeman; 1995.

24 Berdanier CD. Op. cit.

25 Stryer L. Op. cit.

26 Food and Nutrition Board of the National Academy of Sciences, National Research Council. *Recommended Dietary Allowances.* 10th ed. Washington, DC: National Academy Press; 1989.

27 Berdanier CD. Op. cit.

28 Mathews CK, Van Holde KE. Op. cit.

29 Berdanier CD. Op. cit. (see 23)

30 Jenkins DJA, Jenkins AL. The glycemic index, fiber, and the dietary treatment of hypertriglyceridemia and diabetes. *J Am Coll Nutr.* 1987;6:11–17.

31 Read NW, Eastwood MA. Gastrointestinal physiology and function. In: Schweizer TF, Edwards CA, eds. *Dietary Fibre. A Component of Food.* London: Springer-Verlag; 1992:103-117; and Brand-Miller JC. Importance of glycemic index in diabetes. *Am J Clin Nutr.* 1994;59(suppl):747S–752S.

32 Berdanier CD. Op. cit.

33 O'Brien T, Nguyen TT, Zimmerman BR. Hyperlipidemia and diabetes mellitus. *Mayo Clin Proc.* 1998;73:969–976.

34 Anderson JW, Geil PB. Nutritional management of diabetes mellitus. In: Shils ME, Olson JA, Shike M., Ross AC, eds. *Modern Nutrition in Health and Disease.* 9th ed. Philadelphia: Lippincott Williams & Wilkins; 1999:1365–1394.

35 Ibid.

36 Ibid.

37 Franz MJ. Managing obesity in patients with comorbidities. *J Am Diet Assoc.* 1998;98(suppl):S39-S43.; and Burke JP, Haffner SM, Gaskill SP, Williams KL, Stern MP. et al. Reversion from type 2 diabetes to nondiabetic status, influence of the 1997 American Diabetes Association criteria. *Diabetes Care.* 1998;21:1266–1270.

38 Pickup JC, Williams, G, eds. *Textbook of Diabetes.* 2nd ed. Malden, MA, Blackwell Science, Ltd.; 1997.

39 American Diabetes Association. Clinical practice recommendations 1997. *Diabetes Care.* 1997;20(suppl):1044–1045.

40 American Diabetes Association. Op. cit., pp. 1045, 1997.

41 U.S. Department of Health and Human Services. *The Surgeon General's Report on Nutrition and Health.* DHHS (PHS) Publication No. 88-50210. Washington, DC: US Government Printing Office; 1988.

42 Food and Nutrition Board of the National Academy of Sciences, National Research Council. *Recommended Dietary Allowances.* 10th ed. Washington, DC: National Academy Press; 1989.

43 US Departments of Agriculture and Health and Human Services. *Nutrition and Your Health: Dietary Guidelines for Americans.* 5th ed. Home and Garden Bulletin No. 232. Washington, DC: US Government Printing Office; 2000.

44 American Dietetic Association. Position of The American Dietetic Association: Health implications of dietary fiber. *J Am Diet Assoc.* 1997;97:1157–1159.

45 US Department of Agriculture, Agricultural Research Service. *Data Tables: Results from USDA's 1994–96 Continuing Survey of Food Intakes by Individuals and 1994–96 Diet and Health Knowledge Survey.* On: 1994–96 Continuing Survey of Food Intakes by Individuals and 1994096 Diet and Health Knowledge Survey, CD-ROM, NTIS Accession Number PB98-500457; 1997.

46 Ibid.

47 Gurr M. *Nutritional and Health Aspects of Sugars: Evaluation of New Findings.* Washington DC: International Life Sciences Institute; 1995.

48 Glinsmann WH, Park YK. Perspective on the 1986 Food and Drug Administration Assessment of Carbohydrate Sweeteners: Uniform definitions and recommendations for future assessments. *Am J Clin Nutr.* 1995;62(suppl):161S–169S.

49 US Department of Agriculture. *Food Guide Pyramid: A Guide to Daily Food Choices;* Washington, DC: US Government Printing Office; 1992.

50 Giboney M, Sigman-Grant M, Stanton JL, Keast DR. Consumption of sugars. *Am J Clin Nutr.* 1995;62(suppl):178S–194S.

51 Schiffman SS. Aspartame and susceptibility to headache. *New Engl J Med.* 1987;317:1181; and Renwick AG. Acceptable daily intake and the regulation of intense sweeteners. *Food Additive and Contaminants.* 1990;7:463–475.

52 Levine GV, Zehner LR, Saunders JP, Beadle JR. Sugar substitutes: their energy values, bulk characteristics and potential health benefits. *Am J Clin Nutr.* 1990;62(suppl):1161S–1168S.

53 Gurr M. Op. cit.

54 Anderson JW, Smith BS, Gustafson NJ. Health benefits and practical aspects of high-fiber diets. *Am J Clin Nutr.* 1994;59(suppl): 1242S–1247S.

55 Ibid.

56 Burke JP, Haffner SM, Gaskill SP, Williams KL, Stern MP. Reversion from type 2 diabetes to nondiabetic status. Influence of the 1997 American Diabetes Association criteria. *Diabetes Care.* 1998;21:1266–1270.

57 Burn J, Chapman PD, Bishop DT, Mathers J. Diet and cancer prevention: the concerted action polyp prevention (CAPP) studies. *Proc Nutr Soc.* 1998;57:183–186.

58 Slattery ML, Boucher KM, Caan BJ, et al. Eating patterns and risk of colon cancer. *Am J Epidemiol.* 1998;148:4–16.

59 World Health Organization. Op. cit.

60 Fuchs CS, et al. Dietary fiber and the risk of colorectal cancer and adenoma in women. *N Engl J Med.* 1999; 340:169–176.

61 Anderson JW, Smith BS, Gustafson NJ. Op. cit.

62 Anderson JW. Short-chain fatty acids and lipid metabolism. In: Cummings JH, Rombeau JL, Sakata T, eds. *Physiological and Clinical Aspects of Short Chain Fatty Acids.* New York: Cambridge University Press; 1995:509–523.

63 Jacobs DR, Meyer KA, Kushi LH, Folsom AR. Whole-grain intake may reduce the risk of ischemic heart disease death in postmenopausal women: the Iowa Women's Health Study. *Am J Clin Nutr.* 1998;68:248–257.

64 O'Keefe SJ. Nutrition and gastrointestinal disease. *Scand J Gastroenterol.* 1996;220(suppl):52–59.

65 Gordon DT, Stoops D, Ratliff V. Dietary fiber and mineral nutrition. In: Kritchevsky D, Bonfield C, eds. *Dietary Fiber in Health and Disease.* St. Paul, MN: Eagan Press; 1995:267–293.

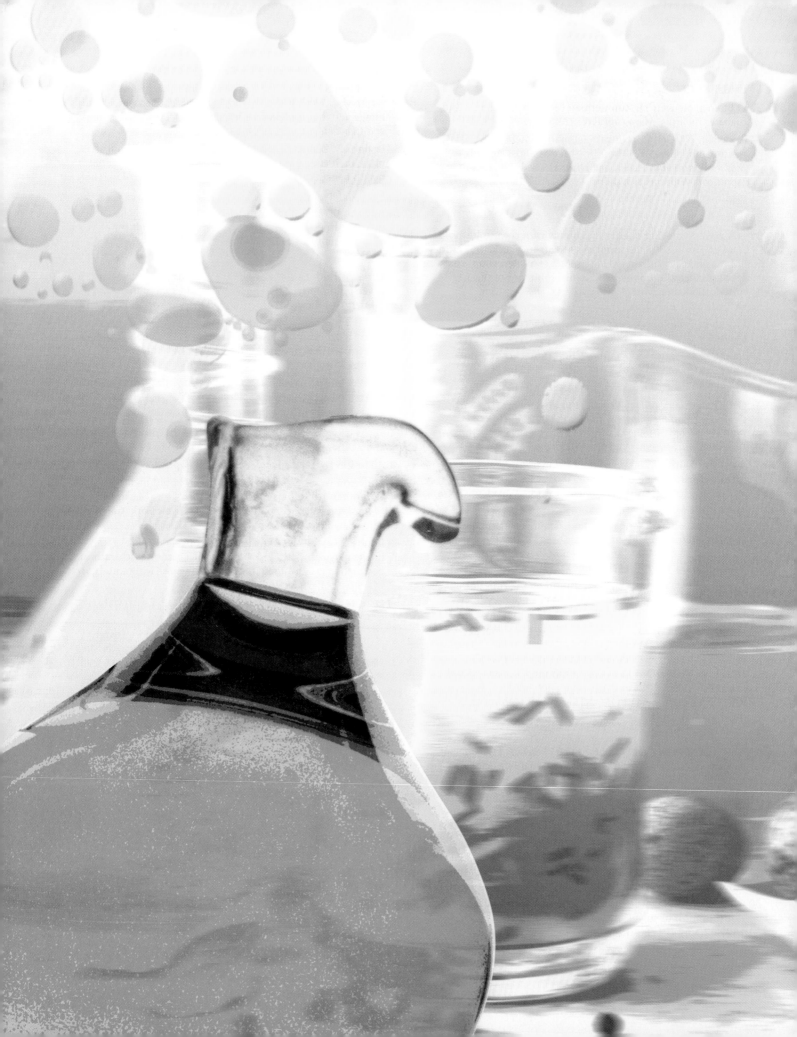

Chapter 5

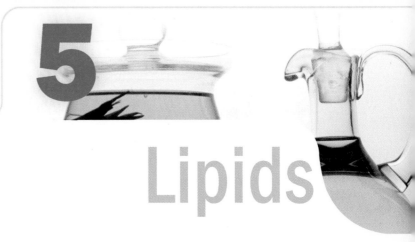

Lipids

Think About It

1 How important is fat to the foods you think of as tasty?

2 Can one have too little body fat?

3 What's your take on the differences between fat and cholesterol?

4 What's your understanding of "good" versus "bad" cholesterol?

Fyi for your Information

This chapter's FYI boxes include practical information on the following topics:

• Fats on the Health Food Store Shelf

• Which Spread for Your Bread?

• Does "Reduced Fat" Reduce Calories? That Depends on the Food

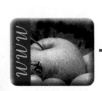

The web site for this book offers many useful tools and is a great source for additional nutrition information for both students and instructors. Visit the site at nutrition.jbpub.com for information on lipids. You'll find exercises that explore the following topics:

• Olestra: Snack Without the Guilt?

• Fat, Low-fat, No Fat?

• Fat Intake and Cancer

• Around the World with Lipids

What About Bobbie?

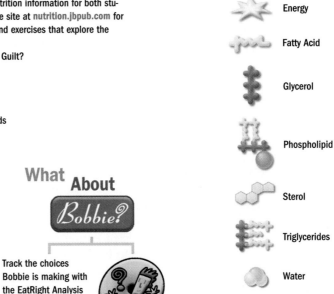

Track the choices Bobbie is making with the EatRight Analysis software.

Key to Illustrations

Chylomicron

Energy

Fatty Acid

Glycerol

Phospholipid

Sterol

Triglycerides

Water

Methyl end   Acid (carboxyl) end

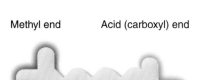

A generic fatty acid

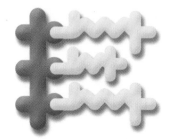

A generic triglyceride

hydrophobic Insoluble in water.

lipophilic Attracted to fat and fat solvents; fat soluble.

hydrophilic [high-dro-FILL-ik] Readily interacting with water (literally, "water-loving"). Hydrophilic compounds are polar and soluble in water.

lipophobic Adverse to fat solvents; insoluble in fat and fat solvents.

phospholipid A compound that consists of a glycerol molecule bonded to two fatty acid molecules and phosphate group with a nitrogen-containing component. Phospholipids have both hydrophilic and hydrophobic regions that make them good emulsifiers.

sterols A category of lipids that includes cholesterol. Sterols are hydrocarbons with several rings in their structures.

fatty acid Compounds containing a long hydrocarbon chain with a carboxyl group (COOH) at one end and a methyl group (CH₃) at the other end.

chain length The number of carbons that a fatty acid contains. Foods contain fatty acids with chain lengths of 4 to 24 carbons, and most have an even number of carbons.

Consider two friends, Maria and Rachel, both on weight-loss diets. Maria swears by a new diet program that allows you to eat all the fat you want, but no high-carbohydrate "starchy" foods, and it's working—she's already lost 10 pounds! Then there's Rachel, whose goal in life is an intake of zero grams of fat. She's fat-obsessed—always buying "fat-free" this or that, and driving her friends nuts with information about the number of fat grams in everything they eat. As you listen to the two of them compare dieting stories, you start to wonder which one has the right approach to fat consumption, or even if there is a right approach. On the one hand, it seems that every day you hear more about Americans' high-fat diets and high rates of obesity and heart disease. On the other hand, is a "no-fat" diet healthy? Are all the low-fat and no-fat products really better choices nutritionally?

Fat is an essential nutrient. Although our bodies are very good at making and storing fat in the form of triglycerides, our bodies cannot make some types of fatty acids (a component of triglycerides) so these must come from the diet. Triglycerides, the fats we associate with fried foods, cream cheese, vegetable oil, and salad dressing, are one type of a larger group of compounds called lipids. Cholesterol, another lipid, is familiar to most Americans, but many people don't realize that their bodies make cholesterol and that dietary cholesterol makes only a small contribution to the total amount in the body. All lipids have important roles, but at the same time, too much triglyceride or too much cholesterol can lead to heart and circulatory problems.

Fats contribute greatly to the flavor and texture of foods. When you take out the fat, sometimes you have to boost the flavor with sugar, sodium, or other additives in order to have a tasty product. This means that fat-free foods sometimes aren't any lower in calories than the regular food—so Rachel can't eat the whole box of fat-free cookies and still expect to lose weight!

Once you have an idea of the role of lipids in the body and in foods, you'll be able to apply the principles of moderation, balance, and variety in selecting a healthful, enjoyable diet with neither too much nor too little fat.

What Are Lipids?

The term *lipids* applies to a broad range of organic molecules that dissolve easily in organic solvents such as alcohol, ether, or acetone, but are much less soluble in water. Lipids generally are **hydrophobic** (averse to water, literally "water fearing") and **lipophilic** (soluble in fat and fat solvents, literally "fat loving"). In contrast, water-soluble substances

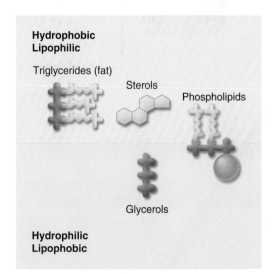

Hydrophobic
Lipophilic

Triglycerides (fat)

Sterols

Phospholipids

Glycerols

Hydrophilic
Lipophobic

are, not surprisingly, **hydrophilic** (attracted to water, "water loving") and **lipophobic** (averse to fat solvents, "fat fearing"). Lipids vary in their solubilities, some being very hydrophobic and others less so. The main classes of lipids found in foods and in the body are triglycerides, phospholipids, and sterols.

Triglycerides are the largest category of lipids. In the body, fat cells store triglycerides in adipose tissue. In foods, we call triglycerides "fats and oils," with fats usually being solid and oils being liquid at room temperature. Overall, however, the choice of terminology—*fat, triglyceride, oil*—is somewhat arbitrary, and the terms are often used interchangeably. In this chapter, when we use the word *fat*, we are referring to *triglycerides*.

About 2 percent of dietary lipids are **phospholipids.** They are found in foods of both plant and animal origin, and the body also makes those that it needs. Unlike other lipids, phospholipids are soluble in both fat and water. These versatile molecules play crucial roles as major constituents in cell membranes, and in blood and body fluids where they help keep fats suspended in these watery fluids.

Only a small percentage of our dietary lipids are **sterols,** yet one infamous member, cholesterol, generates much public concern. The body makes cholesterol, which is an important component of cell membranes and a precursor in the synthesis of sex hormones, adrenal hormones (e.g., cortisol), vitamin D, and bile acids.

Lipids share similar functional properties, solubility, and transport mechanisms although the composition and structure of individual molecules varies. Fatty acids are common components of both triglycerides and phospholipids and are often attached to cholesterol.

Fatty Acids Are Key Building Blocks

Fatty acids determine the characteristics of a fat, such as whether it is solid or liquid at room temperature. Fatty acids that are not joined to another compound, such as the glycerol of a triglyceride, are sometimes called "free" fatty acids, to emphasize that they are unattached. Some free fatty acids have their own distinct flavor. Butyric acid is the fatty acid that gives butter its flavor (see **Figure 5.1**). Caproic, caprylic, and capric acids, all named after the Greek word for goat, have the undesirable "goaty" flavors and odors their names suggest; they may be present as free fatty acids in spoiled foods, contributing to a strong unpleasant odor.

Although there are many kinds of fatty acids, they are basically chains of carbon atoms with an organic acid (carboxyl) group (—COOH) at one end and a methyl group (—CH₃) at the other end.

Chain Length

Fatty acids differ in **chain length** (the number of carbons in the chain). Foods contain fatty acids with chain lengths of 4 to 24 carbons, and most have an even number of carbons. They are grouped as short-chain (< 6 carbons), medium-chain (6–10 carbons), and long-chain (12 or more carbons) fatty acids. (See **Figure 5.2**.) The shorter the carbon chain, the

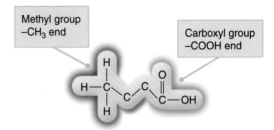

Figure 5.1 **Butyric acid.** Butyric acid is found in butter fat. Like all fatty acids, it has a methyl end (–CH₃) and an acid (carboxyl) end (–COOH).

Methyl group –CH₃ end

Carboxyl group –COOH end

Butyric acid

For simplicity in most of these pictures the hydrogens are omitted from all but the end carbons

Short-chain fatty acid (2-4 carbons)

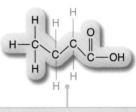

Butyric C4:0

Medium-chain fatty acid (6-10 carbons)

Caprylic C8:0

Long-chain fatty acid (12 or more carbons)

Palmitic C16:0

Figure 5.2 **Fatty acid chain lengths.** Fatty acids can be classified by their chain length as short, medium, long, and very-long chain fatty acids.

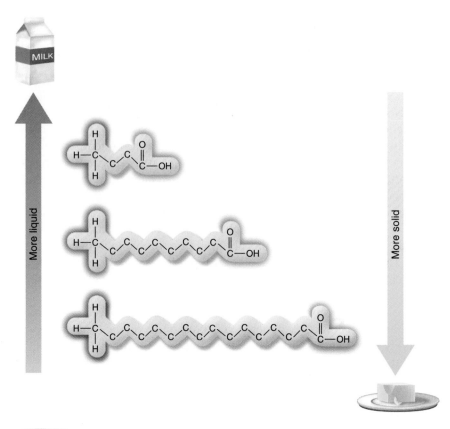

Figure 5.3 **Fatty acid chain lengths and liquidity.** As chain length increases, fatty acids become more solid at room temperature.

Figure 5.4 **Fatty acid nomenclature.** The carbons are identified by their location in the chain. While some disciplines count from the alpha carbon, nutritionists count from the omega carbon.

Methyl (–CH₃) end

Acid (–COOH) end

Omega carbon

Omega end

Alpha end

saturated fatty acid A fatty acid completely filled by hydrogen with all carbons in the chain linked by single bonds.

unsaturated fatty acid The carbon chain contains one or more double bonds. Hydrogen, oxygen, or some other atom can attach easily to a double bond.

monounsaturated fatty acid The carbon chain contains one double bond.

polyunsaturated fatty acid The carbon chain contains two or more double bonds.

more liquid the fatty acid (the lower its melting point). (See **Figure 5.3.**) Shorter fatty acids are also more water-soluble, a property that affects their absorption in the digestive tract.

Each carbon in these chains can be numbered for identification, but it's important to know from which end the counting begins. In organic chemistry, the scientific naming of fatty acids counts from the carbon at the acid (—COOH) end. This carbon is the *alpha* carbon, and the carbon at the methyl (—CH₃) end is the *omega* carbon. They are named after the first and last letters of the Greek alphabet, respectively (See **Figure 5.4.**). Nutritionists identify double-bond locations by their location relative to the omega carbon, as you'll see later.

Saturation

Within a fatty acid chain, each carbon atom has four bonds. When a carbon is joined to adjacent carbons with single bonds (—C—C—C—), it still has two bonds available for other atoms, such as hydrogen atoms. If all the carbons in the chain are joined with single bonds and the remaining bonds are filled with hydrogen, the fatty acid is called a **saturated fatty acid.** It is fully loaded (saturated) with hydrogen.

However, if adjoining carbons are connected by a double bond (C=C), there are two fewer bonds holding hydrogen, so the chain is not saturated with hydrogen. This is an **unsaturated fatty acid.** A fatty acid with one double bond is a **monounsaturated fatty acid (MUFA);** one with two or more double bonds is a **polyunsaturated fatty acid (PUFA). Figure 5.5** illustrates the three types of fatty acids.

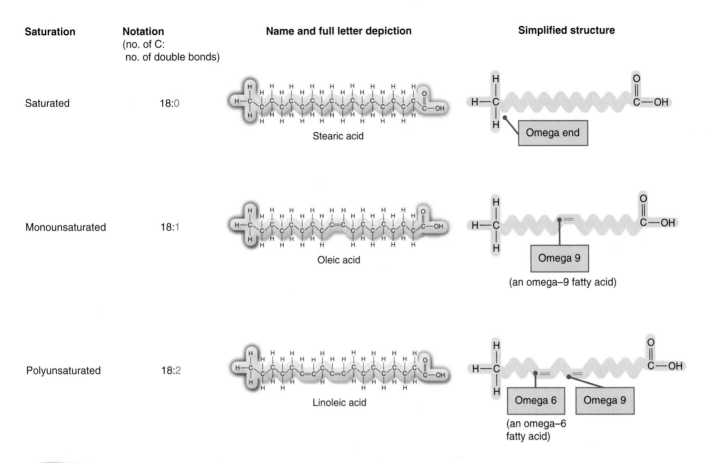

Saturation	Notation (no. of C: no. of double bonds)	Name and full letter depiction	Simplified structure
Saturated	18:0	Stearic acid	Omega end
Monounsaturated	18:1	Oleic acid	Omega 9 (an omega–9 fatty acid)
Polyunsaturated	18:2	Linoleic acid	Omega 6 Omega 9 (an omega–6 fatty acid)

Figure 5.5 **Saturated, monosaturated, and polyunsaturated fatty acids.** Hydrogens saturate the carbon chain of a saturated fatty acid. Unsaturated fatty acids are missing some hydrogens and have one (mono) or more (poly) carbon-carbon double bonds.

Foods never contain only unsaturated or only saturated fatty acids. Food fats are a mixture of fatty acid types, so it is technically wrong to refer to a particular food fat as a "saturated fat." However, food fats with more unsaturated fatty acids typically have a lower melting point and are more likely to be liquid at room temperature. Foods rich in saturated fatty acids tend to be solid at room temperature and have a higher melting point. (See **Figure 5.6.**) For example, the 18-carbon saturated fatty acid, stearic acid, is abundant in chocolate and meat fats, both of which are solid at room temperature. The major fatty acid of olive oil is 18-carbon monounsaturated oleic acid. Olive oil is a thick liquid at room temperature, but may solidify under refrigeration. The major fatty acid of soybean oil is an 18-carbon fatty acid with two double bonds called linoleic acid, and soybean oil is a thin liquid at room temperature. And 18-carbon *alpha*-linolenic acid, a fatty acid with three double bonds, is abundant in flaxseed oil, a very thin liquid at room temperature.

Key Concepts: *The term lipids refers to a group of organic molecules that are soluble in organic solvents, and less soluble in water, including triglycerides, phospholipids, and sterols. Fatty acids are key structural components of both triglycerides and phospholipids, and are sometimes attached to cholesterol. Fatty acids are carbon chains of various lengths. Fatty acids with no double bonds between carbon atoms are called saturated, while those with at least one double bond are unsaturated fatty acids.*

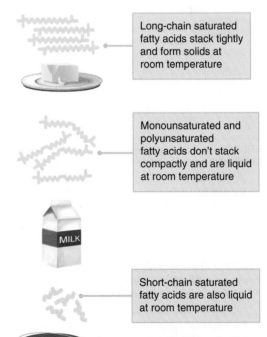

Long-chain saturated fatty acids stack tightly and form solids at room temperature

Monounsaturated and polyunsaturated fatty acids don't stack compactly and are liquid at room temperature

Short-chain saturated fatty acids are also liquid at room temperature

Figure 5.6 **Liquid or solid at room temperature?** Short-chain and unsaturated fatty acids cannot pack tightly together and tend to be more liquid than long-chain saturated fatty acids.

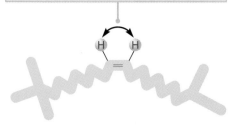

These two neighboring hydrogens repel each other, causing the carbon chain to bend

Cis form (bent)

These two hydrogens are already as far apart as they can get

Trans form (straighter)

Figure 5.7 *Cis-* and *trans-* fatty acids. Fatty acids with the bent *cis* form are more common in food than the *trans* form. Trans fatty acids are most commonly found in hydrogentated fats, such as those in stick margarine, shortening and deep-fat fried foods.

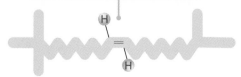

Geometric and Positional Isomers

Otherwise identical unsaturated fatty acids can exist in different geometric forms, or isomers. In most naturally occurring unsaturated fatty acids, the hydrogens next to double bonds are on the same side of the carbon chain. This is called a *cis* formation. The carbon chain of a *cis* **fatty acid** is bent. If the double bond is altered, moving the hydrogens across from each other, the formation is called *trans* and the carbon chain is straighter. (See **Figure 5.7.**) There are small amounts of *trans* **fatty acids** in cow's milk, but the commercial process of **hydrogenation,** adding hydrogens where some of the double bonds are located in the unsaturated fatty acid, creates most of our dietary trans fatty acids. Most trans fatty acids are monounsaturated, but a small number are fatty acids with two double bonds. *Trans* fatty acids have become a health concern because they have been implicated in raising blood cholesterol levels.

The position of double bonds also can move during commercial hydrogenation and during milk production by dairy cattle. Although present in only trace amounts in cow's milk, the positional isomer called **conjugated linoleic acid** (CLA) is being studied for potential positive health effects.

Omega-3, Omega-6, and Omega-9 Fatty Acids

The location of the double bond closest to the omega (methyl) end of the fatty acid chain identifies a fatty acid's family. Oleic acid has one double bond, at carbon 9 (counting from the omega end of the chain) and is classified as an **omega-9 fatty acid.** Linoleic acid has double bonds at carbon-6 and carbon-9 but is an **omega-6 fatty acid,** because the first double bond occurs at carbon 6. **Omega-3 fatty acids** such as alpha-linolenic acid have a double bond at carbon 3, plus two or more double bonds. (See **Figure 5.8.**) All of these fatty acids can be burned for energy. However, when the body uses them to synthesize new compounds, the omega-3, omega-6, and omega-9 classes behave quite differently.

Nonessential and Essential Fatty Acids

The body is a good chemist, synthesizing most fatty acids as it needs them. The liver adds carbons in a process called **elongation** to build storage and structural fats, to manufacture the fat in breast milk, or to make fatty acids

cis fatty acids The hydrogens surrounding a double bond are both on the same side of the carbon chain, causing a bend in the chain. Most naturally occurring unsaturated fatty acids are cis fatty acids.

trans fatty acids In trans fatty acids, the hydrogens surrounding a double bond are on opposite sides of the carbon chain. The bent carbon chain straightens out, and the fatty acid becomes more solid.

hydrogenation [high-dro-jen-AY-shun] A chemical reaction in which hydrogen atoms are added to carbon-carbon double bonds, converting them to single bonds. Hydrogenation of monounsaturated and polyunsaturated fatty acids reduces the number of double bonds they contain, thereby making them more saturated.

conjugated linoleic acid A polyunsaturated fatty acid in which the position of the double bonds has moved, so that a single bond alternates with two double bonds.

omega-9 fatty acid Any polyunsaturated fatty acid in which the first double bond starting from the methyl (CH_3) end of the molecule lies between the 9th and 10th carbon atoms.

omega-6 fatty acid Any polyunsaturated fatty acid in which the first double bond starting from the methyl (CH_3) end of the molecule lies between the 6th and 7th carbon atoms.

omega-3 fatty acid Any polyunsaturated fatty acid in which the first double bond starting from the methyl (CH_3) end of the molecule lies between the 3rd and 4th carbon atoms.

elongation Addition of carbon atoms to fatty acids to lengthen them into new fatty acids.

desaturation Insertion of double bonds into fatty acids to change them into new fatty acids.

nonessential fatty acid The fatty acids that your body can make when they are needed. It is not necessary to consume them in the diet.

essential fatty acids Those the body needs but cannot synthesize, and which must be obtained from diet.

eicosanoids A class of hormone-like substances formed in the body from long-chain fatty acids.

for use in other compounds. The body also synthesizes oleic acid, an omega-9 fatty acid, by removing hydrogens from carbons 9 and 10 of saturated stearic acid, thus creating a double bond at carbon 9. This process is called **desaturation.** Oleic acid can be elongated further and desaturated to create other necessary fatty acids.

Because your body can make saturated and omega-9 fatty acids, it is not essential to get them in your diet. We therefore call them **nonessential fatty acids.** (Do not confuse "nonessential" with "unimportant." Your body ensures an adequate supply of nonessential fatty acids by making them when they are needed.)

Our bodies cannot produce carbon-carbon double bonds before the ninth carbon from the methyl end, so we cannot manufacture certain fatty acids such as omega-6 linoleic or omega-3 alpha-linolenic acids. They must come from food, so they're called **essential fatty acids (EFA).** (See **Figure 5.9.**)

Building Eicosanoids, Omega-3 and Omega-6 Fatty Acids

You metabolize most of the fatty acids you eat to supply your energy needs, but a small proportion become crucial chemical regulators. The **eicosanoids** (also called prostanoids) are one such group of regulators. These signaling molecules are called eicosanoids because they contain 20 or more carbons (*eikosi* is the Greek word for "twenty"). They have profound localized effects through their influence on inflammatory processes, blood vessel dilation and constriction, blood clotting, and more. Because they don't circulate through the body as hormones do, scientists sometimes call eicosanoids "local" hormones. Eicosanoids were first identified in the 1960s and their chemistry is a relatively new area of research.[1]

Eicosanoids are made from unsaturated long-chain fatty acids from membrane phospholipids or circulating free fatty acids. The liver elongates these fatty acids 2 carbons at a time until the carbon chains have 20 or 22 carbons. Elongation alternates with desaturation. Once the fatty acid reaches

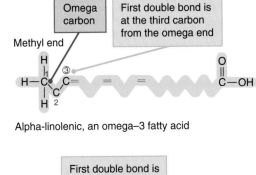

Alpha-linolenic, an omega–3 fatty acid

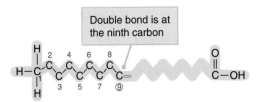

Linoleic, an omega–6 fatty acid

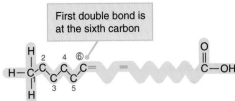

Oleic, an omega–9 fatty acid

Figure 5.8 **Omega-3, omega-6, and omega-9 fatty acids.** Unsaturated fatty acids can be classified by counting from the omega carbon to the location of the first double bond.

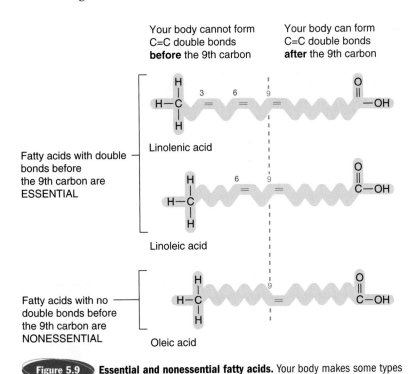

Figure 5.9 **Essential and nonessential fatty acids.** Your body makes some types of fatty acids, but others are essential in your diet.

Table 5.1 Omega-6 to Eicosanoids

Linoleic acid	**(18:2)**
desaturation	
Gamma-linolenic acid	(18:3)
elongation	
Dihomo-gamma-linolenic acid	(20:3)
desaturation	
Arachidonic acid	(20:4)
elongation	
Eicosanoids	**(22:4)**

- thromboxanes
- prostaglandins
- leukotrienes

Table 5.2 Omega-3 to Eicosanoids

Alpha-linolenic acid	**(18:3)**
desaturation	
	(18:4)
elongation	
	(20:4)
desaturation	
EPA (eicosapentaenoic acid)	(20:5)
elongation	
Eicosanoids	**(22:5)**

- thromboxanes
- prostaglandins
- leukotrienes

desaturation	
DHA (docosahexaenoic acid)	(22:6)

linoleic acid [lin-oh-LAY-ik] An essential omega-6 fatty acid that contains 18 carbon atoms and 2 carbon-carbon double bonds (18:2).

alpha-linolenic acid [Al-fah-lin-oh-LEN-ik] An essential omega-3 fatty acid that contains 18 carbon atoms and 3 carbon-carbon double bonds (18:3).

glycerol [GLISS-er-ol] An alcohol that contains 3 carbon atoms, each of which has an attached hydroxyl group (OH). It forms the backbone of mono-, di-, and triglycerides.

20 carbons, the body can convert it to one or more of the eicosanoids, such as thromboxanes, prostaglandins, prostacyclins, lipoxins, and leukotrienes. Eicosanoids can have opposing physiologic effects depending on whether they are derived from an omega-3, omega-6, or omega-9 fatty acid. Here, we will concentrate on eicosanoids derived from the essential fatty acids, that is, from the omega-3s and omega-6s, over which we probably have the most dietary control and where most interest currently lies.

The omega-6s: **Linoleic acid,** an 18-carbon essential fatty acid with two double bonds (18:2), is our main dietary omega-6 fatty acid. In a sequence of elongation and desaturation steps, our bodies convert linoleic acid to arachidonic acid, a 20-carbon fatty acid with 4 double bonds (20:4). To simplify a very complex picture, a series of eicosanoids are then formed from arachidonic acid, and these eicosanoids have the overall effect of constricting blood vessels, promoting blood clotting, and promoting inflammation. (See **Table 5.1.**)

The omega-3s: **Alpha-linolenic acid** is an 18-carbon essential fatty acid with 3 double bonds (18:3). It can ultimately be elongated and desaturated to EPA (eicosapentaenoic acid), with 20 carbons and 5 double bonds (20:5), and DHA (docosahexaenoic acid) with 22 carbons and 6 double bonds (22:6). However, for these reactions to take place, it must compete with the omega-6s (and even with polyunsaturated *trans* fatty acids) for the same enzymes, so only a portion of alpha-linolenic acid is converted to EPA and DHA. The eicosanoids derived from EPA have the overall effect of dilating blood vessels, discouraging blood clotting, and reducing inflammation. (See **Table 5.2.**) Because of these properties, omega-3 fatty acids have gained interest as a potential factor in reducing risk for vascular disease.[2]

Key Concepts: *Unsaturated fatty acids can have cis or trans double bonds. The body can make many of the fatty acids it needs, but cannot make linoleic or alpha-linolenic acids, so these are dietary essentials. The body can elongate and desaturate essential fatty acids to form other important compounds such as eicosanoids.*

Triglycerides

Triglycerides are the major lipid in both the diet and the body. Triglycerides add flavor and texture (and calories!) to foods and are an important source of the body's energy.

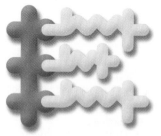

A generic triglyceride

Triglyceride Structure

A triglyceride is three fatty acids attached to a molecule of glycerol. Both in food and in the body, most fatty acids exist as part of a triglyceride molecule. Alone, **glycerol** is a thick, smooth liquid often used in the food industry. Chemically it is an alcohol, a simple 3-carbon molecule with an alcohol (hydroxyl) group (—OH) at each carbon. Glycerol is the backbone of a triglyceride. It is always the same, whereas the fatty acids attached to it can vary considerably. Chemically speaking, a triglyceride is an **ester,** a combination of an alcohol and a fatty acid. An ester forms when a hydrogen and an oxygen from the fatty acid's carboxyl (acid) group combine with a hydrogen

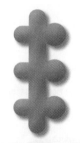

A generic glycerol

from the alcohol's hydroxyl (alcohol) group. This is called a condensation reaction because it produces a molecule of water. The altered fatty acid and alcohol are now chemically joined by an ester linkage. The process itself is called **esterification.**

Esterification produces triglycerides, **diglycerides**—two fatty acids attached to a glycerol, and **monoglycerides**—one fatty acid attached to glycerol. **Figure 5.10** illustrates the formation of a triglyceride. Our foods contain relatively small amounts of mono- and diglycerides, mostly as food additives used for their emulsifying or blending qualities.

Triglyceride Functions

Although some of us, like Rachel at the beginning of this chapter, think of fat as something to avoid, fat is a key nutrient with important body functions. **Figure 5.11** shows the functions of triglycerides.

Energy Source

Fat is a rich and efficient source of calories. Under normal circumstances, dietary and stored fat supply about 60 percent of the body's resting energy needs. Like carbohydrate, fat is *protein-sparing;* that is, fat is burned for energy, sparing valuable proteins for their important roles as muscle tissue, enzymes, antibodies, and other functions. Different body tissues preferentially use different sources of calories. Glucose is virtually the sole fuel for the brain except during prolonged starvation, and fat is the preferred fuel of muscle tissue at rest (see **Figure 5.12**). During physical activity, glucose and glycogen join fat in supplying energy.

High-fat foods are higher in calories than high-protein or high-carbohydrate foods. One gram of fat contains 9 kilocalories, compared to only 4 kilocalories in a gram of carbohydrate or protein, or 7 kilocalories per gram of alcohol. For example, a tablespoon of corn oil (pure fat) has 120 kilocalories while a tablespoon of sugar (pure carbohydrate) has only 50 kilocalories.

Fat's caloric density is especially important when energy needs are high. An infant, for example, who needs ample energy for fast growth, but whose

ester A chemical combination of an organic acid (e.g., fatty acid) and an alcohol. When hydrogen from the alcohol combines with the acid's hydrogen and oxygen, water is released and an ester linkage is formed. A triglyceride is an ester of three fatty acids and glycerol.

esterification [e-ster-ih-fih-KAY-shun] A condensation reaction in which an organic acid (e.g., fatty acid) combines with an alcohol with the loss of water, creating an ester.

diglyceride A molecule of glycerol combined with two fatty acids.

monoglyceride A molecule of glycerol combined with one fatty acid.

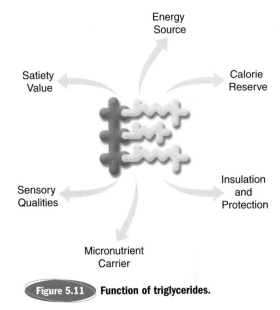

Figure 5.11 Function of triglycerides.

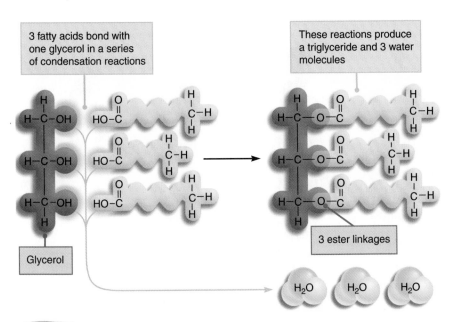

Figure 5.10 **Forming a triglyceride.** Condensation reactions attach three fatty acids to a glycerol backbone to form a triglyceride. These reactions release water.

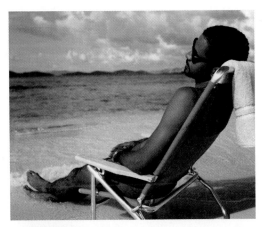

Figure 5.12 **Fat is a potent energy source.** Fat is your muscle's preferred fuel when at rest.

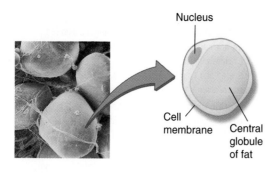

Nucleus

Cell membrane

Central globule of fat

Figure 5.13 **Fat is an efficient storage medium.** Evolution has selected fat, rather than glycogen, as its primary energy storage medium. A gram of fat stores more than six times as much energy as a gram of glycogen. If a 155 pound man (with 20 pounds of fat) could store all his energy reserves as glycogen and none as fat, he would weigh 255 pounds!

adipocyte A fat cell.

adipose tissue Body fat tissue.

visceral fat Fat stores that cushion body organs.

subcutaneous fat Fat stores under the skin.

lanugo [lah-NEW-go] Soft, downy hair that covers a normal fetus from the fifth month but is shed almost entirely by the time of birth. It also appears on semi-starved individuals who have lost much of their body fat, serving as insulation normally provided by body fat.

bioavailability A measure of the degree to which a nutrient becomes available to the body after ingestion and thus is available to the tissues.

lycopene One of a family of plant chemicals, the carotenoids. Others in this big family are alpha-carotene and beta-carotene.

stomach can hold only a limited amount of food, needs the high fat content of breast milk or infant formula to get enough calories. When inappropriately put on a low-fat diet, infants and young children do not grow and develop properly. Other people with high energy needs are athletes, those who are physically active in their jobs, or people regaining weight lost due to illness.

Of course, fat's caloric density has a negative side. In practical terms, 9 kilocalories per gram translates to about 115 to 120 kilocalories per tablespoon of pure fat (e.g., vegetable oil). That makes it very easy to get too many fat calories, and dietary fat in excess of a person's energy needs is a major contributor to obesity.

Energy Reserve

We store excess dietary fat as body fat to tide us over periods of caloric deficit. Fat's caloric density comes in handy for this task, storing energy away in a small space. The fat is stored inside fat cells called **adipocytes,** which form body fat tissue, technically called **adipose tissue.** (See **Figure 5.13.**) Hibernating animals have perfected this process; the fat stores they build in autumn can see them through a winter's fast.

The body possesses complex mechanisms for freeing triglycerides and fatty acids and delivering them when and where they are needed for energy. Cells then break down these lipids to release energy stored in their chemical bonds.

Insulation and Protection

Fat tissue accounts for about 15 to 30 percent of a person's body weight. Part of this is **visceral fat,** adipose tissue around organs that remains relatively inert until called upon to release stored energy. Meanwhile, it serves an important function by cushioning and shielding delicate organs, especially the kidneys. Women have extra fat, most noticeably in the breasts and hips, to help shield reproductive organs and to guarantee adequate calories during pregnancy. Other fat tissue is **subcutaneous,** lying under the skin, where it protects and insulates the body. Perhaps nowhere is fat's structural role more dramatic than in the brain, which is 60 percent fat.[3] **Figure 5.14** shows the primary areas of fat storage in women and men.

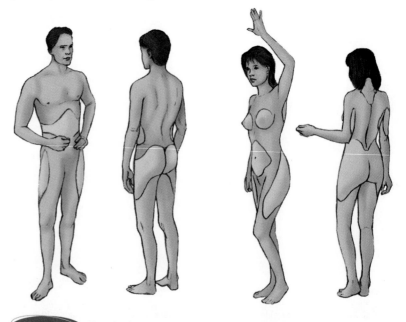

Figure 5.14 **Sites for fat storage differ for men and women.**

Can one have too little body fat? Just ask someone whose body fat has been depleted by illness. It hurts to sit and it hurts to lie down. For people without enough body fat, cool temperatures are intolerable and even room temperature may be uncomfortably cool. Women stop menstruating and become infertile. Children stop growing. Skin deteriorates from pressure sores or from fatty acid deficiency and may become covered with fine hair called **lanugo.** Illness, involuntary starvation, and famine can deplete fat to this extent, as can excessive dieting and exercise.

Carrier of Fat-Soluble Compounds

As you can see in **Figure 5.15,** dietary fats dissolve and transport micronutrients such as fat-soluble vitamins and fat-soluble phytochemicals like carotenoids. Phytochemicals, although not essential (their lack will not cause a deficiency disease), have emerged as contributors to optimal health.

Dietary fats carry other fat-soluble substances through the digestive process, improving their intestinal absorption or **bioavailability.**[4] For example, the body absorbs more **lycopene,** the healthful red-colored phytochemical in tomatoes, if the tomatoes are served with oil or salad dressing. People who suffer from fat malabsorption disorders risk deficiency of fat-soluble micronutrients, so many must use supplements.

Removing a food's lipid portion—for example, removing butterfat from milk—also removes fat-soluble vitamins. In the case of most dairy products, vitamin A is usually replaced. But the natural vitamin E of whole wheat (vitamin E is in the germ) is not replaced after the lipid-rich germ portion of wheat grain is removed during refinement to white flour. Fat-soluble vitamins may be destroyed in fat processing; for example, some vitamin E is lost in processing vegetable oils.

Sensory Qualities

As a food component or as an ingredient, fat contributes greatly to the flavor, odor, and texture of food (see **Figure 5.16**). Simply put, it makes food taste good. Flavorful volatile chemicals are dissolved in the fat of a food; heat sends them into the air, producing mouth-watering odors that pique appetites. Fats have a rich, satisfying feeling in the mouth. In liquid form, they're uniquely efficient at stimulating taste buds.[5] Fats make baked goods tender and moist. And fats can be heated to high temperatures for frying, which seals in flavors and cooks food quickly. These are all good qualities, but too good for many people who find high-fat foods irresistible and eat too much of them. Alas, fat's most appealing attributes are also serious drawbacks to maintaining a healthful diet.

Triglycerides in Food

Dietary triglycerides are found in a variety of fats and oils, and in foods that contain them such as salad dressing or baked goods. Some food fats are obvious, such as butter, margarine, cooking oil, and fat along a cut of meat or under the skin of chicken. Other food fats are found in baked goods, snack foods, nuts, and seeds.

Fats and oils are complex mixtures, but we often categorize them simplistically by their saturation—saturated, monounsaturated, or polyunsaturated—

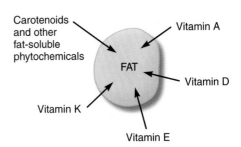

Figure 5.15 **Fat is a micronutrient carrier.** Fat holds more than just energy. It also carries important nutrients, such as fat-soluble vitamins and carotenoids.

Quick Bites

The Marvelous Storage Efficiency of Fat

Why do you think we don't store all our extra energy as readily available glycogen? It would take more than six pounds of glycogen to store the same energy as one pound of fat. Just imagine how much bulkier we would be! How cumbersome it would be to move about! That's why only a very small portion of the body's energy reserve is glycogen.

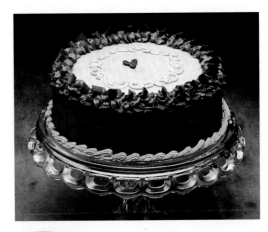

Figure 5.16 Fat imparts a rich, sensory quality to food.

SATURATED FATS AND OILS

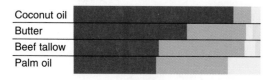

Coconut oil
Butter
Beef tallow
Palm oil

MONOUNSATURATED OILS

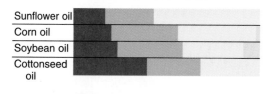

Olive oil
Canola oil
Peanut oil
Safflower oil

POLYUNSATURATED OILS

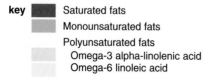

Sunflower oil
Corn oil
Soybean oil
Cottonseed oil

key
Saturated fats
Monounsaturated fats
Polyunsaturated fats
Omega-3 alpha-linolenic acid
Omega-6 linoleic acid

Figure 5.17 **The diversity of fats.**
Source: Adapted from *Nutrition Today*, 31(3) May/June 1996.

depending on their overall fatty acid content. (See **Figure 5.17**.) Canola oil, for example, is often classified as a monounsaturated fat, since its fatty acids are mostly monounsaturated oleic acid; however, 10 percent of its fatty acids are the essential alpha-linolenic acid. While these classifications are useful, they do not always tell the whole story. For example, saturated stearic acid appears to affect blood cholesterol differently from saturated palmitic acid. As we've seen, omega-3 and omega-6 fatty acids also behave differently in the body, even though both classes are polyunsaturated. Their food sources often differ as well.

Sources of Omega-3 Fatty Acid

Generally 18-carbon polyunsaturated fatty acids are found in plant foods. Soybean oil, canola oil, and walnuts are contributors of alpha-linolenic acid, the essential omega-3 fatty acid. However, the most generous source is flaxseed (or linseed) oil, which is more than 50 percent alpha-linolenic. The longer chain omega-3s, EPA and DHA are found in fatty fish (e.g., salmon, tuna, and mackerel) and in fish oil supplements. These should not be taken without medical supervision because of their potent effects;[6] see the FYI feature "Fats on the Health Store Shelf."

Sources of Omega-6 Fatty Acid

Good sources of the 18-carbon, omega-6 fatty acid linoleic acid include seeds, nuts, and the richest source, common vegetable oils. Arachidonic acid, a 20-carbon omega-6 fatty acid, found in some meats, is less common. **Table 5.3** lists the omega-3 fatty acids in some foods.

Table 5.3 **Omega-3 Fatty Acids in Selected Foods**

	18:3 (mg)	20:5 (EPA) (mg)	22:6 (DHA) (mg)
1 tbsp canola oil	1,302		
1 tbsp soybean oil	925		
1 tbsp walnut oil	1,414		
2 tbsp wheat germ	104		
3 oz beef brisket	306		
3 oz canned sockeye salmon (fatty fish)		418	564
3 oz cooked mackerel (fatty fish)		555	1,016
3 oz flounder (lean fish)		207	219
3 oz cooked shrimp		145	122
1 tbsp cod liver oil		938	1,492
1 tbsp salmon oil		1,771	2,480

Fish and seafood also contain small amounts of 18:3, which are not included on this table.

It sounds like a lot of omega-3. But remember, these are milligrams! Dietary fat is usually measured in grams. The 267 milligrams (0.267 g) of EPA and DHA in a serving of shrimp is not much in relation to a diet that has 50+ grams of fat and is a bit less than half the recommendation for daily intake.

Sources: Based on data from US Department of Agriculture, Agricultural Research Service, 1998. USDA Nutrient Database for Standard Reference. Release 13 November 1999; and Kris-Etherton PM, Taylor DS, Yu-Poth S, et al. Polyunsaturated fatty acids in the food chain in the United States. Am J Clin Nutr. 2000;71(suppl):179S–188S.

Commercial Processing of Fats

In nature, almost all fats exist in combination with other macronutrients: they generally occur along with starches in plant foods, and with proteins in animal foods. In earlier times, the only concentrated fats and oils available to people were obtained by very simple processing: rendering fats from meats and poultry; skimming or churning the butterfat from milk; skimming the oil from ground nuts; or pressing a few oil-rich plant parts such as coconuts or olives.

Technology that came into use in the 1920s allowed production of pure vegetable oils.[7] By efficiently removing edible oil from its source, processing has increased the availability of calories worldwide. Processing reduces waste and prevents spoilage during normal use and storage. It does that by inhibiting the destructive processes of hydrolysis and oxidation.

Hydrolysis Products that contain unrefined fats and oils also contain enzymes that hydrolyze oil by splitting fatty acids from triglycerides. Free fatty acids then perpetuate the damaging hydrolysis. Refining destroys the hydrolytic enzymes and removes most free fatty acids.

Oxidation When an unsaturated fat comes in contact with air, oxygen atoms can attach at each of its double-bond sites. The result is oxidative rancidity. Oxidized fats damage body tissues, particularly blood vessels,[8] but fortunately people avoid these bad-tasting rancid fats.

The more unsaturated an oil (the more double bonds it has), the more vulnerable it is to **oxidation.** Oxidation is speeded by light and by small amounts of metals, which are typically removed during refining. Naturally occurring vitamin E inhibits oxidation, and that's why it and other antioxidants are often added to oils.

oxidation Oxygen attaches to the double bonds of unsaturated fatty acids. Rancid fats are oxidized fats.

Unfortunately, processing also has a negative side. To achieve stability and uniform taste, potentially healthful phospholipids, plant sterols, and other phytochemicals are removed, and a significant portion of the natural vitamin E is lost. Oils have become so familiar that we often forget they are highly processed, highly refined foods. Further processing of oils into solid fats such as margarine or shortening also produces some undesirable changes.

Hydrogenation To get a liquid vegetable oil to act like a solid fat, it must be at least partially hydrogenated. Hydrogenation involves breaking some of the double bonds in unsaturated fatty acids and adding hydrogen. This process produces a harder, more saturated fat, one that is more effective for making baked goods and snack foods, and one that spreads like butter. (Most of us recoil at the thought of putting pure corn oil on toast!) While hydrogenation protects the fat from oxidation and rancidity, it also changes some of the double bonds in the fat's structure to the trans configuration. This, combined with the increase in saturated fatty acids has led many to wonder if margarine is indeed a better alternative to butter. (See the FYI feature "Which Spread for Your Bread?")

Key Concepts: *Triglycerides are formed when a glycerol molecule combines with three fatty acids. Dietary triglycerides add texture and flavor to food and are a concentrated source of calories. The body stores excess calories as adipose tissue. While storing energy, adipose tissue also insulates the body and cushions its organs. The fats in food carry valuable fat-soluble nutrients into the body and help with their absorption.*

phosphate group A chemical group (−PO₄) on a larger molecule, where the phosphorus is single bonded to each of the 4 oxygens, and the other bond of one of the oxygens is attached to the rest of the molecule. Often hydrogen atoms are attached to the oxygens. Sometimes there are double bonds between the phosphorus and an oxygen.

Phospholipids

Phospholipids are similar to triglycerides in that they contain both glycerol and fatty acids. However, important differences in their structure make phospholipids entirely different in terms of function. Phospholipids are synthesized by the body and not needed in the diet.

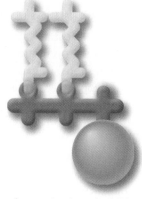

A generic phospholipid

Phospholipid Structure

Phospholipids have a chemical structure similar to that of triglycerides, except one of the fatty acids is replaced by another compound. Phospholipids are diglycerides—two fatty acids attached to a glycerol backbone. A **phosphate group** with a nitrogen-containing component occupies the third attachment site.

The phosphate/nitrogen component of phospholipids is hydrophilic, so a phospholipid's structure makes it compatible with both fat and water: fats are attracted to the fatty acids in its diglyceride area, while the phosphate and its attachment attract water-soluble substances. **Figure 5.18** shows the structure of a phospholipid.

Phospholipid Functions

Because they have both hydrophobic and hydrophilic regions, phospholipids are ideal emulsifiers (compounds that help keep fats suspended in a water-soluble environment) and are often used in foods to keep oil and water mixed. This same property makes phospholipids a perfect structural element for cell membranes—able to communicate with the watery environments of blood and cell fluids, yet with a lipid portion that allows other lipids to enter and exit cells.

Cell Membranes

Phospholipids are major components of cell membranes. Cell membranes are a double layer of phospholipids that selectively allow both fatty and water-soluble substances into the cell. (See **Figure 5.19**.) They also provide

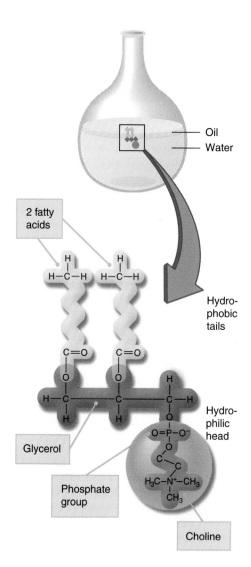

Figure 5.18 **Phospholipid.** A phospholipid is soluble in both oil and water.

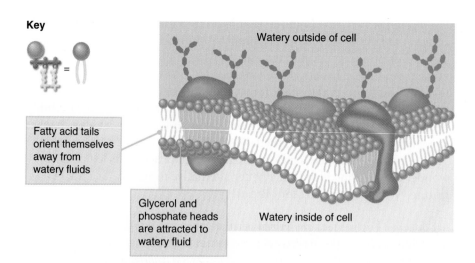

Figure 5.19 **Cell membranes are phospholipid bilayers.** Although proteins and other substances are embedded in cell membranes, these membranes primarily consist of phospholipids.

a temporary store of fatty acids, donating them for short-term energy needs or for synthesis into regulatory chemicals (e.g., eicosanoids). Phosphatidylcholine (a phospholipid), whose **choline** is the precursor to the major neurotransmitter acetylcholine, plays an especially important role in nerve cells. By keeping fatty acids, choline, and other biologically active substances bound in phospholipids and freeing them only as needed, the body is able to regulate them closely.

Lipid Transport

The ability of phospholipids to combine both fatty and water-soluble substances comes in handy throughout the body. In the stomach, dietary phospholipids help break fats into tiny particles for easier digestion. In the intestine, phospholipids from bile continue emulsifying. And in the fluid environment of blood, phospholipids coat the surface of the lipoproteins that carry lipid particles to their destinations in the body.

Emulsifiers (Lecithins)

In the body and in foods of animal origin, phosphatidylcholine is also called **lecithin.** However, for food additives or supplements, the term *lecithin* is used for a mix of phospholipids derived from plants (usually soybeans). Understandably, this inconsistent terminology has caused confusion.

Lecithins are used by the food industry as emulsifiers to combine two ingredients that don't ordinarily mix, such as oil and water. (See **Figure 5.20.**) In high-fat powdered products (e.g., dry milk, milk replacers, and coffee creamers), lecithins help to mix hydrophobic compounds with water. Lecithins in salad dressing, chili, and sloppy-joe mixes increase dispersion and reduce fat separation. Lecithin is even added to chewing gum to increase shelf-life, prolong flavor release, and prevent the gum from sticking to teeth and dental work.

Phospholipids in Food

Phospholipids occur naturally throughout the plant and animal world, although in small amounts relative to triglycerides. They are most abundant in egg yolks, liver, soybeans, and peanuts. Naturally occurring phospholipids are often lost when foods are processed, but other phospholipids are

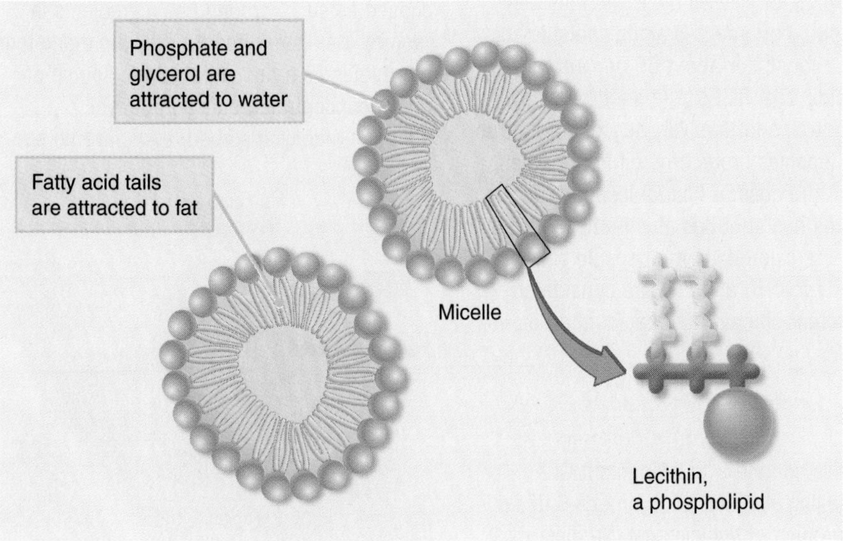

choline A nitrogen-containing compound that is part of the phospholipid lecithin. Choline is also part of the neurotransmitter acetylcholine. The body synthesizes choline from the amino acid methionine.

lecithin In the body, a phospholipid with the nitrogenous component choline. In foods, lecithin is a blend of phospholipids with different nitrogenous components.

Quick Bites

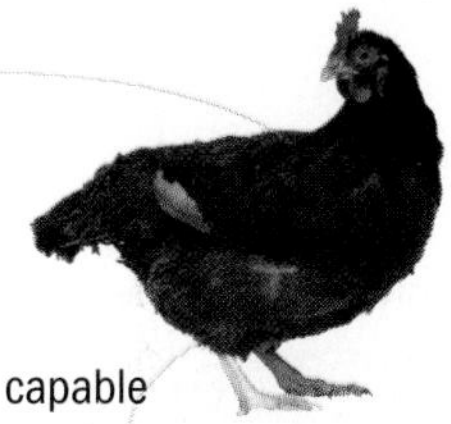

The Power of Yolk

A single raw egg yolk is capable of emulsifying many cups of oil. Cooks take advantage of the natural emulsifying ability of egg yolk phospholipids to emulsify and stabilize preparations like mayonnaise (oil and vinegar emulsion) or hollandaise sauce (butter and lemon juice emulsion). Food producers use phospholipid emulsifiers in processed foods, which today provide much of our intake.

Figure 5.20 **Lecithins and emulsification.** Lecithins form water-soluble packages called *micelles* that suspend fat-soluble compounds in watery mediums. In a micelle, the lecithins form into a water-soluble ball with a fatty core. The hydrophilic head of each lecithin molecule points outward in contact with the watery medium, while the hydrophobic tails point inward in contact with the fatty core.

Phosphate and glycerol are attracted to water

Fatty acid tails are attracted to fat

Micelle

Lecithin, a phospholipid

frequently used as food additives. Overall, a typical diet contains only about two grams per day. However, phospholipids are not a dietary essential because your body can readily synthesize them from available raw materials.

Key Concepts: Phospholipids are diglycerides (glycerol + 2 fatty acids) with a molecule containing a phosphate/nitrogen group attached at the third attachment point of glycerol. This structure gives the phospholipid hydrophobic and hydrophilic regions, contributing to its functional properties. Phospholipids are major components of cell membranes, and act as emulsifiers. Phospholipids also store fatty acids for release into the cell, and they are a source of choline. Phospholipids are not needed in the diet because the body can synthesize them.

Sterols

Although classified as lipids, sterols are quite different from triglycerides and phospholipids, both in structure and function. The best known sterol is cholesterol.

Sterol Structure

While triglycerides and phospholipids have fingerlike structures, sterols are hydrocarbons with a multiple-ring structure (see **Figure 5.21**). Like triglycerides, sterols are lipophilic and hydrophobic. Unlike triglycerides and phospholipids, most sterols contain no fatty acids.

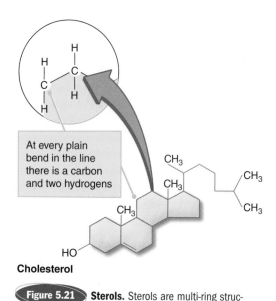

At every plain bend in the line there is a carbon and two hydrogens

Cholesterol

Figure 5.21 **Sterols.** Sterols are multi-ring structures. Because of its role in heart disease, cholesterol has become the best known sterol.

Think
About it
3

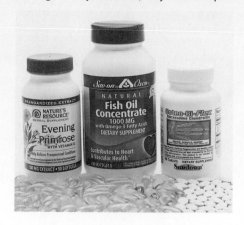

Fyi Fats on the Health Store Shelf

FOR YOUR INFORMATION

Many claims made for lipid products sold as supplements may not hold up under scientific scrutiny. You may not even recognize these products as lipids, especially because their long, complicated names are often abbreviated. The amount of lipid and calories in most of these products is quite small.

EPA and DHA in Fish Oil Capsules

These omega-3 fatty acids are thought to help lower blood pressure, reduce inflammation, reduce blood clotting, and lower high serum triglyceride levels.[1] They were thought to help psoriasis, but studies proved disappointing.[2] EPA (eicosapentaenoic acid) and DHA (docosahexaenoic acid) usually make up only about one-third of the fatty acids in fish oil capsules, and research studies often use multiple doses. These should not be taken without close medical supervision, because their blood-thinning properties can cause bleeding. Because fish oil is highly unsaturated, antioxidant vitamins are included to prevent oxidation. Another problem, though not health related, is that fish oil capsules often leave a fishy aftertaste.

Flaxseed Oil Capsules

Flaxseed oil, or linseed oil, is an unusually good source of omega-3 alpha-linolenic acid, which accounts for about 55 percent of its fatty acids. Like fish oil, flaxseed oil is highly unsaturated, and thus very susceptible to rancidity. Capsules protect the oil from oxygen, but limit the dose. A half-tablespoon of canola oil has about as much omega-3, but adds more calories than a capsule of flaxseed oil. DHA and EPA are considered more potent omega-3 fatty acids than alpha-linolenic.

GLA in Borage, Evening Primrose, or Black Currant Seed Oil Capsules

These oils contain 9 to 24 percent GLA (gamma-linolenic acid), the omega-6 desaturation product of linoleic acid. Studies of GLA's effects on skin diseases, heart conditions, and other disorders have been disappointing.[3]

Medium-Chain Triglycerides Oil

Medium-chain triglycerides (MCT) can be purchased as such, or found as ingredients in "sports" drinks and foods. They are marketed to athletes as a noncarbohydrate source of quick, concentrated energy; however, although readily absorbed, they have no spe-

Cholesterol Functions

Because of the publicity generated by its role in **atherosclerosis** (heart disease), **cholesterol** is the best-known sterol. But cholesterol is a necessary, important substance in the body; it becomes a problem only when excessive amounts accumulate in the blood. Like phospholipids, it is a major structural component of all cell membranes and is especially abundant in nerve and brain tissue. In fact, most cholesterol resides in body tissue, not in the blood serum or plasma that is routinely tested for cholesterol levels.

High cholesterol blood levels are common, but it is also possible to have undesirably low cholesterol levels. Although less common, very low levels (usually defined as less than 160 mg/dl) are associated with some kinds of stroke; increased lung, liver, and behavioral illnesses; and reduced immunity.[9] However, researchers have not yet determined whether low cholesterol causes these conditions or results from them. For people with AIDS or cancer, declining cholesterol levels often indicate that their condition is worsening.[10]

Cholesterol is important not only in cell membranes, but also as a precursor molecule. For example, vitamin D is synthesized from cholesterol. Cholesterol is the precursor of five major classes of sterol hormones: progestins, glucocorticoids, mineralocorticoids, androgens, and estrogens. (See **Figure 5.22.**) Progesterone is essential for maintaining a healthy pregnancy. Glucocorticoids (such as cortisol) increase the formation of

cholesterol [ko-LES-te-rol] A waxy lipid (sterol) whose chemical structure contains multiple hydrocarbon rings.

atherosclerosis [ath-e-roh-scle-ROH-sis] The deposition of fatty plaques inside artery walls. Medium and large arteries acquire yellowish deposits (atheromatous plaques) composed of cholesterol, fat, cellular debris, and calcium. These plaques cause vessel walls to become thick and hardened.

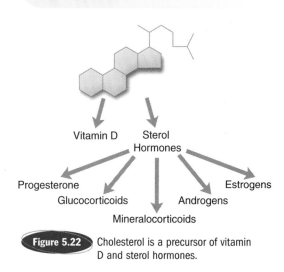

Figure 5.22 Cholesterol is a precursor of vitamin D and sterol hormones.

---

cific performance benefits. A tablespoon of MCT contains about 100 kilocalories.

Lecithin Oil or Granules

Lecithin supplements are derived from soybeans, and are a mixture of phospholipids. They are often promoted as emulsifiers that lower cholesterol, but since dietary phospholipids are broken down by the enzyme lecithinase in the intestine, they cannot have this effect. They may be useful as a source of choline. Since choline is the precursor of acetylcholine (a neurotransmitter), lecithin is promoted for treating Parkinson's and Alzheimer's diseases, which are associated with low levels of acetylcholinein the brain. Unfortunately, these efforts have met with little success.[4]

Monolaurin Capsules

Monolaurin is an ester of lauric acid, a 12-carbon fatty acid found in coconut oil. Lauric acid is said to have anti-infective effects, but the amount in these capsules is probably too small to be significant.

CLA

Conjugated linoleic acid (CLA) is linoleic acid with only one saturated bond between its two double bonds. It is promoted as an aid for reducing body fat, among other claims, but the effects of supplementation are largely unstudied.

DHEA

Dehydroepiandrosterone (DHEA) is a testosterone precursor formed from cholesterol. It is present in the body in large quantities during adolescence, peaks in the 20s, and gradually declines with age. Many elderly people have low levels, and levels also dip during serious illnesses. With only a few exceptions, attempts to use DHEA for illnesses or to slow aging have been disappointing. Researchers generally use doses many times greater than those in over-the-counter supplements, levels that may cause hairiness in women, and, more seriously, a risk of liver problems.[5]

Shark Liver Oil and Squalene Capsules

Squalene, an intermediary compound in the synthesis of cholesterol in the body, and shark liver oil, which contains squalene, are said to help liver, skin, and immune function. The basis for these claims is unclear.

1 Connor SL, Connor WE. Are fish oils beneficial in disease prevention and treatment? *Am J Clin Nutr.* 1997;66:S1020-S1031.

2 Soyland E, et al. Effect of dietary supplementation with very-long-chain n-3 fatty acids in patients with psoriasis. *N Engl J Med.* 1993;328:1812-1816.

3 Berth-Jones J, Graham-Brown RAC. Placebo-controlled trial of essential fatty acid supplementation in atopic dermatitis. *Lancet.* 1993;341:1557-1560.

4 Mauron J, Leathwood P. Dietary phosphatidylcholine as a precursor of brain acetylcholine. In: Horisberger H, Bracco U, eds. *Lipids in Modern Nutrition.* New York: Raven Press; 1987:133-145.

5 Khaw KT. Dehydroepiandrosterone, dehydroepiandrosterone sulphate and cardiovascular disease. *J Endocrinol.* 1996;150:S149-S153.

liver glycogen and the breakdown of fat and protein. Mineralocorticoids (primarily aldosterone) help control blood pressure. Androgens (such as testosterone) promote the development of male sex characteristics, and estrogens promote the development of female sex characteristics. When testosterone is synthesized from cholesterol, an intermediate called DHEA (dehydroepiandrosterone) is formed. DHEA has become a popular nutritional supplement, marketed with the largely unfulfilled promise that it will boost potency and restore youth.

The liver uses cholesterol to manufacture bile acids, which are secreted in bile. The gallbladder stores and concentrates the bile. On demand, the gallbladder releases the bile into the small intestine where the bile acids emulsify dietary fats.

Cholesterol Synthesis

The body can synthesize cholesterol; therefore, it is not needed in the diet. While the liver manufactures most of the cholesterol in your body, and the intestine contributes appreciable amounts, all cells are believed to synthesize some cholesterol. In fact, your body produces at least 1,000 milligrams of cholesterol per day, far more than is found in the average diet.

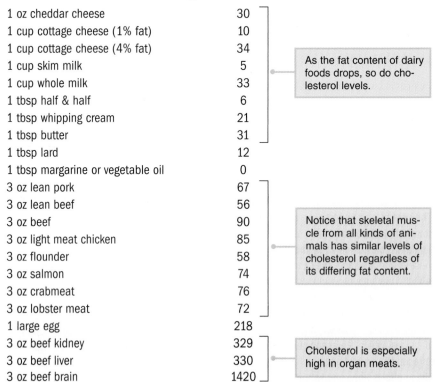

Table 5.4 **Cholesterol in Selected Foods (in milligrams)**

Approximate Cholesterol

1 oz cheddar cheese	30
1 cup cottage cheese (1% fat)	10
1 cup cottage cheese (4% fat)	34
1 cup skim milk	5
1 cup whole milk	33
1 tbsp half & half	6
1 tbsp whipping cream	21
1 tbsp butter	31
1 tbsp lard	12
1 tbsp margarine or vegetable oil	0
3 oz lean pork	67
3 oz lean beef	56
3 oz beef	90
3 oz light meat chicken	85
3 oz flounder	58
3 oz salmon	74
3 oz crabmeat	76
3 oz lobster meat	72
1 large egg	218
3 oz beef kidney	329
3 oz beef liver	330
3 oz beef brain	1420

As the fat content of dairy foods drops, so do cholesterol levels.

Notice that skeletal muscle from all kinds of animals has similar levels of cholesterol regardless of its differing fat content.

Cholesterol is especially high in organ meats.

The values here give only a general idea of amounts in foods. Cholesterol values are quite variable, differing by times of the year, the animal's origin, species or breed, processing, and more. One thing is always true, though: cholesterol is never found in plant foods.

Source: Based on figures from US Department of Agriculture, Agricultural Research Service, 1999. USDA Nutrient Database for Standard Reference, Release 13.

This attests to cholesterol's biological importance. In the lens of the eye, which has a high concentration of cholesterol, on-site cholesterol synthesis may be essential for preventing cataracts.[11] Animal studies suggest that the brain makes almost all the cholesterol incorporated into it during development.[12] Increasing dietary cholesterol reduces synthesis somewhat, but not by an equivalent amount.[13] Less cholesterol is produced when we eat frequent small meals rather than a few large meals. Fasting markedly reduces cholesterol production.[14]

Sterols in Food

Cholesterol occurs only in foods of animal origin. It is distributed based on its biological roles: it is highest in brain, high in liver and other organ meats, and moderate in muscle tissue. Because it is fat soluble, it is found in the butterfat portion of dairy products. Egg yolks are high in cholesterol, with about 218 milligrams per large egg (the egg white contains no cholesterol), and breast milk is moderately high, suggesting the importance of cholesterol during early growth and development.[15] **Table 5.4** lists the amounts of cholesterol in some common foods.

Aside from cholesterol and vitamin D, there are few dietary sterols of nutritional significance. Whale liver and plants contain the cholesterol precursor **squalene.** Although whale liver is not a common item in U.S. grocery stores, squalene capsules are sold as dietary supplements with the unproved claim that squalene speeds healing. Plants contain a number of other sterols (phytosterols) that are poorly absorbed. **Phytosterols** are of current interest because they reduce intestinal absorption of cholesterol, and have recently been introduced as a cholesterol-lowering food ingredient.

Key Concepts: Sterols are hydrocarbons with a distinctive ring structure. Cholesterol is the best known sterol; other sterols are hormones or hormone precursors. Cholesterol is an important precursor compound and is a key component of cell membranes. High levels of blood cholesterol are a heart disease risk. Cholesterol is found only in foods of animal origin, and because the body can make all it needs, cholesterol is not a dietary essential.

Digestion and Absorption

Like the other macronutrients (carbohydrates and proteins), most lipids are broken into smaller compounds for absorption in the gastrointestinal tract. However, because lipids generally are not water soluble and digestive secretions are all water based, the body has to treat lipids a bit differently to digest them.

Digestion of Triglycerides and Phospholipids

Triglycerides are not water soluble, and the enzymes needed to digest them are found in a watery environment; therefore, preparing triglycerides for digestion is a more elaborate process than for either carbohydrates or proteins. But don't worry! Your digestive system is equal to the task. Physical actions (chewing, peristalsis, and segmentation), combined with various emulsifiers allow digestive enzymes to do their work.

In the mouth, a combination of chewing and the work of lingual lipase gets the digestive process rolling, with the small amount of dietary phospholipid providing emulsification. In the stomach, gastric lipase joins in, and the stomach's churning and contractions keep the fat dispersed.

squalene A cholesterol precursor found in whale liver and plants.

phytosterols Sterols found in plants. Phytosterols are poorly absorbed by humans and reduce intestinal absorption of cholesterol. They recently have been introduced as a cholesterol-lowering food ingredient.

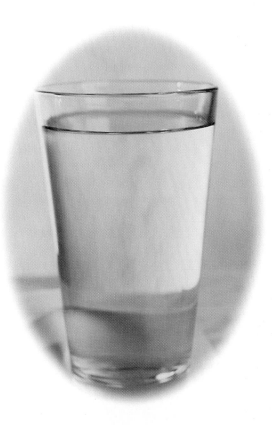

Diglycerides that form in the breakdown process become emulsifiers, too. After two to four hours in the stomach, about 30 percent of dietary triglycerides have been broken down to diglycerides and free fatty acids.[16]

Fat in the small intestine stimulates the release of the hormones cholecystokinin (CCK) and secretin from duodenal cells. CCK signals the gallbladder to contract, sending bile down the bile duct and into the duodenum. Secretin signals the pancreas to release pancreatic juice rich in pancreatic lipase, which joins the bile just before entering the duodenum where they mix with the watery chyme.

Bile contains a large quantity of bile salts and the phospholipid lecithin. These components are the key elements that emulsify fat, breaking globules into smaller pieces so that water-soluble pancreatic lipase can attack the surface. This emulsification process increases the total surface area of fats by as much as 1,000-fold.[17] Many common household detergents remove grease with this same action of emulsification.

As bile breaks up clumps of triglycerides into small pieces and keeps them suspended in solution, pancreatic lipase breaks off one fatty acid at a time. Pancreatic juice contains enormous amounts of pancreatic lipase—enough to digest all accessible triglycerides within minutes. When the lipase has completed its work, most of the dietary triglycerides have been split into monoglycerides and free fatty acids. (See **Figure 5.23**.)

Bile salts surround the products of fat digestion, forming **micelles**—water-soluble globules with a fatty core. The micelles transport the monoglycerides and free fatty acids through the watery intestinal environment to the brush border of the intestinal mucosal cells for absorption.

Phospholipid digestion follows a similar pathway, with phospholipases as well as other lipases participating in the process and with the added release of the phospholipid's phosphate and nitrogen components.

micelles Tiny emulsified fat packets that can enter enterocytes. The complexes are composed of emulsifier molecules oriented with their hydrophobic part facing inward and their hydrophilic part facing outward toward the surrounding aqueous environment.

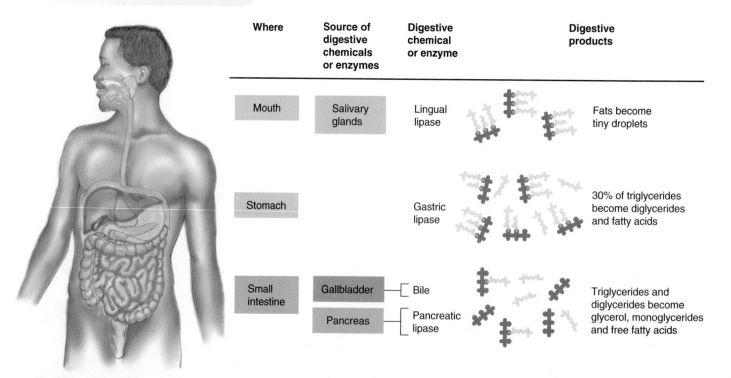

Where	Source of digestive chemicals or enzymes	Digestive chemical or enzyme		Digestive products
Mouth	Salivary glands	Lingual lipase		Fats become tiny droplets
Stomach		Gastric lipase		30% of triglycerides become diglycerides and fatty acids
Small intestine	Gallbladder	Bile		Triglycerides and diglycerides become glycerol, monoglycerides and free fatty acids
	Pancreas	Pancreatic lipase		

Figure 5.23 **Triglyceride digestion.** Most triglyceride digestion takes place in the small intestine.

Digestibility

Normally, triglyceride digestion and absorption are very efficient. It is abnormal to find more than 6 or 7 percent of ingested lipids still intact in fecal matter. Production of fatty stools, called **steatorrhea,** indicates fat malabsorption, a condition that may follow radiation therapy or digestive surgery and often accompanies diseases of malabsorption such as cystic fibrosis or Crohn's disease.

Triglycerides of medium-chain fatty acids (medium-chain triglycerides, or MCT) often are used in products developed for people with fat malabsorption.[18] Medium-chain fatty acids—those with 6 to 12 carbons—are more water-soluble than longer chain fatty acids, and thus more readily emulsified with less need for bile. Because the fatty acid chains are shorter, MCTs are digested more easily. They are hydrolyzed more easily and quickly and absorbed more efficiently.

Breast milk is easily digestible. It is rich in medium-chain fatty acids and contains its own lipase, which enhances fat digestion despite the immaturity of the baby's digestive system. Some free medium-chain fatty acids released by hydrolysis are even absorbed directly through the baby's stomach lining.

Short-chain fatty acids, with the exception of butyric acid in milk fat, are almost never found in foods. Instead, they are produced by bacteria in the colon from undigested food, especially from soluble fiber. These fatty acids enter the cells of the large intestine (**enterocytes**) where they can be used for energy. A lack of short-chain fatty acids, which can occur when prolonged and exclusive intravenous feeding bypasses bacterial activity, is thought to damage intestinal cells, and nutritionists are studying short-chain fatty acid supplements for these cases. Some research also suggests butyric acid stimulates colon cells to suppress cancer growth, a finding that helps explain how dietary fiber may discourage colon cancer.[19]

Lipid Absorption

Most fat absorption takes place in the duodenum or jejunum of the small intestine. Micelles carry the monoglycerides and long-chain fatty acids to the surfaces of the microvilli in the brush border, even penetrating the recesses between individual microvilli. Here, the monoglycerides and long-chain fatty acids immediately diffuse into the intestinal cells (enterocytes). The unabsorbed bile salts return to the interior of the small intestine to ferry another load of monoglycerides and fatty acids. In the last section of the small intestine (the ileum), bile salts are absorbed. They return via the portal vein to the liver where they are once again secreted into the bile. This bile recycling pathway—the liver to the intestine and the intestine to the liver—is called enterohepatic circulation. Figure 3.11 in Chapter 3 illustrates enterohepatic circulation.

As monoglycerides and fatty acids pass into the intestinal cells, they re-form into triglycerides. Most of the triglycerides, as well as cholesterol, and phospholipids join protein carriers to form a **lipoprotein.** When this assemblage leaves the intestinal cell, it is called a **chylomicron.** The chylomicrons make their way to the central lacteal of the villi, where they enter the lymph system, to be propelled through the thoracic duct and emptied into veins in the neck.

steatorrhea Production of stools with an abnormally high amount of fat.

enterocytes Intestinal cells.

lipoprotein Complexes that transport lipids in the lymph and blood. They consist of a central core of triglycerides surrounded by a shell composed of proteins, cholesterol, and phospholipids. The various types of lipoproteins differ in size, composition, and density.

chylomicron [kye-lo-MY-kron] A large lipoprotein particle formed in intestinal cells following the absorption of dietary fats. A chylomicron has a central core of triglycerides and cholesterol surrounded by phospholipids and proteins.

Absorption of glycerol and of short-chain and medium-chain fatty acids is more direct. They are absorbed directly into the bloodstream rather than forming triglycerides and entering the lymph system. These fatty acids can diffuse directly into the capillaries of the villi because they are more water soluble than longer chain fatty acids. Figure 5.24 illustrates the absorption of triglycerides.

One or two hours after you eat, dietary fat begins to appear in the bloodstream. Fat levels peak after three to five hours and fats are generally cleared by 10 hours. That's why health professionals instruct people to fast for 12 hours before having blood drawn for lipid testing.

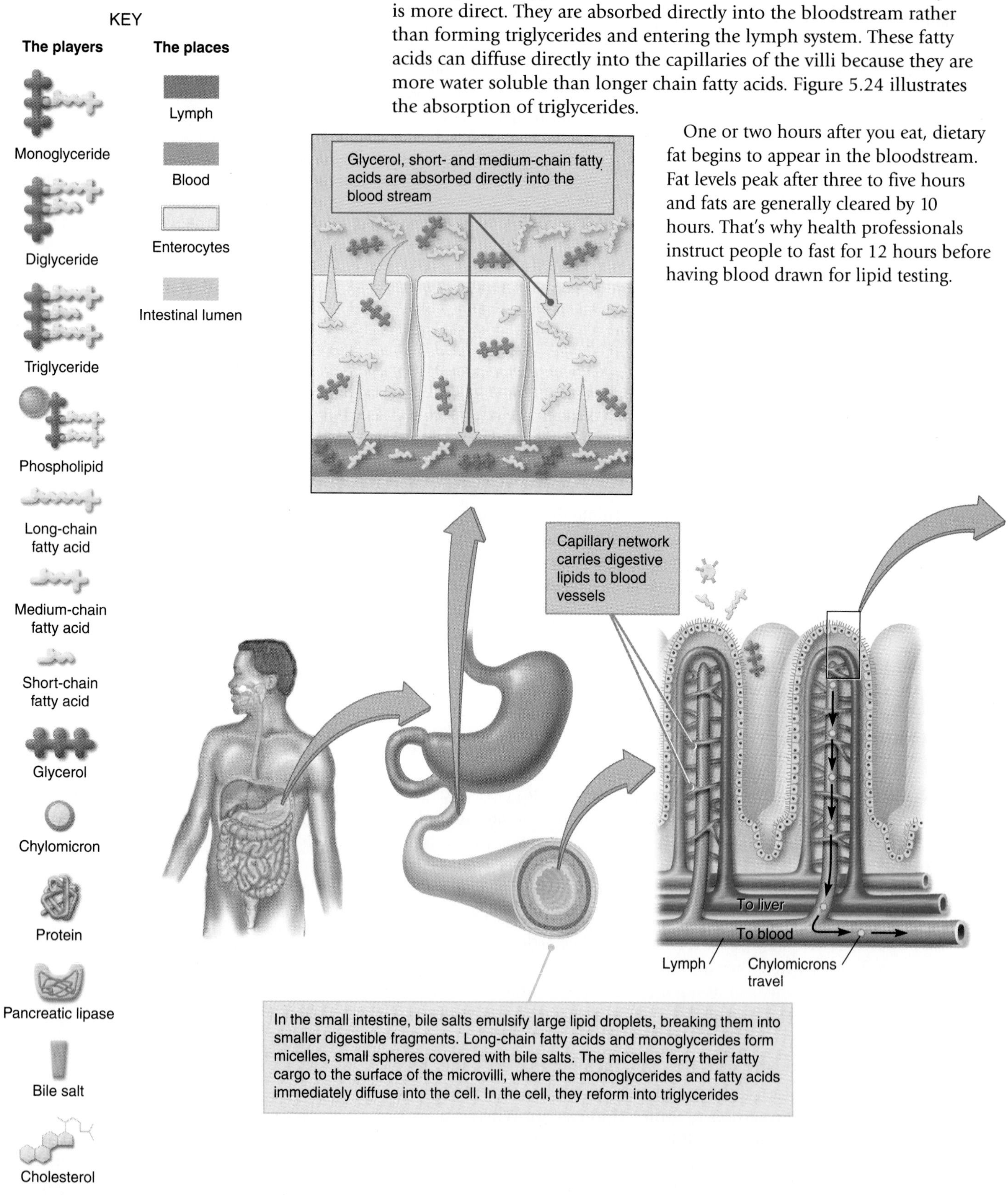

KEY

The players

- Monoglyceride
- Diglyceride
- Triglyceride
- Phospholipid
- Long-chain fatty acid
- Medium-chain fatty acid
- Short-chain fatty acid
- Glycerol
- Chylomicron
- Protein
- Pancreatic lipase
- Bile salt
- Cholesterol

The places

- Lymph
- Blood
- Enterocytes
- Intestinal lumen

Glycerol, short- and medium-chain fatty acids are absorbed directly into the blood stream

Capillary network carries digestive lipids to blood vessels

To liver

To blood

Lymph

Chylomicrons travel

In the small intestine, bile salts emulsify large lipid droplets, breaking them into smaller digestible fragments. Long-chain fatty acids and monoglycerides form micelles, small spheres covered with bile salts. The micelles ferry their fatty cargo to the surface of the microvilli, where the monoglycerides and fatty acids immediately diffuse into the cell. In the cell, they reform into triglycerides

Figure 5.24 **Absorption of triglycerides.** The products of triglyceride digestion are absorbed in the small intestine.

Digestion and Absorption of Sterols

Digestion does little to change cholesterol and other sterols, which are poorly absorbed compared to triglycerides. Cholesterol may be esterified (attached to a fatty acid) prior to absorption. When there is dietary fat in the intestine, cholesterol absorption increases. When there are plenty of plant sterols and dietary fiber in the intestine, especially soluble fiber from fruits, vegetables, oats, peas, and beans, cholesterol absorption decreases. Overall, only about 50 percent of dietary cholesterol is absorbed, and that proportion falls as cholesterol intake increases. Because soluble fiber binds bile acids and cholesterol, and carries them out of the colon, health professionals often recommend eating foods rich in soluble fiber to lower blood cholesterol.

Key concepts: *Digestion breaks most lipids down into glycerol, free fatty acids, monoglycerides, and, in the case of phospholipids, a nitrogenous compound. Long-chain fatty acids and monoglycerides are absorbed primarily into the lymphatic system from the small intestine; glycerol, short-chain, and medium-chain fatty acids are absorbed directly into the blood. Sterols are mostly unchanged by digestion and their absorption is relatively poor.*

Quick Bites

How do cholesterol-lowering medications work?

*O*ne class of cholesterol-lowering medications, the "bile-acid sequestrants," works by combining bile acid and cholesterol in the intestine to form compounds that the body cannot absorb. Since this cholesterol is then lost in the feces, cholesterol must be taken from the blood to make more bile, thus lowering the blood cholesterol level.

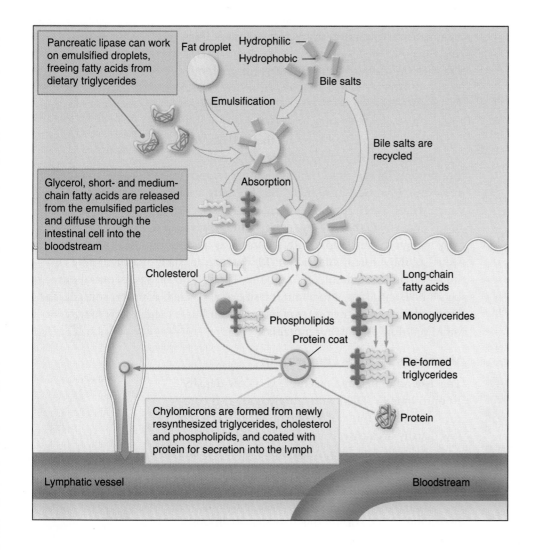

Lipids in the Body

The digestive tract is not the only place where lipids need special handling to move in a water-based environment. To be transported around the body in the bloodstream, lipids must be specially packaged into lipoprotein carriers.

Lipoproteins have a core of triglycerides and cholesterol esters (cholesterol linked to fatty acids) surrounded by a shell of phospholipids with embedded proteins and cholesterol. They can transport water-insoluble (hydrophobic) lipids through the watery environment of the bloodstream. There are several main classes of lipoproteins, and many subclasses. These differ mainly by size, density, and the composition of their lipid cores. In general, as the percentage of triglyceride drops, the density increases. A lipoprotein with a small core that contains little triglyceride is much more dense than a lipoprotein with a large core composed mostly of triglycerides. To get a feel for relative sizes, different lipoproteins can be compared to a huge beach ball, a softball, a baseball, a golf ball, and a $^3/_4$-inch steel ball bearing. (See **Figure 5.25.**)

Chylomicrons

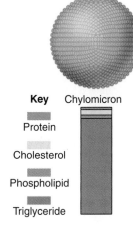

Key Chylomicron

Protein

Cholesterol

Phospholipid

Triglyceride

Chylomicrons formed in the intestinal tract enter the lymphatic system, travel through the thoracic duct, and flow into the bloodstream at the jugular veins of the neck. As they enter the bloodstream, chylomicrons are large, fatty lipoproteins—think of a beach ball three to six feet in diameter. Chylomicrons are about 90 percent fat, but as they circulate through the capillaries, they gradually give up their triglycerides. An enzyme located on the capillary walls, called **lipoprotein lipase,** attacks the chylomicrons and removes triglyceride, breaking it into free fatty acids and glycerol. These components enter adipose cells, as needed, where they are reassembled into triglycerides. Alternatively, they may remain in circulation, with the free fatty acids bound to albumin, a water-soluble protein. After about 10 hours, little is left of a circulating chylomicron but cholesterol-rich remnants. It's like the air was let out of our beach ball, shrinking it to about the size of a $4^1/_2$-inch diameter softball. The liver picks up these chylomicron remnants and uses them as raw material to build very-low-density lipoproteins.

Very-Low-Density Lipoprotein

The liver and intestines assemble **very-low-density lipoproteins (VLDLs)** with a triglyceride-rich core—for relative size, think of a softball. VLDL has a very low density because it is nearly two-thirds fat. As with chylomicrons, lipoprotein lipase splits off and hydrolyzes triglycerides from VLDL as it circulates through the capillaries of the bloodstream. As VLDL loses triglycerides, it becomes denser, gradually becoming an IDL, or intermediate-density lipoprotein. Our softball has shrunk to about the size of a $2^3/_4$-inch diameter baseball.

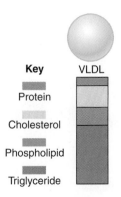

Key VLDL

Protein

Cholesterol

Phospholipid

Triglyceride

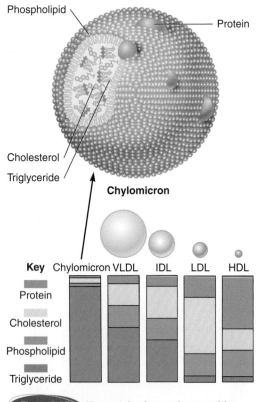

Phospholipid

Protein

Cholesterol

Triglyceride

Chylomicron

Key Chylomicron VLDL IDL LDL HDL

Protein

Cholesterol

Phospholipid

Triglyceride

Figure 5.25 **Lipoprotein sizes and composition.** Lipoproteins become less dense as they increase in size. LDL is about double the size of HDL. VLDL is about 60 times larger than HDL. Chylomicrons range from 500–1000 times larger than HDL.

Intermediate-Density Lipoproteins

Intermediate-density lipoproteins (IDLs) are about 40 percent fat. As IDL travels through the bloodstream, it acquires cholesterol from another lipoprotein (HDL, see below) and circulating enzymes remove some phospholipids. IDL returns to the liver, where liver cells convert it to low-density lipoprotein.

Low-Density Lipoprotein

Low-density lipoproteins (LDLs) deliver cholesterol to body cells, which use it to synthesize membranes, hormones, and other vital compounds. LDL is more than half cholesterol and cholesterol esters; triglycerides make up only 6 percent. For a relative size, think of a golf ball (about $1\frac{5}{8}$ inches in diameter).

Low-density lipoprotein binds to a special receptor on the cell wall. The cell engulfs and ingests the LDL via endocytosis. Inside the cell, LDL is broken into its component parts, releasing its load of cholesterol.

Liver cells also have LDL-receptors that bind LDL and control blood cholesterol levels.[20] Saturated fats appear to block these receptors, which explains why saturated fats tend to raise blood cholesterol levels.[21] A lack of LDL-receptors reduces the uptake of cholesterol, forcing it to remain in circulation at dangerously high levels.

Low-density lipoprotein also is picked up by scavenger receptors. These are a different type of receptor, one that has a particular affinity for altered (oxidized) LDL. When smoking, diabetes, high blood pressure, or infections injure blood vessel walls, the body's emergency repair system swings into action. It mobilizes white blood cells, which travel to the site of the injury where they bury themselves in the blood vessel wall. Certain white blood cells with scavenger receptors bind and ingest LDL. As LDL degrades, it releases its cholesterol. Over several years, this process leads to an accumulation of cholesterol and the development of plaque that thickens and narrows the artery, a condition known as atherosclerosis. Because elevated LDL levels are associated with atherosclerosis and heart disease, LDL-cholesterol has acquired the nickname of "bad cholesterol." The antioxidant vitamin E and several carotenoids reduce the oxidation of LDL and may interfere with scavenger uptake, thus preventing plaque buildup.

High-Density Lipoprotein

High-density lipoproteins (HDLs) are made by the liver and intestines. HDL is about 5 percent triglyceride, similar to LDL. On the other hand, HDL is only about 20 percent cholesterol, much less than LDL, which is more than 50 percent cholesterol. HDL has a higher protein content than any other lipoprotein. For a relative size, think of a steel ball bearing about $\frac{3}{4}$ inches in diameter.

High-density lipoprotein roams the bloodstream scavenging for cholesterol. It picks up cholesterol released by dying cells and from cell membranes as they are renewed. HDL also picks up cholesterol from arterial plaques, reducing their accumulation. HDL hands off cholesterol to other

Key — IDL
Protein
Cholesterol
Phospholipid
Triglyceride

Key — LDL
Protein
Cholesterol
Phospholipid
Triglyceride

Key — HDL
Protein
Cholesterol
Phospholipid
Triglyceride

intermediate-density lipoprotein (IDL) The lipoprotein formed when lipoprotein lipase strips some of the triglycerides from VLDL. Containing about 40 percent triglycerides, this lipoprotein is more dense than VLDL and less dense than LDL. Also called a VLDL-remnant.

low-density lipoprotein (LDL) The cholesterol-rich lipoprotein that results from the breakdown and removal of triglycerides from intermediate-density lipoprotein in the blood.

high-density lipoprotein (HDL) The blood lipoprotein that contains high levels of protein and low levels of triglycerides. Synthesized primarily in the liver and small intestine, HDL picks up cholesterol released from dying cells and other sources and transfers it to other lipoproteins.

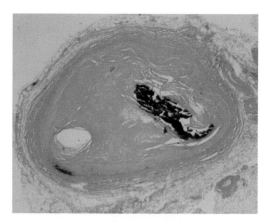

Plaque buildup in a coronary artery.

Think About It
4

lipoproteins, especially IDL, which return the cholesterol to the liver for recycling. HDL appears to have a protective influence against atherosclerosis, and thus has earned the nickname "good cholesterol." Low HDL levels increase risk for atherosclerotic heart disease, while high HDL levels have a protective effect. About 1 percent of the population who have extremely high HDL levels have extremely low rates of heart disease and stroke.[22]

Key Concepts: *Lipoprotein carriers transport lipids in the blood. Chylomicrons, formed in the intestinal mucosal cells, transport lipids from the digestive tract into circulation. VLDL carries lipids from the liver to the other body tissues, delivering triglycerides, and gradually becoming IDL. The liver takes up IDL and assembles LDL, the main carrier of cholesterol. High blood levels of LDL, the "bad cholesterol," have been shown to be a risk factor for heart disease. Circulating HDL picks up cholesterol and sends it back to the liver for recycling or excretion. A relatively high level of HDL, the "good cholesterol," reduces risk for heart disease.*

Lipids in the Diet

Now that you know something about lipids and their importance in the body, you can see that Rachel's no-fat approach to life has serious flaws. However, too much dietary fat can contribute unwanted calories, and high intake of fat has been linked to heart disease. Read on for a discussion of the recommended amounts and balance of lipids in a healthful diet.

Recommended Intakes

Most health policy agencies recommend reducing intake of total fat, saturated fat, and cholesterol. As interest in the relationship between fat intake and health grew in the 1970s and 1980s, the American Heart Association (AHA), the National Cholesterol Education Program (NCEP) of the National Institutes of Health, and the *Dietary Guidelines for Americans* set specific target levels for intake of lipids. **Figure 5.26** shows the consensus recommendations.

The Daily Values on food labels reflect these recommendations. Based on a 2,000-kilocalorie diet, the Daily Value for fat is 65 grams (29 percent of calories), for saturated fat is 20 grams (9 percent of calories), and for cholesterol is 300 milligrams. The NCEP suggests all healthy Americans 2 years of age and older follow these recommendations. Other groups suggest phasing in the reduction in fat intake up to the age of 5 years.[23]

Are we meeting fat intake goals? Dietary surveys, including the large National Health and Nutrition Examination Survey of 1988–94 (NHANES III), report that average fat intake is 34 percent of calories, down from 36 percent 10 years earlier and down markedly from 45 percent in 1965. See "What About Bobbie?" (page 175) to see how to calculate the percentage of calorie intake from fat.

Although percent calories from fat dropped, average calorie intake increased, which means Americans actually are consuming more total grams of fat. Desserts, hamburgers, and french-fried potatoes are the largest contributors to fat intake, according to the NCEP.[24] While fat intake from meats has fallen markedly since 1970, fat from salad and cooking oils and shortenings has risen dramatically.[25]

Released in 2000, new AHA guidelines focus on overall eating patterns rather than specific percentages of dietary fat—an approach similar to the 2000 *Dietary Guidelines for Americans*. The four main goals of the new guidelines are to help Americans: 1) Achieve an overall healthy eating pattern;

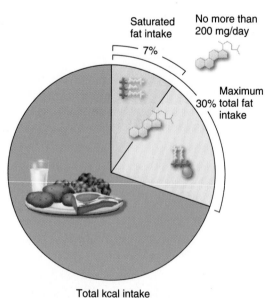

Saturated fat intake

No more than 200 mg/day

7%

Maximum 30% total fat intake

Total kcal intake

Figure 5.26 **Recommended fat intake.** Public health groups recommend that we limit our total fat intake to no more than 30 percent of our total calories. Our saturated fat intake should supply no more than one-third of our fat calories.

2) Achieve and maintain an appropriate body weight; 3) Achieve and maintain a desirable blood cholesterol profile; 4) Achieve and maintain a desirable blood pressure. One of the most significant changes in the new guidelines is a recommendation to consume two weekly servings of fatty fish, such as tuna or salmon.

Essential Fatty Acid Requirements

Although too much fat in the diet is not healthful, we still need to get enough fat to meet our need for essential fatty acids. To fulfill our need for omega-6 fatty acids, linoleic acid should provide about 2 percent of our calories. Average U.S. consumption is much more than that. Two teaspoons of corn oil, which is a little over half linoleic acid, would supply more than 2 percent of the calories in a 2,000-kilocalorie diet.

We know less about requirements for omega-3 fatty acids because science has only recently recognized their importance. Researchers suggest that we should eat a minimum of 3 grams of omega-3 fatty acids each day (about 1.3 percent of calories for a 2,000-kilocalorie diet).[26] The recommended ratio of omega-3 fatty acids to omega-6 fatty acids in the diet is 1:2.3.[27] To meet these recommendations for omega-3 fatty acids, we would need about 1 ounce of vegetable oil per day and 4 meals each week that contained fatty fish; that would be a three-fold increase in U.S. fish consumption! **Figure 5.27** gives an overview of the dietary sources of fatty acids.

Omega-6 and Omega-3 Imbalance

Before commercial processing, large quantities of vegetable oils were unavailable, so the omega-6 linoleic acid was hard to come by. There was a small amount in whole grains, and smaller amounts in fruits and vegetables, and these contained very small amounts of omega-3s. Today, linoleic acid is widely available. In contrast, availability of omega-3s in the food supply has increased very little over time. In fact, some were even removed from foods to discourage rancidity. As a result, the ratio of omega-3 to omega-6 in the American diet has fallen. The low intake of omega-3 fatty

AHA Dietary Guidelines

The guidelines are designed to assist individuals in achieving and maintaining:

A Healthy Eating Pattern Including Foods from All Major Food Groups

- Consume a variety of fruits and vegetables and grain products including whole grains.
- Include fat-free and low-fat dairy products, fish, legumes, poultry, and lean meats.

A Healthy Body Weight

- Match intake of energy to overall energy needs; limit consumption of foods with a high caloric density and/or low nutritional quality.
- Maintain a level of physical activity that achieves fitness and balances energy expenditure with energy intake; for weight reduction, expenditure should exceed intake.

A Desirable Blood Cholesterol and Lipoprotein Profile

- Limit the intake of foods with a high content of saturated fatty acids and cholesterol.
- Substitute grains and unsaturated fatty acids from vegetables, fish, legumes, and nuts.

A Desirable Blood Pressure

- Limit the intake of salt to < 6 grams per day.
- Limit alcohol consumption.
- Maintain a healthy body weight and a dietary pattern that emphasizes vegetables, fruits, and low-fat or fat-free dairy products.

Source: *Circulation.* 2000;102:2296–2311.

TYPE	SOURCE
Basic Fatty Acids	
Saturated fats	Animal products (including dairy products), palm and coconut oils and cocoa butter.
Polyunsaturated fats	Sunflower, corn, soybean, and cottonseed oils
Monounsaturated fats	Most nuts and olive, canola, peanut, and safflower oils.
Trans-fatty Acids	Stick margarine (not soft or liquid margarine) and many fast foods and baked goods.

Essential Fatty Acids	
Omega-3 fatty acids	
Alpha-linolenic acid	Canola oil, soybeans, olive oil, many nuts (e.g., walnuts, peanuts, filberts, pistachios, pecans, almonds), seeds, and purslane (a green, leafy vegetable).
Docosahexaenoic and eicosapentaenoic acids	Fish such as mackerel, tuna, salmon, herring, trout, and cod liver oil. The fish with the lowest amount of total fat include Atlantic cod, haddock, and pink salmon. Other fish high in omega-3 but also high in total fat are sardines and bluefish. Human milk.
Omega-6 fatty acids	
Linoleic acid	Plants (flax) and some vegetable oils (soybean and canola oil).
Omega-9 fatty acids	Olive oil.

Figure 5.27 **Overview of dietary sources of fatty acids.**
Source: *Scientific American.* Cancer smart, July, 1998;4(3).

acids in relation to the high intake of omega-6 fatty acids has caused concerns about an unhealthy imbalance.

Role of Fat Substitutes

The food industry has responded to the public health challenge to make low-fat, low-calorie goodies that still taste good. There are now more than 15 categories of **fat substitutes**, and more than 5,000 fat-reduced foods have made it to the marketplace.[28]

Fat Substitutes: What are they made of?

Some fat substitutes are carbohydrates: generally starches and fibers like vegetable gums, cellulose, maltodextrins, and Oatrim. Some are more digestible than others, but all provide far fewer than the 9 kilocalories per gram of fat. They also incorporate extra water into foods by binding with it, which further dilutes calories. With their moist, thick textures, they mimic fat's richness and smooth "mouth feel."

Other substitutes have proteins as their raw ingredients. Food manufacturers modify egg whites and whey from milk so they are thick and smooth and hold water. This protein and water combination cuts calories because it

---

Fyi Which Spread for Your Bread?

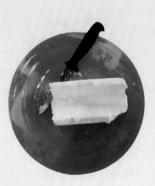

Okay, it's time to see if you can put some of your new knowledge about lipids to work. You're standing in front of the dairy case ready to pick out the best spread. But, wow! So many choices. Of course, there's butter, the traditional spread, wholesome, natural and creamy; sometimes there's just no substitute for the real thing. Margarine is the choice of many, and has come to be more familiar than butter to some consumers. Then what's this "vegetable oil spread"? Here's one that says it "helps promote healthy cholesterol levels."

Butter

When it comes to heart-health, butter has some serious disadvantages: (1) It's high in cholesterol-raising saturated fat, (2) it contains cholesterol, and (3) like other fats, it's high in calories.

Here are the facts: one tablespoon of butter provides the following:
- 100 kcals
- 11 g fat
- 8 g saturated fat
- 30 mg cholesterol
- 85 mg sodium
- 8% Daily Value for vitamin A

The ingredients are simple: "cream, salt, annatto (added seasonally)." Annatto is a natural coloring (a carotenoid) that is used to keep the color of butter consistent, despite what dairy cows might have been grazing on.

If you like the taste of butter, but want a bit less saturated fat and cholesterol, you can buy "whipped butter." The ingredients are the same, with the exception of incorporated air, and the reduction in calories, fat, saturated fat, cholesterol, and sodium is 30 to 40 percent.

Margarine

Margarine was developed to be a substitute for butter. Made from vegetable oils, it appears to be more healthful; as a plant-derived food, it's certainly cholesterol free, and vegetable oils contain more unsaturated fatty acids than butter. Inconveniently, though, unsaturated oils are liquid, and without extra processing, margarine would run right off any slice of bread. Hydrogenated oils are needed to produce a spreadable consistency. But, as you know, hydrogenation increases the number of saturated and *trans* fatty acids in a fat, and both of these are associated with higher blood cholesterol levels.

Looking at the label of a standard stick margarine, you'll find the following per tablespoon:
- 100 kcals
- 11 g fat
- 2 g saturated fat
- 3.5 g polyunsaturated fat
- 3.5 g monounsaturated fat
- 0 mg cholesterol
- 115 mg sodium
- 10 % Daily Value for vitamin A

So compared to butter, we have the same amount of calories and fat (a fact unknown to many consumers!), less saturated fat and cholesterol, and a bit more sodium and vitamin A. The PUFA and MUFA content of butter is not listed, because these are not required elements of the Nutrition Facts label.

Turning to the list of ingredients, we find "liquid soybean oil, partially hydrogenated soybean oil, water, whey, salt, soy lecithin, and vegetable mono- and diglycerides (emulsifiers), sodium benzoate (a preservative),

has fewer calories per gram than fat. Like other proteins, however, these substitutes are denatured by high heat, and this limits their usefulness. The protein-based product Simplesse was used commercially in frozen desserts, but was not well accepted.

The most high-tech fat replacers—and the most controversial—are the lipids (or "fat-based" substitutes, as the industry calls them). This group includes Olean and the poorly digested Caprenin and Salatrim (or Benefat). Caprenin is a blend of medium-chain fatty acids and a 22-carbon fatty acid. Salatrim is primarily a blend of 18-carbon stearic acid and short-chain fatty acids. The fatty acids are arranged on glycerol in a way that inhibits digestion. They provide about half the calories of fat, though this is only an estimate because people differ in their ability to digest them. They are used in reduced-fat candies and baked goods.

One advantage of lipid-based fat substitutes is their ability to withstand heat. That's fortunate for **olestra** (Olean), because few food ingredients have had to "take as much heat." Technically, olestra is a sucrose poly-ester: sucrose (instead of glycerol) is the "backbone" molecule, with six to eight fatty acids attached (instead of triglyceride's three). (See **Figure 5.28**.) The number and arrangement of fatty acids and the length and saturation of

fat substitutes Compounds that imitate the functional and sensory properties of fats, but contain less available energy than fats.

olestra A fat substitute that can withstand heat and is stable at frying temperatures. Olestra, whose trade name is Olean, is a sucrose polyester: Sucrose (instead of glycerol) is the "backbone" molecule, with 6 to 8 fatty acids attached (instead of triglyceride's three). The fatty acid arrangement prevents hydrolysis by digestive lipases, so the fatty acids are not absorbed.

vitamin A palmitate, beta carotene (color)." Nothing terribly unusual, especially now that you know what lecithin and mono- and diglycerides are.

Spreads and Other Butter Imitators

Beyond the traditional stick margarine, there is a growing number of "light," "soft," "whipped," "squeeze," and "spread" products. These items do not fit the legal definition of "margarine," and so the term vegetable oil spread is generally used. In terms of ingredients, these products have more liquid oil and water, and less partially hydrogenated oils. More emulsifiers may be needed, along with flavors (including salt) and colors. The result typically is fewer calories, less saturated fat, and still no cholesterol.

Some products tout the inclusion of canola or olive oil for more healthful MUFA. Others indicate "no trans fatty acids" and have no hydrogenated oils on the list. Two new spreads, and at least one in development, contain plant sterols that reduce intestinal absorption of cholesterol.[1] More expensive than most spreads, these products have been treading a thin regulatory line between food regulations and dietary supplement regula-

tions. A third product, still under development, will contain the soluble fiber psyllium, also meant to lower cholesterol absorption.[2]

Cholesterol-lowering Margarines

Stanols are plant sterols similar in structure to cholesterol. Ingested plant sterols compete with and inhibit cholesterol absorption. Studies show that consumption of stanols reduces total blood cholesterol levels and LDL cholesterol levels.[3] HDL cholesterol levels increased or remained unchanged.[4] The new "cholesterol-lowering" margarines, Benecol and Take Control, contain plant sterols. Consumption of 3 grams of stanol per day, which is equivalent to three pats of margarine, can effectively improve lipid profiles and may reduce cardiovascular risk.[5]

Making Choices

The spread you choose may depend on your purpose. There are times, and foods, where nothing but real butter will do. If you've ever tried baking cookies with a soft, reduced-fat spread, you know the outcome...and probably will use butter, margarine, or vegetable shortening next time.

Remember, your goal is to limit total fats as well as saturated and *trans* fatty acids. Using

less butter or margarine overall will do that. Choosing a margarine or spread with liquid vegetable oil as the first ingredient (meaning that the amount of hydrogenated oil is less) will reduce not only saturated fat, but *trans* as well. Moderation is the key—making choices that consider your whole diet will help you stay in line with heart-healthy recommendations.

1 Haumann BF. Widening array of spread awaits shoppers. *Inform.* Jan 1998;6-13.

2 Ibrahim Y. Rocky path to market for edible foe of cholesterol. *New York Times.* Jan 31, 1999;Sect D:4 (col. 1).

3 Jones PJ, Ntanios FY, Raeini Sarjaz M, Vanstone CA. Cholesterol-lowering efficacy of a sitostanol-containing phytosterol mixture with a prudent diet in hyperlipidemic men. *Am J Clin Nutr.* Jun 1999;69: 1144-1150; and Gylling H, Miettinen TA. Cholesterol reduction by different plant stanol mixtures and with variable fat intake. *Metabolism.* May 1999;48:575-580; and Jones PJ, MacDougall DE, Ntanios F, Vanstone CA. Dietary phytosterols as cholesterol-lowering agents in humans. *Can J Physiol Pharmacol.* Mar 1997;75:217-227.

4 Gylling H, Miettinen TA. Cholesterol reduction by different plant stanol mixtures and with variable fat intake. *Metabolism.* May 1999;48:575-580.

5 Jones PJ, MacDougall DE, Ntanios F, Vanstone CA. Dietary phytosterols as cholesterol-lowering agents in humans. *Can J Physiol Pharmacol.* Mar 1997;75:217-227.

[Fyi] Does "Reduced Fat" Reduce Calories? That Depends on the Food.

Reducing fat intake is a common dietary recommendation, one that can help reduce risk for heart disease, cancer, and obesity. Given that fat is our most concentrated source of calories, we expect a reduced-fat or low-fat food would have fewer calories than it's unmodified counterpart. But is this always true?

Sometimes low-fat and fat-free foods make a big difference in calories.*

Food	Kcalories
1 oz American cheese	105
1 oz reduced-fat cheese product	75
2 oz bologna	180
2 oz fat-free bologna	40
1 tbsp mayonnaise	100
1 tbsp low-fat mayonnaise/dressing	25

But, sometimes they make almost no difference at all**

Food	Kcalories
½ cup canned vegetable soup	80
½ cup fat-free vegetable soup	90
2 chocolate cookies (30 g)	140
2 reduced-fat chocolate cookies (30 g)	120
2 tbsp peanut butter	190
2 tbsp reduced-fat peanut butter	190
3 oz country-style steak-fried potatoes	110
3 oz low-fat steak-fried potatoes	110
2 tbsp butterscotch caramel topping	130
2 tbsp fat-free caramel topping	130

Many fat-reduced products contain added sugar. Although sugar has fewer calories per gram than fat, the amount added may negate any difference in calories. If fat is your concern, low-fat or fat-free makes sense. But if you're trying to reduce fat *and* calories, modified products may not be a big help. So, be a smart shopper—check the label before you check out with a cartload of fat-free foods.

Sources:

* Adapted from Food Insight, Sep/Oct 1997;2–3. Published by the International Food Information Council, Washington, D.C.

** Adapted from Tufts University Health & Nutrition Letter, March 1998;4–5. Published by Tufts University, Medford, Mass.

Nutrition Facts

Serving Size: 1 Tbsp (14g)
Servings: 32

Calories 100
    Fat Cal 100

Amount/serving

	%DV
Total Fat 11g	17%
Saturated Fat 1.5g	8%
Cholesterol 5mg	2%
Sodium 80mg	3%
Total Carbohydrate 0g	0%
Protein 0g	

* Percent Daily Values (DV) are based on a 2,000 calorie diet.

INGREDIENTS: SOYBEAN OIL, WHOLE EGGS AND EGG YOLKS, WATER, VINEGAR, SALT, SUGAR, LEMON JUICE, NATURAL FLAVORS, CALCIUM DISODIUM SULFATE EDTA USED TO PROTECT QUALITY.

Regular mayonnaise

Nutrition Facts

Serving Size: 1 Tbsp (14g)
Servings: 32

Calories 50
    Fat Cal 45

Amount/serving

	%DV
Total Fat 5g	8%
Saturated Fat 1g	4%
Cholesterol 5mg	2%
Sodium 115mg	5%
Total Carbohydrate 0g	0%
Protein 0g	

* Percent Daily Values (DV) are based on a 2,000 calorie diet. Not a significant source of dietary fiber, vitamin A, vitamin C, calcium, and iron.

INGREDIENTS: WATER, SOYBEAN OIL, VINEGAR, FOOD STARCH-MODIFIED*, EGG YOLKS, SUGAR, SALT, SUGAR, LEMON JUICE, MUSTARD FLOUR, XANTHAN GUM*, BETA-CAROTENE (COLOR)*, AND NATURAL FLAVORS, POTASSIUM SORBATE, AND CALCIUM DISODIUM SULFATE EDTA USED TO PROTECT QUALITY.

*INGREDIENTS NOT FOUND IN MAYONNAISE.

Light mayonnaise

each fatty acid determine the characteristics of the sucrose polyester. This allows manufacturers to vary properties such as melting point and consistency, to make it appropriate for each intended use. The fatty acid arrangement prevents hydrolysis by digestive lipase, so the fatty acids are not absorbed. This makes olestra calorie-free, even though its fatty acids give it the flavor and cooking performance of fat. It is stable even at frying temperatures.

The Olestra Controversy: Are Fat Substitutes Safe?

Carbohydrate- and protein-based fat substitutes have raised few safety concerns. Most safety issues center around olestra, which aroused controversy long before it received FDA approval as a food additive in January 1996. The approval process itself was controversial,[29] and olestra continues to evoke strong, conflicting opinions.[30]

Unfortunately, olestra acts as a solvent for fat-soluble nutrients. This means that when it leaves the body unabsorbed, it carries these nutrients with it. The manufacturer replaces fat-soluble vitamins, but critics counter that healthful phytochemicals like the carotenoids are lost and not replaced.

Since olestra is not absorbed, it can cause symptoms of fat malabsorption in some people—diarrhea, gas, and cramps. The FDA requires a label warning: "This Product Contains Olestra. Olestra may cause abdominal cramping and loose stools. Olestra inhibits the absorption of some vitamins and other nutrients. Vitamins A, D, E, and K have been added." Olestra critics want this label displayed more prominently and want the warning to be more explicit about nutrient loss; olestra proponents disagree.

The FDA, concerned about malabsorption and nutrient loss, has limited olestra's use to just a few snack foods. Critics would like to see olestra eliminated altogether, while the industry wants usage expanded. The average olestra intake among users is expected to be about 10 grams daily, the amount in a one-ounce serving of snack chips. This intake would save about 80 kilocalories daily. Heavy snackers who eat olestra products are expected to get about 20 grams. Market surveillance (as mandated by the FDA) is under way to determine actual olestra consumption, its effect on body weight and calorie intake, and incidence of adverse reactions.[31]

Some consumers have complained about digestive symptoms after eating olestra-containing chips, but that could be the "power of suggestion" brought on by adverse publicity and the label warning. In fact, in a large double-blind study of volunteers pitting olestra-containing chips against regular chips, more people had indigestion after eating the regular chips. Will using olestra subtly encourage people to eat more? In another study, when subjects ate unlabeled olestra-containing potato chips, they ate fewer total calories and less fat than when they ate unlabeled regular potato chips. But when they knew the chips they were eating were fat-free, the subjects ate more.[32] If consumers eat too much olestra-containing snacks, they may be more likely to suffer side effects.

Do Fat Substitutes Save Calories? Do They Reduce Total Fat Intake?

Considering the American population as a whole, the answer to these questions seems to be no. American fat and calorie intake has not decreased over the past few years, a time when the fat-substitute market has been growing rapidly. It is clear that fat substitutes won't help if people treat them simply as an excuse to eat more. Nor should "low-fat foods" be confused with "low-calorie foods"; the calories saved by eating low-fat foods are often negligible.[33]

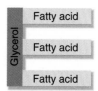

A triglyceride has three fatty acids attached to a glycerol backbone

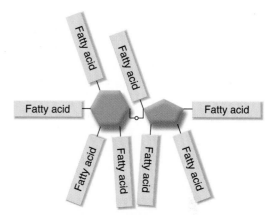

Olestra has six to eight fatty acids attached to a sucrose backbone

Figure 5.28 **The structure of olestra is unlike the structure of a triglyceride.** Although Olestra imparts triglyceride-like qualities to food, your digestive enzymes cannot break it down.

Key Concepts: *Americans are making progress toward meeting dietary goals of no more than 30 percent of calories from fat, no more than 10 percent of calories from saturated fats, and no more than 300 milligrams of cholesterol daily. It appears, though, that progress has slowed over the past few years, with more people eating more fat and calories, despite the increased availability of a wide variety of fat substitutes and lower fat foods.*

Lipids and Health

Moderation and balance are the keys to a healthful diet. When diets are consistently high in fat, several problems emerge. High-fat diets are typically high in calories, and contribute to weight gain and obesity. High intakes of fat and saturated fat increase risk for heart disease, and high-fat diets have been weakly linked to several types of cancer. The dietary recommendations discussed above suggest levels of fat intake that should reduce risk for these conditions.

Obesity

obesity Excessive accumulation of body fat leading to a body weight in relation to height that is substantially greater than some accepted standard.

Obesity is defined as the excessive accumulation of body fat leading to a body weight in relation to height that is substantially greater than some accepted standard (see Chapter 8, "Energy Balance and Weight Management"). The National Institutes of Health estimates that 55 percent of American adults are overweight or obese, and the rates are climbing, especially among children and teens.

Eating large amounts of dietary fat contributes to this obesity epidemic (See **Table 5.5.**) Fat is a dense source of calories, it makes food taste good, and it's often unnoticed or "hidden" in restaurant and convenience foods. Standard advice to Americans trying to maintain or attain normal weight usually includes cutting back on fats and fatty foods, along with increasing physical activity and eating fewer kilocalories. For more on obesity and weight management, see Chapter 8.

Heart Disease

In the early 1960s high blood cholesterol, or **hypercholesterolemia,** was identified as a principal risk factor for **cardiovascular disease,** along with

Table 5.5 **Fat Can Markedly Increase Calories in Food**

	Approximate Calories	Approximate Fat (g)
4 oz fried potatoes	209	9.4
4 oz boiled potatoes	98	0.1
$\frac{1}{2}$ c creamed cottage cheese	108	4.7
$\frac{1}{2}$ c 1% low fat cottage cheese	82	1.2
$\frac{1}{2}$ c green beans + 1 tsp butter	69	5.9
$\frac{1}{2}$ c green beans without butter	18	0.1
3 oz T-bone steak, untrimmed	253	18.0
3 oz T-bone steak, trimmed	182	8.8
$\frac{1}{2}$ c vanilla ice cream	150	8.0
$\frac{1}{2}$ c low fat vanilla ice cream	100	2.0

Source: Based on data from U.S. Department Of Agriculture, Agricultural Research Service, 1999. USDA Nutrient Database for Standard Reference. Release 13.

smoking and high blood pressure. Around the same time, it became clear that changes in diet could affect blood cholesterol levels and therefore change that risk factor. The concepts, as they were then understood, seemed simple: artery disease and heart attack were often caused by atherosclerosis, the buildup of fatty plaques inside the artery wall. High blood cholesterol was associated with atherosclerosis, and diet could affect blood cholesterol levels.

Recently, the picture has become more complicated. A high blood cholesterol level usually leads to more specific testing for HDL and LDL levels. High LDL cholesterol levels are now known to pose a greater risk than high total cholesterol, with some kinds of LDL being more dangerous than others. Low HDL cholesterol levels are also considered a risk factor for heart disease, as are high levels of triglycerides and other newly discovered blood lipids.[34] For example, lipoprotein a (Lp(a)) is a low-density lipoprotein that at high levels seems especially harmful, preventing the normal breakup of blood clots that cause heart attack or stroke. Lp(a) is associated with heart attack, but it's still unclear if and how it is influenced by diet.[35] Some viral and bacterial infections may also damage blood vessels, thus initiating atherosclerosis.[36]

In May 2001, the National Cholesterol Education Program (NCEP) of the National Heart, Lung and Blood Institute (NHLBI) released new guidelines for reducing heart disease risk. Changes from earlier guidelines include (1) treating high cholesterol more aggressively in people with diabetes, (2) a cholesterol test every 5 years for all adults over age 20, (3) defining low HDL as being less than 40 mg/dL compared to the earlier value of 35 mg/dL, (4) intensifying the use of nutrition, physical activity, and weight control in the treatment of elevated blood cholesterol, (5) identifying a "metabolic syndrome" of risk factors linked to insulin resistance, which often occur together and dramatically increase risk of heart attack, and (6) more aggressive treatment for elevated triglycerides.[37] **Table 5.6** shows triglyceride levels and levels of total and LDL cholesterol considered desirable, borderline high, and high according to the new guidelines.

hypercholesterolemia High blood cholesterol (total cholesterol).

cardiovascular disease (CVD) General term for all disorders affecting the heart and blood vessels.

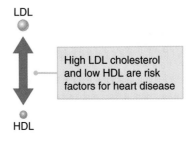

LDL

High LDL cholesterol and low HDL are risk factors for heart disease

HDL

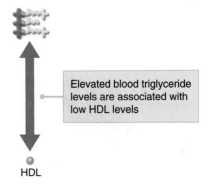

Elevated blood triglyceride levels are associated with low HDL levels

HDL

Table 5.6 Adult Blood Cholesterol and Triglyceride Levels

	TOTAL CHOLESTEROL		*LDL CHOLESTEROL*
Desirable	< 200	Optimal	< 100
Borderline-high	200–239	Near Optimal/above optimal	110–129
High	≥ 240	Borderline high	130-159
		High	160-189
		Very High	≥ 190

Note: All units are mg/dL.

Adult Triglyceride Levels

Normal	< 150 mg/dL
Borderline-high	150-159
High	200-499
Very high	≥ 500

Sources: National Cholesterol Education Program. *Third report of the expert panel on detection, evaluation, and treatment of high blood cholesterol in adults (adult treatment panel III).* NIH publication 01-3305, May 2001.

NCEP Tips for Healthful Eating Out

- Choose restaurants that have low-fat, low-cholesterol menu items.
- Don't be afraid to ask for foods that follow your eating pattern.
- Select poultry, fish, or meat that is broiled, grilled, baked, steamed, or poached rather than fried.
- Choose lean deli meats like fresh turkey or lean roast beef instead of higher fat cuts like salami or bologna.
- Look for vegetables seasoned with herbs or spices rather than butter, sour cream, or cheese. Ask for sauces on the side.
- Order a low-fat dessert like sherbet, fruit ice, sorbet, or low-fat frozen yogurt.
- Control serving sizes by asking for a small serving, sharing a dish, or taking some home.
- At fast-food restaurants, go for grilled chicken and lean roast beef sandwiches or lean plain hamburgers (but remember to hold the fatty sauces), salads with low-fat salad dressing, low-fat milk, and low-fat frozen yogurt. Pizza topped with vegetables and minimum cheese is another good choice.

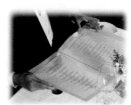

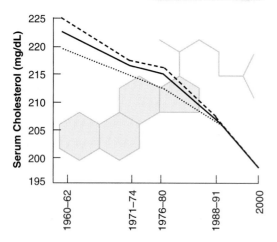

Key
.... men
- - - - women
——— total

Figure 5.29 **Trends in age-adjusted mean serum cholesterol.**
Source: CDC, NCHS, NHESI, NHANES I, NHANES II, NHANES III (Phase 1, 1988–91).

Reducing Risk of Heart Disease: Lifestyle Factors

Some of the risks for development of atherosclerosis are beyond our control—like being male and/or getting older. But we can control many risks. Avoiding or quitting smoking is a positive step toward reducing risk. Managing weight and controlling blood pressure are other steps we can take. Health experts also stress the importance of physical activity for keeping weight normal, and for overall heart health.[38]

Reducing Risk of Heart Disease: Dietary Factors

Some years ago, many health experts were advising people to emphasize polyunsaturated oils in their diets. Health experts seldom give this advice today. When saturated fat is replaced with omega-6 rich polyunsaturated oils like corn oil, total cholesterol and LDL cholesterol may decrease, but so does healthful HDL cholesterol. The polyunsaturated fatty acids in vegetable oils also oxidize easily, and provide too much omega-6 fatty acid in relation to omega-3. New research shows that monounsaturated fats like olive oil, previously thought to have little effect on cholesterol, are now known to lower total and LDL cholesterol without lowering HDL.[39]

Earlier diet advice also emphasized minimizing dietary cholesterol—few egg yolks, no liver or organ meats, and no seafood (the amount of cholesterol in seafood was later found to have been overestimated). Lowering cholesterol intake does help some people, but for most, the result is variable and less effective than lowering intake of saturated fats.

Today, nutritionists recommend lowering total fat intake, lowering saturated fat, and keeping body weight normal. Within total fat limits, monounsaturated oils should be the fat source of choice. Reducing dietary cholesterol is a good idea for those who do respond to such a change. Eating fruits, vegetables, legumes, and grains that contain soluble fiber helps lower cholesterol levels, too. These foods also have antioxidant nutrients and B vitamins such as folic acid that may also reduce the risk of heart disease.

Since its inception in 1985, the National Cholesterol Education Program (NCEP) has made population-wide dietary recommendations. Here are their latest recommendations:

- Choose foods low in saturated fat.
- Choose foods low in total fat.
- Choose foods high in starch and fiber.
- Choose foods low in cholesterol.
- Be more physically active.
- Maintain a healthy weight, and lose weight if you are overweight.

Beyond Cholesterol

Just when it seems the role of diet in heart disease is clear, new questions arise to confuse the picture. It's true that death from coronary heart disease has fallen dramatically, by more than 50 percent over the past 30 years. That drop seems related to a 28 percent drop in hypercholesterolemia from 1976 to 1994 (See **Figure 5.29**.) which in turn parallels a reduced consumption of cholesterol and percentage of calories from fat.[40]

But have less fat and cholesterol made us more heart healthy? Or do falling death rates reflect better treatment of heart attacks and existing heart disease? Although the weight of evidence supports preventive efforts including diet, several studies suggest that treatment, rather than prevention, has been the more important factor in reducing deaths from heart disease.[41]

Since most heart attacks occur in people with average to moderately high blood cholesterol, researchers are exploring other factors that may produce these heart attacks.[42] They also are exploring why many people with high blood cholesterol don't develop heart disease. Looking beyond fat and cholesterol, researchers have found that other important dietary factors are involved.

Antioxidants There is much good evidence for the oxidation theory, which has become widely accepted. In the blood, oxygen can damage low-density lipoproteins. Once oxidized, they are deposited in the inner layer of the blood vessels, and the atherosclerotic process begins.[43] A diet high in vitamin E and other antioxidants appears to inhibit oxidation and subsequent atherosclerosis.[44]

Homocysteine High levels of the amino acid homocysteine may contribute to heart disease by promoting atherosclerosis, excessive blood clotting, or blood vessel rigidity. Folic acid and vitamins B_6 and B_{12} are all important in the metabolism of homocysteine, reducing destructive levels. Scientists believe that a diet rich in these vitamins helps prevent blood vessel damage from homocysteine.[45]

Dietary Omega-3 Fatty Acids In the 1970s a study of the Inuits (Greenland Eskimos) focused attention on the beneficial physiologic influence of EPA and DHA, the omega-3 fatty acids in fish fats.[46] Researchers were puzzled: here was a population with a high intake of fat, saturated fat, and cholesterol from marine mammals and fish. Yet they had little evidence of atherosclerosis. The Inuits were compared to Danes among whom atherosclerosis was common, and whose diet was similarly high in fat, but from meats and dairy products. It became clear the high EPA and DHA content of fish in the Inuit diet had a protective effect, discouraging blood cells from clotting and from sticking to artery walls. Population studies of other cultures yielded fairly consistent results. The Japanese, for example, with their generous fish intake, had low rates of atherosclerosis. A considerable number of observational and intervention studies have pointed in the same direction, some showing that as few as two or three servings of fish weekly can be protective.

Interest in omega-3 fatty acids has expanded recently. Research shows that omega-3s can modestly lower blood pressure, and can help lower elevated blood triglycerides.[47] In addition to their circulatory effects, they may also help some chronic inflammatory conditions such as rheumatoid arthritis,[48] asthma,[49] or psoriasis. Research in these areas has sometimes disappointed,[50] and despite their low rates of heart disease, Greenland Eskimos are at higher risk for hemorrhagic types of strokes due to reduced blood clotting. All in all, however, there are enough positive results to encourage further study and recommend regular consumption of fish for EPA and DHA, as well as plant foods with alpha-linolenic acid.[51]

Soluble Fiber As described in Chapter 4, soluble fibers bind to bile acids in the gastrointestinal tract, so these bile acids are excreted in the feces rather than recycled and reused. Additional bile acids then must be made from cholesterol, lowering the total amount in the body. In addition, soluble fibers can be fermented by intestinal bacteria, and the resulting short-chain fatty acids have been linked to reduced cholesterol synthesis.[52]

The French Paradox How can the French eat rich cheeses and fatty meats but still have low rates of heart disease? The focus is on their intake of red

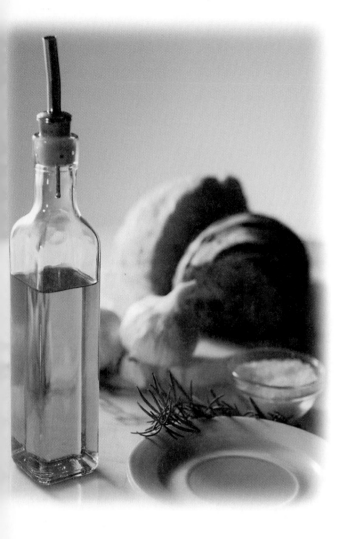

wine and grapes, both rich in antioxidant phytochemicals.[53] There's understandable reluctance to recommend wine, even a small glass daily, but grapes and other purple fruits and vegetables contain the same phytochemicals as red wine. The French diet is evidence that fruits and vegetables help reduce the risk of heart disease.

The Mediterranean Diet How can Greeks, Turks, and others around the Mediterranean eat a diet high in fat but still have low rates of heart disease? The focus here is on the source of the fat—olive oil. Their diet pattern—ample fresh fruits, vegetables, pasta and grains, small amounts of meat and poultry, and generous use of olive oil—has gained support among some nutritionists.[54]

Other Phytochemicals Along with antioxidants, other plant chemicals affect heart disease risk. Two widely studied phytochemical groups are isoflavones in soybeans and lignans in flax seed, whole grains, and some fruits. These are also referred to as phytoestrogens—plant compounds with hormone-like effects. In November 1999, the FDA approved a health claim for food labels about the role of soy protein in reducing the risk of coronary heart disease. The proposal was based on studies showing that 25 grams of soy protein per day has a cholesterol-lowering effect.[55]

Cancer

The evidence linking dietary fat to cancer is inconclusive. The case looks strong when we compare cancer rates of countries: overall cancer rates are generally higher in countries with high fat intake, and lower in countries where people eat less fat. But in population studies within those countries, the evidence linking fat to cancer is weaker. The Nurses' Health Study followed more than 121,000 women for 14 years and found no evidence that higher total fat intake was associated with an increased risk of breast cancer.[56] These results call into question theories that link dietary fat with other cancers. Red meat intake, but not total fat, may be related to colon cancer, and animal fats may be related to prostate cancer. Calorie intake may be a more important factor than fat intake.[57]

Development of Cancer

Cancer develops in a multistage process that occurs over many years. There are typically three phases of development:

1. *initiation,* when something alters a cell's genetic structure and prepares it to act abnormally during later stages

2. *promotion,* a reversible stage when a chemical or other factor encourages initiated cells to become active, and

3. *progression,* when promoted cells multiply and may invade surrounding healthy tissue

Evidence suggests that between 30 and 40 percent of cancers are due to poor food choices and physical inactivity, although the role of nutrition and diet in cancer development is complex. Some dietary factors may act as promoters; many others may have protective roles, blocking the cellular changes in one of the developmental stages.

When cancer is chemically induced in the rodents traditionally used as research subjects, high intake of fat, calories, and omega-6 fatty acids all appear to promote tumor growth.[58] Just how relevant these studies are to humans is unclear, and any conclusions about the relationship between dietary fats and cancer remain controversial.

Diet and Cancer Risk Reduction

Strategies for reducing cancer risk include a moderately low-fat diet and increased consumption of fruits and vegetables and whole grains. Sounds familiar, right? The same antioxidant properties that may reduce atherosclerosis can also affect cancer development. In addition to having antioxidant effects, nutrients and other phytochemicals may inhibit multiplication of cancer cells, alter enzymes, inhibit the conversion of chemicals into toxins, and alter hormone metabolism.

The report *Food, Nutrition and the Prevention of Cancer: A Global Perspective* presents guidelines for reducing the risk of cancer.[59] These recommendations were based on 4,500 research studies and contributions from more than 120 individuals, organizations, and peer reviewers. The "Advice to Individuals" concerning diet includes the following statements. Reducing fat intake is just one of many recommendations.

1. Choose predominantly plant-based diets rich in a variety of vegetables and fruits, legumes, and minimally processed starchy staple foods.

2. Avoid being underweight or overweight and limit weight gain during adulthood to less than 5 kg (11 lb).

3. If occupational activity is low or moderate, take an hour's brisk walk or similar exercise daily, and also exercise vigorously for a total of at least one hour each week.

4. Eat 400 g to 800 g (15–30 oz), or five or more portions (servings) a day of a variety of vegetables and fruits, all year round.

5. Eat 600 g to 800 g (20–30 oz), or more than seven portions (servings) a day of a variety of cereals (grains), legumes, roots, tubers, and plantains. Select minimally processed foods. Limit consumption of refined sugar.

6. Alcohol consumption is not recommended. Limit alcoholic drinks to fewer than two drinks per day for men and one for women.

7. Limit intake of red meat to less than 80 g (3 oz) daily. Fish, poultry, and meat from nondomesticated animals is preferable to red meat.

8. Limit consumption of fatty foods, particularly those of animal origin. Choose modest amounts of appropriate vegetable oils.

9. Limit consumption of salted foods and use of cooking and table salt. Use herbs and spices to season foods.

10. Do not eat food that, as a result of prolonged storage at ambient temperatures, is liable to contamination with mycotoxins (toxins produced by molds).

11. Use refrigeration and other appropriate methods to preserve perishable foods.

12. When levels of additives, contaminants, and other residues conform to proper regulations, their presence in food and drink is not known to be harmful. However, unregulated or improper use can be a health hazard, and this applies particularly in economically developing countries.

Quick Bites

What does the color of beef fat reveal?

Yellow-tinged fat indicates that a steer was grass fed, white fat suggests that the animal was fed corn or cereal grain, at least during its final months. Thus, steak surrounded by pearly white fat should be more tender and, consequently, more expensive.

13. Do not eat charred food. For meat and fish eaters, avoid burning meat juices. Consume the following only occasionally: meat and fish grilled (broiled) in a direct flame; cured or smoked meats.

14. For those who follow these recommendations, dietary supplements are probably unnecessary, and possibly unhelpful, for reducing cancer risk.

Key Concepts: Excessive fat intake has been linked to obesity, heart disease, and cancer. There is a major public heath effort to reduce intake of fat, saturated fat, and cholesterol. Cholesterol-lowering diets have changed over the years, with somewhat less emphasis on reducing dietary cholesterol, and more on reducing fats and saturated fats, and increasing fruits, vegetables, and whole grains. The evidence linking dietary fats with cancer is less clear, but many other dietary factors are important in reducing risk.

Label [to] **Table**

The Nutrition Facts panel shown here highlights all of the lipid-related information you can find on a food label. Look to the top of the label where it states that this product contains 35 Calories from Fat. Do you know how you can estimate this number from another part of the label? Recall (or look to the bottom of the label) that each gram of fat contains 9 kilocalories. If this food item has 4 grams of fat, then it should make sense that there are approximately 36 kilocalories provided by fat. In this case, because the manufacturer listed only 35 you can assume that the 4 grams fat on the label is rounded up from the actual total fat content of 3.9 grams (3.9 grams of fat × 9 kilocalories per gram = 35 kilocalories of fat).

Total Fat is the second thing you'll see along with saturated fat. Recall that fats are classified into 3 types: saturated, monounsaturated, and polyunsaturated. Manufacturers are required to list only saturated fat on the label but they can voluntarily list the others. Using this food label, you can estimate the amount of unsaturated fat by simply looking at the highlighted sections. There are 4 total grams of fat and 2.5 of them are saturated. That means the remaining 1.5 grams are either polyunsaturated or monounsaturated. Without even knowing what food item this label represents, you can decipher that it contains more saturated fat than unsaturated fat (2.5g vs. 1.5g). This is typical of a food that contains fat from an animal source or tropical oil.

Do you see the 6% to the right of "Total Fat"? This does not mean that the food item contains 6% of its calories from fat. In fact, this food item contains 23% of its calories from fat (35 fat kcal ÷ 154 total kilocalories = .23, or 23% fat). The 6% refers to the Daily Values found below. You can see that a person who consumes 2,000 kcalories per day could consume up to 65 grams of fat per day. This product contributes just 4 grams per serving, which is 6% of that amount (4 ÷ 65 = .06, or 6%). Note that the % Daily Value for saturated fat is 12% which means that just a few servings of this food can contribute quite a bit of saturated fat to your diet. Cholesterol is also highlighted on this label (20 mg) along with its Daily Value contribution (7%).

Nutrition Facts

Serving Size: 1 cup (248g)
Servings Per Container: 4

Amount Per Serving

Calories 154   Calories from fat 35

	% Daily Value*
Total Fat 4g	6%
Saturated Fat 2.5g	12%
Cholesterol 20mg	7%
Sodium 170mg	7%
Total Carbohydrate 19g	6%
Dietary Fiber 0g	0%
Sugars 14g	
Protein 11g	

Vitamin A 4%	•	Vitamin C 6%
Calcium 40%	•	Iron 0%

* Percent Daily Values are based on a 2,000 calorie diet. Your daily values may be higher or lower depending on your calorie needs:

		Calories:	2000	2,500
Total Fat	Less Than		65g	80g
Sat Fat	Less Than		20g	25g
Cholesterol	Less Than		300mg	300mg
Sodium	Less Than		2,400mg	2,400mg
Total Carbohydrate			300g	375g
Dietary Fiber			25g	30g

Calories per gram:
Fat 9 • Carbohydrate 4 • Protein 4

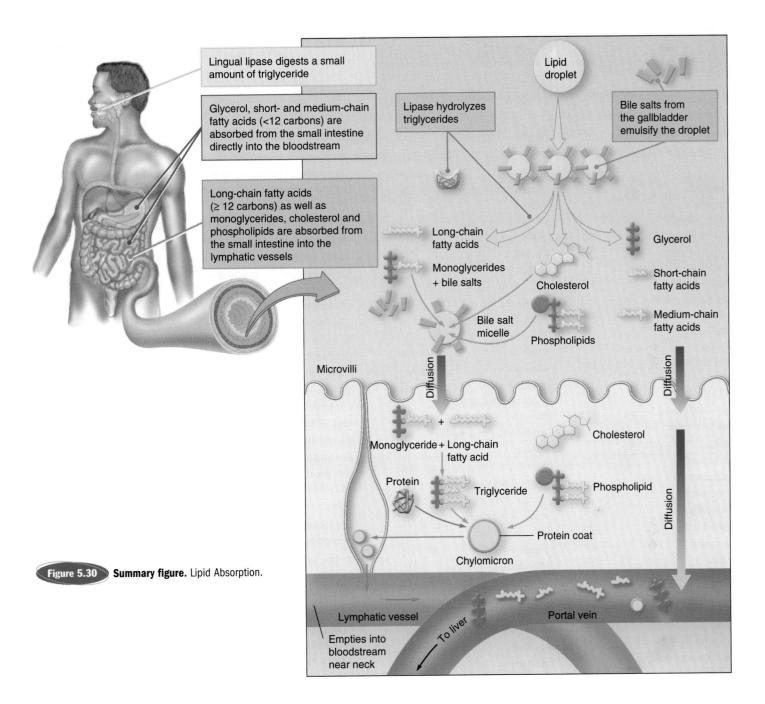

Lingual lipase digests a small amount of triglyceride

Glycerol, short- and medium-chain fatty acids (<12 carbons) are absorbed from the small intestine directly into the bloodstream

Long-chain fatty acids (≥ 12 carbons) as well as monoglycerides, cholesterol and phospholipids are absorbed from the small intestine into the lymphatic vessels

Lipid droplet

Lipase hydrolyzes triglycerides

Bile salts from the gallbladder emulsify the droplet

Long-chain fatty acids

Monoglycerides + bile salts

Cholesterol

Glycerol

Short-chain fatty acids

Medium-chain fatty acids

Bile salt micelle

Phospholipids

Microvilli

Diffusion

Diffusion

Monoglyceride + Long-chain fatty acid

Cholesterol

Protein

Triglyceride

Phospholipid

Diffusion

Protein coat

Chylomicron

Lymphatic vessel

To liver

Portal vein

Empties into bloodstream near neck

Figure 5.30 **Summary figure.** Lipid Absorption.

LEARNING *Portfolio*

c h a p t e r   5

Key Terms

	page		page
adipocyte	144	lanugo [lah-NEW-go]	144
adipose tissue	144	lecithin	149
alpha-linolenic acid [Al-fah-lin-oh-LEN-ik]	142	linoleic acid [lin-oh-LAY-ik]	142
atherosclerosis [ath-e-roh-scle-ROH-sis]	151	lipophilic	136
bioavailability	144	lipophobic	136
cardiovascular disease (CVD)	167	lipoprotein	155
chain length	136	lipoprotein lipase (LPL)	158
cholesterol [ko-LES-te-rol]	151	low-density lipoprotein (LDL)	159
choline	149	lycopene	144
chylomicron [kye-lo-MY-kron]	155	micelles	154
cis fatty acids	140	monoglyceride	143
conjugated linoleic acid	140	monounsaturated fatty acid	138
desaturation	140	nonessential fatty acid	140
diglyceride	143	obesity	166
eicosanoids	140	olestra	163
elongation	140	omega-3 fatty acid	140
enterocytes	155	omega-6 fatty acid	140
essential fatty acids	140	omega-9 fatty acid	140
ester	143	oxidation	147
esterification [e-ster-ih-fih-KAY-shun]	143	phosphate group	148
fat substitutes	163	phospholipid	136
fatty acid	136	phytosterols	153
glycerol [GLISS-er-ol]	142	polyunsaturated fatty acid	138
high-density lipoprotein (HDL)	159	saturated fatty acid	138
hydrogenation [high-dro-jen-AY-shun]	140	squalene	153
hydrophilic [high-dro-FILL-ik]	136	steatorrhea	155
hydrophobic	136	sterols	136
hypercholesterolemia	167	subcutaneous fat	144
intermediate-density lipoprotein (IDL)	159	trans fatty acids	140
		unsaturated fatty acid	138
		very-low-density lipoprotein (VLDL)	158
		visceral fat	144

Study Points

➤ Lipids are a group of compounds that are soluble in organic solvents but not in water. Fats and oils are part of the lipids group.

➤ There are three main classes of lipids: triglycerides, phospholipids, and sterols.

➤ Fatty acids—long carbon chains with methyl and carboxyl groups on the ends—are components of both triglycerides and phospholipids, and are often attached to cholesterol.

➤ Saturated fatty acids have no double bonds between carbons in the chain, monounsaturated fatty acids have one double bond, and polyunsaturated fatty acids have more than one double bond.

➤ Two polyunsaturated fatty acids, linoleic acid and alpha-linolenic acid, are essential; they must be supplied in the diet. Phospholipids and sterols are made in the body and do not have to be supplied in the diet.

➤ Essential fatty acids are elongated and desaturated in the process of making "local hormones" called eicosanoids. These compounds regulate many body functions.

➤ Triglycerides are food fats and storage fats. They are composed of glycerol and three fatty acids.

➤ In the body, triglycerides are an important source of energy. Stored fat provides an energy reserve.

➤ Phospholipids are made of glycerol, two fatty acids, and a phosphate group with a nitrogen-containing component.

➤ Phospholipids are components of cell membranes and lipoproteins. Their unique affinity for both fat and water allows them to be effective emulsifiers in foods and in the body.

➤ Cholesterol is found in cell membranes and is used to synthesize vitamin D, bile acids, and steroid hormones. High levels of blood cholesterol are associated with heart disease risk.

➤ Most sources recommend that Americans consume no more than 30 percent of calories as fat, no more than 7 percent of calories as saturated fat, and no more than 200 milligrams of cholesterol each day.

➤ Diets high in fat and saturated fat tend to increase blood levels of LDL cholesterol and increase risk for heart disease.

➤ Excess fat in the diet is linked to obesity, heart disease, and some types of cancer.

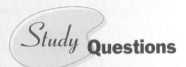
Study Questions

1. **How is it that different oils can contain a mixture of polyunsaturated, monounsaturated and saturated fats?**

2. **What does the hardness or softness of a lipid typically signify?**

3. **What is the most common form of lipid found in food?**

4. **What are the positive and negative consequences of hydrogenating a fat?**

5. **List the many functions of triglycerides.**

6. **Describe the difference between LDL and HDL in terms of cholesterol and protein composition.**

7. **List the recommendations for intake of fat, saturated fat, polyunsaturated fat, monounsaturated fat, and cholesterol.**

8. **What foods contain cholesterol?**

9. **Name the two essential fatty acids.**

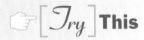
[Try] This

The Fat = Fullness Challenge

The goal of this experiment is to see whether fat affects your desire to eat between meals. Do this experiment for two consecutive breakfasts. Each meal is to include only the foods included below. Try to eat normally for the other meals of the day and eat around the same time of day. Each of these breakfasts has approximately the same calories but one has a high percentage of them from fat, the other from carbohydrate. After each breakfast, take note of how many hours pass before you feel hungry again.

Day 1 (~455 kcal)

One 3-oz bagel with 3 tbsp of jelly

Day 2 (~460 kcal)

2 eggs fried with minimal (< ¹/₂ tbsp) amount of butter/margarine

2 pieces of whole wheat bread with 1 tbsp of butter/margarine or ²/₃ tbsp of peanut butter

The Salad Dressing Experiment

You can learn a lot from oil-and-vinegar dressing! The purpose of this experiment is twofold. First, you will understand better what it means to say that lipids are insoluble (or not water soluble). Second, you will be able to experience how fat acts based on its density. Go to your local grocery store and purchase a seasoning packet for Italian (oil and vinegar) dressing. Make sure you also purchase the amount of oil (any type is fine) and vinegar (any type is fine) you need based on the directions. Once home, prepare the dressing. Shake the dressing as if you were to pour it on a salad and then let it stand. What happens to the dressing? What explains this action? Once the dressing settles, which ingredient is found on top—the oil or the vinegar? What property of fat explains this?

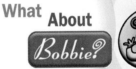
What About Bobbie?

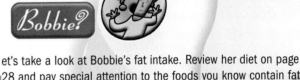

Let's take a look at Bobbie's fat intake. Review her diet on page 28 and pay special attention to the foods you know contain fat. Do you think she ate above or below the recommended 30 percent of total calories from fat? Did she eat more saturated or unsaturated fat? How about her cholesterol intake? Do you think she came in below the guideline?

Bobbie's total fat intake was 98 grams. Here are the foods that contributed the most fat:

Food	Fat (g)
Meatballs	17
Salad dressing	14
Tortilla chips	11
Pizza	11
Garlic bread	10
Cream cheese	8
Mayonnaise	7

Bobbie's diet has 36 percent of its calories from fat, which is higher than the recommended intake of 30 percent or less of total calorie intake. Here's how to calculate this:

$$98 \text{ g fat} \times 9 \text{ kcal/g} = 882 \text{ kcal fat}$$

$$882 \text{ kcal fat} \div 2{,}440 \text{ total kcal} = 0.36, \text{ or } 36\% \text{ kcal from fat}$$

What About

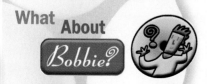

Are you surprised her fat intake is so high? Her intake doesn't look too unusual but you can see how the "extras" along the way add up. Look at the list of fat-containing foods again. Do you think her diet is higher in saturated or unsaturated fat? Well, three of the foods listed are animal products (meatballs, pizza, and cream cheese) so you know they contribute to the amount of saturated fat. Both the tortilla chips and garlic bread contain a mixture of saturated and unsaturated fats and the Italian dressing contains mostly unsaturated fat. Her overall saturated fat intake is 32 grams. That's about 12 percent of her caloric intake, which is almost in line with the guideline of less than 10 percent saturated fat intake. So even though her fat intake is slightly higher than recommended, her mix of saturated and unsaturated fats is very close to the guidelines. If Bobbie wanted to lower her saturated fat and total fat intake, what changes could she make? Here are some suggestions:

Bobbie can lower her saturated fat intake by:

- topping her bagel with peanut butter instead of cream cheese.
- decreasing the number of meatballs on her pasta.
- snacking on pizza less often.

Bobbie can lower her overall fat intake by:

- using cream cheese on only half her bagel and using jelly on the other half.
- using only mustard on her sandwich, not mustard and mayonnaise.
- reducing the amount of tortilla chips she eats by half and having a piece of fruit in their place.
- reducing the amount of Italian dressing she puts on her salad, 2 tbsp contains almost 140 kilocalories!
- having a plain piece of bread with dinner, not the garlic bread made with butter or margarine.

In terms of cholesterol, how do you think Bobbie did? She consumed 263 milligrams in this day, which is under the recommended upper limit of 300 milligrams. If she follows the above tips to lower her saturated fat intake, she'll find her overall cholesterol intake will be cut in half!

References

1 Samuelsson B. Identification of a smooth muscle-stimulating factor in bovine brain. *Biochem Biophys Acta.* 1964;84:218–219.

2 Connor WE. Importance of *n*-3 fatty acids in health and disease. *Am J Clin Nutr.* 2000;71(suppl):171S–175S.

3 Crawford MA. The role of essential fatty acids in neural development: implications for perinatal nutrition. *Am J Clin Nutr.* 1993;57:S703–S710.

4 Erdman JW, Bierer TL, Gugger ET. Absorption and transport of carotenoids. *Ann NY Acad Sci.* 1993;691:76–85.

5 Bilger B. The flavor of fat. *The Sciences.* Nov/Dec 1997:10.

6 National Cholesterol Education Program (NCEP). *Detection, Evaluation, and Treatment of High Blood Cholesterol in Adults.* Washington (DC): National Institutes of Health; 1993.

7 Wan PJ, Hron RJ. Extraction solvents for oilseeds. *Inform.* 1998;9(7):707–709.

8 Seidner DL. Clinical uses for omega-3 polyunsaturated fatty acids and structured triglycerides. *Support Line* (a newsletter of the Dietitians in Nutrition Support) June 1994;16(3):7–11.

9 Neaton JD, Blackburn H, Jacobs D, et al. Serum cholesterol level and mortality findings for men screened in the Multiple Risk Factor Intervention Trial. Multiple Risk Factor Intervention Trial research group. *Arch Intern Med.* 1992;152:1490–1500.

10 Cheblowski RT, Grosvenor M, Lillington L. Dietary intake and counseling, weight management, and the course of HIV infection. *J Am Diet Assoc.* 1995;95:428–432.

11 Cendella RJ. Cholesterol and cataracts. *Surv Opthalmol.* Jan 1996 40:4, 320–337.

12 Morell P, Jurevics H. Origin of cholesterol in myelin. *Neurochem Res.* Apr 1996;21:463–470.

13 Jones PJH. Regulation of cholesterol biosynthesis by diet in humans. *Am J Clin Nutr.* 1997;66:438–446.

14 Ibid.

15 Strauss E. One-eyed animals implicate cholesterol in development. *Science.* 1998;280:1528–1529.

16 Jones PJH, Kubow S. Lipids, sterols and their metabolites. In: Shils ME, Olson JA, Shike M, Ross CA, eds. Modern Nutrition in Health and Disease. 9th ed. Philadelphia: Lippincott Williams & Wilkins; 1999:67-94.

17 Guyton AC, Hall JE. *Textbook of Medical Physiology.* 9th ed. Philadelphia: WB Saunders; 1996.

18 Holt PR, Hashim SA, Van Itallie TB. Treatment of malabsorption syndrome and exudative enteropathy with synthetic medium chain triglycerides. *Am J Gastroenterol.* 1965;43:549–559.

19 Archer SY, Meng S, Shei A, et al. p21(WAF1) is required for butyrate-mediated growth inhibition of human colon cancer cells. *Proc Nat Acad Sci USA.* 1998;95:6791–6796.

20 Brown MS, Goldstein JL. A receptor-mediated pathway for cholesterol homeostasis. *Science.* 1986;232:34–47.

21 Dietschy JM, Turley SD, Spady DK. Role of liver in the maintenance of cholesterol and low density lipoprotein homeostasis in different animal species, including humans. *J Lipid Res.* 1993;34:1637–1659.

22 National Cholesterol Education Program. Op. cit.

23 Williams CL, Bollella M, Boccia L, et al. Dietary fat and children's health. *Nutrition Today.* 1998;33(4):144–155.

24 High blood cholesterol: what's known, what's new, what's ahead. *Heart Memo.* Summer 1998;5–17.

25 US Department of Agriculture, Economic Research Service. *Food Review.* Sept/Dec 1997.

26 Kris-Etherton PM, Taylor DS, Yu-Poth S, et al. Polyunsaturated fatty acids in the food chain in the United States. *Am J Clin Nutr.* 2000;71(suppl):179S–188S.

27 Ibid.

28 Calorie Control Council. Consumer demand for less fat remains strong. *Calorie Control Commentary.* Fall 1996;3.

29 Blackburn H. Olestra and the FDA. *N Engl J Med.* 1996;334:1996.

30 Jacobsen M, Corcoran L. Olestra. *Nutrition Action Healthletter* Mar 1998;9–11; and Callaway CW. Role of fat-modified foods in the American diet. *Nutrition Today.* 1998;33(4):156–163.

31 Kristal AR, Patterson RE, Neuhouser ML, et al. Olestra Postmarketing Surveillance Study: Design and baseline results for the sentinel site. *J Am Diet Assoc.* 1998;98:1290–1296.

32 Miller DL, Casteollanos VH, Shide DJ, et al. Effect of fat-free potato chips with and without nutrition labels on fat and energy intakes. *Am J Clin Nutr.* 1998;68:282–290.

33 Are reduced-fat foods keeping Americans healthier? *Tufts University Health & Nutrition Letter.* 1998;16(1):4–5.

34 Hoeg JM. Evaluating coronary heart disease risk. *JAMA.* 1997;277:1387–1390.

35 Bostrom AG, Cupples A, Jenner JL. Elevated plasma lipoprotein(a) and coronary heart disease in men aged 55 years and younger: a prospective study. *JAMA.* 1996;276:544–548.

36 Mlot C. Chlamydia linked to atherosclerosis. *Science.* 1996;272:1422; and Zhou YF, Leon MB, Waclawiw MA, et al. Association between prior cytomegalovirus infection and the risk of restonsis after coronary atherectomy. *N Engl J Med.* 1996;335:624–630.

37 National Cholesterol Education Program. *Third report of the expert panel on detection, evaluation, and treatment of high blood cholesterol in adults (adult treatment panel III).* NIH publication 01-3305, May 2001.

38 Ibid.

39 Kris-Etherton PM, Pearson TA, Wan Y, et al. High-monounsaturated fatty acid diets lower both plasma cholesterol and triacylglycerol concentrations. *Am J Clin Nutr.* 1999;70:1009–1015.

40 National Cholesterol Education Program. Second report of the expert panel on detection, evaluation, and treatment of high blood cholesterol in adults Washington (DC). Washington, DC: National Institutes of Health; 1993.

41 Rosamond WD, Chambless LE, Folsom AR, et al. Trends in the incidence of myocardial infarction and in mortality due to coronary heart disease, 1987 to 1994. *N Engl J Med.* 1998;339:861–867.

42 National Heart, Lung, and Blood Institute. Emerging risk factors—science's agenda for the next century. *Heart Memo.* Summer 1998:15.

43 Witzum JL. The oxidation hypothesis of atherosclerosis. *Lancet.* 1994;344:793–795.

44 Hodis HN, Mack WJ, LaBree L, et al. Serial coronary angiographic evidence that antioxidant vitamin intake reduces progression of coronary artery atherosclerosis. *JAMA.* 1995;273:1849–1854.

45 Epstein FH. Homocysteine and atherothrombosis. *N Engl J Med.* 1998;338:1042–1060.

46 Bang HO, Dyerberg J. The composition of food consumed by Greenlandic Eskimos. *Acta Med Scand.* 1973;200:69–73.

47 Harris WS. N-3 Fatty acids and serum lipoproteins: human studies. *Am J Clin Nutr.* 1997;65:S1645–1654.

48 Adam O. Review, anti-inflammatory diet in rheumatic diseases. *Euro J Clin Nutr.* 1995;49:703–717.

49 Lewis RA, Austen K, Soberman RJ. Leukotrienes and other products of the 5-lipoxygenase pathway. *N Engl J Med.* 1990;323;645–655.

50 Soyland E, Funk J., Rajka G., et al. Effect of dietary supplementation with very-long-chain n-3 fatty acids in patients with psoriasis. *N Engl J Med.* 1993;328:1812–1816.

51 Neaton JD, Blackburn H, Jacobs D, et al. Serum cholesterol level and mortality findings for men screened in the Multiple Risk Factor Intervention Trial. Multiple Risk Factor Intervention Trial research group. *Arch Intern Med.* 1992;152:1490–1500.

52 Anderson JW. Short-chain fatty acids and lipid metabolism. In: Cummings JH, Rombeau JL, Sakata T, eds. *Physiological and Clinical Aspects of Short Chain Fatty Acids.* New York: Cambridge University Press; 1995:509–523.

53 Drewnowski A, Henderson SA, Shore AB. Diet quality and dietary diversity in France: implications for the French paradox. *J Am Diet Assoc.* 1996;96:663–669.

54 Katan MB, Grundy SM, Willett WC. Beyond low fat diets. *N Engl J Med.* 1997;337:563–566.

55 FDA Talk Paper. New Health Claim Proposed for Relationship of Soy Protein and Coronary Heart Disease. November 10, 1998, Food and Drug Administration, US Department of Health and Human Services, Rockville, MD.

56 Holmes, MD, Hunter DJ, Colditz, GA, et al., Association of dietary intake of fat and fatty acids with risk of breast cancer. *JAMA.* 1999; 281:914–920.

57 Katan MB, Grundy SM, Willett WC. Op. cit.

58 Jonnalagadda SS, Mustad VA, Shaomei Y, et al. Effects of individual fatty acids on chronic diseases. *Nutrition Today.* 1996;31(3):90–107.

59 World Cancer Research Fund/American Institute for Cancer Research. *Food, Nutrition and the Prevention of Cancer: A Global Perspective.* Washington, DC: American Institute for Cancer Research; 1997.

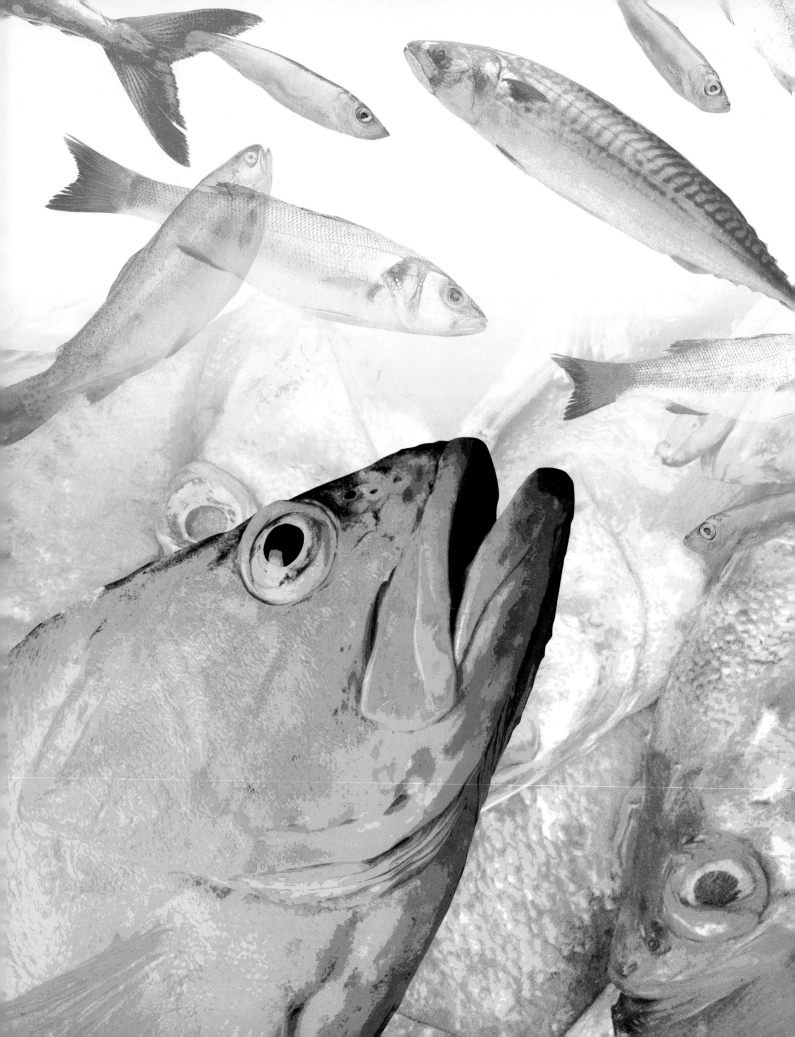

Chapter 6

Proteins and Amino Acids

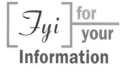

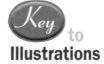

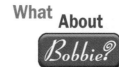

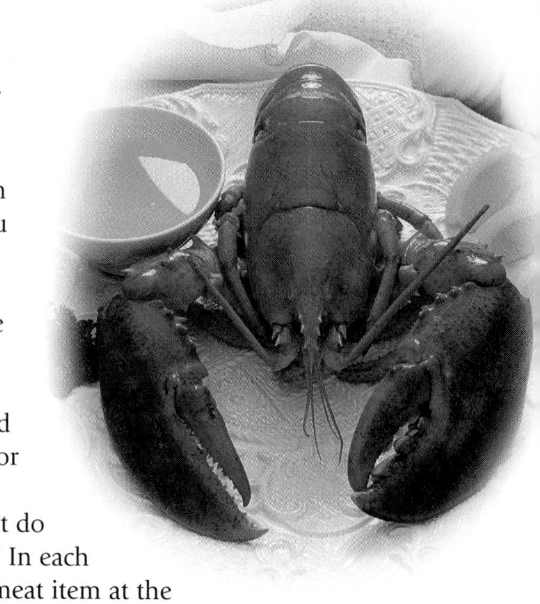

*T*hink of your favorite meal—perhaps a holiday feast, the foods you always ask for on your birthday, or something from a special restaurant. What are you imagining? If you are like most Americans, you have probably conjured up something along the lines of steak and baked potato; a lobster feast with corn on the cob; turkey with dressing, mashed potatoes, and all the trimmings; or maybe something more simple, a juicy hamburger and fries. What do all these meals have in common? In each case you may have thought of a meat item at the center of the plate, surrounded by various grain or vegetable accompaniments. From a young age, we're told that meat is an important source of protein and that protein helps us grow big and strong. Many traditional ways of eating in the United States emphasize meat as the most important part of the meal, and protein as the most important nutrient. But do such meals conform to your body's needs? Would a different style of eating be more healthful? For example, what about adding a small amount of meat to a stir-fry of vegetables over rice? Or what about eliminating meat from the diet? What makes the most sense nutritionally?

From the body's perspective, protein is certainly extremely important. Protein is part of every cell; it is needed in thousands of chemical reactions, and keeps us "together" structurally. But, as you are about to learn, the human body is so good at using the protein we feed it that our actual needs for dietary protein are relatively small—meat doesn't need to be at the center of the plate to keep you healthy!

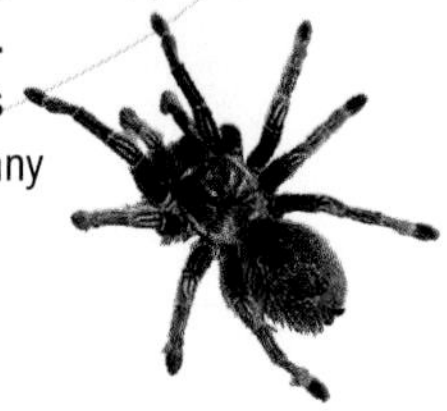

Why Is Protein Important?

The word *protein* was coined by the Dutch chemist Gerardus Mulder in 1838, and comes from the Greek word *protos*, meaning "of prime importance." Mulder discovered that proteins are a major component of all plant and animal tissues, second only to water. Today we know that these intricately constructed molecules are vital to many aspects of health and play an integral role in every living cell. Our bodies constantly assemble, break down, and use proteins, so we count on our diet to provide enough protein each day to replace what is being used. When we eat more protein than we need, the excess is either used to make energy or stored as fat.

Most people associate protein with animal foods like beef, chicken, fish, or milk. However, plant foods such as dried beans and peas, grains, nuts, seeds, and vegetables also provide protein. Many protein-rich plant foods are also rich in vitamins and minerals. These plant foods usually are low in fat and calories.

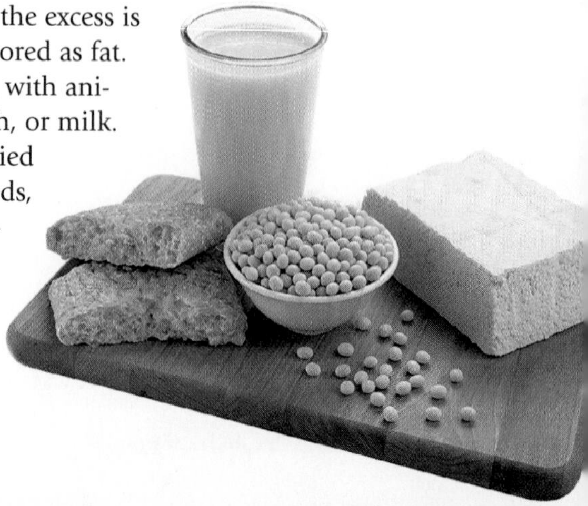

Quick Bites

A Bugburger Anyone?

*D*id you know that bugs provide 10 percent of the protein consumed worldwide? What creepy crawler would you choose for your dinner plate? A grasshopper is 15 to 60 percent protein. Pound for pound, spiders have more protein than any other bug.

People living in poverty may suffer from a shortage of both protein and energy in the diet. When the diet lacks protein, the body breaks down body tissue such as muscle and uses it as a protein source. This causes loss, or **wasting**, of muscle, organs, and other tissues. Protein deficiency also increases susceptibility to infection, and impairs digestion and absorption of nutrients. In the United States and other industrialized countries, most people are able to get more than enough protein to meet their physiological needs. In fact, a more common problem in these areas is excess intake of protein.

Amino Acids: The Building Blocks of Protein

Just as glucose is the basic building block of carbohydrates, amino acids are the basic building blocks of protein. Proteins are sequences of amino acids. Your body has 20 different amino acids to choose from when building these sequences. Nine of these amino acids are called **essential amino acids** because your body cannot make them and must get them in the diet. Your body can manufacture the remaining 11, called **nonessential amino acids**, when enough nitrogen, carbon, hydrogen, and oxygen are available. Nonessential amino acids do not need to be supplied in your diet. **Table 6.1** lists the essential, nonessential, and conditionally essential amino acids.

Sometimes, certain nonessential amino acids can become essential. Tyrosine and cysteine are both considered **conditionally essential amino acids**. Under normal circumstances, your body makes tyrosine from the essential amino acid phenylalanine, and cysteine from the essential amino acid methionine. When your intake of phenylalanine and methionine is low, however, your body needs tyrosine and cysteine from your diet to free phenylalanine and methionine for protein formation.

As you learned in Chapter 4, people with the disease phenylketonuria (PKU) must control their consumption of phenylalanine, a component of the artificial sweetener aspartame. PKU is a genetic disorder that impairs phenylalanine metabolism. People with PKU lack sufficient amounts of an enzyme that converts phenylalanine to tyrosine, so tyrosine becomes an essential amino acid. People with PKU must carefully monitor the amount of phenylalanine in their diets so they have enough to support growth and

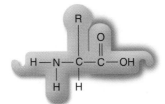

Table 6.1 Essential, Nonessential, and Conditionally Essential Amino Acids

Essential	Nonessential	Conditionally Essential
Histidine	Alanine	
Isoleucine	Arginine	Arginine
Leucine	Asparagine	
Lysine	Aspartic acid	
Methionine	Cysteine	Cysteine
Phenylalanine	Glutamic acid	
Threonine	Glutamine	Glutamine
Tryptophan	Glycine	
Valine	Proline	
	Serine	
	Tyrosine	Tyrosine

wasting The breakdown of body tissue such as muscle and organ for use as a protein source when the diet lacks protein.

essential amino acid An amino acid the body cannot make at all or cannot make enough of to meet physiological needs. Essential amino acids must be supplied in the diet.

nonessential amino acid An amino acid the body can make if supplied with adequate nitrogen. Nonessential amino acids do not need to be supplied in the diet.

conditionally essential amino acid An amino acid that is normally made in the body (nonessential) but becomes essential under certain circumstances, such as during critical illness.

Figure 6.1 **Structure of an amino acid.** All amino acids have a similar structure. Attached to a carbon atom is a hydrogen (H) shown here but not in later illustrations of amino acids, an amino group ($-NH_2$), an acid group ($-COOH$) and a side group (R). The side group gives each amino acid its unique identity.

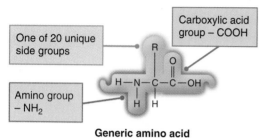

Carboxylic acid group – COOH

One of 20 unique side groups

Amino group – NH_2

Generic amino acid

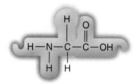

Glycine

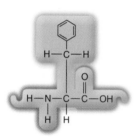

Phenylalanine

Figure 6.2 **Forming a peptide bond.** Imagine a row of people facing forward with their hands joined—the right hand joined to the left hand. Similarly, when two amino acids join together, the carboxyl group of one amino acid is matched with the amino group of another. A condensation reaction forms a peptide bond and releases water.

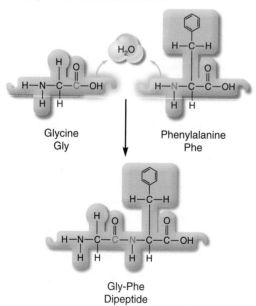

H_2O

Glycine
Gly

Phenylalanine
Phe

Gly-Phe
Dipeptide

maintenance of body tissue, but not too much. Excess phenylalanine and byproducts of its abnormal metabolism (called phenylketones) can build up in the body and contribute to irreversible brain damage.[1] Because foods that have aspartame contain phenylalanine, they can be dangerous for people with PKU. Without treatment, the IQ of individuals with PKU averages about 40; however, those who are treated starting at birth have IQs in the normal range.

Other amino acids also can become essential under certain circumstances. The amino acid glutamine is the main fuel for rapidly dividing cells and plays a key role in transporting nitrogen between organs.[2] Although normally considered nonessential, glutamine can become essential after trauma or during periods of critical illness that increase the body's need for it.[3] The amino acid arginine can also become essential during conditions of illness or severe physiological stress.[4]

Amino Acids Are Identified by Their Side Groups

Amino acids (with the exception of proline) uniformly consist of a central carbon atom chemically bonded to one hydrogen atom (H), one carboxylic acid group ($-COOH$), one amino (nitrogen-containing) group ($-NH_2$), and one side group unique to each amino acid (R). The side group gives each amino acid its identity. It can vary from a simple hydrogen atom, as in glycine, to a complex ring of carbon and hydrogen atoms, as in phenylalanine. The side groups mean that amino acids differ in shape, size, composition, electrical charge, and pH. When amino acids are linked to form a protein, these characteristics work together to determine that protein's specific function. **Figure 6.1** shows the structure of an amino acid.

Key Concepts: *Amino acids, which consist of a central carbon atom bonded to a hydrogen, a carboxyl group, an amino group, and a side group, are the building blocks of protein. Essential amino acids cannot be made by the body and must be supplied in the diet. Nonessential amino acids can be made in the body, given an adequate supply of nitrogen, carbon, hydrogen, and oxygen.*

Protein Structure: Unique Three-Dimensional Shapes and Functions

Proteins are very large molecules. Their chains of linked amino acids twist, fold, or coil into unique shapes. Just as we combine letters of the alphabet in different sequences to form an infinite variety of words, the body combines amino acids in different sequences to form a nearly infinite variety of proteins. For this reason, protein molecules are more diverse than either carbohydrates or lipids.

Amino Acid Sequence

Amino acids link in specific sequences to form strands of protein (often called peptides) up to hundreds of amino acids long. One amino acid is joined to the next by a **peptide bond**. To form a peptide bond, the carboxyl ($-COOH$) group of one amino acid bonds to the amino ($-NH_2$) group of another amino acid, releasing water (H_2O) in the process. (See **Figure 6.2**.) A **dipeptide** is two amino acids joined by a peptide bond, while a **tripeptide** is three amino acids joined by peptide bonds. The term **oligopeptide** refers to a chain of 4 to 10 amino acids, while a **polypeptide** contains more than 10 amino acids.[5] Proteins in the body and in the diet are long polypeptides, most with hundreds of linked amino acids.

Protein Shape

As its amino acids are assembled in the cell's cytoplasm, each protein chain assumes a unique three-dimensional shape that derives from the sequence and properties of its amino acids. The three-dimensional shape of a protein determines its function and its interaction with other molecules. For example, **Figure 6.3** illustrates the unique folded and twisted shape of **hemoglobin**, the iron-carrying protein in red blood cells. In the lungs, hemoglobin binds oxygen and releases carbon dioxide. Hemoglobin delivers oxygen to other tissues and picks up carbon dioxide for the return trip to the lungs.

Some amino acids carry electrical charges and therefore are attracted to the charged ends of water molecules (**hydrophilic amino acids**). In a watery environment, hydrophilic amino acids orient themselves on the outside of the folded protein chain in close contact with water molecules. Other amino acids are electrically neutral and do not interact with water (**hydrophobic amino acids**). In a watery environment, hydrophobic amino acids fold to the inside of the protein molecule. The amino acid cysteine, which has sulfur atoms in its side group, sometimes will chemically bond to another cysteine in the chain, creating a **disulfide bridge**, which helps stabilize the protein's structure.

peptide bond The bond between two amino acids formed when a carboxyl (–COOH) group of one amino acid joins an amino (–NH₂) group of another amino acid, releasing water in the process.

dipeptide Two amino acids joined by a peptide bond.

tripeptide Three amino acids joined by peptide bonds.

oligopeptide Four to 10 amino acids joined by peptide bonds.

polypeptide More than 10 amino acids joined by peptide bonds.

hemoglobin [HEEM-oh-glow-bin] The oxygen-carrying protein in red blood cells that consists of four heme groups and four globin polypeptide chains. The presence of hemoglobin gives blood its red color.

hydrophilic amino acids Amino acids that are attracted to water (water-loving).

hydrophobic amino acids Amino acids that are repelled by water (water-fearing).

disulfide bridge A bond between the sulfur components of two sulfur-containing amino acids that helps stabilize the structure of protein.

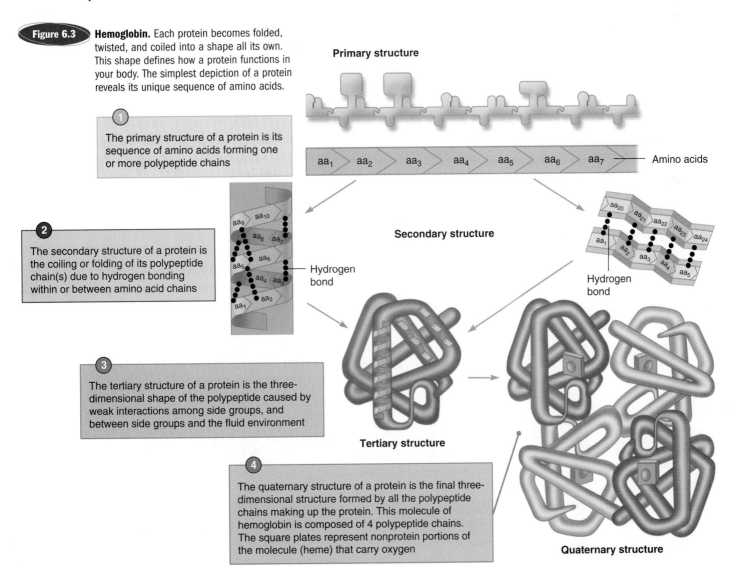

Figure 6.3 **Hemoglobin.** Each protein becomes folded, twisted, and coiled into a shape all its own. This shape defines how a protein functions in your body. The simplest depiction of a protein reveals its unique sequence of amino acids.

Primary structure

1 The primary structure of a protein is its sequence of amino acids forming one or more polypeptide chains

aa₁ aa₂ aa₃ aa₄ aa₅ aa₆ aa₇ — Amino acids

Secondary structure

2 The secondary structure of a protein is the coiling or folding of its polypeptide chain(s) due to hydrogen bonding within or between amino acid chains

Hydrogen bond

Hydrogen bond

3 The tertiary structure of a protein is the three-dimensional shape of the polypeptide caused by weak interactions among side groups, and between side groups and the fluid environment

Tertiary structure

4 The quaternary structure of a protein is the final three-dimensional structure formed by all the polypeptide chains making up the protein. This molecule of hemoglobin is composed of 4 polypeptide chains. The square plates represent nonprotein portions of the molecule (heme) that carry oxygen

Quaternary structure

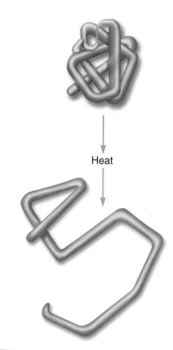

Heat

Figure 6.4 **Denaturation.** Heat, pH, oxidation and mechanical agitation are some of the forces that can destabilize a protein, causing it to unfold and lose its functional shape.

denaturation An alteration in the three-dimensional structure of a protein resulting in an unfolded polypeptide chain that usually lacks biological activity.

Protein Denaturation: Destabilizing a Protein's Shape

Acidity, alkalinity, heat, alcohol, oxidation, and agitation can all disrupt the chemical forces that stabilize a protein's three-dimensional shape, causing it to unfold and lose its shape (denature), as shown in **Figure 6.4**. Since a protein's shape determines its function, denatured proteins lose their ability to function properly.

If you've ever cooked an egg, you've witnessed protein **denaturation**. As the egg cooks some of its protein bonds break. As these proteins unfold, they bump into and bind to each other. Eventually, as these interconnections increase, the liquid egg coagulates to form a solid. Egg white proteins denature and stiffen as they are whipped, and milk proteins denature and curdle when acid is added.

If an egg is eaten raw, its avidin protein can bind to the B vitamin biotin in the digestive tract, making the vitamin unavailable for absorption. Cooking the egg denatures the avidin, and destroys its affinity for biotin. Denaturation is the first step in breaking down protein for digestion. Stomach acids denature protein, uncoiling the structure into a simple amino acid chain that digestive enzymes can start breaking apart.

Key Concepts: *Proteins are large molecules made up of amino acids joined in various sequences. Amino acids are joined by peptide bonds. Each protein assumes a unique three-dimensional shape depending on the sequence of its amino acids and properties of their side groups. Acid, alkaline, heat, alcohol, and agitation can disrupt chemical forces that stabilize proteins, causing the proteins to denature, or lose their shape.*

Functions of Body Proteins

The human body contains thousands of different proteins, each with a specific function determined by its unique shape. They act as enzymes, speeding up chemical reactions, and as hormones, which are a kind of chemical

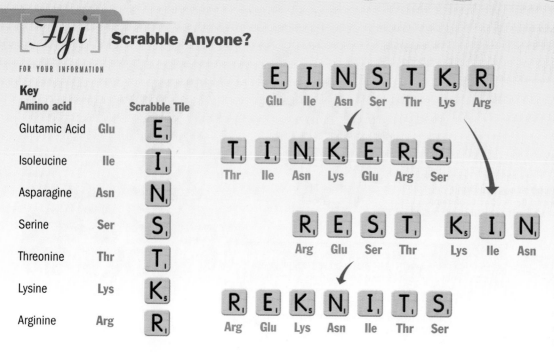

messenger. Antibodies made of protein protect us from foreign substances. Proteins maintain fluid balance by pumping molecules across cell membranes and attracting water. They maintain the acid and base balance of body fluids by taking up or giving off hydrogen ions as needed. Finally, proteins transport many key substances such as oxygen, vitamins, and minerals to target cells throughout the body. **Figure 6.5** illustrates the functions of proteins in the human body.

Structural and Mechanical Functions

Structures such as bone, skin, and hair owe their physical properties to unique proteins. **Collagen**, which appears microscopically as a densely packed long rod, is the most abundant protein in mammals, and gives skin and bone their elastic strength. Hair and nails are made of **keratin**, which is another dense protein made of coiled helices. Protein is essential for building these anatomical structures; therefore, protein deficiencies during a child's development can be disastrous. **Figure 6.6** shows structural proteins.

Motor proteins are exactly what their name implies—proteins that turn energy into mechanical work. In fact, these proteins are the final step in converting our food into physical work. When you bike down a road or up a mountain, you are using your stored food energy to power minuscule molecular motors in your muscles. These molecular motors slide muscle proteins past each other, causing muscles to contract. As you pump the pedals, proteins turn that energy bar you ate into work! Similarly, specialized motor proteins are involved in a variety of processes including cell division, muscle contraction, and sperm swimming.

Quick Bites

How to Beat the Stiffest Egg Whites

Whenever you want the greatest possible lightness or fluffiness, beat egg whites alone. A single drop of yolk or fat may reduce the foam's maximum volume by as much as two-thirds. Also avoid plastic bowls because plastics tend to retain fatty material on their surfaces.

collagen The most abundant fibrous protein in the body, it is the major constituent of connective tissue, forms the foundation for bones and teeth, and helps maintain the structure of blood vessels and other tissues.

keratin A water-insoluble fibrous protein that is the primary constituent of hair, nails, and the outer layer of the skin.

motor proteins Proteins that use energy and convert it into some form of mechanical work. Motor proteins are active in processes such as dividing cells, contracting muscle, and swimming sperm.

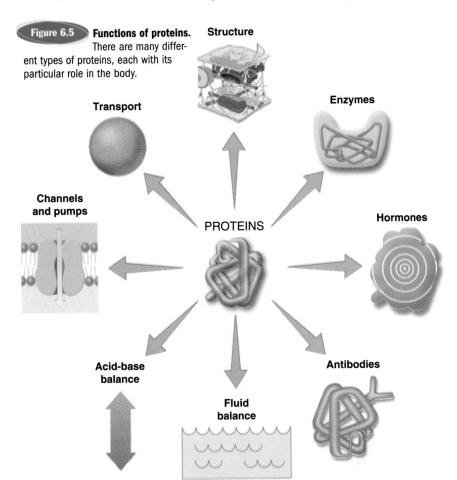

Figure 6.5 **Functions of proteins.** There are many different types of proteins, each with its particular role in the body.

Structure

Transport

Enzymes

Channels and pumps

PROTEINS

Hormones

Acid-base balance

Fluid balance

Antibodies

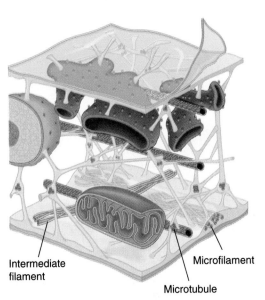

Intermediate filament

Microfilament

Microtubule

Figure 6.6 **Structural proteins.** Proteins provide structure to all cells including hair, skin, nails, and bone. As part of muscle, they transform energy into mechanical movement.

antibody [AN-tih-bod-ee] A large blood protein produced by B lymphocytes in response to exposure to a particular antigen (e.g., a protein on the surface of a virus or bacterium). Each type of antibody specifically binds to and helps eliminate its matching antigen from the body. Once formed, antibodies circulate in the blood and help protect the body against subsequent infection.

immune response A coordinated set of steps, including production of antibodies, that the immune system takes in response to an antigen.

intracellular fluid The fluid in the body's cells, it usually is high in potassium and phosphate and low in sodium and chloride. It constitutes about two-thirds of total body water.

extracellular fluid The fluid located outside of cells. It is composed largely of the liquid portion of the blood (plasma) and the fluid between cells in tissues (interstitial fluid), with fluid in the GI tract, eyes, joints, and spinal cord contributing a small amount. It constitutes about one-third of body water.

interstitial fluid [in-ter-STISH-ul] The fluid between cells in tissues. Also called intercellular fluid.

intravascular fluid The fluid portion of the blood (plasma) contained in arteries, veins, and capillaries. It accounts for about 15 percent of the extracellular fluid.

Enzymes

Enzymes are proteins that catalyze chemical reactions without being used up or destroyed in the process. (See **Figure 6.7A** and **B**.) Every cell contains thousands of types of enzymes, each with its own purpose. During digestion, for example, enzymes help break down carbohydrates, proteins, and fats into monosaccharides, amino acids, and fatty acids for absorption into the body. Enzymes release energy from these nutrients to fuel thousands of body processes. Enzymes also trigger the reactions that build muscle and tissue.

Our foods also contain enzymes, which cooking inactivates, or denatures. Stomach acid denatures the enzymes in raw foods. You may notice special purified enzymes being sold as supplements to enhance digestion. Most of the time, stomach acid denatures these enzymes so they are unable to function in the intestinal tract. However, some enzyme supplements are coated with a special substance to protect them from stomach acid. For example, a specially coated tablet form of the enzyme lactase can help people with lactose intolerance. Coated enzymes temporarily help break down foods in the small intestine but eventually are digested themselves.

Hormones

Hormones are chemical messengers that are made in one part of the body but act on cells in other parts of the body. (See **Figure 6.8**.) Many are proteins with important regulatory functions. Insulin, for example, is a protein hormone that plays a key role in regulating the amount of glucose in the blood. It is released from the pancreas in response to a rise in blood glucose levels and functions to lower those levels. (See Chapter 4.)

People with type 1 diabetes must take insulin injections to control blood sugar. Insulin cannot be taken as a pill, because if it were, it would be denatured and digested just like any other protein.

Thyroid-stimulating protein (TSH) and leptin are two other protein hormones. The pituitary gland produces TSH, which stimulates the thyroid gland to produce the hormone thyroxine. Thyroxine, a modified form of

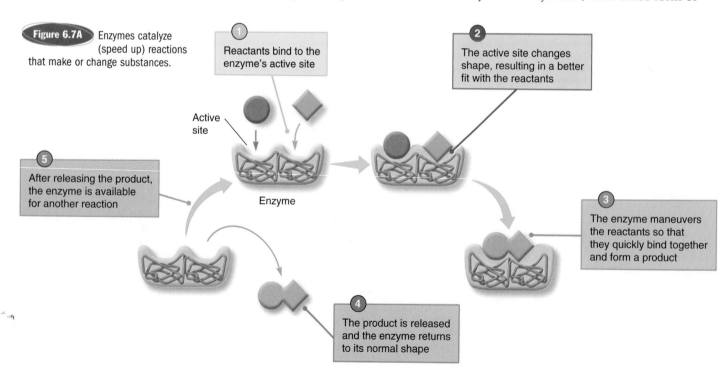

Figure 6.7A Enzymes catalyze (speed up) reactions that make or change substances.

Active site

1 Reactants bind to the enzyme's active site

2 The active site changes shape, resulting in a better fit with the reactants

Enzyme

3 The enzyme maneuvers the reactants so that they quickly bind together and form a product

5 After releasing the product, the enzyme is available for another reaction

4 The product is released and the enzyme returns to its normal shape

the amino acid tyrosine, increases the body's metabolic rate. Leptin is produced by fat cells and plays an important role in body weight regulation.[6] For more information on leptin, see Chapter 8, "Energy Balance, Body Composition, and Weight Management."

Immune Function

Proteins play an important role in the immune system, which is responsible for fighting infection and invasion by foreign substances. (See **Figure 6.9**.) **Antibodies** are blood proteins that attack and inactivate bacteria and viruses that cause infection. When your diet does not contain enough protein, your body cannot make as many protein antibodies as it needs. Your immune response is weakened and your risk of infection and illness increases. Each protein antibody has a specific shape that allows it to attack and destroy a specific foreign invader. Once your immune system learns how to make a certain kind of antibody, your body can protect itself by quickly making that antibody the next time the same germ invades.

Viruses, such as those that cause the common cold, take over cells in order to replicate. In a series of steps known as the **immune response**, your body mobilizes its defenses. As part of the defense strategy, you produce protein antibodies that bind to the viruses, marking them for destruction. Even when the viruses are gone, special cells retain a memory of this virus so that a faster immune response can be mounted against future invasions. When people are immunized for a disease like measles or mumps, they are actually getting a small amount of dead or inactivated virus in the injection. The dead virus cannot cause infection, but it does cue the body to make antibodies to the disease.

Fluid Balance

Fluids in the body are **intracellular** (inside cells) or **extracellular** (outside cells). There are two types of extracellular fluid—**intercellular**, or **interstitial**, (between cells) and **intravascular** (in the blood). These interior and exterior fluid levels must stay in balance for body processes to work properly.

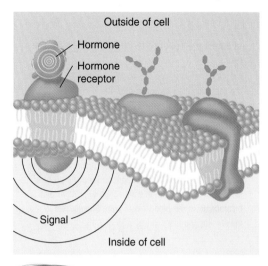

Figure 6.8 **Hormones.** Hormones are formed in one part of the body and carried in the blood to a different location where they signal cells to alter activities.

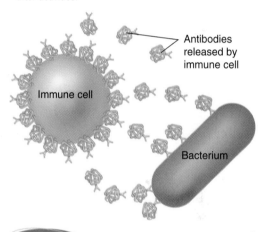

Figure 6.9 **Proteins and the immune system.** Protein antibodies are a crucial line of defense against invading bacteria and viruses.

Figure 6.7B Enzymes catalyze reactions that break down molecules.

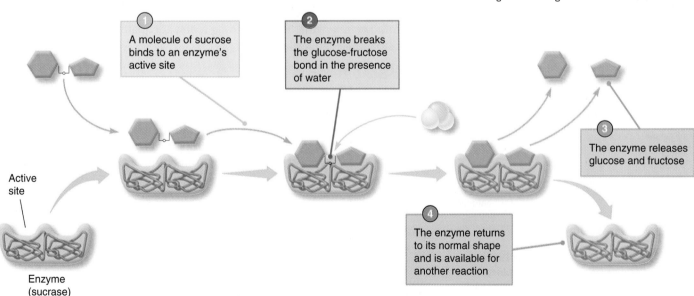

1. A molecule of sucrose binds to an enzyme's active site

2. The enzyme breaks the glucose-fructose bond in the presence of water

3. The enzyme releases glucose and fructose

4. The enzyme returns to its normal shape and is available for another reaction

Active site

Enzyme (sucrase)

edema Swelling caused by the build up of fluid between cells.

pH Unit for expressing the acidity of a solution, based on the contribution of hydrogen ions. The pH scale ranges from 0 to 14, with a value of 7 representing neutral pH at which the concentrations of H+ and hydroxyl ions (OH−) are equal. A pH lower than 7 is acidic; a pH higher than 7 is alkaline.

buffer A compound or mixture of compounds that can take up and release hydrogen ions to keep the pH of a solution constant. The buffering action of proteins and bicarbonate in the bloodstream plays a major role in maintaining the blood pH at 7.35 to 7.45.

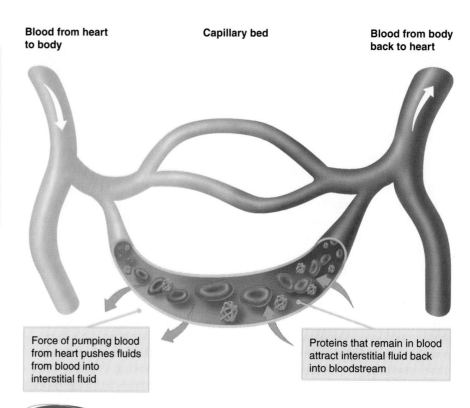

Blood from heart to body

Capillary bed

Blood from body back to heart

Force of pumping blood from heart pushes fluids from blood into interstitial fluid

Proteins that remain in blood attract interstitial fluid back into bloodstream

Figure 6.10 **Proteins in the blood.** Blood proteins attract fluid into capillaries. This counteracts the force of blood pressure, which forces fluid out.

Proteins in the blood help to maintain appropriate fluid levels in the vascular system. (See **Figure 6.10**.) The force of the heart's beating pushes fluid and nutrients from the capillaries out into the fluid surrounding the cells. But blood proteins like albumin and globulin are too large to leave the capillary beds. These proteins remain in the capillaries, where they attract fluid. This provides a balancing and partially counteracting force that keeps fluid in the circulatory system.

If the diet does not have enough protein to maintain normal levels of blood proteins, fluid will leak into the surrounding tissue and cause swelling, also called **edema**. Children with protein malnutrition often suffer from severe edema. Reestablishing a diet adequate in protein and energy will allow the edema to subside.

Acid-Base Balance

Using a scale of 0 to 14, **pH** is a measure of the concentration of hydrogen ions in a substance. The higher the concentration of hydrogen ions, the lower the pH. Acids, with a high concentration of hydrogen ions, have a pH lower than 7; bases, with a low concentration of hydrogen ions, have a pH higher than 7. The lower the pH, the stronger the acid. The higher the pH, the stronger the base. The body works hard to keep the pH of the blood near 7.4, or nearly neutral. We can tolerate only small fluctuations in blood pH without disastrous physiological consequences. Only a few hours with a blood pH above 8.0 or below 6.8 will cause death.

Proteins help maintain stable pH levels in body fluids by serving as buffers; they pick up extra hydrogen ions when conditions are acidic, and they donate hydrogen ions when conditions are alkaline. (See **Figure 6.11**.) If proteins are not available to **buffer** acidic or alkaline substances, the blood can become too acidic or too alkaline, resulting

The measure of hydrogen ions in a substance

pH

14

Alkalosis

Ideal blood pH   7.4

Blood pH range

6.8

Acidosis

0

Bases

Acids

Proteins can either donate or accept hydrogen ions to maintain stable pH levels

High hydrogen ion concentration = low pH

Figure 6.11 **Proteins help maintain stable pH levels.** Proteins act as buffers. When conditions are acidic, they pick up extra hydrogen ions. When conditions are alkaline, they donate hydrogen ions.

in either **acidosis** or **alkalosis**. Both conditions can be serious; either can cause proteins to denature, and this can lead to coma or death.

Transport Functions

Many substances pass in and out of cells via proteins that cross cell membranes and act as channels and pumps. Channels allow substances to flow rapidly through the membranes by passive diffusion and require no input of energy. Pumps (active transporters), in contrast, must use energy to drive the transport of substances across membranes. More than one-third of the energy your body consumes at rest is used by sodium-potassium protein pumps that control cell volume and nerve impulses and drive the active transport of sugars and amino acids.[7] **Figure 6.12** shows a transmembrane protein.

Proteins also act as carriers, transporting many important substances in the bloodstream for delivery throughout the body (see **Figure 6.13**). Lipoproteins, for example, package proteins with lipids so that lipid particles can be carried in the blood. Other proteins carry fat-soluble vitamins and certain other vitamins and minerals. Since protein carries vitamin A in the blood, protein deficiency contributes to vitamin A deficiency. The protein transferrin carries iron in the blood. In the liver, iron is stored as part of ferritin, a different protein.

Source of Energy and Glucose

Although your body preferentially burns carbohydrate and fat for energy, if necessary it can use protein for energy or to make glucose. Thus carbohydrate and fat are protein-sparing: they spare amino acids from being burned for energy and allow them to be used for protein synthesis.

If the diet does not provide enough energy to sustain vital functions, the body will sacrifice its own protein from enzymes, muscle, and other tissues to make energy and glucose for use by the brain, lungs, and heart. This is what happens in cases of starvation. (See Chapter 7, "Metabolism.")

When the body uses its own protein for energy, it first breaks the protein into individual amino acids. To release energy from an amino acid, the body first removes the nitrogen group—a process called **deamination**. To make energy or glucose, it can use the remaining carbon, hydrogen, and oxygen compounds.

If the diet contains more protein than is needed for protein synthesis, most of the excess is converted to glucose or stored as fat. Thus, people who take protein supplements or eat high-protein diets in hopes of increasing muscle mass may instead be expensively adding to their body fat.

This review of protein functions illustrates the diversity of proteins' roles. Clearly, protein is of "prime importance," just as the Greeks believed. For proteins to perform all these functions, the diet must provide adequate amounts of protein components. In addition, the body needs adequate energy from carbohydrates and fats, and adequate digestibility of protein foods.

Key Concepts: In the body, proteins perform numerous vital functions that are determined by each protein's shape. As enzymes, they speed up chemical reactions; as hormones, they are chemical messengers. Protein antibodies protect the body from infection and illness; proteins also maintain fluid balance and acid-base balance, and transport substances throughout the body. If needed, protein can also be used as a source of energy or glucose.

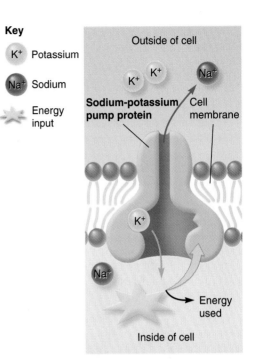

Key
K+ Potassium
Na+ Sodium
Energy input

Figure 6.12 **A transmembrane protein.** Proteins form channels and pumps that help move substances in and out of cells.

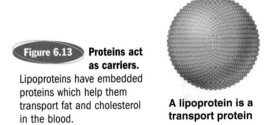

Figure 6.13 **Proteins act as carriers.** Lipoproteins have embedded proteins which help them transport fat and cholesterol in the blood.

A lipoprotein is a transport protein

acidosis An abnormally low blood pH (below about 7.35) due to increased acidity.

alkalosis An abnormally high blood pH (above about 7.45) due to increased alkalinity.

deamination The removal of the amino group ($-NH_2$) from an amino acid.

Protein Digestion and Absorption

Before your body can make a body protein from food protein, it must digest and absorb the protein you eat. **Figure 6.14** shows the breakdown of protein so the body can absorb and digest it.

Protein Digestion

The first step in using dietary protein is digesting its long polypeptide chains into amino acids. Like the other energy-yielding nutrients, digestion requires enzymes from a number of sources. Digestion of protein begins in the stomach.

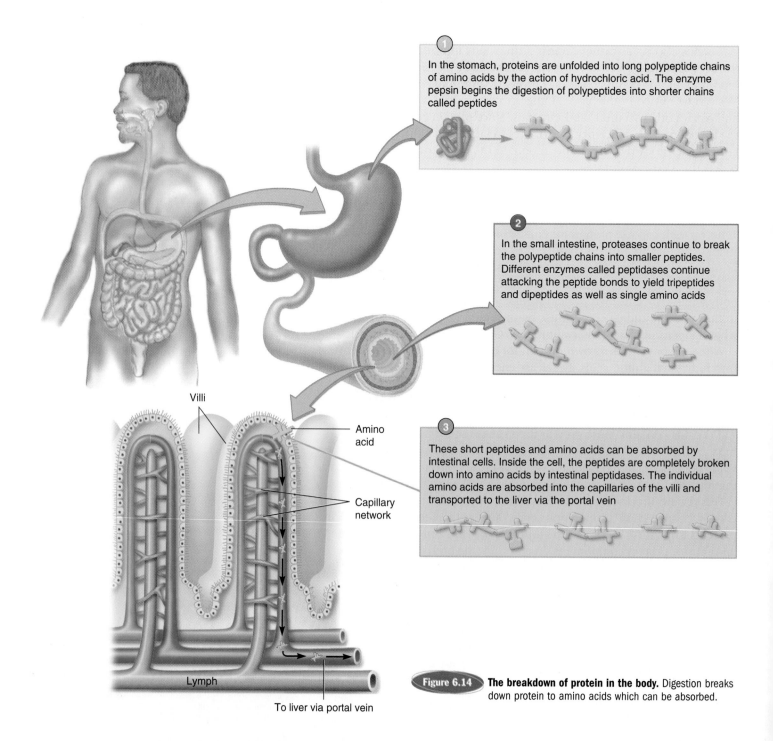

1. In the stomach, proteins are unfolded into long polypeptide chains of amino acids by the action of hydrochloric acid. The enzyme pepsin begins the digestion of polypeptides into shorter chains called peptides

2. In the small intestine, proteases continue to break the polypeptide chains into smaller peptides. Different enzymes called peptidases continue attacking the peptide bonds to yield tripeptides and dipeptides as well as single amino acids

3. These short peptides and amino acids can be absorbed by intestinal cells. Inside the cell, the peptides are completely broken down into amino acids by intestinal peptidases. The individual amino acids are absorbed into the capillaries of the villi and transported to the liver via the portal vein

Villi

Amino acid

Capillary network

Lymph

To liver via portal vein

Figure 6.14 **The breakdown of protein in the body.** Digestion breaks down protein to amino acids which can be absorbed.

In the Stomach

In the stomach, hydrochloric acid (HCl) denatures a protein, unfolding it and making the amino acid chain more accessible to the action of enzymes. Glands in the stomach lining produce the proenzyme pepsinogen, an inactive **precursor** of the enzyme pepsin. When pepsinogen comes in contact with hydrochloric acid, it is converted to the active enzyme pepsin. Gastric juices must be acidic for this enzyme to be active; it is most active at a (very acidic) pH of 2.5 and is inactive at a pH above 5.0. Gastric glands secrete hydrochloric acid at a pH of approximately 0.8. Once the acid is mixed with the gastric contents, the pH of the gastric juices falls to 2.5—the ideal medium for pepsin activity. By the time dietary protein leaves the stomach, pepsin has broken it down into individual amino acids and peptides of various lengths. Pepsin is responsible for about 10 to 20 percent of protein digestion.[8]

In the Small Intestine

From the stomach, amino acids and polypeptides pass into the small intestine, where most protein digestion takes place. In the small intestine, **proteases** (protein-digesting enzymes) break down large peptides into smaller peptides. If a cell produces active forms of proteases, it will digest itself and break down its own cellular protein. However, cells employ a protective strategy. They produce and secrete most proteases as **proenzymes**, inactive forms of the enzymes, for later activation. This delayed activation protects the integrity of the cell.

Both the pancreas and the small intestine make digestive proenzymes. The pancreas makes **trypsinogen** and **chymotrypsinogen**, which are secreted into the small intestine in response to the presence of protein. Here, these proenzymes are cleaved into their active forms, **trypsin** and **chymotrypsin**, respectively. These activated proteases break polypeptides into smaller peptides. Pancreatic enzymes completely digest only a small percentage of proteins into individual amino acids; most of the proteins at this point are dipeptides, tripeptides, and still larger polypeptides.

The final stages of protein digestion take place on the surface of the intestine's lining, and require enzymes secreted by the intestinal lining cells. Brush border (microvilli) **peptidases** react with intestinal fluids that come in contact with the cell surface and split the remaining larger polypeptides into tripeptides, dipeptides and even some all the way into amino acids. These smaller units are transported across the microvilli membranes into the cell. Inside the cell many other peptidases specifically attack the linkages between the amino acids. Within minutes, these peptidases digest virtually all the remaining dipeptides and tripeptides into individual amino acids for absorption into the bloodstream.

Undigested Protein

Any parts of proteins that are not digested and absorbed in the small intestine continue on through the large intestine and pass out of the body in the feces. Normally the body efficiently digests and absorbs protein. Diseases of the intestinal tract, however, decrease the efficiency of absorption and increase protein losses in the feces.[9] People with **celiac disease**, for example, cannot properly digest gluten—a protein found in wheat, rye, and oats. Unless treated with a gluten-free diet, people with celiac disease show poor growth, weight loss, and other symptoms resulting from poor absorption of protein and other nutrients. People who suffer from **cystic fibrosis** have fewer protein-digesting enzymes than normal in the small intestine, resulting in poor digestion and absorption of protein and other nutrients.[10]

precursor A substance that is converted into another active substance. Enzyme precursors are also called proenzymes.

protease An enzyme that breaks down protein into peptides and amino acids.

proenzyme An inactive precursor of an enzyme.

trypsin/trypsinogen A protease produced by the pancreas that is converted from the inactive proenzyme form (trypsinogen) to the active form (trypsin) in the small intestine.

chymotrypsin/chymotrypsinogen A protease produced by the pancreas that is converted from the inactive proenzyme form (chymotrypsinogen) to the active form (chymotrypsin) in the small intestine.

peptidases Enzymes that act on small peptide units by breaking peptide bonds.

celiac disease [SEA-lee-ak] A disease that involves an inability to digest gluten, a protein found in wheat, rye, oats, and barley. If untreated, it causes flattening of the villi in the intestine, leading to severe malabsorption of nutrients. Symptoms include diarrhea, fatty stools, swollen belly, and extreme fatigue.

cystic fibrosis An inherited disorder that causes widespread dysfunction of the exocrine glands resulting in chronic lung disease, abnormally high levels of electrolytes (e.g., sodium, potassium, chloride) in sweat, and deficiency of pancreatic enzymes needed for digestion.

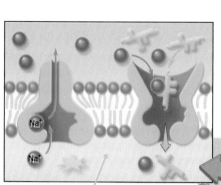

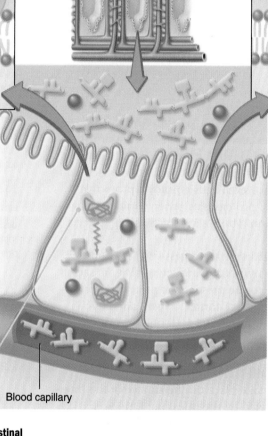

Active transport
Peptides and most amino acids are actively transported into the cell by a sodium co-transport strategy. First, energy is used to pump sodium out of the cell. A special transport protein in the cell membrane allows the sodium to reenter the cell when accompanied by an amino acid. The sodium "drags" the amino acid along during reentry. There are five structural types of amino acids and a unique transport protein has been identified for each one

Facilitated diffusion
Some amino acids can enter the cell directly via facilitated diffusion. A membrane protein undergoes a conformational change to help the amino acid enter the cell. No energy is required. All the amino acids use facilitated diffusion to leave the cell and enter the bloodstream

Peptidases
Within the intestinal cell, enzymes called peptidases attack the remaining peptide bonds, completing the breakdown of tripeptides and dipeptides to individual amino acids

Blood capillary

Figure 6.15 **Protein absorption into an intestinal cell.** Intestinal cells use active transport and facilitated diffusion to absorb amino acids.

Amino Acid and Peptide Absorption

Absorption of some amino acids requires active transport while others are absorbed via facilitated diffusion. Although the active transport process is the same for amino acids as it is for glucose and galactose, amino acids and monosaccharides use different transport proteins.

Although there are several active transport mechanisms, similar amino acids share the same active transport system. The amino acids leucine, isoleucine, and valine, for example, all depend on the same carrier molecule for absorption. Normally proteins in foods supply a mix of many amino acids, so amino acids that share the same transport system are absorbed fairly equally. If a person consumes a large amount of one particular amino acid, however, absorption of other amino acids that share the same transport system will be deficient. Thus, if you take a supplement of one amino acid, you may be interfering with absorption of another amino acid from your diet.

Most protein absorption takes place in the cells that line the duodenum and jejunum. (See **Figure 6.15.**) After they are absorbed, most amino acids and the few absorbed peptides are transported via the portal vein to the liver and then released into general circulation. Some amino acids remain in the

Think
About It
2

intestinal cells and are used to synthesize intestinal enzymes and new cells. More than 99 percent of protein enters the bloodstream as individual amino acids. Peptides are rarely absorbed, and whole proteins that escape digestion hardly ever are. The absorption of only a few molecules of whole protein can cause a severe allergic reaction or immune dysfunction.[11]

Key Concepts: *Protein digestion begins in the stomach, where the enzyme pepsin breaks proteins into smaller peptides. Digestion continues in the small intestine, where proteases break polypeptides into smaller peptide units, which are then absorbed into cells where additional enzymes complete digestion to amino acids. Key enzymes are pepsin in the stomach, and trypsin and chymotrypsin from the pancreas. Proteases (protein-digesting enzymes) are synthesized and secreted as inactive proenzymes. This is so cells do not digest themselves.*

Proteins in the Body

Once in the bloodstream, amino acids are transported throughout the body and are available for synthesizing cellular proteins. Cells build the proteins they need by using peptide bonds to link amino acids.

Protein Synthesis

Genetic material in the nucleus of every cell is the blueprint for the thousands of proteins needed to perform life functions. Cells store this genetic material in the form of long coiled molecules of **DNA** (deoxyribonucleic acid) in each cell's nucleus.

To synthesize a protein, the cell uses a specific length of the DNA in the cell nucleus, called a gene, as a pattern to make a special type of ribonucleic acid (RNA) called **messenger RNA (mRNA).** This mRNA carries the code for the sequence of amino acids needed in the protein. The mRNA leaves the nucleus of the cell and attaches itself to one of the **ribosomes,** or protein-making machines, in the cell's cytoplasm.

Another type of RNA, **transfer RNA (tRNA),** then gathers the necessary amino acids from cell fluid and carries them to the mRNA, where enzymes bind each amino acid to the growing protein chain. During protein synthesis, thousands of tRNAs each carry their own specific amino acid to the site of protein synthesis, but only one mRNA controls the sequencing of amino acids for a given protein.

The third type of RNA, **ribosomal RNA (rRNA),** is the major component of ribosomes. For many years, scientists assumed that rRNA served primarily as a structural framework for protein synthesis and had little catalytic function. With the discovery that RNA in general can play many catalytic roles, scientists now believe that rRNA has a major role in directing protein synthesis. **Figure 6.16** illustrates protein synthesis.

Just as one missing part of a car can stop an entire auto assembly line, so can one missing amino acid stop synthesis of an entire protein in the cell. If a nonessential amino acid is missing during protein synthesis, the cell will either make that amino acid or obtain it from the liver via the bloodstream, and protein synthesis will continue. If an essential amino acid is missing, the body may break its own protein down to supply the missing

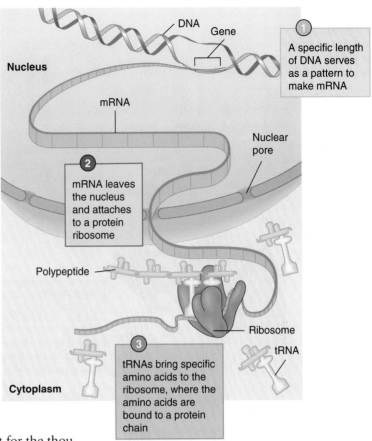

Figure 6.16 **Protein synthesis.** Ribosomes are our protein synthesis factories. mRNA carries manufacturing instructions from DNA in the cell nucleus to the ribosomes. tRNA collects amino acids in the correct sequence and rRNA in the ribosome directs protein synthesis.

DNA (Deoxyribonucleic Acid) The carrier of genetic information. Specific regions of each DNA molecule, called genes, act as blueprints for the synthesis of proteins.

messenger RNA (mRNA) Long, linear single-stranded molecules of ribonucleic acids formed from DNA templates that carry the amino acid sequence of one or more proteins from the cell nucleus to the cytoplasm where the ribosomes translate mRNA into proteins.

ribosomes Cell components composed of protein located in the cytoplasm that translate messenger RNA into protein sequences.

transfer RNA (tRNA) A type of ribonucleic acid that is composed of a complementary RNA sequence and an amino acid specific to that sequence. Inserts the appropriate amino acid when the messenger RNA sequence and the ribosome call for it.

ribosomal RNA (rRNA) A type of ribonucleic acid that is a major component of ribosomes. It provides a structural framework for protein synthesis and orchestrates the process.

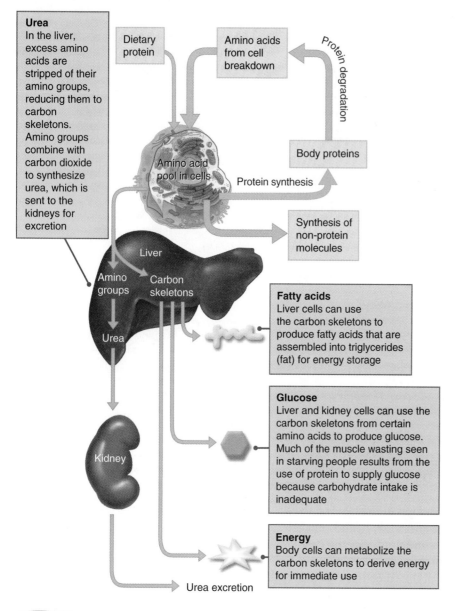

Urea
In the liver, excess amino acids are stripped of their amino groups, reducing them to carbon skeletons. Amino groups combine with carbon dioxide to synthesize urea, which is sent to the kidneys for excretion

Dietary protein

Amino acids from cell breakdown

Protein degradation

Body proteins

Amino acid pool in cells

Protein synthesis

Liver

Amino groups

Carbon skeletons

Urea

Kidney

Synthesis of non-protein molecules

Fatty acids
Liver cells can use the carbon skeletons to produce fatty acids that are assembled into triglycerides (fat) for energy storage

Glucose
Liver and kidney cells can use the carbon skeletons from certain amino acids to produce glucose. Much of the muscle wasting seen in starving people results from the use of protein to supply glucose because carbohydrate intake is inadequate

Energy
Body cells can metabolize the carbon skeletons to derive energy for immediate use

Urea excretion

Figure 6.17 **Protein turnover.** Cells draw upon their amino acid pools to synthesize new proteins. These small pools turn over quickly, and must be replenished by amino acids from dietary protein and degradation of body protein. Dietary protein supplies about one-third and the breakdown of body protein supplies about two-thirds of the roughly 300 grams of body protein synthesized daily. When dietary protein is inadequate, increased degradation of body protein replenishes the amino acid pool. This can lead to the breakdown of essential body tissue.

amino acid pool The amino acids in body tissues and fluids that are available for new protein synthesis.

protein turnover The constant synthesis and breakdown of proteins in the body.

amino acid. If a missing essential amino acid is unavailable, protein synthesis halts, and the partially completed protein is broken down into individual amino acids for use elsewhere in the body.

Genetic defects in DNA can also cause problems in protein synthesis. People who have sickle-cell anemia have a defect in the amino acid sequencing of their hemoglobin. A genetic error causes the substitution of the amino acid valine for glutamic acid in two locations in the protein chain. This simple error causes the shape of hemoglobin to change so much that the red blood cell becomes stiff and sickle-shaped instead of soft and disk-shaped. This faulty protein cannot carry oxygen efficiently, so it causes serious medical problems.

The Amino Acid Pool and Protein Turnover

Cells throughout the body constantly and simultaneously synthesize and break down protein. When cells break down protein, the protein's amino acids return to circulation. (See **Figure 6.17**.) These available amino acids, found throughout body tissues and fluids, are collectively referred to as the **amino acid pool**.[12] Some of these amino acids may be used for protein synthesis; others may have their amino group removed and be used to produce energy or nonprotein substances such as glucose.

The constant recycling of proteins in the body is known as **protein turnover**.[13] Each day, more amino acids in your body are recycled than are supplied in your diet. Of the approximately 300 grams of protein synthesized by the body each day, 200 grams are made from recycled amino acids. This remarkable recycling capacity is the reason we need so little protein in our diet compared to carbohydrate and fat. In a healthful diet, only 10 to 15 percent of our daily calories must come from protein, whereas carbohydrate should supply about 55 to 60 percent and fat no more than 30 percent.

Synthesis of Nonprotein Molecules

Amino acids have roles other than as components of peptides and proteins; they are precursors of many molecules with important biological roles. Your body makes nonprotein molecules from amino acids and the nitrogen they contain. The vitamin niacin, for example, is made from the amino acid tryptophan. Precursors of DNA, RNA, and many coenzymes derive in part from amino acids. Your body also uses amino acids to make **neurotransmitters**, chemicals that send signals from nerve cells to other parts of the body. Serotonin, which helps regulate mood, is made from tryptophan. Norepinephrine and epinephrine (also called noradrenaline and adrenaline, respectively), which ready the body for action, are neurotransmitters made from tyrosine. Your body also uses tyrosine to make melanin, a skin pigment, and a hormone called thyroxin, which helps regulate metabolism. The simple amino acid glycine combines with many toxic substances to make less harmful substances that the body can excrete. Your body uses the amino acid histidine to make histamine, a potent vasodilator (dilates blood vessels) and a culprit in allergic reactions.

Protein and Nitrogen Excretion

Cells break down and recycle amino acids. Amino acid breakdown yields amino groups ($-NH_2$). This NH_2 molecule is unstable and quickly converts to ammonia (NH_3). However, ammonia is toxic to cells, so it is expelled into the bloodstream as a waste product and is carried to the liver. In the liver, an amino group and an ammonia group react with carbon dioxide through a series of reactions (known collectively as the **urea** cycle) to generate urea and water. The nitrogen-rich urea is transported from the liver by way of the bloodstream to the kidneys, where it is filtered from the blood and sent to the bladder for excretion in the urine. Small amounts of other nitrogen-containing compounds, such as ammonia, uric acid, and creatinine, are also excreted in the urine. Some nitrogen is also lost through skin, sloughed off GI cells, mucus, hair and nail cuttings, and body fluids.

Nitrogen Balance

Because nitrogen is excreted as proteins are recycled or used, we can use the balance of nitrogen in the body to evaluate whether the body is getting enough protein. (See **Figure 6.18**.) We can estimate the balance of nitrogen, and therefore protein, in the body by comparing nitrogen intake to the sum of all sources of nitrogen excretion (urine, feces, skin, hair, and body fluids).[14]

If nitrogen intake exceeds nitrogen excretion, the body is said to be in **positive nitrogen balance**. Positive nitrogen balance means that the body is adding protein, as is the case for growing children, pregnant women, or

neurotransmitter A substance released at the end of a stimulated nerve cell that diffuses across a small gap and binds to another nerve cell or muscle cell, stimulating or inhibiting it.

urea The main nitrogen-containing waste product in mammals. Formed in liver cells from ammonia and carbon dioxide, urea is carried via the bloodstream to the kidneys, where it is excreted in the urine.

positive nitrogen balance Nitrogen intake exceeds the sum of all sources of nitrogen excretion.

$$\text{nitrogen balance} = \text{grams of nitrogen intake} - \text{grams of nitrogen output}$$

Figure 6.18 Protein (nitrogen) balance.

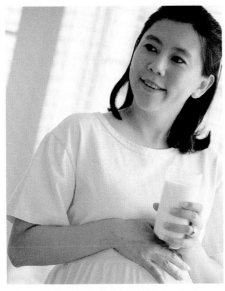

A pregnant woman is adding protein so she has a positive nitrogen balance.

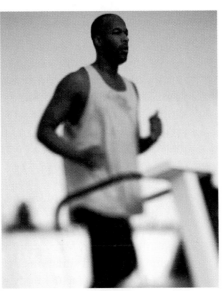

A healthy person who is neither gaining nor losing protein is in nitrogen equilibrium.

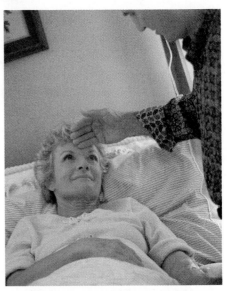

A person who is severely ill and losing protein has a negative nitrogen balance.

negative nitrogen balance Nitrogen intake is less than the sum of all sources of nitrogen excretion.

nitrogen balance Nitrogen intake minus the sum of all sources of nitrogen excretion.

nitrogen equilibrium Nitrogen intake equals the sum of all sources of nitrogen excretion; nitrogen balance equals zero.

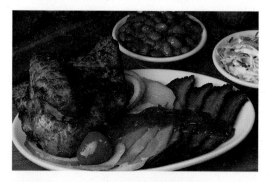

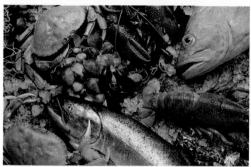

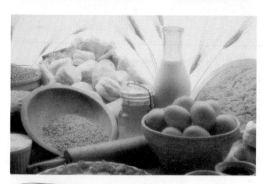

Figure 6.19 Protein sources.

Convert weight to kg
(pounds ÷ 2.2)
Multiply kg by 0.8 = Protein RDA in g

Male, 19–24 years old, 72 kg (158 lb)
72 kg × 0.8 g/kg = 58 g protein

Female, 19–24 years old, 58 kg (128 lb)
58 kg × 0.8 g/kg = 46 g protein

people recovering from protein deficiency or illnesses. If nitrogen excretion exceeds nitrogen intake, the body is in **negative nitrogen balance**. This means that the body is losing protein. People who are starving or on extreme weight-loss diets or who suffer from fever, severe illnesses, or infections are in a state of negative nitrogen balance. If nitrogen intake equals nitrogen excretion, **nitrogen balance** is zero and the body is in **nitrogen equilibrium**. Healthy adults are in nitrogen equilibrium, which means their dietary protein intake is adequate to maintain and repair tissue. They have no net gain or loss of body protein and they simply excrete excess dietary protein.

Key Concepts: *The information that allows a cell to make a particular protein is stored in cellular DNA. Three forms of RNA—mRNA, tRNA, and rRNA—are needed to build body proteins. Cells throughout the body constantly synthesize and break down protein simultaneously, a process known as protein turnover. Nitrogen-containing end products of protein metabolism are excreted in urine via the kidneys. Comparison of nitrogen intake (from dietary protein) to nitrogen excretion gives a measure of nitrogen balance and indicates protein status in the body.*

Proteins in the Diet

Many government and health organizations have made recommendations about the amount of protein in a healthful diet, just as they have for other nutrients. Meat, eggs, milk, legumes, grains, and vegetables are all sources of protein. Fruits contain minimal amounts and, along with fats, are not considered protein sources. **Figure 6.19** shows some good sources of protein.

Recommended Intakes of Protein

The World Health Organization (WHO) bases its requirements for essential amino acids on nitrogen balance studies published in the 1950s.[15] These requirements are minimum levels used to develop nutrition and policy interventions around the world. Newer methods of measuring amino acid requirements suggest some of the WHO values for specific amino acids may be too low.[16] In the United States, the Recommended Dietary Allowance (RDA, see Chapter 2) is the accepted dietary standard for protein. RDAs are set to meet the nutritional needs of most healthy people, but most people actually require somewhat less protein than the RDA. RDA values also assume people are consuming adequate energy and other nutrients to allow their bodies to use dietary protein for protein synthesis, rather than for energy. Other countries, such as Canada, make recommendations similar to the RDAs.

People older than 2 years should get 30 percent or less of their energy intake from fat and about 55 percent or more of their energy intake from carbohydrate.[17] That leaves about 10 to 15 percent of energy to come from protein, an amount that is usually higher than the RDA. Protein currently provides about 15 percent of the average American's energy intake.[18]

Adults

For adults, the RDA for protein intake is 0.8 grams per kilogram of body weight.[19] In clinical situations that require precise assessments, ideal body weight (rather than actual body weight) is typically used to determine protein needs. The RDA for adults translates into a daily protein recommendation of 58 grams for the average male and 46 grams for the average female

Think
About It

3

in the 19-to-24 age group. Because average body weights are slightly higher in adults older than 25, their RDAs are slightly higher (63 g for males and 50 g for females). When calculated as a percentage of average energy intake, the protein RDA for adults provides about 8 to 11 percent of energy intake.

Other Life Stages

Infants 0 to 6 months of age require 2.2 grams of protein per kilogram body weight, the highest protein need relative to body weight of any time of life (see **Table 6.2**). Protein requirements gradually fall throughout childhood and adolescence until a person reaches adult body size, at an average of age 15 to 18 for females and age 19 to 24 for males.

Both pregnancy and lactation (production of breast milk) increase a woman's need for protein. The RDA for pregnant women is 60 grams (an increase of about 10 g to 15 g) while the RDA during initial lactation is 65 grams. Most American women already consume more than enough protein to support pregnancy and lactation.

Some nutritionists suggest that people older than 50 should consume up to 1.2 grams of protein per kilogram body weight. Although elderly people on average have less lean body mass to maintain than younger people, the body becomes less efficient at digesting, absorbing, and using protein as it ages.[20] (See **Figure 6.20**.) The current RDA for this age group is still 0.8 grams per kilogram, although this may change in upcoming DRI revisions.

Physical Stress

Severe physical stress can increase the body's need for protein. Infections, burns, fevers, and surgery all increase protein losses, and the diet must replace that lost protein. A severe infection can increase protein requirements by one-third. Severe burns can increase requirements two to four times. Less severe physical stressors, such as a viral illness with a mild fever lasting only a few days, rarely increase protein requirements. Muscle-building activities, such as intense weight training, increase protein need much less than most people think and the typical American diet supplies an ample amount of protein, even for bodybuilders. (See the FYI feature "Do Athletes Need More Protein?")

Protein Consumption in the United States

According to data from the U.S. Department of Agriculture's *1994–1996 Continuing Survey of Food Intake by Individuals*,[21] the average American consumes 75 grams of protein daily. Protein intakes meet or exceed the protein RDA for every age and gender group, except for women age 70 and older, where average protein intake falls just three grams short of the RDA. If you remember that an RDA value is adequate for practically all people in an age and gender group, an *average* intake slightly below the RDA is not of any real concern. (See Chapter 2 for more on RDAs.)

Key Concepts: *Infants, who are growing rapidly, have the highest protein needs relative to body weight. The Recommended Dietary Allowance (RDA) for protein declines from 2.2 grams per kilogram for infants 0 to 6 months old to 0.8 grams per kilogram for adults. Pregnancy, physical changes in old age, and severe physical stress all can alter protein requirements. Americans currently consume about 15 percent of their energy as protein, and obtain an average of 75 grams of protein daily—an amount that exceeds the RDA for almost all age and gender categories.*

Table 6.2 Protein RDA for Infants, Children, and Teens

Age	Protein RDA (g/kg body weight)
0–6 months	2.2
6 months–1 year	1.6
1 to 3 years	1.2
4 to 6 years	1.1
7 to 10 years	1.0
11 to 14 years	1.0
15 to 18 years (males)	0.9
15 to 18 years (females)	0.8

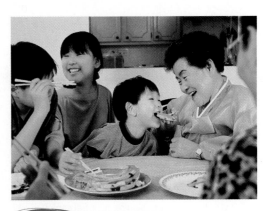

Figure 6.20 Protein needs change as we age.

Quick Bites

Mother's Milk

Because it contains less protein, and in particular less casein protein, infants digest human milk more readily than cows' milk. Milks high in casein protein tend to form curds (clumps) in the stomach upon exposure to stomach acid. These tough curds are hard for digestive enzymes to break apart.

complete protein A protein that supplies all of the essential amino acids in the proportions the body needs. Also known as high-quality proteins.

incomplete protein A protein that lacks one or more essential amino acids. Also called low-quality proteins.

complementary protein Two or more incomplete food proteins whose assortment of amino acids make up for, or complement, each other's lack of specific essential amino acids so that the combination provides sufficient amounts of all the essential amino acids.

Protein Quality

Although both animal and plant foods contain protein, the quality of protein in these foods differs. Foods that supply all the essential amino acids in the proportions needed by the body are called **complete**, or **high-quality proteins**. Foods that lack adequate amounts of one or more essential amino acids are called **incomplete**, or low-quality, proteins.

When a variety of foods provide ample dietary protein, protein quality of foods is not a primary dietary concern. But wherever protein or energy intake is marginal, or when only one or a few plant foods are the main protein sources in the diet, protein quality becomes critical for good health.

Complete Proteins

Animal foods generally provide complete protein; that is, they provide all the essential amino acids in approximately the right proportions. One exception is gelatin, a protein derived from animal collagen that lacks the essential amino acid tryptophan.

FOR YOUR INFORMATION

Do Athletes Need More Protein?

Athletes are not only pumping iron these days, they're also pumping protein supplements in hopes of building muscle and improving performance. Look inside many sports magazines and you'll see ads for protein or amino acid supplements targeted to athletes. You cannot force your body to build muscle by pumping in more protein than you need, any more than you can make your car run faster by adding more gas to a full tank. Extra protein does not build muscles; only regular workouts fueled by a mix of nutrients does.

Protein Requirements for Athletes

Many people assume that because muscle fibers are protein, building muscle must require protein. This is only partially true. The heavy resistance-type exercise that is needed to stimulate muscle growth must first be fueled by glucose and fatty acids (glucose will be the predominant fuel). Little protein is used as a fuel source in resistance-type exercise. However, studies show that when men consume the RDA for protein (0.8 g/kg body weight) and engage in heavy resistance exercise, they go into negative nitrogen balance.[1] Further studies estimate the actual protein needs during resistance training as approximately 1.7 to 1.8 grams per kilogram. For endurance athletes, less protein is used

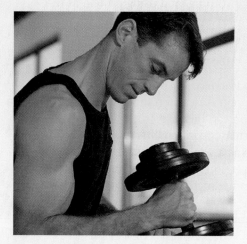

for muscle building, but more protein is used as a fuel source. The net effect is that protein needs of endurance athletes are estimated at 1.2 to 1.4 grams per kilogram.

Does this mean the serious athlete has to head for the protein shelves of the local health food store? Since Americans, on average, consume almost twice as much protein as they need, most athletes already get enough protein. An athlete in training (let's make him 70 kg) might consume up to 5,000 kilocalories per day. Even if his diet contained only 10 percent of calories as protein (on the low side in our meat-loving society), he would be getting about 126 grams of protein daily, about 1.8 grams per kilogram. It is unlikely that an athlete would not be able to meet his or her protein needs from a normal, mixed diet, even one that follows the Food Guide Pyramid recommendations.

Risks of Supplements

So, maybe there's no benefit to taking protein or amino acid supplements, but there's no harm either, right? This isn't necessarily true. If excess protein means excess calories, this adds weight as fat, not muscle, and that can slow down your performance. Purified protein supplements can contribute to calcium losses and therefore harm bone health. Excess protein means excess nitrogen that must be excreted, a risk for dehydration if fluid intake is not monitored. Supplements of single amino acids can interfere with absorption of other amino acids and can alter neurotransmitter activity. Contamination of the amino acid L-tryptophan led to devastating illness and ban of this supplement until recently.[2]

So, if you are a weekend athlete, there's no need to increase the protein in your diet, and no reason to expect that doing so will help your performance. If you are a competitive athlete, choosing adequate calories from a wide variety of foods will probably ensure an adequate protein intake, even at levels recommended for strength training. Supplements are unnecessary, expensive, and may disrupt normal protein balance in the body. Play it safe, choose a healthful diet to fuel your exercise.

1 Lemon PWR. Is increased dietary protein necessary or beneficial for individuals with a physically active lifestyle? *Nutr Rev.* 1996;54:S169–S175.

2 Herbert V. L-tryptophan. *Nutr Today.* Mar/Apr 1992;27.

Red meats, poultry, fish, eggs, milk, and milk products (all animal foods) contain complete protein. More than 20 percent of these foods' energy content is protein. Protein provides about 80 percent of the energy in water-packed tuna. The protein isolated from soybeans also provides a complete, high-quality protein equal to that of animal protein.[22] Although soy protein contains a lower proportion of the amino acid cysteine than animal protein, the amount of soy typically consumed provides all the amino acids in sufficient amounts to meet the body's needs. Moreover, soybeans contain no cholesterol or saturated fat and soy protein actually lowers blood lipid levels, reducing the risk of heart disease.[23]

Americans, on the average, obtain about 65 percent of their protein intake from animal foods.[24] (See **Table 6.3.**) In other parts of the world, animal proteins play a smaller role. In Africa and East Asia, for example, animal foods provide only 20 percent of protein intake.[25]

Complementary Proteins

With the exception of soy protein, the protein in plant foods is incomplete; that is, it lacks one or more essential amino acids and does not match the body's amino acid needs as closely as animal foods do. Although the protein in one plant food may lack certain amino acids, the protein in another plant food may be a **complementary protein** that completes the amino acid pattern. So the protein of one plant food can provide the essential amino acid(s) that the other plant food is missing. **Table 6.4** lists some examples of complementary food combinations.

For example, grain products such as pasta are low in the essential amino acid lysine but high in the essential amino acids methionine and cysteine. Legumes such as kidney beans are low in methionine and cysteine but high in lysine. In a dish that combines these foods, such as a pasta-kidney bean salad, the protein from pasta complements the protein from kidney beans, so together they provide a complete protein. Generally, when you combine grains with legumes, or legumes with nuts or seeds, you will get complete, high-quality protein.

Small amounts of animal foods can also complement the protein in plant foods. For example, Asians often flavor rice with small amounts of beef, chicken, or fish, complementing the protein in the rice. Americans eat breakfast cereal with milk, which complements the protein in the cereal.

Protein complementation is important only for people who consume little to no animal proteins. For these people, a wide variety of plant protein sources is the key to obtaining adequate amounts of all the essential amino acids. When protein and energy intake are adequate, there is no need to plan complementary proteins at each meal.[26] Complementary proteins may still need to be combined in the same meal for infants and very young children.[27]

Boosting your intake of plant protein foods can provide benefits. High-protein plant foods are usually rich in vitamins, minerals, and dietary fiber. Plant foods contain no cholesterol and little fat, and they usually cost less than animal foods high in protein. Lentil loaf, for example, is substantially cheaper to make than meat loaf.

Evaluating Protein Quality

A high-quality protein (1) provides all the essential amino acids in the amounts the body needs, (2) provides enough other amino acids to serve as nitrogen sources for synthesis of nonessential amino acids, and (3) is easy to digest. If a food protein contains the right proportion of amino acids but cannot be digested and absorbed, it is useless to the body.

Table 6.3 Top Ten Sources of Protein in the United States

Rank	Food	% of Protein Contributed
1	beef	18
2	poultry	14
3	milk	9
4	yeast bread	7
5	cheese	6
6	fish/shellfish*	4
7	eggs	3
8	pork, fresh	3
9	ham	3
10	pasta	2

* Does not include tuna.
Source: 1989–1991 Continuing Survey of Food Intake by Individuals.

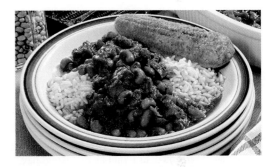

Table 6.4 Examples of Complementary Food Combinations

Beans and rice

Beans and corn or wheat tortillas

Rice and lentils

Rice and black-eyed peas

Pea soup with bread or crackers

Garbanzo beans (chick peas) with sesame paste

Pasta with beans

Peanut butter on bread

[*Fyi*] High-Protein Plant Foods

FOR YOUR INFORMATION

Of the top ten sources of protein in the American diet, only two sources—yeast breads and pasta—are plant-based (see Table 6.3). Lentils, a dense source of plant protein, don't even make the list. Yet look at the comparison between the nutritional profile of lentils and the profile of beef in **Table A**.

Table A: How Do Lentils Stack Up Against Beef?

	Cooked lentils	Lean broiled sirloin
Amount	1 cup	5 ounces
Energy	230 kcals	315 kcals
Protein	18 grams	47 grams
Fat	1 gram	12 grams
Cholesterol	0	139 milligrams
Carbohydrate	40 grams	0
Dietary fiber	9 grams	0
Percent calories from fat	4%	34%

When we consider these two foods in light of the *Dietary Guidelines for Americans* (see Chapter 2), it's no contest. To reduce fat, saturated fat, and cholesterol, and to increase complex carbohydrates and fiber, the lentils win hands down! With all that lentils have going for them, you'd think more Americans would be eating them. Yet dried beans, peas, and lentils combined contribute less than 1 percent of the daily protein intake of Americans, while beef contributes 17.7 percent.

High-protein plant foods also contribute complex carbohydrates, dietary fiber, and vitamins and minerals to the diet. Since these plant foods contain little fat, they are nutrient dense; that is, they provide a high amount of protein and nutrients relative to their energy contribution.

Sources of Plant Protein

Grains and grain products, legumes (lentils and dried beans and peas such as kidney beans or chickpeas), starchy vegetables, and nuts and seeds all provide protein (**Table B**). A serving of a grain product or starchy vegetable provides an average of 3 grams of protein, a serving of legumes provides about 10 grams of protein, and a serving of vegetables provides about 2 grams of protein. Although a serving of these foods contains less protein than a serving of meat, you can eat more plant protein foods for fewer calories.

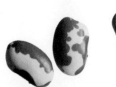

Complementing Plant Proteins

It's important to remember that plant proteins lack one or more of the essential amino acids needed to build body proteins, so individual plant proteins need to complement each other. A simple rule to remember in complementing plant proteins is that combining grains and legumes or combining legumes and nuts or seeds provides complete, high-quality protein.

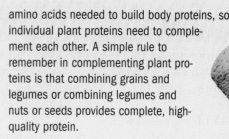

Soy Protein

The protein in soybeans is a notable exception to the rule that most plant proteins are not complete. Soy provides complete, high-quality protein comparable to that in animal foods. In addition, soybeans provide no saturated fat or cholesterol, and are rich in

Table B: Plant Sources of Protein

Plant Protein Source	Grams of Protein	Kilocalories
GRAIN PRODUCTS		
1 whole wheat bagel (3")	6	157
1 whole English muffin, mixed grain	6	155
1 large flour tortilla (10")	6	234
1 cup cooked spaghetti	7	197
1 cup cooked brown rice	5	216
1 cup cooked oatmeal	6	145
2 slices whole wheat bread	6	138
1/2 cup low-fat granola	5	213
STARCHY VEGETABLES		
1 cup cooked corn	5	177
1 cup baked hubbard squash	5	103
1 medium baked potato with skin	4	228
LEGUMES		
1/2 cup tofu	10	97
1 cup lentils	18	230
1 cup cooked kidney beans	15	225
VEGETABLES		
1 cup cooked broccoli	5	44
1 cup cooked cauliflower	2	29
1 cup cooked Brussels spouts	4	61
NUTS AND SEEDS		
2 tablespoons peanut butter	8	190
1/4 cup peanuts	9	208
1/4 cup sunflower seeds	7	208

Source: USDA Nutrient Database for Standard Reference, Release 13, 1999.

isoflavonoids—phytochemicals that help reduce risk of heart disease and cancer and improve bone health.

Isoflavonoids act as antioxidants, protecting cells and tissues from damage. One specific isoflavonoid, genistein, inhibits growth of both breast and prostate cancer cells in the laboratory. Isoflavonoids protect low-density lipoprotein cholesterol (the kind of cholesterol associated with greater risk of heart disease) from oxidation. Oxidized low-density lipoprotein cholesterol contributes to the plaque buildup in arteries. The isoflavones in soybeans also act as phytoestrogens, helping to protect older women from cardiovascular disease and osteoporosis. Soy foods that contain most or all of the bean, such as soy milk, sprouts, flour, and tofu, are the best sources of these phytochemicals.

It is easy to incorporate a variety of soy foods into your diet. Tofu, tempeh, ground soy, soy milk, soy flour, and textured soy protein are soy-based products that can be included in many meals and snacks (**Table C**).

The nutritional benefits of plant protein sources such as soy foods and other legumes, grains, and vegetables deserve a closer look. Most Americans would benefit from emphasizing plant protein foods in their diet. Next time you plan to make meat loaf, make lentil loaf instead.

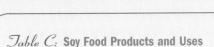

Table C: **Soy Food Products and Uses**

Tofu A solid cake of curdled soymilk similar to soft cheese. Tofu comes in hard and soft varieties. It absorbs flavors of the foods it is mixed with. Soft tofu can be substituted for cheese in pasta dishes, stuffed in large shell pasta, blended with fruit, or used to make pie filling. Hard tofu can be used in salads, shish-ka-bobs and in place of meat in stir-fry or mixed dishes.

Tempeh Tempeh is a flat cake made from fermented soybeans. It has a mild flavor and chewy texture. Tempeh can be grilled, included in sandwiches, or combined in casseroles.

Meat Analogs Meat analogs are meat alternatives made primarily of soy protein. Flavored and textured to resemble chicken, beef, and pork, and can be substituted for meat in mixed dishes, pizza, tacos, or sloppy joes.

Soymilk Soymilk is the liquid of the soybean. It comes in regular and low-fat versions and in different flavors. Soymilk can be used plain or substituted for regular milk on cereals, in hot cocoa, puddings, or desserts.

Soy Flour Soy flour is made from roasted soybeans ground into flour. Soy flour can replace up to one-quarter of the regular flour in a recipe.

Textured Soy Protein Textured soy protein resembles ground beef. It can be rehydrated and substituted for ground beef in any recipe.

Quick Bites

Paleolithic Protein

Didn't our ancestors eat a lot of meat too? Researchers estimate that hunter/gatherer populations' diets were about one-third meat and two-thirds vegetable. The meat from wild game, however, averages only one-seventh the fat of domesticated beef (about 4g of fat per 100g of wild meat, compared to 29g of fat per 100g of domestic meat). In addition, compared to the meat at your local supermarket, the fat contained in game animals that graze on the free range has five times as much polyunsaturated fat.

$$\text{Chemical score*} = \frac{\text{mg of the essential amino acid in food}}{\text{mg of the essential amino acid in reference protein}}$$

*For a percent value, multiply this result by 100.

$$\text{Protein Efficiency Ratio (PER)} = \frac{\text{Weight gain in grams}}{\text{Protein intake in grams}}$$

$$\text{Net Protein Utilization (NPU)} = \frac{\text{Nitrogen retained}}{\text{Nitrogen intake}} \times 100$$

We can measure protein quality in many ways, but any assessment of protein quality requires, at the least, information about the amino acid composition of the food protein. Protein quality might be assessed to plan a special diet or develop a new product such as infant formula.

Chemical, or Amino Acid, Scoring

A simple way to determine a food's protein quality is to compare its amino acid composition to that of a reference pattern of amino acids. This method is referred to as **chemical scoring**, or **amino acid scoring**. The amino acid composition of the reference pattern closely reflects the amounts and proportions of amino acids humans need. Currently, researchers are using the pattern of amino acids required by preschool children as the reference.[28] If a protein meets the amino acid needs of growing preschool-aged children, then it should also meet the needs of almost all other segments of the population.

For each of the nine essential amino acids, researchers take the number of milligrams of the amino acid in a food and divide it by the number of milligrams of that amino acid in the reference pattern. The result is multiplied by 100 to convert the figure to a percent value. For example, if a food contains only 65 percent of the lysine in the reference, the chemical score for the amino acid lysine is 65. The amino acid with the lowest score is the **limiting amino acid** (the amino acid present in the smallest amount relative to biological need). The chemical score of the food protein is the score of its limiting amino acid.

Protein Efficiency Ratio

Protein efficiency ratio (PER) measures amino acid composition *and* accounts for digestibility. Researchers compare the weight gain of growing animals fed a test protein with the weight gain of growing animals fed a high-quality reference protein (e.g., casein, the main protein in cow's milk). Thus, this method measures how well the body can use the test protein, which reflects amino acid composition, digestibility, and availability. The PER is used to determine the protein quality of infant formulas.

Net Protein Utilization

Net protein utilization (NPU) measures how much dietary protein the body actually uses. Scientists carefully measure the nitrogen content of a test food, and then give the food to laboratory animals as their sole protein source. They then measure the animals' nitrogen excretion to determine how much of the food's nitrogen content was retained. The more nitrogen the animal retains from a food, the higher the protein quality of that food—that is, the more efficiently the animal was able to use the food protein to make body proteins.

Biological Value

The **biological value (BV)** method determines how much of the nitrogen absorbed from a particular food protein is retained by the body for growth and/or maintenance. Nitrogen retention is a function of absorption (if it's not absorbed, it can't be retained) so measuring nitrogen absorption is a key element of this method. In general, if a protein has an essential amino acid composition similar to our needs, that protein will be more efficiently retained by the body.

Determining biological value is a tedious process because the key measures of urinary and fecal nitrogen output must be measured while subjects (human or animal) are consuming the test protein and again while they are on a nitrogen-free diet. The final value expresses nitrogen retention as a percentage of nitrogen absorption. Egg protein has a biological value of 100. This means that all the absorbed egg protein is retained by growing laboratory animals (100 percent). The biological value of the protein in corn is 60, meaning only 60 percent of the absorbed corn protein (and not all of it is absorbed) is retained for use by the body.

$$\text{Biological Value (BV)} = \frac{\text{Nitrogen retained}}{\text{Nitrogen absorbed}} \times 100$$

Protein Digestibility Corrected Amino Acid Score

The **Protein Digestibility Corrected Amino Acid Score (PDCAAS)** accounts for both the amino acid composition of a food and the digestibility of the protein. The first step in determining PDCAAS is the same used to determine the chemical score—divide the amount of the limiting amino acid by the amount of the same amino acid in the reference pattern. Then, instead of multiplying by 100 to get a percent figure, multiply by the percentage of digestible food protein. This will produce a score between 0 and 1. Egg protein provides all the amino acids preschool children need (the reference standard) and is fully digested, so it has a PDCAAS of 1.0.

$$\text{PDCAAS} = \text{Chemical Score} \times \begin{array}{c} \text{\% digestibility of} \\ \text{the protein} \end{array}$$

Thus, if a protein food has a chemical score of 0.70 based on its limiting amino acid, and 80 percent of the protein in that food is digestible, the PDCAAS score would be 80 percent of 0.70, or 0.56. The PDCAAS value of isolated soybean protein is 0.99. The scores for beef, canned chickpeas (garbanzo beans), and whole wheat are 0.92, 0.66, and 0.40, respectively.

The U.S. Food and Drug Administration (FDA) has recognized the PDCAAS as the official method for determining the protein quality of most food.[29] If the %DV for protein is listed on a food label, it must be based on the food's PDCAAS. It would be misleading to say that, for example, 8 grams of protein from tuna and 8 grams from kidney beans would contribute equally to amino acid needs; even though the amount of protein per serving might be the same, the %DV would be different for these two foods. For baby foods and infant formulas, the PER method is used to determine protein quality.

Key Concepts: *In general, animal foods provide complete protein that contains the right mix of all the essential amino acids. With the exception of soybean protein, plant foods contain incomplete protein, lacking in one or more amino acids. Plant foods can be combined to complement each other's amino acid patterns. Researchers use many methods to determine protein quality, including chemical analysis of amino acid content and biological measures of the protein's digestibility, retention in the body, or its ability to support growth.*

Estimating Your Protein Intake

By this time, you may be wondering how much protein you consume in a typical day. To be accurate, you would need an inconvenient and expensive chemical analysis of your food intake. Instead, you can estimate your protein intake using more readily available information. First, food labels list the quantity of protein (in grams) in a serving of food. If you have a label for every food you consume, just add up the grams.

Another way to estimate your protein intake is to use the food exchange lists found in **Figure 2.4** and **Appendix B**. In the exchange lists, one starch exchange provides an average of 3 grams of protein, one milk exchange provides 8 grams, one vegetable exchange provides 2 grams, and one meat exchange provides 7 grams. Fruit and fat exchanges contribute 0 protein. You can also use food composition tables or computer software to calculate your protein intake.

chemical scoring A method to determine the protein quality of a food by comparing its amino acid composition to that of a reference protein. Also called amino acid scoring.

amino acid scoring A method to determine the protein quality of a food by comparing its amino acid composition to that of a reference protein. Also called chemical scoring.

limiting amino acid The amino acid in shortest supply during protein synthesis. Also the amino acid in the lowest quantity when evaluating protein quality.

protein efficiency ratio (PER) Protein quality calculated by comparing the weight gain of growing animals fed a test protein with growing animals fed a high-quality reference protein. It depends on both the digestibility and amino acid composition of a protein.

net protein utilization (NPU) Percentage of ingested protein nitrogen retained by the body. It measures the amount of dietary protein the body uses.

biological value (BV) The extent to which protein in a food can be incorporated into body proteins, BV is expressed as the percentage of the absorbed dietary nitrogen retained by the body.

protein digestibility corrected amino acid score (PDCAAS) A measure of protein quality that takes into account the amino acid composition of the food and the digestibility of the protein. Calculated by multiplying the amino acid score by the percentage of the digestible food protein.

protein hydrolysate A protein that has been treated with acid or enzymes to break it down into amino acids and polypeptides.

As a reference point, if you consume the minimum number of servings recommended in the Food Guide Pyramid (see Chapter 2), you will get an ample amount of protein—more than enough to meet most people's protein needs.

Proteins and Amino Acids as Additives and Supplements

Proteins contribute to the structure, texture, and taste of food. They are often added to foods to enhance these properties. The milk protein casein is added to frozen dessert toppings. Gelatin is added to yogurt and fillings. **Protein hydrolysates**—protein that has been broken down into amino acids and polypeptides—are added to many foods as thickeners, stabilizers, or flavor enhancers.

Amino acids are also used as additives. Monosodium glutamate (sodium bound to the amino acid glutamic acid) is a flavor enhancer added to many foods. The artificial sweetener aspartame is a dipeptide composed of aspartic acid and phenylalanine.

Protein and amino acid supplements are sold to dieters, athletes, and people who suffer from certain diseases. Despite a lack of scientific evidence, people buy the amino acid lysine for cold sores and the amino acid tryptophan in hopes that it will relieve pain, depression, and sleep disorders. A number of protein powders and amino acid cocktails are marketed with the claims that they enhance muscle building and exercise performance. Although the anecdotal evidence (stories from friends and health food store clerks) for these products may be convincing, few scientific studies back up these claims. Remember, muscle work builds muscle strength and size, and muscles prefer carbohydrate to fuel this type of work.

There are no documented health benefits from consuming large amounts of individual amino acids, and the risks are unknown. An excess of a single amino acid in the digestive tract can impair absorption of other amino acids that use the same carrier for absorption. This could cause a deficiency of one or more amino acids and an unhealthy excess of the supplemented amino acid.

Key Concepts: You can use food labels or exchange list values to estimate your protein intake. Eating a diet that follows the Food Guide Pyramid will supply adequate amounts of protein. Supplements of protein or amino acids are rarely necessary and might be harmful.

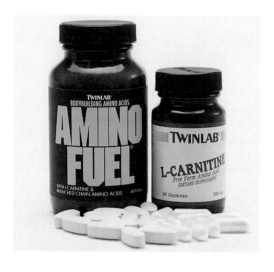

The Pros and Cons of Vegetarianism

What did Socrates, Plato, Albert Einstein, Leonardo da Vinci, William Shakespeare, Charles Darwin, and Mahatma Gandhi have in common? They all advocated a vegetarian lifestyle.[30] George Bernard Shaw, vegetarian, famous writer, and political analyst of the early 1900s, wrote, "A man fed on whiskey and dead bodies cannot do the finest work of which he is capable."[31]

Meat-eaters often contend that vegetarian diets do not provide enough protein and other essential nutrients, but this is not necessarily the case. With careful planning, a diet that contains no animal products can be nutritionally complete and also offer many health benefits. Poorly planned vegetarian diets, however, can pose health risks.

Why People Become Vegetarians

In parts of the world where food is scarce, vegetarianism is not a choice but a necessity. Where food is abundant, people choose vegetarianism for many reasons.

Table 6.5 Religious Groups with Vegetarian Dietary Practices

Religious Group	Dietary Practices
Buddhism	Some sects lacto-vegetarian, other sects vegan
Hinduism	Generally lacto-vegetarian, but mutton or pork eaten occasionally
Seventh-Day Adventists	Lacto-ovo vegetarian emphasizing whole-grain foods. Also avoid alcohol, tobacco, and caffeine.

People may choose a vegetarian diet because of religious beliefs, concern for the environment, a desire to reduce world hunger and make better use of scarce resources, an aversion to eating another living creature, or concerns about cruelty to animals. Still others become vegetarians because they believe it is healthier for them. The number of vegetarians in the United States has doubled in the last 10 years. Today, more than 12 million Americans consider themselves vegetarian.[32] **Table 6.5** shows three religious groups and their vegetarian practices.

Types of Vegetarians

Although all vegetarians share the practice of not eating meat and meat products, they differ greatly in specific dietary practices. Lacto-ovo-vegetarians use animal products such as milk, cheese, and eggs, but abstain from eating the flesh of animals. Vegans eat no animal-based foods and usually avoid products such as cosmetics made with animal-based ingredients. Fruitarians eat only raw fruit, nuts, and green foliage.

Some people eat a semi-vegetarian diet, avoiding red meats but eating small amounts of chicken or fish. The Mediterranean diet, known for reducing the risk of heart disease, is a semi-vegetarian diet rich in grains, pasta, vegetables, cheeses, and olive oil supplemented with small amounts of chicken and fish. **Table 6.6** lists the types of vegetarian diets and the foods typically included and excluded.

Zen macrobiotic diets are mostly vegan and stress whole grains, locally grown vegetables, beans, sea vegetables, and soups. Extreme Zen macrobiotic diets can be very limited, such as a diet of primarily brown rice.

Health Benefits of Vegetarian Diets

Vegetarian diets usually contain less fat, saturated fat, and cholesterol than nonvegetarian diets. Vegetarian diets that emphasize fresh fruits and vegetables contain higher amounts of antioxidants such as beta-carotene and vitamins C and E, which protect the body from cell and tissue damage. Fruits and vegetables also contain dietary fiber and phytochemicals—substances that are not essential in the diet but that can have important health effects.

On average, vegetarians have lower blood cholesterol levels and are less likely to develop heart disease than nonvegetarians. Vegetarian diets low in fat and saturated fat combined with other healthy lifestyle habits can

Prophetic Eggs

Can an egg predict the future? In Trinidad and Tobago, people say you can tell the future by the shape an egg white makes when added to warm water on Good Friday.

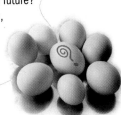

Table 6.6 Types of Vegetarian Diets

Type	Animal Foods Included	Foods Excluded
Semi-vegetarian	Dairy products, eggs, chicken, fish	Red meats (beef, pork)
Pesco-vegetarian	Dairy products, eggs and fish	Beef, pork, poultry
Lacto-ovo-vegetarian	Dairy products, eggs	Any animal flesh
Lacto-vegetarian	Dairy products	Eggs, all animal flesh
Ovo-vegetarian	Eggs	Dairy products and animal flesh
Vegan	None	All animal products
Fruitarian	None	All foods except raw fruits, nuts, and green foliage

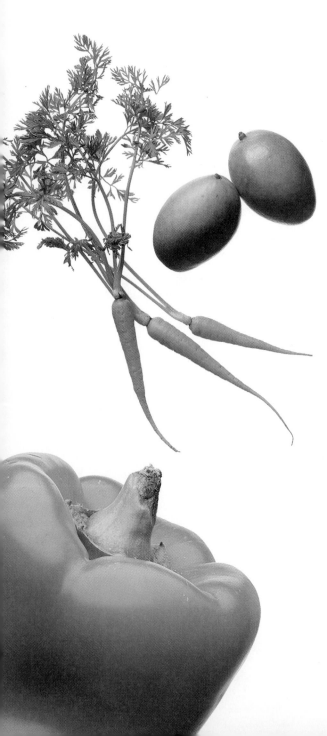

reverse the clogging of arteries that eventually can lead to heart attack or stroke.[33]

Vegetarians usually weigh less for their height than nonvegetarians, partly because their diets provide less energy and partly because of other healthful lifestyle factors such as regular exercise. High blood pressure occurs less frequently among vegetarians than among nonvegetarians, regardless of body weight or sodium intake.

Certain cancers such as breast and colon cancers occur less frequently in vegetarians than in nonvegetarians. The high dietary fiber intake typical in vegetarian diets may protect against colon cancer, while the lower estrogen levels of vegetarian women may protect against breast cancer.[34]

Health Risks of Vegetarian Diets

Although vegetarian diets offer many health benefits, certain types of vegetarian diets pose some unique nutritional risks. The more limited the vegetarian diet, the more likely are nutritional problems. Lacto-ovo-vegetarian diets that contain a variety of foods generally are nutritionally adequate but can be high in fat and cholesterol. However, iron content may be low if the diet contains large amounts of milk products.

Vegan diets tend to be low in iron, zinc, calcium, vitamin D, vitamin B_6, and vitamin B_{12}. The best sources of these nutrients are animal foods—red meat for iron and zinc, fortified milk for calcium and vitamin D, chicken for vitamin B_6, and any animal foods for B_{12}. Plant foods contain a form of iron called non-heme iron that is not as well absorbed as the heme-iron in animal foods. Since vitamin C aids iron absorption in the body, however, the higher vitamin C intakes of vegetarians may offset the lower iron intakes to some degree. Because high-protein intake increases calcium losses, vegans—who have a lower protein intake—may need less calcium than nonvegetarians.

Vegans tend to have higher intakes of phytates (found in whole grains, bran, and soy products), oxalates (found in spinach, rhubarb, and chocolate), and tannins (found in tea). These compounds can bind minerals, making them less available to the body for absorption.

Very limited vegan diets, such as fruitarian diets or extreme Zen macrobiotic diets, pose the greatest nutritional risks. These diets are likely to be deficient in many essential nutrients.

Although vegetarian diets may be adequate for most people, vegetarian diets must be planned carefully for people in periods of rapid growth—infants, young children, and women who are pregnant or breastfeeding.

Dietary Recommendations for Vegetarians

Vegetarians can follow a modified version of the Food Guide Pyramid to help plan meals (**Figure 6.21**). Vegetarians who include milk, milk products, and eggs in their diet can easily meet their nutritional needs for protein and other essential nutrients but must take care to choose low-fat milk products and limit eggs to avoid excess saturated fat and cholesterol.

Since grains, vegetables, and legumes (dried beans and peas) all provide protein, vegans who eat a variety of foods also can meet their protein needs easily. Although most plant foods do not contain complete protein, eating complementary plant protein sources during the same day adequately meets the body's needs for protein production.

Vegans who avoid all animal products must supplement their diets with a reliable source of vitamin B_{12}, such as fortified soy milk. Although bacteria in some fermented foods and in the knobby growths of some seaweeds produce vitamin B_{12}, most vegans do not eat enough seaweeds and fermented foods to meet their vitamin B_{12} needs.

The American Dietetic Association gives the following nutritional guidelines for vegetarians:

1. Choose a variety of foods, including whole grains, vegetables, fruits, legumes, nuts, seeds and, if desired, dairy products and eggs.

2. Choose whole, unrefined foods often and minimize intake of highly sweetened, fatty, and heavily refined foods.

3. Choose a variety of fruits and vegetables.

4. If animal foods such as dairy products and eggs are used, high-fat dairy foods and eggs should be limited in the diet because of their saturated fat content and because their frequent use displaces plant foods in some vegetarian diets.

5. Vegans should include a regular source of vitamin B_{12} in their diets along with a source of vitamin D if sun exposure is limited.

6. Solely breast-fed infants should have supplements of iron after the age of 4 to 6 months and, if sun exposure is limited, a source of vitamin D. Breast-fed vegan infants should have vitamin B_{12} supplements if the mother's diet is not fortified.

7. Do not restrict dietary fat in children younger than 2 years. For older children, include some foods higher in fat (eggs, nuts, seeds, nut and seed butters, avocados, and vegetable oils) to help meet nutrient and energy needs. [35]

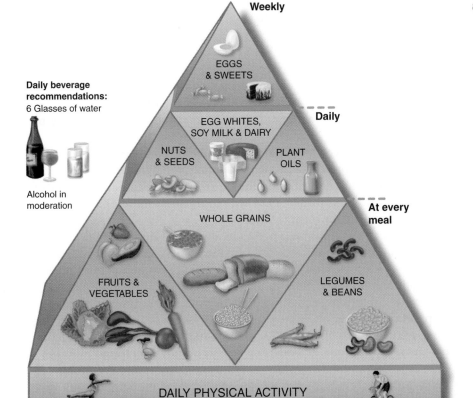

Figure 6.21 **Vegetarian Food Guide Pyramid.** With careful planning, a diet that lacks animal products can be nutritionally complete. **Source:** © 2000 Oldways Preservation & Exchange Trust.

Weekly

EGGS & SWEETS

Daily beverage recommendations: 6 Glasses of water

Alcohol in moderation

EGG WHITES, SOY MILK & DAIRY

Daily

NUTS & SEEDS

PLANT OILS

WHOLE GRAINS

At every meal

FRUITS & VEGETABLES

LEGUMES & BEANS

DAILY PHYSICAL ACTIVITY

Key Concepts: *Vegetarian diets eliminate animal products to various degrees. Lacto-ovo-vegetarians include milk and eggs in their diets, while vegans eat no animal foods. Vegetarian diets tend to be low in fat and high in fiber and phytochemicals, which may help reduce chronic disease risks. Careful diet planning is necessary for vegans and growing children to ensure that all their nutrient needs are met.*

The Health Effects of Too Little or Too Much Protein

Because protein plays such a vital role in so many body processes, protein deficiency can wreak havoc in numerous body systems. A lack of available protein means insufficient amounts of essential amino acids, which stops the synthesis of body proteins.

Protein deficiency occurs when energy and/or protein intake is inadequate. Adequate energy intake spares dietary and body proteins so they can be used for protein synthesis. Without adequate energy intake, the body burns dietary protein for energy rather than using it to make body proteins. Protein deficiency can occur even in people who eat seemingly adequate amounts of protein if the protein they eat is of poor quality or cannot be absorbed.

Although protein deficiency is widespread in poverty-stricken communities and in some nonindustrialized countries, most people in industrialized countries face the opposite problem—protein excess. Although the RDA for a 70-kilogram (154-pound) person is 56 grams, the average American man consumes approximately 105 grams of protein daily and the average woman 65 grams. And many meat-loving Americans eat far more.

Many researchers suggest that high protein intakes pose significant health risks. Links to heart disease, cancer, and osteoporosis have been suggested. However, the independent effects of high protein intake are difficult to determine, since high protein intake often goes hand in hand with high intakes of saturated fat and cholesterol.

Protein-Energy Malnutrition

protein-energy malnutrition (PEM) A condition resulting from long-term inadequate intakes of energy and protein that can lead to wasting of body tissues and increased susceptibility to infection.

A deficiency of protein, energy, or both in the diet is called **protein-energy malnutrition**, or PEM. Protein and energy intake are difficult to separate because diets adequate in energy usually are adequate in protein, and diets inadequate in energy inhibit the body's use of dietary protein for protein synthesis.

Although it can occur at all stages of life, PEM is most common during childhood, when protein is needed to support rapid growth. It is the most common form of malnutrition in the world, affecting an estimated 500 million children worldwide.[36] PEM symptoms can be mild or severe and exist in either acute or chronic forms.

Protein-energy malnutrition occurs in all parts of the world but is most common in Africa, South and Central America, East and Southeast Asia, and the Middle East. In industrialized countries, PEM occurs most often in populations living in poverty, in the elderly, and in hospitalized patients with other conditions such as anorexia nervosa, AIDS, cancer, or malabsorption syndromes.[37]

We see two forms of severe PEM: kwashiorkor and marasmus. Sometimes people have symptoms of both. Researchers do not understand fully why PEM causes symptoms of kwashiorkor in some people and symptoms of marasmus in others.[38] Historically, kwashiorkor was thought to result from inadequate intake of protein but adequate intake of energy. Marasmus was thought to result from inadequate intake of both protein and energy. Now researchers know that the lines between these two diseases are not so clear and that protein deficiency rarely develops with adequate energy intake.

Researchers believe that kwashiorkor develops from acute PEM, while marasmus develops from chronic PEM. Some researchers also believe that kwashiorkor is an abnormal adaptation to PEM, whereas marasmus is a normal adaptation. Other factors, such as infections or toxins in the diet, may trigger the development of kwashiorkor rather than marasmus.[39] See **Figure 6.22** for signs and symptoms of kwahshiorkor and marasmus.

Kwashiorkor

The term *kwashiorkor* is a Ghanian word that describes the "evil spirit which infects the first child when the second child is born." In many cultures, babies are breast-fed until the next baby comes along. When it does, the first baby is weaned from nutritious breast milk and placed on a watered-down version of the family's diet. In areas of poverty, this diet is often low in protein, or the protein is not absorbed easily.

The symptom of kwashiorkor that sets it apart from marasmus is edema, or swelling of body tissue, usually in the feet and legs. Lack of blood proteins reduces the force that keeps fluid in the bloodstream, and instead, fluid leaks out into the tissues. The belly can also become bloated from both edema and accumulation of fat in the liver, since no proteins are available to transport the fat. Other features of kwashiorkor include stunted weight and height, increased susceptibility to infection, dry and flaky skin, and sometimes skin sores, dry and brittle hair, and changes in skin color. Since the energy deficit is usually not as severe (or as long-standing) in kwashiorkor as in marasmus, people with kwashiorkor may still have some body fat stores left.

Kwashiorkor usually develops in children between 18 and 24 months of age, about the time weaning occurs. Its onset can be rapid and is often triggered by an infection or illness that increases the child's protein needs. In hospital settings, kwashiorkor can develop in situations where protein needs are extremely high (trauma, infection, burns) but dietary intake is poor.

Marasmus

Marasmus is derived from the Greek word *marasmos*, which means "withering" or "to waste away." It develops more slowly than kwashiorkor and results from chronic PEM. Protein, energy, and nutrient intake are all grossly inadequate, depleting body fat reserves and severely wasting muscle tissue, including vital organs like the heart. Growth slows or stops, and children are both short and very thin for their age. Metabolism slows and body temperature drops as the body tries to conserve energy. Children with marasmus are apathetic, often not even crying in an effort to conserve energy. Their hair is sparse and falls out easily. Because muscle and fat are used up, a child with marasmus often looks like a frail, wrinkled elderly person.

Marasmus occurs most often in infants and children 6 to 18 months of age who are fed diluted or improperly mixed formulas. Because this is a time of rapid brain growth, marasmus can permanently stunt brain development and lead to learning disabilities. Marasmus also occurs in adults during cancer and starvation, including the self-imposed starvation of the eating disorder known as anorexia nervosa.

Nutritional Rehabilitation

In order to recover, people with PEM need gradual and careful refeeding to correct protein, energy, fluid, and vitamin and mineral imbalances.[40] People with PEM are often dehydrated and have low body potassium stores as a

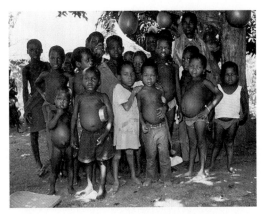

(a)

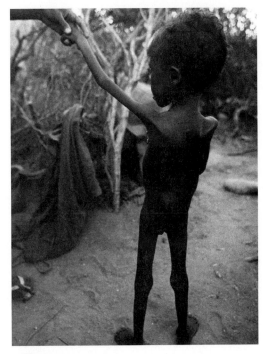

(b)

Figure 6.22 **Kwashiorkor and marasmus.**
(a) Edema in the feet and legs and a bloated belly are symptoms of kwashiorkor. (b) Children with marasmus are short and thin for their age and can appear frail and wrinkled.

result of diarrhea. These imbalances in fluids and electrolytes are corrected first in order to raise blood pressure and strengthen the heart. Once these imbalances have been corrected, the patient receives protein and other nutrients in small amounts that are gradually increased as tolerated.

Excess Dietary Protein

In industrialized countries, an excess of protein and energy is more common than a deficiency. Although not as severe or life-threatening, high protein intake can also cause health problems (see **Figure 6.23**). Therefore, the National Research Council recommends that protein intakes not exceed twice the amount recommended in the RDAs.[41]

Kidney Function

Since the kidneys must excrete the products of protein breakdown, high protein intake can strain kidney function and is especially harmful for people with kidney disease or diabetes.

To prevent dehydration, it is important to drink plenty of fluids to dilute the byproducts of protein breakdown for excretion. Human infants should not be fed unmodified cow's milk until they are at least one year of age because the high protein concentration in cow's milk combined with an immature kidney system can cause fluid losses and dehydration.

Mineral Losses

High protein intake can cause the body to excrete more calcium, contributing to bone mineral losses and increasing the risk of osteoporosis, a disease that causes bones to become porous and brittle. Animal proteins trigger greater calcium losses than plant proteins because animal proteins are especially rich in sulfur-containing amino acids, which are acidic and tend to draw calcium out of the body.[42]

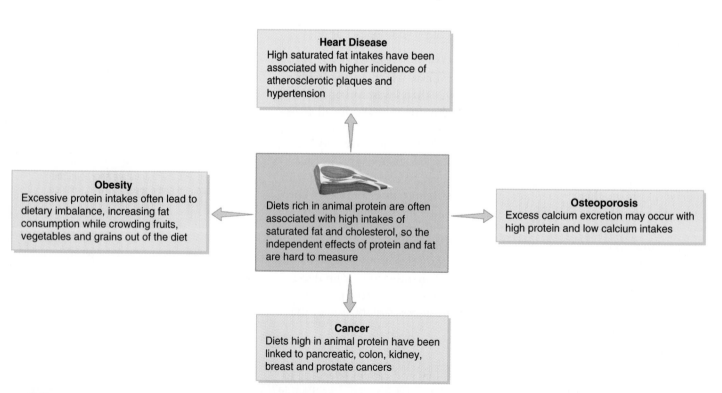

Heart Disease
High saturated fat intakes have been associated with higher incidence of atherosclerotic plaques and hypertension

Obesity
Excessive protein intakes often lead to dietary imbalance, increasing fat consumption while crowding fruits, vegetables and grains out of the diet

Diets rich in animal protein are often associated with high intakes of saturated fat and cholesterol, so the independent effects of protein and fat are hard to measure

Osteoporosis
Excess calcium excretion may occur with high protein and low calcium intakes

Cancer
Diets high in animal protein have been linked to pancreatic, colon, kidney, breast and prostate cancers

Figure 6.23 **Excess protein.** In developed countries, excess protein and energy are a greater problem than protein deficiency.

If a person meets the Adequate Intake level (AI) for calcium, the calcium losses caused by high protein intake may not be significant. Indeed, the AI for calcium is set high to offset the high protein intake of Americans. However, the calcium intake of many people, especially women, falls short of the AI, while their protein intake typically exceeds the RDA.

Obesity

High-protein foods are also often high in fat. A diet high in fat and protein may provide too much energy, contributing to obesity. Large amounts of high-protein foods will displace fruits, vegetables, and grains—foods that contain fewer calories. Some researchers have recently suggested that high dietary protein intake alters hormones and the body's response to hormones, including leptin, which regulates feeding centers in the brain to reduce food intake.[43] Some studies suggest that because of this effect on hormones, a high protein intake early in life increases the risk of obesity later in life.[44]

Heart Disease

Research has linked high intake of animal protein to high blood cholesterol levels and increased risk of heart disease. Foods high in animal protein, however, are also high in saturated fat and cholesterol. The role that protein plays in the development of heart disease independent of its association with fat is less clear. Soy protein foods, which contain no saturated fat or cholesterol, have been shown to lower blood cholesterol levels and reduce risk for heart disease.[45]

Cancer

Some studies suggest a link between a diet high in animal protein foods and an increased risk for certain types of cancers.[46] Cancer of the colon, breast, pancreas, and prostate have been linked to high protein and fat intake. As with obesity and heart disease, however, the independent effects of protein and fat are difficult to separate.

Key Concepts: *Protein deficiency and protein excess both pose health risks. Protein and energy malnutrition (PEM) is the most common form of malnutrition in the world. PEM can manifest itself in two forms: kwashiorkor and marasmus. Among other symptoms, kwashiorkor is distinguished by edema, or swelling of the tissues. Marasmus results from chronic PEM and is distinguished by severe wasting of body fat and muscles. Excess dietary protein intake may contribute to loss of bone calcium, obesity, heart disease, and certain forms of cancer.*

Label [to] **Table**

Have you ever visited a health food store and noticed all the protein powders, amino acid supplements, and high protein bars? Do you believe claims like "protein boosts your energy level" or "amino acid X helps you build muscle" or "protein shakes are the best pre-workout fuel"? You know from this chapter that protein is an important nutrient and it's used to build and repair tissue. But do you need one of these supplements? Before reaching into your wallet, check out the Nutrition Facts of this protein powder and determine whether it's a good buy.

Take a look at this label and note how far down protein is on the list of nutrients. This de-emphasized placement of protein was intentional to try to get consumers to de-emphasize protein in their diets. You may recall that most Americans eat more protein than they need, and because much of that protein comes from animal foods, they are also getting excess saturated fat. Unlike most nutrients, it doesn't show the %DV. Although there is a DV for protein (50 grams), manufacturers must first determine a food protein's quality by the PDCAAS method before they can determine %DV. Manufacturers are not required to give the %DV for protein.

Do protein and amino acid supplements do what they claim to do? In terms of building muscle, exercise physiologists agree that it takes consistent muscle work (i.e., weight lifting) and a healthy diet that meets the body's calorie needs. It does not depend on extra protein. In fact, muscles use carbohydrate and fat for fuel, not protein, so these other nutrients are more important for effective workouts.

In terms of protein's ability to boost your energy level, recall that anything with calories (carbohydrates, proteins, and fats) provides the body with "energy." In fact, unlike carbohydrates and fats, only a small amount of protein is used for energy expenditure. Research shows that the best thing to eat prior to a workout is carbohydrate, not protein, because carbohydrate provides glucose to the muscle cells. Review this label again. What percentage of this protein powder's calories is from protein?

kcalories 154

Protein   11 grams X 4 kcalories per gram
**   = 44 protein kcalories**

$44 \div 154 = 0.28$ or 28% protein kcalories

Surprise! Surprise! Only one quarter of the powder's calories are protein anyway, so it's OK as a pre-workout fuel not because of its protein content but because of its ample carbohydrate!

Nutrition Facts

Serving Size: 2 scoops
Servings Per Container: 18

Amount Per Serving

Calories 154   Calories from fat 35

	% Daily Value*
Total Fat 4g	6%
Saturated Fat 2.5g	12%
Cholesterol 20mg	7%
Sodium 170mg	7%
Total Carbohydrate 17g	6%
Dietary Fiber 0g	0%
Sugars 14g	
Protein 11g	

Vitamin A 4%	•	Vitamin C 6%
Calcium 40%	•	Iron 0%

* Percent Daily Values are based on a 2,000 calorie diet. Your daily values may be higher or lower depending on your calorie needs:

	Calories:	2000	2,500
Total Fat	Less Than	65g	80g
Sat Fat	Less Than	20g	25g
Cholesterol	Less Than	300mg	300mg
Sodium	Less Than	2,400mg	2,400mg
Total Carbohydrate		300g	375g
Dietary Fiber		25g	30g

Calories per gram:
Fat 9   •   Carbohydrate 4   •   Protein 4

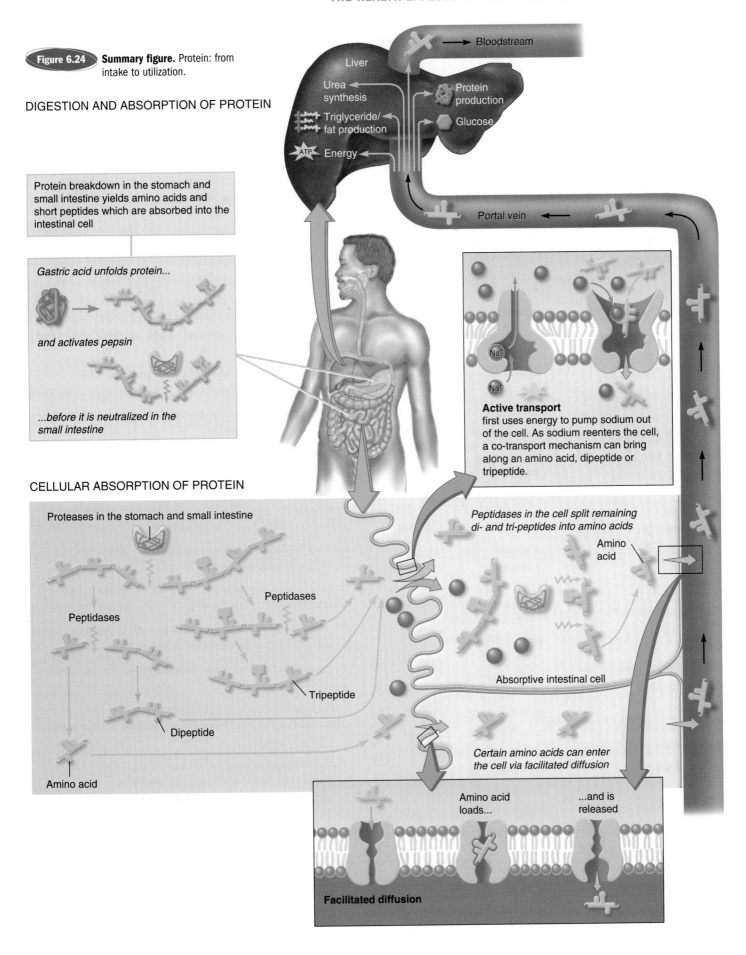

Figure 6.24 **Summary figure.** Protein: from intake to utilization.

DIGESTION AND ABSORPTION OF PROTEIN

Bloodstream

Liver

Urea synthesis

Protein production

Triglyceride/ fat production

Glucose

ATP Energy

Portal vein

Protein breakdown in the stomach and small intestine yields amino acids and short peptides which are absorbed into the intestinal cell

Gastric acid unfolds protein...

and activates pepsin

...before it is neutralized in the small intestine

Active transport
first uses energy to pump sodium out of the cell. As sodium reenters the cell, a co-transport mechanism can bring along an amino acid, dipeptide or tripeptide.

Na⁺

Na⁺

CELLULAR ABSORPTION OF PROTEIN

Proteases in the stomach and small intestine

Peptidases

Peptidases

Tripeptide

Dipeptide

Amino acid

Peptidases in the cell split remaining di- and tri-peptides into amino acids

Amino acid

Absorptive intestinal cell

Certain amino acids can enter the cell via facilitated diffusion

Amino acid loads...

...and is released

Facilitated diffusion

LEARNING *Portfolio* chapter 6

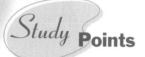

Key Terms

Study Points

> Many vital compounds are proteins, including enzymes, hormones, transport proteins, and regulators of both acid-base and fluid balance.

> Proteins are long chains of amino acids.

> Amino acids are composed of a central carbon atom bonded to hydrogen, carboxyl, amino and side groups.

> At least 20 amino acids are important in human nutrition; nine of these amino acids are considered essential (must come from the diet) while the body can make the other eleven (non-essential) amino acids.

> The amino acid sequence of a protein determines its shape and function.

> Denaturing of proteins changes their shape and therefore their functional properties.

> Protein digestion begins in the stomach through the action of hydrochloric acid and the enzyme pepsin.

> Proteins are completely digested in the small intestine and absorbed by facilitated diffusion and active transport.

> Dietary protein is found in meats, dairy products, legumes, grains and vegetables.

> In general, animal foods contain higher quality protein than is found in plant foods.

> Protein needs are highest when growth is rapid, such as during infancy, childhood, and adolescence.

> The protein intake of most Americans exceeds their RDA.

> Protein deficiency is most common in developing countries and results in the conditions known as marasmus and kwashiorkor.

> Protein excess is also harmful and may affect risk for osteoporosis, heart disease, and cancer.

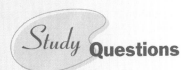

Study Questions

1. **List the functions of body proteins.**

2. **Describe the differences among essential, nonessential, and conditionally essential amino acids.**

3. **Among the nutrient molecules, which element is unique to protein and how does it fit into the basic structure of an amino acid?**

4. **Why are most plant proteins considered incomplete?**

5. **What are complementary proteins? List three examples of food combinations that contain complementary proteins.**

6. **What health effects occur if you are protein deficient?**

7. **How is protein related to immune function?**

8. **Describe a vegan diet.**

9. **List the potential health benefits of a vegetarian diet.**

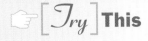 [Try] **This**

The Sweetness of Nutrasweet

The purpose of this experiment is to see the effect of high temperatures on the dipeptide known as NutraSweet (aspartame). Make a cup of hot tea (or coffee) and add one packet of Equal (one brand of aspartame). Stir and taste the tea; note its sweetness. Reheat the tea (via a microwave or stovetop) so that it boils for 30 to 60 seconds. After the tea cools, taste it. Does it still taste sweet? Why or why not?

The Vegetarian Challenge

The purpose of this activity is to eat a completely vegetarian diet for one day. Begin by making a list of your typical meals and snacks. Once the list is complete, review each food item and determine if it contains animal products. Cross off items that contain animal products and circle the remaining vegan-friendly options. Double-check the circled list with a friend or roommate. You may have missed something! Create a full day's worth of meals and snacks using your circled foods as well as additional vegan options. Make sure your menu looks complete and nutritionally balanced. Try to stick to this menu for at least one day. Pay attention to deviations you make and whether these are vegan food choices.

What About Bobbie?

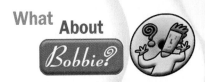

Take a minute to review Bobbie's food intake with a special eye on protein. How do you think she did? Do you think she's lower or higher than her RDA? Let's first calculate her protein RDA. Since Bobbie weighs 155 pounds, her protein RDA is as follows:

155 pounds ÷ 2.2 pounds = 70.5 kilograms
70.5 kilograms X 0.8 grams protein = 56.40 grams

Her protein intake is 97 grams. This is quite high compared to her RDA! Are you surprised to learn she eats twice as much protein as she needs? Her diet doesn't look that high in protein, does it? Here are the foods that contribute the most protein to her diet:

Food	Protein Grams
Turkey breast	9
Meatballs	23
Bagel	7
Spaghetti	10
Pizza	12

Another way to evaluate Bobbie's protein intake is in terms of calories. If her total protein intake is 97 grams, then 388 kilocalories come from protein. Remember, her total kilocalorie intake is 2,440, which means protein comprises 16 percent. General guidelines recommend that 10 to 15 percent of energy come from protein.

So what's the deal? Is Bobbie eating way too much protein or just the right amount? Using her RDA as a guide, you'd say she's overconsuming protein, but based on her calories, she's doing just fine. To get to the bottom of this you're going to have to look a little closer. The real issue here is her calorie intake. If you check the RDA table (page i) to see the recommended calorie intake for a 19-year-old woman, you'll see that it's 2,200 kilocalories. So the bigger issue here is that Bobbie may be consuming too many calories. Even though she ate approximately 16 percent as protein, because her calorie intake was high, her total protein intake was high too. Can you calculate what her protein grams should have been if she actually consumed close to the energy RDA?

15% of 2,200 kcalories = 330 protein kcalories
330 protein kcalories ÷ 4 calories per gram = 82 grams

So, Bobbie's protein RDA is 51 grams per day; yet, based on the general protein recommendation of 15 percent of calories, she could consume up to 82 grams. The 51-gram-per-day recommendation based on Bobbie's body weight is more accurate than the 82-gram-per-day recommendation based on the RDA for energy (calories). If you remember the review of Bobbie's diet in the carbohydrate chapter, it should now make sense that she should consume less protein and eat more fruits and vegetables.

References

1 Nelson JE, Moxness KE, Jensen MD, Gastineau, CF. *Mayo Clinic Diet Manual: A Handbook of Nutritional Practices.* 7th ed. St. Louis: Mosby; 1994.

2 Griffiths RD, Jones C, Palmer TE. Six-month outcome of critically ill patients given glutamine-supplemented parenteral nutrition. *Nutrition.* 1997;13:295–302.

3 Van der Hulst RR, von Meyenfeldt MR, Soeters PB. Glutamine: an essential amino acid for the gut. *Nutrition.* 1996;12:S78–S81.

4 Alexander JW, Ogle CK, Nelson JL. Diets and infection: composition and consequences. *World J Surg.* 1998;22:209–212.

5 Voet D, Voet JG. *Biochemistry.* 2nd ed. New York: Wiley; 1995.

6 Schwartz M, Seeley RJ. The new biology of body weight regulation. *J Am Diet Assoc.* 1997;97:54-58; and Considine RB, Sinha MK, Heiman ML, et al. Serum immunoreactive-leptin concentrations in normal-weight and obese humans. *N Eng J Med.* 1996;334:292-295.

7 Stryer L. *Biochemistry.* 4th ed. New York: WH Freeman; 1995.

8 Guyton A, Hall J. *Textbook of Medical Physiology.* 9th ed. Philadelphia: WB Saunders; 1996.

9 Sardesai VM. *Introduction to Clinical Nutrition.* New York: Marcel Dekker; 1998.

10 Ibid.

11 Guyton A, Hall, J. Op. cit.

12 Matthews DE. Proteins and amino acids. In: Shils ME, Olson JA, Shike M, Ross AC, eds. *Modern Nutrition in Health and Disease.* 9th ed. Philadelphia: Lippincott Williams & Wilkins; 1999:11-48.

13 Suryawan A, Hawes JW, Harris RA, et al. A molecular model of human branched-chain amino acid metabolism. *Am J Clin Nutr.* 1998;68:72–81.

14 Matthews DE Op. cit.

15 Food and Agricultural Organization, World Health Organization, United Nations University. *Energy and Protein Requirements.* Rome: Food and Agricultural Organization; 1985.

16 Basile-Filho A, Beaumier L, El-Khoury E, et al. Twenty-four-hour L-[1-¹³C] tyrosine and L-[3,3-²H₂] phenylalanine oral tracer studies at generous, intermediate, and low phenylalanine intakes to estimate aromatic amino acid requirements in adults. *Am J Clin Nutr.* 1998;67:640–659; and Kurpad AV, El-Khoury E, Beaumier L, et al. An initial assessment, using 24-h [¹³C] leucine kinetics, of the lysine requirement of healthy adult Indian subjects. *Am J Clin Nutr.* 1998;67:58–66.

17 US Department of Health and Human Services (USDHHS). *The Surgeon General's Report on Nutrition and Health.* DHHS (PHS) publication 88-50210. Washington, DC: US Government Printing Office; 1988.

18 McDowell MA, Briefel RR, Alaimo K, et al. *Energy and macronutrient intake of persons ages 2 months and over in the United States: Third National Health and Examination Survey, Phase 1, 1988–91. Advance data from vital and health statistics.* No 255. Hyattsville, MD: National Center for Health Statistics; 1994.

19 Food and Nutrition Board of the national Academy of Sciences, National Research Council. *Recommended Dietary Allowances.* 10th ed. Washington, DC: National Academy Press; 1989.

20 Millward DJ, Roberts SB. Protein requirements of older individuals. *Nutr Res Rev.* 1996;9:67–87.

21 US Department of Agriculture, Agricultural Research Service. *Data Tables: Results from USDA's 1994–96 Continuing Survey of Food Intakes by Individuals and 1994–96 Diet and Health Knowledge Survey.* On: 1994–96 Continuing Survey of Food Intakes by Individuals and 1994–96 Diet and Health Knowledge Survey, CD-ROM, NTIS accession no. PB98-500457; 1997.

22 Young VR. Soy protein in relation to human protein and amino acid nutrition. *J Am Diet Assoc.* 1991;91:828–835.

23 Anderson JW, Johnstone RM, Cook-Newell ME. Meta-analysis of the effects of soy protein intake on serum lipids. *N Engl J Med.* 333:276–282, 1995.

24 Young VR, Pellett PL. Plant proteins in relation to human protein and amino acid nutrition. *Am J Clin Nutr.* 1994;59:1203S–1212S.

25 Ibid.

26 Young VR, Pellett PL. Loc. cit.; and American Dietetic Association. Position of the American Dietetic Association: vegetarian diets. *J Am Diet Assoc.* 1997;97:1317–1321.

27 Dwyer JT. Nutritional consequences of vegetarianism. *Ann Rev Nutr.* 1991;11:61–91.

28 Protein quality evaluation, Report of the Joint FAO/WHO Expert Consultation, FAO Food and Nutrition Paper 51. Rome: Food and Agriculture Organization of the United Nations; 1991; and Sarwar G, McDonough RE. Evaluation of protein digestibility-corrected amino acid score method for assessing protein quality of foods. *J Assoc Official Analytic Chem.* 1990;73:347–356.

29 Protein quality evaluation, Report of the Joint FAO/WHO Expert Consultation, Op. cit.; and Sarwar G, McDonough RE. Loc. cit.

30 Ballenntine R. *Transition to Vegetarianism: An Evolutionary Step.* Honesdale, PA: Himalayan International Institute of Yoga Science and Philosophy; 1987; and Null G. *The Vegetarian Handbook: Eating Right for Total Health.* New York: St. Martin's; 1987.

31 Null G. Op. cit.

32 Gustafson N. *Vegetarian Nutrition.* 2nd ed. Eureka, CA: Nutrition Dimension; 1997.

33 Gould KL, Ornish D, Scherwitz L, et al. Changes in myocardial perfusion abnormalities by positron emission tomography after long-term intense risk factor modification. *JAMA.* 1995;274:894–901.

34 American Dietetic Association. *Position of the American Dietetic Association: Vegetarian Diets.* 1997;97:1317–1321.

35 Ibid.

36 Latham MC. Protein-energy malnutrition. In: Brown ML, ed. *Present Knowledge in Nutrition.* Washington, DC: International Life Sciences Institute-Nutrition Foundation; 1990.

37 Swail WS, Samour PQ, Babineau TJ, Bistrian BR. A proposed revision of current ICD-9-CM malnutrition code definitions. *J Am Diet Assoc.* 1996;96:370–373.

38 Manary MJ, Broadhead RL, Yarasheski KE. Whole-body protein kinetics in marasmus and kwashiorkor during acute infection. *Am J Clin Nutr.* 1998;67:1205–1209.

39 Jelliffe DB, Jelliffe EFP. Causation of kwashiorkor: toward a multifactorial consensus. *Pediatrics.* 1992;90:110–112.

40 Hoffer LJ. Metabolic consequences of starvation. In: Shils ME, Olson JA, Shike M, Ross AC, eds. *Modern Nutrition in Health and Disease.* 9th ed. Philadelphia: Lippincott Williams & Wilkins; 1999:645-665.

41 Ibid.

42 Itoh R, Nishiyama N, Suyama Y. Dietary protein intake and urinary excretion of calcium: a cross-sectional study in a healthy Japanese population. *Am J Clin Nutr.* 1998;67:438–444.

43 Rolland-Cachera MR, Deheeger M, Bellisle F. Nutrient balance and body composition. *Reprod Nutr Dev.* 199737:727–734; and Schwartz M, Seeley RJ. The new biology of body weight regulation. *J Am Diet Assoc.* 1997;97:54–58.

44 Parizkova J, Rolland-Cachera MF. High proteins early in life as a predisposition for later obesity and further health risks. *Nutrition.* 1997;13:818–819.

45 Anderson JW, Johnstone RM, Cook-Newell ME. Meta-analysis of the effects of soy protein intake on serum lipids. *N Engl J Med.* 1995;333:276–282.

46 Giovannuci E. Intake of fat, meat, and fiber in relation to colon cancer in men. *Cancer Res.* 1994;54:2390.

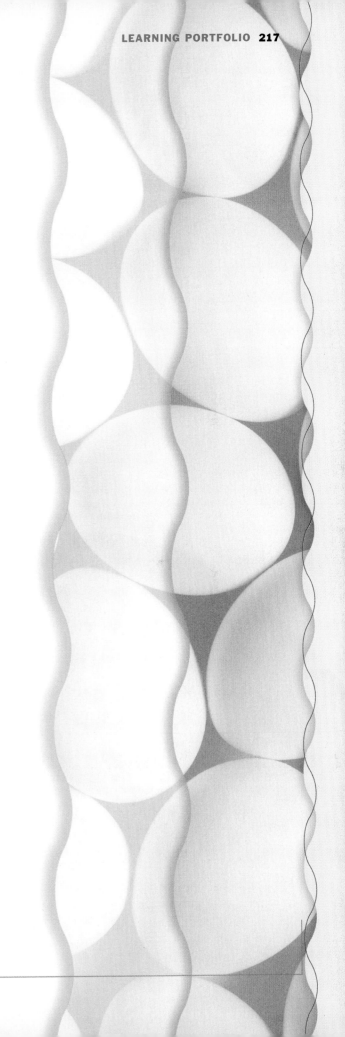

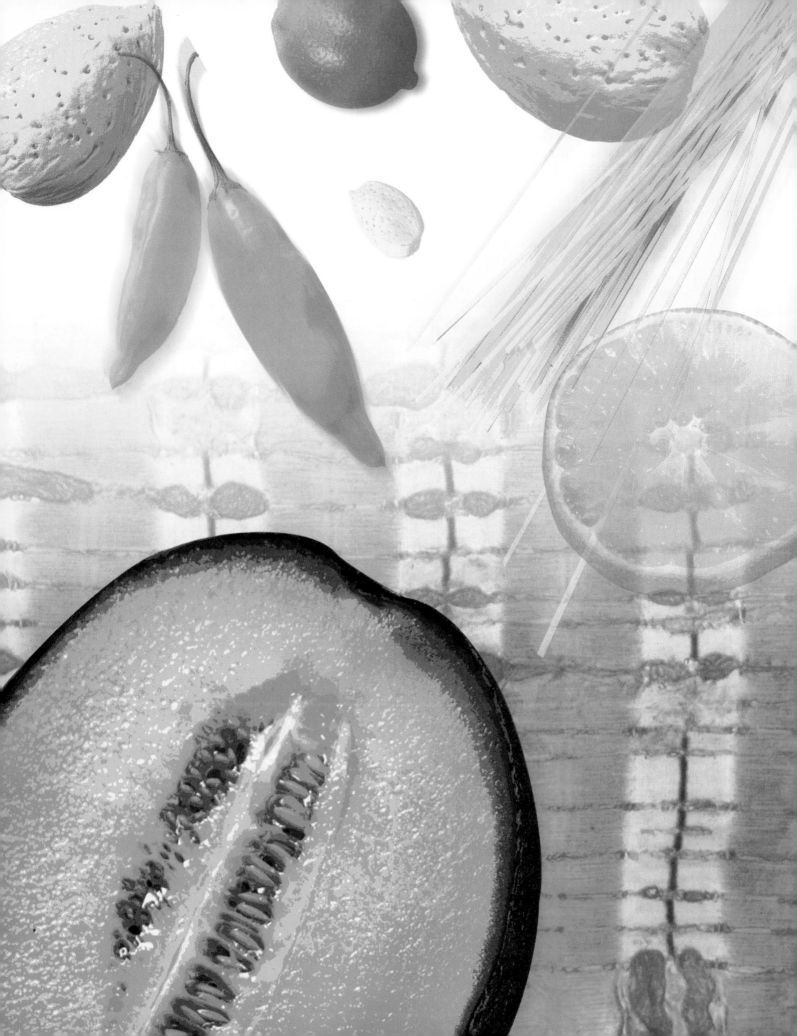

Chapter 7

Metabolism

Think About It

1. You are driving on "the energy highway." You stop at the tollbooth. What kind of currency do you need to pay the toll?

2. When you think of "cell power," what comes to mind?

3. What do you think is meant by the saying: "Fat burns in a flame of carbohydrate"?

4. When it comes to fasting, what's your body's first priority?

Fyi for your Information

This chapter's FYI boxes include practical information on the following topics:
- Do Carbohydrates Turn Into Fat
- Key Intersections Direct Metabolic Traffic
- Metabolic Profiles of Important Sites

The web site for this book offers many useful tools and is a great source for additional nutrition information for both students and instructors. Visit the site at nutrition.jbpub.com for information on metabolism. You'll find exercises that explore the following topics:
- Mitochondria Malfunctions
- Deadly Dinitrophenol
- The Ketosis Diet
- The Citric Acid Cycle (Krebs cycle)

What About *Bobbie?*

Track the choices Bobbie is making with the EatRight Analysis software.

Key to Illustrations

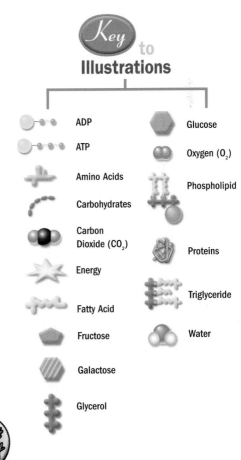

ADP	Glucose
ATP	Oxygen (O₂)
Amino Acids	Phospholipid
Carbohydrates	
Carbon Dioxide (CO₂)	Proteins
Energy	
Fatty Acid	Triglyceride
Fructose	Water
Galactose	
Glycerol	

EXTRACTION OF ENERGY

Protein
(amino acids)

Carbohydrates

Fats
(fatty acids)

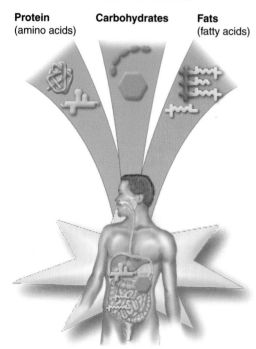

Molecular building blocks

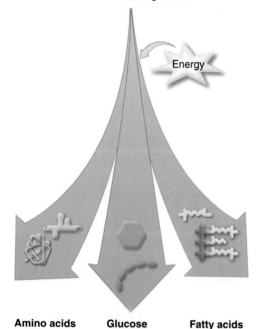

Energy

Amino acids
Body protein

Glucose
Glycogen

Fatty acids
Lipids

BIOSYNTHESIS

Figure 7.1 **Metabolism.** Cells use metabolic reactions to extract energy from food and to form building blocks for biosynthesis.

*Y*our body is a wonderfully efficient factory. It accepts raw food materials, burns some to generate power, uses some to produce finished goods, routes the rest to storage, and discards waste and by-products. The stored inventory is kept fresh through constant turnover—production processes continually draw it down and the inflow of raw materials constantly replenishes it.

Do you ever wonder how your biological factory responds to changing supply and demand? In normal circumstances, it is humming along nicely with all processes in balance. When supply exceeds demand, your body stores excess raw materials in inventory. When supply fails to meet demand, your body draws on these stored materials to meet its needs. Your biological factory never stops and even though a storage or energy-production process may dominate, all your factory operations are active to some extent at all times.

Collectively, these processes are known as **metabolism**. (See **Figure 7.1**.) While some metabolic reactions break down molecules to extract energy, others synthesize building blocks to produce new molecules. To carry out metabolic processes, thousands of chemical reactions occur every moment in cells throughout your body—the most active metabolic sites include your liver and muscle cells.

Energy: Fuel for Work

To operate, machines need energy. Cars use gasoline for fuel, factory machinery uses electricity, and windmills rely on wind power. So what about you? All cells require energy to sustain life. Even during sleep your body uses energy for breathing, pumping blood, maintaining body temperature, delivering oxygen to tissues, removing waste products, synthesizing new tissue for growth, and repairing damaged or worn-out tissues. When awake, you need additional energy for physical movement (such as standing, walking, talking) and for the digestion and absorption of foods.

Where does the energy come from to power your body's "machinery"? The forms of energy in biological systems are heat, mechanical, electrical, and chemical. Our cells get their energy from **chemical energy** held in the molecular bonds of carbohydrates, fats, and protein—the energy nutrients—as well as alcohol. This chemical energy originates as light energy from the sun. Green plants use light energy to make carbohydrate in a process called **photosynthesis**. In photosynthesis, carbon dioxide (CO_2) from the air combines with water (H_2O) from the earth to form a carbohydrate, usually glucose ($C_6H_{12}O_6$), and oxygen (O_2). Plants store glucose as starch and release oxygen into the atmosphere. Plants like corn, peas, squash, turnips, potatoes, and rice store especially high amounts of starch in their edible parts. In the glucose molecule, the chemical bonds between the carbon (C) and hydrogen (H) atoms hold energy from the sun.[1]

Within any system (including the universe) the total amount of energy is constant. While energy can change from one form to another and move from one location to another, the system never gains or loses energy. This principle, the first law of thermodynamics, is known as the conservation of energy.

Transferring Food Energy to Cellular Energy

Although burning food releases energy as heat, we cannot use heat to power the many cellular functions that maintain life. Rather than using combustion, we transfer energy from food to a form that our cells can use. (See **Figure 7.2**.) This transfer is not completely efficient; we lose roughly half of the total food energy as heat[2] as our bodies extract energy from food in three stages:

Stage 1: Digestion, absorption, and transportation. Digestion breaks food down into small subunits—simple sugars, fatty acids, monoglycerides, glycerol, and amino acids—that the small intestine can absorb. The circulatory system then transports these nutrients to tissues throughout the body.

metabolism All chemical reactions within organisms that enable them to maintain life. The two main categories of metabolism are catabolism and anabolism.

chemical energy Energy contained in the bonds between atoms of a molecule.

photosynthesis The process by which green plants use radiant energy from the sun to produce carbohydrates (hexoses) from carbon dioxide and water.

STAGES IN THE EXTRACTION OF ENERGY FROM FOOD

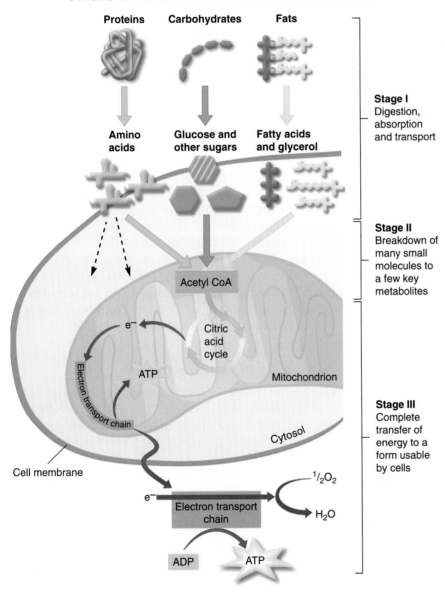

Figure 7.2 **Energy extraction from food.** In the first stage, the body breaks down food into amino acids, sugars, and fatty acids. In the second stage, cells degrade these molecules to a few simple units, such as acetyl CoA, that are pervasive in metabolism. In the third stage, the oxygen-dependent reactions of the citric acid cycle and electron transport chain liberate large amounts of energy in the form of ATP.

CATABOLIC REACTIONS

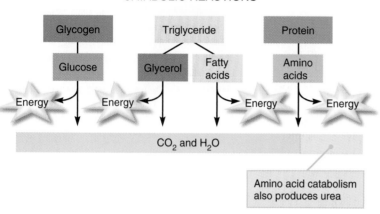

Amino acid catabolism
also produces urea

ANABOLIC REACTIONS

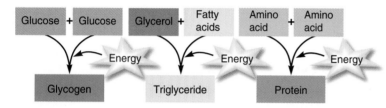

Figure 7.3 **Catabolism and anabolism.** Catabolic reactions break down molecules and release energy and other products. Anabolic reactions consume energy as they assemble complex molecules.

Stage 2: Breakdown of the many small molecules to a few key metabolites. Inside individual cells, chemical reactions convert simple sugars, fatty acids, glycerol, and amino acids to a few key **metabolites** (products of metabolic reactions). This process liberates a small amount of usable energy.

Stage 3: Transfer of energy to a form that cells can use. The complete breakdown of metabolites to carbon dioxide and water liberates large amounts of energy. As we extract available energy from food, the reactions during this stage are responsible for more than 90 percent of the transformation to a form of energy our bodies can use.

What Is Metabolism?

Metabolism is a general term that encompasses all chemical changes that occur in living organisms. The term **metabolic pathway** describes a series of chemical reactions that either break down a large compound into smaller units (**catabolism**) or build more complex molecules from smaller ones (**anabolism**).[3] For example, when you eat bread or rice, the GI tract breaks down the starch into glucose units. Tissue cells can further catabolize these glucose units to release energy for activities such as muscle contractions. On the other hand, anabolic reactions take available glucose molecules and assemble them into glycogen for storage. **Figure 7.3** illustrates catabolism and anabolism.

Metabolic pathways are never completely inactive. Their activity ebbs and flows in response to internal and external events. Imagine, for example, that your instructor keeps you late and you have only five minutes to get to your next class! As you hustle across campus, your body ramps up energy production to fuel the demand created by your rapidly contracting muscles.

The Cell Is the Metabolic Processing Center

Cells are the "work centers" of metabolism. (See **Figure 7.4**.) Although our bodies are made up of different types of cells (e.g., liver cells, brain cells, kidney cells, muscle cells, etc.), they have a similar structure. The basic animal

metabolite Any substance produced during metabolism.

metabolic pathway A series of chemical reactions that either break down a large compound into smaller units (catabolism) or synthesize more complex molecules from smaller ones (anabolism)

catabolism [ca-TA-bol-iz-um] Any metabolic process whereby cells break down complex substances into simpler, smaller ones.

anabolism [an-A-bol-iz-um] Any metabolic process whereby cells convert simple substances into more complex ones.

cell The basic structural unit of all living tissues, which has two major parts—the nucleus and cytoplasm

nucleus The primary site of genetic information in the cell, enclosed in a double-layered membrane. The nucleus contains the chromosomes, and is the site of messenger RNA (mRNA) and ribosomal RNA (rRNA) synthesis, the "machinery" for protein synthesis in the cytosol.

cytoplasm The cytoplasm is the material of the cell, excluding the cell nucleus and cell membranes. The cytoplasm includes the fluid cytosol, the organelles, and other particles.

cytosol The fluid inside the cell membrane, excluding organelles. The cytosol is the site of glycolysis and fatty acid synthesis.

organelle Various membrane-bound structures that form part of the cytoplasm. Organelles, including mitochondria and lysosomes, perform specialized metabolic functions.

mitochondria (mitochondrion) The sites of aerobic production of ATP, where most of the energy from carbohydrate, protein, and fat is captured. Called the powerhouse of the cell, the mitochondria contain two highly specialized membranes, an outer membrane and a highly folded inner membrane, that separate two compartments, the internal matrix space and the narrow intermembrane space. A human cell contains about 2,000 mitochondria.

cell is divided roughly into two parts—the cell **nucleus** and a membrane-enclosed space called the **cytoplasm**. As we zoom in for a closer look, we see that a fluid called the **cytosol** fills the cytoplasm. Floating in the cytosol are many **organelles**, small units that perform specialized metabolic functions. A large number of these—the capsule-like **mitochondria**—are power generators that contain many important energy-producing pathways.

Organelles

Endoplasmic reticulum (ER)
- An extensive membrane system extending from the nuclear membrane.
- Rough ER: The outer membrane surface contains ribosomes, the site of protein synthesis.
- Smooth ER: Devoid of ribosomes, the site of lipid synthesis.

Golgi apparatus
- A system of stacked membrane-encased discs.
- The site of extensive modification, sorting and packaging of compounds for transport.

Lysosome
- Vesicle containing enzymes that digest intracellular materials and recycle the components.

Mitochondrion
- Contains two highly specialized membranes, an outer membrane and a highly folded inner membrane. Membranes separated by narrow intermembrane space. Inner membrane encloses space called mitochondrial matrix.
- Often called the powerhouse of the cell. Site where most of the energy from carbohydrate, protein and fat is captured in ATP (adenosine triphosphate).
- About 2,000 mitochondria in a cell.

Ribosome
- Site of protein synthesis.

Nucleus
- Contains genetic information in the base sequences of the DNA strands of the chromosomes.
- Site of RNA synthesis — RNA needed for protein synthesis.
- Enclosed in a double-layered membrane.

Cytoplasm
- Enclosed in the cell membrane and separated from the nucleus by the nuclear membrane.
- Filled with particles and organelles which are dispersed in a clear fluid called cytosol.

Cytosol
- The fluid inside the cell membrane.
- Site of glycolysis and fatty acid synthesis.

Cell membrane
- A double layered sheet, made up of lipid and protein, that encases the cell.
- Controls the passage of substances in and out of the cell.
- Contains receptors for hormones and other regulatory compounds.

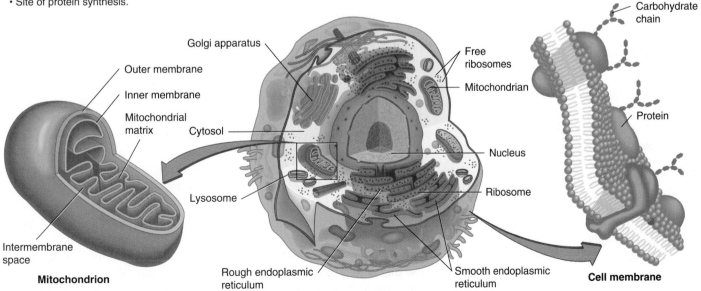

Golgi apparatus

Outer membrane

Inner membrane

Mitochondrial matrix

Cytosol

Lysosome

Intermembrane space

Mitochondrion

Rough endoplasmic reticulum

Free ribosomes

Mitochondrian

Nucleus

Ribosome

Smooth endoplasmic reticulum

Carbohydrate chain

Protein

Cell membrane

Figure 7.4 **Cell structure.** Liver cells, brain cells, kidney cells, muscle cells, etc., all have a similar structure.

cofactor A compound required for an enzyme to be active. Cofactors include coenzymes and metal ions such as iron (Fe^{2+}), copper (Cu^{2+}), and magnesium (Mg^{2+}).

coenzyme An organic compound, often a B vitamin derivative, that combines with an inactive enzyme to form an active enzyme. Coenzymes associate closely with these enzymes, allowing them to catalyze certain metabolic reactions in a cell.

ATP (adenosine triphosphate) [ah-DEN-oh-seen try-FOS-fate] A high-energy compound that is the main direct fuel that cells use to synthesize molecules, contract muscles, transport substances, and perform other tasks.

NADH The reduced form of nicotinamide adenine dinucleotide (NAD^+), this coenzyme, derived from the B vitamin niacin, acts as an electron carrier in cells, and undergoes reversible oxidation and reduction.

$FADH_2$ The reduced form of flavin adenine dinucleotide (FAD), this coenzyme, derived from the B vitamin riboflavin, acts as an electron carrier in cells and undergoes reversible oxidation and reduction.

NADPH The reduced form of nicotinamide adenine dinucleotide phosphate, this coenzyme, derived from the B vitamin niacin, acts as an electron carrier in cells, undergoing reversible oxidation and reduction. The oxidized form is $NADP^+$.

biosynthesis Chemical reactions that form simple molecules into complex biomolecules, especially carbohydrate, lipids, protein, nucleotides, and nucleic acids.

ADP (adenosine diphosphate) The compound produced upon hydrolysis of ATP, and used to synthesize ATP. Composed of adenosine and two phosphate groups.

pyrophosphate Inorganic phosphate. This high-energy phosphate group is an important component of ATP, ADP, and AMP.

Enzymes, which are catalytic proteins, speed up chemical reactions in metabolic pathways. Many enzymes are inactive unless combined with certain smaller molecules called **cofactors**, which usually are derived from a vitamin or mineral. Vitamin-derived cofactors are also called **coenzymes**. All the B vitamins form coenzymes used in metabolic reactions. (For more on coenzymes see Chapter 10, "Water-Soluble Vitamins.")

Key Concepts: *Metabolism refers to the many reactions that take place in cells to build tissue, produce energy, break down compounds, and do other cellular work. Anabolism refers to reactions that build compounds, such as protein or glycogen. Catabolism is the breakdown of compounds to yield energy. Mitochondria, the powerhouses of cells, contain many of the breakdown pathways that produce energy.*

Who Are the Key Energy Players?

Certain compounds have recurring roles in metabolic activities. **Adenosine triphosphate, ATP,** is the fundamental energy molecule used to power cellular functions, so it is known as the universal energy currency. Two other molecules, **NADH** and **$FADH_2$,** are important couriers that carry energy for the synthesis of ATP. A similar energy carrier, **NADPH,** delivers energy for **biosynthesis**.

Think About It

1

ATP: Adenosine Triphosphate

To power biosynthesis and other cellular processes, your body must convert the energy in food to a readily usable form. Some processes, such as the complete breakdown of glucose and fatty acids, release energy, and others, such as building glucose from other compounds, consume energy. The universal energy currency, ATP, usually powers energy-consuming processes and kick-starts many energy-releasing processes. Remember that making large molecules from smaller ones, like constructing a building from bricks, requires energy.

Production of ATP is the fundamental goal of metabolism's energy-producing pathways. Similar to the saying "All roads lead to Rome," you could say that, with few exceptions, energy-producing pathways lead to ATP.

The ATP molecule has three phosphate groups attached to adenosine, which is an organic compound. Because the bonds between the phosphate groups store a tremendous amount of energy, ATP is an energy-rich molecule. (See **Figure 7.5.**) Breaking a high-energy phosphate bond releases energy to power biological work. When a metabolic reaction breaks the first phosphate bond, it breaks down ATP to **adenosine diphosphate (ADP)** and **pyrophosphate (P_i)**. Breaking the remaining phosphate bond releases an equal amount of energy and breaks down ADP to **adenosine monophosphate (AMP)** and P_i.

ATP and ADP are interconvertible because the reaction can proceed in either direction, as **Figure 7.6** shows. As energy is extracted from carbohydrate, protein, and fat, ADP binds P_i to form ATP and capture energy in the new high-energy phosphate bond. When the reaction flows in the opposite direction, ATP releases P_i to form ADP while breaking one high-energy phosphate bond. This liberated energy can power biological activities such

---

as motion, active transport across cell membranes, biosynthesis, and signal amplification.

The body's pool of ATP is a small, immediately accessible energy reservoir rather than a long-term energy reserve. The typical lifetime of an ATP molecule is less than one minute and ATP production increases or decreases in direct relation with energy needs. A person at rest uses about 40 kilograms of ATP in 24 hours (an average rate of about 28 g/min). In contrast, strenuous exercise can use as much as 500 grams per minute! On average, you turn over your body weight in ATP every day.[4]

The molecule **guanosine triphosphate (GTP)** is similar to ATP and contains the same amount of available energy. Like ATP, GTP contains high-energy phosphate bonds and three phosphate groups, but they are linked to guanosine rather than adenosine. Energy-rich GTP molecules are crucial for vision and they supply part of the power necessary to synthesize protein and glucose. GTP is readily converted to ATP.

NADH and FADH₂

When breaking down nutrients, metabolic reactions release high-energy electrons. Further reactions transfer energy from these electrons to the

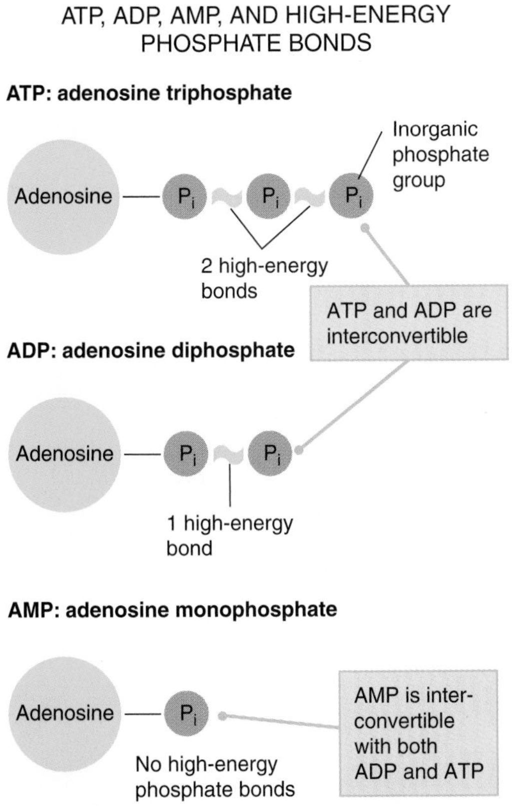

AMP (adenosine monophosphate) Hydrolysis product of ADP and of nucleic acids. Composed of adenosine and one phosphate group.

GTP (guanosine triphosphate) A high-energy compound, similar to ATP, but with three phosphate groups linked to guanosine.

ATP   Adenosine–P~P~P

GTP   Guanosine–P~P~P

ATP, ADP, AMP, AND HIGH-ENERGY PHOSPHATE BONDS

ATP: adenosine triphosphate

Adenosine — P$_i$ ~ P$_i$ ~ P$_i$ — Inorganic phosphate group

2 high-energy bonds

ATP and ADP are interconvertible

ADP: adenosine diphosphate

Adenosine — P$_i$ ~ P$_i$

1 high-energy bond

AMP: adenosine monophosphate

Adenosine — P$_i$

No high-energy phosphate bonds

AMP is interconvertible with both ADP and ATP

Figure 7.5 Your body can readily use the energy in high-energy phosphate bonds. During metabolic reactions, phosphate bonds form or break to capture or release energy.

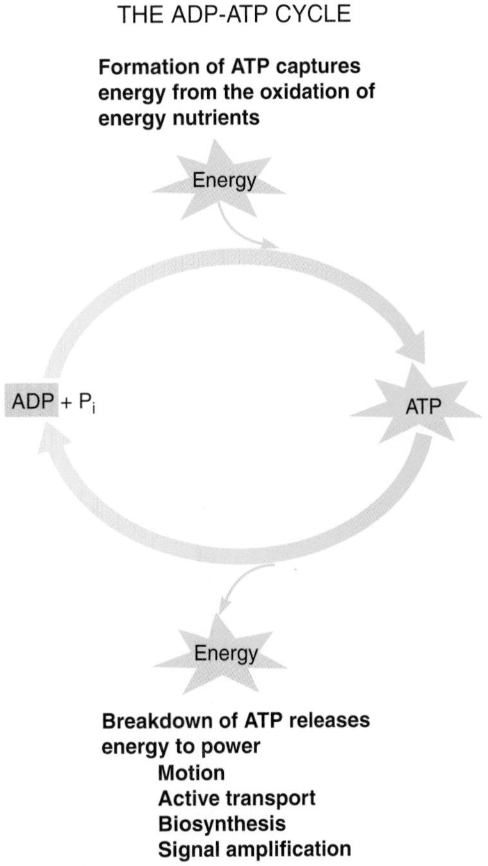

THE ADP-ATP CYCLE

Formation of ATP captures energy from the oxidation of energy nutrients

Energy

ADP + P$_i$ → ATP

Energy

Breakdown of ATP releases energy to power
Motion
Active transport
Biosynthesis
Signal amplification

Figure 7.6 When extracting energy from nutrients, the formation of ATP from ADP + P$_i$ captures energy. Breaking a phosphate bond in ATP to form ADP + P$_i$ releases energy for biosynthesis and work.

$$NAD^+ + 2H^+ \leftrightarrow NADH + H^+$$
NADH carries two high-energy electrons

$$FAD + 2H^+ \leftrightarrow FADH_2$$
FADH₂ carries two high-energy electrons

$$NADPH + H^+ \leftrightarrow NADP^+ + 2H^+$$
NADPH releases energy for biosynthesis when converted to NADP⁺.

high-energy bonds of ATP. (See **Figure 7.7**.) To reach the site of ATP production, high-energy electrons hitch a ride on special molecular carriers. One major electron acceptor is **nicotinamide adenine dinucleotide (NAD⁺)**, a derivative of the B vitamin niacin. The metabolic pathways have several energy-transfer points where an NAD⁺ accepts two high-energy electrons and two **hydrogen ions** (two protons [2H⁺]) to form NADH + H⁺. For simplicity, the "+ H⁺" is often dropped when talking about NADH.

The other major electron acceptor is **flavin adenine dinucleotide (FAD)**, a derivative of the B vitamin riboflavin. When FAD accepts two high-energy electrons, it picks up two protons (2H⁺) and forms FADH₂.

NADPH

Energy powers the assembly of building blocks into complex molecules of carbohydrate, fat, and protein. NADPH, an energy-carrying molecule similar to NADH, delivers much of the energy these biosynthetic reactions require. The only structural difference between NADPH and NADH is the presence or absence of a phosphate group. Although both molecules are energy carriers, their metabolic roles are vastly different. Whereas the energy carried by NADH primarily produces ATP, nearly all the energy carried by NADPH drives biosynthesis. When a reaction transforms NADPH into NADP⁺ (nicotinamide adenine dinucleotide phosphate), NADPH releases its cargo of two energetic electrons.

Key Concepts: *ATP is the energy currency of the body. NADH and FADH₂ are hydrogen and electron carriers important in the production of ATP. NADPH is also a hydrogen and electron carrier, but is involved in anabolic processes.*

NAD⁺ (nicotinamide adenine dinucleotide) The oxidized form of nicotinamide adenine dinucleotide, this coenzyme, derived from the B vitamin niacin, acts as an electron carrier in cells, undergoing reversible oxidation and reduction. The reduced form is NADH.

hydrogen ion Also called a proton, this lone hydrogen has a positive charge (H⁺). It does not have its own electron, but it can share one with another atom.

FAD (flavin adenine dinucleotide) A coenzyme synthesized in the body from riboflavin, it undergoes reversible oxidation and reduction and thus acts as an electron carrier in cells. FAD is the oxidized form; FADH₂ is the reduced form.

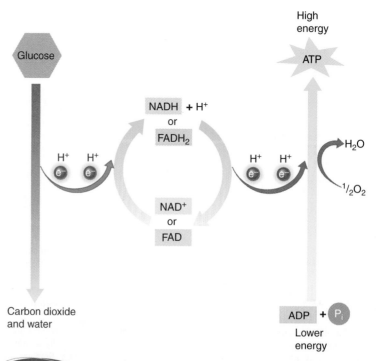

ENERGY TRANSFER

Figure 7.7 **Energy transfer.** As energy moves from glucose to ATP, molecules become high-energy or low-energy as they collect and transfer high-energy electrons and hydrogen ions.

Breakdown and Release of Energy

The complete catabolism of carbohydrate, protein, and fat for energy occurs via several pathways. Although each nutrient follows a different initial path, they eventually share two important catabolic pathways—the citric acid cycle and the electron transport chain. This section first describes the pathways that catabolize glucose. Then it discusses the steps that start the breakdown of fat and protein.

Extracting Energy from Carbohydrate

Cells obtain usable energy from carbohydrate via four main pathways: glycolysis, pyruvate to acetyl CoA, the citric acid cycle, and the electron transport chain. (See **Figure 7.8**.) Although glycolysis and the citric acid cycle produce small amounts of energy, the electron transport chain is the major ATP production site.

Glycolysis

Glycolysis is an **anaerobic** process; that is, it does not require oxygen. In the cytosol, this sequence of reactions breaks down glucose into **pyruvate** while producing a relatively small amount of energy.

The reactions of the glycolytic pathway convert each six-carbon glucose molecule into two three-carbon pyruvate molecules. While glycolysis both consumes and releases energy, it produces more than it uses. During the early stages, glycolysis needs two ATP to drive reactions. In the later stages, various reactions produce energy-rich molecules of NADH and release four ATP. The glycolysis of one glucose molecule yields a net of two NADH and two ATP, along with the two pyruvates. (See **Figure 7.9**.)

Although most glycolytic reactions can flow in either direction, some are irreversible, one-way reactions. These one-way reactions prevent glycolysis from running backward.

What about the other simple sugars, fructose and galactose? The breakdown of fructose and galactose is similar to that of glucose. These sugars are broken down mainly by glycolysis in liver cells and normally are not available to other tissues.[5] Although they enter glycolysis at intermediate points, the result is the same. One molecule of glucose, fructose, or galactose produces two NADH, a net of two ATP and two pyruvate. The pyruvate molecules easily pass from the cytosol to the interior of mitochondria, the cell's power generators, for further processing.

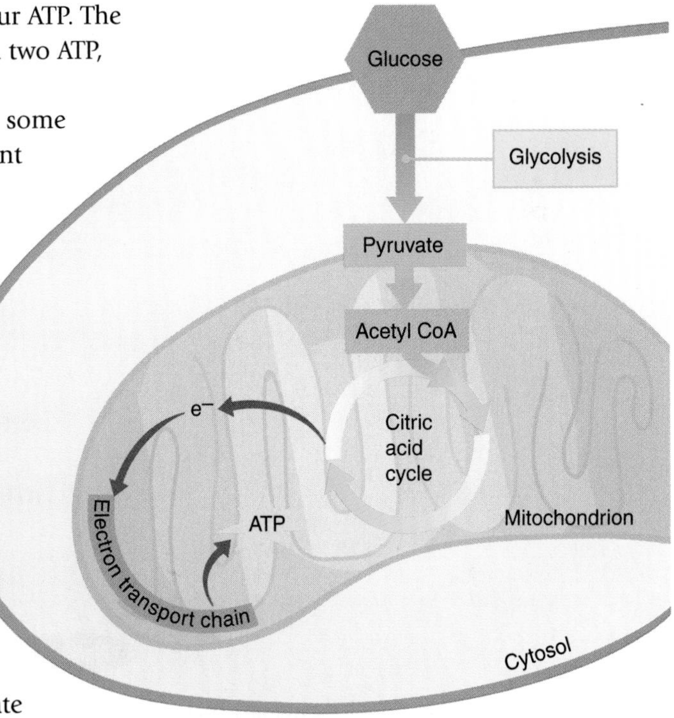

Pyruvate to Acetyl CoA

When a cell requires energy and oxygen is readily available, an **aerobic** reaction in the mitochondria irreversibly converts pyruvate to **acetyl CoA** while producing CO_2 and one energy-rich molecule of NADH. (See **Figure 7.10**.) To form acetyl CoA, this reaction removes one carbon from the three-carbon pyruvate and adds **coenzyme A**, a molecule derived from the B vitamin pantothenic acid. Together, the two pyruvate molecules from glycolysis produce two NADH and two acetyl CoA molecules.

glycolysis [gligh-COLL-ih-sis] The anaerobic metabolic pathway that breaks a glucose molecule into two molecules of pyruvate and yields two molecules of ATP and two molecules of NADH. Glycolysis occurs in the cytosol of a cell.

anaerobic [AN-ah-ROW-bic] Referring to the absence of oxygen or the ability of a process to occur in the absence of oxygen.

pyruvate The three-carbon compound that results from glycolytic breakdown of glucose. Pyruvate, the salt form of pyruvic acid, also can be derived from glycerol and some amino acids.

aerobic [air-ROW-bic] Referring to the presence or need of oxygen. The complete breakdown of glucose, fatty acids, and amino acids to carbon dioxide and water occurs only via aerobic metabolism. The citric acid cycle and electron transport chain are aerobic pathways.

acetyl CoA A key intermediate in the metabolic breakdown of carbohydrates, fatty acids, and amino acids. It consists of a two-carbon acetate group linked to coenzyme A, which is derived from pantothenic acid.

coenzyme A Coenzyme A is a cofactor derived from the vitamin pantothenic acid.

Figure 7.8 **Obtaining energy from carbohydrate.** The complete oxidation of glucose uses four major metabolic pathways: glycolysis, pyruvate to acetyl CoA, the citric acid cycle, and the electron transport chain. Glycolysis takes place in the cytosol. The remaining reactions take place in the mitochondria.

Quick Bites

When Glycolysis Goes Awry

Red blood cells do not have mitochondria, so they rely on glycolysis as their only source of ATP. They use ATP to maintain the integrity and shape of their cell membranes. A defect in red blood cell glycolysis can cause a shortage of ATP, which leads to deformed red blood cells. Destruction of these cells by the spleen leads to a type of anemia called hemolytic anemia.

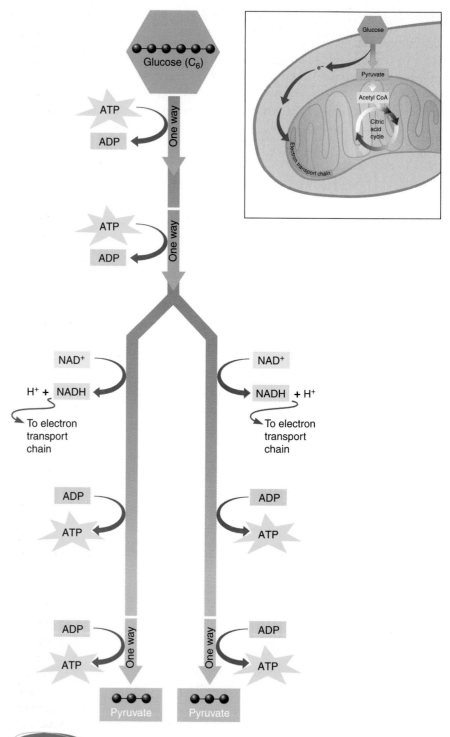

Figure 7.9 **Glycolysis.** The glycolysis of one glucose molecule yields two pyruvate molecules, a net of two ATP and two NADH. Glycolytic reactions do not require oxygen and critical steps are irreversible.

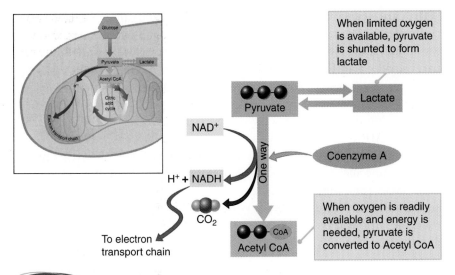

When limited oxygen is available, pyruvate is shunted to form lactate

When oxygen is readily available and energy is needed, pyruvate is converted to Acetyl CoA

lactate The ionized form of lactic acid, a three-carbon acid. It is produced when insufficient oxygen is present in cells to oxidize pyruvate.

citric acid cycle The metabolic pathway occurring in mitochondria in which the acetyl portion (CH_3COO-) of acetyl CoA is oxidized to yield two molecules of carbon dioxide and one molecule each of NADH, $FADH_2$, and GTP. Also known as the Krebs cycle and tricarboxylic acid cycle.

oxaloacetate A four-carbon intermediate compound in the citric acid cycle. Acetyl CoA combines with free oxaloacetate in the mitochondria forming citrate and beginning the cycle.

Figure 7.10 **Pyruvate to acetyl CoA.** When oxygen is readily available, each pyruvate formed from glucose yields one acetyl CoA and one NADH.

If oxygen is not readily available, a condition that occurs in contracting muscle cells, pyruvate cannot form acetyl CoA. Instead, pyruvate is rerouted to form **lactate**, another three-carbon compound. Lactate is an alternative fuel that muscle cells can use or that liver cells can convert to glucose. When oxygen again becomes readily available, lactate reenters the aerobic pathways. It converts back to pyruvate, which irreversibly forms acetyl CoA. You will learn more about lactate production, cycling, and use in Chapter 13, "Sports Nutrition."

Although pyruvate passes easily between the cytosol and the mitochondria, the mitochondrial membrane is impervious to acetyl CoA. The acetyl CoA produced from pyruvate is trapped inside the mitochondria, ready to enter the citric acid cycle.

Citric Acid Cycle

For further processing, acetyl CoA can enter the **citric acid cycle**. This circular pathway is an elegant set of reactions that occur in the mitochondria. It begins when the two-carbon acetyl CoA combines with the four-carbon compound **oxaloacetate** to yield the six-carbon compound citrate (citric acid). This first step frees coenzyme A. This coenzyme A leaves the cycle, becoming available to react with another pyruvate and form a new acetyl CoA. As the citric acid cycle proceeds, reactions transform citrate into a sequence of intermediate compounds. These reactions also remove two carbons and release them in two molecules of CO_2. Since acetyl CoA added two carbons to the cycle and the cycle releases two carbons as CO_2, there is no net gain or loss of carbon atoms. The final step in the citric acid cycle regenerates oxaloacetate.

The citric acid cycle produces most of the energy-rich molecules that ultimately generate ATP. For each acetyl CoA entering the cycle, one complete "turn" produces three NADH, one $FADH_2$, and one GTP. Since the breakdown of one glucose molecule yields two molecules of acetyl CoA, the citric acid cycle "turns" twice for each glucose molecule and produces twice these amounts (i.e., six NADH, two $FADH_2$ and two GTP).

The citric acid cycle goes by many names. It may be called the **Krebs cycle** after Sir Hans Krebs, the first scientist to explain its workings, who was awarded the Nobel Prize in 1953 for his work. It also may be called the **tricarboxylic acid (TCA) cycle** because a tricarboxylic acid (citrate) is formed in the first step. Most nutritionists use the term citric acid cycle. **Figure 7.11** shows an overview of the citric acid cycle.

In addition to producing energy-rich NADH and $FADH_2$ to power the generation of ATP, the citric acid cycle is an important source of building blocks for the biosynthesis of amino acids and fatty acids. Many of the cycle's intermediate molecules may be used for biosynthesis rather than the completion of the cycle. For example, oxaloacetate may be converted to glucose or to amino acids for protein synthesis. Without an alternative supply of oxaloacetate, the citric acid cycle stops. Fortunately, oxaloacetate can be synthesized directly from pyruvate, easily replenishing the citric acid cycle's supply.

Quick Bites

The Latest ATP Count

The number of ATP (or GTP) formed directly in glycolysis and the citric acid cycle is unequivocally known, but the ATP formed from NADH and $FADH_2$ in the electron transport chain is less certain. Old estimates credited NADH from the citric acid cycle with 3 ATP and $FADH_2$ with 2 ATP. The best current estimates are 2.5 and 1.5, respectively. "Hence, about 30 ATP are formed when glucose is completely oxidized to CO_2; this value supersedes the traditional estimate of 36 ATP." —Lubert Stryer, Professor of Biochemistry, Stanford University

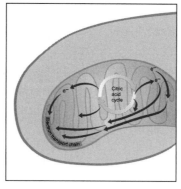

The citric acid cycle produces 3 NADH and 1 $FADH_2$ which carry pairs of high-energy electrons to the electron transport chain. It also forms one GTP which is readily converted to 1 ATP.

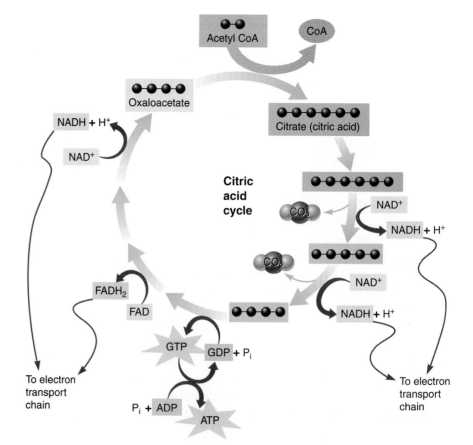

Figure 7.11 **The citric acid cycle.** This circular pathway conserves carbons as it accepts one acetyl CoA and yields two CO_2, three NADH, one $FADH_2$ and one GTP (readily converted to ATP).

Electron Transport Chain

The final step in glucose breakdown is a sequence of linked reactions that take place in the **electron transport chain**, an organized series of carrier molecules located in the inner **mitochondrial membrane**. This pathway produces most of the ATP available from glucose. Because the mitochondrion is the site of both the citric acid cycle and the electron transport chain, it truly is the energy powerhouse of the cell.

The carriers NADH and $FADH_2$ now deliver their high-energy cargo. NADH produced in the mitochondria by the citric acid cycle delivers its high-energy electrons to the beginning of the chain. In the inner mitochondrial membrane, these electrons are passed along a chain of linked reactions, giving up energy along the way to power the final production of ATP. At the end of the electron transport chain, oxygen accepts the energy-depleted electrons and reacts with hydrogen to form water. This formation of ATP coupled to the flow of electrons along the electron transport chain is called **oxidative phosphorylation** because it requires oxygen, and it phosphorylates ADP (joins it to P_i) to form ATP. (See **Figure 7.12**.)

Without an oxygen "basket" at the end to accept the energy-depleted electrons, the transport of electrons down the chain would halt, stopping ATP production. Without ATP, there is no power for our body's essential functions. If our oxygen supply is not rapidly restored, we die.

What about $FADH_2$? The high-energy electrons from $FADH_2$ enter the electron transport chain at a later point than the electrons from NADH. Since they travel through fewer reactions, the electrons from $FADH_2$ generate fewer ATP.

Historically, it was thought that NADH from the citric acid cycle produced 3 ATP and $FADH_2$ produced 2 ATP. Biochemists have revised the estimates of the net amount of ATP generated by the electron transport chain.[6] They now think that each pair of electrons carried by NADH from the citric acid cycle generates about 2.5 ATP and each $FADH_2$ generates 1.5 ATP.

What about the NADH from glycolysis? Remember that glycolysis takes place in the cytosol, while the citric acid cycle and electron transport chain are in the mitochondria. NADH in the cytosol cannot penetrate the outer mitochondrial membrane. Instead, cytosolic NADH transfers its high-energy electrons to special carrier molecules that shuttle them across the outer mitochondrial membrane and deliver them to the electron transport chain. The electron transport chain accepts delivery of the electrons either at the beginning (like NADH from the citric acid cycle) or farther along   (like

electron transport chain An organized series of carrier molecules—including flavin mononucleotide (FMN), coenzyme Q, and several cytochromes—that are located in mitochondrial membranes and shuttle electrons from NADH and $FADH_2$ to oxygen, yielding water and ATP.

mitochondrial membrane The mitochondria are enclosed by a double shell separated by an intermembrane space. The outer membrane acts as a barrier and gatekeeper, selectively allowing some molecules to pass through while blocking others. The inner membrane is where the electron transport chains are located.

oxidative phosphorylation Formation of ATP from ADP and P_i coupled to the flow of electrons along the electron transport chain.

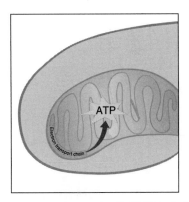

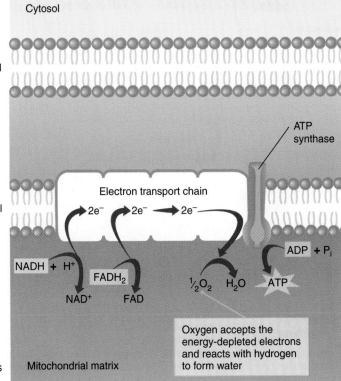

Cytosol

Outer mitochondrial membrane

Inner mitochondrial membrane

ATP synthase

Electron transport chain

$2e^-$ → $2e^-$ → $2e^-$

NADH + H⁺

NAD⁺

FADH₂

FAD

½O₂ **H₂O**

ADP + Pᵢ

ATP

Mitochondrial matrix

Oxygen accepts the energy-depleted electrons and reacts with hydrogen to form water

Figure 7.12 **Electron transport chain.** This pathway produces most of the ATP available from glucose. Mitochondrial NADH deliver pairs of high-energy electrons to the beginning of the chain. Each of these NADH molecules ultimately produces 2.5 ATP. The pairs of high-energy electrons from $FADH_2$ enter this pathway farther along, so one $FADH_2$ produces 1.5 ATP.

FADH$_2$). The electron pairs from glycolytic NADH (See **Figure 7.13**) generate either 2.5 or 1.5 ATP, depending on where the electrons enter the electron transport chain. Due to this difference, the complete oxidation of a glucose molecule does not always produce the same amount of ATP. (see **Figure 7.14.**)

End Products of Glucose Catabolism

Now you've seen all the steps in glucose breakdown. What has the cell produced from glucose? The end products of complete catabolism are carbon dioxide (CO_2), water (H_2O), and ATP. Both the conversion of pyruvate to acetyl CoA and the citric acid cycle produce CO_2. The electron transport chain produces water. While glycolysis makes small amounts of ATP and the citric acid cycle makes a little as GTP, the electron transport chain generates the vast majority of this universal energy currency. **Table 7.1** summarizes the pathways of glucose metabolism.

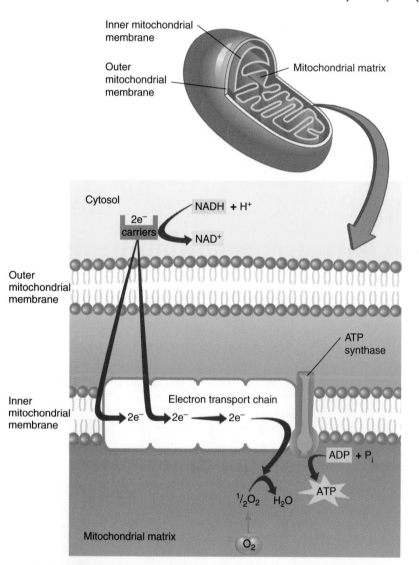

COMPLETE OXIDATION OF GLUCOSE

Pathway	ATP formed by pathway	ATP formed in electron transport chain
Glycolysis (1 Glucose)		
Net 2 ATP (4 produced – 2 used)	2	
2 NADH*		3 to 5
2 Pyruvate to 2 Acetyl CoA		
First pyruvate → Acetyl CoA		
1 NADH		2.5
Second pyruvate → Acetyl CoA		
1 NADH		2.5
Citric Acid Cycle (twice)		
First acetyl CoA → Citric acid cycle		
1 GTP (ATP)	1	
1 FADH$_2$		1.5
3 NADH		7.5
Second acetyl CoA → Citric acid cycle		
1 GTP (ATP)	1	
1 FADH$_2$		1.5
3 NADH		7.5
Subtotal	4	26 to 28
		Total = 30 to 32

*Each NADH formed in the cytosol by glycolysis will produce either 2.5 or 1.5 ATP in the electron transport chain. (See figure 7.13)

Figure 7.13 NADH from glycolysis is in the cytosol and cannot cross the outer mitochondrial membrane. It hands off its high-energy electrons to special carriers that shuttle them across the membrane. The carriers may deliver them at the beginning or farther along the electron transport chain. Depending on the delivery point, each NADH from glycolysis produces 2.5 or 1.5 ATP.

Figure 7.14 **Complete oxidation of glucose.** These metabolic pathways and molecules move energy from glucose to ATP. Complete oxidation of one glucose molecule yields 30 to 32 ATP.

Key Concepts: *The metabolism of glucose to yield energy occurs in several steps. Glycolysis breaks the six-carbon glucose molecule into two pyruvate molecules. Each pyruvate loses a carbon and combines with a coenzyme A to form an acetyl CoA, which then enters the citric acid cycle. Since two acetyl CoAs are formed from a single glucose molecule, the citric acid cycle operates twice. Finally, the NADH and FADH₂ formed in all these pathways carry high-energy electrons to the electron transport chain where ATP and water are produced. When completely oxidized, each glucose molecule yields carbon dioxide, water, and ATP.*

Extracting Energy from Fat

To begin catabolizing fat, the body breaks down triglycerides into their component parts, glycerol and fatty acids. Glycerol, a small three-carbon molecule, carries a relatively small amount of energy and the liver can convert it to pyruvate or glucose. Fatty acids contain nearly all the energy stored in triglycerides.

In the cytosol, a fatty acid must be activated—linked to coenzyme A—before it can enter the breakdown pathways. The breakdown of one ATP molecule to one AMP and two P$_i$ provides the energy to drive this reaction. Although this activation reaction requires only one molecule of ATP, it breaks both of ATP's high-energy phosphate bonds and consumes the energetic equivalent of two ATP (double the amount of energy released from ATP $\rightarrow$ ADP + P$_i$).

Carnitine Shuttle

Without assistance, the activated fatty acid cannot get inside the mitochondria where fatty acid oxidation and the citric acid cycle operate. This entry problem is solved by **carnitine**, a compound formed from the amino acid lysine. Carnitine has the unique task of ferrying fatty acids from the cytosol across the mitochondrial membrane to the interior of the mitochondria. When carnitine is in short supply, the production of ATP slows. Moderate carnitine deficiency in heart or skeletal muscle reduces muscle endurance;

carnitine [CAR-nih-teen] A compound that transports fatty acids from the cytosol into the mitochondria, where they undergo beta-oxidation.

Table 7.1 **Summary of the Major Metabolic Pathways in Glucose Metabolism**

Phase	Location	Type	Summary	Starting Materials	End Products
Glycolysis	Cytosol	Anaerobic	A series of reactions that convert one glucose molecule to two pyruvate molecules.	Glucose, ATP	Pyruvate, ATP, NADH
Pyruvate to acetyl CoA	Mitochondria	Aerobic	Pyruvate from glycolysis combines with coenzyme A to form acetyl CoA while releasing carbon dioxide.	Pyruvate, coenzyme A	Acetyl CoA, carbon dioxide, NADH
Citric acid cycle	Mitochondria	Aerobic	This cycle of reactions degrades the acetyl portion of acetyl CoA and releases the coenzyme A portion. This cycle releases carbon dioxide and produces most of the energy-rich molecules, NADH and FADH₂, generated by the breakdown of glucose.	Acetyl CoA	Carbon dioxide, NADH, FADH₂, GTP
Electron transport chain	Mitochondria (membrane)	Aerobic	As the electrons from NADH and FADH₂ pass along this chain of transport proteins, they release energy to power the generation of ATP. Oxygen is the final electron acceptor and combines with hydrogen to form water.	NADH, FADH₂	ATP, water

more extreme deficiency causes muscular strength to fail more quickly.[7] Based on its role in fatty acid oxidation, carnitine supplements are sold with the claim they act as "fat burners." Research data has shown few benefits from carnitine supplementation in healthy people, with little or no effect on fatty acid oxidation rates or athletic performance.[8]

Beta-Oxidation

> **beta-oxidation** The breakdown of a fatty acid into numerous molecules of the two-carbon compound acetyl coenzyme A (acetyl CoA).

Once in the mitochondria, a process known as **beta-oxidation** disassembles the fatty acid and converts it into several molecules of acetyl CoA. (See **Figure 7.15**.) Starting at the beta carbon of the fatty acid (the second carbon from the acid end), enzymes clip a two-carbon "link" off the end of the chain. Reactions convert this two-carbon link to one acetyl CoA, while also forming one $FADH_2$ and one NADH. In stepwise fashion this process repeats, shortening the chain by two carbons at a time until only one two-carbon segment remains. This final two-carbon link simply becomes one acetyl CoA without producing $FADH_2$ and NADH.

In nature, almost all fatty acids have an even number of carbons. Although they can vary in length from 4 to 26 carbons, they often are 16 or 18 carbons long. If your body encounters an odd-numbered fatty acid, it breaks down this chain in the same way until it reaches a final three-carbon link. Rather than try to clip this link into smaller segments, a reaction joins it with coenzyme A. This three-carbon compound enters the citric acid cycle at a point farther along than acetyl CoA's entry point. Since it skips some of the early citric acid cycle reactions, it has a shorter journey than acetyl CoA and produces two fewer NADH molecules.

The Citric Acid Cycle and Electron Transport Chain Complete Fatty Acid Breakdown

Once the links from the fatty acid chain enter the citric acid cycle as acetyl CoA, the remaining pathways to ATP are identical to those described for glucose. Acetyl CoA enters the citric acid cycle, producing GTP and the electron carriers NADH and $FADH_2$. Then these carriers (and the NADH and $FADH_2$ produced during beta-oxidation) take their high-energy cargo to the electron transport chain.

The end products of fatty acid breakdown are the same as those of glucose breakdown: carbon dioxide, water, and ATP. Because a fatty acid chain typically contains many more carbon atoms than a molecule of glucose does, a single fatty acid produces substantially more ATP. (See **Figure 7.16**.)

Fat Burns in a Flame of Carbohydrate

Acetyl CoA from beta-oxidation can enter the citric acid cycle only when fat and carbohydrate breakdown are synchronized. Without a steady supply of oxaloacetate, acetyl CoA cannot start the citric acid cycle. Conditions like starvation and very-low-carbohydrate diets can deplete oxaloacetate, blocking acetyl CoA from entry. This reroutes the acetyl CoA to form a family of compounds called ketone bodies.

Under normal conditions, each turn of the citric acid cycle reforms oxaloacetate. This does not, however, completely replenish the oxaloacetate supply. Biosynthesis can use some of the intermediate compounds of the citric acid cycle as building blocks for other molecules, thus reducing the supply of oxaloacetate.

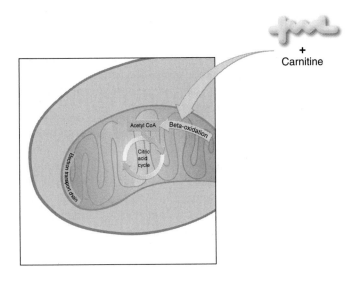

Pathway	ATP yield
Beta oxidation – stearic acid (C18:0)	
8 NADH	20
8 FADH$_2$	12
Citric acid cycle – 9 acetyl CoA	
1 GTP x 9 = 9 GTP	9
3 NADH x 9 = 27 NADH	67.5
1 FADH$_2$ x 9 = 9 FADH$_2$	13.5
Subtotal	122
ATP needed to start beta-oxidation	−2
Net yield	**120**

The grand total:
120 ATP from one molecule of stearic acid

Figure 7.16 The complete oxidation of one 18-carbon fatty acid yields about four times as much ATP as the complete oxidation of one glucose molecule.

BETA-OXIDATION

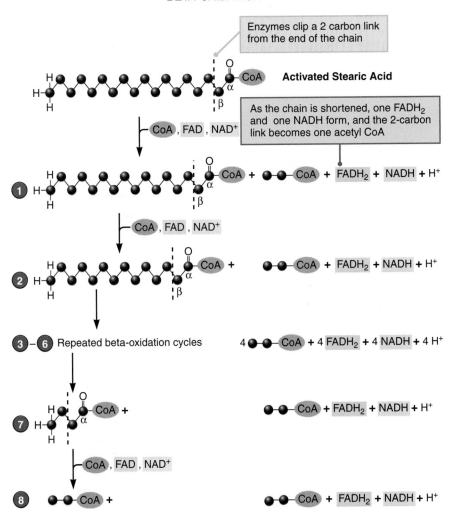

Enzymes clip a 2 carbon link from the end of the chain

Activated Stearic Acid

As the chain is shortened, one FADH$_2$ and one NADH form, and the 2-carbon link becomes one acetyl CoA

CoA , FAD , NAD$^+$

1 CoA + CoA + FADH$_2$ + NADH + H$^+$

CoA , FAD , NAD$^+$

2 CoA + CoA + FADH$_2$ + NADH + H$^+$

3 – 6 Repeated beta-oxidation cycles   4 CoA + 4 FADH$_2$ + 4 NADH + 4 H$^+$

7 CoA +   CoA + FADH$_2$ + NADH + H$^+$

CoA , FAD , NAD$^+$

8 CoA +   CoA + FADH$_2$ + NADH + H$^+$

Total   9 acetyl CoA + 8 FADH$_2$ + 8 NADH + 8 H$^+$

Figure 7.15 **Beta-oxidation.** Beta-oxidation reactions repeatedly clip the two-carbon end off a fatty acid until it is degraded entirely.

For fatty acid oxidation to continue efficiently and unabated, reactions in the mitochondria help ensure a reliable supply of oxaloacetate. These reactions convert some pyruvate directly to oxaloacetate rather than to acetyl CoA. Since carbohydrate (glucose) is the original source of the pyruvate and, hence, this oxaloacetate, scientists coined the adage, *Fat burns in a flame of carbohydrate.*

Key Concepts: *Extracting energy from fat involves several steps. First, triglycerides are separated into glycerol and three fatty acids. Glycerol forms pyruvate and continues along the catabolic pathways to yield a small amount of energy. Beta-oxidation breaks down fatty acids to yield acetyl CoA, NADH, and FADH₂. Acetyl CoA then enters the citric acid cycle. The NADH and FADH₂ produced by beta-oxidation and the citric acid cycle deliver high-energy electrons to the electron transport chain where ATP and water are made. One triglyceride molecule, when completely catabolized, yields water, carbon dioxide, and substantially more ATP than one glucose molecule.*

Extracting Energy from Protein

Because protein has vital structural and functional roles, neither protein nor amino acids is considered a storage medium for energy. The primary and unique role of amino acids is to serve as building blocks for the synthesis of body protein and nitrogen-containing compounds. However, if energy production falters due to a lack of available carbohydrate and fat, protein comes to the rescue. During starvation, for example, the body's energy needs take priority so it breaks down protein.

When the body uses amino acids as an energy source, a process called deamination strips off the amino group (—NH₂), leaving what is called a "carbon skeleton." (See **Figure 7.17**.) The liver quickly converts the amino group to ammonia and then to urea. The kidneys excrete the urea in urine. When you eat more protein than you need, your body excretes the excess nitrogen and uses carbon skeletons to produce energy, glucose, or fat. Much to their dismay, bodybuilders who drink pricey protein drinks in an attempt to build muscle may end up gaining fat instead!

Carbon Skeletons Enter Pathways at Different Points

To extract energy from carbon skeletons, the body uses many of the same breakdown pathways it uses to extract energy from glucose, especially the citric acid cycle and electron transport chain. Unlike glucose, these skeletons enter the pathways at several points. It's a bit like a crowd of people streaming into a concert through five doors rather than one main entrance. The carbon skeleton from each type of amino acid has a unique structure. The number of carbon atoms it contains determine the carbon skeleton's fate, be it pyruvate, acetyl CoA, or one of the intermediates of the citric acid cycle.

If the carbon skeleton of an amino acid becomes pyruvate or a citric acid cycle intermediate, the amino acid is called **glucogenic**. When needed, your body can use these amino acids to form glucose (see the section "Gluconeogenesis"). If the carbon skeleton of an amino acid becomes acetyl CoA (which can be converted to ketone bodies), the amino acid is called **ketogenic** (see the section "Ketogenesis"). Ketone bodies and acetyl CoA cannot be converted to glucose.

End Products of Amino Acid Catabolism

The complete breakdown of an amino acid yields urea, carbon dioxide, water, and ATP. The carbon skeleton's point of entry to the breakdown pathways (see **Figure 7.18**) determines the amount of ATP. Amino acids

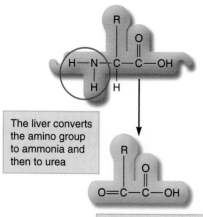

The liver converts the amino group to ammonia and then to urea

The structure of the carbon skeleton determines where it can enter the energy producing pathways.

Figure 7.17 **Deamination.** A deamination reaction strips the amino group from an amino acid.

glucogenic In the metabolism of amino acids, a term describing an amino acid broken down into pyruvate or an intermediate of the TCA cycle; that is, any compound that can be used in gluconeogenesis to form glucose.

ketogenic In the metabolism of amino acids, a term describing an amino acid broken down into acetyl CoA (which can be converted into ketone bodies).

that become pyruvate produce more ATP than amino acids that enter the pathways as acetyl CoA or as a citric acid cycle intermediate.

Key Concepts: *To extract energy from amino acids, first they are deaminated, removing the amino groups. The liver quickly converts these amino groups to urea and sends them to the kidneys for excretion. The structure of the remaining carbon skeletons (amino acids without their amino groups) determines where they enter the catabolic pathways. Some carbon skeletons of amino acids are converted to pyruvate, some to acetyl CoA, and others to intermediate compounds of the citric acid cycle. Complete oxidation of amino acids yields water, carbon dioxide, urea, and ATP.*

Biosynthesis and Storage

The metabolic processes of breakdown and renewal are ongoing operations. While some cells break down carbohydrate, fat, and protein to extract energy, other cells are busy building glucose, fatty acids, and amino acids. When your body needs energy, the breakdown pathways prevail. When it has an excess of nutrients, the biosynthetic pathways are dominant. Both processes are active to some extent at all times, but each one ebbs and flows in response to your body's needs.

Amino acid oxidation
The amount of ATP that an amino acid produces depends upon where it enters the breakdown pathways.

Biosynthesis from amino acids
Some (glucogenic) amino acids can form glucose. Other (ketogenic) amino acids can form acetyl CoA (and thus ketone bodies) but not glucose. A few amino acids can form either glucose or acetyl CoA.

Figure 7.18 Metabolic pathways can break down amino acids for energy or use carbon skeletons for biosynthesis.

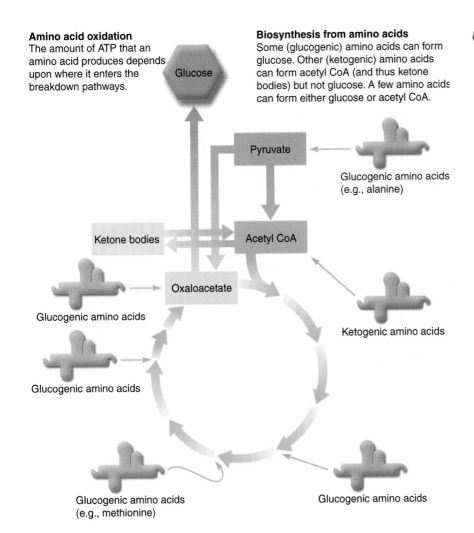

Glucose

Pyruvate

Glucogenic amino acids
(e.g., alanine)

Ketone bodies

Acetyl CoA

Glucogenic amino acids

Oxaloacetate

Ketogenic amino acids

Glucogenic amino acids

Glucogenic amino acids
(e.g., methionine)

Glucogenic amino acids

gluconeogenesis [gloo-ko-nee-oh-JEN-uh-sis]
Synthesis of glucose within the body from noncarbohydrate precursors such as amino acids, lactic acid, and glycerol. Fatty acids cannot be converted to glucose.

Cori cycle The circular path that regenerates NAD⁺ and glucose when oxygen is low and lactate and NADH build up in excess in muscle tissue.

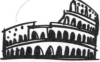

Quick Bites

Sweet Origins

The word *gluconeogenesis* is derived from the Greek words *glyks* meaning "sweet," *neo* meaning "new," and *genesis* meaning "origin" or "generation."

Making Carbohydrate (Glucose)

Your body sets a high priority on maintaining an adequate amount of glucose circulating in the bloodstream. **Table 7.2** shows the amount of energy, in kilocalories, that a typical 70-kilogram man has available. Blood glucose is the primary source of energy for your brain, central nervous system, and red blood cells, and they need a constant supply. In fact, while you're at rest, your brain consumes about 60 percent of the energy consumed by your entire body.

The brain stores little glucose—only about 8 kilocalories. About 140 kilocalories of glucose circulate in the blood or are stored in adipose tissue. Your primary carbohydrate stores are in the form of glycogen. Muscle tissue holds about 1200 kilocalories of glycogen, and the liver stores another 400 kilocalories.

Gluconeogenesis: Pathways to Glucose

Liver and kidney cells can remake glucose from pyruvate using a clever strategy called **gluconeogenesis** (See **Figure 7.19**). Gluconeogenesis and glycolysis share many reactions, albeit in opposite directions. Yet some glycolytic reactions are irreversible so gluconeogenesis is *not* simply a reversal of glycolysis. To make glucose from pyruvate, the gluconeogenic pathways flow back through energy-consuming detours that bypass these irreversible steps.

During intense exercise or when there is a lack of dietary carbohydrate, gluconeogenesis becomes an important source of glucose. Your body can use gluconeogenic pathways to make glucose from noncarbohydrate sources.

The major precursors of glucose are lactate, amino acids, and glycerol. Although some lactate is continually formed and degraded, lactate production becomes substantial in exercising muscle. Low oxygen levels in actively contracting muscle cells inhibit the conversion of pyruvate to acetyl CoA. Gluconeogenesis in the liver converts some of the lactate back to glucose via the **Cori cycle**. Gluconeogenesis also can draw upon glucogenic amino acids from dietary protein and cellular amino acid pools. During starvation, the breakdown of skeletal muscle becomes an important source of glucogenic amino acids. Your body also can break down triglycerides to yield glycerol and fatty acids. Although it can make a small amount of glucose from glycerol, it cannot make glucose from fatty acids.

Your liver is the major site of gluconeogenesis, accounting for about 90 percent of glucose production. Your kidneys make the rest.

Key Concepts: *Your body can make glucose from pyruvate, lactate, glucogenic amino acids, and glycerol but not from fatty acids. While most gluconeogenesis takes place in the liver, the kidneys are responsible for about 10 percent of glucose synthesis.*

Table 7.2 **Available Energy (kcal) in a Typical 70-kg man**

Organ	Glucose or Glycogen	Triglycerides	Mobilizable Proteins
Blood	60	45	0
Liver	400	450	400
Brain	8	0	0
Muscle	1,200	450	24,000
Adipose tissue	80	135,000	40

Source: Adapted from Stryer L. *Biochemistry.* New York: WH Freeman; 1995.

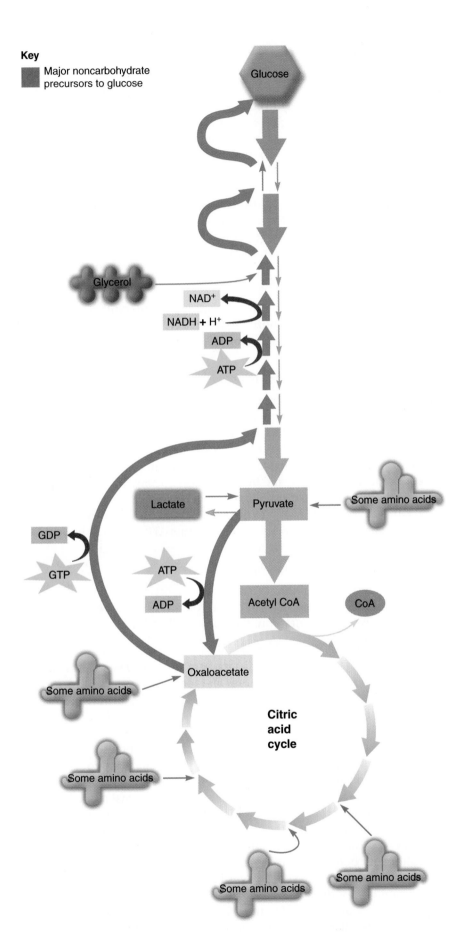

Key

Major noncarbohydrate precursors to glucose

Figure 7.19 **Gluconeogenesis.** Liver and kidney cells make glucose from pyruvate by way of oxaloacetate. Gluconeogenesis is NOT the reverse of glycolysis. Although these pathways share many reactions, albeit in the reverse direction, gluconeogenesis must detour around the irreversible steps in glycolysis.

glycogenesis The formation of glycogen from glucose.

glycogenolysis The breakdown of glycogen to glucose.

lipogenesis [lye-poh-JEN-eh-sis] Synthesis of fatty acids, primarily in liver cells, from acetyl CoA derived from the metabolism of alcohol and some amino acids.

Storage: Glucose to Glycogen

Our main storage form of glucose is glycogen, a branched-chain polysaccharide made of glucose units (see Chapter 4, "Carbohydrate"). Both the liver and muscle store glycogen. Liver glycogen serves as a glucose reserve for the blood, and muscle glycogen supplies glucose to exercising muscle tissue. Glycogen stores are limited, so fasting or strenuous exercise can deplete them rapidly.

A pathway called **glycogenesis** assembles glucose molecules into branched chains for storage as glycogen. When the body needs glucose, a different series of reactions known as **glycogenolysis** breaks down the glycogen chains into individual glucose molecules. In muscle, these glucose molecules enter glycolysis and continue along the metabolic pathways to produce ATP. In the liver, glycogenolysis yields glucose that moves into the bloodstream to maintain glucose blood levels.

Making Fat (Fatty Acids)

Acetyl CoA is the most important ingredient in fatty acid synthesis. Compounds that can be metabolized to form acetyl CoA can feed fatty acid synthesis. Such precursors include ketogenic amino acids, alcohol, and fatty acids themselves.

Lipogenesis: Pathways to Fatty Acids

When the body has a plentiful supply of energy (ATP) and abundant building blocks, a process called **lipogenesis** builds long-chain fatty acids. While you can think of fatty acid synthesis as a reassembly of two-carbon links supplied by acetyl CoA, lipogenesis is *not* the reversal of beta-oxidation. These are different sets of reactions that take place in different locations—fatty acid synthesis occurs in the cytosol and beta-oxidation operates inside the mitochondria. Another important distinction is that beta-oxidation releases energy, and fatty acid synthesis requires energy. In beta-oxidation, reactions deliver high-energy electrons to NADH for ultimate ATP synthesis. In lipogenesis, NADPH supplies energy to power the synthesis of fatty acids.

Storage: Fatty Acids to Triglycerides

On the endoplasmic reticulum, which is a type of organelle in the cell, the body assembles surplus fatty acids and glycerol into triglycerides. Adipose tissue stores these triglycerides until the body needs them.

From Dietary Energy to Stored Triglyceride

When you eat a high-fat diet, most dietary fatty acids head straight to your fat stores. Your body continuously stores and mobilizes fat in response to its energy status. When your body is at rest or performing low-intensity activities, it prefers to use fat as fuel. When you overeat, your body uses adipose tissue as a long-term energy storage depot.

If you eat more protein than your tissues can use, your body converts most of the excess protein to fat. Interestingly, your body does not readily form excess carbohydrate into fatty acids. In research studies, massive overfeeding of carbohydrate in normal men caused only minimal amounts of fat synthesis. So are carbohydrates calorie "free"? Unfortunately not. The first law of thermodynamics—the conservation of energy—is still intact. Although excess carbohydrate may not dramatically increase fat synthesis, it does shift your body's fuel preferences so it burns more carbohydrate and fewer fatty acids.[9] Since your body is burning less fat, it can send a greater proportion of dietary fat to fat stores. Although there is minimal conversion of carbohydrate to fat, this "fat-sparing" shift in fuel use still leads to the accumulation of fat in adipose tissue. See **Table 7.3**.

Quick Bites

Why didn't my cholesterol levels drop?

Your body can make cholesterol from acetyl CoA by way of ketones. In fact, all 27 carbons in synthesized cholesterol come from acetyl CoA. The rate of cholesterol formation is highly responsive to cholesterol levels in cells. If levels are low, the liver makes more. If levels are high, synthesis decreases. This is why dietary cholesterol in the absence of dietary fat often has little impact on cholesterol blood levels.

Table 7.3 **Summary of Energy Yield and Interconversions**

Dietary Nutrient	Yields Energy?	Convertible to Glucose?	Convertible to Amino Acids and Body Proteins?	Convertible to Fat?
Carbohydrate (glucose, fructose, galactose)	Yes	Yes	Yes, can yield nonessential amino acids when amino groups are available	Insignificant
Fat (triglycerides)				
Fatty acids	Yes, large amounts	No	No	Yes
Glycerol	Yes, small amounts	Small amounts	Yes (see carbohydrate)	Insignificant
Protein (amino acids)	Yes, generally not much (see starvation in text)	Yes, if insufficient carbohydrate is available	Yes	Yes
Alcohol (ethanol)	Yes	No	No	Yes

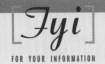

Do Carbohydrates Turn into Fat? Marc Hellerstein, M.D., Ph.D.

FOR YOUR INFORMATION

Thirty years ago, Dr. Jules Hirsch and his colleagues addressed this question indirectly. They found that the composition of fatty acids in adipose tissue closely resembled the subjects' dietary fat intake. Moreover, when they put these subjects on controlled diets of different fatty acid composition for six months, adipose fatty acids slowly changed to reflect the new dietary fatty acid composition. These studies concluded that "we are what we eat" with regard to body fat and that fatty acid synthesis is minimal at best.

The body's ability to make fat from carbohydrate is called *de novo lipogenesis* (DNL). Numerous studies using a technique called indirect calorimetry have shown that net DNL is absent or very low in humans under most dietary conditions, even after a large carbohydrate meal. But could there be concurrent synthesis *and* use of fat that results in no net change?

Concurrent DNL and burning of fatty acids is called *futile cycling*. About 25 to 28 percent of the carbohydrate energy is lost during the inefficient conversion to fatty acids. Does this costly conversion really happen? New stable isotopic methods have helped answer this question.

Direct Evidence

Direct evidence from stable isotopic methods show that DNL is minimal in normal (nonobese, nondiabetic, nonoverfed) men. DNL represents less than 1 gram of saturated fat per day, whether the subjects are given large meals, intravenous glucose, or a liquid diet.

Do any circumstances stimulate DNL? Dr. Jean-Marc Schwarz gave fructose and glucose orally to lean and obese subjects. The dietary fructose increased DNL up to twentyfold compared with equal calorie loads of glucose. Nevertheless, fat synthesis still represented only a small percentage of the fructose load given (< 5%). Dr. Scott Siler has shown that drinking alcohol stimulates DNL. Again, however, only a small percentage (< 5%) of the alcohol was converted to fat; the great majority was released from the liver as acetate.

My laboratory studied the effect of five to seven days of carbohydrate overfeeding or underfeeding in normal men. Fat synthesis by the liver was highly sensitive to the degree of dietary carbohydrate excess. In fact, we could determine exactly which diet a person was eating by measuring DNL. Even so, the absolute amount of fat synthesis remained low, even on massively excessive carbohydrate intakes. DNL may be a sensitive *signal*

of excess carbohydrate in the diet, but it is not a quantitatively important route for excess carbohydrate disposal.

Other conditions yield similar findings. Very-low-fat diets (10% of energy as fat; 70% as carbohydrate) stimulate lipogenesis, but, again, not a large amount. In young women, lipogenesis increases during the follicular phase of the menstrual cycle, but the amount is small, representing only one to two pounds of extra fat per year. A high rate of DNL has been documented in humans only under conditions of massive carbohydrate overfeeding - for example, 5,000 to 6,000 carbohydrate calories per day for more than a week.

Are carbohydrate calories "free"?

Alas, we still become fatter if we overeat carbohydrate. At rest, our bodies normally burn fat as our primary fuel source. An excess of dietary carbohydrate energy causes a fat-sparing shift in fuel selection as it markedly reduces the use of fat to fuel the body. Dietary fat makes a beeline for body fat storage rather than being burned to release energy. Thus, excess dietary carbohydrate is not "free" when the diet also contains fat, because the carbohydrate spares fat use.

Dr. Hellerstein is Professor of Medicine at the University of California, San Francisco, and Professor of Nutritional Sciences at the University of California at Berkeley.

Source: Healthline.

ketone [KEE-tone] Ketones are organic compounds that contain a chemical group consisting of C=O (a carbon-oxygen double bond) bound to two hydrocarbons. Pyruvate and fructose are examples of ketones. Acetone and acetoacetate are both ketones and ketone bodies. While beta-hydroxybutyrate is not a ketone, it is a ketone body.

ketogenesis The process in which excess acetyl CoA from fatty acid oxidation is converted into the ketone bodies acetoacetate, beta-hydroxybutyrate, and acetone.

Key Concepts: *When cells have plentiful ATP and the diet supplies an excess of energy, they make fatty acids and triglycerides. Cells use energy carried by NADPH to power the synthesis of fatty acids from acetyl CoA building blocks. Glycerol and fatty acids are assembled into triglycerides on the endoplasmic reticulum.*

Making Ketone Bodies

Ketone bodies (sometimes incorrectly called **ketones**) include three compounds—acetoacetate, beta-hydroxybutyrate, and acetone. Acetoacetate and beta-hydroxybutyrate are acids, so they are sometimes referred to as keto acids. You may recognize the term *acetone*, which also is a common solvent. In fact, you can smell the strong odor of acetone on the breath of people with high levels of ketone bodies in their blood; their breath smells like nail polish remover!

Your body makes and uses small amounts of ketone bodies at all times. Although long considered to be just an emergency energy source or the result of an abnormal state like starvation or uncontrolled diabetes, ketone bodies are normal, everyday fuels. In fact, your heart and kidneys prefer the ketone body acetoacetate to glucose as a fuel source.[10]

Ketogenesis: Pathways to Ketone Bodies

Your body derives ketone bodies from the metabolism of fat. When the amount of available carbohydrate is insufficient to support normal fatty acid breakdown, ketone bodies enter the picture. The liver makes ketone bodies from acetyl CoA molecules by a process called **ketogenesis**. (See **Figure 7.20**.)

Ketogenesis is highly active when fatty acid oxidation in the liver produces such an abundance of acetyl CoA that it overwhelms the available supply of oxaloacetate. Unable to enter the citric acid cycle, the excess acetyl CoA is shunted to ketone body production. When a person has uncontrolled diabetes or is actually starving, ketone bodies help provide emergency energy to all body tissues, especially the brain and the rest of the CNS. Other than glucose, ketone bodies are your central nervous system's only effective fuel.[11] (See "Special States" section for more detail on starvation and diabetes mellitus.) After the liver makes ketone bodies from acetyl CoA molecules, the ketone bodies travel to other tissues via the blood-

Figure 7.20 Ketogenesis. For acetyl CoA from fatty acid oxidation to enter the citric acid cycle, fat and carbohydrate metabolism must be synchronized. When acetyl CoA cannot enter the citric acid cycle it is shunted to form ketone bodies.

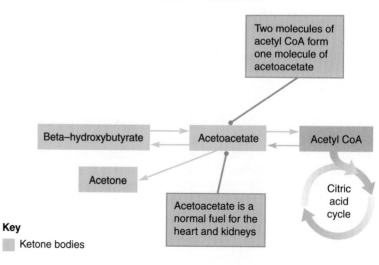

KETONE BODY FORMATION

Two molecules of acetyl CoA form one molecule of acetoacetate

Beta–hydroxybutyrate Acetoacetate Acetyl CoA

Acetone

Acetoacetate is a normal fuel for the heart and kidneys

Citric acid cycle

Key
Ketone bodies

stream. Tissue cells can convert the ketone bodies back to acetyl CoA for ATP production via the citric acid cycle and electron transport chain. [12]

To dispose of excess ketone bodies, your kidneys excrete them in urine and your lungs exhale them. If this removal process cannot keep up, ketone bodies accumulate in the blood—a condition known as **ketosis**. During ketosis, blood levels of the keto acids acetoacetate and beta-hydroxybutyrate rise, altering the blood's acid-base (pH) balance. Known as **ketoacidosis**, this condition can cause brain damage and eventually death.[13] Ketoacidosis is particularly dangerous in uncontrolled type 1 diabetes mellitus. During a short fast, blood concentrations of keto acids usually do not rise substantially.

Given time, your body can adapt to a very high-fat diet and avoid ketosis. Eskimos, for example, sometimes live almost entirely on fat but do not develop ketosis. Even brain cells can adapt to derive 50 to 75 percent of their fuel from ketone bodies (principally beta-hydroxybutyrate) after a few weeks of a low supply of glucose, the preferred fuel.[14]

Key Concepts: *While some ketone bodies are made and used for energy all the time, a lack of available carbohydrate accelerates ketone body production. The ketone bodies acetoacetate, beta-hydroxybutyrate, and acetone can be made from any precursor of acetyl CoA: pyruvate, fatty acids, glycerol, and certain amino acids. Ketone bodies become an important fuel source during starvation, uncontrolled diabetes mellitus, and high-fat/very-low-carbohydrate diets. In type 1 diabetes mellitus, an accumulation of ketone bodies can acidify the blood, a dangerous condition known as ketoacidosis.*

Making Protein (Amino Acids)

Your body rebuilds proteins from a pool of amino acids in your cells. But how is that amino acid pool replenished? Your diet supplies some amino acids, the breakdown of body proteins supplies some, and cells make some. During protein synthesis, your cells can make nonessential amino acids and retrieve essential amino acids from the bloodstream. Your cells cannot make essential amino acids, so if a cell lacks one and your diet doesn't supply it, protein synthesis stops. The cell breaks down this incomplete protein into its constituent amino acids, which are returned to the bloodstream (see Chapter 6, "Proteins" for more details of protein synthesis).

Biosynthesis: Making Amino Acids

Since there are many types of amino acids, with different structures, your body uses many different pathways to synthesize nonessential amino acids. Each pathway is short, involving just a few steps, one of which adds an amino group to the carbon skeleton. Pyruvate and other intermediates of glycolysis and the citric acid cycle supply the carbon skeletons.

To make nonessential amino acids, the body transfers the amino group from one amino acid to a new carbon skeleton; a process called **transamination (Figure 7.21)**. To make the amino acid alanine, for example, pyruvate swipes an amino group from the amino acid glutamic acid to yield alanine and alpha-ketoglutaric acid. Transamination requires several enzymes. One group of enzymes, the aminotransferases, is derived from the B vitamin pyridoxine (B$_6$). Although vitamin B$_6$ deficiency is rare, a lack of B$_6$ will inhibit amino acid synthesis and impair protein formation.

ketoacidosis Acidification of the blood caused by a buildup of ketone bodies. It is primarily a consequence of uncontrolled type 1 diabetes mellitus and can be life threatening.

transamination [TRANS-am-ih-NAY-shun] The transfer of an amino group from an amino acid to a carbon skeleton to form a different amino acid.

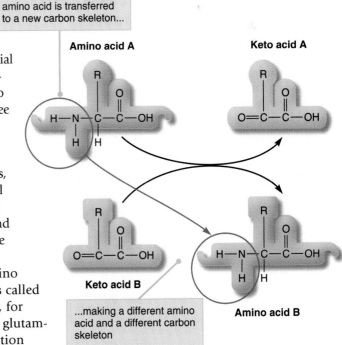

The amino group from one amino acid is transferred to a new carbon skeleton...

Amino acid A

Keto acid A

Keto acid B

...making a different amino acid and a different carbon skeleton

Amino acid B

Figure 7.21 **Transamination.** A transamination reaction transfers the amino group from one amino acid to form a different amino acid.

Key Concepts: *Proteins are made from combinations of essential and nonessential amino acids. The body synthesizes nonessential amino acids from pyruvate, other glycolytic intermediates, and compounds from the citric acid cycle. To form amino acids, transamination reactions transfer amino groups to carbon skeletons.*

Regulation of Metabolism

Just as the cruise control on your car regulates its speed within a narrow range, your body tightly controls the reactions of your metabolic pathways. Whether highly or minimally active, each pathway proceeds at just the right speed, not too fast and not too slowly.

How does your body achieve this remarkable control? While a number of strategies operate simultaneously, certain hormones are the master regulators.

Hormones of Metabolism

Hormones are chemical messengers that help determine whether metabolic processing favors catabolic (breakdown) or anabolic (building) pathways. The major regulatory hormones are insulin, glucagon, cortisol, and epinephrine.

The pancreas secretes insulin, the leader of the storage (anabolic) team. Its mission is to decrease the amount of glucose in the blood, so it promotes carbohydrate use and storage (as glycogen). Since insulin stimulates the use of glucose over fat, its actions are *fat-sparing*. In addition, insulin promotes fat storage in adipose tissue, cellular uptake of amino acids, and

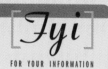

Key Intersections Direct Metabolic Traffic

PYRUVATE IS PIVOTAL

Pyruvate is a pivotal point in the metabolic pathways. How does it select a path? What determines its destination? When ATP levels are low, cellular energy is in short supply, so the metabolic pathways flow toward the production of ATP. Depending on oxygen availability, low ATP routes pyruvate to acetyl CoA or lactate. When ATP is abundant, cells have ample energy so the biosynthetic pathways prevail as pyruvate is converted to oxaloacetate or the amino acid alanine, oxaloacetate is converted to glucose and stored as glycogen.

To Acetyl CoA

When cells need ATP and have readily available oxygen, they rapidly convert pyruvate to acetyl CoA. This irreversible reaction commits the carbons of carbohydrates to oxidation by the citric acid cycle or to the biosynthesis of lipids. Acetyl CoA cannot be converted to glucose.

To and from Lactate

When cells need ATP but lack readily available oxygen, they reroute most pyruvate to form lactate. Although this route is always at least minimally active, it prevails when oxygen levels are low. Reversible reactions convert pyruvate to lactate, so these substances are interconvertible. For more about lactate and its various fates, see the feature "Lactate Is Not a Metabolic Dead End" in Chapter 13. The reaction that converts pyruvate to lactate uses energy carried by NADH, so it also produces NAD⁺. This regeneration of NAD⁺ is critical to continued glycolysis. Anaerobic conditions cut off the supply of NAD⁺ from other sources, so without the NAD⁺ generated in the production of lactate, glycolysis would stop.

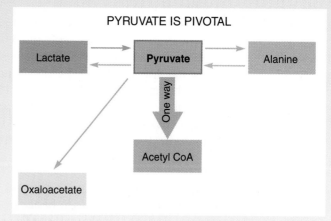

The demand for ATP and the availability of oxygen determine pyruvate's destination.

To Oxaloacetate

Cells also can convert pyruvate to oxaloacetate, another pivotal molecule. Oxaloacetate can react with acetyl CoA to start the citric acid cycle when ATP is needed, or provide the building blocks to make glucose.

Oxaloacetate is essential for acetyl CoA's entry into the citric acid cycle. A steady supply of oxaloacetate is critical to the citric acid

assembly of these amino acids into proteins. Insulin also inhibits the breakdown of body proteins.

The pancreas also secretes glucagon, the leader of the breakdown (catabolic) team. Glucagon's mission is to increase the amount of glucose in circulation, so it stimulates the breakdown of liver glycogen. The adrenal glands secrete two other members of the breakdown team—the hormones cortisol and epinephrine. Cortisol promotes the breakdown of amino acids for gluconeogenesis and helps increase the activity of enzymes driving gluconeogenic reactions.[15] Epinephrine stimulates the conversion of glycogen to glucose in muscle, leading to an increase in available glucose.

The actions of each team ebb and flow in response to the levels of available nutrients.[16] While both the storage and breakdown teams are always active, storage dominates in times of plenty and breakdown dominates in times of need.

Key Concepts: *Hormones and other factors regulate the balance of anabolic and catabolic pathways in energy metabolism. The hormone insulin stimulates glycogen, protein, and triglyceride synthesis, while glucagon, along with cortisol and epinephrine, stimulates breakdown of glycogen and triglycerides.*

Special States

Now you can put your new knowledge of metabolism to work by evaluating case studies of special physiological states: feasting, fasting, stress, diabetes mellitus, and exercising. What happens to your metabolism under these

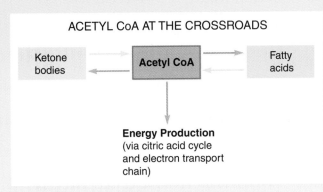

Acetyl CoA sits at a key intersection of carbohydrate and fatty acid breakdown pathways.

cycle's efficient extraction of energy from fatty acids. Carbohydrate feeds the pool of oxaloacetate as reactions break down carbohydrate to pyruvate and irreversibly convert the pyruvate to oxaloacetate. Cells can also make glucose from this oxaloacetate and store energy in the branched glucose chains of glycogen.

When cells have abundant ATP, they restrict the activities of certain enzymes, thus slowing the entry of acetyl CoA into the citric acid cycle. This reroutes the acetyl CoA into energy-storage pathways to form fatty acids in order to store energy as fat.

To and from Alanine

Since a reversible process converts pyruvate to the amino acid alanine, pyruvate and alanine are interconvertible. Although alanine is the only amino acid made from pyruvate, many other amino acids can be converted to pyruvate. Thus, pyruvate is located at a major junction of amino acid and carbohydrate metabolism.

ACETYL CoA AT THE CROSSROADS

Acetyl CoA, like pyruvate, stands at a pivotal point in metabolism. The breakdown pathways for glucose, fatty acids, and some amino acids converge at acetyl CoA. Once formed, what are acetyl CoA's options? It cannot return to pyruvate or make glucose, but acetyl CoA can enter major energy-producing and biosynthetic pathways. The body's energy status determines the predominant route.

To Energy Production

When cells need ATP and have oxaloacetate available, acetyl CoA enters the citric acid cycle for the ultimate production of ATP by the electron transport chain.

To and from Ketone Bodies

When the production of oxaloacetate does not match acetyl CoA production, acetyl CoA cannot enter the citric acid cycle so the metabolic pathways shunt acetyl CoA to form ketone bodies.

To and from Fatty Acids

When energy is abundant, acetyl CoA molecules become building blocks for fatty acid chains. The body assembles these fatty acid chains into triglycerides and stores them in adipose tissue.

situations? Read on to find out which states stimulate breakdown and which stimulate biosynthesis.

Feasting

You're stuffed. You just ate a huge holiday dinner: two servings of turkey with a big ladle of gravy and ample servings of dressing, mashed potatoes, caramelized sweet potatoes, green peas, and two bread rolls. To top it off, you ate a piece of pumpkin pie with whipped cream. You meant to stop there; you loudly proclaimed, "I'm so full I can't eat another bite!" But eventually your grandmother convinced you to taste her special pecan pie. Gosh, that was good! But now you are lying prostrate on the couch, tight and bloated, with your belt loosened. Your feasting may be finished for now, but your body's work has just begun.

Your meal led to a huge influx of carbohydrate, fat, and protein—a plentiful supply for your tissues and far more energy than you need to be a couch potato. The influx of food triggers the rapid secretion of the storage hormone insulin and inhibits the release of the breakdown hormones glucagon, cortisol, and epinephrine. Insulin is sometimes called the "hormone of plenty" because when energy is abundant, it promotes the replenishment of energy stores (glycogen and fat), the synthesis of protein, and the maintenance and repair of tissues. Its suppression of glucagon and cortisol reduces the rate of breakdown.

The storage hormone insulin signals your cells to "store, store, store!" Consequently, much of your holiday dinner will wind up stored as fat. The surplus carbohydrate first enters glycogen stores, until it fills that limited storage medium. In the short term, excess carbohydrate primarily readjusts your body's fuel preferences.[17] In a fat-sparing shift, your body maximizes its use of carbohydrate and minimizes its use of fat, thus promoting fat storage in adipose tissues.[18]

What happens to the surplus fat and protein? Fat is the perfect energy storage package for both. While a minor amount produces some ATP, nearly all excess dietary fat heads to the adipose storage depot. Excess protein, beyond what's needed to replenish the overall body pool of amino acids, follows the metabolic pathways to fat storage. (See **Figure 7.22**.)

The Return to Normal

Within a few hours of this frenzied bout of storage, the amount of glucose circulating in the bloodstream drops to the fasting level. This level (70 to 110 mg/dL) is the amount of glucose healthy people have in their blood three to four hours after eating. The level of amino acids in the blood returns to baseline and the secretion of insulin slows.

As insulin levels decline and the level of blood glucose continues to fall, the pancreas secretes the breakdown hormone glucagon. Glucagon broadcasts the orders "release the glucose!" and swings into action to counteract falling blood glucose levels. It stimulates the breakdown of liver glycogen to glucose, which is released into the bloodstream. Glucagon also stimulates the production of glucose from amino acids and hinders energy storage by inhibiting synthesis of glycogen and fatty acids. Should blood glucose levels continue to fall, the adrenal glands secrete epinephrine, which signals the liver to further increase its release of glucose into the bloodstream.

FEASTING

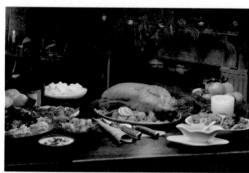

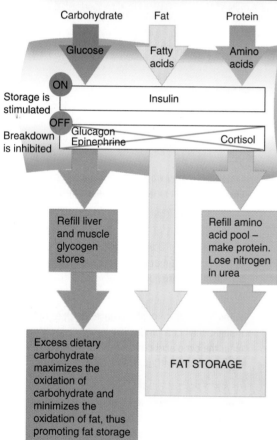

Figure 7.22 **Feasting.** Your body deals with a large influx of energy-yielding nutrients by increasing cellular uptake of glucose and promoting fat storage.

Epinephrine also stimulates the breakdown of muscle glycogen to form glucose, which is used directly by muscle tissue for a "fight-or-flight" response to danger; this glucose does not enter the bloodstream. If low blood glucose levels persist for hours or days, the pituitary and adrenal glands join the battle by secreting growth hormone and cortisol, respectively. These hormones cause most cells to shift their fuel usage from glucose to fatty acids. Cortisol also promotes the breakdown of amino acids for gluconeogenesis and helps increase the activity of enzymes driving gluconeogenic reactions.[19] All breakdown hormones work in concert to maintain blood glucose levels and ensure a constant supply of glucose for the central nervous system and red blood cells[20]—until it is time to attack the leftovers!

Key Concepts: *Feasting, or taking in too many calories, stimulates anabolic processes such as glycogen and triglyceride synthesis. Insulin is the key hormone that promotes synthesis and storage of glycogen and fat.*

Fasting

Feasting on a holiday dinner floods your body with excess energy that it busily stores for future use. On the other hand, fasting and starvation deprive your body of energy, so it must employ an opposing strategy—the mobilization of fuel. (See **Figure 7.23**.) Whether starvation occurs in a child during a famine, a young woman with anorexia nervosa, a patient with AIDS wasting syndrome, or a person intentionally fasting, their bodies respond in the same way.

Some people deprive themselves of food for a purpose—weight loss, political protest, religious fasting, or an attempt to "cleanse" their bodies. The cleansing motivation is ironic, since fasting actually unleashes damaging toxins to circulate throughout the body. Over time, fat stores accumulate environmental toxins, such as DDT, PCBs, and benzene.[21] In the case of PCBs, despite the fact that Congress banned their use decades ago, more than 9 out of 10 Americans still have traces in their body fat.[22] When bound in adipose tissue, toxins are relatively harmless. But fasting breaks down adipose tissue and releases these toxins, giving them a second chance to damage cells. While the body's detoxification center—the liver—and the intestines remove a small portion of these liberated toxins, the balance remain in circulation where they can wreak havoc.

Survival Priorities and Potential Energy Sources

Starvation confronts your body with several dilemmas. Where is it going to get energy to fuel survival needs? What should it burn first—fat, protein, or carbohydrate? Should it adjust its fuel preferences over time? How can it conserve its energy reserves? Which tissues should it sacrifice to ensure survival?

Your body's first priority is to preserve glucose-dependent tissue: red blood cells, brain cells, and the rest of the central nervous system. Your brain will not tolerate even a short interruption in the supply of adequate energy. Within hours, your body depletes its carbohydrate reserves, so your body sacrifices readily available circulating amino acids to make glucose and ATP.

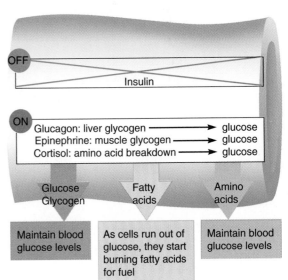

Figure 7.23 **Fasting.** During a short fast, cells first break down liver glycogen to maintain blood glucose levels. They also burn fatty acids and ramp up the production of glucose from amino acids.

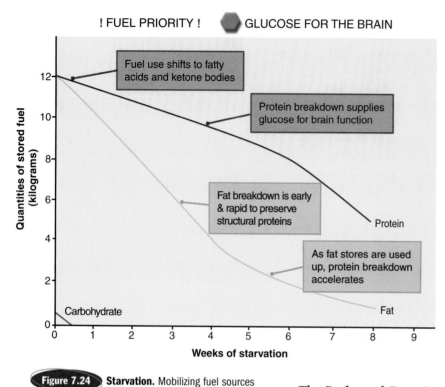

! FUEL PRIORITY !   GLUCOSE FOR THE BRAIN

Fuel use shifts to fatty acids and ketone bodies

Protein breakdown supplies glucose for brain function

Fat breakdown is early & rapid to preserve structural proteins

As fat stores are used up, protein breakdown accelerates

Protein

Carbohydrate

Fat

Quantities of stored fuel (kilograms)

Weeks of starvation

Figure 7.24 **Starvation.** Mobilizing fuel sources during starvation.

Your body's second priority is to maintain muscle mass. In the face of danger, we rely on our ability to "fight or flee." This survival mechanism requires a large muscle mass, so we can move quickly and effectively. Your body grudgingly uses muscle protein for energy and breaks it down rapidly only in the final stages of starvation. (See **Figure 7.24.**)

While your body stores most of its energy reserve in adipose tissue, triglycerides are a poor source of glucose. Although your body can make a small amount of glucose from the glycerol backbone, it cannot make any glucose from fatty acids. This means your body's primary energy stores—fat—are incompatible with your body's paramount energy priority—glucose for your brain. To meet this metabolic challenge, your body's antistarvation strategies include a glucose-sparing mechanism. It shifts to fatty acids and ketone bodies to fuel its needs. In time, even your brain adapts as most, but not all, of its cells come to rely on ketone bodies for fuel.

The Prolonged Fast: In the Beginning

What happens during the fasting state? Let's take a metabolic look at Fasting Frank, a political activist determined to make a dramatic statement. Frank begins fasting at sundown, planning only to drink water and consume no other foods or liquids.

The first few hours are no different from your nightly fast between dinner and breakfast. As blood glucose drops to fasting baseline levels, the storage team retreats and the breakdown team swings into action. Increased secretion of the hormone glucagon stimulates the breakdown of liver glycogen to glucose. The liver's gluconeogenic pathways become highly active as they begin churning out glucose from circulating amino acids. The liver pours glucose into the bloodstream to supply other organs and altruistically shifts to fatty acids for its own energy needs. Since insulin is in retreat, glucose tends to remain in the bloodstream rather than enter liver and muscle cells. Faced with a diminishing supply of glucose, muscle cells also start burning fatty acids. After about 12 hours, the battle to maintain a constant supply of blood glucose exhausts nearly all carbohydrate stores.[23]

The First Few Days

During the next few days, fat and protein are the primary fuels. To preserve structural proteins, especially muscle mass, Frank's body first turns to easily metabolized amino acids. It breaks them down and uses some components to produce ATP and others as building blocks for gluconeogenesis. Glucogenic amino acids, especially alanine, furnish about 90 percent of the brain's glucose supply. As Frank's body breaks down triglycerides for fuel, the glycerol portion supplies the remaining 10 percent.

The Early Weeks

As starvation continues, Frank's body initiates several energy-conservation strategies. It ratchets down its energy use by lowering body temperature, pulse rate, blood pressure, and basal metabolism. He becomes lethargic, reducing the amount of energy expended in activity. Frank also begins to have detectable signs of mild vitamin deficiencies as his body depletes its small reserves of vitamin C and most B vitamins.

If Frank's body continued to rapidly break down protein, he would survive less than three weeks. To avoid such a quick demise, protein breakdown slows drastically and gluconeogenesis by the liver drops by two-thirds or more.[24] To pick up the slack, his body doubles the rate of fat catabolism to supply fatty acids for fuel and glycerol for glucose. The liver gives priority to the ketogenic pathways and starts pouring ketone bodies into the bloodstream. Ketone bodies are an important glucose-sparing energy source for the brain and red blood cells. After about 10 days of fasting, ketone bodies meet most of the nervous system's energy needs. Yet some brain cells can use only glucose. To maintain a small, but essential, supply of blood glucose, protein breakdown crawls along, supplying amino acids for gluconeogenesis. **Figure 7.25** shows how the body reacts to starvation by readjusting its selection of fuel.

Several Weeks of Fasting

After several weeks of fasting, Frank is increasingly susceptible to disease and infection. His severe micronutrient deficiencies add to his overall poor health.

The average person has about three weeks of fat stores and the rate of fat depletion is fairly constant. As the later stages of starvation exhaust the final fat stores, the body turns again to protein, its sole remaining fuel source. Normally, Frank's body breaks down about 30 to 55 grams of protein each day, but now it accelerates the rate to several hundred grams daily. You can see some of the effects of accelerated protein breakdown in starving children suffering from kwashiorkor. The loss of blood proteins causes the swollen limbs and bulging stomachs that typify this type of protein-energy malnutrition (PEM). (For more detail on PEM see Chapter 6.)

The End Is Near

In the final stage of protein depletion, the body deteriorates rapidly. You can see the severe muscle atrophy and emaciation in photos of Holocaust victims. Their bodies sacrificed muscle tissue in an attempt to preserve brain tissue. Even organ tissues were not spared. The final stage of starvation attacks the liver and intestines, greatly depleting them. It moderately depletes the heart and kidneys, and even mounts a small attack on the nervous system. Amazingly, starving people can cling to life until they lose about half their body proteins, after which death generally occurs.

How long can a person survive total starvation? Several years ago, some Irish prisoners starved themselves to death—the average time from the start of fast to death was 60 days.[25] Most people survive total starvation for one to three months. Starvation survival factors include:

- **Starting percentage of body fat**—ample adipose tissue prolongs survival.
- **Age**—middle-aged people survive longer than children and the elderly.
- **Sex**—women fare better due to a higher proportion of body fat.
- **Energy expenditure levels**—increased activity leads to an earlier demise.

Key Concepts: *Fasting, or underconsumption of energy (calories), favors catabolic pathways. The body first obtains fuel from stored glycogen, then from stored fat and functional proteins. The body adapts to using more and more ketone bodies as fuel because limited carbohydrate is available. Larger stores of fat in adipose tissue extend survival time during starvation. In prolonged starvation, the body catabolizes muscle tissue to continue minimal production of glucose from amino acids.*

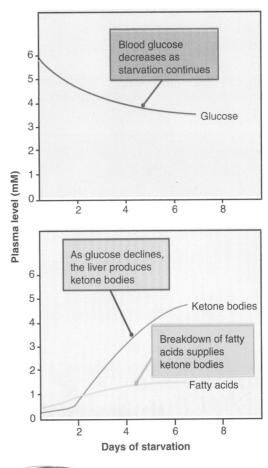

Figure 7.25 Shifting fuel selection during starvation.

Psychological Stress

Our bodies respond to stress in the same way they respond to danger; we mobilize for "fight or flight." In primitive times, this response would culminate in rapid physical movement. In modern times, there often is no such outlet. Also, the discrete short-term triggering event, like an attack by a lion, has been largely replaced by a never-ending assault from noise, overcrowding, competition, and economic pressures. Today, many people suffer from chronic stress—a condition that scientists have linked to several diseases such as hypertension and heart disease that are common in the modern world.

When we are stressed, our bodies increase the availability of biological building blocks and ramp up energy production, especially in muscle tissues that are related to movement. Stress hormones, including epinephrine, cortisol, growth hormone, and glucagon, stimulate the breakdown of glycogen and the production of glucose. The elevated levels of blood glucose and increased metabolic rate provide energy to help us to respond to threats—real or perceived.

Cells prepare for action by taking up glucose at a near maximal rate. This slows the assimilation of new glucose. When the danger passes, cells need

---

Metabolic Profiles of Important Sites

Brain

What powers your brain? Glucose! But brain cells cannot store glucose, so they need a constant supply. Your brain uses about 120 grams of glucose daily, which corresponds to a dietary energy intake of about 420 kilocalories. When your body's at rest, your brain accounts for about 60 percent of your glucose use.[1]

What happens during starvation? When glucose is in short supply, the liver comes to the rescue by converting fatty acids to ketone bodies. Ketone bodies are a critical source of replacement fuel that augments the supply of glucose to the brain.

Still, some brain cells can use only glucose. These cells survive by breaking down amino acids to make glucose via gluconeogenesis.[2]

Muscle

Muscle can use a variety of fuels—lactate, fatty acids, ketone bodies, glucose, and pyruvate. Unlike your brain, muscle stores large amounts of carbohydrate fuel—about 1,200 kilocalories in the form of glycogen. This represents about three-fourths of the glycogen in your body. To fuel bursts of activity, muscle cells readily obtain glucose from glycogen.[3]

When your muscles actively contract, they rapidly deplete available oxygen, thus inhibiting the production of ATP via the aerobic breakdown pathways. ATP formed during glycolysis becomes the primary fuel. Muscle cells use the pyruvate from glycolysis to form lactate. The lactate travels to the liver, which converts it to glucose. The glucose returns to your muscle cells and undergoes anaerobic glycolysis. Known as the Cori cycle, this pathway rapidly produces ATP while shifting part of the metabolic burden from your muscles to your liver.

While fatty acids are the primary fuel for muscles at rest, glycogen and glucose fuel short intense activity, such as when you are sprinting to arrive at class on time. During prolonged exercise, such as running a marathon, fatty acid oxidation kicks in to help out. Fatty

acids can directly supply energy or form ketone bodies to augment the fuel supply.

Your muscle cells are major sites for glycolysis, beta-oxidation, and the common aerobic breakdown pathways—the citric acid cycle and the electron transport chain.

Adipose Tissue

Adipose tissue is your body's primary energy storage depot. A 55-kilogram (121-pound) woman with 25 percent body fat (a healthy body composition) stores about 105,000 kilocalories in adipose tissue, enough energy to

higher than normal amounts of insulin to return blood glucose to baseline levels. This condition, called glucose intolerance, is a known complication of chronic stress.[26]

Diabetes and Obesity

In type 1 diabetes mellitus, a lack of insulin limits the cellular uptake of glucose. The starving, glucose-deprived cells signal the liver to make more glucose. This combination of limited uptake and increased production causes abnormally high blood glucose levels. The starving cells turn to fatty acids for energy. Inside the cells, the increased rate of fatty acid oxidation, along with a lack of glucose, leads to the production of ketone bodies. In untreated type 1 diabetes mellitus, ketone bodies rapidly accumulate, causing ketosis and a characteristic smell of acetone on the breath. The blood becomes acidic and the condition of a person with untreated type 1 diabetes mellitus can progress quickly to coma and death.

Obese people and individuals with type 2 diabetes mellitus often have only mildly elevated blood glucose levels, elevated fasting insulin levels, and glucose intolerance. Although insulin levels are adequate, their cells have difficulty taking up glucose, possibly due to a problem with insulin

---

run 40 marathons! Your liver assembles fatty acids into triglycerides and sends them to adipose tissue for storage. Eighty to 90 percent of the volume of an adipose cell is pure triglyceride.[4]

To supply fatty acids for energy production, adipose cells break down triglycerides to glycerol and free fatty acids.

Liver

Most substances absorbed by your intestines eventually pass through the liver, the body's main metabolic factory. This versatile organ performs glycolysis, gluconeogenesis, beta-oxidation, lipogenesis, ketogenesis, and cholesterol synthesis.

Your liver can store up to 400 kilocalories of glucose as glycogen. When blood glucose levels are low, the liver breaks down stored glycogen to glucose or makes glucose from noncarbohydrate precursors. Several sources pitch in to provide glucose building blocks: muscle supplies lactate and the amino acid alanine; adipose tissue supplies glycerol; and your diet supplies glucogenic amino acids.

The liver is the traffic cop for lipid metabolism. When energy is abundant, the liver directs fatty acids to storage. When energy is scarce, the liver breaks down fatty acids to form ATP. If an inadequate amount of carbohydrate blocks the entry of acetyl CoA into the citric acid cycle, the liver redirects fatty acids to ketone bodies.

Kidney

Your kidneys are important disposal systems of metabolic wastes. Without rapid elimination, these wastes can build up to toxic levels. When your liver deaminates amino acids (removes amino groups), a cooperative effort eliminates the released nitrogen. Your liver captures the nitrogen in urea, which it releases into the bloodstream. The kidneys filter out the urea and excrete it in urine.

The kidneys can make glucose (gluconeogenesis) from amino acids and other precursors. During prolonged starvation, the kidneys produce glucose in amounts that rival production by the liver![5]

Heart

Your heart relies on an interesting mix of fuels. Rather than glucose, which it uses only in small amounts, your heart relies on free fatty acids, lactate, and ketone bodies. During normal conditions, free fatty acids supply the bulk of its energy.[6] When glucose is in short supply, your heart makes a special effort to spare its use. It uses ketone bodies, then free fatty acids, and finally glucose as its fuel source.[7] During heavy exercise, your body releases large amounts of lactate into the bloodstream. Compared to other types of tissue, your heart is particularly capable of using lactate to supply the energy it needs.[8]

Red Blood Cells

Just like the brain, red blood cells rely primarily on glucose for fuel. In red blood cells, glycolysis and the pentose phosphate pathway (an alternative energy-producing pathway), extract energy from glucose. Since red blood cells have no mitochondria, these cells do not contain the pathways for beta-oxidation, citric acid cycle, or electron transport chain.

The pentose phosphate pathway generates the NADPH that is critical for a red blood cell's health. Energy carried by NADPH helps maintain cell membrane pliability and ion transport capabilities. NADPH also helps preserve iron in the cell's hemoglobin and prevent premature breakdown of the cell's proteins.[9]

1 Stryer L. *Biochemistry*. 4th ed. New York: WH Freeman; 1995.
2 Guyton AC, Hall JE. *Textbook of Medical Physiology*. 9th ed. Philadelphia: WB Saunders; 1996.
3 Stryer L. Op. cit.
4 Guyton AC, Hall JE. Op. cit.
5 Ibid.
6 Schaap FG, van der Vusse GJ, Glatz JF. Fatty acid-binding proteins in the heart. *Mol Cell Biochem*. 1998;180:1–2, 43–51.
7 Murray RK, et al. *Harper's Biochemistry*. 24th ed. Stamford, CT: Appleton & Lange; 1996.
8 Guyton AC, Hall, JE. Op. cit.
9 Ibid.

receptors. Because some glucose is entering the cell, ketosis is less common among those with type 2 diabetes. (For more details on diabetes, see Chapter 4.)

Exercise

Exercise not only increases muscle fitness, it also increases "cell fitness" by enhancing the ability of cells to take up glucose. In fact, regular exercise often can reduce a diabetic's need for insulin.

The duration and intensity of exercise changes the mix of fuels your body uses. At rest, it predominantly uses fat. During short-term, high-intensity exercise, fuel use shifts to carbohydrate. In long-term exercise, such as running a marathon, elite runners use a mix of carbohydrate and fat.[27] (For more information on fuel use during exercise, see Chapter 13.)

Key Concepts: Chronic psychological stress can cause glucose intolerance, so that a person needs more insulin for glucose to enter cells. In uncontrolled diabetes mellitus, cells react much like they do in starvation. Untreated type 1 diabetes mellitus can cause a dangerous accumulation of ketone bodies and acidification of the blood. Exercise enhances glucose uptake. Depending on the duration and intensity of exercise, your body chooses different mixes of metabolic fuels.

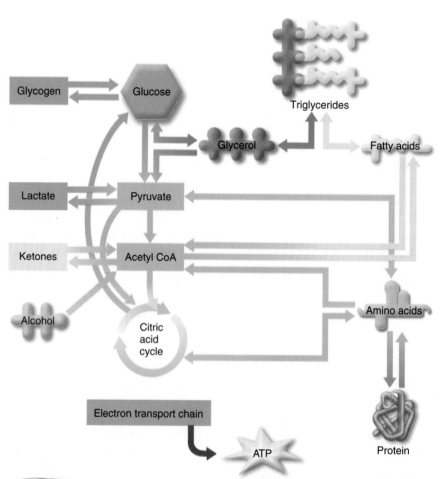

Figure 7.26 **Summary figure.** Like traveling a maze of city streets, molecules move through a network of breakdown and biosynthetic pathways. Not all pathways are available to a molecule. Just as traffic lights and one-way streets regulate traffic flow, cellular mechanisms control the flow of molecules in metabolic pathways. These mechanisms include hormones, irreversible reactions, and the location of the reactions in the cell.

LEARNING *Portfolio* chapter 7

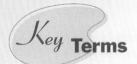

Key Terms

Study Points

➤ Energy is necessary to do any kind of work. The body converts chemical energy from food sources—carbohydrates, proteins, and fats—into a form usable by cells.

➤ Anabolic reactions (anabolism) build compounds. These reactions require energy.

➤ Catabolic reactions (catabolism) break compounds into smaller units. These reactions produce the energy.

➤ Adenosine triphosphate, ATP, is the energy currency of the body.

➤ NADH, FADH₂, and NADPH are important carriers of hydrogen and high-energy electrons. NADH and FADH₂ are used in making ATP, while NADPH is used in biosynthetic reactions.

➤ Cells extract energy from carbohydrate via four main pathways: glycolysis, pyruvate to acetyl CoA, the citric acid cycle, and the electron transport chain.

➤ The citric acid cycle and electron transport chain require oxygen. Glycolysis does not.

➤ The electron transport chain produces more ATP than the other catabolic pathways.

➤ To extract energy from fat, first triglycerides are separated into glycerol and fatty acids. Next, beta-oxidation breaks down the fatty acids to yield acetyl CoA, NADH, and FADH₂. The acetyl CoA enters the citric acid cycle, producing more NADH and FADH₂. The NADH and FADH₂ deliver their high-energy electrons to the electron transport chain to make ATP.

➤ To extract energy from an amino acid, first it is deaminated (the amino group is removed). Depending on the structure of the remaining carbon skeleton, it enters the catabolic pathways as pyruvate, acetyl CoA, or a citric acid cycle intermediate. The citric acid cycle and the electron transport chain complete the production of ATP.

➤ The liver converts the nitrogen portion of amino acids to urea, which the kidney excretes.

➤ Tissues differ in their preferred source of fuel. The brain, nervous system, and red blood cells rely primarily on glucose, while other tissues use a mix of glucose, fatty acids, and ketone bodies as fuel sources.

➤ When carbohydrate is available, glucose can be stored as glycogen in liver and muscle tissue.

➤ Glucose can be produced from the noncarbohydrate precursors glycerol and some (glucogenic) amino acids, but not from fatty acids.

➤ The hormone insulin regulates metabolism by favoring anabolic pathways. It promotes the uptake of glucose by cells, thus removing it from the bloodstream.

➤ Glucagon, cortisol, and epinephrine stimulate catabolic pathways. These hormones promote the breakdown of glycogen to glucose and of amino acids to make glucose via gluconeogenesis. The breakdown of liver glycogen increases the amount of glucose in the blood.

➤ Feasting, or overconsumption of energy, leads to glycogen and triglyceride storage.

➤ Fasting, or underconsumption of energy, leads to the mobilization of liver glycogen and stored triglycerides. Starvation, the state of prolonged fasting, leads to protein breakdown as well and can be fatal.

Study Questions

1. What is the "universal energy currency"? Where is most of it produced?

2. Name the two energy-equivalent molecules that contain three phosphates as part of their structure. What makes these two molecules different? How many high-energy phosphate bonds do they contain?

3. In the catabolic pathways, what two molecules are major electron acceptors? After they accept electrons, what electron carriers do they become? What is the primary function of the electron carriers?

4. How many pyruvate molecules does glycolysis produce from one glucose molecule? What does the oxidative step after glycolysis produce? What does the citric acid cycle produce from a single glucose molecule?

5. What two-carbon molecules does beta-oxidation form as it "clips" the links of a fatty acid chain? What other molecules important to the production of ATP does beta-oxidation produce?

6. What dictates whether an amino acid is considered ketogenic or glucogenic?

7. What are ketone bodies and when are they produced?

8. Name the three tissues where energy is stored. Which contains the largest store of energy?

9. Define gluconeogenesis and lipogenesis. Under what conditions do they predominantly occur? What are their primary inputs and outputs?

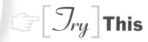 *Try* **This**

Comparing Fad Diets

The purpose of this exercise is to have you evaluate two fad diets in regard to their metabolic consequences. The two diets, Cabbage Soup and Super Protein, are described below. Once you've reviewed them, please answer the following questions.

Will these diets result in weight loss? On the seventh day of each of these diets, which of the following metabolic pathways will be working?

- Glycogenolysis
- Lipolysis
- Gluconeogenesis
- Cori cycle

Diet 1: The Cabbage Soup Diet

A person following the Cabbage soup diet only eats a water-based soup made out of cabbage and a few other vegetables. Three to four meals per day of this restricted diet supplies approximately 500 kilocalories per day. It is devoid of protein and fat and gets its calories from the small amount of carbohydrate in the vegetables.

Diet 2: The Super Protein Diet

In the Super Protein Diet a person can eat an unlimited amount of protein-rich foods like meat, poultry, eggs, and seafood. However, no added fats or carbohydrates are allowed. The average person can consume about 1,400 kilocalories if he or she eats 3 or 4 small meals a day.

Fasting for Ketones

The purpose of this experiment is to see if a day without eating will cause your body to produce measurable ketones in your urine. Before starting your fast, check with your physician. Go to your local pharmacy and ask the pharmacist for urine ketone strips (often called Keotstix). Bring them home and read the directions. Before you start your one-day fast, test your urine to see if it has a detectable amount of ketones. Start your 24-hour fast (or as long as you can go without food or calorie-containing fluids) and test your urine at 6-hour intervals. Do you detect a color change on the strips as the day goes on? Why? What has happened metabolically as the day progresses?

Remember to drink lots of water!

References

1 Alberts B, ed., Bray D, Lewis J, Raff M, Roberts K, Watson JD. *Molecular Biology of the Cell*. 3rd ed. New York: Garland; 1994.

2 Stipanuk MH. *Biochemical and Physiological Aspects of Human Nutrition*. Philadelphia: WB Saunders; 2000.

3 Murray RK, Granner DK, Mayes PA, Rodwell VW. *Harper's Biochemistry*. 24th ed. Stamford, CT: Appleton & Lange; 1996.

4 Stryer L. *Biochemistry*. 4th ed. New York: WH Freeman; 1995.

5 Stipanuk MH. Op. cit.

6 Campbell MK. *Biochemistry*. 3rd ed. Philadelphia: Saunders College Publishing; 1999; and Stryer L. Op. cit.

7 Burge B. Carnitine in energy production. *Healthline*. July 1999.

8 Hawley JA, Brouns F, Jeukendrup A. Strategies to enhance fat utilization during exercise. *Sports Med*. 1998;25:4, 241–257; and Brass EP, Hiatt WR. The role of carnitine and carnitine supplementation during exercise in man and individuals with special needs. *J Am Coll Nutr*. 1998;17:3, 207–215.

9 Hellerstein MK, Schwartz JM, Neese RA. Regulation of hepatic de novo lipogenesis in humans. *Ann Rev Nutr*. 1996;16:527–557.

10 Stryer L. Op. cit.

11 Stein, JH. Internal Medicine. 4th ed. St. Louis, MO: Mosby-Yearbook; 1994.

12 Murray RK, et al. Op. cit..

13 Anderson JW. Prevention and management of diabetes mellitus. In: Shils ME, Olson JA, Shike M, Ross AC. *Modern Nutrition in Health and Disease*. 9th ed. Philadelphia: Lippincott Williams & Wilkins; 1999:1365-1394.

14 Guyton AC, Hall JE. *Textbook of Medical Physiology*. 9th ed. Philadelphia: WB Saunders; 1996.

15 Murray RK, et al. Op. cit.

16 Griffin JE, Ojeda SR. *Textbook of Endocrine Physiology*. 3rd ed. New York: Oxford University Press; 1996.

17 Shah M, Garg A. High-fat and high-carbohydrate diets and energy balance. *Diabetes Care*. 1996;19:10, 1142–1152.

18 Stubbs RJ, Prentice AM, James WP. Carbohydrates and energy balance *Ann NY Acad Sci* 1997;819:44–69.

19 Murray RK, et al. Op. cit.

20 Guyton AC, Hall JE. Op. cit.

21 Scheele JS. A comparison of the concentrations of certain pesticides and polychlorinated hydrocarbons in bone marrow and fat tissue. *Sci Total Environ*. 1998;221:2-3, 201–204.

22 Gower T. The fasting cure. *Health*. April 1999:61–63.

23 Guyton AC, Hall JE. Op. cit.

24 Ibid.

25 Ganong WF. *Review of Medical Physiology*. 18th ed. Stamford, CT: Appleton & Lange; 1997.

26 Summers RL, Woodward LH, Sanders DY, Hall JE. Graphic analysis for the study of metabolic states. *Adv Physiol Ed*. 1996;15:1, S81–S87.

27 Stryer L. Op. cit.

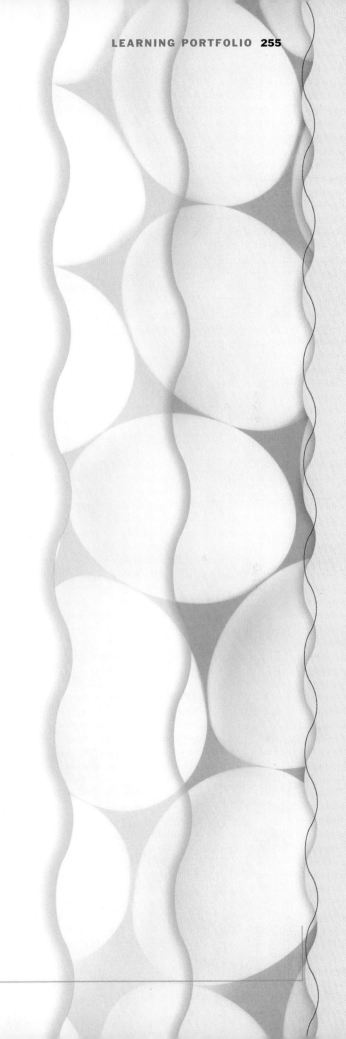

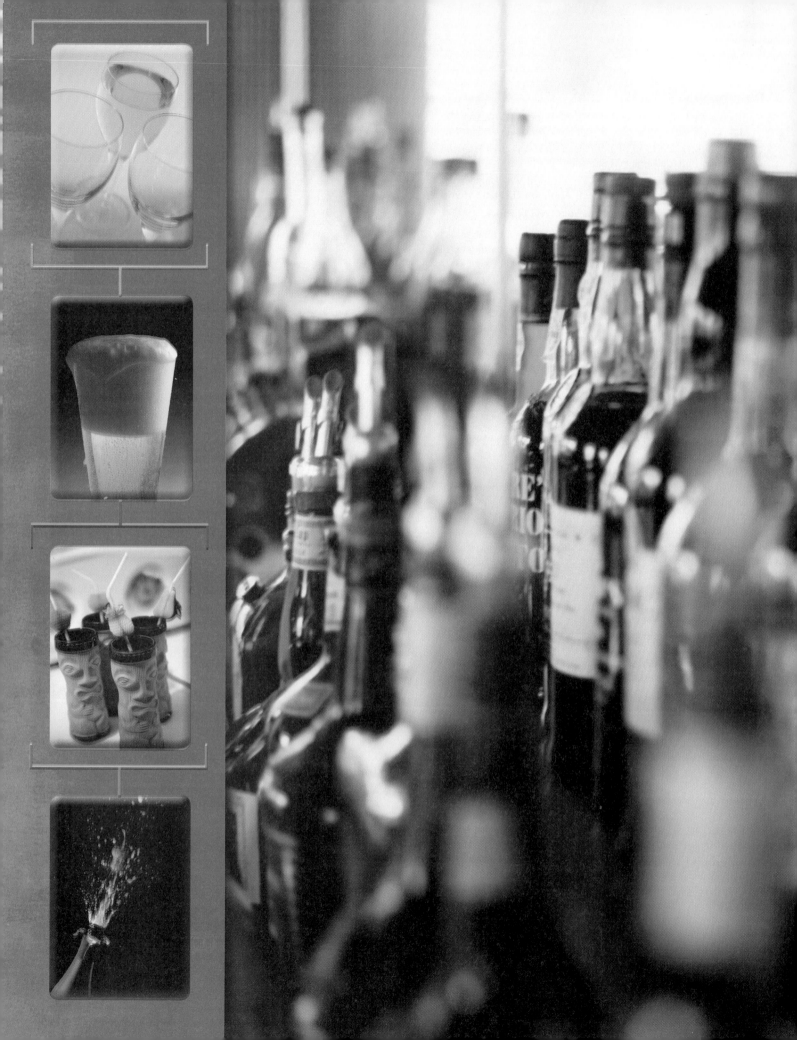

Spotlight on Alcohol

Think About It

1 Have you ever thought of alcohol as a poison?

2 In a word or two, how would you describe alcohol? Is it a nutrient?

3 What's your impression of the alcohol content of wine compared to that of beer? How about compared to vodka?

4 After a night of drinking and carousing, your friend awakens with a splitting headache and asks you for a pain reliever. What would you recommend?

Fyi for your Information

This chapter's FYI boxes include practical information on the following topics:
- College Drinking Culture
- Myths About Alcohol

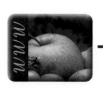

The web site for this book offers many useful tools and is a great source for additional nutrition information for both students and instructors. Visit the site at **nutrition.jbpub.com** for information on alcohol. You'll find exercises that explore the following topics:
- The Legal Age Around the World
- Time to Hand Over the Car Keys?
- Diabetics and Alcohol
- The Culture of Alcohol

Key to Illustrations

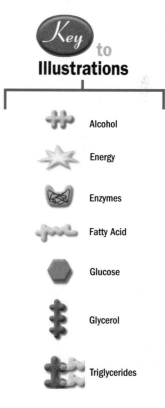

Alcohol

Energy

Enzymes

Fatty Acid

Glucose

Glycerol

Triglycerides

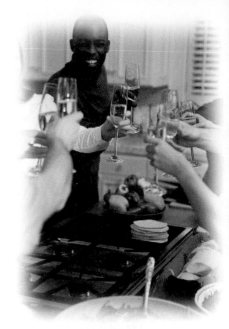

*T*hink about alcohol. What image comes to mind: Champagne toasts? Elegant gourmet dining? Hearty family meals in the European countryside? Or do you think of wild parties? Or sick, out-of-control drunks? Violence? Car accidents? Broken homes? No other food or beverage has the power to elicit such strong, disparate images—images that reflect both the healthfulness of alcohol in moderation, the devastation of excess, and the political, social, and moral issues surrounding alcohol.

Alcohol has a long and somewhat checkered history. More drug than food, alcoholic beverages produce pharmacologic effects in the body while providing little, if any, nutrient value other than energy. Yet alcohol is an important component in the study of nutrition for several reasons. Alcohol is common to the diets of many people. In moderation, it may have significant health benefits, yet even small quantities can raise risks for birth defects and breast cancer. In large amounts, it interferes with nutrient intake and utilization and causes significant damage to every organ system in the body. The *Dietary Guidelines for Americans* advise us, "If you drink alcohol, do so in moderation."

For most people, alcohol consumption is a pleasant social activity. Moderate alcohol use is not harmful for most adults. Nonetheless, many people have serious trouble with drinking. Heavy drinking can increase the risk for certain cancers. It can also cause liver cirrhosis, brain damage, and harm to the fetus during pregnancy. In addition, drinking increases the risk of death from automobile crashes, recreational accidents, and on-the-job accidents and also increases the likelihood of homicide and suicide.

History of Alcohol Use

Alcohol has had a prominent role throughout history. Old religious and medical writings frequently recommend its use, although with warnings for moderation. Thanks to alcohol's antiseptic properties, fermented drinks were safer than water during the centuries before modern sanitation, especially as people moved to towns and villages where water supplies were contaminated. Even mixing alcohol with dirty water afforded some protection from bacteria.[1]

At a time when life was filled with physical and emotional hardships, people valued alcohol for its analgesic and euphoric qualities. People relied on it to lift spirits, ease boredom, numb hunger, and dull the discomfort, even pain, of daily routine. Before the twentieth century, it was one of the few painkillers available in the Western world.

In sharp contrast to our contemporary employment standards, drinking was often encouraged at the worksite. Workers might be given alcohol as an inducement to do boring, painful, or dangerous jobs. Distilled spirits, beers, and wines accompanied sailors and passengers on all long voyages, supplying relatively pathogen-free fluid and calories. In fact legend has it that even the Puritans, a group known for rigid morality, disembarked at Plymouth Rock because their beer supply on board was depleted.[2]

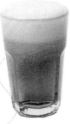

Quick Bites

Preferred Beverages

*B*eer is the national beverage of Germany and Britain. Wine is the national beverage of Greece and Italy.

alcohol Common name for ethanol or ethyl alcohol (CH_3CH_2OH). As a general term, it refers to any organic compound with one or more hydroxyl (–OH) groups.

ethanol Chemical name for drinking alcohol, a two-carbon compound with one hydroxyl group. Also known as ethyl alcohol.

ethyl alcohol See ethanol.

methanol The simplest alcohol, a one-carbon compound with one hydroxyl group. Also known as methyl alcohol and wood alcohol.

methyl alcohol See methanol.

wood alcohol Common name for methanol.

blood-brain barrier The barrier created by tight junctions between the cells that make up the blood capillaries in the brain.

The Chemistry and Character of Alcohol

An **alcohol** is an organic compound that has one or more hydroxyl (—OH) groups (also called alcohol groups) in its structure. A compound name that ends in *ol* usually indicates an alcohol structure. For example, tocopherol is the alcohol form of vitamin E, retinol is the alcohol form of vitamin A, and glycerol is the alcohol that forms the backbone of triglycerides and phospholipids.

Forms of Alcohol

Outside of chemistry class, the term *alcohol* usually refers to the specific alcohol compound in beer, wine, and spirits. Its technical name is **ethanol**, or **ethyl alcohol**, a two-carbon compound with one hydroxyl group (see **Figure SA.1**). Ethanol is commonly abbreviated to "EtOH," shorthand often preferred by health professionals. In this chapter, when we use the term *alcohol*, we are referring to ethanol.

Not all alcohols are safe to drink. The simplest alcohol is **methanol**, also called **methyl alcohol** or **wood alcohol**, a solvent used in paints and for woodworking. Some years ago, down-on-their-luck alcoholics thought they had discovered a way to save money—wood alcohol used at that time to heat chafing dishes was intoxicating but considerably cheaper than beer or wine. Unfortunately, methanol caused blindness and death. Methanol is no longer used in these products, but methanol poisoning from other sources still occurs.[3] Today, methanol is used in a number of consumer products, including paint strippers, duplicator fluid, model airplane fuel, and dry gas. Most windshield washer fluids are 50 percent methanol.

Alcohol (ethanol) is a small molecule. Consequently, unlike starch, protein, and fat, it requires no digestive breakdown to be absorbed, and gastrointestinal absorption is quick and easy. Because of alcohol's unusual ability to cross the **blood-brain barrier**, it affects the brain directly. The blood-brain barrier prevents the passage of many compounds from the blood into the brain, and vice versa.

Organic Solvent

Fats and other lipophilic substances dissolve in alcohol. Thus, alcohol is used to extract fat-soluble flavors (vanilla extract, for example) and as a carrier of medications. Ethanol can also dissolve microbial cell membranes and, until it was replaced by inedible isopropyl alcohol, ethanol was used as a topical disinfectant. Unfortunately alcohol can irritate and damage human cells, making it a potent toxin.

Boiling Point

Alcohol boils at 172°F (78°C), a much lower temperature than water, thereby allowing the distillation of pure alcohol. Many cooks use alcoholic beverages as an ingredient. During cooking, alcohol evaporates. When heated long enough, alcohol dissipates almost entirely, leaving behind the flavors that were in the alcohol product.

Alcohol: Is It a Nutrient?

Alcohol eludes easy classification. Like fat, protein, and carbohydrate, metabolized alcohol provides energy. Laboratory experiments in the nineteenth century demonstrated that upon oxidation pure alcohol releases 7 kilocalories per gram, but many people doubted it actually produced energy in the body. These doubts were the basis of the controversial

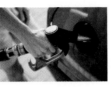
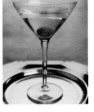

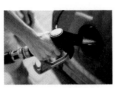
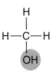

Methanol
(wood alcohol)

Methanol is an alcohol used as an alternative car fuel and in paint strippers, duplicator fluid and model airplane fuels.

Ethanol
(ETOH)

Ethanol is the alcohol in beer, wine and liquor.

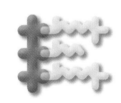
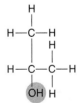

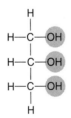

Glycerol

Glycerol is the alcohol that forms the backbone of triglyceride molecules.

Isopropanol
(rubbing alcohol)

Isopropanol is an alcohol that is used as a disinfectant or solvent, and in making many commercial products.

Figure SA.1 Alcohols. Ethanol is not the only alcohol people consume. When people eat fat, they consume the alcohol glycerol. Consuming the alcohol methanol or isopropanol can be deadly.

conclusion that alcohol was not food and formed part of the early argument for Prohibition. (See **Figure SA.2**.) However, energy researchers Atwater and Benedict did a series of famous direct calorimetry experiments and showed that alcohol did indeed produce 7 kilocalories per gram in the body—findings that were a great disappointment to the Temperance Movement because it showed alcohol was a food.[4]

But alcohol's status as a nutrient is more questionable. It is certainly different from any other substance in the diet. It provides energy but is not essential, performing no necessary function in the body. Unlike the nutrients, alcohol is not stored in the body. It provides calories, but chronic overconsumption does not usually lead to obesity. And for no nutrient are the dangers of overconsumption so dramatic and the window of safety so narrow. In the small amounts most people usually consume, alcohol acts as a drug, producing a pleasant euphoria. For some people, it is addictive with the characteristics of tolerance, dependence, and withdrawal symptoms. Certainly alcohol is a substance available in the diet, but it does *not* meet the definition of a nutrient.

Key Concepts: *Alcohol, or more specifically the compound ethyl alcohol, is a small organic molecule that has been part of people's diets for thousands of years. Although it provides calories, alcohol performs no essential function in the body and, therefore, is not a nutrient.*

Quick Bites

Nutrients in Beer?

Most of the carbohydrate used in the production of alcohol is converted to ethanol. In beer, however, some carbohydrate remains, along with a little protein and some vitamins. So while it is technically correct to say there are nutrients in beer, amounts are small when beer is consumed at recommended low levels.

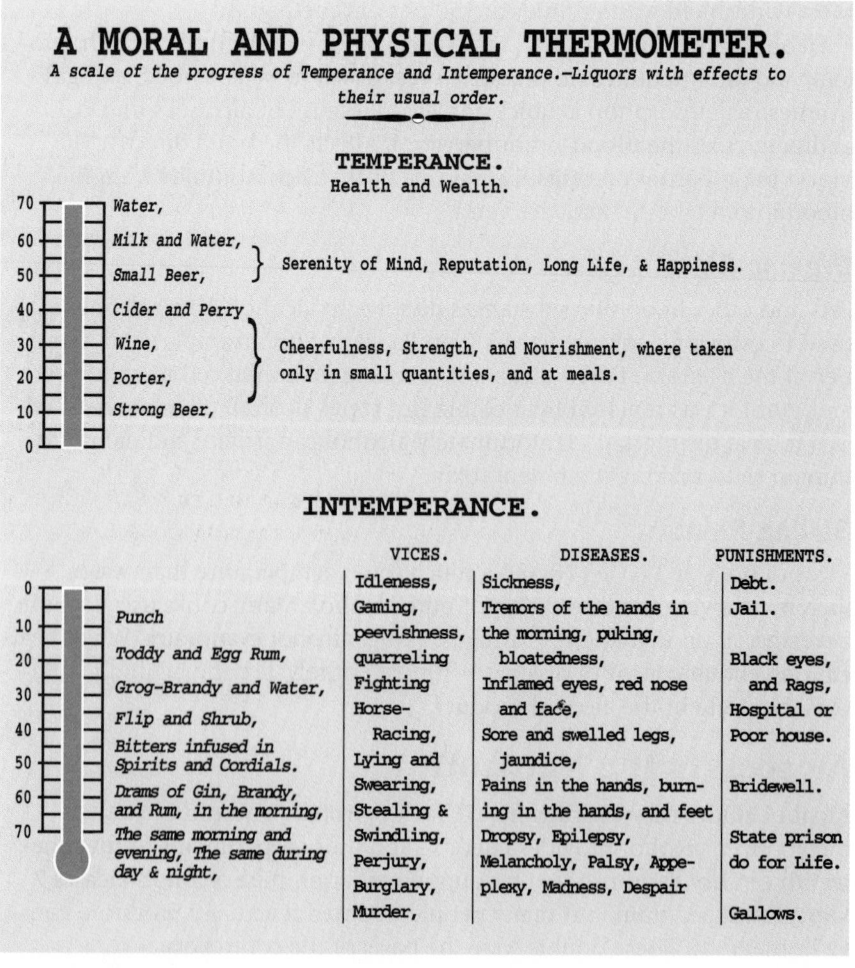

Figure SA.2 **A moral and physical thermometer of temperance and intemperance.**
Created by physician and political figure Benjamin Rush (1745–1813).
Source: Reprinted with permission from *Quarterly Journal of Studies on Alcohol*, vol 4, pp. 321–341, 1943 (presently *Journal of Studies on Alcohol*), Copyright Journal of Studies on Alcohol, Inc., Rutgers Center of Alcohol Studies, Piscataway, NJ 08854.

Formation or Production of Alcohol and Its Sources

When yeast cells metabolize sugar to energy, they produce alcohol and carbon dioxide by a process called fermentation. If little oxygen is present, these cells produce more alcohol and less carbon dioxide. **Figure SA.3** shows living yeast cells.

Fermentation can occur spontaneously in nature—it requires only sugar, water, a warm environment, and yeast (whose spores are present in air and soil). Human experience with alcohol probably began at least 10,000 years ago with spontaneously fermented fruits or honey. It's reasonable to assume that humans have always had small quantities of alcohol in their diets since all humans possess the enzymes to metabolize at least minimal amounts of alcohol.[5] Very small amounts of alcohol are even produced by our intestinal flora.

Humans learned to make wine from fruits, mead from honey, and beer from grain, probably about 5,000 years ago. In some areas, people made alcohol-containing dairy products. Using simple yeast fermentation, they could not produce beverages with alcohol levels above 16 percent—the point at which alcohol kills off the yeast, halting alcohol production. Later, seventh-century Egyptian chemists discovered how to use distillation to capture concentrated alcohol, which could be added to drinks to boost alcohol content. Distilled alcoholic beverages (such as rum, gin, and whiskey) are called spirits, liquor, or hard liquor.

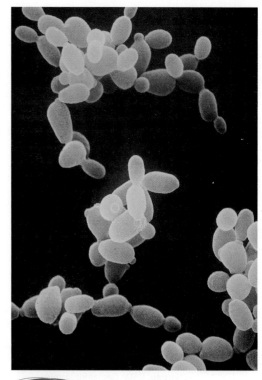

Figure SA.3 A yeast plant micrograph.

Beer, wine, and liquor have different alcohol levels: most beer is up to 5 percent alcohol although some beers exceed 6 percent; wine is 8 to 15 percent alcohol; and hard liquor is typically 35 to 45 percent alcohol. Beer and wine are labeled with the percentage of alcohol, but hard liquor is labeled by "proof," which is twice the alcohol percentage (an 80 proof whiskey is 40 percent alcohol).

Pure alcohol, a clear, colorless liquid used in chemistry labs, is 95 percent alcohol. (Even "pure" alcohol contains some water.) The beverage closest to pure alcohol is vodka, which is alcohol and water and almost nothing else; gin is similar but flavored with juniper berries. Scotch, rum, rye, whiskeys, and other liquors have residual flavor traces of the grain from which they were fermented or flavors introduced during storage. All liquors, however, contain little of nutritional value besides energy. Beer and wine do contain unfermented carbohydrates and a trace of protein but, like liquor, have negligible minerals. With the exception of niacin in beer, alcoholic beverages have negligible vitamins as well. **Table SA.1** shows the amount of calories in various alcoholic beverages.

Think About It **3**

Table SA.1 Calories and Alcohol in Selected Beverages

Beverage	Serving Size	Kcalories	Alcohol (g)
Light beer	12 fl oz	99	11.3
Beer	12 fl oz	146	12.8
White table wine	4.5 fl oz	90	12.3
Red table wine	4.5 fl oz	95	12.3
Dessert wine	4.5 fl oz	203	20.2
Distilled beverages (gin, rum, vodka, whiskey)			
80 proof	1.5 fl oz	97	14.0
86 proof	1.5 fl oz	105	15.1
90 proof	1.5 fl oz	110	15.9
94 proof	1.5 fl oz	116	16.7
100 proof	1.5 fl oz	124	17.9
Coffee liqueur, 53 proof	1.5 fl oz	175	11.9
Bloody Mary cocktail	4 fl oz	92	11.1
Daiquiri cocktail	4 fl oz	224	27.8
Whiskey sour cocktail	4 fl oz	163	20.1
Tequila sunrise cocktail	4 fl oz	137	11.6
Piña colada cocktail	4 fl oz	233	12.4

Sources: US Department of Agriculture, Agricultural Research Service. 1999. USDA Nutrient Database for Standard Reference, Release 13. Nutrient Data Laboratory Home Page, http://www.nal.usda.gov/fnic/foodcomp, accessed 5/26/00; and Pennington JAT. *Bowes and Church's Food Values of Portions Commonly Used.* 17th ed. Philadelphia: Lippincott-Raven; 1998.

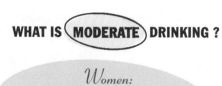

WHAT IS MODERATE DRINKING ?

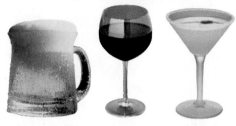

Women:
No more than **1** drink a day

Men:
No more than **2** drinks a day

COUNT AS A DRINK...

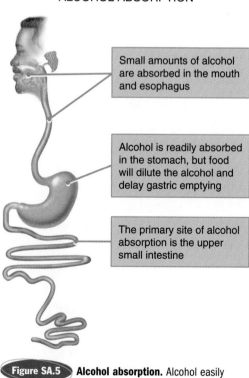

12 ounces
of regular beer

5 ounces
of wine

1.5 ounces
of 80-proof
distilled spirits

Figure SA.4 **What is moderate drinking?**
Source: USDA Center for Nutrition Policy and Promotion.

ALCOHOL ABSORPTION

Small amounts of alcohol are absorbed in the mouth and esophagus

Alcohol is readily absorbed in the stomach, but food will dilute the alcohol and delay gastric emptying

The primary site of alcohol absorption is the upper small intestine

Figure SA.5 **Alcohol absorption.** Alcohol easily diffuses in and out of cells, so most alcohol is absorbed unchanged.

Distillation can yield more than just ethanol. Traces of other volatile compounds, such as methanol, evaporate and then condense in the distillate. These are called congeners. These biologically active compounds help to create the distinctive taste, smell, and appearance of alcoholic beverages such as whiskey, brandy, and red wine. But congeners are also suspected of causing or contributing to hangovers, and they may play a role in alcohol's relationship to cancer.[6]

One serving of alcohol, or a **standard drink**, is generally defined as 12 ounces of beer, 4 to 5 ounces of wine, or $1\frac{1}{2}$ ounces (a "jigger") of liquor. All contain roughly 15 grams (one measured tablespoon) of pure alcohol. (See **Figure SA.4**.) Most health professionals who speak of "moderate alcohol intake" usually mean no more than one (for women) or two (for men) servings in a day.[7] Moderate intake is *not* an average of seven drinks per week, when there are six days of abstinence followed by seven drinks in one night! That's **binge drinking** and it's dangerous.

Key Concepts: *Alcohol is formed when yeast ferments sugars to yield energy. Distillation methods produce concentrated solutions, with up to 95 percent alcohol. A typical serving of beer, wine, or distilled spirits contains about 15 grams of alcohol.*

Alcohol Absorption

Absorption of alcohol begins immediately in the mouth and esophagus where small quantities enter the bloodstream. Although alcohol absorption continues in the stomach, the small intestine efficiently absorbs most of the alcohol consumed.[8] (See **Figure SA.5**.)

You've heard it before: "Don't drink on an empty stomach." Eating before or with a drink impedes the rush of alcohol into the bloodstream in several ways. Food, especially if it contains fat, delays gastric emptying into the small intestine, where absorption is faster. The delay also provides a longer opportunity for oxidizing stomach enzymes to work. And food dilutes the stomach contents, lowering the concentration of alcohol and its rate of absorption.

fermentation The anaerobic conversion of various carbohydrates to carbon dioxide and an alcohol or organic acid accompanied by production of ATP.

congeners Biologically active compounds that include nonalcoholic ingredients as well as other alcohols such as methanol. Congeners contribute to the distinctive taste and smell of the beverage and may increase intoxicating effects and subsequent hangover.

standard drink One serving of alcohol (about 15 g) defined as 12 ounces of beer, 4 to 5 ounces of wine, or 1.5 ounces of liquor.

binge drinking Consuming excessive amounts of alcohol in short periods of time.

acetaldehyde A toxic intermediate compound (CH_3CHO) formed by the action of enzyme systems during the metabolism of alcohol.

alcohol dehydrogenase The enzyme that catalyzes the oxidation of ethanol and other alcohols.

aldehyde dehydrogenase The enzyme that catalyzes the conversion of acetaldehyde to acetate with the concurrent reduction of NAD^+ to NADH.

fatty liver Accumulation of fat in the liver, a sign of increased fatty acid synthesis.

About 80 to 95 percent of alcohol is absorbed unchanged. However, some oxidation does proceed in the digestive tract, mainly in the stomach, and products of this metabolism join alcohol as it diffuses into the gut cells.[9] These products travel via the portal circulation directly to the liver, where most alcohol metabolism takes place. When all goes well, metabolism achieves two goals: energy production and protection from the damaging effects of alcohol and its even more toxic metabolite **acetaldehyde**.

Alcohol Metabolism

The body cannot store potentially harmful alcohol, so the body works extra hard to get rid of it. To prevent alcohol from accumulating and destroying cells and organs, the body quickly metabolizes it and removes it from the blood. The liver selectively metabolizes alcohol before other compounds and has alternative pathways to handle excess consumption. Alcohol is metabolized in three stages:

1. Alcohol is first converted to acetaldehyde, a toxic and highly reactive substance.

2. Acetaldehyde is then rapidly converted to acetate and then acetyl CoA.

3. Acetyl CoA either enters the citric acid cycle or is made into fatty acids.

Metabolizing Small Amounts of Alcohol

Alcohol dehydrogenase (ADH) is a zinc-containing enzyme that catalyzes the conversion of small to moderate amounts of alcohol to acetaldehyde, a toxic substance. (See **Figure SA.6**.) To avoid toxic buildup, another enzyme, **aldehyde dehydrogenase (ALDH)**, quickly and effectively converts acetaldehyde to acetate. People differ in their ability to eliminate toxic acetaldehyde and small amounts of it are found in the blood of intoxicated people.[10]

Dehydrogenases in the gastrointestinal tract and the liver are responsible for almost all alcohol metabolism. Probably about 4 to 9 percent, possibly as much as 20 percent, of alcohol is changed to acetaldehyde in the digestive tract.[11] Gastrointestinal aldehyde dehydrogenase does not completely convert acetaldehyde to acetate. The remaining acetaldehyde is more destructive than alcohol itself and can damage the gut mucosa.[12]

The metabolic reactions that convert alcohol to acetaldehyde and acetaldehyde to acetate consume NAD⁺ while forming NADH. Acetate combines with coenzyme A to form acetyl CoA. The conversion of NAD⁺ to NADH and the resulting buildup of NADH dramatically slows the citric acid cycle, blocking the entry of acetyl CoA into this pathway. In the competition for the limited supply of NAD⁺, the detoxification of alcohol always takes priority over the operation of the citric acid cycle. This slowed citric acid cycle can process little acetyl CoA, be it from alcohol, carbohydrate, or fat. As a result, cells route most of the acetyl CoA to the synthesis of fatty acids, which are assembled into fat.

Fat accumulation in the liver can be seen after a single bout of heavy drinking, and fatty acid synthesis accelerates with chronic alcohol consumption. Fatty liver is the first stage of liver destruction in alcoholics.

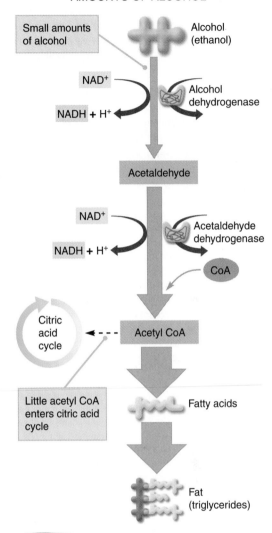

METABOLIZING SMALL TO MODERATE AMOUNTS OF ALCOHOL

Figure SA.6 **Metabolizing alcohol.** The metabolism of alcohol inhibits the citric acid cycle and primarily forms fat.

Quick Bites

Alcohol Aversion Therapy

In alcohol aversion therapy, the medication disulfiram (Antabuse) deliberately blocks the conversion of toxic acetaldehyde to acetate (acetic acid). Even small amounts of alcohol trigger the highly unpleasant Antabuse-alcohol reaction, which includes a throbbing headache, breathing difficulties, nausea, copious vomiting, flushing, vertigo, confusion, and a drop in blood pressure.

Quick Bites

How to Shock Your Surgeon

*I*f a former alcoholic neglects to disclose past alcohol use before undergoing surgery, the surgeon could be in for a big surprise. Even if the patient is now a teetotaler, his MEOS could still act like that of an alcoholic—still operating at the faster speed it formerly needed to process alcohol quickly. The overactive MEOS would deplete anesthesia much quicker than expected. Theoretically, the patient could wake up in the middle of surgery, much to the shock of the surgeon. That's why anesthesiologists and surgeons ask their patients about alcohol use, past and present.

Microsomal Ethanol-Oxidizing System (MEOS)
An energy-requiring enzyme system in the liver that normally metabolizes drugs and other foreign substances. When the blood alcohol level is high, alcohol dehydrogenase cannot metabolize it fast enough, and the excess alcohol is metabolized by MEOS.

Metabolizing Large Amounts of Alcohol

Large amounts of alcohol can overwhelm the alcohol dehydrogenase system, the usual metabolic path. As alcohol builds up, the body identifies it as foreign and routes it into the primary overflow pathway, the **Microsomal Ethanol-Oxidizing System (MEOS)**. The liver ordinarily uses the MEOS bypass pathway to metabolize drugs and detoxify "foreign" substances. Chronic heavy drinking appears to activate MEOS enzymes, which may be responsible for transforming the pain reliever acetaminophen into chemicals that can damage the liver. (See **Figure SA.7**.)

The MEOS pathway uses different enzymes from the alcohol dehydrogenase system and when transforming alcohol into acetaldehyde, it oxidizes NADPH to NADP (rather than reducing NAD^+ to NADH). If this pathway is repeatedly exposed to large doses of alcohol, its capacity and processing speed increase.

THE MEOS OVERFLOW PATHWAY

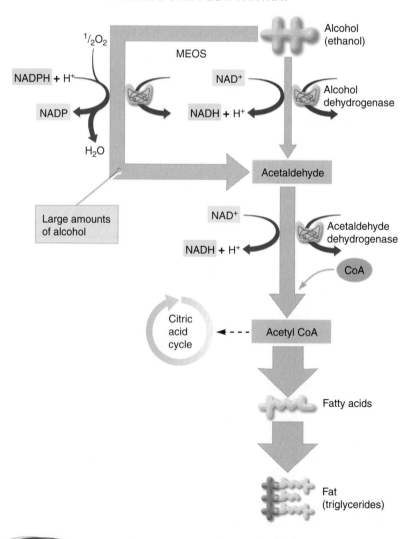

Figure SA.7 **The MEOS overflow pathway.** Large amounts of alcohol can overwhelm its typical metabolic route, so excess alcohol enters an overflow pathway called the Microsomal Ethanol-Oxidizing System (MEOS).

Removing Alcohol from Circulation

Despite its multiple alcohol-processing pathways, the liver can metabolize only a certain amount of alcohol per hour, regardless of the amount in the bloodstream. The rate of alcohol metabolism depends on several factors, including the amount of metabolizing enzymes in the liver, and varies greatly between individuals. In general, after one standard drink, the amount of alcohol in the drinker's blood (blood alcohol concentration, or BAC) peaks in 30 to 45 minutes. (See **Figure SA.8.**) When absorption exceeds the liver's capacity, a bottleneck is created and alcohol enters the systemic circulation. Alcohol diffuses rapidly, dispersing equally into all body fluids, including cerebrospinal fluid and the brain and, during pregnancy, into the placenta and fetus. About 10 percent of circulating alcohol is lost in urine, through the lungs, and through skin. Consequently, urine tests and breathalyzer tests both reflect concentrations of blood alcohol as well as alcohol levels in the brain, and can indicate how much a person's mental and motor functions may be impaired. Excessive alcohol consumption deprives the brain of oxygen. The struggle to deal with an overdose of alcohol and lack of oxygen eventually causes the brain to shut down functions that regulate breathing and heart rate. This shutdown leads to a loss of consciousness and in some cases coma and death. When a drinker passes out, the body is actually protecting itself: when you lose consciousness, you can't add more alcohol to your system. When you hear of an **alcohol poisoning** death, it usually is the result of consuming such a large quantity of alcohol in such a short period of time that the brain of the victim was overwhelmed. Heart and lung functions shut down and the person died.

alcohol poisoning An overdose of alcohol. The body is overwhelmed by the amount of alcohol in the system and cannot metabolize it fast enough.

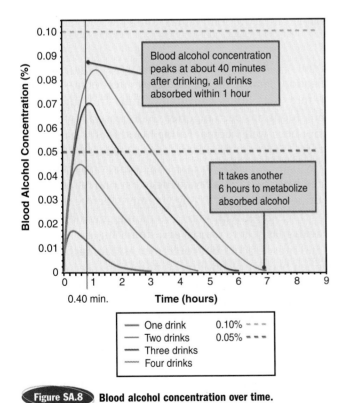

Figure SA.8 Blood alcohol concentration over time.

Source: National Institute on Alcohol Abuse and Alcoholism. Alcohol Alert No. 35. PH371; January 1997. http://silk.nih.gov/silk/niaaa1/publication/aa35.htm. Accessed 10/11/00.

Hangover Symptoms

Constitutional—fatigue, weakness, and thirst

Pain—headache and muscle aches

Gastrointestinal—nausea, vomiting, and stomach pains

Sleep and biological rhythms—decreased sleep, decreased dreaming when asleep

Sensory—vertigo and sensitivity to light and sound

Cognitive—decreased attention and concentration

Mood—depression, anxiety, and irritability

Sympathetic hyperactivity—tremor, sweating, increased pulse, and blood pressure

Possible Contributing Factors

Direct effects of alcohol
- Dehydration
- Electrolyte imbalance
- Gastrointestinal disturbances
- Low blood sugar
- Sleep and biological rhythm disturbances

Alcohol withdrawal

Alcohol metabolism (i.e., acetaldehyde toxicity)

Nonalcohol factors
- Compounds other than alcohol in beverages, especially the congener methanol
- Use of other drugs, especially nicotine
- Personality traits such as neuroticism, anger, and defensiveness
- Negative life events and feelings of guilt about drinking
- Family history for alcoholism

Figure SA.9 Hangover causes and symptoms.

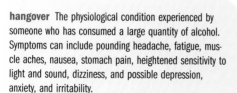

Quick Bites

Ancient Hangover Helpers

According to the Ancient Persians, eating five almonds could prevent a hangover. The Romans and Greeks had a different solution: celery.

hangover The physiological condition experienced by someone who has consumed a large quantity of alcohol. Symptoms can include pounding headache, fatigue, muscle aches, nausea, stomach pain, heightened sensitivity to light and sound, dizziness, and possible depression, anxiety, and irritability.

The Morning After

After a night of drinking, the drinker may suffer from a pounding headache, fatigue, muscle aches, nausea, and stomach pain as well as a heightened sensitivity to light and noise—a **hangover** in full force. The sufferer may be dizzy, have a sense that the room is spinning, and may be depressed, anxious, and irritable. Usually a hangover begins within several hours after the last drink, when the blood alcohol level is dropping. Symptoms normally peak about the time the alcohol level reaches zero and they may continue for an entire day.[13]

What causes a hangover? Scientists have identified several causes of the painful symptoms of a hangover. (See **Figure SA.9**.) Alcohol causes dehydration, which leads to headache and dry mouth. Alcohol directly irritates the stomach and intestines, contributing to stomach pain and vomiting. The sweating, vomiting, and diarrhea that can accompany a hangover cause additional fluid loss and electrolyte imbalance. Alcohol's hijack of the metabolic process diverts liver activity away from glucose production and can lead to low blood sugar (hypoglycemia), causing lightheadedness and lack of energy. Alcohol also disrupts sleep patterns, interfering with the dream state and contributing to fatigue. In general, the greater the amount of alcohol consumed, the more likely a hangover will strike. However, some people experience a hangover after only one drink, while some heavy drinkers do not have hangovers.[14]

In addition, factors other than alcohol may contribute to the hangover. A person with a family history of alcoholism has increased vulnerability to hangover. Mixing alcohol and drugs is suspected of increasing the likelihood of a hangover. The congeners in most alcoholic beverages can contribute to more vicious hangovers. Research shows that gin and vodka, beverages that contain less of these biologically active compounds, cause fewer headaches.[15]

Treating a Hangover

So what can you do about a hangover? Few treatments have undergone rigorous, scientific investigation. Time is the most effective treatment—symptoms usually disappear in 8 to 24 hours. Consuming fruits, fruit juices, or other fructose-containing foods has been reported to decrease a hangover's intensity, but this has not been well studied. Eating bland foods that contain complex carbohydrates, such as toast or crackers, can combat low blood sugar and possibly nausea. Sleep can ease fatigue and drinking nonalcoholic, noncaffeinated beverages can alleviate dehydration (caffeine is a diuretic and increases urine production). Taking vitamin B_6 before drinking may reduce the severity of hangover symptoms.[16] Certain medications can relieve symptoms. Antacids may relieve nausea and stomach pains. Aspirin may reduce headache and muscle aches but could increase stomach irritation. Avoid acetaminophen because alcohol metabolism enhances its toxicity to the liver.[17] People who drink three or more alcoholic beverages a day should avoid all over-the-counter pain relievers and fever reducers. These heavy drinkers may have an increased risk of liver damage and stomach bleeding from medicines that contain aspirin, other salicylates, acetaminophen (Tylenol), ibuprofen (Advil), naproxen sodium (Aleve), or ketoprofen (Orudis KT and Actron).[18]

People with hangovers should avoid "the hair of the dog that bit you," a remedy that calls for drinking more alcohol. Additional drinking only enhances the toxicity of the alcohol previously consumed and extends the recovery time.

Think About It

4

Individual Differences in Alcohol Metabolism

Individuals vary in their ability to metabolize alcohol and acetaldehyde and thus differ in their susceptibility to inebriation, to hangover, and, in the long term, to addiction and organ damage.

The result of individual differences is easiest to see in acute responses to alcohol. For example, when people of Asian descent drink alcohol, about half experience flushing around the face and neck, probably as a result of high blood acetaldehyde levels.[19] These individuals lack gastric alcohol dehydrogenase and have an inefficient form of hepatic aldehyde dehydrogenase. This may explain why their ancestors depended on boiled water (for teas) as a source of safe fluid. In contrast, Europeans are able to metabolize larger quantities of alcohol, and historically have relied on fermentation to produce fluids that were safer to drink.[20]

Elderly people often find their tolerance for alcohol is less than it used to be. Due to decreased tolerance, the effects of alcohol, such as impaired coordination, occur at lower intakes in the elderly than in younger people whose tolerance increases with increased consumption. This reduced tolerance is compounded by an age-related decrease in body water, so that blood alcohol concentrations in older people are likely to rise higher after drinking.[21]

Women and Alcohol

Men and women respond differently to alcohol. (See **Figure SA.10**.) Blood alcohol rises faster in women, so they become more intoxicated than men at an equivalent dose of alcohol.[22] Accordingly, moderate drinking is usually defined as "two standard drinks for men and one for women."[23] Women also metabolize alcohol more slowly than men. Various factors are responsible for alcohol's greater effect on women:

Body size and composition. Women on average are smaller than men and have smaller livers, and therefore have less capacity for metabolizing alcohol. Women also have lower total body water and higher body fat than men of comparable size. After alcohol is consumed, it diffuses uniformly into all body water, both inside and outside cells. Because of their smaller quantity of body water, after drinking equivalent amounts of alcohol women have higher concentrations of alcohol in their blood than men.

Less enzyme activity. For nonalcoholics, alcohol dehydrogenase (the primary enzyme involved in the metabolism of alcohol) is 40 percent less active in the stomachs of women than of men.[24] This contributes to higher blood alcohol concentrations and lengthens the time needed to metabolize and eliminate alcohol.

Chronic alcohol abuse. This exacts a greater physical toll on women than on men. Female alcoholics have death rates 50 to 100 percent higher than those of male alcoholics. Further, a greater percentage of female alcoholics die from suicides, alcohol-related accidents, circulatory disorders, and cirrhosis of the liver.

Key Concepts: *Alcohol does not need to be digested prior to absorption and moves easily across the GI tract lining into the bloodstream. Once alcohol is absorbed, the liver metabolizes it. The primary metabolic enzymes are alcohol dehydrogenase and aldehyde dehydrogenase. When large amounts of alcohol are consumed, some is metabolized by the MEOS pathway. There are a number of genetic and gender differences in the amount and activity levels of alcohol-metabolizing enzymes.*

Body composition

Women have a higher percentage of fat than men (size for size women have less water than men to dilute alcohol).

Less enzyme activity

Alcohol dehydrogenase, the primary enzyme involved in the metabolism of alcohol, is up to 40% less active in women than in men.

Body size

Women are smaller on average than men (smaller livers and less total water).

Hormonal fluctuations

Women typically have a heightened response to alcohol which is increased when they are about to have their periods, or when taking birth control pills.

Figure SA.10 **Women and men respond differently to alcohol.**

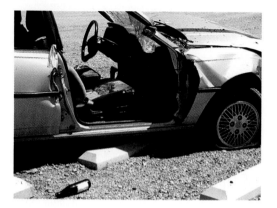

When Alcohol Becomes a Problem

Alcohol affects every organ system in the body. In the short term, small amounts of alcohol change the levels of neurotransmitters in the brain, reducing inhibitions and physical coordination. In the long term, chronic intake of large amounts of alcohol damages the heart, liver, GI tract, and brain. When a pregnant woman drinks, alcohol can have a devastating effect on the development of her baby.

Alcohol in the Brain and the Nervous System

Alcohol diffuses readily into the brain, and because a small amount is absorbed from the mouth directly into circulating blood, its effects can be almost immediate, reaching the brain in as little as one minute after consumption. **Figure SA.11** shows the effects alcohol has on the brain.

Because alcohol is fat soluble, it easily can cross the protective fatty membrane of nerve cells. There, it disrupts the brain's complex system for communicating between nerve cells. Neurotransmitters that excite nerve cells and those that inhibit nerve cells are thrown out of balance. Excess of some neurotransmitters produces sleepiness; high levels of others cause a loss of coordination; an imbalance of others impairs judgment and mental ability; and still other neurotransmitters perpetuate the desire to keep drinking, even when it's clearly time to stop. Changes in these messengers are suspected of leading to addiction and symptoms of alcohol withdrawal.[25] In the short run, they probably contribute to a hangover.

Alcohol's short-term effects are dose related. One or two drinks typically bring alcohol blood levels to 0.04 percent and usually cause only mild, pleasant changes in mood and release of inhibitions. With more drinks and rising blood alcohol levels, coordination, judgment, reaction time, and vision are increasingly impaired. In some states and Canadian provinces it is illegal for a person whose blood level of alcohol has reached or exceeds 0.08 percent to drive a motor vehicle. **Table SA.2** shows the effects various amounts of alcohol have on mood and behavior.

The acute effect of a large alcohol load—swallowed accidentally by children, for example—is hypoglycemia (low blood sugar) severe enough to kill.[26] Binge drinking, especially following several days of little food, also can be deadly. The lack of food depletes glycogen stores, and heavy drinking suppresses gluconeogenesis. The resulting severe hypoglycemia is a medical emergency with the potential for coma and death.

Figure SA.11 **Effects of alcohol on the brain.** As blood alcohol concentration rises, different parts of the brain are affected.

Blood alcohol concentration

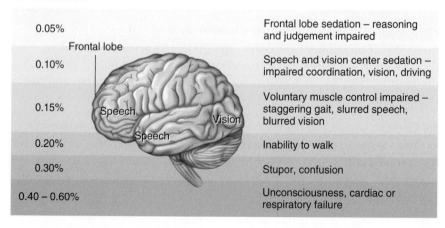

Blood alcohol concentration	Effect
0.05%	Frontal lobe sedation – reasoning and judgement impaired
0.10%	Speech and vision center sedation – impaired coordination, vision, driving
0.15%	Voluntary muscle control impaired – staggering gait, slurred speech, blurred vision
0.20%	Inability to walk
0.30%	Stupor, confusion
0.40 – 0.60%	Unconsciousness, cardiac or respiratory failure

Chronic alcoholism produces many different mental disorders. Malnutrition is a probable factor in most of these, even when diet appears adequate. After years of drinking, brain cells become permanently damaged and unable to metabolize nutrients properly.

Alcohol's Effect on the Gastrointestinal System

Years of heavy drinking and ongoing contact with alcohol and acetaldehyde eventually damage the gastrointestinal system, which in turn discourages eating, compromises absorption of protective nutrients, and leaves the digestive lining even more vulnerable to damage as the vicious cycle continues.

 Table SA.2 Alcohol Impairment Chart

This chart is intended as a guide, not a guarantee.
IMPAIRMENT BEGINS WITH YOUR FIRST DRINK.
FOR SAFETY'S SAKE, NEVER DRIVE AFTER DRINKING!

Men

BODY WEIGHT IN POUNDS

DRINKS	100	120	140	160	180	200	220	240	
	APPROXIMATE BLOOD ALCOHOL PERCENTAGE								
1	.04	.03	.03	.02	.02	.02	.02	.02	IMPAIRMENT BEGINS
2	.08	.06	.05	.05	.04	.04	.03	.03	DRIVING SKILLS
3	.11	.09	.08	.07	.06	.06	.05	.05	SIGNIFICANTLY
4	.15	.12	.11	.09	.08	.08	.07	.06	AFFECTED
5	.19	.16	.13	.12	.11	.09	.09	.08	POSSIBLE CRIMINAL PENALTIES
6	.23	.19	.16	.14	.13	.11	.10	.09	
7	.26	.22	.19	.16	.15	.13	.12	.11	LEGALLY INTOXICATED
8	.30	.25	.21	.19	.17	.15	.14	.13	
9	.34	.28	.24	.21	.19	.17	.15	.14	CRIMINAL PENALTIES
10	.38	.31	.27	.23	.21	.19	.17	.16	

Subtract .01% for each 40 minutes of drinking.
One drink is 1.25 oz. of 80 proof liquor, 12 oz. of beer, or 5 oz. of table wine.

Women

BODY WEIGHT IN POUNDS

DRINKS	90	100	120	140	160	180	200	220	240	
	APPROXIMATE BLOOD ALCOHOL PERCENTAGE									
1	.05	.05	.04	.03	.03	.03	.02	.02	.02	IMPAIRMENT BEGINS
2	.10	.09	.08	.07	.06	.05	.05	.04	.04	DRIVING SKILLS
3	.15	.14	.11	.10	.09	.08	.07	.06	.06	SIGNIFICANTLY AFFECTED
4	.20	.18	.15	.13	.11	.10	.09	.08	.08	POSSIBLE CRIMINAL PENALTIES
5	.25	.23	.19	.16	.14	.13	.11	.10	.09	
6	.30	.27	.23	.19	.17	.15	.14	.12	.11	LEGALLY INTOXICATED
7	.35	.32	.27	.23	.20	.18	.16	.14	.13	
8	.40	.36	.30	.26	.23	.20	.18	.17	.15	
9	.45	.41	.34	.29	.26	.23	.20	.19	.17	CRIMINAL PENALTIES
10	.51	.45	.38	.32	.28	.25	.23	.21	.19	

Note: Data supplied by the Pennsylvania Liquor Control Board.

Source: The National Clearinghouse for Alcohol and Drug Information, Substance Abuse and Mental Health Services Administration. http://lcb.state.pa.us/edu/adult-Chart.htm, accessed 10/20/00.

[*Fyi*] College Drinking Culture

FOR YOUR INFORMATION

From car crashes to alcohol poisonings—the culture of drinking on many college campuses puts students at grave risk. An overwhelming number of college students, many of whom are below the minimum legal drinking age, use alcohol. The findings of a recent, nationwide survey are typical of studies on campus drinking: more than 80 percent of college students had had at least one drink of alcohol during the 30 days preceding the survey and nearly half (47 percent) of student drinkers say that they drink to get drunk.[1] Such figures are averages for all campuses, however, and mask variability among schools. There is little drinking in some schools, a troubling level in many others.[2]

Binge Drinking

Binge drinking is especially worrisome, and it is widespread on college campuses. What is binge drinking? *Binge drinking* is defined as the consumption of at least five drinks in a row for men or four drinks in a row for women. Approximately 2 of 5 (44 percent) of students report binge drinking behaviors and about 1 of 4 (23 percent) report bingeing frequently, three or more times in a two-week period. Frequent binge drinkers average more than 14 drinks per week and account for more than two-thirds of the alcohol consumed by college students.[3] College binge drinkers may drink not for sociability, but solely and purposefully to get drunk.

Binge drinkers often do something they later regret—argue with friends, make fools of themselves, get sick, engage in unplanned (and often unprotected) sexual activity, or drive drunk. Afterward they may forget where they were or what they did, but the consequences of the binge remain. These consequences may include alienated friends, a hangover, and embarrassment. Or the consequences could be much more serious, such as sexually transmitted disease, hospitalization, permanent injury, rape, pregnancy, and death.

Abstaining

There is a polarizing trend in college drinking with binge drinkers at one end and abstainers at the other. The number of college students who do not drink alcohol is rising and now is nearly equal to the number of colleges students who frequently binge. About 1 of 5 (19 percent) students report consuming no alcohol within the past year.[4]

The Campus Drinker

Researchers have looked closely at the students who are binge drinkers. The findings tend to agree on the following characteristics:

- *Ethnicity.* Studies suggest that college students who are members of racial and/or ethnic minorities drink less than white students.[5]
- *Age.* Younger students are more likely than older students to binge drink and to have alcohol-related problems.[6]
- *Past alcohol use.* Binge drinking during high school, especially among men, is strongly predictive of binge drinking in college.[7]
- *Athletic participation.* Despite the perception that competitive athletes are health conscious, athletes may be more likely than other students to binge drink.[8]
- *Personality characteristics.* Heavy drinking and alcohol-related problems during college are associated with psychological factors such as impulsiveness, depression, anxiety, or early deviant behavior. A family history of alcohol abuse is another risk factor.[9]
- *Group and peer influence on drinking behavior.* "But my friends drink more than I do" is a common refrain. Students often believe that they drink less than others and generally overestimate how much their peers drink. This exaggerated perception leads to greater personal consumption.
- *Drinking in groups.* Group influence can exaggerate any behavior, and drinking is no exception.[10]
- *Serving oneself.* The convenience of self-serve also boosts alcohol consumption.[11]
- *Fraternities and sororities.* Fraternity and sorority members drink greater amounts of alcohol and more frequently than other groups on campus.[12]

Some students have a romanticized notion of heavy drinking. The image of the macho drinker, the urbane and sophisticated drinker, or the creative artistic drinker may hold special appeal to the student with a poor self-image.

Binge Drinkers and Problem Behaviors

Interestingly, students who are frequent binge drinkers or who report specific alcohol-related problems do not see themselves as problem drinkers.[13] Yet these students are more likely than their classmates to

- damage property.
- have unprotected sex.
- drink and drive.
- have trouble with authorities.
- perform poorly in classes.
- miss classes.
- have hangovers.
- get injured.[14]

Heavy drinking on campus creates problems for all students. In colleges where significant binge drinking goes on, classmates are more often insulted or humiliated; their property is damaged more often; and they receive more unwanted sexual advances—all as a result of their peers' drinking. Classmates of binge drinkers are more likely to have their studies disturbed or to have to take care of a drunken student.[15]

Interventions

Many campuses have alcohol abuse prevention programs as well as treatment programs. Treatment must often start with helping students recognize that their drinking is a problem. Group programs are very helpful for students, just as they are for other populations. However, other innovative treatments are also helping students. The Alcohol Skills Training Program focuses on monitoring and moderating one's own drinking. The goal is reduction of alcohol use, not necessarily abstinence. Heavy-drinking students who took the course said one year later they were drinking less, compared with similar students who took a more traditional alcohol education course. A single individual motivational session for heavy-drinking freshmen has also helped reduce alcohol-related problems during the first two years of college.[16]

Many questions remain about college binge drinking: What is the best way to keep students from heavy drinking, and to intervene effectively when they do binge drink? How can we prevent students from harming themselves and others, from squandering the opportunities of a college education, from becoming addicted to alcohol? Questions on social policy must be explored, too, and answered honestly. For example, does prohibiting alcohol on campus cause students to drive in search of a drink? How effective are restrictions on alcohol advertising? Do restrictions interfere with the rights of students who are 21 and older? To what degree must schools act as surrogate parents? The questions are difficult, but the answers are crucial.

1 Wechsler H, Lee JE, Kuo M, Lee H. College Binge drinking in the 1990s: a continuing problem. *J Am Coll Health.* 2000;48(10):99–210.

2 Wechsler H, Dowdall GW, Davenport A, Rimm EB. A gender-specific measure of binge drinking among college students. *Am J Public Health.* 1995;7:982–985.

3 Wechsler H, Lee, JE, Kuo M, Lee H. Op. cit.

4 Ibid.

5 Ibid.

6 Ibid.

7 Ibid.

8 Wechsler H, Nelson T, Weitzman E. From knowledge to action: how Harvard's college alcohol study can help your campus design a campaign against student alcohol abuse. *Change.* In press.

9 Baer, JS, Kivlahan DR, Marlatt GA. High-risk drinking across the transition from high school to college. *Alcoholism: Clin Experiment Res.* 1995;19(1):54–61.

10 Marlatt GA, Baer JS, Larimer M. Preventing alcohol abuse in college students: a harm-reduction approach. In: Boyd GM, Howard J, Zucker RA, eds. *Alcohol Problems among Adolescents: Current Directions in Prevention Research.* Hillsdale, NJ: Lawrence Erlbaum Associates; 1995:147–172.

11 Geller ES, Russ NW, Altomari MG. Naturalistic observations of beer drinking among college students. *J Appl Behav Anal.* 1986;19(4):391–396; and Geller ES, Kalsher MJ. Environmental determinants of party drinking: bartenders versus self-service. *Environ Behav.* 1990;22(1):74–90.

12 Wechsler H, Dowdall GW, Davenport A, Rimm, EB. Op. cit.; and Marlatt GA, Baer JS, Larimer, M. Op. cit.; and Baer, JS, Kivlahan DR, Marlatt, GA. Op. cit.

13 Presley CA, Meilman PW, Cashin JR, Lyerla R. *Alcohol and Drugs on American College Campuses: Use, Consequences, and Perceptions of the Campus Environment.* Vol. 3. 1991–1993. Carbondale, IL: Core Institute; 1996.

14 Wechsler H, Lee JE, Kuo M, Lee H. Op. cit.

15 Ibid.

16 Marlatt GA, Baer JS, Larimer M. Op. cit.

esophagitis Inflammation of the esophagus.
gastritis Inflammation of the stomach.

Chronic irritation from alcohol and acetaldehyde erodes protective mucosal linings, causing inflammation and release of destructive free radicals. **Esophagitis** (inflammation of the esophagus), esophageal stricture (closing), and swallowing difficulties are common among alcoholics. When the stomach repeatedly is exposed to alcohol at high concentrations, **gastritis** (inflammation of the stomach) often develops. Alcoholics frequently have diarrhea and malabsorption, evidence of intestinal damage. The mouth, throat, esophagus, stomach, and small and large intestines are all at greatly increased risk of cancer. Smoking dramatically multiplies this risk.

Alcohol and the Liver

Metabolizing and detoxifying alcohol is almost entirely the responsibility of the liver. So it's not surprising that too much drinking hurts the liver more than any other site in the body. In the United States, heavy alcohol use is considered the most important risk factor for chronic liver disease. During the 1980s, alcoholic fatty liver, acute alcoholic hepatitis, and alcoholic cirrhosis together accounted for 46 percent of deaths from chronic liver disease and 49 percent of hospitalizations for liver disease.[27]

The earliest evidence of liver damage is fat accumulation, which can appear after only a few days of heavy drinking. Fatty liver (see **Figure SA.12**) recedes with abstinence but persists with continued drinking. Is fatty liver in and of itself harmful? The answer is controversial among liver researchers, with some experts suggesting it's a benign condition. However, studies show 5 to 15 percent of people with alcoholic fatty liver who continue to drink develop liver fibrosis (excessive fibrous tissue) or cirrhosis (scarring) in only 5 to 10 years.[28] The abundance of accumulated fat is vulnerable to peroxidation and production of destructive compounds, including free radicals.

Fat accumulation is one of several factors resulting in alcoholic liver disease. Accumulation of NADH may be another. With regular, high intakes of alcohol, alcohol and acetaldehyde continually irritate and inflame the liver, producing alcoholic hepatitis (persistent inflammation of the liver) in 10 to 35 percent of heavy drinkers. The inflammatory process also generates free radicals that batter away at liver cells. The destruction of liver cells becomes self-perpetuating, especially if antioxidant nutrients are unavailable to help break the cycle. If intestinal damage has also occurred, toxins, including those produced by bacterial flora, may be able to cross the intestinal barrier into circulation and worsen inflammation.[29]

Alcoholic hepatitis may be treatable, but it's often fatal. Alcoholic hepatitis also predisposes to liver cancer and cirrhosis, conditions that are usually fatal. With continued inflammation, the liver makes excessive collagen and becomes fibrous (fibrotic liver disease) and scarred (cirrhosis). This ultimately kills liver cells by choking off tiny blood vessels that nourish liver cells. About 10 to 20 percent of heavy drinkers develop cirrhosis.[30]

Dietary manipulations may be helpful in liver disease, but abstinence is the cornerstone of therapy. Reducing dietary fats reduces hepatic fat accumulation somewhat. Adequate micronutrients and a healthful balance of macronutrients probably speed recuperation from liver diseases in their earlier stages.[31] In late-stage liver disease, dietary restrictions, often of proteins, may slow disease progression or improve symptoms. One thing is clear, however: at any stage of alcoholic liver disease, popping nutrient supplements will not substitute for abstinence, and may be detrimental.

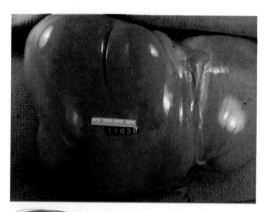

Figure SA.12 Fatty liver.

Quick Bites

Are alcoholics more likely to get food poisoning?

When alcohol inhibits the breakdown of another toxin, the effect can be dramatic. Consider seafood toxins, for example. The alcoholic who sits down for a good fish dinner should be extra careful about seafood because alcoholic liver disease makes him 200 times more likely to die from *Vibrio vulnificus*, a bacterium found in raw oysters. Alcohol also accentuates the symptoms of *ciguatera*, or "fish poisoning," a relatively common food poisoning in tropical areas where people eat large fish from infected waters.

Fetal Alcohol Syndrome

Fetal alcohol syndrome is perhaps alcohol's saddest result. The severely affected victims of the syndrome have a variety of congenital defects: mental retardation, coordination problems, and heart, eye, and genitourinary malformations, as well as low birth weight and slowed growth rate. Most apparent are characteristic facial abnormalities. Severe cases of fetal alcohol syndrome are rare, but subtle damage with one or two abnormalities, sometimes called "fetal alcohol effects," is probably much more widespread. Symptoms of the syndrome may not emerge until months after birth and are apt to go undiagnosed.[32] This disorder, a major cause of mental retardation in the United States, is preventable.

Alcohol is especially damaging in the early weeks of pregnancy, before a woman may know she is pregnant. It crosses the placenta into the tiny body of the fetus, where its effects are grossly magnified. Both the congeners in alcoholic beverages and the associated disturbed metabolism of vitamin A and folic acid, nutrients clearly required for fetal growth and development, can interfere with embryonic development.[33]

In contrast to other disorders brought about by chronic, excessive drinking, the quantity of alcohol that causes fetal alcohol syndrome may be relatively small. A safe level during pregnancy is not known; therefore, pregnant women should abstain from alcohol consumption. Unlike most other alcohol-related diseases, fetal alcohol damage does not require chronic intake. A binge, even several drinks at a party, at the wrong moment of pregnancy can cause problems. However, population studies show that babies with neurodevelopmental problems are more common among women who drink more frequently during pregnancy.[34]

Official health advisories issued in 1981, 1990, and 1995 warn women against drinking alcohol if they are pregnant or considering becoming pregnant. Labels on alcoholic beverages must carry a warning label for pregnant women. Yet government surveys estimate that consumption

> **fetal alcohol syndrome** A set of physical and mental abnormalities observed in infants born to women who abuse alcohol during pregnancy. Affected infants exhibit poor growth, characteristic abnormal facial features, limited hand-eye coordination, and mental retardation.

[Fyi] Myths About Alcohol

FOR YOUR INFORMATION

Poor alcohol, so misunderstood. Myths and misunderstandings just keep circulating about alcohol. Some of these statements are partly true, but most are completely false. You may have heard some of the following:

- *Alcohol is a stimulant.* No. It's actually a depressant, but its initial depressing effect on inhibitions and judgment may make it seem stimulating.
- *Alcohol keeps you warm.* Partly true. It dilates blood vessels near the body's surface, giving a feeling of warmth. But as body heat escapes, alcohol cools the inner body.

- *Alcohol is an aphrodisiac.* Partly true. By suppressing inhibitions, it may loosen behavior. However, sexual function is often compromised by alcohol.
- *Most alcoholics live on skid row.* No. The highly visible skid-row alcoholic represents only a minority of alcoholics.
- *Beer is a source of vitamins.* Partly true. Beer does contain a fair amount of niacin. But you'd need about 1 liter to fulfill niacin requirements. Levels of other vitamins are much lower.
- *Alcohol helps you sleep.* No. Alcohol disrupts sleep patterns, leading to a restless, unsatisfying sleep.

- *Laboratory animals love to drink.* No. Alcohol is usually given by tube feeding because most animals refuse to drink it willingly.
- *It's good to have a beer before breastfeeding.* No. Alcohol may be relaxing and allow milk to flow more readily, but alcohol concentrations in breastmilk are similar to those in the mother's blood. Alcohol reduces milk production by reducing the intensity of the infant's suckling.

increased between 1991 and 1995. In 1995, 16 percent of pregnant women consumed alcohol, and 3.5 percent did so frequently.[35] **Figure SA.13** shows alcohol consumption by women of childbearing age.

Key Concepts: *Alcohol affects every organ system of the body. In the brain and nervous system, alcohol is a depressant. In the GI tract, alcohol damages cells of the esophagus and stomach and increases the risk for GI cancers. The liver is most affected by alcohol consumption, culminating in alcoholic hepatitis and cirrhosis after years of alcohol abuse. Alcohol intake during pregnancy can have devastating effects on fetal development.*

Alcoholics and Malnutrition

In the United States, where food is plentiful and fortification of foods with vitamins and minerals is common, overt nutrient deficiencies are rare—except among alcoholics. The results of their poor diet interact with the results of alcohol's toxicity—which include diarrhea, malabsorption, liver malfunction, bleeding, bone marrow changes, and hormonal changes—to worsen malnutrition. In general, the more a person drinks, the worse the malnutrition. (See **Figure SA.14**.)

Poor Diet

Disordered eating is common among heavy drinkers, especially among alcoholic women.[36] Factors responsible for the poor diet of alcoholics are much easier to identify than to correct. Economic factors include poverty, lack of cooking facilities, and homelessness. Anxiety, depression, loneliness, and isolation are all characteristic of alcoholism, and all contribute to loss of appetite. So can physical pain. Lack of interest in food is common. There may be an aversion to many specific foods, or to eating in general, especially after the experience of diarrhea, painful indigestion, or difficulty swallowing.

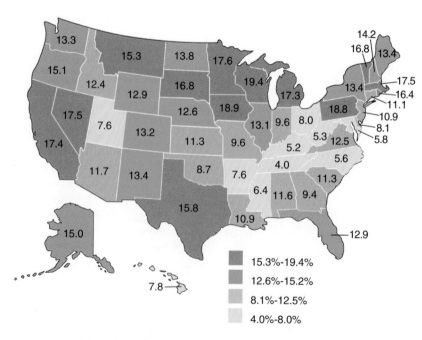

Figure SA.13 **Prevalence of frequent alcohol consumption among women of childbearing age (18–44 years).**
Source: Alcohol consumption among pregnant and childbearing-aged women. *MMWR.* 1997;46:346–350.

Legend:
- 15.3%-19.4%
- 12.6%-15.2%
- 8.1%-12.5%
- 4.0%-8.0%

* Consumption of an average of seven or more drinks per week or five or more drinks on at least one occasion during the preceding month.

Heavy drinkers who get about half their calories from alcohol cannot eat enough to obtain adequate vitamins and minerals. Severely malnourished alcoholics often have multiple deficiencies.

Vitamin Deficiencies

Inadequate intake, poor absorption, increased vitamin destruction in the body, and urinary losses all contribute to vitamin deficiencies in the alcoholic. Alcohol also interferes with the conversions of vitamin precursors to active forms.

Folate, thiamin, and vitamin A are most often affected by alcoholism. Folate deficiency contributes to malabsorption, anemia, and nerve damage—all of which worsen malnutrition. Vitamin A deficiency also creates a vicious cycle by damaging gastrointestinal epithelium and by compromising immunity, leaving the victim susceptible to infections. Thiamin deficiency contributes to classic diseases of alcoholism: the brain damage of Wernicke-Korsakoff syndrome, polyneuropathy (nerve inflammation), and cardiomyopathy (heart inflammation). Alcoholics can have overt scurvy from vitamin C deficiency. Vitamin B_6 and vitamin B_{12} deficiencies are less common.

Alcohol metabolism competes with the normal metabolism of vitamins and other nutrients. For example, ethanol competes successfully with retinol for dehydrogenase.[37] Retinol (vitamin A) can use that enzyme for its conversion to other active forms of vitamin A, and the disruption of its metabolism is probably one way alcohol increases cancer risk. The same disruption may produce fetal birth defects when pregnant women drink.

Alcohol-induced fat malabsorption and metabolic abnormalities contribute to depletion of fat-soluble vitamins A, D, E, and K. Blood-clotting factors drop with depleted vitamin K, increasing risk of bleeding and anemia. Vitamin E deficiency is not generally recognized as a complication of alcoholism, but its depletion due to fat malabsorption is possible. Optimal vitamin E is necessary to quench free radicals generated during alcohol metabolism.[38]

Mineral Deficiencies

Alcoholics are commonly deficient in minerals such as calcium, magnesium, iron, and zinc. Alcohol itself does not seem to affect their absorption. Rather, fluid losses and an inadequate diet are the primary culprits. Magnesium deficiency causes "shakes" similar to that seen in alcohol withdrawal. Chronic diarrhea and loss of epithelial tissue (caused by skin rashes or sloughing off the digestive lining) may seriously deplete zinc, a mineral needed for immune function. In cases of bleeding, especially gastrointestinal blood loss, iron levels fall.

But not all minerals are lower in heavy drinkers than in nondrinkers. Unless there's bleeding, a heavy drinker's iron levels tend to be higher than normal in the blood and liver, potentially contributing to harmful lipid peroxidation—the production of unstable lipid molecules that contain excess oxygen. Copper and nickel may also be elevated in advancing disease, but the reason and the effects are unclear.[39]

The Macronutrients and Body Weight

Animal experiments can demonstrate a number of ways alcohol alters digestion and metabolism of carbohydrate, fat, and protein, but the relevance to humans at usual levels of intake is not certain. Alcohol interferes

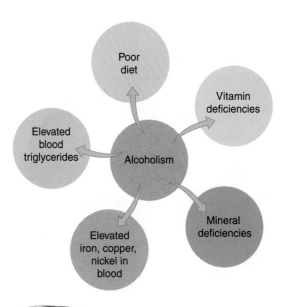

Figure SA.14 **Alcoholism and malnutrition.** Alcoholics' poor diets interact with alcohol's toxicity to worsen their malnutrition.

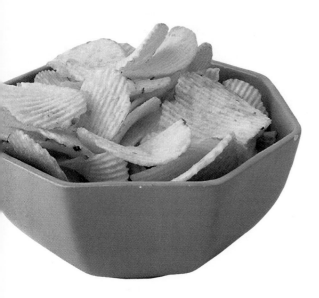

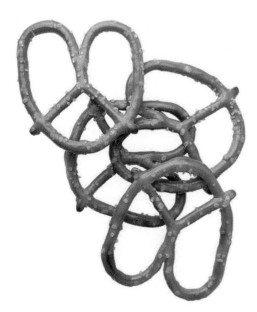

with amino acid absorption, but its direct overall effect on protein balance appears minimal. It inhibits gluconeogenesis and lowers blood sugar, probably contributing to hangovers, and at the most extreme, causing acute, potentially lethal hypoglycemia if a person who drinks heavily neglects to eat.[40]

Alcohol's most dramatic effect is on fats. You have seen that alcohol causes fatty liver. In the blood, excess alcohol has the undesirable effect of raising triglyceride levels, often significantly. Hyperlipidemia (high blood fats) is common among heavy drinkers. Abstinence and a balanced diet can usually return blood lipids to normal.[41] On the other hand, moderate alcohol use increases protective high-density lipoproteins (HDL, or "good cholesterol"), an important factor in alcohol's relationship to the reduced risk for coronary artery disease.

Although alcohol has a relatively high caloric value, alcohol consumption does not necessarily result in increased body weight. While some studies report weight gain,[42] other studies show that when chronic heavy drinkers substitute alcohol for carbohydrates in their diets, they lose weight and weigh less than their nondrinking counterparts. Furthermore, when chronic heavy drinkers eat an otherwise normal diet, they do not gain weight.[43] Some possible explanations for this seeming paradox are (1) the high levels of alcohol consumed by alcoholics are metabolized mainly by the MEOS backup pathway, which is less efficient and loses more energy as heat than other alcohol-metabolizing pathways;[44] (2) with so much alcohol to handle, the liver is unable to efficiently process fats; (3) energy-producing mitochondria are permanently damaged;[45] and (4) energy is lost from malabsorbed nutrients, especially fat.

Key Concepts: *Alcohol interferes with normal nutrition by reducing the intake of nutrient-dense foods and by affecting the absorption, metabolism, and excretion of many vitamins and minerals. Although alcohol contains a significant number of calories (7 kcal/g), during alcohol metabolism excess intake often is wasted as heat, and the weight gain that accompanies high intakes is less than might be expected from the calorie content.*

Does Alcohol Have Benefits?

Can a potentially harmful drink like alcohol play a role in a healthful diet? The consensus of health experts is that it can—but not for everyone. The question continues to arouse much debate, however, and even those supporting alcohol's usefulness often have reservations. Public health statements on alcohol are typically accompanied by plenty of "ifs" and "buts."

Good, fairly consistent epidemiological evidence suggests that low to moderate drinking reduces mortality among populations.[46] (**Table SA. 3** gives the official definitions of levels of drinking.) Tracked against alcohol intake, death rates typically follow what statisticians describe as a "U-shaped curve." Mortality rates for people who drink slightly or moderately are lower than for people who rarely or never drink. The lowest rate is seen in people who consume one drink per week. Increasing the number of drinks confers no additional benefit. As the number of drinks increases, the mortality rate rises. People who consume two drinks per day have about the same mortality rate as nondrinkers.[47] Beyond three drinks per day, the death rate rises dramatically.[48] Alcohol's primary benefit is to raise protective HDL cholesterol levels. It may also inhibit formation of blood clots, but this connection is less clear.[49] In addition, alcohol may have subjective benefits like stress relief and relaxation.

In most studies, wine, beer, and spirits appear equally protective. Recent findings of reduced rates of nonfatal heart attacks among exclusive beer drinkers support the view that protective benefits of moderate drinking are due to the alcohol itself rather than other substances in alcoholic beverages.[50] However, international comparisons that highlight unexpectedly low rates of heart disease in France, despite a high-fat diet (the **French paradox**), suggest red wine may have a unique protective effect. However, the apparent benefits of red wine may result from overall healthier behavior

French paradox The phenomenon that French people have a lower incidence of heart disease than people whose diets contain comparable amounts of fat. Part of the difference has been attributed to the regular and moderate drinking of red wine.

Table SA.3 How Much Is Too Much?

Term	Criterion
Moderate drinking (NIAAA)	Men: ≤ 2 drinks per day Women: ≤ 1 drink per day Over 65: ≤ 1 drink per day
At-risk drinking (NIAAA)	Men: > 14 drinks per week or > 4 drinks per occasion Women: > 7 drinks per week or > 3 drinks per occasion
Alcohol abuse (APA)	Maladaptive pattern of alcohol use leading to clinically significant impairment or distress, manifested within a 12-month period by one or more of the following: • Failure to fulfill role obligations at work, school, or home. • Recurrent use in hazardous situations. • Legal problems related to alcohol. • Continued use despite alcohol-related social or interpersonal problems. • Symptoms have never met criteria for alcohol dependence.
Alcohol dependence (APA)	Maladaptive pattern of alcohol use leading to clinically significant impairment or distress, manifested within a 12-month period by three or more of the following: • Tolerance (either increasing amounts used or diminished effects with the same amount). • Withdrawal (withdrawal symptoms or use to relieve or avoid symptoms). • Use of larger amounts over a longer period than intended. • Persistent desire or unsuccessful attempts to cut down or control use. • Great deal of time spent obtaining or using or recovering from use. • Important social, occupational, or recreational activities given up or reduced. • Use despite knowledge of alcohol-related physical or psychological problems.
Hazardous use (WHO)	Person at risk for adverse consequences.
Harmful use (WHO)	Use resulting in physical or psychological harm.

Note: NIAAA = National Institute on Alcohol Abuse and Alcoholism; APA = American Psychiatric Association; WHO = World Health Organization.
Source: O'Connor PG, Schottenfeld RS. Patients with alcohol problems. *N Engl J Med.* 1998;338(9):593. Copyright © 1998 Massachusetts Medical Society. All rights reserved.

of people who drink red wine; a direct connection between red wine and health benefits remains unproved.[51] Nevertheless, recognizing that alcohol generally confers moderate protection, and the possibility that wine has a particular benefit, the Bureau of Alcohol Tobacco and Firearms recently granted permission for wine labels to include one of the following statements:

> The proud people who made this wine encourage you to consult your family doctor about the health effects of wine consumption.

> To learn the health effects of wine consumption, send for the Federal Government's Dietary Guidelines for Americans...[52]

Public health agencies and organizations caution against inappropriate drinking. (See **Figure SA.15**.) While low to moderate alcohol use may have some benefit, these groups advise people to discuss their alcohol intake with their doctors, and they urge moderation (see **Table SA.3**). Public health officials also point out the numerous groups who should not drink any alcohol:

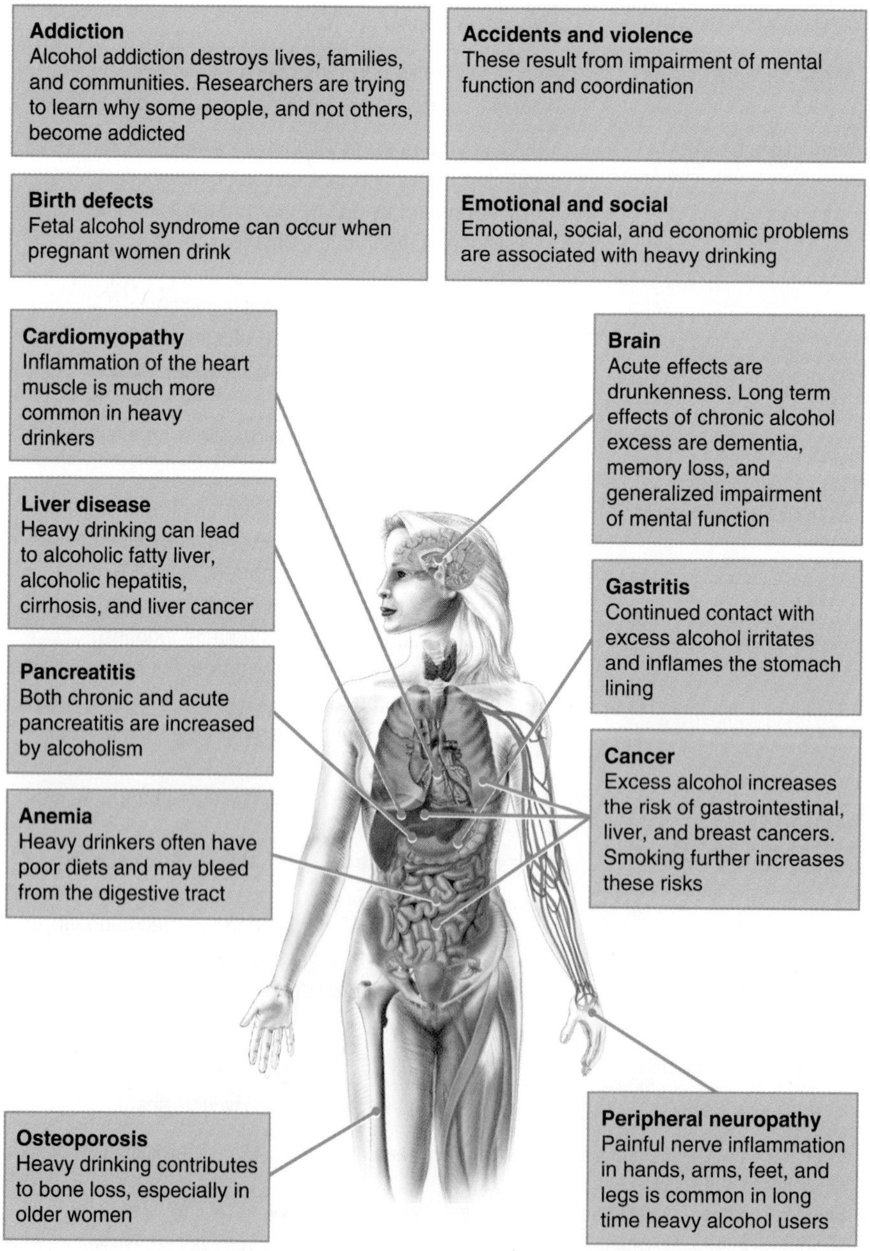

Figure SA.15 **Summary figure: harmful effects of alcohol.** Because excess alcohol reaches all parts of the body, it causes a wide array of physical problems. Here are some of the ways alcohol can harm.

Addiction
Alcohol addiction destroys lives, families, and communities. Researchers are trying to learn why some people, and not others, become addicted

Accidents and violence
These result from impairment of mental function and coordination

Birth defects
Fetal alcohol syndrome can occur when pregnant women drink

Emotional and social
Emotional, social, and economic problems are associated with heavy drinking

Cardiomyopathy
Inflammation of the heart muscle is much more common in heavy drinkers

Brain
Acute effects are drunkenness. Long term effects of chronic alcohol excess are dementia, memory loss, and generalized impairment of mental function

Liver disease
Heavy drinking can lead to alcoholic fatty liver, alcoholic hepatitis, cirrhosis, and liver cancer

Gastritis
Continued contact with excess alcohol irritates and inflames the stomach lining

Pancreatitis
Both chronic and acute pancreatitis are increased by alcoholism

Cancer
Excess alcohol increases the risk of gastrointestinal, liver, and breast cancers. Smoking further increases these risks

Anemia
Heavy drinkers often have poor diets and may bleed from the digestive tract

Osteoporosis
Heavy drinking contributes to bone loss, especially in older women

Peripheral neuropathy
Painful nerve inflammation in hands, arms, feet, and legs is common in long time heavy alcohol users

- children and adolescents
- people on certain medications
- people who have an alcohol-related illness or another illness that will be worsened by alcohol
- people who will be driving or operating machinery
- pregnant women or women who may be in the early weeks of pregnancy and don't know they are pregnant
- people with a personal or strong family history of alcoholism[52]

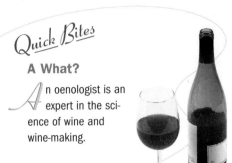

Quick Bites

A What?

An oenologist is an expert in the science of wine and wine-making.

Key Concepts: *Although alcohol has the potential to reduce risk for heart disease, most health organizations recommend moderate to no drinking. It is too early in the scientific investigation of alcohol's benefits to recommend alcohol intake for all adults. Some people, such as pregnant women, should not drink alcohol at all.*

Label [to] Table

Have you ever wondered how much protein, carbohydrate, and fat are in a can of beer? If you've ever looked at a beer label, you know it's quite different from a food label. Look at the following information from a can of light beer and see if you can calculate the calories from carbohydrate, fat, and protein.

Serving size = 12 fl oz

Calories = 105 (kcal)

Carbohydrate = 5 g

Protein = 0.7 g

Fat = 0 g

First, to figure out how many calories come from the three macronutrients, multiply the number of grams by their respective calorie contribution per gram:

5 g carbohydrate × 4 kcal/g = 20 kcal from carbohydrates

0.7 g protein × 4 kcal/g = 2.8 kcal from protein

0 g fat × 9 kcal/g = 0 kcal from fat

Uh oh. Is this adding up correctly? So far we have accounted for only 23 of the 105 kilocalories in this beer. Where are the other 82 kilocalories? Don't forget that many of the calories in beer come from alcohol, and it's easy to calculate just how many grams are in this can of light beer. Remember alcohol has 7 kcalories per gram so the remaining 82 kilocalories come from 12 grams of alcohol (82 ÷ 7 = 11.7).

So, for the 105 kilocalories this beer provides, you get very little (if any) protein, carbohydrate, or fat. Instead, a majority of the calories come from alcohol. This holds true for the micronutrients as well—beer contains negligible amounts of vitamins or minerals.

This is why people say alcoholic beverages have only "empty calories." They provide calories, but almost no nutrient value!

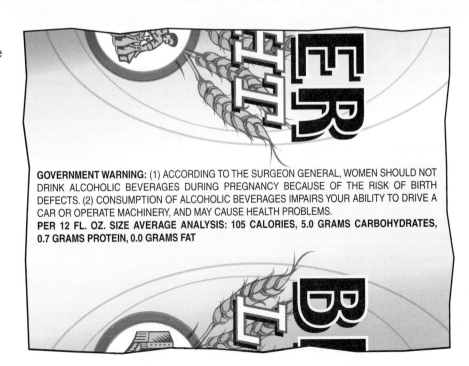

GOVERNMENT WARNING: (1) ACCORDING TO THE SURGEON GENERAL, WOMEN SHOULD NOT DRINK ALCOHOLIC BEVERAGES DURING PREGNANCY BECAUSE OF THE RISK OF BIRTH DEFECTS. (2) CONSUMPTION OF ALCOHOLIC BEVERAGES IMPAIRS YOUR ABILITY TO DRIVE A CAR OR OPERATE MACHINERY, AND MAY CAUSE HEALTH PROBLEMS.
PER 12 FL. OZ. SIZE AVERAGE ANALYSIS: 105 CALORIES, 5.0 GRAMS CARBOHYDRATES, 0.7 GRAMS PROTEIN, 0.0 GRAMS FAT

LEARNING *Portfolio*

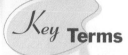

Key Terms

	page		page
acetaldehyde	263	fermentation	262
alcohol	258	fetal alcohol syndrome	273
alcohol dehydrogenase	263	French paradox	277
alcohol poisoning	264	gastritis	272
aldehyde dehydrogenase	263	hangover	266
binge drinking	262	methanol	258
blood-brain barrier	258	methyl alcohol	258
congeners	262	Microsomal Ethanol-Oxidizing	
esophagitis	272	System (MEOS)	263
ethanol	258	standard drink	262
ethyl alcohol	258	wood alcohol	258
fatty liver	263		

> Malnutrition among alcoholics is common due to poor food choices and alcohol's interference with the absorption, metabolism, and excretion of nutrients.

> Fetal alcohol syndrome is one of the most devastating consequences of alcohol consumption; and it is preventable.

> Moderate alcohol consumption has been linked to reduced risk of heart disease.

> The potential benefits of moderate alcohol consumption may be related to effects on lipoprotein levels and the antioxidant components of beverages such as wine.

> Health organizations recommend moderate to no alcohol consumption.

Study Points

> Alcohol, or ethyl alcohol, is a small organic compound with one hydroxyl (alcohol) group attached to two carbons.

> As an organic solvent, alcohol can dissolve fats and other lipids.

> Alcohol provides seven kilocalories per gram but no essential function for the body; therefore, alcohol is not a nutrient.

> Alcohol requires no digestion and is absorbed easily all along the gastrointestinal tract.

> Most of the acetyl CoA produced from alcohol is routed to the synthesis of fatty acids; fatty liver is apparent even after one night of binge drinking.

> Different rates of alcohol metabolism can be attributed to different levels of the alcohol metabolizing enzymes; these differences are due to genetic and gender variations.

> Alcohol affects all organs in the body, but the most obvious effects are in the brain and the nervous system, the GI system, and the liver.

Study Questions

1. How much alcohol is in a standard drink of beer, of wine, and of liquor?

2. List the ways food helps to delay or avoid inebriation.

3. Where does alcohol metabolism take place?

4. What are the three stages of alcohol metabolism?

5. What causes "fatty liver" in an alcoholic?

6. What causes a hangover? Is there any way to relieve one?

7. Among health authorities, what is the consensus about drinking alcohol?

8. List some factors that affect our ability to metabolize alcohol.

9. Why do health-care professionals advise pregnant women not to drink alcohol?

10. List the positive and the negative effects of alcohol.

👉 [*Try*] **This**

Cruising through the Medicine Cabinet

This exercise will increase your awareness of the amounts of alcohol in over-the-counter medications. Look through your medicine cabinet and check the ingredient lists of all the products there. In particular, take a close look at any mouthwash or cough syrup. Which products contain alcohol? How much? What do you think its purpose is in these medicines? ✍

References

1 Roe DA. *Alcohol and the Diet.* Westport, CT: AVI Publishing; 1979.

2 Ibid.

3 Mittal BV, Desai AP, Khade KR. Methyl alcohol poisoning: an autopsy study of 28 cases. *J Postgrad Med.* 1991;37:9–13.

4 Roe DA. Op. cit.

5 Vallee BL. Alcohol in the Western world. *Scientif Amer.* June 1998;80–85.

6 Swift R, Davidson D. Alcohol hangover: mechanisms and mediators. *Alcohol Health Res World.* 1998;22(1): 54–60.

7 USDA Center for Nutrition Policy and Promotion. Does alcohol have a place in a healthy diet? *Nutr Insights.* August 1997;4.

8 Seitz HK, Oneta CM. Gastrointestinal alcohol dehydrogenase. *Nutr Rev.* 1998;56:52–60.

9 Ibid.

10 Swift R, Davidson D. Op. cit.

11 Seitz HK, Oneta CM. Op.. cit.

12 Ibid.

13 Swift R, Davidson D. Op. cit.

14 Ibid.

15 Ibid.

16 Wiese JG, Slipak MG, Browner WS. The Alcohol Hangover. *Ann Intern Med* 2000;132:897–902.

17 Swift R, Davidson D. Op. cit.

18 Nordenberg T. "An aspirin a day…" just another cliché? *FDA Consumer.* March-April 1999; 15–17.

19 Steinmetz CG, Xie P, Weiner H, et al. Structure of mitochondrial aldehyde dehydrogenase: the genetic component of ethanol aversion. *Br J Psychiatry.* 1996;168:762–767.

20 Vallee BL. Op. cit.

21 National Institute on Alcohol Abuse and Alcoholism (NIAAA). *Alcohol Alert: Alcohol and Aging.* April 1998;40.

22 NIAAA. *Alcohol Alert: Moderate Drinking.* April 1992;16.

23 USDA Center for Nutrition Policy and Promotion. Op. cit.

24 Swift R, Davidson D. Op. cit.

25 Valenzuela CF. Alcohol and neurotransmitter interactions. *Alcohol Health Res World.* 1997;21:108–148.

26 Bradford DE. Alcohol and the young child. *Alcohol Alcohol* 1984;19:173–175.

27 Deaths and hospitalizations from chronic liver disease and cirrhosis—United States, 1980–1989. *MMWR.* 1993;41:969–973.

28 Teli MR, Day CP, Burt AD, et al. Determinants of progression to cirrhosis or fibrosis in pure alcoholic fatty liver. *Lancet.* 1995;346:987–990.

29 NIAAA. *Alcohol Alert: Alcohol and the Liver: Research Update.* 1998;42.

30 Ibid.

31 Teli MR, Day CP, Burt AD, et al. Op. cit.

32 Identification of children with fetal alcohol syndrome and opportunity for referral of their mother for primary prevention, Washington, 1993–1997. *MMWR.* 1998;47:861–864.

33 Roe DA. Op. cit.

34 Alcohol consumption among pregnant and childbearing-aged women—United States, 1991 and 1995. *MMWR.* 1997;46:346–350.

35 Ibid.

36 Lilenfeld LR, Kaye WH. The link between alcoholism and eating disorders. *Alcohol Health Res World.* 1996;20:94–99.

37 Seitz HK, Oneta CM. Op. cit., and Wang XD. Chronic alcohol intake interferes with retinoid metabolism and signaling. *Nutr Rev.* 1999;57:51–59.

38 Feinman L, Lieber CS. Nutrition and diet in alcoholism. In: Shils ME, Olson JA , Shike M, Ross CA, eds. *Modern Nutrition in Health and Disease.* 9th ed. Philadelphia: Lippincott Williams & Wilkins; 1999:1523–1542.

39 Ibid.

40 Ibid.

41 Ibid.

42 NIAAA. *Alcohol Alert: Alcohol Metabolism.* 1997;35.

43 Ibid.

44 Suter PM, Hassler E, Vetter MD. Effects of alcohol on energy metabolism and body weight regulation: is alcohol a risk factor for obesity? *Nutr Rev.* 1997;55:157–171.

45 Lands WE. Alcohol and energy intake. *Am J Clin Nutr.* 1995;62:5 suppl, 1101–1106S.

46 Klatsky AL. Is it the drink or the drinker? Circumstantial evidence only raises a probability. *Am J Clin Nutr.* 1999;69:2–3.

47 Gazino JM, et. al. Light-to-moderate alcohol consumption and mortality in the Physicians' Health Study enrollment cohort. *J Am Coll Cardiol.* 2000;35:1, 96–105.

48 Pearson TA. Alcohol and heart disease. *Circulation.* 1996;94:3023–3025.

49 Klatsky AL. Op. cit.

50 Bobak M, Skodova Z, Marmot M. Effect of beer drinking on risk of myocardial infarction: population based case-control study. *BMJ.* 2000;320:1378-1379.

51 Tjonneland A, Gronbaek M, Stripp C, Overvad K. Wine intake and diet in a random sample of 48763 Danish men and women. *Am J Clin Nutr.* 1999;69:49–54.

52 *Treasury Announces Actions Concerning Labeling of Alcoholic Beverages.* Press release from US Treasury Department, Bureau of Alcohol Tobacco and Firearms. February 5, 1999.

53 Pearson TA. Op. cit.

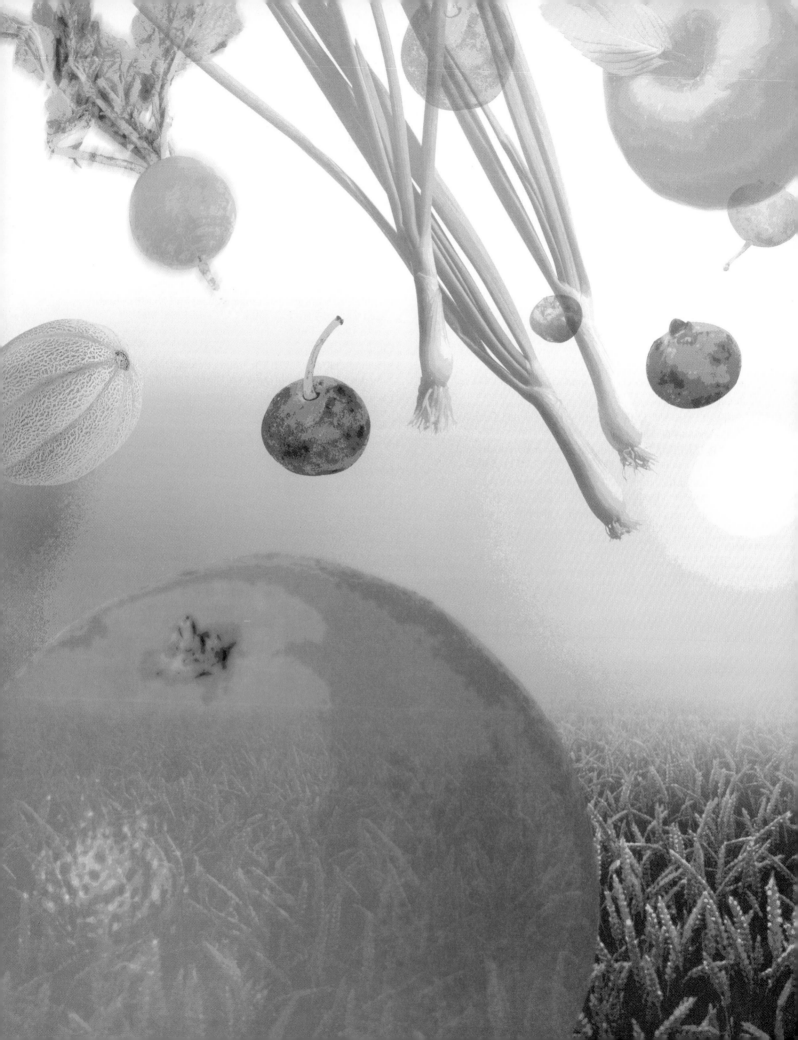

Chapter 8

Energy Balance, Body Composition, and Weight Management

Think About It

1 How often do you reject dessert after a big meal?

2 When it comes to body-fat distribution, are you an apple or a pear?

3 How much time do you spend talking with your friends about weight?

4 What does it mean if you are metabolically fit?

Fyi for your Information

This chapter's FYI boxes include practical information on the following topics:

• What's Neat about NEAT?

• Mark's Energy Balance

• High Protein Diets for Weight Loss: Helpful or Harmful?

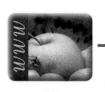

The web site for this book offers many useful tools and is a great source for additional nutrition information for both students and instructors. Visit the site at **nutrition.jbpub.com** for information on energy balance, body composition, and weight management. You'll find exercises that explore the following topics:

• Leptin in Mice and Humans

• Weighing In

• Calculating Your Health

• BMI Calculator

• Childhood Obesity

• Bariatric Surgery

Key to Illustrations

 Carbon Dioxide (CO_2)

 Water (H_2O)

What About Bobbie?

Track the choices Bobbie is making with the EatRight Analysis software.

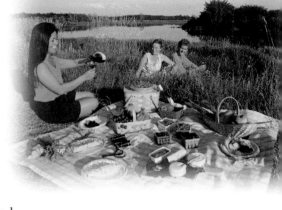

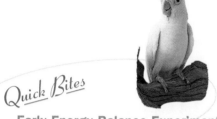

*Y*our body is in the energy exchange business. Here's how it works. You pay for the energy you expend with energy from the food in your diet. If you do a fairly good job of balancing input and output, your body does the rest—maintaining energy equilibrium and keeping your weight steady. But suppose you give your body more energy than it can handle? Your body banks the excess energy as fat, and you gain weight. If your "account" grows too big, you become obese. Losing that extra weight—withdrawing the fat from your account—is not always easy.

An average adult consumes 2,200 to 3,000 kilocalories per day. In one year, that adds up to 803,000 to 1,095,000 kilocalories! Yet, amazingly, most people maintain roughly the same weight during their working lives despite such a huge intake of energy over time.

Whether or not they are aware of their energy intake and expenditure, people who maintain a relatively constant weight are in energy equilibrium. Thanks to your body's ability to match intake and expenditure, this regulation occurs automatically—within limits.

Energy balance is the relationship between energy intake and energy output. **Energy intake** is the amount of calories you take in through consumption of carbohydrate, protein, fat, and alcohol. **Energy output** is the energy you use primarily for basic body functions, physical activity, and the processing of food. If you take in more energy than your body needs, you store the surplus as fat—the major energy reserve, and as glycogen—the short-term energy/carbohydrate reserve. **Positive energy balance** leads to weight gain. On the other hand, when your energy intake is less than needed, your body uses stores of glycogen and fat for fuel (along with body protein if the deficit is extreme) and body weight goes down, a **negative energy balance**. Thus, body weight change reflects overall energy balance.

Most adults maintain close to **energy equilibrium**—a balance of intake and output that results in little or no change in weight over time. Your body can be in energy equilibrium even if your energy intake is very high, as long as expenditure also is high. Conversely, your body can be in energy equilibrium when you don't expend much energy, as long as your intake also is low. Positive energy balance often happens around major holidays when overeating and inactivity generally prevail. It also occurs, appropriately, during pregnancy and other times of growth when the body purposefully increases energy stores. Starvation is an example of negative energy balance. **Figure 8.1** shows three people with different ratios of energy intake to energy expenditure.

Key Concepts: *Energy balance is the relationship between energy intake and energy output. Energy intake is the amount of calories contained in the diet. Energy output is the amount of fuel used mainly for basic body functions, the processing of food, and physical activity.*

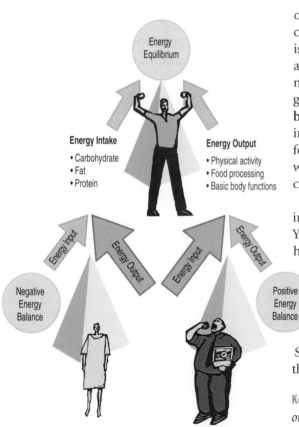

Figure 8.1 **Energy balance.**

Energy In

We can measure the energy content of a food with a **bomb calorimeter**, which **Figure 8.2** shows. Inside a sealed chamber, the food is completely burned and sensors measure the amount of heat produced by its combustion. Your body is not as efficient as a bomb calorimeter. It does not completely digest all food and it is unable to oxidize nitrogen. When calculating the amount of energy your body can extract from food, the number of calories released by combustion in a bomb calorimeter is adjusted downward to:

4 kcal per gram pure carbohydrate
4 kcal per gram pure protein
9 kcal per gram pure fat
7 kcal per gram pure alcohol

If we know a food's carbohydrate, fat, and protein content, we can use these numbers to estimate its calorie content.

Regulation of Food Intake

The body attempts to closely regulate food consumption to maintain energy balance. This intricate process involves internal cues—interactions and feedback mechanisms among hormones and hormone-like compounds and organ systems—and external cues—stimuli in the eating environment including the sight, smell, and taste of food. The complex interplay of internal and external cues ensures adequate food intake for survival. On the other hand, this complexity makes it difficult to isolate specific factors that cause overeating and obesity or disordered eating.

Hunger, Satiation, and Satiety

Internal cues, or sensations, influence eating behavior through three processes. (See **Figure 8.3**.) The first, **hunger**, prompts eating ("I'm hungry").

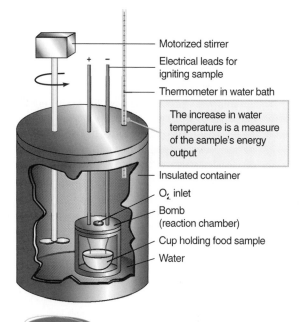

The increase in water temperature is a measure of the sample's energy output

Figure 8.2 A bomb calorimeter.

energy balance The balance in the body between amounts of energy consumed and expended.

energy intake The caloric or energy content of food provided by the sources of dietary energy: carbohydrate (4 kcal/g), protein (4 kcal/g), fat (9 kcal/g), and alcohol (7 kcal/g).

energy output The use of calories or energy for basic body functions, physical activity, and processing of consumed foods.

positive energy balance Periods of time in which energy intake exceeds energy expenditure, resulting in an increase in body energy stores and weight gain.

negative energy balance Periods of time in which energy intake is lower than energy expenditure, resulting in depletion of the body's energy stores and weight loss.

energy equilibrium A balance of energy intake and output that results in little or no change in weight over time.

bomb calorimeter An instrument used to measure the energy content of a food.

hunger The internal, physiological drive to find and consume food. Unlike appetite, hunger is often experienced as a negative sensation, often manifesting as an uneasy or painful sensation.

HUNGER, SATIATION, AND SATIETY

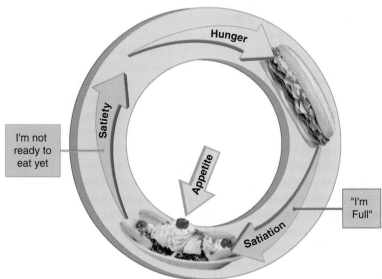

Figure 8.3 Hunger, satiation, and satiety are internal cues that influence eating behavior.

satiation Feeling of satisfaction and fullness that terminates a meal.

satiety The effects of a food or meal that delays subsequent intake. Feeling of satisfaction and fullness following eating that quells the desire for food.

appetite A psychological desire to eat that is related to the pleasant sensations often associated with food.

hypothalamus [high-po-THAL-ah-mus] A region of the brain involved in regulating hunger and satiety, respiration, body temperature, water balance, and other body functions.

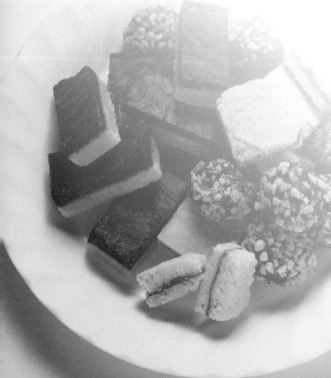

The second, **satiation**, terminates a meal ("I'm full"). The third, **satiety**, determines the interval between meals ("I'm not yet ready to eat again").

Appetite

Complicating the picture of hunger, satiation, and satiety is **appetite**. The distinction between hunger and appetite is crucial for understanding what we eat and why. Hunger is the physiological need for food. Appetite is the psychological desire to eat and is related to pleasant sensations associated with food. In this sense, hunger is the more basic drive, while appetite is a reflection of eating experiences. When a person is truly hungry, any food will do, whereas appetite frequently involves the desire for a specific food or type of food, often in the absence of hunger. For example, after a big meal of steak, potato, salad, and bread, you probably wouldn't want additional helpings. But you might be tempted by the dessert cart! That's appetite. At times, we are hungry but have no appetite or interest in food, such as when we are sick or under the influence of certain medications. Hunger and appetite work in tandem to ensure adequate nourishment.

Key Concepts: *If we know the macronutrient composition of a food, we can estimate the number of kilocalories based on the factors 4, 4, 9, and 7 kilocalories per gram for carbohydrate, protein, fat, and alcohol, respectively. The basic regulation of food intake is controlled by sensations of hunger, a physiological drive to eat; satiation, feelings of satisfaction that lead to ending a meal; and satiety, continued feelings of fullness that delay the start of the next feeding. Appetite is the psychological urge to eat, and often has no relation to hunger.*

Control by Committee

What, then, stimulates hunger, satiation, and appetite? Early theories focused on the stomach as the eating control center. In the 1950s, scientists thought the brain's **hypothalamus** controlled food intake because they had discovered that stimulating one part of the hypothalamus caused voracious eating, and stimulating another part caused refusal to eat. Thus, they concluded that a hypothalamic abnormality caused obesity. Since then, other areas of the brain have been implicated either as sensors of nutritional status or as neural centers that interact to control our selection and consumption of food. Today, we know the brain is only one of several sites in the body that influence our eating decisions.[1]

Composition of the Diet

Among the energy-yielding nutrients, protein seems to have the strongest satiating effect. Recent studies suggest that the energy density (kcal/g) of the diet is a major influence on satiation and satiety independent of the diet's macronutrient content.[2] Energy-dense diets (e.g., high-fat, low-fiber diets) tend to delay satiation and encourage overeating. One explanation is that people tend to eat a fairly constant amount of food.[3] The fiber content of the diet also affects energy density[4], satiation, and satiety. Soluble fibers tend to enhance satiety by slowing gastric emptying, and the bulking properties of insoluble fibers seem to enhance satiation. Other influences include the variety of foods consumed, the palatability of the diet,[5] and possibly the glycemic index.[6]

Circulating Nutrients

As we've seen in previous chapters, ingested nutrients are broken down, absorbed, and circulated to the liver. The liver acts as a sensor, monitoring circulating nutrient levels and signaling the brain when levels are high or low. Eating behavior, however, appears to have only weak links to blood levels of specific nutrients. Overall energy availability is a more important regulator than circulating nutrient levels. Other probable regulating factors include products of the liver's metabolism of nutrients and the heat generated by the metabolism of food.

Gastrointestinal Sensations

As food fills your stomach and small intestine, they become distended and trigger the transmission of signals to the brain. These signals stimulate a sense of fullness, suppressing the urge to eat.[7]

The passage of a reasonable amount of food through the mouth satisfies hunger—even if the food never reaches the stomach. When researchers fed large amounts of food to a person with a hole in the esophagus, hunger decreased even though the food was diverted outside the body and did not come into contact with the rest of the GI tract. During the process of tasting, salivating, chewing, and swallowing the brain probably measures the passage of food, much like a water meter measures the flow of water. After a certain amount of food passes through the mouth, hunger diminishes for 20 to 40 minutes.[8]

Temperature

While exposure to cold tends to increase the amount we eat, exposure to heat tends to reduce it. This is probably the result of interactions between the systems in the hypothalamus that regulate body temperature and food intake. Increased food intake in cold temperatures is an important survival mechanism; it increases the metabolic rate, which helps generate heat, and increases fat stores that provide insulation to reduce heat loss.[9]

Neurological and Hormonal Factors

Hormones, **neuroendocrine** (hormone-like) factors, and some drugs (including appetite suppressants) influence eating behavior through their direct or indirect effects on brain neurotransmitters.[10] Some hormones—cortisol, glucagon, insulin, and the gastrointestinal hormones secretin and cholecystokinin,[11]—have a short-term effect on eating behavior. In the brain, insulin appears to suppress food intake by inhibiting the synthesis of **neuropeptide Y (NPY)**,[12] a recently identified neuroendocrine factor that is a potent stimulator of food intake. A drop in insulin levels activates NPY. Within the hypothalamus, NPY triggers an integrated response that leads to decreased energy expenditure, increased food intake, and obesity.[13] NPY appears to stimulate a general desire to eat, rather than a specific desire for energy or a given macronutrient.[14]

The hormone **leptin** also appears to have a major role in regulating food intake. Fat cells produce this hormone, which tells the central nervous system just how much fat the body is storing. Leptin interacts with leptin receptors in the hypothalamus, where animal studies show that it suppresses appetite and increases energy expenditure.[15] When obese experimental animals that do not produce leptin are given the hormone, their weight normalizes. (See **Figure 8.4**.) A few rare cases of genetic leptin deficiency or abnormal leptin receptors have been identified in humans with profound overeating and weight gain. On the other hand, common human obesity is associated with increased, not decreased, leptin levels.[16]

neuroendocrine Related to cells that produce a hormone in response to a neural stimulus. These cells may be part of an endocrine gland, like the pancreas and adrenal glands, or may be neurons in the brain.

neuropeptide Y (NPY) A neurotransmitter widely distributed throughout the brain and peripheral nervous tissue. NPY activity has been linked to eating behavior, depression, anxiety, and cardiovascular function.

leptin A hormone produced by adipose cells that signals the amount of body fat content and influences food intake.

Quick Bites

Why do we have hunger pangs?

When the stomach has been without food for at least three hours, intense stomach contractions can begin, sometimes lasting two to three minutes. Healthy young people have the strongest contractions, due to good muscle tone in the GI tract. After 12 to 24 hours, contractions of an empty stomach can cause painful hunger pangs.

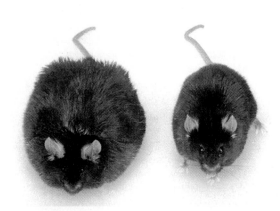

Figure 8.4 **Leptin and obesity in mice.**

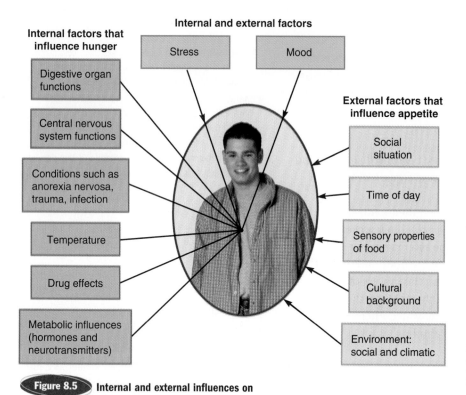

Internal factors that influence hunger

- Digestive organ functions
- Central nervous system functions
- Conditions such as anorexia nervosa, trauma, infection
- Temperature
- Drug effects
- Metabolic influences (hormones and neurotransmitters)

Internal and external factors

- Stress
- Mood

External factors that influence appetite

- Social situation
- Time of day
- Sensory properties of food
- Cultural background
- Environment: social and climatic

Figure 8.5 Internal and external influences on hunger and appetite.

Quick Bites

Brrr! Shivering Away Calories

Cold weather increases energy needs. Shivering alone can increase the RMR by 2.5 times. Although shivering bodies use both fat and carbohydrate, carbohydrates are the preferred fuel. In addition, people with less body fat shiver more in the cold.

total energy expenditure The total of the resting energy expenditure (REE), energy used in physical activity, energy used in processing food (TEF), and adaptive thermogenesis (minor) expressed in kilocalories per day.

resting energy expenditure (REE) The minimum energy needed to maintain basic physiological functions (e.g., heartbeat, muscle function, and respiration).

basal metabolic rate (BMR) A clinical measure of resting energy expenditure performed upon awakening, 10 to 12 hours after eating, and 12 to 18 hours after significant physical activity. Often used interchangeably with RMR.

resting metabolic rate (RMR) A clinical measure of resting energy expenditure performed three to four hours after eating or performing significant physical activity. Often used interchangeably with BMR.

lean body mass The portion of the body exclusive of stored fat, including muscle, bone, connective tissue, organs, and water.

Environmental and Social Factors

External factors and cues also affect food intake. Food's sensory properties—flavor, texture, color, temperature, and presentation—influence its appeal. The aroma of freshly baked bread or the warmth and softness of chocolate chip cookies right out of the oven encourage us to consume more than our hunger dictates!

Time of day, social circumstances, and cultural preferences also influence our appetite. (See **Figure 8.5**.) Many Americans would find pancakes, bacon, and eggs appealing at breakfast, but they would reject a ham sandwich, macaroni and cheese, or chicken stir-fry for their morning meal. Cultural backgrounds and social situations strongly define what we find acceptable or unacceptable as food or as part of a meal (e.g., chips and pretzels for snacks at a party, but not for a formal dinner). For more on cultural influences, see Chapter 1.

Key Concepts: *Many factors in the digestive tract, central nervous system, and general circulation interact to influence feeding behavior. The brain, especially the hypothalamus, receives signals from all over the body about energy status. Two factors currently being studied intensively are neuropeptide Y—a factor that stimulates feeding—and the hormone leptin. External factors also influence what we eat. Time of day, season of the year, social circumstances, and cultural traditions, as well as the food itself can enhance or suppress appetite.*

Energy Out: Uses of Fuel

Energy output, or expenditure, is the amount of fuel the body uses. It has three major components:

1. energy to maintain basic physiological functions such as breathing and blood circulation,
2. energy to process the food we eat, and
3. energy for physical activity.

Other energy costs include growth, body temperature maintenance in cold environments, physical trauma, fever, psychological stress, and drug metabolism. The sum of all energy expended is the **total energy expenditure (TEE)**. **Figure 8.6** illustrates the major components of energy expenditure.

Major Components of Energy Expenditure

Energy Expenditure at Rest

For most people, the major portion of expended energy goes to maintain basic body functions: heartbeat, respiration, nervous function, muscle tone, body temperature, and so on. This minimum energy necessary to sustain life is called the **resting energy expenditure (REE)**. The rate of energy expended at rest (as kcal/hr or kcal/d) is measured as either the **basal metabolic rate (BMR)** or the **resting metabolic rate (RMR)**. Researchers measure BMR under the following conditions:

1. the person is lying at rest,
2. the person just awoke from a normal overnight sleep,
3. 10 to 12 hours have elapsed since the person's last meal, and
4. no physical activity has taken place—usually for 12 to 18 hours since the last extreme bout.

The RMR differs slightly from the BMR. Researchers usually measure RMR three to four hours after a person eats or does significant physical work. BMR and RMR are virtually interchangeable; it's just that the ideal conditions for BMR are harder to meet. For this reason, in the remainder of this text we will use the terms *resting metabolic rate (RMR)* and *resting energy expenditure (REE)*.

Factors That Affect RMR. Over time, your RMR varies less than 5 percent. However, among different people, RMR can vary by as much as 25 percent; individual differences in muscle and organ mass account for most of this variation. Resting muscles and organ tissue make the greatest contribution to RMR because they have greater metabolic activity than other tissue such as fat. (See **Table 8.1**.) Muscles, organs, bones, and fluids make up most of the **lean body mass**—the total mass of the body that isn't fat. Differences in lean body mass explain 60 to 80 percent of the variation in resting metabolic rate among individuals.[17] As a result, an extremely muscular person with a large lean body mass has a higher resting energy expenditure than someone who weighs the same but has a higher proportion of body fat.

Age, sex, degree of muscle development, and, of course, body size are the primary influences on a person's lean body mass. (See **Figure 8.7**.) In the aging adult, lean body mass tends to decrease while body fatness rises, resulting in a RMR reduction of about 2 to 3 percent per decade.[18] However, declining lean body mass does not account fully for the age-related decline in RMR, which also may reflect declining organ function.[19] Keeping physically active as we age helps slow loss of lean tissue and discourages gain of fat, thus maintaining a higher RMR.

Women tend to be smaller than men, and pound for pound they generally have less lean body mass. Yet even when differences in lean body mass are taken into account, a man's metabolic rate is still about 50 kilocalories per day higher than that of a woman.[20] The reason is unclear, but this difference

Table 8.1	Approximate Energy Expenditure of Organs in Adults
Organ	**Percentage of RMR**
Liver	29
Brain	19
Heart	10
Kidney	7
Skeletal muscles (at rest)	18
Remainder (including bone)	17
	100

Source: Mahan LK, Escott-Stump S. *Krause's Food, Nutrition and Diet Therapy.* 10th ed. Philadelphia: WB Saunders; 2000:20. Reprinted by permission of the publisher.

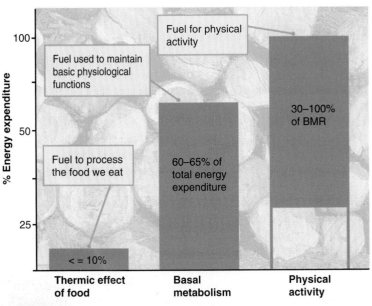

Figure 8.6 Major components of energy expenditure.

Increase RMR

- Total body weight
- Large body surface area
- Hot and cold ambient temperature
- Fever
- Hyperthyroidism
- Stress
- Caffeine
- Smoking
- Increased lean body mass
- Rapid growth
- Pregnancy and lactation

- Genetics
- Some medications

- Aging
- Female gender
- Fasting / starvation
- Hypothyroidism
- Sleep

Decrease RMR

Figure 8.7 Factors that affect RMR.

is consistent throughout the lives of men and women. RMR also varies during the menstrual cycle, fluctuating from the low point about one week before ovulation to the high point just before the onset of menstruation.[21]

Together, body composition, age, fitness, sex, and genetics account for 80 to 90 percent of the variation in the metabolic rate. Other factors may be less consistent, of shorter duration, or limited to individual situations. During sleep, RMR falls about 10 percent. RMR relative to lean body mass rises during periods of rapid growth, such as in infancy and adolescence. Hormones, especially thyroxine (thyroid hormone) and norepinephrine help regulate metabolic rate. Inadequate thyroxine production (hypothyroidism) can slow the metabolic rate; excess thyroxine (hyperthyroidism) can increase the metabolic rate. Physical stress increases the metabolic rate, probably in response to changes in norepinephrine levels. Fever increases RMR by about 7 percent for each degree of temperature over 98.6°F. Environmental temperature also affects the metabolic rate. During exposure to cold, RMR increases. As ambient temperatures rise above normal, RMR first decreases and then plateaus. At much higher temperatures, RMR increases. During starvation, the metabolic rate declines as the body slows basic functions to conserve energy and prolong survival. Finally, some variation in RMR has been attributed to unknown genetic factors.[22]

Key Concepts: Energy expenditure has three major components: fuel for basic body functions, fuel to process the food we eat, and fuel that supports physical activity. Factors that affect resting energy expenditure include body composition, age, fitness, sex, genetics, stage of growth, hormone levels, fever, and nutritional status.

Energy Expenditure for Physical Activity

Physical activity is more than just exercise and sport. It includes work and leisure activities, other general daily activities, even fidgeting. The energy expended in physical activity typically ranges from 30 to 100 percent of the RMR.[23] Energy cost depends on the activity's duration, type (whether it is

---

[*Fyi*] What's Neat About NEAT?

FOR YOUR INFORMATION

It seems Jan only has to look at food to gain weight. Yet her same-size friend Molly doesn't seem to gain weight no matter what she eats. Both eat about the same amount of calories and get about the same amount of exercise. So what's missing? Recent research suggests that fidgeting and movements such as posture adjustments may be part of the answer.

Studies in the early 1900s were the first to suggest that weight gained in response to overeating wasn't proportional to the extra calories ingested. Following experiments on himself, the German scientist Neumann coined the term "luxuskonsumption" to describe his observation that excess calories did not result in weight gain and therefore must be lost as

heat.[1] Further studies supported this idea, showing wide individual variation in response to overfeeding. Some suggest that the ease of weight gain is genetically based.[2]

A recent study at the Mayo Clinic attributes differences in weight gain in response to overfeeding to a mechanism described as NEAT: Non-Exercise Activity Thermogenesis.[3] According to the researchers, NEAT is "the thermogenesis (heat production) that accompanies physical activities other than volitional (intentional) exercise, such as the activities of daily living, fidgeting, spontaneous muscle contraction, and maintaining posture when not recumbent."

In the NEAT study, 16 volunteers (12 men and 4 women) were given an extra 1,000 kilo-

calories per day—roughly equivalent to two double cheeseburgers—for a period of 8 weeks. Prior to the overfeeding, careful measurements were made over a two-week period to determine maintenance energy requirements. Physical activity during the study was controlled, and meals were provided only through the Mayo Clinic General Clinical Research Center. Questionnaires and interviews were done to assure compliance.

The average weight gained by the study participants was 4.7 kilograms (10.3 lb), but some gained as much as 7.2 kilograms (15.8 lb), while others added only 1.4 kilograms (3.1 lb). The theoretical expected weight gain from an 8-week excess of 56,000 kilocalories,

walking, running, or typing, for example), and intensity. **Table 8.2** shows the amounts of energy expended in some specific activities. Body size affects energy cost, too—it takes more energy to move a bigger mass, so a large person expends more calories per minute than a smaller person doing the same activity. Fitness level has an effect, as well. Individuals who are fit exercise more efficiently, with lower energy costs. However, they will be able to exercise with greater intensity and duration, burning more calories overall.

Even though you feel worn out after studying hard for an exam, mental activity uses little energy. However, if you can't seem to sit still when studying, fidgeting may be a significant contributor to your energy output. The recently coined term **NEAT** stands for **nonexercise activity thermogenesis**, which is the energy associated with fidgeting, maintenance of posture, and similar contributors to energy expenditure.[24]

Energy Expenditure to Process Food

After we eat, our bodies expend energy to digest, absorb, and metabolize nutrients—processes that generate heat. This energy output is collectively called the **thermic effect of food (TEF)**. The TEF is lowest for fat and highest for protein. Converting excess protein and carbohydrate to energy stores (fat and glycogen) requires more energy than the efficient process of simply storing excess dietary fat as body fat. TEF peaks about one hour after eating and normally dissipates within five hours. For a typical mixed diet, TEF accounts for approximately 10 percent or less of total energy expenditure. It's possible to increase the TEF by altering the macronutrient composition of the diet, but not by much—only about 50 kilocalories or so daily.

Key Concepts: *An individual's fitness level, weight, and the duration, type, and intensity of activity affect the amount of energy expended in physical activity. The thermic effect of food is the energy needed to process the food we eat and is influenced by the amount and mix of nutrients in the diet.*

> **nonexercise activity thermogenesis (NEAT)** The output of energy associated with fidgeting, maintenance of posture, and other minimal physical exertions.
>
> **thermic effect of food (TEF)** The energy used to digest, absorb, and metabolize energy-yielding foodstuffs. It constitutes about 10 percent of total energy expenditure but is influenced by various factors. Also called dietary-induced thermogenesis (DIT) and meal-induced thermogenesis (MIT).

---

would be 7.3 kilograms (16.0 lb) to 9.1 kilograms (20.0 lb)—more than the maximum weight gain of any participant!

After accounting for RMR, TEF, and energy expended in physical activity, the remaining energy expenditure was attributed to NEAT. The amount of energy expended as NEAT varied among the participants by nearly 800 kilocalories per day. Participants with higher NEAT were resistant to weight gain, suggesting that people who can effectively activate NEAT tend not to gain weight, even with overeating. Further, this suggests that obesity may be related to an ineffective activation of NEAT.

Leptin levels do not appear to regulate NEAT. The participants' leptin levels were related to their changes in body fat but not to changes in their energy expenditure as NEAT.[4]

So is the take-home message, "fidget more, stand up straight, and you won't gain weight?" Not exactly. The researchers did not account for factors such as the extra energy needed to move a higher body weight in activity. In addition, they relied on self-reports and pedometers that lack precision and accuracy.[5] Attributing the entire difference in energy expenditure to NEAT ignores heat production by brown adipose tissue, a type of fat tissue that tends to "waste" energy.[6] Clearly, though, there are mechanisms in some individuals that tend to resist weight gain, and further studies may help to identify and quantify NEAT.

1 Neumann RO. Experimentalle Beitrage zur Lehre von dem taglichen Nahrungsbedarf der Menschen unter besonder Berucksichtigung der notwendigen Eisewissmenge. *Arch Hyg.* 1902;45:1–2.

2 Bouchard C, Tremblay A, Despres JP, et al. The response to long-term overfeeding in identical twins. *N Engl J Med.* 1990;322:1477–1482.

3 Levine JA, Eberhardt NL, Jensen MD. Role of nonexercise activity thermogenesis in resistance to fat gain in humans. *Science.* 1999;283:212–214.

4 Levine JA, Eberhardt NL, Jensen MD. Leptin responses to overfeeding: relationship with body fat and nonexercise activity thermogenesis. *J Clin Endocrinol Metab.* 1999;84:2751–2754.

5 Ravussin E, Danforth E. Beyond sloth – physical activity and weight gain. *Science.* 1999;283:184–185.

6 Napoli R, Horton ES. Energy Requirements. In: Ziegler EE, Filer LJ, eds. *Present Knowledge in Nutrition.* 7th ed. Washington, DC: ILSI Press; 1996; and Levine JA, Eberhardt NL, Jensen MD. Loc. cit.

Table 8.2 Amount of Energy Expended in Specific Activities

			Kcal/hr at Different Body Weights				
Description	kcal/hr/kg	kcal/hr/lb	*50 kg* *110 lb*	*57 kg* *125 lb*	*68 kg* *150 lb*	*80 kg* *175 lb*	*91 kg* *200 lb*
Aerobics							
light	3.0	1.36	150	170	205	239	273
moderate	5.0	2.27	250	284	341	398	455
heavy	8.0	3.64	400	455	545	636	727
Bicycling							
leisurely <10 mph	4.0	1.82	200	227	273	318	364
light 10–11.9 mph	6.0	2.73	300	341	409	477	545
moderate 12–13.9 mph	8.0	3.64	400	455	545	636	727
fast 14–15.9 mph	10.0	4.55	500	568	682	795	909
racing 16–19 mph	12.0	5.45	600	682	818	955	1091
BMX or mountain	8.5	3.86	425	483	580	676	773
Daily Activities							
sleeping	1.2	0.55	60	68	82	95	109
studying, reading, writing	1.8	0.82	90	102	123	143	164
cooking, food preparation	2.5	1.14	125	142	170	199	227
Home Activities							
house painting, outside	4.0	1.82	200	227	273	318	364
general gardening	5.0	2.27	250	284	341	398	455
shoveling snow	6.0	2.73	300	341	409	477	545
Running							
jogging	7.0	3.18	350	398	477	557	636
running 5 mph	8.0	3.64	400	455	545	636	727
running 6 mph	10.0	4.55	500	568	682	795	909
running 7 mph	11.5	5.23	575	653	784	915	1045
running 8 mph	13.5	6.14	675	767	920	1074	1227
running 9 mph	15.0	6.82	750	852	1023	1193	1364
running 10 mph	16.0	7.27	800	909	1091	1273	1455
Sports							
Frisbee, ultimate	3.5	1.59	175	199	239	278	318
hacky sack	4.0	1.82	200	227	273	318	364
wind surfing	4.2	1.91	210	239	286	334	382
golf	4.5	2.05	225	256	307	358	409
skateboarding	5.0	2.27	250	284	341	398	455
rollerblading	7.0	3.18	350	398	477	557	636
soccer	7.0	3.18	350	398	477	557	636
field hockey	8.0	3.64	400	455	545	636	727
swimming, slow to moderate laps	8.0	3.64	400	455	545	636	727
skiing downhill, moderate effort	6.0	2.73	300	341	409	477	545
skiing cross country, moderate effort	8.0	3.64	400	455	545	636	727
tennis, doubles	6.0	2.73	300	341	409	477	545
tennis, singles	8.0	3.64	400	455	545	636	727
Walking							
strolling <2 mph, level	2.0	0.91	100	114	136	159	182
moderate pace ~3 mph, level	3.5	1.59	175	199	239	278	318
brisk pace ~3.5 mph, level	4.0	1.82	200	227	273	318	364
very brisk pace ~4.5 mph, level	4.5	2.05	225	256	307	358	409
moderate pace ~3 mph, uphill	6.0	2.73	300	341	409	477	545

Source: Adapted from Nieman, DC. *Exercise Testing and Prescription.* 4th ed. Mountain View, CA: Mayfield Publishing; 1999.

The Measurement of Energy Expenditure

Calorimetry, the measurement of energy expenditure, helps us understand individual differences in energy expenditure and the effects of environmental conditions, as well as age, sex, exercise, and other factors.

A Brief History of Calorimetry

Antoine Lavoisier, an eighteenth-century French chemist, was the first to study food combustion in the body. He theorized that just as a burning candle needs oxygen and releases heat, organisms need oxygen to live and release heat as they combust food.

Lavoisier built the first **calorimeter**, quite an achievement at that time. A calorimeter consists of a chamber within a chamber. The inner chamber is large enough to house an animal or human; the outer chamber is sensitive to temperature changes that occur in the inner one. Lavoisier packed ice into a sealed pocket around the inner chamber (his studies were possible only in winter when ice was plentiful), then placed it inside the outer chamber, which was insulated to shield it from the outside environment. As the animal in the inner chamber used energy, it produced heat that melted the ice. By collecting the resulting water and measuring its volume, Lavoisier could accurately calculate the amount of heat the animal produced.

Direct and Indirect Calorimetry

Lavoisier's technique illustrates the principles of **direct calorimetry**. When your body combusts food, it captures some energy while losing the rest as heat. This heat loss is proportional to the body's total energy use and can be measured directly using a chamber like that of Lavoisier. Modern chambers dispense with the ice and instead measure the temperature change in a surrounding layer of water.

Direct calorimetry is expensive and complex. The chamber must be large enough to accommodate a person, yet maintain the precision to measure the relatively small changes of temperature. Since the advent of alternative methods, direct calorimetry is no longer widely used.

Indirect calorimetry is easier and less expensive than direct calorimetry. It is "indirect" because energy production (as heat) is not measured directly. Instead energy expenditure is estimated from a person's oxygen consumption and carbon dioxide production. (See **Figure 8.8**.) Burning (oxidizing) fuel consumes oxygen and produces carbon dioxide in proportion to the amount of fuel burned and the amount of energy released.

For indirect calorimetry, a technician collects respiratory gases. For short periods of rest or exercise, expired air can be collected using a face mask,

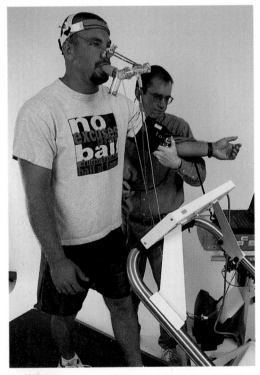

Figure 8.8 Measuring energy expended in physical activity.

calorimetry [kal-oh-RIM-eh-tree] The measurement of the amount of heat given off by an organism. It is used to determine total energy expenditure.

calorimeter A device used to measure quantities of heat generated by various processes.

direct calorimetry Determination of energy use by the body by measuring the heat released from an organism enclosed in a small insulated chamber surrounded by water. The rise in the temperature of the water is directly related to the energy used by the organism.

indirect calorimetry Determination of energy use by the body without directly measuring the production of heat. Methods include gas exchange, the measurement of oxygen uptake and/or carbon dioxide output, and the doubly labeled water method.

doubly labeled water A method for measuring daily energy expenditure over extended time periods, typically 7 to 14 days, while subjects are living in their usual environment. Small amounts of water that is isotopically labeled with deuterium and oxygen-18 (^2H_2O and $H_2{}^{18}O$) are ingested. Energy expenditure can be calculated from the difference between the rates at which the body loses each isotope.

isotopes [EYE-so-towps] Forms of an element in which the atoms have the same number of protons but different numbers of neutrons.

Quick Bites

Double-Checking Dietary Recall

When researchers used the doubly labeled water method to check the validity of food diaries and dietary recalls, they found that obese people underreport their energy intake by 20 to 50 percent and lean people underreport by 10 to 30 percent. Energy expenditure in the obese subjects was normal relative to their body size.

mouthpiece, or canopy system. For periods of 24 hours or longer, the person stays inside a metabolic chamber, which measures the gas exchange. This cumbersome apparatus makes indirect calorimetry impractical for use during physically demanding activities or normal living conditions.

Doubly Labeled Water

A relatively new and easier technique to measure total energy expenditure is called **doubly labeled water**. (See **Figure 8.9**.) Rather than measuring respiratory gases, this indirect calorimetry technique relies on measuring the **isotopes** (a form of an element with a higher than usual atomic mass, but the same characteristics of the usual element) of hydrogen and oxygen in excreted water and carbon dioxide. A person swallows a small quantity of two kinds of water, one labeled with the hydrogen isotope deuterium ($^2H_2$), and the other labeled with an isotope of oxygen (oxygen-18, or ^{18}O). Both isotopes occur naturally and are nonradioactive. The body excretes oxygen-18 as part of water ($H_2{}^{18}O$) and carbon dioxide ($C^{18}O_2$). It excretes deuterium only as part of water (^2H_2O). Scientists use the difference between the rate of deuterium loss and ^{18}O loss to calculate carbon dioxide output and determine the total energy expenditure.

The doubly labeled water technique is noninvasive and unobtrusive. The subjects can stay in their normal environment and perform normal activities during the testing period, which typically lasts 7 to 14 days or longer.

The doubly labeled water method is emerging as the "gold standard" against which other methods are compared. For best accuracy, doubly labeled water studies should last at least 14 days. Unfortunately, the doubly labeled water technique is not widely available, and it's expensive—the ^{18}O isotope costs about $500 for a 70-kilogram adult, and the analytic equipment is costly. So the technique is not suited to large-scale studies. It has other limitations as well: it cannot give information about individual days, individual activities, or day-to-day variability.

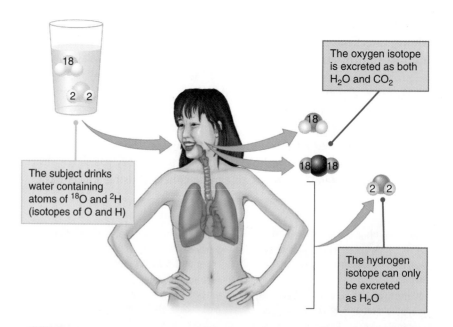

The oxygen isotope is excreted as both H_2O and CO_2

The subject drinks water containing atoms of ^{18}O and ^2H (isotopes of O and H)

The hydrogen isotope can only be excreted as H_2O

Figure 8.9 **Doubly labeled water.** When using doubly labeled water, scientists measure the excretion rates of the two isotopes to calculate carbon dioxide output and determine total energy expenditure.

Key Concepts: *Energy expenditure can be measured using direct or indirect calorimetry. Direct calorimetry measures heat production by the body, which is proportional to total energy use. Indirect calorimetry measures oxygen consumption and carbon dioxide production, from which energy use can be calculated. A third technique, the doubly labeled water method, is gaining acceptance as the "gold standard" for determining energy expenditure.*

Estimating Total Energy Expenditure

Directly measuring a person's total energy expenditure requires sophisticated equipment that is inaccessible to all but a few people in research settings. To determine the energy needs of most people, nutritionists must rely on calculated estimates.

We still use the classic equations that Harris and Benedict developed nearly 100 years ago to estimate REE. The **Harris-Benedict equations** are based on age, height, weight, and sex.[25] One drawback is that they can overestimate the resting energy expenditure, especially for obese people.[26] (See Appendix H for the conversion factors for kilograms and centimeters.)

More recent equations based on larger groups of subjects estimate REE from age, sex, and body weight.[27] (See **Table 8.3**.) These equations deliver estimates for a wide range of ages, including children and older people. Height is excluded because it was not found to influence the results appreciably.

For a quick and easy REE estimate, the abbreviated method provides good estimates for adults. However, it dramatically underestimates children's REE and somewhat overestimates older people's REE. The use of 1.0 kilocalorie per kilogram for men compared to 0.9 kilocalories per kilogram for women reflects their different body compositions. Men have proportionally more lean body mass, so they burn more calories per kilogram of body weight.

Energy expended in physical activity can be estimated as a multiple of REE based on a person's general activity level (see **Table 8.4**). The activity level for most of the U.S. population falls in the light or moderate categories.

The thermic effect of food is about 10 percent of the sum of REE plus energy expended in physical activity. Summation of the three estimated components—REE, physical activity, and TEF—delivers the estimated total energy expenditure. See the FYI feature "Mark's Energy Balance" for specific examples of these estimates.

Harris-Benedict equation An equation used to estimate REE based on a person's age, weight, height, and sex.

Harris-Benedict Equations

For adult men
$$REE = 66 + 13.7W + 5.0H - 6.8A.$$

For adult women
$$REE = 655 + 9.6W + 1.8H - 4.7A.$$

W = weight in kilograms
H = height in centimeters
A = age

Abbreviated Method to Estimate REE

For adult men
$$REE = weight~(kg) \times 1.0~kcal/kg \times 24~hr$$
$$REE = weight~(kg) \times 1.0 \times 24$$

For adult women
$$REE = weight~(kg) \times 0.9~kcal/kg \times 24~hr$$
$$REE = weight~(kg) \times 0.9 \times 24$$

Table 8.3 **Estimating REE from Body Weight, Sex, and Age**

Age (yr)	REE Males	REE Females
0–3	$(60.9 \times wt) - 54$	$(61.0 \times wt) - 51$
3–10	$(22.7 \times wt) + 495$	$(22.5 \times wt) + 499$
10–18	$(17.5 \times wt) + 651$	$(12.2 \times wt) + 746$
18–30	$(15.3 \times wt) + 679$	$(14.7 \times wt) + 496$
30–60	$(11.6 \times wt) + 879$	$(8.7 \times wt) + 829$
>60	$(13.5 \times wt) + 487$	$(10.5 \times wt) + 596$

Note: Body weight is in kg and REE is kcal per day.

Table 8.4 **Estimating Energy Expended in Physical Activity**

Percentage of REE	Activity Level	Description
20–30%	Sedentary	Mostly resting with little or no activity
30–45%	Light	Occasional unplanned activity, e.g., going for a stroll
45–65%	Moderate	Daily planned activity, such as brisk walks
65–90%	Heavy	Daily workout routine requiring several hours of continuous exercise
90–120%	Exceptional	Daily vigorous workouts for extended hours; training for competition

body composition The chemical or anatomical composition of the body. Commonly defined as the proportions of fat, muscle, bone, and other tissues in the body.

RDA for Energy

The tenth edition of the *Recommended Dietary Allowances* includes values for energy.[28] Unlike the RDAs for protein, vitamins, and minerals, those for energy represent *average* needs of individuals. If RDA values for energy were set like those for the other nutrients (at ~2 standard deviations *above* the mean), the energy RDA would greatly overestimate most people's energy needs. The energy RDAs are 2,200 kilocalories per day for females 19 to 50 years old, and 2,900 kilocalories per day for males 19 to 50 years old. These values assume light to moderate activity levels, and average weights of 55 kilograms (121 lb) for women and 70 kilograms (154 lb) for men.

Body Composition: Understanding Fatness and Weight

Body weight reflects a person's energy balance, yet many people have a distorted notion of their weight—thinking they're too fat when they are not, or thinking their weight is just fine, when it isn't. While it's simple to step onto a scale, weight alone does not tell the whole story because **body composition** is more important than weight in determining health risks. For example, an individual with a high weight for height may have excess adipose tissue and be considered obese, or he may be very fit and muscular and have no weight-related health risk.

Assessing Body Weight

Weight Tables

For a given height (and usually sex), weight tables provide a narrow range of body weights that are associated with good health and "acceptable" appearance. Some tables also take bone structure into account by including adjustments for frame size. Weight tables are quick, easy, and cheap,

---

[*Fyi*] Mark's Energy Balance

FOR YOUR INFORMATION

Mark, a college student, kept a one-day food and activity record. He consumed 3,000 kilocalories. His day included the typical activities of daily living (sleeping, small amounts of meal preparation, showering, etc.), studying, and briskly walking to and from class. He did not participate in any exercise class or fitness activities. Do you think Mark was in energy equilibrium or imbalance on the day he kept his food record? To find out, let's calculate his energy output by estimating his resting energy expenditure, energy expended in physical activity, and thermic effect of food.

Mark's characteristics are

Weight = 180 lb   180 ÷ 2.2 = 81.82 kg

Height = 6' 0"   72 x 2.54 = 182.88 cm
   (72 in.)

Age = 20 yr   BMI = 24.5 kg/m²

Activity = light to moderate

We can use the abbreviated equation to estimate Mark's *Resting Energy Expenditure (REE)*:

To estimate REE of adult men:
weight × 1.0 kcal/kg × 24 hr
Mark's REE = 81.82 kg × 1.0 kcal/kg × 24 hr
   REE = 1,964 kcal

Mark's *overall activity level* was light to moderate. Using Table 8.4, we find energy expended in this level of physical activity is about 45% of REE.

Mark's physical activity = 45% of 1,964 kcal
   Physical activity = 884 kcal

We can calculate Mark's *thermic effect of food* as 10 percent of the sum of his REE and physical activity expenditures:

Mark's TEF = 0.1 x (1,964 kcal + 884 kcal)
   TEF = 285 kcal

but they ignore body composition, fail to consider other measures of health and fitness, and foster a mentality that there is such a thing as "perfect weight."

Some weight tables rely on statistics from the Metropolitan Life Insurance Company, which identified the weights associated with the greatest longevity. The resulting tables contain "desirable weight" ranges based on height, sex, and body frame size. However, the data underlying these tables have several limitations. First, the data reflect only people who purchased insurance, so some population segments are underrepresented. Second, they do not take age into account. Also, the data were recorded when people bought the insurance, and were not updated to include weight changes over time; therefore, they may not actually represent the weights associated with longevity.

Body Mass Index

Body mass index (BMI), also known as the **Quetelet index**, correlates reasonably well with body fatness and health risks.[29] To determine your BMI, accurately measure your height without shoes and your weight with minimal clothing. Then use these numbers in the equation to calculate your BMI.

In 1998 the National Institutes of Health released the first federal guidelines on the identification, evaluation, and treatment of overweight and obesity.[30] These guidelines define obesity in adults as a BMI greater than 30 kg/m². Overweight is defined as 25 kg/m² to 29.9 kg/m². A normal range is generally considered to be 19 kg/m² to 24.9 kg/m². BMI under 19 kg/m² is considered underweight. The Dietary Guidelines for Americans suggest that we should "Aim for a Healthy Weight" and defines healthy weight as a BMI from 18.5 to 25 kg/m².[31] **Figure 8.10** shows the recommended weights.

body mass index (BMI) Body weight (in kilograms) divided by the square of height (in meters), expressed in units of kg/m². Also called Quetelet index.
Quetelet index see body mass index.

To calculate BMI

$$BMI = \frac{weight\ (kg)}{height\ (m)^2}, \text{ or}$$

$$BMI = \frac{weight\ (lb)}{height\ (in)^2} \times 704.5.$$

Now we can add it all up to estimate his *total energy expenditure.*

Mark's TEE = 1,964 kcal + 884 kcal + 285 kcal
TEE = 3,133 kcal

How do the results from other REE estimation methods compare to the abbreviated method? Using the *Harris-Benedict equation,*

REE[HB] = 66 + (13.7 × 81.82) + (5.0 × 182.88) − (6.8 × 20)
REE[HB] = 1,965 kcal (essentially the same as 1,964 kcal)

Harris-Benedict Equations
For adult men, REE[HB] = 66 + (13.7 × weight) + (5.0 × height) − (6.8 × age)
For adult women, REE[HB] = 655 + (9.6 × weight) + (1.8 × height) − (4.7 × age)

Using the equation table and Mark's *body weight, sex, and age* (see **Table 8.3**),
REE[ET] = (15.3 x 81.82) + 679
REE[ET] = 1,931 kcal (close to 1,964 kcal)

Equation Table for Estimating REE (Table 8.3)
For men age 18–30,
REE[ET] = (15.3 × weight) + 679

How does Mark's *energy balance* measure up?

Energy input	Energy output
Calories consumed	REE + physical activity + TEF
3,000 kcal	3,133 kcal

Mark's energy output this day slightly exceeds his energy intake by 133 kilocalories. If this imbalance continued, he would notice a slow, subtle weight loss.

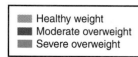

- Healthy weight
- Moderate overweight
- Severe overweight

Directions: Find your weight on the bottom of the graph. Go straight up from that point until you come to the line that matches your height. Then look to find your weight group.

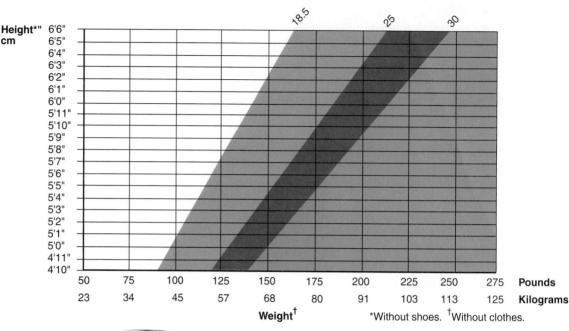

*Without shoes. †Without clothes.

Figure 8.10 **Are you at a healthy weight?** BMI measures weight in relation to height. The BMI ranges shown above are for adults. They are not exact ranges of healthy and unhealthy weights. However, they show that health risk increases at higher levels of overweight and obesity. Even within the healthy BMI range, weight gains can carry health risks for adults. **Source:** *Report of the Dietary Guidelines Advisory Committee on the Dietary Guidelines for Americans*, 2000, page 3.

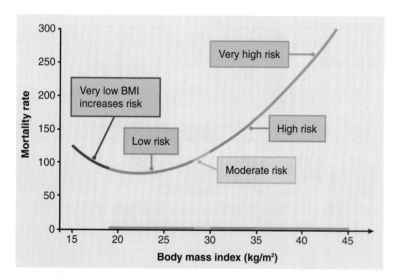

Figure 8.11 **BMI and mortality.** People with a very low or high BMI have a higher relative mortality.

Correlating BMI with health risk produces a J-shaped curve: those with low BMI (<20 kg/m^2) have a higher relative mortality, as do those with a high BMI (30 kg/m^2 to 35 kg/m^2). Mortality rates then rise more steeply after BMI exceeds 35 kg/m^2. (See **Figure 8.11**.)

Although BMI is an improvement over weight measures for indicating excessive body fatness, BMI still has a limited ability to distinguish between muscle weight and excess fat weight. A classic example is the heavy football player or bodybuilder with a large muscle mass who has a BMI greater than 30 kg/m^2 but is not obese. The NIH guidelines and Dietary Guidelines for Americans also suggest evaluating risk factors associated with obesity such as high blood pressure, high blood cholesterol, family history of obesity-related disease, or excess abdominal fat (measured by waist circumference) before recommending weight loss or other treatment.

It has been suggested that BMI should not be used with children because they are still growing.[32] In the United States, BMI declines from birth until about age 4 to 6 years and then gradually increases through adolescence.[33] A committee of pediatric obesity experts concluded that BMI-for-age can be used as a screening tool for obesity[34] and recently, age- and sex-specific definitions of overweight and obesity based on BMI have been established using international data.[35]

Revised pediatric growth charts released in 2000 include sex-specific percentile curves for BMI for children aged 2 to 20 years.[36] A BMI-for-age at or above the 95th percentile indicates the need for further evaluation and possible treatment. Further evaluation may also be indicated if the child's

BMI-for-age is at or above the 85th percentile and is accompanied by other risk factors (mentioned above).[37] A child with a BMI-for-age that is below the fifth percentile is considered underweight.

Key Concepts: Body composition is a key element in determining energy expenditure and risk of disease. Measures of weight and height are used to identify overweight and obesity, but height-weight tables do not address body composition. Weight and height measures can be used to calculate BMI, which is a better assessment tool. Elevated BMIs in adults or children can increase health risks.

Assessing Body Fatness

Body composition is the relative amount of fat and lean body mass. Body composition measures help eliminate the need to guess if excess weight is muscle or fat. Also, such measures can signal when "normal" weight is actually excess fluid or fat masking wasted muscles and organs. The desirable range of body fat in adult women is 20 to 25 percent of total body weight and in men, 12 to 20 percent. When body fat exceeds 30 percent in women or 25 percent in men the risk of chronic disease rises dramatically. There are several indirect methods for measuring body composition and each has shortcomings.

Densitometry is the measure of body density (body mass divided body volume). Since fat and lean tissues have different densities, if we know the person's volume and weight, we can calculate the ratio of fat to lean body mass. The density of fat doesn't vary; however, hydration status, age, sex, and ethnicity all influence the density of lean body mass. For example, bone loss in the elderly leads to a lower density of lean body mass.

Densitometry and Underwater Weighing

Underwater weighing, also called **hydrostatic weighing**, is a common densitometry method for research studies. A seated person is submerged fully in water and weighed, as **Figure 8.12** illustrates. Body density is calculated using the above-water weight, the submerged weight, and the quantity of water displaced during submersion. Underwater weighing often is impractical because it requires a special water tank and other nonportable, expensive equipment. The subject must exhale completely, submerge without taking a breath, and remain motionless until the water is still and the scale is steady—clearly not the experience for everyone!

Densitometry and Air Displacement

Air displacement is more practical to measure than water displacement. With a newly developed device, the **BodPod**, densitometric determinations have become faster and easier. A person sits in a sealed chamber of known volume and displaces a certain volume of air. This technique is similar to underwater weighing, but researchers use air displacement, rather than water displacement, to calculate body density. **Figure 8.13** shows an air displacement chamber.

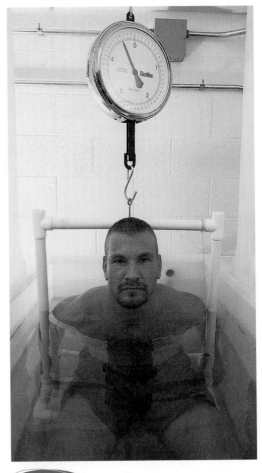

Figure 8.12 Underwater weighing.

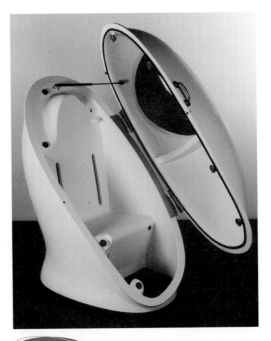

Figure 8.13 BodPod.

densitometry A method for estimating body composition from measurement of total body density.

hydrostatic weighing Determining body density by measuring the volume of water displaced when the body is fully submerged in a specialized water tank. Also called underwater weighing.

underwater weighing See hydrostatic weighing.

BodPod A device used to measure the density of the body based on the volume of air displaced as a person sits in a sealed chamber of known volume.

dual energy x-ray absorptiometry (DEXA)
A technique originally developed to measure bone density now also used to measure body composition.

total body water All of the water in the body, including intracellular and extracellular water, and water in the urinary and GI tracts.

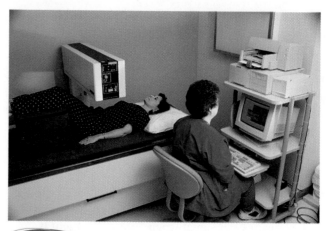

Figure 8.14 DEXA (dual-energy x-ray absorptiometry scan).

The Fattest Mammals

Among mammals, humans carry the largest percentage of weight as body fat.

Dual Energy X-Ray Absorptiometry

Dual energy x-ray absorptiometry (DEXA) is a relatively new technique that originally was used to measure bone density. Today, researchers also use it to analyze body composition by differentiating bone, other lean tissue, and fat.[38] A person undergoing a DEXA scan lies on a padded table while an x-ray detector above scans from head to foot, producing a two-dimensional image of tiny dots, or pixels (**Figure 8.14**). Although the DEXA scan is an excellent technique, its accuracy in obese people and the effects of tissue thickness and hydration status on scan accuracy are unclear. Furthermore, the instrument is expensive and not practical for everyday use in the field.

Isotope Dilution

Researchers can directly measure **total body water** and use this quantity to estimate lean body mass. The subject swallows a known quantity and concentration of isotopically labeled water. Unlike doubly labeled water, which uses and compares two isotopes, this technique uses a single isotope to label the water. After three or four hours, it is assumed that the labeled water is fully mixed in the body's water pool. The researcher takes a sample of body water (e.g., from plasma, saliva, or urine), measures the concentration of the isotopes, and calculates the total volume of body water. Based on the assumption that lean body mass is 73 percent water, researchers can estimate the total lean body mass. Unfortunately, this assumption does not hold true for all people; the amount of water in lean body mass can vary, especially in the elderly. Obesity and dehydration from severe exercise and use of diuretics or laxatives also may influence the results.

Skinfold Thickness

As you learned in Chapter 2, skinfold thickness is often used to measure body fatness. Typically, more than half of body fat is right under the skin, and the percentage increases as body weight increases.[39]

A special caliper is used to measure skinfold thickness at several sites on the body, typically over the triceps muscles on the back of the upper arm, just below the shoulder blade, near the navel, and over the hips. Predictive equations then estimate regional and total body fatness.

Because of its simplicity, and the relatively low cost (< $500 for calipers), skinfold anthropometry has become popular in health clubs and weight-control programs. Skinfold measures are also widely used in large population studies. Done correctly, body composition estimates from skinfolds correlate well with those from underwater weighing, but an inexperienced or careless measurer can easily make large errors. Skinfold thicknesses are especially useful in tracking the changes in subcutaneous fat distribution in an individual over time. They usually work better for monitoring malnutrition, rather than for identifying overweight and obesity.

Bioelectrical Impedance Analysis

Bioelectrical impedance analysis (BIA) measures the rate at which a small electric current flows through the body between electrodes placed on the wrist and ankle. (See **Figure 8.15**.) Fat doesn't conduct electricity well; it resists, or impedes, the current. In contrast, electrolyte-containing fluids readily conduct a current. These fluids are found mostly in lean body tissues so the leaner the person, the less the resistance. From the impedance reading, the researcher calculates total body water and then estimates total lean body mass and body fatness.

Compared to underwater weighing, results of BIA usually are as good as and often slightly better than skinfold measurements in assessing body fatness.[40] Just as in the isotope dilution method, age, obesity, and altered hydration can affect the accuracy of BIA results. Despite its limitations, bioelectrical impedance is accepted as a valuable tool for measuring body composition in field studies. The equipment is easily portable and only moderately expensive ($2,500–$8,000), making the technique popular at upscale health clubs and weight-loss centers. Similar to BIA, total body electrical conductivity (TOBEC) is an acceptably accurate measure of conductivity, but is less widely used because the equipment is expensive.

Computed Tomography and Magnetic Resonance Imaging

Although **computed tomography (CT)** and **magnetic resonance imaging (MRI)** are primarily medical diagnostic techniques, researchers can use them to distinguish and quantify body tissues. CT scans use x-ray beams to produce highly detailed cross-sectional images of body tissues (**Figure 8.16**), and MRI technology uses a magnetic field and radio-frequency waves to produce both cross-sectional images and chemical analysis of body tissues. But CT and MRI are costly techniques limited to research settings, and CT scans entail exposure to radiation.

Near-Infrared Interactance

Near-infrared interactance uses the principle that materials of different composition absorb, reflect, or transmit infrared light at different rates. A probe acts as an infrared transmitter and detector. Placed on the biceps muscle, it transmits infrared light through the skin and detects the amount reflected. Analysis of the transmitted and reflected values can estimate body composition. The method, though instantly popular in health clubs and athletic departments, has not yet been validated and appears to overestimate body fat in lean subjects and underestimate fatness in the obese. Experts do not currently recommend it for body composition assessment.[41]

Key Concepts: *Body fatness can be assessed by several methods. Underwater weighing uses the principle of density to determine relative amounts of fat-free and fat mass. Skinfold measures assess the thickness of fat deposits directly underneath the skin. Bioelectrical impedance (BIA) uses differences in resistance to an electric current to determine amounts of lean tissue. More sophisticated techniques such as dual energy x-ray absorptiometry (DEXA), isotope dilution, CT and MRI scans more accurately assess body composition; however, their expense may limit their usefulness on a large scale.*

bioelectrical impedance analysis (BIA) Technique using the resistance of tissue to the flow of an alternating electric current to estimate amounts of total body water, lean tissue mass, and total body fat.

computed tomography (CT) The gathering of anatomical information from cross-sectional images generated by a computer synthesis of x-ray data.

magnetic resonance imaging (MRI) Medical imaging technique that uses a magnetic field and radiofrequency radiation to generate anatomical information.

near-infrared interactance The measurement of body composition using infrared radiation. It is based on the principle that substances of different densities absorb, reflect, or transmit infrared light at different rates.

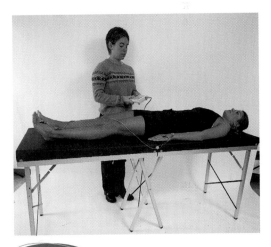

Figure 8.15 Bioelectrical impedance.

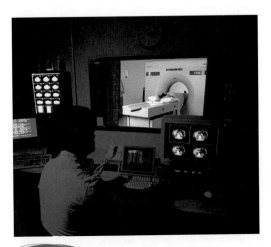

Figure 8.16 CT scans produce detailed cross-sectional images.

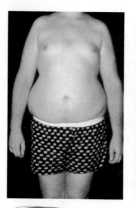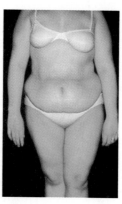

Figure 8.17 Body fat distribution.

Body Fat Distribution

Just as body weight doesn't tell the whole story in determining obesity and health risk, body fatness may also give an incomplete picture. The location of fat—**body fat distribution**—can also be a risk factor, independent of total body fat.[42] The "pear shape," or **gynoid** obesity more common in women, has fat distributed predominantly around the hips and thighs. The "apple shape," or **android** obesity typical of men, has extra fat distributed higher up, around the abdomen. The apple pattern of fat distribution is associated with a decidedly greater health risk than the pear pattern of fat distribution. **Figure 8.17** shows the apple-shaped and pear-shaped distributions of fat.

Excess abdominal fat appears to raise blood lipid levels, which in turn interferes with insulin function. Consequently, it has been linked to high blood lipids, glucose intolerance and insulin resistance, and high blood pressure; it increases risk of heart disease and diabetes mellitus. The risks exist for both men and women who have excess abdominal fat. In fact, android obesity may indicate an increased breast cancer risk for women.[43]

Waist Circumference

Waist circumference is used to assess abdominal fatness. *The Dietary Guidelines for Americans* suggests that if your waist measurement increases, you are probably gaining fat. NIH clinical guidelines suggest that for people with a BMI of 25 kg/m² to 34.9 kg/m², a waist circumference of larger than 40 inches in men or larger than 35 inches in women is a sign of increased health risk. When BMI is 35 kg/m² or higher, waist circumference measures lose their power to predict health risks.

Key Concepts: *Distribution of body fat is important in evaluating risk of disease. Excess body fat around the abdomen (even with normal to slightly elevated BMI) is associated with higher disease risk. Waist circumference can be used to assess body fat distribution.*

When Energy Balance Goes Awry

Despite its intricate system of regulating energy balance, the body's ability to maintain a normal weight can be overwhelmed, resulting in overweight, obesity, or underweight.

Overweight is generally defined as a BMI greater than 25 but less than 30, or body weight that is 10 to 20 percent above desirable weight or the recommended weight range in a height-weight table. Technically, it is an excess of a total body weight that includes all body tissues—fat, bone muscle, water, and so on.

Obesity is generally defined as a BMI greater than or equal to 30, or a body weight that is 20 percent or more above the recommended weight range in a height-weight table. The definition of obesity assumes an excess of body fat.

Underweight is generally defined as 15 to 20 percent or more below desirable weight for height. This condition is much less common than overweight and obesity and may result from an underlying illness. We will discuss underweight briefly at the end of this chapter.

Health Risks of Overweight and Obesity

Overweight and obesity are major public health challenges. In 1998, 55 percent of the adult American population was estimated to be overweight or obese (BMI ≥ 25).[44] Obese people are at higher risk for heart disease,

body fat distribution The pattern of fat distribution on the body.

gynoid obesity Excess storage of fat located primarily in the buttocks and thighs. Also called gynecoid obesity.

android obesity [AN-droyd] Excess storage of fat is located primarily in the abdominal area.

waist circumference The waist measurement, as a marker of abdominal fat content, can be used to indicate health risks.

overweight Body weight in relation to height that is greater than some accepted standard but less than that defined as obesity.

obesity Excessive accumulation of body fat leading to a body weight in relation to height that is substantially greater than some accepted standard.

underweight Body weight in relation to height that is less than some accepted standard.

the leading cause of death in the United States, and for stroke, diabetes, hypertension, some forms of cancer, gallbladder and joint diseases, and psychosocial problems. The longer obesity persists, the higher the risks. Table 8.5 lists the effects that being overweight could have on your health.

The blood lipid levels that typically accompany obesity—high serum triglycerides, low high-density lipoproteins, and a high ratio of low-density lipoproteins to high-density lipoproteins—increase the risk for atherosclerosis.[45] Even a person who is only mildly to moderately obese has an elevated risk of coronary heart disease. However, modest weight loss (about 10 percent of body weight) reduces risk.

Type 2 diabetes, the most common form of diabetes in the United States, is three times more likely to develop in people who are obese, especially if they have abdominal ("apple") obesity. Obesity increases insulin resistance and compromises glucose tolerance. Diabetes in turn is a risk factor for heart disease, kidney disease, and vascular problems. Again, modest levels of weight reduction can improve glucose tolerance.

Weight loss lowers blood pressure in overweight people. Overweight people are two to six times more likely to develop hypertension,[46]

Quick Bites

Where's the fat?

The location of excess abdominal fat may hold information about health risks. Within the abdomen, visceral fat—fat surrounding the organs may be more harmful than subcutaneous fat—fat under the skin. Only imaging can distinguish between the two.

Table 8.5   **What Are the Risks of Being Overweight?**

Hypertension

Overweight people are more likely to have high blood pressure, a major risk factor for heart disease and stroke, than people who are not overweight.

Heart Disease and Stroke

Hypertension, very high blood levels of cholesterol and triglycerides (blood fats) can lead to heart disease and often are linked to being overweight. Being overweight also contributes to angina (chest pain caused by decreased oxygen to the heart) and sudden death from heart disease or stroke without any signs or symptoms.

Diabetes

Overweight people are twice as likely to develop type 2 diabetes as people who are not overweight. Type 2 diabetes is a major cause of early death, heart disease, kidney disease, stroke, and blindness.

Cancer

Several types of cancer are associated with being overweight. In women, these include cancer of the uterus, gallbladder, cervix, ovary, breast, and colon. Overweight men are at greater risk for developing cancer of the colon, rectum, and prostate. For some types of cancer, such as colon or breast, it is not clear whether the increased risk is due to the extra weight or a high-fat and high-calorie diet.

Sleep Apnea

Sleep apnea is a serious condition that is closely associated with being overweight. Sleep apnea can cause a person to stop breathing for short periods during sleep and to snore heavily. Sleep apnea may cause daytime sleepiness and even heart failure. The risk for sleep apnea increases with higher body weights. Weight loss usually improves sleep apnea.

Osteoarthritis

Extra weight appears to increase the risk of osteoarthritis by placing extra pressure on weight-bearing joints and wearing away the cartilage (tissue that cushions the joints) that normally protects them. Weight loss can decrease stress on the knees, hips, and lower back and may improve the symptoms of osteoarthritis.

Gout

Gout is a joint disease caused by high levels of uric acid in the blood. Uric acid sometimes forms into solid stone or crystal masses that become deposited in the joints. Gout is more common in overweight people and the risk of developing the disorder increases with higher body weights.

Note: *Over the short term, some weight loss diets may lead to an attack of gout in people who have high levels of uric acid or who have had gout before. People who have a history of gout should check with their doctors or other health professionals before trying to lose weight.*

Gallbladder Disease

Gallbladder disease and gallstones are more common if you are overweight. Your risk of disease increases as your weight increases. It is not clear how being overweight may cause gallbladder disease.

Weight loss itself, particularly rapid weight loss or loss of a large amount of weight, can actually increase your chances of developing gallstones. Modest, slow weight loss of about one pound a week is less likely to cause gallstones.

Source: NIH Publication No. 98-4098 May 1998.

sleep apnea Periods of absence of breathing during sleep.

probably due to increased resistance in the peripheral blood vessels, changes in the way the kidneys handle sodium, and other changes in kidney function.

The risk of cancer also increases with obesity, but the exact reason is unknown. Diet is a probable factor; the same diet pattern that contributes to obesity (high calorie, high-fat, low-fiber, low in fruits and vegetables) may also be a cancer risk. Inactivity increases cancer risk, especially for breast cancer. Obese people also have higher levels of hormones that influence development of some cancers; obese women have more endometrial, gallbladder, cervical, and ovarian cancers.[47]

Obese people are more likely to have obstructive **sleep apnea**, in which the airway collapses during sleep and breathing stops for a short spell. Typically, the individual wakes up, gasps for air, begins breathing again, and then falls asleep until the airway collapses again and the cycle repeats; this pattern causes fragmented sleep. Sleep apnea is an independent risk factor for future cardiovascular events such as heart attack and stroke. Modest weight loss alleviates sleep apnea, improves sleep quality, and reduces daytime drowsiness.[48]

Key Concepts: *Health problems from excess body fatness are a major concern. Obesity is a risk factor for many chronic diseases including heart disease, cancer, hypertension, and diabetes. In many cases, a modest amount of weight loss (~10 percent) can improve symptoms and disease management.*

The Prevalence of Overweight and Obesity

The prevalence of obesity has increased at an alarming rate and obesity is now a worldwide public health problem.[49] Obesity has become so common throughout the world that it is beginning to emerge as the most important contributor to ill health—displacing undernutrition and infectious diseases.[50] Not only is obesity prevalent in Europe and the Americas, it is on the rise in Southeast Asia. Over the past two decades, Japan and China have seen a marked increase in overweight and obesity. In the Middle East, the United Arab Emirates now recognizes obesity as a major public health problem.[51]

The goal of *Healthy People 2010* is to cut the prevalence of obesity to no more than 15 percent of adults and 5 percent of children and adolescents. In the United States, overweight and obesity increased dramatically during the 1980s, when the rate jumped from one of every four Americans to one of three, according to data from the 1980 and the 1991 surveys of the National Health and Nutrition Examination Studies (NHANES).[52] The most recent NHANES III surveys, conducted from 1988 to 1994, report that 59.4 percent of men and 50.7 percent of women in the United States are overweight or obese.[53] If we keep it up, the entire adult population will be overweight or obese by the year 2030! The escalating problem is blamed on overconsumption of plentiful, tasty, and energy-dense foods, along with decreased physical activity.

People's weight management efforts have increased along with the increase in overweight, obesity, and societal emphasis on thinness. In the NHANES III survey, 30 percent of males and 53 percent of females reported they had tried to lose weight in the past 12 months. More than 50 million Americans are expected to go on a diet this year, and while some will be successful, statistics tell us that 95 percent of those who lose weight will gain it back. Every year, about 8 million Americans enroll in some kind of structured weight-loss program, and many more spend their hard-earned

Quick Bites

Island Obesity

Some of the most obese people in the world live in the islands of Micronesia. Among these populations, the Naurus are the most obese.

money on diet books, pills, videos, and supplements; the diet industry rakes in about $30 billion to $50 billion every year! According to one study, adults trying to lose weight spend about six months out of the year doing so, mostly with diet and exercise.[54]

Children and adolescents are also concerned about weight. In studies of grade-school girls from various socioeconomic backgrounds, 28 to 40 percent reported that they sometimes dieted or were very often worried about being fat.[55]

Key Concepts: *Worldwide, the number of overweight or obese people has increased markedly in recent years. At the same time, more people are engaging in weight control efforts and at younger ages.*

Early Theories of Weight Regulation

What causes obesity? The basics of energy balance tell us that weight gain is a result of positive energy balance: energy intake is greater than energy output. So what happens when energy regulation goes awry and results in obesity? Several theories have emerged over time.

Fat Cell Theory

According to the **fat cell theory**, the number and size of fat cells in the body help determine how easily a person gains or loses fat weight. People with an above-average number of fat cells, **hypercellular obesity**, may have been born with them or may have developed them at certain critical times because of overeating. In **hypertrophic obesity**, fat cells are larger than normal. Fat cells continue to expand as they fill with more fat; when their capacity is reached, the body generates more cells. (See **Figure 8.18.**) If body fat increases from three to five times the normal amount (which usually occurs by 40 percent or more overweight), fat tissue is likely to have both bigger fat cells and more of them, a condition termed **hyperplasia**.

Even with weight loss, the number of fat cells does not decline (though presumably some could be removed by liposuction). Fat cells do get smaller, but beyond a certain point, they resist further shrinking and the body strives to refill them with fat. The fat cell theory provides an explanation of why weight loss is difficult and weight regain is easy for some obese people, but not why they became obese in the first place.

Set Point Theory

For most people, body fat and body weight remain constant over long periods despite fluctuations in food intake and activity. The set point model of body weight regulation builds on this observation. The body maintains a certain weight by its own internal controls, even if that weight is too high, and it actively resists weight change. The **set point theory** assumes that there is an active regulatory system to keep the body at its set point. However, many people experience significant weight changes during adulthood, so if set points do exist, they vary over a wide range of weights and can be changed. The set point theory has been challenged as too simplistic, and there is little science to support it.

Other Early Theories

Based on dietary recalls and other self-reporting, obese people often seem to eat too little to justify their weight. So other mechanisms, hormonal or metabolic, were thought to cause their obesity. Some researchers hypothesized that obesity resulted from an imbalance in the hypothalamus.

fat cell theory The theory that the quantity of fat stored in the body is a result of the number and size of fat cells.

hypercellular obesity Obesity due to an above-average number of fat cells.

hypertrophic obesity Obesity due to an increase in the size of fat cells.

hyperplasia (hyperplastic obesity) Obesity due to an increase in both the size and number of fat cells.

set point theory A theory that a regulatory mechanism operates to keep a certain variable (e.g., body temperature, weight) at a constant value called the set point.

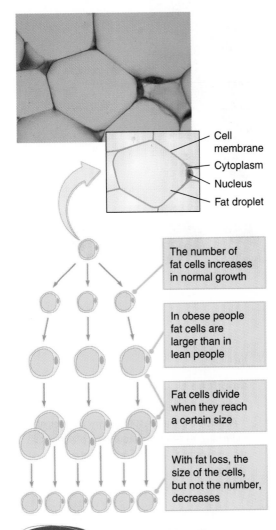

- Cell membrane
- Cytoplasm
- Nucleus
- Fat droplet

The number of fat cells increases in normal growth

In obese people fat cells are larger than in lean people

Fat cells divide when they reach a certain size

With fat loss, the size of the cells, but not the number, decreases

Figure 8.18 **The formation of fat cells.**

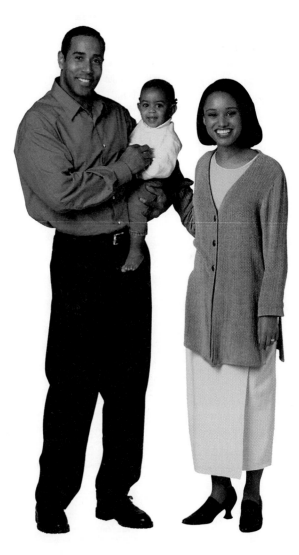

Experiments showed that this explanation is an oversimplification.[56] Hypothyroidism was also thought to be an important contributor to obesity but is now recognized as relatively rare. Underreporting of food intake is a widely recognized problem in studies that assess dietary intake.[57] Yet again, this is an incomplete explanation for obesity.

Key Concepts: *Many theories have been proposed to explain obesity. These include the fat cell theory that obesity is related to too many fat cells and enlarged fat cells; the set point theory that obese individuals are "programmed" to carry a certain amount of weight; and other theories, all largely discounted today.*

Current Thinking about Obesity

We now recognize that obesity probably involves alterations in the interactions of several regulatory mechanisms—the brain and its neurotransmitters, the gut and its peptides, the liver and its metabolic processes, the adipose tissue and its secreted proteins, and endocrine hormones. These mechanisms interact with sociocultural and environmental factors, exercise patterns, and biological factors of heredity, age, and sex.

Heredity and Genetic Factors

Investigation of the molecular markers of obesity has barely begun, but the research is promising. So far scientists have identified several genes that when damaged or dysfunctional can cause obesity or increase its likelihood.

Hereditary patterns of obesity, on the other hand, have been observed for some time. It is clear that when both parents are morbidly obese (body weight 100 percent above normal), the probability that their children will be obese is high (80 percent); whereas when neither parent is obese, the probability that their children will be obese is relatively low (less than 10 percent). However, about 25 to 30 percent of obese individuals have normal-weight parents.[58]

To what extent are family patterns environmental versus hereditary? Because of the interplay between genetics and the environment, the hereditary component is difficult to estimate. Environment and sociocultural influences interact closely with heredity to produce obesity. Best estimates are that genes alone generally account for 50 to 90 percent of the variation in the amounts of stored body fat.[59]

Sociocultural Influences

Social factors have long been recognized as important influences on the development of obesity. Our culture also influences our perception of appropriate body weight. Idealization of thinness creates unhealthy pressures to diet. At the same time, the abundance of high-calorie, highly palatable food, and the social enjoyment of eating create pressures to overeat. **Table 8.6** summarizes social characteristics that are key predictors of weight.

Age and Lifestyle

Both men and women gain the most weight between 25 and 34 years of age. Weight tends to increase slowly thereafter and then decline in the years after age 55.[60] People are most concerned about body weight and appearance in adolescence and young adulthood. These concerns decline with maturity and are replaced by concerns about weight as it relates to health. In the elderly, the need to maintain weight often becomes important.

Exercise patterns also influence the development of obesity, which is generally associated with reduced physical activity. The extent to which obesity

Quick Bites

American Obesity Epidemic

Experts estimate that more than half of Americans are at least somewhat overweight, and nearly 30 percent of adults are obese. Adults who engage in at least 30 minutes of exercise per day are less likely to be obese, but only 22 percent of adults meet this standard.

leads to physical inactivity is unclear; however, excessive television viewing is linked to obesity in children.

Sex

In general, males and females set different weight standards for themselves. Beginning in grade school, boys are less likely than girls to consider themselves overweight; in fact males of all ages accept some degree of overweight. Boys typically are more concerned about becoming taller and more muscular. By early adulthood, the number of men who want to increase their weight about equals the number who want to lose weight, whereas almost all females want to lose weight. As adults, males tend to see themselves as overweight at higher weights, while females describe themselves as overweight when they are closer to a desirable body weight. (See **Figure 8.19.**) Adult women feel thin only when they are below 90 percent of desirable body weight, whereas men rate themselves as thin until they are as high as 105 percent of a desirable body weight.[61]

Although women try harder than men to avoid overweight or to slim down,[62] they often develop obesity after pregnancy and at menopause. In pregnancy, fat stores increase to meet the energy demands of lactation.

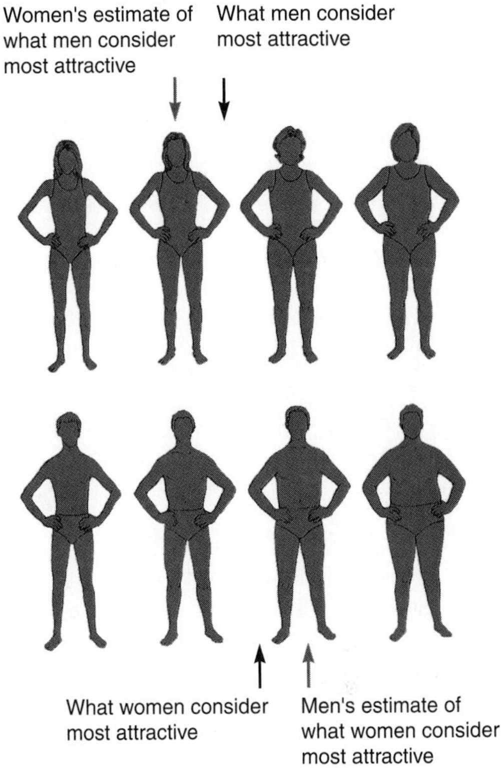

Table 8.6 **Sociocultural Influences on Obesity**

Social Contexts

Culture	People in developed societies have more body fat than those in developing societies.
History	Fatness is increasing in the United States, but idealized weights are decreasing.

Social Characteristics

Age and lifestyle	Fatness increases during adulthood, declines in the elderly.
Sex	Obesity is more prevalent in women than in men.
Race and ethnicity	Obesity is more prevalent in African American, Hispanic, Native American, and Pacific Islander women.

Socioeconomic status

Income	Obesity is more prevalent in lower-income women.
Education	Less-educated women have a higher incidence of obesity.
Occupational prestige	Obesity is more prevalent in women (people) in less prestigious jobs.
Employment	Women who are not employed have a higher incidence of obesity.
Household composition	Older people who live with others have a higher incidence of obesity.
Marriage	Married men have a higher incidence of obesity.
Residence	Rural women have a higher incidence of obesity.
Region	People residing in the South have a higher incidence of obesity.

Source: Adapted with permission from Dalton S., Body weight terminology, definitions, and measurements. In: Dalton, S ed. *Overweight and Weight Management: The Health Professional's Guide to Understanding and Practice.* Gaithersburg, MD: Aspen; 1997:314.

Figure 8.19 What men and women consider attractive.
Source: Data compiled from Fallon A, Rozin P. Sex differences in perceptions of desirable body shape. *Journal of Abnormal Psychology.* 1985;94:102–105; and Kalat J. *Introduction to Psychology.* 5th ed. Belmont, CA: Wadsworth;1999.

restrained eating An eating pattern in which a person avoids food as long as possible, and then gorges on food.

binge eating Consumption of a very large amount of food in a brief period of time (e.g., 2 hr) accompanied by a loss of control over how much and what is eaten.

weight cycling Repeated periods of gaining and losing weight; also called yo-yo dieting.

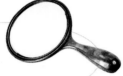

Quick Bites

Mirror, Mirror, on the Wall

A recent study demonstrated that college students and supermarket shoppers ate less in front of a mirror, spreading less full-fat cream cheese on bagelettes and less full-fat margarine on bread than when there was no mirror. The researchers speculated that the mirror decreased food consumption by increasing self-awareness, providing an external reality check on the amount of food a person was consuming. Mirrors had no effect on the consumption of low-fat or nonfat products, perhaps because people did not perceive these products to be unhealthy.

Many women retain this extra weight after they give birth and become heavier with each child.

Race and Ethnicity

In the United States the prevalence of obesity and attitudes toward it differ among racial and ethnic groups. Black and Latina women are more likely to be overweight than white women.[63] As cultures, African Americans, Hispanic Americans, Native Americans, and Pacific Islanders typically value thinness less than white Americans do.[64]

Socioeconomic Status

American women of lower socioeconomic status are more likely to be obese, and their tendency to become overweight with age is more pronounced. The stigma of obesity can impede upward mobility for them. Rural women tend to be heavier than women who live in metropolitan areas, and Southern women are most likely to be overweight.[65]

Employment

Some studies suggest that employed women are thinner than women who are not in the labor force.[66] Employers tend to hire people of normal weight rather than overweight or obese people. Working outside the home also provides income that some women can use for healthier food choices, physical activity programs, and health care; on the other hand, there is less time to prepare healthful meals and get routine exercise. Changing jobs, losing a job, or retiring often changes eating patterns and subsequently body weight.

Psychological Factors

Do overweight and obese people experience greater distress than thinner people? And do they overeat in response? Research results are conflicting. Certain obese subgroups, however, may be more prone to emotional eating than others; these subgroups include **restrained eaters** and **binge eaters**.[67]

Restrained Eaters Some people try to reduce their calorie intake by fasting or avoiding food as long as possible—usually by skipping meals or delaying eating—or by severely restricting the types of food they eat. Then, like a dam that bursts, environmental or emotional stress can trigger a complete release of inhibitions toward eating (disinhibition) and the person overeats. Although this pattern does not occur in all obese binge eaters, the "fast, then binge" behavior is common in obese people who chronically attempt to lose weight.[68] This pattern also occurs in "normal" weight women who perceive themselves as fat. These "restrained" eating patterns appear to be passed on from mother to daughter.[69]

Binge Eaters A binge eater compulsively overeats, sometimes for days on end. Some people binge only at night, consuming most of their excess calories between 6 P.M. and the time they go to sleep. Binge eating is common among people enrolled in weight-loss programs—estimates of the prevalence range from 23 to 46 percent.[70] People who binge are more likely to be emotional eaters or have psychological problems than those who do not binge. For more information about binge eating, see the "Spotlight on Eating Disorders."

Weight Cycling **Weight cycling** is a pattern of losing and regaining weight, over and over again. You might expect this behavior to be harmful, harder on the body than overweight itself. However, researchers have found little evidence of that, and most experts conclude that the potential benefits of weight loss for obese individuals outweigh the potential risks of weight cycling.[71]

Key Concepts: Hereditary factors are important in the development of obesity, explaining up to 50 to 90 percent of the variation of body weight. Sex, age, and sociocultural factors such as socioeconomic status, employment status, marital status, and having children also are related to weight. Overly restrained eating may result in episodes of overeating and weight gain. Binge eating is common among people in weight-loss programs.

weight management The adoption of healthful and sustainable eating and exercise behaviors that reduce disease risk and improve well-being.

Weight Management

The numerous factors that lead to obesity are interrelated and different for every person. Approaches to weight management are just as complex and to be effective they must be tailored to the individual. As you continue reading, keep in mind the following definition of **weight management** from The American Dietetic Association, noting there is no mention of weight loss or ideal weight.

> *Weight management is the adoption of healthful and sustainable eating and exercise behaviors indicated for reduced disease risk and improved feelings of energy and well-being.[72]*

The Evolution of Weight Management

Our understanding of obesity, its causes, and its treatment has changed over time. Until recently many cultures associated obesity with prosperity and good health. In the latter part of the twentieth century, however, Westernized cultures generally have moved away from such beliefs.

In the seventeenth century obesity was attributed to an imbalance of biochemical functions, or a "mechanical malfunction." By the nineteenth century, excessive fat cells were blamed. In the beginning of the twentieth century, obesity was attributed to "glandular malfunction." A classic paper in 1930 by Newburgh and Johnston, "Endogenous Obesity—A Misconception," challenged that view. They said obesity was an overabundance of energy stored in adipose tissue, the result of (1) human weakness and moral laxity and (2) insufficient physical activity.[73] In the 1940s, obesity was said to be evidence of psychological problems. During these years, concern about body weight was gaining momentum and with it interest in how to lose weight. In 1942, the Metropolitan Life Insurance Company published its first weight tables, based on the relationship of weight to life span.

In the 1940s self-help groups such as TOPS (Take Off Pounds Sensibly) and the noncommercial forerunner of Weight Watchers appeared. They were founded with the idea that failed willpower could be countered with inspiration, encouragement, and group support. In 1960 Overeaters Anonymous adapted the "12-step" spirituality-based approach used to treat alcoholism and developed a program to overcome compulsive overeating.

Commercial programs appeared in the 1950s and 1960s. These included Weight Watchers, followed by Diet Center, Jenny Craig, Nutri-System, and similar programs. Many sell prepackaged foods and sometimes supplements, in addition to holding group support meetings. Low-calorie meal-replacement beverages also became available; however, the popular liquid protein-sparing diets of the 1970s resulted in cardiac abnormalities and some deaths. In the 1980s Jane Fonda's exercise videos urged followers to "go for the burn," and the fitness movement was born.

The weights of celebrity models often molded popular notions about desirable weight. In the early 1960s, as today, thin was "in." (At that time, the trendsetter was supermodel Twiggy, who at 5 feet, 7 inches, weighed 98 pounds.) Between 1959 and today, the number of diet and exercise articles

Quick Bites

People Persuasion

The best predictor of the amount of food eaten at a given time is the amount of people present. Studies show that meals eaten with other people last longer and tend to have 44 percent more calories than those eaten alone.

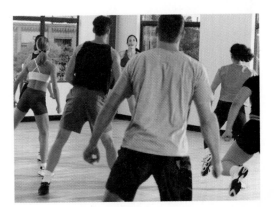

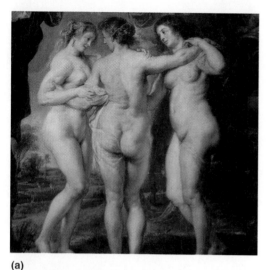

(a)

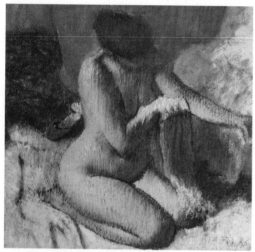

(b)

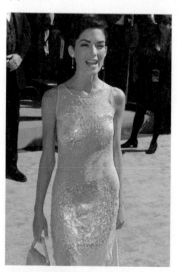

(c)

Figure 8.20 **Society's changing standards of beauty.** (a) Ruben's *The Three Graces*, 1639. (b) Degas's *After the Bath*, 1896, (c) Actress Lara Flynn Boyle, 1999.

in women's magazines escalated, and diet books became best sellers. Dieting became an institution with its own magazines, television shows, camps and resorts, and weight-loss gurus. **Figure 8.20** shows various levels of fatness, all of which were considered beautiful at one time.

The first research on behavioral control of overeating was published in 1967[74] and sparked interest in behavior modification. Initially behavioral approaches neglected nutrition and exercise; they focused solely on identifying and changing eating habits. The expectation was that behavior would change in 10 to 20 weeks, and weight loss would follow. This low-tech approach was disappointing, but the high-tech ones haven't worked too well either. Surgery and anti-obesity drugs have limited success, and the FDA has banned some diet aids because of health risks.

With so many disappointments, so many failures, a backlash against dieting has emerged, despite obesity's link to health risks. The antidiet advocates' rallying cry is, "Diets don't work!" While acknowledging that severe obesity is dangerous, they argue for size acceptance and challenge the notion that mild obesity is unhealthful.

A new view of obesity evolved in the 1990s—obesity as a complex disorder with multiple contributing factors. (See **Figure 8.21**.) Emphasis has shifted from simple weight loss to improving overall health, with fitness more important than a number on the scale. Dietary recommendations emphasize moderation and a balanced diet that is low in fat and high in healthful foods. Behavior change is still an important part of weight management, but change is seen as an ongoing process that requires new skills for maintaining a healthy lifestyle over the long run. The requirement for vigorous exercise has been relaxed; moderate exercise for improving fitness, regardless of weight, is now stressed.

We now understand there are limitations to what a person can weigh or look like. While not abandoning efforts to achieve good health, the desire to lose weight should be balanced by self-acceptance. We recognize that futile attempts to achieve an "ideal" body shape and weight may undermine self-esteem and be emotionally or physically harmful.

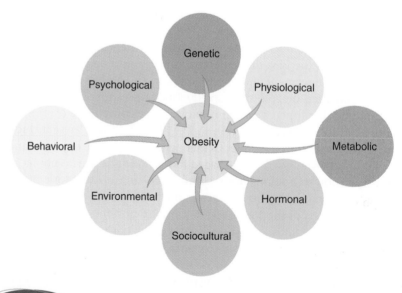

Figure 8.21 Multiple factors contribute to obesity.

Key Concepts: *Theories about causes of obesity and appropriate methods of treatment have changed over the years. Currently, the focus is on improving health through weight management by establishing healthy eating and exercise patterns and accepting the limitations of heredity.*

Components of Weight Management

A long-term approach to weight management includes a balanced diet of moderate caloric intake, adequate exercise, cognitive-behavioral strategies for changing habits and behavior patterns, and attention to balancing self-acceptance and the desire for change. **Figure 8.22** shows the necessary components of an effective program to treat obesity.

Diet Composition

To lose weight, our dietary choices must provide fewer calories than we expend. Long-term weight management means adopting a lifelong eating strategy, rather than a short-term "diet." Gradual weight loss resulting from small changes in energy intake, such as a reduction of 200 to 300 kilocalories each day, is more successful in long-term weight control than a drastic diet of only 1,000 to 1,200 kilocalories per day. Eliminating one can of regular soda from your daily routine would reduce your energy intake by about 150 kilocalories. Eating half a serving of fries instead of a whole serving would save another 100 kilocalories. Changes in diet need to be small but sustainable, and should focus on the balance of food groups suggested by the Food Guide Pyramid.

What specific roles do protein, carbohydrate, and fat play in obesity and weight loss? Over the years, each has been targeted as either the cause of obesity or the solution to successful weight loss. For example, in the 1950s and 1960s weight-loss diets advocated high protein and restricted carbohydrates.[75] But high-protein diets tend to be high in fat, as well. Every few years, these high-fat or high-protein diets reappear with a new name, usually with the claims "new" or "revolutionary." (Their many food restrictions, despite promises of "all you can eat," result in low energy intakes that produce the weight loss.) At the May, 2000 National Nutrition Summit, the USDA announced plans for a coordinated nutrition research program to look at the long- and short-term health and nutrition effects of various types of popular diets.[76]

Several large surveys of the relationship between diet composition and body weight have found that higher fat intakes and fewer complex carbohydrates are associated with excess body fat.[77] Many people have gotten the message to reduce dietary fat, but in their enthusiasm they have forgotten to manage total energy intake. They have replaced excessive fats with excessive carbohydrates and have neglected to limit portions. Portion guidelines from the Food Guide Pyramid or Exchange Lists for Meal Planning can help reduce overall food intake.

Physical Activity

Regular physical activity is a vital component of weight management. Physical activity promotes fitness and good health. At the same time, it discourages overeating by reducing stress, produces positive feelings that reinforce self-worth and a sense of accomplishment, and often includes pleasant socialization.

Both anaerobic activity (e.g., slow sit-ups and lifting weights) and aerobic activity (e.g., brisk walking, swimming, jumping rope, jogging) are helpful. Aerobic activity burns calories directly, and anaerobics are best for building

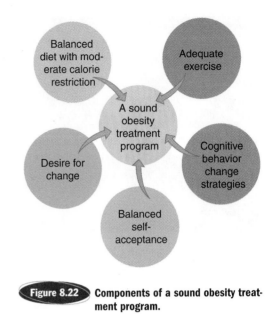

Figure 8.22 Components of a sound obesity treatment program.

Quick Bites

The Beverly Hills Diet

The *Beverly Hills Diet*, introduced in 1980, begins with ten days of fruit and water only. Many dieters reported an unpleasant side effect—diarrhea.

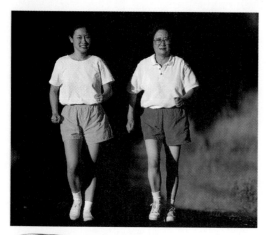

Figure 8.23 Weight management through lifetime habits.

ABC model of behavior A behavioral model that includes the external and internal events that precede and follow the behavior. The "A" stands for antecedents, the events that precede the behavior ("B"), which are followed by consequences ("C") that positively or negatively reinforce the behavior.

muscle mass, the metabolically active tissue that raises resting energy expenditure. Review **Table 8.2** to see how activity affects energy burning.

The approach of "going for the burn" and "no pain, no gain" (the mottoes of aerobics movement during the 1970s and 1980s) is neither necessary nor desirable. Instead regular exercise of moderate intensity—any activity that expends four to seven kcalories per minute—provides substantial health benefits. An exercise program designed for the long run must be enjoyable and convenient, and must fit into the daily routine. Some ways to increase activity include walking the dog an extra half hour daily, climbing a stairway instead of taking an elevator, walking instead of using transportation, and taking up a hobby like bicycling. (See **Figure 8.23**.)

Cognitive-Behavioral Change

Stress management can be an important part of weight management.[78] The **ABC model of behavior (Figure 8.24)** is a tool that helps you cope with daily stresses and their impact on eating behavior.

The ABC model helps manage events that trigger behaviors and factors that reinforce them. The "A" part of the model, *antecedents*, are the events that precede the behavior and trigger it. Overeating, is a possible *behavior*, the "B" part of the model. The *consequences*, or "C," follow and reinforce the "B." The "C" may be desirable, such as relief from stress, or undesirable, such as guilt or weight gain. The "C" may be immediate or, like weight gain, occur in the future; the consequences with the greatest influence are those that occur immediately.

Identifying the cues (A) that trigger overeating is the first step to changing or avoiding these triggers. You might remove problem foods from the house or avoid the grocery store's candy aisle. New antecedents can trig-

---

High-Protein Diets for Weight Loss: Helpful or Harmful?

High-protein weight-loss diets are in style again. Browse through the weight-loss section of any major bookstore and you will find books like *Protein Power, Dr. Atkins' New Diet Revolution, Sugar Busters*, and *Enter the Zone*. All these books promote variants of a high-protein diet for weight loss.

These diets revisit an idea that was popular in the 1970s (and has historical roots dating back nearly 200 years) that carbohydrates (starches and sugars) make us fat. Proponents of high-protein diets point to the fact that throughout the high-carb, low-fat 1980s and early 1990s and with the explosion of fat-free foods, Americans got fatter. They fail to note that although the percentage of calories from fat decreased, Americans

ate more total calories and exercised less— a recipe for weight gain.

Common Myths about High Protein Intake for Weight Loss

1. *Myth:* Early humans existed on a diet that was high in protein, and our bodies are still tuned to eat this way.
   Fact: Early humans were more gatherers than hunters. They subsisted on a diet of primarily nuts, seeds, fruits, and vegetables occasionally supplemented with meat. Early humans also had a life expectancy about half that of ours today.[1]
2. *Myth:* Dietary protein cannot be converted into body fat.
   Fact: Excess energy from fat, alcohol,

and protein is converted to fat and stored in the body's fat cells.

3. *Myth:* High-protein diets result in quick and permanent weight loss.
   Fact: High-protein diets may result in quick weight loss, but it is seldom permanent. Initial weight loss on high-protein diets come from loss of body fluids. Later weight loss comes from both fat and muscle tissue. Because unsupervised high-protein diets don't teach lifestyle change or reflect people's usual eating patterns, weight is usually quickly regained when the diet is stopped.

4. *Myth:* You can eat all you want on a high-protein diet and still lose weight.

ger positive behaviors (for example, putting exercise clothes by the door to prompt exercise).

You can affect the behavior of overeating (B) by using **positive self-talk** to encourage a new behavior and avoiding excuses and rationalizations to eat something inappropriate.

Positive consequences (C) help to reinforce new behaviors. You could sign a contract with a friend that rewards you for deciding not to overeat. Rewards such as time for physical activity not only reinforce behavior but also develop fitness. **Table 8.7** summarizes cognitive-behavioral tools for changing habits and behavior patterns.

Balancing Acceptance and Change

Behavior change for obesity management must be complemented by acceptance. Self-acceptance helps self-esteem and improves general satisfaction with life. It is destructive to be overly concerned with body weight and shape, or for people to have unattainable goals of idealized physical appearance. But self-acceptance should not be confused with complacency or a do-nothing approach that ignores health risks.

What is a reasonable expectation for weight management? One proposal is a modest weight-loss goal of roughly 10 percent, enough to produce health benefits and perhaps to encourage continued success. (See **Figure 8.25**) Another goal is to restore and maintain a "natural weight," a body weight that is naturally appropriate given the limitations of heredity. To attain this weight, some experts would abandon dieting altogether; they propose learning to use the body's hunger and satiation signals to regulate eating. Another approach to the "natural weight" goal is to focus on routinely eating a structured but balanced diet of moderate calories and getting adequate exercise; then accept whatever weight results.

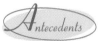

Antecedents

Her mouth starts watering as she passes by a bakery with delicious sights and aromas.

Behavior

She purchases many pastries intending some for later. Despite this resolve, she succumbs to the need for instant gratification, immediately eating them all.

Consequences

She regrets her behavior and feels guilty. Overeating may leave her feeling ill and nauseated.

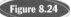 **Figure 8.24** The ABC model of eating behavior.

positive self-talk Constructive mental or verbal statements made to one's self to change a belief or behavior.

Fact: Anyone who "goes on a diet" becomes more conscious of what he or she eats, and generally eats less. High-protein, low-carbohydrate diets can also induce a state of ketosis, which tends to reduce appetite. Also, sample diet plans from high-protein books are generally low in calories.

But, do they work?

Some people who have tried high-protein weight-loss diets report dramatic weight loss on a diet that allows abundant amounts of steak, bacon, and eggs. However, rapid initial weight loss from the depletion of glycogen stores may come at a price: constipation, nausea, weakness, dehydration, and fatigue are common side effects. While ketosis may

suppress appetite, it also gives the breath a fruity odor. Also, a diet that ignores much of the USDA Food Guide Pyramid limits the intake of many vitamins and minerals—a fact the authors of many plans address by recommending supplements. But, supplements don't provide fiber or the many phytochemicals found in fruits and vegetables. Diets that contain 60 percent or more of calories from fat may contain more cholesterol and saturated fat than is recommended for heart health.

The Best Diet to Follow

Is there a "best" diet? If there were, we wouldn't have so many diet books vying for our attention and money! Our knowledge of people's nutrient needs still points to the Pyramid for guidance; the best diet empha-

sizes fruits, vegetables, and grains, not high-protein foods. And although weight loss may be the goal of many, weight maintenance is the key to reducing health risks of obesity. Weight maintenance requires permanent changes to eating habits, and more important, increased physical activity. So, instead of a walk through the diet book aisle, save your money and improve your health with a fitness walk through the mall.

1 Eaton SB, Shostak M, Konner, M. *The Paleolithic Prescription.* New York: Harper & Row; 1988.

metabolic fitness The absence of all metabolic and biochemical risk factors associated with obesity.

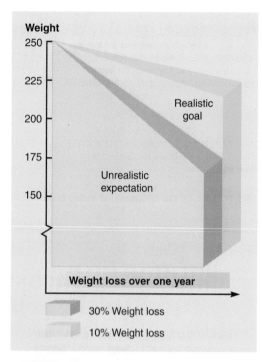

Figure 8.25 Expectations and reasonable weight goals.

BASIC TENETS OF SIZE ACCEPTANCE

- Human beings come in a variety of sizes and shapes. We celebrate this diversity as a positive characteristic of the human race.
- There is no ideal body size, shape, or weight that every individual should strive to achieve.
- Every body is a good body, whatever its size or shape.
- Self-esteem and body image are strongly linked. Helping people feel good about their bodies and about who they are, can help motivate and maintain healthy behaviors.
- Appearance stereotyping is inherently unfair to the individual because it is based on superficial factors which the individual has little or no control over.
- We respect the bodies of others even though they might be quite different from our own.
- Each person is responsible for taking care or his/her body.
- Good health is not defined by body size; it is a state of physical, mental, and social well-being.

People of all sizes and shapes can reduce their risk of poor health by adopting a healthy lifestyle.

Source: Excerpted from *Basic Tenets of Health at Every Size*, developed by dietitians and nutritionists who are advocates of size acceptance; their efforts coordinated by James P. Ikeda, MA, Rd, Nutrition Education Specialist, Department of Nutritional Sciences, University of California, Berkeley.

For people who eat healthfully and get adequate exercise as part of their healthy lifestyle, their weight as measured by a scale should not be a primary concern.[79] Indeed, overweight and even obese people with healthy lifestyles who focus on being physically fit may reduce their risk for heart disease, diabetes, and other chronic ailments. Besides, weight is not a good indicator of body fatness or health.

Metabolic Fitness

Some health experts are now suggesting that weight goals be replaced by the goal of achieving **metabolic fitness**,[80] especially for those who have difficulty achieving or maintaining recommended weight or BMI levels. The aim of metabolic fitness is the absence of metabolic or biochemical risk

Table 8.7 Cognitive-Behavioral Tools for Changing Behavior

Tool	Description
Self-monitoring	Prospectively recording information about behavior to identify the antecedents (what precedes and elicits a particular action), the behaviors of interest (usually eating behavior), and the consequences (the thoughts, feelings, and reactions that accompany the behavior of interest).
Environmental management	Avoiding or changing cues that trigger undesirable behavior (e.g., not driving by the doughnut shop, putting the cookie jar out of sight), or instituting new cues to elicit new behaviors (e.g., putting your walking shoes by the door as a reminder to exercise); also called "stimulus control."
Alternate behaviors	Learning new ways of responding to old cues or circumstances that can't be changed or avoided (e.g., taking a walk when you get upset instead of getting something to eat.)
Reward	Giving yourself, or arranging to be given, rewards for engaging in desired behaviors.
Negative reinforcement	Arranging to give up something desirable (e.g., money) or to endure something undesirable (e.g., wash your friend's car) for engaging in unwanted behaviors.
Social support	Getting others to participate in or otherwise provide emotional and physical support of your weight-management efforts.
Cognitive coping	Reducing negative self-talk, increasing positive self-talk, and challenging beliefs that undermine your resolve and contribute to negative emotions; setting reasonable goals and avoiding "thinking traps."
Managing emotions	Using reframing, disengagement, imagery, and self-soothing to reduce or manage negative emotions.
Relapse prevention and recovery	Identifying high-risk situations that pose a hazard for relapsing, and learning to recover from small indiscretions before they become major relapses.

Source: Adapted from Nash JD. *The New Maximize Your Body Potential.* Palo Alto, CA: Bull Publishing Company; 1997. Used with permission.

factors associated with obesity. These risk factors include high cholesterol (especially when HDL cholesterol is low), high triglyceride level, elevated blood glucose, insulin resistance, high blood pressure, and elevated fatty acids synthesis. Adult weight gain greater than 18 kilograms (about 40 pounds) and upper-body fat distribution in obese persons are also deemed to be risk factors.[81] Individuals are considered metabolically fit if these risk factors are at normal levels. Abnormal levels put the individual at greater risk for coronary heart disease, diabetes, gout, hypertension, and associated conditions. People can lower or even normalize these risk factors through modest weight loss (5 to 10 percent of initial body weight) achieved by a low-fat, reduced-calorie diet and a moderate increase in physical activity (e.g., walking 30 minutes a day, no fewer than five days a week). Recent research shows that just increasing physical activity levels can improve metabolic fitness.[82]

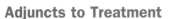

Key Concepts: *Successful weight management involves healthful food choices and regular physical activity. Identifying cues that precede overeating can help a person make behavior changes. Long-term weight management should include self-acceptance and enhanced self-esteem. Goals of idealized body size and shape should be replaced with goals that promote good health and a lifetime of fitness. Behavior changes should focus on metabolic outcomes that improve blood lipids and blood pressure rather than on achievement of a specific weight.*

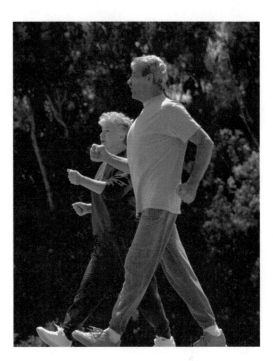

Adjuncts to Treatment

Anti-Obesity Prescription Drugs

The pharmaceutical industry has long been searching for a "magic bullet" to cure obesity. Now that it's clear that obesity involves multiple factors, the focus is on drugs with multiple mechanisms and drugs to be used in conjunction with proper diet and exercise.[83] The stories of Redux and Fen-Phen illustrate that there are no easy solutions to overweight. Fen-Phen is actually two prescription drugs, Pondimin (fenfluramine) and Ionamin (phentermine), that in combination suppress appetite by increasing brain serotonin more than if used alone. Although these drugs had been on the market for more than 20 years, they had never been tested or approved for use together. In 1996 a similar appetite suppressant, Redux (dexfenfluramine), was approved. Doctors wrote millions of prescriptions, many for people with little or no need to lose weight. The excitement was short-lived. These drugs were found to be the likely cause of heart valve problems, so Pondimin (Fen) and Redux were withdrawn from the market. The FDA did not request withdrawal of phentermine (Phen).[84]

Redux had been approved for short-term use for serious obesity; like Pondimin, it had not been studied or approved as part of a combination. Thus the misuse of these drugs may have contributed to their danger. The phentermine half of Fen-Phen is now sometimes combined with the antidepressant Prozac (creating Phen-Pro), a drug combination that has not been proved safe or effective.

Another prescription appetite suppressant, Meridia (sibutramine), was brought to market in 1998. Meridia boosts serotonin and norepinephrine but is believed to be safer than Redux.[85] Like all prescription drugs, Meridia can have side effects, in this case increased blood pressure and heart rate.

Xenical (orlistat), approved in 1999, is a lipase inhibitor—it blocks fat absorption by up to 30 percent. A low-fat diet is needed with Xenical, or the unabsorbed fat can produce diarrhea and flatulence. Fat-soluble nutrients are lost when taking this drug, and vitamin supplementation is necessary.

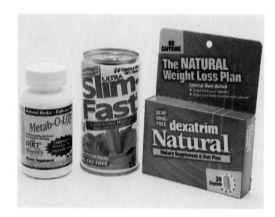

Over-the-Counter Drugs and Dietary Supplements

Nonprescription (over-the-counter or OTC) weight-loss pills may contain caffeine, phenylpropanolamine, benzocaine, or fiber. Caffeine, a stimulant and diuretic, and phenylpropanolamine suppress appetite. Benzocaine numbs the tongue, reducing taste sensations, thus discouraging eating. Pills with fiber theoretically fill the stomach and provide a feeling of fullness. Although moderately effective, fiber pills can lead to dehydration; much of the lost weight is water, which is easily regained when the pills are stopped.

Numerous dietary supplements are marketed for weight loss, with names like "Weight Away." Common ingredients include chromium picolinate, chitosan, hydroxycitric acid (HCA), ephedra, and St. John's wort. In fact, the combination of ephedra and St. John's wort has been marketed as an "herbal fen-phen." Few studies have been done on the efficacy of these products for weight loss, and what little evidence exists does not support the claims. In addition, ephedra (also known as ma huang) is dangerous to people with hypertension, heart disease, or diabetes. Over-the-counter medicines and dietary supplements are no substitute for exercise and healthful eating in the pursuit of long-term weight control. There is no quick, easy way to lose weight.

Self-Help Books and Manuals

Some people respond well to simple information provided in an easy-to-understand format. Good, well-researched self-help manuals and books can help these people.[86] However, each year dozens of dubious diet books reach the market. Here are some flags to spot them:

1. Unbalanced diet patterns. The recommended pattern should not stray too far from the USDA Food Pyramid guidelines (see Chapter 2).

2. Claims of a "scientific breakthrough" or promises of "quick and easy" weight loss. There is no magic when it comes to weight management.

3. Irrational food instructions: food restrictions (e.g., no fruits), illogical overemphasis of some foods (e.g., five grapefruits daily), and irrational food patterns (e.g., don't mix red and green foods). Such restrictions set the stage for feelings of deprivation and binge eating.

4. The promise of a cure for some disease along with weight loss. That's not only a waste of money, it's dangerous.

Self-Help Groups

Self-help groups, often led by lay people, help many people cope with their weight. Such groups reduce the isolation and alienation some obese people experience and can provide a community in which there is understanding and acceptance of shared experience.

Commercial Programs

Commercial weight-loss programs provide group or individual counseling, and group support. Some sell prepackaged foods or nutritional supplements. Some companies employ dietitians, health educators, psychologists, or physicians to develop and guide the program at the corporate level.

Several commercial programs, such as Optifast, Medifast, New Directions, and Health Management Resources (HMR), use **very-low-calorie diets (VLCD)** as the initial phase of treatment. These liquid diets are high in protein, supplemented with all needed vitamins and minerals, but provide only 400 to 800 kilocalories per day. The body responds

Quick Bites

Letter on Corpulence

The first popular diet book in the United States was published in the early 1800s. Called *Bantry's Letter on Corpulence*, the book advocated restricting intake of carbohydrates.

very-low-calorie diet (VLCD) A diet supplying 400 kilocalories per day to 800 kilocalories per day, that includes adequate high-quality protein, little or no fat, and little carbohydrate.

like it would to starvation, adjusting fluid and electrolyte balance, metabolic activities, hormone levels, and organ functions. When such diets were first introduced in the 1970s, several deaths resulted from cardiac abnormalities. As a result, VLCD should only be undertaken with close medical supervision. The refeeding and maintenance phases of these programs are very important in terms of weight maintenance. However, many people drop out once they reach their weight-loss goal and before learning how to adjust their eating habits for long-term weight maintenance.

In early 1999, the Federal Trade Commission (FTC) issued guidelines encouraging commercial programs to release the following information to potential clients:

- staff training and education
- risks of overweight and obesity
- risks of their products or program
- cost
- program outcomes such as success and failure rates

Consumers should obtain this information before registering for a weight-loss program and should think twice about any program that does not willingly provide it.

Professional Private Counselors

Private counselors can be physicians, psychotherapists, nutritionists, or dietitians. They provide individualized weight management and the support and attention that obese people may need. Physicians can also prescribe medication and monitor its safety and effectiveness. Carefully scrutinize the training and credentials of private counselors before committing to any program.

Surgery

Morbid obesity—body weight that exceeds 100 percent of normal and poses a clear health risk—can sometimes be successfully treated surgically. Surgery should be a last-ditch effort, used when all legitimate, less invasive methods have failed. The most common procedures reduce stomach size by creating a smaller, upper stomach or "pouch." As a result, the patient can eat very few calories at one time.[87] Gastric bypass is another surgical procedure that limits food intake. Following this surgery, digestion and absorption of caloric foods is inhibited, but so is absorption of some micronutrients—an obvious drawback. (See **Figure 8.26**.)

The long-term effectiveness of gastric surgery depends on how patients manage their eating. They can defeat the procedure by consuming high-calorie drinks or semisolid foods that overcome stomach size. With time the pouch stretches, allowing more solid foods, but by then, it is hoped that healthy eating habits have been established. These patients are likely to need life-long medical supervision.

Liposuction is a cosmetic surgical procedure that removes fat to reshape the body. Although the procedure removes some fat cells, the body still has billions of other fat cells ready to store extra fat. Thus, liposuction is not an effective way to attain significant or long-term weight loss. Liposuction should not be used casually. The procedure has risks such as blood clots, perforation injuries, skin and nerve damage, and unfavorable drug reactions.

Quick Bites

Diet Revolution?

The *Diet Revolution* first promoted by Dr. Atkins in 1972 centered on putting dieters into a state of ketosis by consuming few carbohydrates. In 1973 the American Medical Association called the diet dangerous and required Atkins to testify before the U.S. Senate Select Committee on Nutrition.

morbid obesity Obesity characterized by body weight exceeding 100 percent of normal; a condition so severe it often requires surgery.

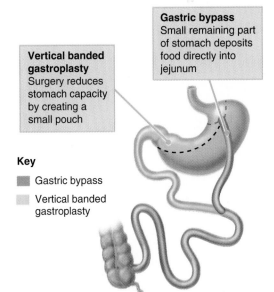

Gastric bypass Small remaining part of stomach deposits food directly into jejunum

Vertical banded gastroplasty Surgery reduces stomach capacity by creating a small pouch

Key
- Gastric bypass
- Vertical banded gastroplasty

Figure 8.26 **Gastric surgery in obesity treatment.** In vertical-banded gastroplasty, surgery reduces the size of the stomach. A gastric bypass routes food to the jejunum, bypassing the duodenum and most of the stomach.

Quick Bites

**The Fletcherism Fad:
Chew Until You...**

At the turn of the twentieth century, a retired businessman named Horace Fletcher started a dietary craze known as "Fletcherism." Calling the mouth "Nature's Food Filter," he believed that the sense of taste and the urge to swallow are perfect guides to nutrition. Although he recommended chewing food at least 50 times before swallowing, preferably until tasteless, he far exceeded this by once chewing a piece of onion 722 times. His philosophy did lead to some weight loss; people adhering to Fletcherism cut back on energy intake due to the additional mechanical effort of chewing.

Key Concepts: *Prescription and over-the-counter drugs to lose weight have varying effectiveness. Drugs have potential side effects and must be used with caution and medical supervision. Books and commercial programs can help some individuals. However, consumers should always proceed with caution before spending money. Surgical intervention is an aggressive approach to weight management and should be considered a last resort for those who are morbidly obese. Liposuction removes fat cells from specific parts of the body but is not considered an effective approach to weight control.*

Underweight

From a public health standpoint, underweight is much less of a problem than obesity, but for underweight people, it can be troublesome and frustrating. Underweight is defined as 15 to 20 percent or more below desired weight for height, or a BMI under 19 kg/m^2.

When underweight is simply an inherited pattern, and diet and other health behaviors are fine, health risk is not a concern. Health is an issue when underweight is the result of undernutrition; deficits in protein and micronutrients as well as energy can cause disorders ranging from fatigue to compromised immune function.

Causes and Assessment

The causes of underweight are as diverse as those of overweight. They include the following:

- altered response to hunger, appetite, satiety, and external cues, described earlier in this chapter
- factors in eating disorders such as distorted body image, compulsive dieting, and compulsive overexercising
- metabolic and hereditary factors
- prolonged psychological and emotional stress
- addiction to alcohol and street drugs
- bizarre diet patterns, or diets that are inadequate

Underweight can be a sign of underlying disease, cancer for example, and plays a role in its diagnosis. Illness can speed up metabolic rate, spoil the appetite, or interfere with digestion. Correcting the underweight helps improve the quality of life.

Laboratory tests, skinfold thicknesses and other anthropometric measures, and body fat assessments are especially useful in determining cause and need for treatment of underweight people.

Weight Gain Strategies

The basic goal is to create positive energy balance. Here are some strategies:

- Have small frequent meals with nutrient-dense and energy-dense foods and beverages.
- Drink fluids at the end of the meal or, better yet, between meals.
- Use high-calorie weight-gain beverages and foods.
- Use timers or other cues (similar to the ABC model on page 313, but with a different goal) to prompt eating.
- Use a balanced vitamin/mineral supplement to ensure deficiency does not contribute to poor appetite.

Sometimes prescription drugs such as appetite stimulants are helpful. Medication can also speed stomach emptying, improving appetite for the next meal. Digestive enzyme replacements help underweight caused by poor digestion or absorption.

Exercise has a role in weight gain, as well. Simple anaerobic or isometric exercise encourages weight gain as lean body mass rather than fat.

Key Concepts: *Underweight is not as common as overweight. Gaining weight can be difficult, but the basic concepts of energy balance apply.*

Label [to] **Table**

Do you believe by choosing cookies or chips labeled "low-fat" or sticking with certain brand names associated with "diet foods" you are automatically making the right decisions? It may surprise you to know that many low-fat or fat-free products have nearly the same amount of calories as the full-fat versions! After reading this chapter you now know that when it comes to weight loss, total calories are just as important as calories from fat. If you eat a fat-free food, but eat so much of it that your calories are excessive, you will still gain weight. To illustrate this point, let's compare the nutrient labels from some leading cookie manufacturers. The lower fat cookie (on right) claims they are "better for you" and have "50% less fat" compared to regular cookies. Here are the labels:

Regular Cookie	Lower Fat Cookie
Serving 2 cookies (29g)	*Serving 2 cookies (26g)*
Calories 140	*Calories 110*
Calories from fat 50	*Calories from fat 25*
Total Fat 6g	*Total Fat 3g*

True, there is a 50 percent reduction in fat content (6g vs. 3g), which is an important part of the picture. However, take a look at the Total Calories. The lower fat cookies only have 30 fewer kilocalories than the regular cookies, which may be a surprise to those who think they are saving more.

There is another interesting piece of information on these labels, the serving size. At first glance, you may think the serving size of the cookies are the same, two cookies. However after further inspection you can see that the lower fat cookies are slightly smaller. A 10 percent reduction in size/weight is certainly worth noting when you are trying to explain how a product can have fewer calories.

The next time you are in the cookie aisle debating whether you should settle a craving with a low-fat product or its full-fat version, be a smart consumer and read the label before you buy!

Nutrition Facts

Serving Size: 2 cookies (26g)
Servings Per Container: 18

Amount Per Serving

Calories 110   Calories from fat 25

	% Daily Value*
Total Fat 3g	5%
Saturated Fat 0.5g	3%
Polyunsaturated Fat 0g	
Monounsaturated Fat 1g	
Cholesterol 0mg	0%
Sodium 130mg	5%
Total Carbohydrate 20g	7%
Dietary Fiber 0g	0%
Sugars 10g	
Protein 1g	

Vitamin A 0%	•	Vitamin C 0%
Calcium 0%	•	Iron 2%

* Percent Daily Values are based on a 2,000 calorie diet. Your daily values may be higher or lower depending on your calorie needs:

		Calories:	2000	2,500
Total Fat	Less Than		65g	80g
Sat Fat	Less Than		20g	25g
Cholesterol	Less Than		300mg	300mg
Sodium	Less Than		2,400mg	2,400mg
Total Carbohydrate			300g	375g
Dietary Fiber			25g	30g

Lower fat cookie

Nutrition Facts

Serving Size: 2 cookies (29g)
Servings Per Container about 16

Amount Per Serving

Calories 140   Calories from fat 50

	% Daily Value*
	9%
Total Fat 6g	8%
Saturated Fat 1.5g	0%
Cholesterol 0mg	4%
Sodium 105mg	7%
Total Carbohydrate 21g	3%
Dietary Fiber less than 1g	
Sugars 8g	
Protein 2g	

Vitamin A 0%	•	Vitamin C 0%
Calcium 0%	•	Iron 4%

* Percent Daily Values are based on a 2,000 calorie diet. Your daily values may be higher or lower depending on your calorie needs:

		Calories:	2000	2,500
Total Fat	Less Than		65g	80g
Sat Fat	Less Than		20g	25g
Cholesterol	Less Than		300mg	300mg
Sodium	Less Than		2,400mg	2,400mg
Total Carbohydrate			300g	375g
Dietary Fiber			25g	30g

Regular cookie

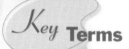

LEARNING *Portfolio* chapter 8

Key Terms

	page
ABC model of behavior	312
android obesity [AN-droyd]	302
appetite	286
basal metabolic rate (BMR)	288
binge eating	308
bioelectrical impedance analysis (BIA) [im-PEE-dance]	301
BodPod	299
body fat distribution	302
body composition	296
body mass index (BMI)	297
bomb calorimeter	285
calorimeter	293
calorimetry [kal-oh-RIM-eh-tree]	293
computed tomography (CT)	301
densitometry	299
direct calorimetry	293
doubly labeled water	294
dual energy x-ray absorptiometry (DEXA)	300
energy balance	285
energy equilibrium	285
energy intake	285
energy output	285
fat cell theory	305
gynoid obesity	302
Harris-Benedict equation	295
hunger	285
hydrostatic weighing	299
hypercellular obesity	305
hyperplasia (hyperplastic obesity)	305
hypertrophic obesity	305
hypothalamus [high-po-THAL-ah-mus]	286
indirect calorimetry	293

	page
isotopes [EYE-so-towps]	294
lean body mass	288
leptin	287
magnetic resonance imaging (MRI)	301
metabolic fitness	314
morbid obesity	317
near-infrared interactance	301
negative energy balance	285
neuroendocrine	287
neuropeptide Y (NPY)	287
nonexercise activity thermogenesis (NEAT)	291
obesity	302
overweight	302
positive energy balance	285
positive self-talk	313
Quetelet index	297
resting energy expenditure (REE)	287
resting metabolic rate (RMR)	288
restrained eating	308
satiation	286
satiety	286
set point theory	305
sleep apnea	304
thermic effect of food (TEF)	291
total body water	300
total energy expenditure	288
underwater weighing	299
underweight	302
very-low-calorie diet (VLCD)	316
waist circumference	302
weight cycling	308
weight management	309

Study Points

➤ Energy balance is the relationship between energy intake and energy output.

➤ The energy content in food can be measured directly using a bomb calorimeter, or estimated using the factors 4 kilocalories per gram for carbohydrate and protein, 9 kilocalories per gram for fat, and 7 kilocalories per gram for alcohol.

➤ Food intake is regulated by hunger, satiation, satiety, and appetite, which are all influenced by complex factors. Hunger is the physiological need to eat. Satiation is the feeling of fullness that leads to termination of a meal. Satiety is the feeling of satisfaction and lack of hunger that determines the interval until the next meal. Appetite is a desire to eat that is influenced by external factors such as flavors and smells and environmental and cultural factors.

➤ Gastrointestinal stimulation, circulating nutrients, neurotransmitters, and hormones signal the brain, especially the hypothalamus, to regulate food intake.

➤ Two recently discovered factors may have major roles in regulating food intake and energy balance: neuropeptide Y, a hormonelike factor that stimulates feeding, and leptin, a hormone produced by fat cells.

➤ The major components of energy expenditure are resting energy expenditure, the thermic effect of food, and energy for physical activity.

➤ Calorimetry is the measurement of energy use, either directly by measuring heat production, or indirectly by determining oxygen intake and carbon dioxide production.

➤ Body composition, age, sex, genetics, and hormonal activity affect the amount of energy used for resting metabolism.

➤ The energy cost of physical activity is affected by the person's size and the intensity and duration of the activity.

➤ Body composition and its relative amounts of fat and lean body mass have a major influence on energy expenditure and risk of chronic disease.

➤ Body mass index, a ratio related to total body fatness and risk of chronic disease, is calculated with height and weight measurements.

➤ The prevalence of obesity and being overweight is escalating worldwide, contributing to chronic disease.

➤ Health risks associated with obesity are more pronounced when excess body fat is in the abdominal region of the body.

➤ We do not understand completely the factors that cause obesity, but experts believe that a complex interaction of hormonal and metabolic factors play a role, along with genetic, sociocultural, and psychological factors.

➤ With the growing evidence that traditional approaches to obesity are generally unsuccessful in the long term, many professionals now promote health and fitness rather than focus on ideal body weight.

➤ Physical activity improves fitness and helps achieve the negative energy balance needed for weight reduction.

➤ Accepting body weight and shape and abandoning unrealistic ideas of thinness are important elements in weight management.

➤ Long-term weight management includes a balanced diet of moderate calorie intake, adequate exercise, cognitive-behavioral strategies for changing habits and behavior patterns, and attention to balancing self-acceptance and the desire for change.

➤ Surgical approaches to weight control should be considered only as a last resort for the morbidly obese.

➤ If the cause is not hereditary, being underweight can pose health problems.

➤ Gaining weight can be difficult for people who are underweight.

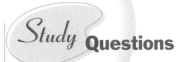

Study Questions

1. Explain the concept of energy balance.

2. List and describe the three main components of energy expenditure

3. Explain the three main factors that dictate energy expenditure in activity.

4. List the techniques for measuring body composition.

5. Obesity is a complex disorder that involves multiple contributors. List the types of factors involved in the development and maintenance of obesity.

6. Using the Body Mass Index (BMI), what values are associated with being underweight, overweight, and obese? Do these vary for men and women?

7. Describe the concept of metabolic fitness.

8. What is the difference between hyperplastic and hypertrophic obesity?

9. What are the four components of a sound approach to weight management?

10. Explain how the ABCs of behavior modification can assist with weight control.

11. Define underweight.

☞ *Try* This

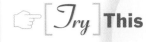

A One-Week Energy Balance Check

The purpose of this exercise is to see if you're in energy balance by monitoring your body weight for one week. Measure your weight on a Monday morning soon after you wake up. Record your weight. Don't change your normal routine of exercise and food intake. One week later weigh yourself again (on a Monday morning just after waking). Did your weight change? If not, your energy intake closely matched your energy output. If so, did you gain or lose weight? What factors do you think contributed to your body weight change? Try repeating this exercise over a longer period of time. Measure and record your weight every Monday morning for six months. What happens? ✋

Increasing Your Energy Output

Physical activity is the most variable component of the energy output side of the energy balance equation. The purpose of this exercise is to increase your calorie expenditure by committing to daily exercise for one week. Make each exercise session 30 minutes long and remember: the longer the duration, the harder the intensity, and the larger the muscle groups involved, the greater the caloric expenditure. Choose an exercise that is comfortable such as walking, jogging, cycling, swimming, or rollerblading. Once your week is complete, ask yourself these questions: How did this week's daily exercise affect my energy balance? Have I gained or lost weight during this week? Did I compensate for the extra calorie expenditure by increasing my calorie intake?

Changing Your Energy Input

Would you like to change your weight by a pound or two? The purpose of this exercise is to reduce or increase your energy input (calorie intake) so that you gain or lose one pound by the end of a week. How? Make only minor adjustments in your usual diet but try to change the energy content for each of your meals by a small amount. Keep a food log and use Appendix A or Eat Right Analysis Software to estimate your calorie total for each of the days. Your goal is to change your calorie total by approximately 500 kilocalorie per day. You should not consume less than 1,500 kilocalorie (for women) or 1,800 kilocalorie (for men) per day. Weigh yourself at the start and at the end of the week. What change, if any, do you see?

What About Bobbie?

Remember, Bobbie is a 20-year-old college sophomore who weighs 155 pounds and is 5'4". She gained 10 pounds her freshman year and would like to lose it because she thinks her ideal weight is more like 145 pounds. She exercises infrequently but likes to walk with her friends and occasionally goes to an aerobics class. How would you suggest she lose the extra 10 pounds? First, let's start by reducing her calorie intake. Here is Bobbie's typical day of eating and a suggested alternative that will save her some calories.

Typical Day	Alternative	Kcalories
BREAKFAST		
1 cinnamon-raisin bagel		
3 Tbsp. light cream cheese	1 Tbsp. light cream cheese	70 saved
Coffee, 2 Tbsp. 2% milk, 2 tsp. sugar		
SNACK		
1 banana		
LUNCH		
2 slices sourdough bread		
2 ounces turkey lunch meat 2 tsp. regular mayo, 2 tsp. mustard, 1 slice tomato, dill pickle, lettuce leaf		
12 oz. diet coke		
Salad 2 C iceberg lettuce with 2 Tbsp. each: shredded carrot, chopped egg, croutons, kidney beans, Italian dressing	1 Tbsp. Italian dressing	70 saved
1 chocolate chip cookie		
SNACK		
1 ½ oz. tortilla chips, ½ C salsa	1 oz. tortilla chips	70 saved
2 C water		
DINNER		
1 ½ C pasta	1 C pasta	100 saved
3 oz. meatballs, 3 oz. spaghetti sauce, 2 Tbsp. parmesan cheese		
1 slice garlic bread,	delete garlic bread	185 saved
½ C green beans	1 C green beans	25 added
1 tsp. butter	delete butter	30 saved
SNACK		
1 slice cheese pizza		
		525 saved
Total		**25 added**

As you can see, small changes in Bobbie's diet can result in a 500-kilocalorie deficit, which will translate to approximately one pound per week of weight loss. This doesn't take into account any extra exercise she might do. So if she starts to work out more regularly, she can make fewer changes in her calorie intake and still lose one pound per week.

References

1 Pribilia BA, Mattes RD. *Neural Influences on Feeding.* Redwood City, CA: Healthline; in press.

2 McCrory MA, Fuss PJ, Saltzman E, Roberts SB. Dietary determinants of energy intake and weight regulation in healthy adults. *J Nutr.* 2000;130:2765–2795.

3 Rolls BJ. The role of energy density in the overconsumption of fat. *J Nutr.* 2000;130(25 Suppl):268S–271S.

4 Burton-Freeman B. Dietary fiber and energy regulation. *J Nutr.* 2000;130:272S–275S.

5 McCrory MA, et al. Op. cit.

6 Ludwig DS. Dietary glycemic index and obesity. *J Nutr.* 2000;130:280S–283S.

7 Guyton AC, Hall JE. *Textbook of Medical Physiology.* 9th ed. Philadelphia: WB Saunders; 1996.

8 Ibid.

9 Ibid.

10 Schwartz MW, Woods SC, Porter D Jr, et al. Central nervous system control of food intake. *Nature.* 2000;404(6):661–671.

11 Smith GP, Gibbs J. Satiating effect of cholecystokinin. *Ann NY Acad Sci.* 1994;713:236–241.

12 Schwartz MW, Seeley RJ. Review of: Seminars in Medicine of the Beth Israel Deaconess Medical Center: neuroendocrine responses to starvation and weight loss. *N Engl J Med.* 1997; 336(25):1802–1811.

13 Ibid.

14 Flood JF, Morley JE. Increased food intake by neuropeptide Y is due to an increased motivation to eat. *Peptides.* 1991;12:1329–1332.

15 Schwartz MW, Baskin DG, Kaiyala KJ, Woods SC. Model for the regulation of energy balance and adiposity by the central nervous system. *Am J Clin Nutr.* 1999;69:584–596.

16 Anderson, GH. Hunger, appetite, and food intake. In: Ziegler EE, Filer LJ, eds. *Present Knowledge in Nutrition.* 7th ed. Washington, DC: ILSI Press; 1996.

17 Ravussin E, Bogardus C. Relationship of genetics, age, and physical fitness to daily energy expenditure and fuel utiliza-

tion. *Am J Clin Nutr.* 1989;49:968–975.

18 Poehlman ET, Berke EM, Joseph JR, Gardner AW, Goran MI. Influence of aerobic capacity, body composition and thyroid hormones on the age-related decline in resting metabolic rate. *Metabolism.* 1992;41:915–921.

19 Mahan LK, Escott-Stump S. *Krause's Food, Nutrition & Diet Therapy.* 10th ed. Philadelphia: WB Saunders; 2000.

20 Bouchard C, ed. *The Genetics of Obesity.* Boca Raton, FL, 1994:135–145.

21 Mahan LK, Escott-Stump. Op. cit.

22 Arciero PJ, Goran MI, Poehlman ET. Resting metabolic rate is lower in women compared to men. *J Appl Physiol.* 1993;75:2514–2520.

23 Ravussin E, Danforth E. Beyond sloth—physical activity and weight gain. *Science.* 1999;283:184–185.

24 Levine JA, Eberhardt NL, Jensen MD. Role of nonexercise activity thermogenesis in resistance to fat gain in humans. *Science.* 1999;283:212–214.

25 Harris JA, Benedict FG. A biometric study of basal metabolism in man. Washington: Carnegie Institute of Washington publication 279; 1919.

26 Mahan LK, Escott-Stump. Op. cit.

27 Food and Nutrition Board, National Research Council, NAS. Energy. *Recommended Dietary Allowances.* 10th ed. Washington, DC: National Academy Press; 1989.

28 Ibid.

29 Rippe JM, Crossley S, Ringer R. Obesity as a chronic disease: modern medical and lifestyle management. In: The Obesity Epidemic: A Mandate for a Multidisciplinary Approach. *J Am Diet Assoc.* October 1998(suppl):S9–S15.

30 Expert Panel on the Identification, Evaluation and Treatment of Overweight in Adults. Clinical guidelines on the identification, evaluation and treatment of overweight and obesity in adults: executive summary. *Am J Clin Nutr.* 1998;68:899–917.

31 US Department of Agriculture, Department of Health and Human Services. *Nutrition and Your Health: Dietary Guidelines for Americans.* Home and Garden Bulletin 232, 5th ed.; 2000.

32 USDA Center for Nutrition Policy and Promotion. *Body Mass Index and Health.* Nutrition Insights series, Insight 16; March 2000. www.usda.gov/cnpp/insights.htm. Accessed 6/3/00.

33 Centers for Disease Control and Prevention. "Body Mass Intake-for-Age." http://www.cdc.gov/nccdphp/dnpa/bmi/bmi-for-age.htm. Accessed 6/4/00.

34 Barlow SE, Dietz WH. Obesity evaluation and treatment: expert committee recommendations. *Pediatrics.* 1998;102, E29 (http://www.pediatrics.org/cgi/content/full/102/3/e29. Accessed 6/3/00.

35 Cole TJ, Bellizzi MC, Flegal KM, Dietz WH. Establishing a standard definition for child overweight and obesity world-

wide: international survey. *BMJ.* 2000;320:1–6.

36 National Center for Health Statistics. "CDC Growth Charts: United States." http://www.cdc.gov/growthcharts. Accessed 8/30/00.

37 Barlow, SE, Dietz WH. Op cit.

38 Pietrobelli A, Formica C, Wang Z, Heymsfield SB. Dual-energy x-ray absorptiometry body composition model: a review of physical concepts. *Am J Physiol.* 1996;34:E941–E951.

39 Pi-Sunyer FX. Obesity. In: Shils ME, Olson JA, Shike M, Ross CA, eds. *Modern Nutrition in Health and Disease.* 9th ed. Philadelphia: Lippincott Williams & Wilkins; 1999:1395–1418.

40 Lee RD, Nieman DC. *Nutritional Assessment.* 2nd ed. St. Louis: Mosby-Year Book; 1996.

41 Ibid.

42 Despres JP, Allard C, Tremblay A, et al. Evidence for a regional component of body fatness in the association with serum lipids in men and women. *Metabolism.* 1985;34:967–973.

43 Ziegler RG. Anthropometry and breast cancer. *J Nutr.* 1997;127(suppl 5):924S–928S.

44 National Institutes of Health. 1998. http://www.nhlbi.nih.gov/nhlbi.htm.

45 Blackburn GL. Effects of weight loss on weight-related risk factors. In: Brownell KD, Fairburn CG, eds. *Eating Disorders and Obesity.* New York: Guilford; 1995:406–410.

46 National High Blood Pressure Education Program (NHBPEP). Working group: report on primary prevention of hypertension. *Arch Intern Med.* 1993;153:186.

47 Pi-Sunyer XF. Medical complications of obesity. In: Brownell KD, Fairburn CG, eds. *Eating Disorders and Obesity.* New York: Guilford; 1995:401–405.

48 Blackburn, GL. Op. cit.

49 Friedman JM. Obesity in the new millennium. *Nature.* 2000; April 6, 2000, vol. 404:632–634.

50 Kopelman PG. Obesity as a medical problem. *Nature.* 2000; April 6, 2000, vol. 404, 635–643.

51 Ibid.

52 Dalton S. Trends in prevalence of overweight in the United States and other countries. In: Dalton, S. ed. *Overweight and Weight Management: The Health Professional's Guide to Understanding and Practice.* Gaithersburg, MD: Aspen; 1997:142–160.

53 National Heart Lung and Blood Institute (NHLBI). Clinical guidelines on the identification, evaluation, and treatment of overweight and obesity in adults. June 1998.

54 Dalton S. Body weight terminology, definitions, and measurements. In: Dalton S, ed. Op. cit., 1–38.

55 Gustafson-Larson AM, Terry RD. Weight-related behaviors and concerns of fourth-grade children. *J Am Diet Assoc.* 1992;92:818–822.

56 Vasselli JR, Maggio CA. Mechanisms of appetite and body weight regulation. In: Dalton S, ed. Op. cit., 187–208.

57 Johansson L, Solvoll K, Bjorneboe G-E A, Drevon CA. Under- and overreporting of energy intake related to weight status and lifestyle in a nationwide sample. *Am J Clin Nutr.*

1998;68:266–274.

58 Bouchard, C. Genetic factors and body weight regulation. In: Dalton S, ed., Op. cit., 161–186.

59 Barsh GS, Faroogi S, O'Rahilly S. Genetics of body-weight regulation. *Nature,* 2000; April 6, 2000, vol. 404, 644–51

60 Williamson DF, Kahn HS, Remington PL, Anda RF. The 10-year incidence of overweight and major weight gain in US adults. *Arch Intern Med.* 1990;150:665–672.

61 Anderson AE. Eating disorders in males. In: Brownell KD, Fairburn CG, eds. *Eating Disorders and Obesity.* New York: Guilford; 1995:177–182.

62 Pliner P, Chaiken S, Flett GL. Gender differences in concern with body weight and physical appearance over the lifespan. *Personal Soc Psychol Bull.* 1990;16:262–273.

63 Kopelman PG. Op. cit.

64 James W. The Epidemiology of Obesity. Chadwick D, Cardew G, eds. *The Origins and Consequences of Obesity.* Chichester: Wiley; 1996:1–16.

65 Sobal J, Troiano R, Frongillo E. Rural-urban differences in obesity. *Rural Sociol.* 1996;61:289–305.

66 Sobal J, Rauschenbach B, Frongillo E. Marital status, fatness, and obesity. *Social Sci Med.* 1992;35:915–923.

67 Faith MS, Allison DB, Geliebter A. Emotional eating and obesity. In: Dalton S, ed. Op. cit., 439–465.

68 Arnow B, Kenardy J, Agras WS. The emotional eating scale: the development of a measure to assess coping with negative affect by eating. *Int J Eat Disorders.* 1995;18:79–90.

69 Cutting TM, Fisher JO, Grimm-Thomas K, and Birch LL. Like mother, like daughter: familial patterns of overweight are mediated by mothers' dietary disinhibition. *Am J Clin Nutr.* 1999;69:608–613.

70 Marcus MD. Binge eating in obesity. In: Fairburn CG, Wilson GT, eds. *Binge Eating: Nature, Assessment, and Treatment.* New York: Guilford;1993:77–96.

71 Kirschenbaum DS, Fitzgibbon ML. Controversy about the treatment of obesity: criticisms or challenges? *Behav Ther.* 1995;26:43–68.

72 Position of The American Dietetic Association on Weight Management. *J Am Diet Assoc.* 1997;97(1):71–74.

73 Newburgh LH, Johnston MW. Endogenous obesity—a misconception. *JAMA.* 1930;3:815–825.

74 Stuart RB. Behavioral control of overeating. *Behav Res Ther.* 1967;5:357–365.

75 Castellanos VH, Rolls BJ. Diet composition and the regulation of food intake and body weight. In: Dalton S, ed. Op. cit., 254–283.

76 USDA news release. "USDA Coordinated Nutrition Research Program on Popular Diets." May 30, 2000. http://www.usda.gov, Accessed 6/5/2000.

77 Miller WC, Niederpruem MG, Wallace JP, Lindeman AK. Dietary fat, sugar, and fiber predict body fat content. *J Am Diet*

Assoc. 1994;94:612–615.

78 Christiano B, Mizes S. Appraisal and coping deficits associated with eating disorders: implications for treatment. *Cognitive Behav Pract.* 1997;4:263–290.

79 Welle S, Forbes GB, Statt M, et al. Energy expenditure under free living conditions in normal-weight and overweight women. *Am J Clin Nutr.* 1992;55:14–21.

80 Campfield LA. Treatment options and the maintenance of weight loss. In: Allison DB, Pi-Sunyer FX, eds. *Obesity Treatment: Establishing Goals, Improving Outcomes, and Reviewing the Research Agenda.* New York: Plenum;1995:93–95.

81 Blackburn GL. Obesity and the metabolic syndrome. 1999. http://www.obesity.org/obmetabolic.htm.

82 Irwin ML, Mayer-Davis EJ, Addy CL, et al. Moderate-intensity physical activity and fasting insulin levels in women: the Cross-Cultural Activity Participation Study. *Diabetes Care.* 2000;23(4):449.

83 Campfield LA. The role of pharmacological agents in the treatment of obesity. In: Dalton S, ed. Op. cit., 466-485.

84 Diet Drugs Off Market. Updates. *FDA Consumer Magazine.* Nov/Dec 1997.

85 Aronne LJ. Modern medical management of obesity: the role of pharmaceutical intervention. *J Am Diet Assoc.* 1998;98:10 (suppl 2):S23–S26.

86 Carter JC, Fairburn CG. Cognitive-behavioral self-help for binge eating disorder: a controlled effectiveness study. *J Consult Clin Psychol.* 1998;66:616–623.

87 Pi-Sunyer FX. Op. cit.

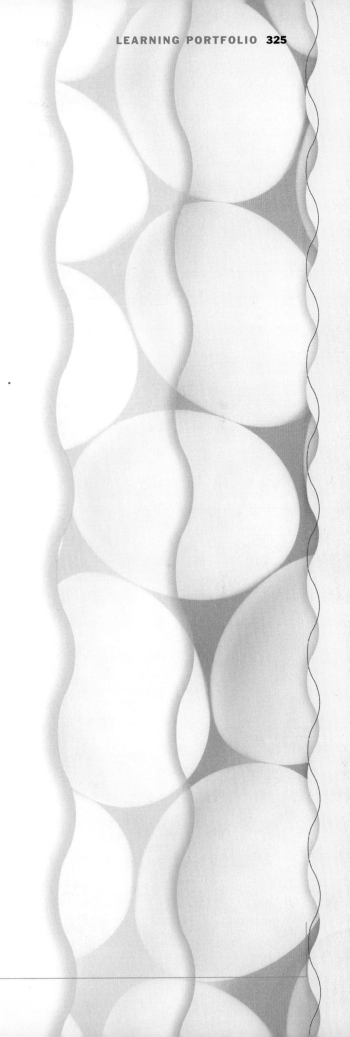

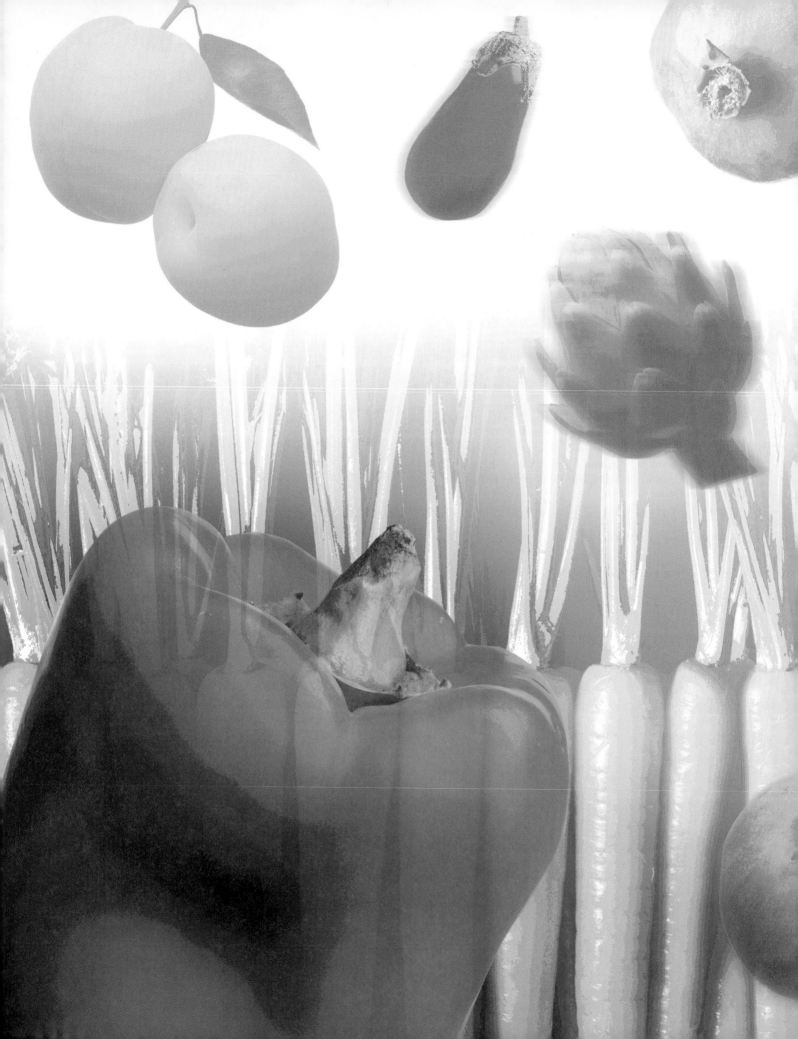

Chapter 9

Fat-Soluble Vitamins

Think About It

1 How do you feel about taking vitamin supplements?

2 Do you prefer vegetables or meat? What food group, if any, supplies most of your vitamin needs?

3 From a well-lighted area, you step into a dark room. Over time, you see details. What's going on?

4 Your grandmother is a strict vegetarian and she seldom goes outdoors. What can you tell her about vitamin D intake?

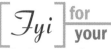
Fyi for your Information

This chapter's FYI boxes include practical information on the following topics:
• A Short History of Vitamins

• Are Megadoses of Vitamin E Appropriate?

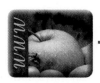

The web site for this book offers many useful tools and is a great source for additional nutrition information for both students and instructors. Visit the site at nutrition.jbpub.com for information on fat-soluble vitamins. You'll find exercises that explore the following topics:
• New Roles for Vitamin A?

• Vitamin D

• Vitamin E in 3-D

• "K" is for Clotting

Key to Illustrations

 Chylomicron

 Fat-Soluble Vitamins

 Free Radical

 LDL

 Lipids/Fats

 Minerals

What About Bobbie?

Track the choices Bobbie is making with the EatRight Analysis software.

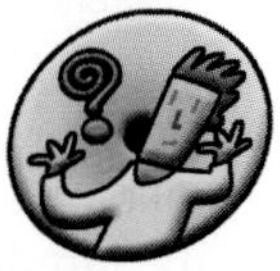

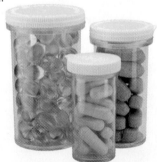

*Y*ou get a panicky call from your sister-in-law—her six-month-old baby is turning orange! She and her husband have done everything the pediatrician told them to do about feeding; just last month they started giving the baby infant cereal, and now have started him on strained baby food. They introduced just one food at a time. In fact, they have only fed him one food other than cereal—carrots. Yes, the baby liked them, so much that he eats two to three jars at each meal! Do you think that could be the problem? But aren't vegetables supposed to be good for you?

Vegetables are healthful foods, and carrots are an important source of many nutrients. Carrots are probably best known as a source of beta-carotene, a vitamin A precursor and the pigment that gives carrots their orange color. Your sister-in-law's baby is eating large quantities of carrots, and the excess beta-carotene circulating in his blood gives the skin a yellow-orange cast. This condition is known as **carotenodermia** and is completely harmless. But, it has probably given at least one or two new parents a scare!

carotenodermia A harmless yellow-orange cast to the skin due to high levels of carotenoids in the bloodstream resulting from consumption of extremely large amounts of carotenoid-rich foods, such as carrot juice.

Understanding Vitamins

Vitamins. Just the word probably makes you think of health and well-being! Children can quickly tell you that fruits and vegetables are good sources of vitamins and can recite some of the best food sources: oranges for vitamin C, carrots for vitamin A, and so on. For many people, however, vitamins have become something to purchase and take in supplement form, not a criterion for choosing foods. Americans spend huge amounts of money, *billions* of dollars each year, on vitamin supplements. Their reasons for taking vitamins are almost as varied as the vitamins themselves—some people take supplements because they "don't eat right." Some take them for extra "insurance," while others look to vitamins to prevent and cure a whole host of conditions from colds to cancer. Is all this money well spent?

To answer this question, you need to consider several aspects of vitamin supplementation. First, survey data indicate few widespread nutrient deficiencies in the United States. From that perspective, people are probably taking many supplements unnecessarily. Another approach is the common sentiment that "if a little is good, more must be better." This misguided belief can lead to problems when applied to vitamin supplementation. Although high doses of some vitamins cause no ill effects, others can have serious, life-long consequences. A third consideration is that research continues to identify relationships between vitamins and reduced risk of some diseases, so some supplementation may be warranted.

These two chapters on vitamins will help you explore some of the implications of too much or too little of a vitamin in the diet and understand the facts about vitamins: what they are, what they do in the body, and which foods contain them. Armed with this information, you will be able to make wise decisions about food and whether to take supplements.

MAJOR ROLES OF VITAMINS

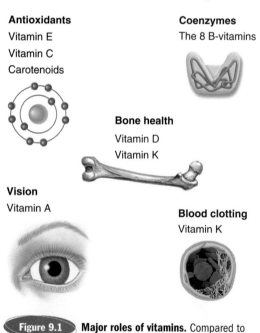

Antioxidants
Vitamin E
Vitamin C
Carotenoids

Coenzymes
The 8 B-vitamins

Bone health
Vitamin D
Vitamin K

Vision
Vitamin A

Blood clotting
Vitamin K

Figure 9.1 **Major roles of vitamins.** Compared to carbohydrate, fat, and protein, the body needs tiny amounts of vitamins. Vitamins, however, are crucial for normal functioning, growth and maintenance of body tissues.

Anatomy of the Vitamins

Although many people think of vitamins as energy boosters, in truth, vitamins do not supply the body with energy in the form of calories—a fact that distinguishes them from fat, carbohydrate, and protein. However, many vitamins regulate the chemical reactions that allow us to obtain energy from those nutrients. Vitamins differ from fat, protein, and carbohydrate in other important ways. For one, the amounts of vitamins a body needs daily—a mere microgram or two in some cases—are infinitesimal compared to the grams of fat, carbohydrate, and protein required each day. Another difference is structural: vitamins are individual units rather than long chains of smaller units.

Like fat, carbohydrate, and protein, however, vitamins are organic (carbon-containing) compounds essential for normal functioning, growth, and maintenance of the body. The functions of vitamins are often interrelated (see **Figure 9.1**), so a deficiency of just one can cause profound health problems.

Fat-Soluble versus Water-Soluble Vitamins

Scientists categorize vitamins based on their solubility. Vitamins A, D, E, and K are lipid-like molecules that are soluble in fat. The B vitamins and vitamin C, on the other hand, are soluble in water. This difference in solubility affects the way the body absorbs, transports, and stores vitamins. **Figure 9.2** illustrates the body's absorption of vitamins.

Figure 9.2 **Absorption of vitamins.** Water-soluble vitamins are absorbed in the intestinal cell and delivered directly to the bloodstream. Fat-soluble vitamins are absorbed with fat.

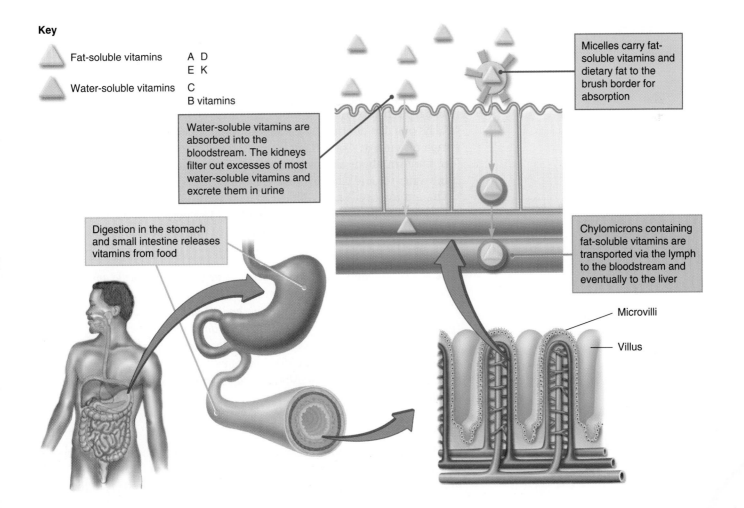

Key

Fat-soluble vitamins — A D / E K

Water-soluble vitamins — C / B vitamins

Micelles carry fat-soluble vitamins and dietary fat to the brush border for absorption

Water-soluble vitamins are absorbed into the bloodstream. The kidneys filter out excesses of most water-soluble vitamins and excrete them in urine

Digestion in the stomach and small intestine releases vitamins from food

Chylomicrons containing fat-soluble vitamins are transported via the lymph to the bloodstream and eventually to the liver

Microvilli

Villus

megadose A dose of a nutrient that is 10 or more times the recommended amount.

provitamin An inactive form of a vitamin that the body can convert into an active useable form. Also referred to as vitamin precursors.

vitamin precursor See provitamin.

retinoids Compounds in foods that have chemical structures similar to vitamin A. Retinoids include the active forms of vitamin A (retinol, retinal, and retinoic acid) and the main storage forms of retinol (retinyl esters).

retinol The alcohol form of vitamin A; one of the retinoids; thought to be the main physiologically active form of vitamin A; interconvertible with retinal.

retinal The aldehyde form of vitamin A; one of the retinoids; the active form of vitamin A in the photoreceptors of the retina; interconvertible with retinol

retinoic acid The acid form of vitamin A; one of the retinoids; formed from retinal but not interconvertible; helps growth, cell differentiation, and the immune system; does not have a role in vision or reproduction.

carotenoids A group of yellow, orange, and red pigments in plants, including foods. Many of these compounds are precursors of vitamin A.

provitamin A Carotenoid precursors of vitamin A in foods of plant origin, primarily deeply colored fruits and vegetables.

Intestinal cells absorb fat-soluble vitamins along with dietary fat. The amount absorbed typically varies from 40 to 90 percent of the amount consumed; efficiency of absorption generally falls as the dietary intake rises above the body's needs. Just like triglycerides and other dietary lipids, lipoproteins carry absorbed fat-soluble vitamins on their journey through the lymph and bloodstream. As chylomicrons move through the blood, cells take up most of the triglycerides and leave behind chylomicron remnants that contain the fat-soluble vitamins. The liver picks up these remnants and either stores the vitamins for future use or repackages them for delivery via the bloodstream to other tissues.

Water-soluble vitamins are dissolved in the watery compartments of foods. Once absorbed, these nutrients travel directly into the bloodstream and then move independently in and around the cells of the body. Unlike fat-soluble vitamins, water-soluble vitamins do not need lipoprotein carriers. Their storage and excretion differs too. While most fat-soluble vitamins accumulate and can be stored indefinitely, the kidneys filter out most excess water-soluble vitamins and excrete them in urine. Two vitamins are exceptions to this general rule: water-soluble vitamin B_{12} is stored more readily than the other water-soluble vitamins, and fat-soluble vitamin K is excreted more readily than the other fat-soluble vitamins.

Storage and Toxicity

Fat-soluble vitamins accumulate in the liver and adipose tissues where they can be drawn upon in times of need. Once these vitamin stores are established, you can go for days, weeks, or even months without consuming more and suffer no ill effects. On the other hand, excessive intake of the fat-soluble vitamins A or D can exceed the body's storage capacity, with toxic effects.

Your body does not store most water-soluble vitamins in appreciable amounts, so they should be a part of your daily diet. Small variations in daily intake typically do not cause problems, however. For example, it takes 20 to 40 days of a diet deficient in the water-soluble vitamin C before deficiency symptoms emerge. Consuming excess water-soluble vitamins usually is harmless, since your body simply excretes the surplus. However, large amounts of some water-soluble vitamins (like vitamin B_6) can cause permanent damage.

Vitamin toxicity is rarely linked to high vitamin intakes from food or to the use of supplements that contain 100 to 150 percent of the recommended amounts. People who take **megadoses** of one or more vitamins run a high risk of toxicity.

Key Concepts: *Vitamins are organic substances needed in minuscule amounts for various roles in regulation of body processes. Two classes of vitamins have been identified: fat-soluble vitamins (A, D, E, and K) and water-soluble vitamins (the B vitamins and vitamin C). Fat-soluble vitamins, which are stored in the liver and fatty tissues of the body, are generally excreted much more slowly than water-soluble vitamins. Because they are stored for long periods, fat-soluble vitamins generally pose a greater risk of toxicity than water-soluble vitamins when consumed in excess.*

Provitamins

Certain vitamins in foods are in inactive forms that the body cannot use directly. These substances are known as **provitamins**, or **vitamin precursors**. Once a provitamin is ingested, the body converts it to the active vitamin form. One familiar provitamin in many fruits and vegetables is beta-carotene (**Figure 9.3**). Once beta-carotene is absorbed, the body converts it to an active form of vitamin A. In fact, beta-carotene is a major source of vitamin A in the diet. When experts calculate vitamin requirements or monitor consumption, they must take provitamins into account.

Vitamins in Foods

What foods do you think of as good sources of vitamins? As mentioned, even very young children know that fruits and vegetables are important in the diet because "they give you vitamins." In fact, vitamins are found in every food group, including the fats and oils that most of us are trying to eat less of. One more reason to include variety in your diet—no one food group, or one choice within a food group is a good source of all vitamins.

The amounts of specific vitamins in a food depend on several factors. For plant foods, whether fruits, vegetables, or grains, the soil content, growing conditions, and maturity at harvest affect the vitamin content. Although an animal's diet can have some impact on animal-derived food, its capacity for absorption and storage keeps the vitamin content fairly consistent.

Generally, the more a food is processed and cooked, the more vitamins it loses. Most food processing (e.g., cooking, milling grain, canning vegetables, and drying fruit) reduces vitamin content. For more information on how to preserve the vitamin content of your foods, see "FYI Fresh, Frozen, or Canned? Raw or Cooked? Selecting and Preparing Foods to Maximize Vitamin Content" in Chapter 10 "Water-Soluble Vitamins."

Key Concepts: All types of foods contain vitamins. Provitamins are vitamin precursors that the body can convert to the active vitamin form. Growing conditions, storage, processing, and cooking all affect the amounts of vitamins in foods.

Vitamin A: The Retinoids

Vitamin A is best known for its role in vision, but it is also crucial for proper growth, reproduction, immunity, and cell differentiation. It helps maintain healthy bones as well as skin and mucous membranes. Vitamin A deficiency not only can destroy vision, it also disrupts numerous functions throughout the body.

Forms of Vitamin A

The body uses three active forms of vitamin A, known collectively as the **retinoids**. These compounds include **retinol**, the alcohol form of vitamin A; **retinal**, the aldehyde form of vitamin A; and **retinoic acid**, the acid form of vitamin A (see **Figure 9.4**). While all three forms have essential functions, retinol is the key player in the vitamin A family. In fact, the standard unit for quantifying the biologic activity of the various forms of vitamin A and its precursors is known as a retinol activity equivalent (RAE).

Your body can easily convert retinol, which is required for reproduction and bone health, to retinal, the form of vitamin A essential for night and color vision. In turn, retinal can reform retinol or it can irreversibly form retinoic acid, which is important for cell growth and differentiation. The interconvertible nature of retinol and retinal allows them to support all the activities of the vitamin A family.

Colorful plant pigments called **carotenoids** are precursors of vitamin A. The body converts some carotenoids, the **provitamin A** compounds, to vitamin A with varying degrees of efficiency. The yellow-orange pigment

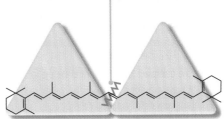

Once beta-carotene is absorbed, it can be cleaved in the middle to yield two molecules of vitamin A

Beta-carotene, a vitamin A precursor

Figure 9.3 **Beta-carotene.** Beta-carotene may be cleaved at different locations, so it may yield less than two molecules of vitamin A. Other provitamin A carotenoids yield less vitamin A than beta-carotene.

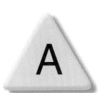

Retinol

Retinal

Retinoic acid

Figure 9.4 **Forms of vitamin A.** Retinol is the alcohol form of vitamin A, retinal is the aldehyde form, and retinoic acid is the acid form.

retinyl esters The main storage form of vitamin A; one of the retinoids. Retinyl esters are retinol combined with fatty acids, usually palmitic acid. Also known as preformed vitamin A.

retinol-binding protein (RBP) A carrier protein that binds to retinol and transports it in the bloodstream from the liver to destination cells.

cornea The transparent outer surface of the eye.

retina A paper-thin tissue that lines the back of the eye and contains cells called rods and cones.

rod cells Light-sensitive cells in the retina that react to dim light and transmit black-and-white images.

cone cells Light-sensitive cells in the retina that are sensitive to bright light and translate it into color images.

beta-carotene can be cleaved into two molecules of retinal and thus has the highest potential vitamin A activity of the provitamin A family. Of all the provitamin A carotenoids, beta-carotene yields the most vitamin A. **Figure 9.5** shows the interconversions and functions of the three active forms of vitamin A.

Storage and Transport of Vitamin A

In well-nourished people, the liver stores more than 90 percent of the body's vitamin A; the remainder is deposited in adipose tissue, lungs, and kidneys.[1] The body stores vitamin A primarily as **retinyl esters**—retinol linked to a fatty acid, usually palmitic acid. Your liver gradually accumulates vitamin A reserves, which reach their peak in adulthood. The liver releases retinol in just the right amounts to maintain normal retinol blood levels. A healthy liver can store up to a year's supply of vitamin A, but taking large doses of vitamin A supplements can exceed this capacity and lead to toxicity.

Many fat-soluble vitamins need carrier proteins to ferry them in the blood to where the body needs them. For instance, **retinol-binding protein (RBP)** carries retinol released by the liver. Once the RBP drops off the retinol to a target cell, the cell can convert retinol to retinal or retinoic acid as needed. Continued production of RBP requires zinc and adequate intake of protein.

Key Concepts: *Vitamin A occurs in three forms in the body: retinol, retinal, and retinoic acid. Each form of the vitamin has specific roles in the body. Most vitamin A is stored by the liver in the form of retinyl esters. Retinol-binding protein carries vitamin A in the bloodstream.*

Functions of Vitamin A

Vitamin A is crucial for vision, for maintaining healthy cells—particularly skin cells—for fighting infections and bolstering immune function, and for promoting growth and development. (See **Figure 9.6**.) In addition, the provitamin A carotenoids may play a role in prevention of cancer and other chronic diseases.

Vitamin A and Vision

When light enters the eye, it passes through the **cornea**, a transparent membrane, and hits the **retina**, the paper-thin tissues that line the back of the eye. The retina contains millions of light-sensitive cells called **rods** and **cones**. The rods react to dim light and process black-and-white images. The cones respond to bright light and translate it into color images. Within both rods and cones, a cascade of reactions converts light into a nerve signal the brain can process so we experience sight.

VITAMIN A INTERCONVERSIONS

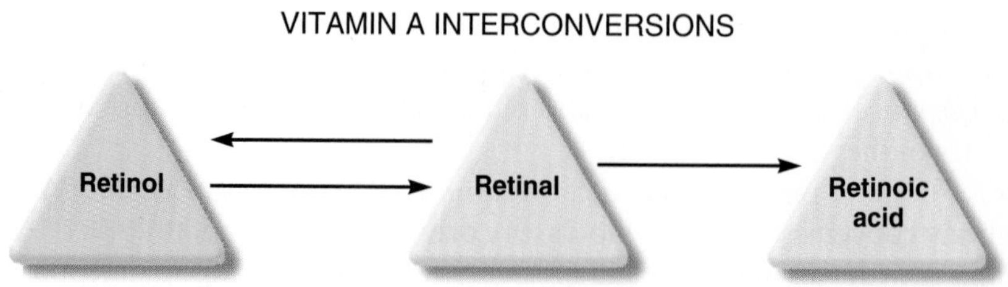

Figure 9.5 **Vitamin A interconversions.** Whereas retinol and retinal are interconvertible, the reaction that forms retinoic acid is irreversible.

Retinol → Retinal → Retinoic acid

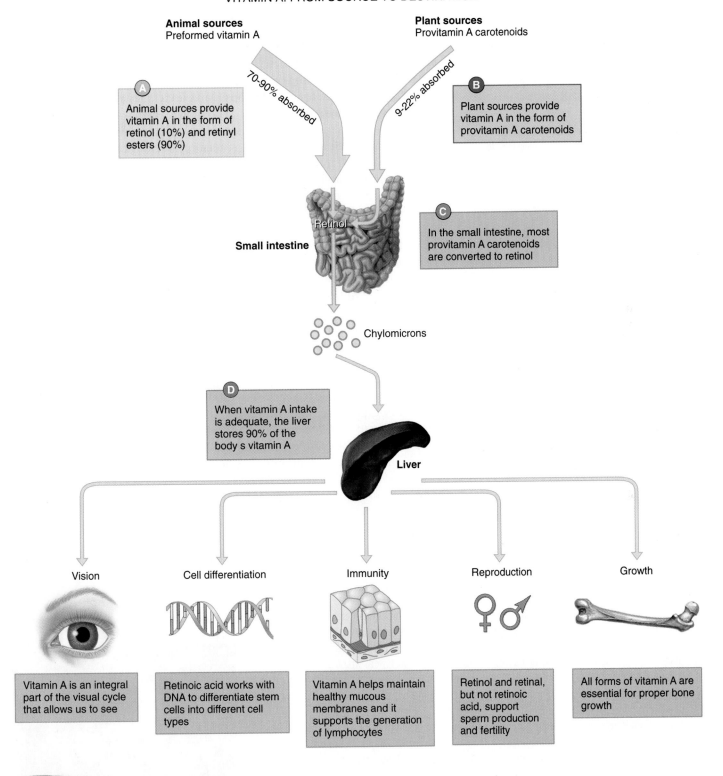

VITAMIN A: FROM SOURCE TO DESTINATION

Animal sources
Preformed vitamin A

Plant sources
Provitamin A carotenoids

70-90% absorbed

9-22% absorbed

A Animal sources provide vitamin A in the form of retinol (10%) and retinyl esters (90%)

B Plant sources provide vitamin A in the form of provitamin A carotenoids

Retinol

Small intestine

C In the small intestine, most provitamin A carotenoids are converted to retinol

Chylomicrons

D When vitamin A intake is adequate, the liver stores 90% of the body s vitamin A

Liver

Vision

Cell differentiation

Immunity

Reproduction

Growth

Vitamin A is an integral part of the visual cycle that allows us to see

Retinoic acid works with DNA to differentiate stem cells into different cell types

Vitamin A helps maintain healthy mucous membranes and it supports the generation of lymphocytes

Retinol and retinal, but not retinoic acid, support sperm production and fertility

All forms of vitamin A are essential for proper bone growth

Figure 9.6 **Vitamin A: from source to destination.** Retinoids from animal foods and carotenoids from plant foods are absorbed from the small intestine and carried by chylomicrons to the liver. Vitamin A plays a crucial role in vision and is essential for proper synthesis, reproduction, and bone growth.

opsin A protein that combines with retinal to form rhodopsin in rod cells.

rhodopsin Found in rod cells, this light-sensitive pigment molecule consists of a protein called opsin combined with retinal.

bleaching process A complex light-stimulated reaction in which rod cells lose color as rhodopsin is split into retinal and opsin.

dark adaptation The process that increases the rhodopsin concentration in your eyes, allowing them to detect images in the dark better.

night blindness The inability of the eyes to adjust to dim light or to regain vision quickly after exposure to a flash of bright light.

How does retinol become a functioning part of the retina? (See **Figure 9.7**.) Retinol is carried in the blood to the retina, where it is converted to retinal. Retinal in turn combines with the protein **opsin** to form a pigment known as **rhodopsin**. Rhodopsin is abundant in rod cells and makes it possible to see in dim light. When light strikes the retina, rod cells undergo a **bleaching process** causing the color of the rod cells to fade. In this transformation, retinal separates from the opsin and undergoes a structural shift, from a "bent," or *cis*, configuration, to a "straightened," or *trans*, configuration. As the retinal detaches, the opsin changes shape as well, disrupting the activities in the cell membrane and generating an electrical impulse. This impulse is relayed to the brain, and you see a black-and-white image. Most of the retinal released in this process is quickly converted back to *trans*-retinol, and then to *cis*-retinal, which spontaneously recombines with opsin. The reformed rhodopsin can respond to light again and begin another cycle.

You've probably had the experience of stepping into a dark room and being unable to see until your eyes adjust. The familiar explanation for this, that you must wait for your pupils to dilate and let in more light, is only part of the story. Your eyes also adapt by changing the amount of available rhodopsin. If you awaken in the middle of the night and turn on a bright light, the light level is blinding until your eyes adjust. Rhodopsin breaks down quickly in bright light, and the reduced supply makes the rod cells less light sensitive. Conversely, when you enter a dark room, your eyes produce rhodopsin to increase their sensitivity to light. Known as **dark adaptation**, the speed of adjustment to dim light is related directly to the amount of vitamin A available to regenerate rhodopsin. People with a vitamin A deficiency experience **night blindness**, the inability of the eyes to adjust to dim light or to regain vision quickly after exposure to a flash of bright light. Due to the lack of vitamin A, rhodopsin regeneration slows dramatically. Although the eyes contain only 0.01 percent of the body's vitamin A, they

Fyi Short History of Vitamins

FOR YOUR INFORMATION

From roughly 1500 B.C.E. to A.D. 1900 there was an empirical understanding that some diseases (which we now call vitamin deficiency diseases) could be cured by eating certain foods. About 400 B.C.E. the Greek physician Hippocrates, following the practice of Arab and Egyptian physicians, prescribed beef liver to people who were unable to see certain stars in the night sky. His maxim was "Let food be thy medicine," but he did not know that beef liver is a rich source of vitamin A, a fat-soluble vitamin necessary for vision.

Similarly, Native Americans knew empirically that extracts of pine needles could prevent or cure scurvy, a condition that includes bleeding gums and loss of energy. In 1753 James Lind, a Scottish surgeon, urged the British navy to include lemon juice in the diet of sailors to prevent scurvy. The navy finally adopted this practice 40 years later. In 1865 they substituted limes, which gave British sailors their nickname "limeys." We now know that the pine needles and citrus fruits provide vitamin C, a water-soluble vitamin whose deficiency causes scurvy.

Many scientists began systematically studying deficiency diseases in the late nineteenth century. They induced "deficiency states" in animals or humans by depriving them of certain foods. The subjects were restored to health when they ate the withheld food. In 1880 the Dutch scientist Christiaan Eijkman, for instance, produced beriberi in chickens by only feeding them polished (white) rice. When

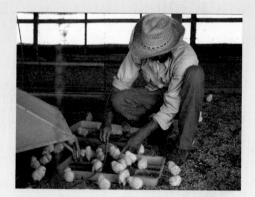

he restored their normal food of unpolished (brown) rice, the chickens quickly recovered. We now know that thiamin, which is removed during polishing, is essential for the health of both man and bird.

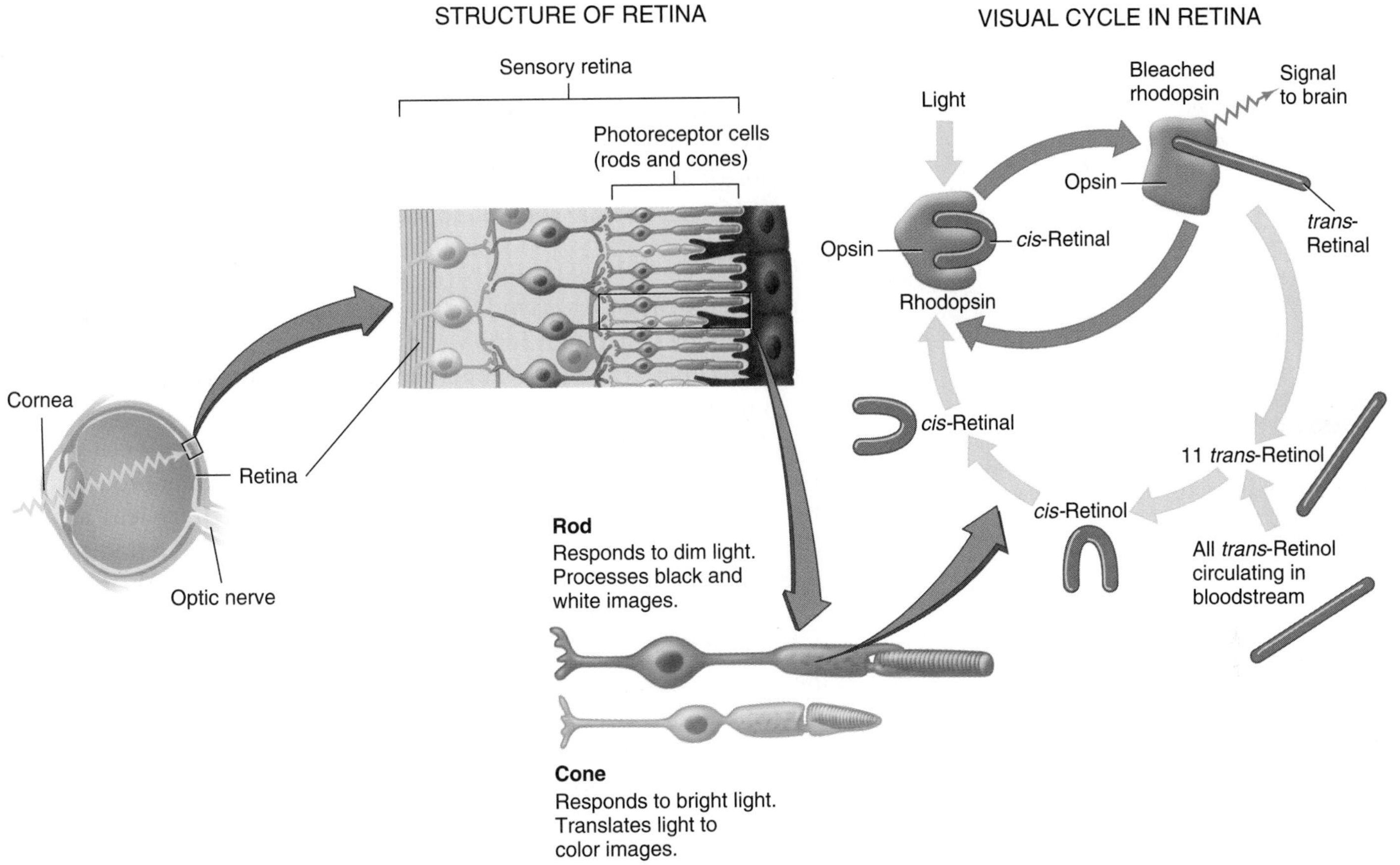

STRUCTURE OF RETINA

VISUAL CYCLE IN RETINA

Rod
Responds to dim light. Processes black and white images.

Cone
Responds to bright light. Translates light to color images.

Figure 9.7 **Vitamin A and the visual cycle.** Rhodopsin is the combination of the protein opsin and vitamin A (retinal). When stimulated by light, opsin changes shape and vitamin A changes from its bent *cis* form to a straighter *trans* form. This sends a signal to the brain and you see an image in black and white. A similar process using a different protein called iodopsin provides color.

In the early twentieth century, scientists began to use chemistry to isolate and identify the critical factors in food that relieved "deficiency states." In 1912, for instance, Casimir Funk isolated a nitrogen-containing compound (an amine) in rice hulls. When given to thiamin-deprived chickens in its pure form, this amine restored the birds to health. Because this compound was required for life (vita) and was nitrogen-containing (amine), Funk coined the term vitamines to describe these essential growth factors. Other vitamines, or vitamins, as they later came to be called, continued to be discovered, purified, and eventually synthesized.

The discovery and naming of vitamins did not proceed without false starts. Some candidate substances did not meet the test of time, and thus we have no vitamins F, G, H, I, or J. On the other hand, vitamin B turned out to be a group of water-soluble vitamins rather than a single vitamin, so today we have eight "B vitamins." The last vitamin to be discovered was vitamin B_{12} and it was not completely synthesized until 1972.

As the vitamins were being isolated and characterized, it became clear that many Americans were not getting enough vitamins, so the National Academy of Sciences established recommended vitamin intakes. Many foods, especially flour and breads, are now fortified or enriched with vitamins.

Today we are exploring the health effects of vitamins beyond simply preventing deficiency diseases. This phase started in 1955, when large doses of niacin were found to lower cholesterol levels. Intense research is exploring vitamin E's potential to slow aging and reduce risks for cancer, heart disease, and cataract formation. Several B vitamins are under investigation for their role in heart disease. Vitamins B_6, folate, and vitamin B_{12} affect the body's levels of the amino acid homocysteine, which recently was identified as an independent risk factor for coronary heart disease.

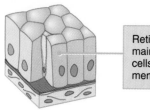

Retinoic acid helps maintain the integrity of cells in the mucous membrane

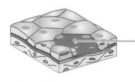

Inadequate retinoic acid impairs the structure and function of these cells

Figure 9.8 **Mucous membrane integrity.** Mucous membranes contain a higher percentage of goblet cells. Without retinoic acid, fewer stem cells become goblet cells and these surfaces become hard and scaly.

iodopsin Color-sensitive pigment molecules in cone cells that consist of opsin-like proteins combined with retinal.

stem cells A formative cell whose daughter cells may differentiate into other cell types.

epithelial cells The millions of cells that line and protect the external and internal surfaces of the body. Epithelial cells form epithelial tissues such as skin and mucous membranes.

epithelial tissues A closely packed layer of epithelial cells that covers the body and lines its cavities.

goblet cells One of the many types of specialized cells that produce and secrete mucus. These cells are found in the stomach, intestines, and portions of the respiratory tract.

Quick Bites

Vitamin A Isn't Just For Eyes

A recent study conducted in Nepal showed that women who took vitamin A supplements during pregnancy had a much lower risk of maternal mortality than those who took a placebo. The researchers concluded that regular and adequate intake of vitamin A or beta-carotene can reduce the risk of pregnancy-related death in areas where vitamin A deficiency is common.

are so sensitive to vitamin A levels that one injection of the vitamin can relieve night blindness within minutes.[2]

Vitamin A is also involved in color vision, as part of the pigment **iodopsin** in cone cells. During color vision, iodopsin undergoes a transformation cycle similar to that of rhodopsin. A lack of vitamin A affects rod cells before it affects cone cells, so as a vitamin A deficiency worsens, night blindness emerges before color blindness.

Vitamin A in Cell Differentiation

Vitamin A's role in vision is crucial, but this function uses only a small fraction of the body's vitamin A supply. A much larger proportion, in the form of retinoic acid, is put to work in normal cell differentiation, the process through which **stem cells** develop into highly specific types of cells with unique functions. Retinoic acid interacts with receptor sites on a cell's DNA—the genetic material that spurs production of particular proteins. When retinoic acid helps activate these receptors in the cell nucleus, stem cells begin transforming into mature differentiated cells. This retinoic acid–dependent differentiation can be seen in **epithelial cells**, the millions of cells that cover and protect the external and internal surfaces of the body. (See **Figure 9.8**.) Epithelial cells form **epithelial tissue**, the largest of which is the skin. The epithelial tissue that lines internal organs includes the mucous membranes of the mouth, nose, stomach, intestine, and eyelids. When epithelial cells differentiate, some develop into mucus-secreting cells (**goblet cells**), and others become different types of mature cells, such as skin cells.[3]

Vitamin A and Immune Function

Vitamin A influences the immune system in important ways. It helps maintain the health of epithelial tissues, the first line of defense against bacterial, parasitic, and viral attack. Vitamin A also supports the generation of T-lymphocytes, important immune cells, maintaining the body's ability to mount an immune response against infectious invaders.[4]

Vitamin A and Reproduction

Although the exact biochemical mechanism is unknown, vitamin A affects both male and female reproductive processes. Both retinol and retinal support reproduction, but retinoic acid does not. In men, vitamin A supports the production of sperm, and in women, it helps maintain fertility, possibly by supporting the production of reproductive tract secretions.

Vitamin A and Bone Health

Vitamin A (retinol, retinal, and retinoic acid) is essential for bone growth. As with the reproductive system, the exact mechanism is unclear, but a lack of vitamin A causes bones to weaken, although they also become thicker than normal. This may be due to a disruption of the bone remodeling process and the failure of immature bone cells to develop properly.

Key Concepts: *Vitamin A plays a crucial role in vision as part of the compound rhodopsin in the rod cells of the retina. When light hits the retina, rhodopsin separates, changes shape, and sends a nerve impulse to the brain. When vitamin A is inadequate, the lack of rhodopsin makes it difficult to see in dim light. Vitamin A is also involved in cell differentiation, growth and development, immune function, reproduction, and bone health.*

Dietary Recommendations for Vitamin A

Similar amounts of dietary retinoids and carotenoids do not provide the same amount of vitamin A. To develop dietary recommendations, scientists reconciled this difference by creating a standardized measurement based on retinol, called **retinol activity equivalents (RAE)**. One retinol activity equivalent is the amount of a given form of vitamin A equal to the activity of one microgram (1/1,000,000 of a gram) of retinol. Using this standard, 12 micrograms (µg) of beta-carotene equal 1 RAE, and 24 micrograms of other carotenoids yield 1 RE. (See **Figure 9.9**.)

You may also see the vitamin A content of dietary supplements expressed as **international units (IU)**. IU is an inexact, outdated measure of vitamin A that was derived using research that did not account for the poor bioavailability, or absorption efficiency, of carotenoids. One IU of vitamin A activity is equal to about 0.3 µg of retinol from animal foods and 3.6 µg of beta-carotene from plant foods.

Most Americans take in adequate amounts of vitamin A and have large stores of the vitamin in their livers. The RDA for vitamin A for males age 14 years and older is 900 micrograms RAE. For females age 14 years and older, the vitamin A RDA is 700 micrograms RAE. Pregnant women should consume slightly more vitamin A (770 micrograms) while lactating women are advised to consume 1,300 micrograms RAE.[5]

1 retinol activity equivalent (RAE) = 1 µg retinol

= 2 µg supplemental beta-carotene

= 12 µg dietary beta-carotene

= 24 µg dietary carotenoids

Figure 9.9 Retinol Equivalents Conversion.

retinol activity equivalents (RAE) A unit of measurement of the vitamin A content of a food. One RAE equals 1 µg of retinol.

international units (IU) An outdated system to measure vitamin activity, this measurement does not consider differences in bioavailability.

preformed vitamin A Retinyl esters, the main storage form of vitamin A. About 90 percent of dietary retinol is in the form of esters, mostly found in foods from animal sources.

Sources of Vitamin A

About half the dietary vitamin A intake comes from animal food sources as **preformed vitamin A**, the retinoids (including retinyl esters, which are the main storage form of vitamin A). The other half of dietary vitamin A intake comes from fruits and vegetables in the form of provitamin A carotenoids, especially beta-carotene. **Figure 9.10** shows foods that are good sources of vitamin A.

Animal foods are the richest sources of retinoids. About 10 percent of vitamin A content is in the form of retinol and the remaining 90 percent is retinyl esters. Liver and fish liver oils (e.g., cod liver oil) are among the top sources. Milk fat (as in whole milk, butter, and other dairy products) also contain vitamin A. Foods fortified with vitamin A (in the form of retinyl palmitate or retinyl acetate) include margarine, some breakfast cereals, and reduced-fat milks. Reduced-fat milks that are not fortified vary greatly in vitamin A content (e.g., unfortified nonfat milk contains no vitamin A). Products, such as yogurt, that are made from reduced-fat or skim milk, are not generally fortified with vitamin A. The body absorbs about 75 percent of dietary retinol and retinyl esters.

The best sources of provitamin A carotenoids are dark-green and yellow-orange vegetables, such as carrots, spinach, broccoli, squash, sweet potatoes, and some orange-colored fruits like cantaloupe, peaches, apricots, and mango. In a varied diet, beta-carotene supplies

VITAMIN A

Daily Value = 5000 IU

Exceptionally good sources			
Beef liver	85 g (3 oz)		30, 689 IU
Carrots, cooked	85 g (~1/2 cup)		20, 871 IU
Sweet potato	110 g (1 small)		18, 759 IU
Chicken liver	85 g (3 oz)		13, 919 IU
Spinach, cooked	85 g (~1/2 cup)		6, 616 IU
Spinach, raw	85 g (~3 cups)		5, 708 IU
Mango, fresh	140 g (~1 cup)		5, 452 IU
Cantaloupe, fresh	140 g (1/4 med. melon)		4, 513 IU
Collards, cooked	85 g (~1/2 cup)		2, 660 IU
Romaine lettuce, raw	85 g (~1 1/2 cups)		2, 210 IU
Oatmeal, instant, fortified, cooked	1 cup		1, 996 IU
Broccoli, cooked	85 g (~1/2 cup)		1, 608 IU
Tomato juice, canned	240 ml (1 cup)		1, 351 IU
Wheat bran flakes cereal	30 g (3/4 cup)		1, 250 IU
Watermelon, fresh	280 g (1/16 melon)		1, 024 IU
Apricot, dried	40 g (~3 Tbsp.)		945 IU
Prunes, dried	40 g (~5 prunes)		795 IU
All bran cereal	30 g (1/2 cup)		750 IU
Corn flakes cereal	30 g (1 cup)		750 IU
Peach, fresh	140 g (2 small)		749 IU
Blackeyed peas	90 g (~1/2 cup)		712 IU
Green beans, cooked	85 g (~3/4 cup)		566 IU
Milk, 1%, 2%, skim	240 ml (1 cup)		500 IU

High: 20% DV or more

Good: 10-19% DV

Figure 9.10 Food sources of vitamin A. Vitamin A is found as retinol in animal foods and as beta-carotene and other carotenoids in plant foods. Some of the best sources are liver, orange and deep-yellow vegetables, and dark-green leafy vegetables. This figure, and others like it in the vitamin and mineral chapters, references the Daily Value standard used on food labels. By law, a food may be labeled a "Good Source" of a nutrient if it contains 10–19% of the Daily Value for that nutrient, and it is a "High Source" if it contains ≥20% of the DV.
Source: U.S. Department of Agriculture, Agricultural Research Service, 1999. USDA Nutrient Database for Standard Reference, Release 13. Nutrient Data Laboratory Home Page, http://www.nal.usda.gov/fnic/foodcomp.

about one-third the total vitamin A, even though the body absorbs this provitamin less efficiently than retinol or retinyl esters. For more information about carotenoids, see "The Carotenoids" section later in this chapter.

Key Concepts: *Intake recommendations for vitamin A are expressed in RAEs (retinol activity equivalents) to account for the differences in bioavailability between retinoids and carotenoids. Current recommendations suggest that adult men consume 900 micrograms RAE each day and the recommendation for adult women is 700 micrograms RAE. Retinol is available from a few animal foods such as liver, fish liver oils, milk fat, and egg yolks. Vitamin A can also be formed from precursor compounds, called carotenoids, which are found in some yellow-orange fruits and in dark-green and yellow-orange vegetables.*

Vitamin A Deficiency

Although dietary deficiency of vitamin A is rare in North America and Western Europe, it is the leading cause of childhood blindness worldwide, especially in Southeast Asia, parts of Africa, and Central and South America. In these regions, vitamin A deficiency typically results from general protein-energy malnutrition in infants and young children. It is estimated that 500,000 preschool children worldwide become blind each year as a result of vitamin A deficiency. (See **Figure 9.11**.)

Although few Americans suffer from a vitamin A deficiency, certain groups are at risk. Newborns, especially premature infants, are at risk because their liver stores of vitamin A are low. Because their diets lack vitamin A–rich foods, impoverished people, particularly children and older adults, may suffer marginal vitamin A status. People with alcoholism or liver disease are at risk because their damaged livers may be incapable of storing much vitamin A. Medicines that alter lipid absorption inhibit vitamin A absorption too. People who have chronic diarrhea, celiac disease, Crohn's disease, cystic fibrosis, or pancreatic insufficiency and other fat-malabsorption conditions may develop vitamin A deficiency over time. In the United States, vitamin A deficiency occurs most often in people who suffer from fat malabsorption syndromes or severely restricted diets as seen in anorexia nervosa. Inadequate intake of zinc also can cause symptoms of vitamin A deficiency because zinc is required for the body to use vitamin A efficiently.

Eyes

Night blindness is an early symptom of vitamin A deficiency, and can be corrected completely with early treatment. As the deficiency worsens, the lack of retinoic acid interferes with the normal differentiation of epithelial cells, and reduces the formation of mucus-secreting goblet cells. As mucus production drops, the cornea and conjunctiva (the outer surface of the eye), and the mucous membrane lining the inner surface of the eyelid become extremely dry. The lack of mucus prevents the eye from washing away dirt and bacteria, thus increasing the likelihood of infection. As the cornea deteriorates, foamy, white triangular patches known as Bitôt's spots develop. Eventually, irreversible scars form on the cornea, which also develops ulcers and sometimes liquefies during the final stages of deterioration. Collectively, these symptoms that progress toward total blindness are known as **xerophthalmia**. Unlike night blindness, which can be reversed with a single dose of vitamin A, corneal drying and scarring usually is permanent.

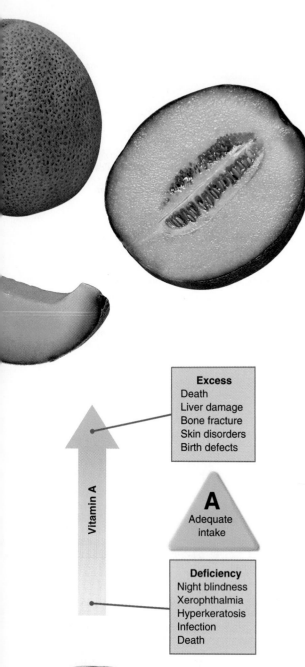

Figure 9.11 **Vitamin A intake.** A broad range of vitamin A intake is adequate and provides for normal function. Too much or too little vitamin A can have serious consequences.

Excess
Death
Liver damage
Bone fracture
Skin disorders
Birth defects

Vitamin A

A
Adequate intake

Deficiency
Night blindness
Xerophthalmia
Hyperkeratosis
Infection
Death

xerophthalmia A condition caused by vitamin A deficiency that dries the cornea and mucous membranes of the eye.

Skin

A lack of retinoic acid shifts the differentiation of epithelial cells toward the production of skin cells. This increased supply packs the skin with extra cells, increasing the density and making the skin hard and scaly. An early symptom of vitamin A deficiency is follicular **hyperkeratosis** or "goose flesh." In this condition, the hair follicles on the skin become plugged with **keratin**, a protein normally present only on the outermost surface of the skin. As a result, the skin becomes rough and bumpy. Sweat glands lose their ability to secrete perspiration. Typically, hyperkeratosis causes thickening of the palms and soles, as well as attacking the flexure areas (elbows, knees, wrists, and ankles) of the skin. In advanced stages the entire body can be involved. Usually, the appearance of hyperkeratotic symptoms in the skin lags behind the development of other symptoms of vitamin A deficiency. When vitamin A is restored, the skin is slower to recover than other affected tissues.[6]

Other Epithelial Cells

Hyperkeratosis affects other types of epithelial cells and disrupts their ability to secrete mucus. This particularly affects the mouth, respiratory tract, urinary tract, female genital tract, seminal vesicles of the testes, and glands of the eyes, making them vulnerable to infection. In men, a vitamin A deficiency halts the production of sperm. Women can become infertile, possibly due to disruptions in the production of reproductive tract secretions.

Hyperkeratinization near sensory receptors causes a loss of taste and smell, which in turn can cause loss of appetite and weight.

Immune Function

When lack of vitamin A leads to dry and dysfunctional epithelial tissues, microorganisms easily can breach the body's defenses. The respiratory tract, mucous membranes, and skin become especially vulnerable to infection. To make things worse, insufficient vitamin A reduces the number of T-lymphocytes, which are important immune cells, and compromises their ability to mount an immune response. Vitamin A deficiency thus leaves a person highly susceptible to bacterial, parasitic, and viral infections. Children with mild vitamin A deficiencies run a high risk of diarrhea, respiratory tract infections, and measles. People with severe vitamin A deficiencies have such impaired immune systems that simple infections may be fatal.[7]

Growth and Other Effects

Vitamin A deficiency retards growth and development, and leads to bone deformities. Teeth may have thin, defective enamel. Kidney stones frequently afflict people with vitamin A deficiency.

Vitamin A Toxicity

Vitamin A toxicity occurs infrequently, but as more people take megadoses of nutritional supplements, the potential for toxic overdoses increases. With the exception of a sustained diet of large amounts of liver or fish oils, food alone generally cannot supply massive amounts of vitamin A. Children tend to be more vulnerable to toxicity and overenthusiastic supplementation of children's diets with vitamin A can be dangerous. Vitamin A toxicity has a wide range of symptoms, both subtle and overt, including fatigue, vomiting, abdominal pain, bone and joint pain, loss of appetite, skin disorders, headache, blurred or double vision, and liver damage, which in turn leads to jaundice. (See Figure 9.11.) Vitamin A toxicity can be fatal! The UL for vitamin A is 3,000 µg per day of retinol.

hyperkeratosis Excessive accumulation of the protein keratin that produces rough and bumpy skin, most commonly affecting the palms and soles, as well as flexure areas (elbows, knees, wrists, ankles). It can affect moist epithelial tissues and impair their ability to secrete mucus. Also called hyperkeratinization.

keratin A sulfur-containing protein normally present in the outermost surface of the skin as well as in hair, nails, and tooth enamel.

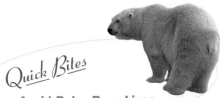

Quick Bites

Avoid Polar Bear Liver

Liver and onions may be your favorite meal, but do not use polar bear liver. Polar bear liver is so rich in vitamin A that a single serving can be toxic for humans

teratogen Any substance that causes birth defects.

Preformed vitamin A, taken in excess, is a known **teratogen**. Birth defects associated with vitamin A toxicity include cleft palate, heart abnormalities, and brain malfunction.[8] Excess vitamin A is most hazardous when taken during the two weeks prior to conception and the first two months of pregnancy. The embryo is undergoing a great deal of cell differentiation and excess amounts appear to interfere with the vitamin's normal support of this process. An acute excess intake of vitamin A as retinol during pregnancy also can cause spontaneous abortions. Pregnant women should avoid prenatal supplements that contain retinol and instead use those that have beta-carotene as the vitamin A source. Pregnant women should take supplements only when their doctors advise them to do so.

Although large doses of beta-carotene (provitamin A) may cause the harmless condition carotenodermia, they do not seem to cause any serious side effects. Conversion of beta-carotene to retinol occurs relatively slowly, and its absorption decreases as dietary intake increases.

Acne Treatment

Up to 90 percent of boys and up to 80 percent of girls experience acne during adolescence, making it the most common skin ailment seen by physicians. The disease has a wide spectrum, ranging from just a few transient pimples to large, chronic, painful nodules that scar when healing.[9]

Retinoic acid is the most commonly prescribed treatment to reduce the formation of blackheads and whiteheads. Retin-A (all-trans-retinoic acid) is available for topical use (applied to the skin). Accutane (13-cis-retinoic acid) is taken orally. Both Retin-A and Accutane increase one's sensitivity to the sun, so sun exposure must be limited to avoid sunburn. More important, these medications, like any large dose of vitamin A, cause birth defects, so any woman who may become pregnant should not take them. Since retinoids accumulate in fat stores, even from topical administration, these medications should be discontinued at least two years before becoming pregnant.

Key Concepts: *Deficiency of vitamin A results in progressive vision loss from temporary night blindness, to reversible blindness, and finally permanent blindness. In addition, the lack of mucus secretions and reduced immune function make the person with vitamin A deficiency vulnerable to infections. Vitamin A toxicity can result from the use of supplements, even with dosages just a few times higher than the RDA. The consequences of vitamin A toxicity during pregnancy are potentially devastating, and pregnant women should avoid both retinol-containing supplements and medications made from retinoids, such as Accutane and Retin-A.*

The Carotenoids

Carotenoids are naturally occurring compounds that give the deep yellow, orange, and red colors to fruits and vegetables such as apricots, carrots, and tomatoes. Carotenoids also are abundant in dark green vegetables, such as spinach, but the even more plentiful green chlorophyll masks the carotenoid colors. Researchers have identified about 600 carotenoids, 50 of which are typically in the U.S. diet, but they have identified only 34 in blood samples and human milk.[10] The major carotenoids are alpha-carotene, beta-carotene, lutein, zeaxanthin, cryptoxanthin, and lycopene. The yellow-orange pigment beta-carotene, which lends its color to cantaloupe, carrots, and squash, is the most common carotenoid.[11] The body can convert alpha-carotene, beta-carotene, and beta-cryptoxanthin to retinol, so they are called

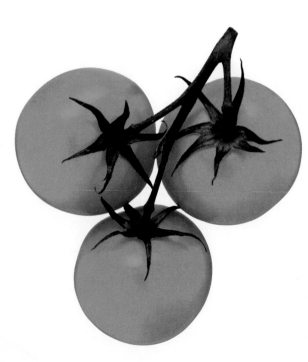

provitamin A carotenoids. Lycopene, lutein, and zeaxanthin have no vitamin A activity, so they are called nonprovitamin A carotenoids.

Functions of Carotenoids

Although carotenoids have diverse biological functions independent of their conversion to vitamin A, there is no evidence that carotenoids are essential nutrients in the technical sense. Because no other specific nutrient functions have been identified for any of the carotenoids, the Food and Nutrition Board has not established DRIs for carotenoids.[12] Yet carotenoids have roles in fighting free radicals, bolstering immune function, enhancing vision, and preventing cancer.

Carotenoids as Antioxidants

Beta-carotene and other carotenoids function as potent antioxidants—substances that can interfere with the damaging effects of **free radicals**, which are highly unstable, reactive compounds. Free radicals can damage both the structure and function of cell membranes, nucleic acids, and electron-dense regions of proteins.[13] This damage may form the biological basis of several acute medical problems, such as premature aging, cancer, atherosclerosis, cataracts, age-related macular degeneration, and an array of degenerative diseases.[14] For more information about free radicals and antioxidants, see the "Vitamin E" section later in this chapter.

free radical A short-lived, highly reactive chemical often derived from oxygen-containing compounds, which can have detrimental effects on cells, especially DNA cell membranes.

Carotenoids and the Immune System

Carotenoids can boost the immune response. Beta-carotene has been shown to enhance certain measures of immune function when taken as a supplement by elderly males[15] and healthy male nonsmokers.[16] Carotenoids also help protect skin from redness and damage following exposure to UV radiation.[17]

Carotenoids and Vision

In the eye, lutein and its close relative zeaxanthin are found in the macula, the central portion of the retina that is responsible for sharp and detailed vision. Scientists believe these carotenoids filter harmful blue light in the macula and scavenge free radicals in retinal tissues.[18] People with the highest intakes of lutein and zeaxanthin also have a decreased risk of cataracts.[19]

Carotenoids and Cancer

Certain carotenoids, including lycopene and beta-carotene, can strengthen growth-regulatory signals between cells. Growth-inhibiting signals from normal cells can help prevent damaged cells from reproducing, especially cells damaged by chemical carcinogens.[20] People with the highest intakes of carotenoid-rich fruits and vegetables and/or high blood levels of specific carotenoids usually have the lowest risk for certain types of cancer. Animal and human studies associate foods rich in specific carotenoids with reduced risks of specific cancers:

- Lycopene may lower the risk of prostate cancer.
- Lutein, zeaxanthin, alpha-carotene, and beta-carotene may lower the risk of lung cancer.
- Beta-carotene may lower the risk of oral cancers.
- Cryptoxanthin may lower the risk of cervical cancer.[21]

These studies focused on foods containing these carotenoids, not carotenoid supplements.

Absorption and Storage of Carotenoids

In foods, fibrous proteins tightly bind carotenoids, so your body absorbs only 20 to 40 percent of what you consume. (See **Figure 9.12**.) This proportion drops even further—to 10 percent or less—as the amount of carotenoids you eat increases. Olestra, the fat substitute in some snack foods, and dietary fiber also reduce carotenoid absorption. Conversely, dietary fat, protein, and vitamin E enhance carotenoid absorption. When dietary fat enters the small intestine, bile is secreted which helps emulsify the fat and enhances the absorption of carotenoids. In fact, when there is a lack of bile, carotenoids are not absorbed.[22] Intestinal cells convert most absorbed carotenoids to vitamin A and deliver the remaining absorbed and unchanged carotenoids to the lymph and eventually the bloodstream, where they circulate bound to lipoproteins.

Although the liver and adipose tissue are the primary carotenoid storage depots, the kidneys, adrenal glands, and other fatty tissues throughout the body also contain carotenoids.[23] Extremely large intakes of carotenoid-rich foods have not been associated with toxic effects but they can have disconcerting results. Carotenoids are strong coloring agents and people who regularly drink carrot juice, for example, may suddenly discover their skin has acquired an orange tinge! They have the harmless condition carotenodermia, just like the baby in the introduction to this chapter.

Sources of Carotenoids

Many fruits and vegetables are rich in carotenoids. Good sources of beta-carotene include apricots, cantaloupe, carrots, leafy green vegetables, pumpkin, sweet potatoes, and winter squash. Because of its yellow-orange color, beta-carotene is added to margarine, gelatin, soft drinks, cake mixes, cereals, and other products. Carrots and pumpkins are rich in alpha-carotene, too. Lutein and zeaxanthin are present in leafy green vegetables, pumpkin, and red pepper. Guava, pink grapefruit, tomatoes and tomato products, and watermelon are good sources of lycopene. Cryptoxanthin is found in mangoes, nectarines, oranges, papaya, peaches, and tangerines.[24]

A few minutes of cooking breaks some of the chemical bonds in food. This helps release carotenoids and makes them easier to absorb. In a study of healthy females, daily consumption of processed carrots and spinach over a four-week period tripled their beta-carotene blood levels compared to their blood levels when they consumed these vegetables raw.[25] Cooked tomato products yield more lycopene than raw tomatoes because heat ruptures plant cell walls, releasing the carotenoid.

Carotenoid Supplementation

More and more people are taking carotenoid supplements. Mixed carotenoid supplements derived from sea algae or palm oil contain a variety of carotenoids including the six major ones. A UL has not been set for beta-carotene or carotenoids. Instead, the Food and Nutrition Board advises against supplementation for the general population and supports existing recommendations for increased consumption of carotenoid-rich fruits and vegetables.

Many scientists have searched for a connection between beta-carotene supplementation and a reduced risk of heart disease, but a consistent association has not emerged.[26] Beta-carotene supplements actually may cause harm to current smokers and people exposed to asbestos.[27] On the other hand, there is a strong link between eating fruits and vegetables rich in beta-carotene and reduced disease rate. In foods there may be beneficial

Quick Bites

And They Called It Cantaloupe

The word *cantaloupe* comes from a papal garden in a small town near Rome named Cantaloupo. One-half of a cantaloupe has 444 RAE as beta-carotene.

Quick Bites

Pizza vs. Tomato Juice

One U.S. study linked intake of tomato sauce, tomatoes, and pizza to lowered risk of prostate cancer. Tomato juice, however, was not protective. That's not surprising. According to John Erdman, Ph.D., of the University of Illinois in Urbana, the cancer-fighting carotenoid found in tomatoes (lycopene) is a fat-soluble substance, so it needs some fat like that found in pizza and most pasta sauces to be absorbed. The lycopene in tomato juice, however, seems to be especially poorly absorbed.

CAROTENOIDS: FROM SOURCE TO DESTINATION

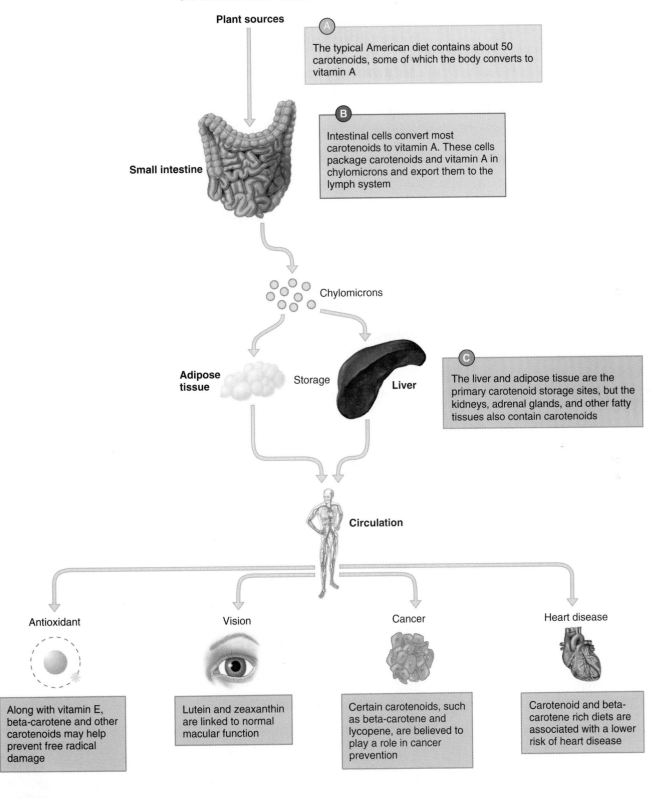

Plant sources

A The typical American diet contains about 50 carotenoids, some of which the body converts to vitamin A

Small intestine

B Intestinal cells convert most carotenoids to vitamin A. These cells package carotenoids and vitamin A in chylomicrons and export them to the lymph system

Chylomicrons

Adipose tissue Storage **Liver**

C The liver and adipose tissue are the primary carotenoid storage sites, but the kidneys, adrenal glands, and other fatty tissues also contain carotenoids

Circulation

Antioxidant

Along with vitamin E, beta-carotene and other carotenoids may help prevent free radical damage

Vision

Lutein and zeaxanthin are linked to normal macular function

Cancer

Certain carotenoids, such as beta-carotene and lycopene, are believed to play a role in cancer prevention

Heart disease

Carotenoid and beta-carotene rich diets are associated with a lower risk of heart disease

Figure 9.12 **Carotenoids: from source to destination.** In the body, the provitamin A carotenoids alpha-carotene, beta-carotene, and beta-cryptoxanthin can be converted to retinol. The nonprovitamin A carotenoids lycopene, lutein, and zeaxanthin have no vitamin A activity. Independent of vitamin A activity, carotenoids can function as antioxidants, and may be involved in normal macular function, and reduced risk of heart disease and cancer.

interactions among naturally occurring beta-carotene, other carotenoids, and other phytochemicals. Additional carotenoids, such as lycopene, lutein, and cryptoxanthin, are now being studied. Although eating carotenoid-rich fruits and vegetables is clearly linked to reduced disease rates, the use of carotenoid supplements is not recommended.

Vitamin D

Sometimes called the sunshine vitamin, vitamin D is unique because, given sufficient sunlight, your body can synthesize all it needs of this fat-soluble nutrient. In fact, it could be argued that vitamin D is technically not a nutrient—it is synthesized and functions like a hormone, and it is not always necessary in the diet. When the ultraviolet rays of the sun strike the skin, they alter a precursor derived from cholesterol, converting it into vitamin D. Although fortified milk and other foods supply vitamin D, your body can make plenty as long as it gets regular exposure to sunlight.

Vitamin D is essential for bone health. In children, it promotes bone development and growth. In adults, it is necessary for bone maintenance. In the elderly, vitamin D helps prevent osteoporosis and fractures. Although severe vitamin D deficiency in children and adults is rare, vitamin D deficiency is widespread among sick people and the elderly.[28]

Forms and Formation of Vitamin D

Vitamin D can be considered either a vitamin or a hormone. Like other vitamins, a lack of dietary vitamin D (coupled with minimal sun exposure) will cause a deficiency. The active form of vitamin D is like a hormone because it is made in one part of the body and regulates activities in other parts. (See **Figure 9.13**.)

Ten compounds, called vitamin D_1 through D_{10}, exhibit **antirachitic** properties; that is, they prevent a childhood bone disease called rickets. The most important of these compounds are D_2 (ergocalciferol) and D_3 (cholecalciferol). Ergocalciferol is found exclusively in plant foods. Cholecalciferol is found in animal foods (eggs and fish oils), but most is synthesized in the skin.

In the skin, ultraviolet (UV) radiation from the sun converts a cholesterol derivative (7-dehydrocholesterol) to cholecalciferol, which then enters the bloodstream and travels to the liver. The liver also receives dietary cholecalciferol and ergocalciferol from chylomicrons. In the liver, cholecalciferol and ergocalciferol are converted into calcidiol and then sent to the kidneys. The kidneys perform the final step—the formation of **calcitriol**, the predominant, active form of vitamin D. The body derives about 90 percent of its calcitriol from the cholecalciferol synthesized in the skin.[29]

Functions of Vitamin D

Vitamin D's primary role is to regulate blood calcium levels. We know that vitamin D is involved in other regulatory processes, which are subjects of current investigations. In fact, vitamin D may have anticancer effects since leukemia cells and breast, lung, cervix, and colon tumor cells contain receptors for calcitriol. Researchers are studying the use of topical vitamin D to treat psoriasis. A gene that regulates vitamin D receptors may predict bone density status in older people. Finally, calcitriol may trigger cell differentiation in certain tissues.

antirachitic Pertaining to activities of an agent used to treat rickets.

calcitriol The active form of vitamin D, it is an important regulator of blood calcium levels.

VITAMIN D: FROM SOURCE TO DESTINATION

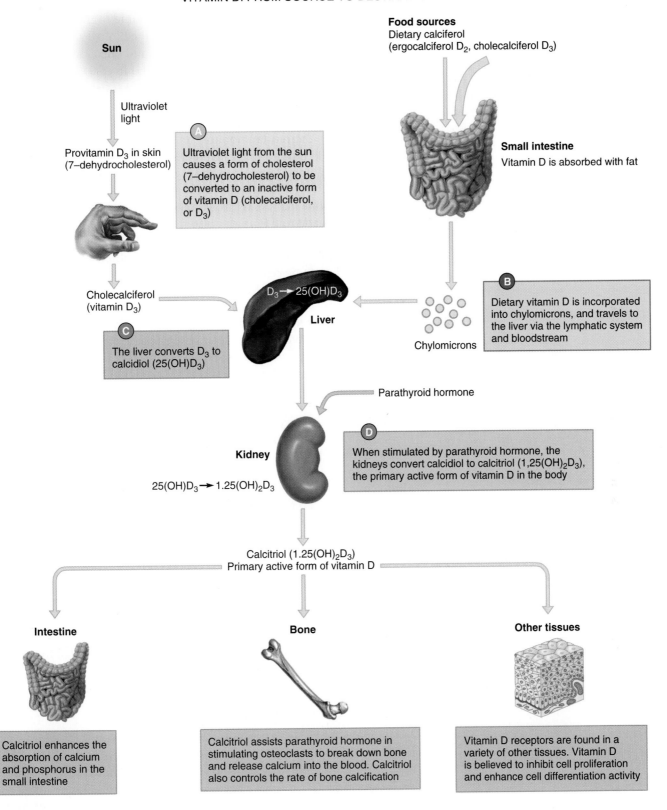

Sun

Ultraviolet
light

Provitamin D$_3$ in skin
(7–dehydrocholesterol)

Cholecalciferol
(vitamin D$_3$)

A Ultraviolet light from the sun
causes a form of cholesterol
(7–dehydrocholesterol) to be
converted to an inactive form
of vitamin D (cholecalciferol,
or D$_3$)

C The liver converts D$_3$ to
calcidiol (25(OH)D$_3$)

Food sources
Dietary calciferol
(ergocalciferol D$_2$, cholecalciferol D$_3$)

Small intestine
Vitamin D is absorbed with fat

B Dietary vitamin D is incorporated
into chylomicrons, and travels to
the liver via the lymphatic system
and bloodstream

Chylomicrons

D$_3$ ➝ 25(OH)D$_3$
Liver

Parathyroid hormone

Kidney

25(OH)D$_3$ ➝ 1.25(OH)$_2$D$_3$

D When stimulated by parathyroid hormone, the
kidneys convert calcidiol to calcitriol (1,25(OH)$_2$D$_3$),
the primary active form of vitamin D in the body

Calcitriol (1.25(OH)$_2$D$_3$)
Primary active form of vitamin D

Intestine

Bone

Other tissues

Calcitriol enhances the
absorption of calcium
and phosphorus in the
small intestine

Calcitriol assists parathyroid hormone in
stimulating osteoclasts to break down bone
and release calcium into the blood. Calcitriol
also controls the rate of bone calcification

Vitamin D receptors are found in a
variety of other tissues. Vitamin D
is believed to inhibit cell proliferation
and enhance cell differentiation activity

Figure 9.13 **Vitamin D: from source to destination.** Vitamin D is unique because, given sufficient sunlight, your body can synthesize al it needs.
Both dietary and endogenous vitamin D must be activated by reactions in the kidneys and liver. Active vitamin D (calcitriol) is important
for calcium balance and bone health, and may have a role in cell differentiation.

parathyroid hormone A hormone secreted by the parathyroid glands in response to low blood calcium. It stimulates calcium release from bone and calcium absorption by the intestines, while decreasing calcium excretion by the kidneys. It acts in conjunction with calcitriol to raise blood calcium. Also called parathormone.

calcitonin A hormone secreted by the thyroid gland in response to elevated blood calcium. It stimulates calcium deposition in bone and calcium excretion by the kidneys, thus reducing blood calcium.

osteoclasts Bone cells that promote bone resorption and calcium mobilization.

osteoblasts Bone cells that promote bone deposition and growth.

Quick Bites

Do you know vitamin D when you see it?

The general terms *vitamin D* and *calciferol* are used to refer to both vitamin D_2 (ergocalciferol) and vitamin D_3 (cholecalciferol), and to any combination of these two compounds.

Regulation of Blood Calcium Levels

The liver and adipose tissue store vitamin D. In times of need, the liver and kidneys convert stored vitamin D to calcitriol, the biologically active form in the body. Calcitriol helps maintain calcium and phosphorus blood levels within a normal range. Calcitriol acts directly and in concert with two other hormones: **parathyroid hormone** (parathormone) from the parathyroid gland, and **calcitonin** from the thyroid gland. These hormones regulate activity in the bone, kidneys, and small intestine to adjust blood calcium levels. Much as a thermostat monitors temperature, receptors in the parathyroid gland monitor the calcium blood level.

When calcium blood levels drop, the parathyroid gland releases parathyroid hormone (PTH). PTH stimulates the activity of **osteoclasts** (bone cells that digest the bone matrix), releasing calcium ions from bone into the bloodstream. Parathyroid hormone also raises blood calcium levels by signaling the kidneys to slow calcium excretion. PTH also stimulates the kidney to activate vitamin D. Calcitriol is released by the kidneys and enhances the action of PTH on bone cells. Calcitriol then stimulates the intestinal cells to make more carrier proteins for calcium transport, enhancing the absorption of calcium from food and thereby helping to elevate blood levels of calcium.

When calcium blood levels are too high, the thyroid gland releases calcitonin and the parathyroid gland decreases its release of PTH. Calcitonin inhibits the activity of osteoclasts, shifting the balance toward the activity of **osteoblasts** (bone-building cells). This net bone-building activity removes calcium ions from the bloodstream and deposits them in new bone. Calcitonin promotes bone growth in children and helps maintain bone health during pregnancy and lactation. Since high levels of calcium in the blood inhibit release of parathyroid hormone, the kidney continues to excrete calcium. In the absence of PTH, the kidney activates little or no calcitriol. In the small intestine, lower calcitriol levels reduce the production of protein carriers for calcium transport, thus reducing calcium absorption.

Even if calcium and phosphorus intakes are adequate, teeth and bones do not calcify normally without calcitriol. Conversely, calcification progresses normally when calcitriol status is adequate even if calcium and phosphorus levels are low. Calcitriol controls the rate of calcification independent of the absolute blood levels of calcium and phosphorus.

Key Concepts: *The best known function of vitamin D, in the active form of calcitriol, is to help regulate blood calcium levels. Calcitriol works with two other hormones, parathyroid hormone and calcitonin, to alter the amount of calcium in the bone, the amount excreted from the kidney, and the amount absorbed from the intestine to keep blood levels in a normal range. It is known that calcitriol has effects on other tissues, but these functions have not been well studied.*

Dietary Recommendations for Vitamin D

Although the body can synthesize vitamin D, scientists still recognize vitamin D as an essential nutrient for most people. Because of the variability of sunlight throughout the year, and some people's limited sun exposure, intake recommendations have been developed. Dietary recommendations are given as Adequate Intake (AI) levels that assume no available vitamin D from skin synthesis.[30]

Infants are born with stores of vitamin D that last about nine months. Beyond that, they must obtain vitamin D via exposure to sunlight, formula, or a supplement administered under the guidance of a physician. Breast milk contains very little vitamin D and is unlikely to meet a baby's needs beyond infancy. Exclusively breast-fed infants who receive little exposure to sunlight need supplemental vitamin D. The AI for infants and children from birth to 18 years is 5 micrograms per day.

In later adulthood, the intake recommendations for vitamin D increase because vitamin D synthesis decreases with aging. For men and women aged 19 through 50 years, the AI for vitamin D is 5 micrograms per day. For people ages 51 through 70, the AI increases to 10 micrograms per day, and for people older than 70, the AI rises to 15 micrograms per day.

As for vitamin A, International Units (IU) rather than micrograms (μg) will be found on supplement labels. The conversion works out to 1 μg = 40 IU. Therefore, 200 IU is the equivalent of the AI for ages 19 through 50.

Sources of Vitamin D

In theory, all of our required vitamin D could be synthesized in the skin when it is exposed to UV light. In fact, the diet may supply only about 10 percent of our needs.[31]

Sunlight and Vitamin D Synthesis

How much exposure to the sun is needed for an adequate supply of vitamin D? It depends on several factors including:

- Time of day—the sun's rays are most intense between 10:00 A.M. and 2:00 P.M.

- Season—the sun is higher in the sky and delivers more radiation during the summer months.

- Environment—80 percent or more of the sun's UV rays penetrate clouds,[32] but ordinary window glass blocks UV radiation.

- Location—sunlight is less intense in the northern and southern latitudes than near the equator. A sun worshiper in Florida receives 50 percent more radiation than one in Maine. (See **Figure 9.14**.)

- Use of sunscreen—sunscreen protects the skin against sun damage, but it also blocks the ultraviolet light necessary for vitamin D synthesis.

- Skin type—light-skinned people absorb UV rays more quickly than dark-skinned people.

A rule of thumb is to expose your hands, face, and arms to the sun for about $\frac{1}{3}$ to $\frac{1}{2}$ the time it would take you to burn.[33] Repeat this exposure two to three times a week to get adequate vitamin D.

Dietary Sources of Vitamin D

Few foods naturally contain vitamin D, so the major dietary sources of the nutrient are vitamin D–fortified milk and other fortified foods such as breakfast cereal. In the United States, milk is fortified with 10 micrograms of vitamin D (400 IU) per quart. Three surveys of the vitamin D content of fortified milk in the United States and Canada suggest that as many as 70 percent of the milk samples did not contain vitamin D in the range of 8 to 12 micrograms. Some samples of nonfat milk contained no vitamin D.[34] Because of this variability, the U.S. Food and Drug Administration now monitors dairies' compliance with vitamin D fortification.

Vitamin D is found in oily fish (e.g., herring, salmon, and sardines) as well as in cod liver oil and other fish oils. Egg yolk, butter, and liver supply various amounts of vitamin D depending on the vitamin D content of the

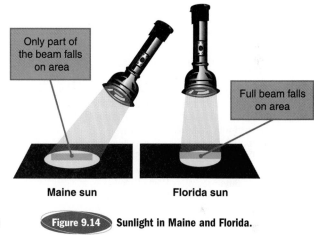

Only part of the beam falls on area

Full beam falls on area

Maine sun **Florida sun**

Figure 9.14 Sunlight in Maine and Florida.

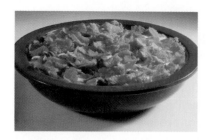

VITAMIN D

Daily Value = 400 IU

Exceptionally good source

Cod liver oil	1 Tbsp.	1,360 IU
Salmon, canned, solids + bones	55 g (2 oz)	343 IU
Sardines, canned, solids + bones	55 g (2 oz)	150 IU
Milk, nonfat	240 ml (1 cup)	98 IU
Milk, 1%, 2% milkfat	240 ml (1 cup)	98 IU
Milk, whole, 3.25% milkfat	240 ml (1 cup)	98 IU
Fortified, ready-to-eat cereals	30 g	40 IU

High: 20% DV or more

Good: 10-19% DV

Figure 9.15 **Food sources of vitamin D.** Only a few foods are naturally good sources of vitamin D. Therefore, fortified foods such as milk and some cereals are important, especially for people with limited exposure to the sun. Units are IU to be consistent with Daily Value definitions.
Source: U.S. Department of Agriculture, Agricultural Research Service, 1999. USDA Nutrient Database for Standard Reference, Release 13. Nutrient Data Laboratory Home Page, http://www.nal.usda.gov/fnic/foodcomp.

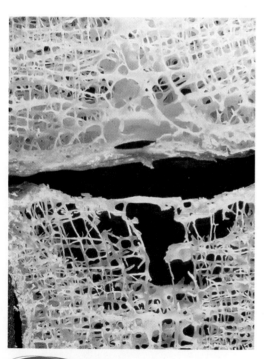

Figure 9.16 **Osteoporosis.** Normal (top) and osteoporotic bone (bottom). The osteoporotic bone is noticeably less dense.

foods consumed by the source animals. Plants are a poor source, so strict vegetarians must get their vitamin D through exposure to sunlight. If sun exposure is not possible, nutritionists may recommend dietary supplements. **Figure 9.15** shows some foods that are sources of vitamin D.

Key Concepts: *Intake recommendations for vitamin D are very small, only 5 micrograms per day for young adults. Needs from the diet increase with age as the ability of the skin to synthesize vitamin D declines. Few foods are naturally good sources of vitamin D, and so most of the dietary intake comes from fortified milk and other fortified foods.*

Vitamin D Deficiency

Long-term deficiency of vitamin D takes a profound toll on the skeleton. When vitamin D is in short supply, the intestines absorb only about 10 to 15 percent of dietary calcium so bones don't get enough of this bone-building mineral.

Rickets and Osteomalacia

In children with vitamin D deficiency, the bones weaken and the skeleton fails to harden. Children with this disease, called **rickets**, often have bowed legs or knocked knees and other skeletal deformities. Although vitamin D fortification of milk has reduced the incidence of rickets in the United States, many children worldwide still suffer from the disease. In the United States, rickets is sometimes seen in children with malabsorption syndromes such as cystic fibrosis. One study found that rickets also occurs among dark-pigmented Alaskan children younger than 2 years old who are breast-fed.[35]

In adults, vitamin D deficiency causes a similar skeletal problem called **osteomalacia**, or "soft bones." Osteomalacia increases the risk for fractures in the hip, spine, and other bones. In addition to preventing adequate calcium absorption, osteomalacia alters the function of the parathyroid gland, boosting calcium losses from the bones. Risk of osteomalacia is high in people who have diseases that affect the stomach, kidneys, gallbladder, liver, or intestine—organs that are involved with the absorption or activation of vitamin D.

Osteoporosis

Along with osteomalacia, vitamin D deficiency is associated with **osteoporosis**, increased bone turnover, and an increased risk of bone fractures.[36] (See **Figure 9.16**.) Administration of vitamin D to elderly people with or without a deficiency slows bone turnover and increases bone density. In elders with low blood levels of cholecalciferol, vitamin D supplementation substantially reduces the risk of osteoporotic fractures, including hip fractures.[37] For more information on osteoporosis see Chapter 11, "Water and Major Minerals," and Chapter 16, "Adult Nutrition."

Who Is Most at Risk for a Vitamin D Deficiency?

In 1998 a pivotal study was published suggesting many more people are deficient in vitamin D than had been suspected. The investigation of nearly 300 patients hospitalized in Boston showed that almost three of five people had too little vitamin D to maintain optimal levels of calcium in their bones.[38]

One explanation for the vitamin D shortfall may be that more people are protecting their skin with sunscreen, which may help prevent skin cancer, but reduces vitamin D synthesis. Any sunscreen with a sun protection factor (SPF) of 8 or more blocks vitamin D synthesis in the skin. The problem worsens with age. Adults older than 65 years have a fourfold decrease in their ability to produce vitamin D_3 via the sun, compared to adults 20 to 30 years old.[39]

Living in a northern region compounds the problem. During the dead of winter, daylight hours are so short and the sunlight is so weak that vitamin D synthesis halts. (See **Figure 9.17**.) Although the same is true for the southern latitudes, little of the world's population lives in this region. Fortunately, the skin of most people under the age of 50 years can make sufficient amounts of vitamin D with just the amount of skin on the hands exposed for 10 to 15 minutes per day during warmer months. Most younger people make and store enough vitamin D during the summer to last through the winter months.

People over age 50 are advised to expose some skin to the sun for about 15 minutes each day during warm months. In the winter, many experts recommend a vitamin supplement. Most multivitamin/mineral supplements contain 10 micrograms (400 IU) of vitamin D. Healthy adults over age 70 should check with their physicians to determine whether more supplemental vitamin D is in order.

Vitamin D Toxicity

Sun exposure does not cause vitamin D toxicity, but high supplement doses can be highly toxic. The Tolerable Upper Intake Level (UL) for adults over 19 years of age is 50 *micrograms* (2,000 IU) per day. Before consuming supplements that contain more than the AI, people should consult a physician.

The hallmark of vitamin D toxicity is **hypercalcemia**—a high concentration of calcium in the blood. This condition affects numerous tissues in the body. Initially, it hampers the kidneys' ability to concentrate urine, causing excessive urination and thirst. Prolonged hypercalcemia can cause the excess calcium in the bloodstream to leave deposits in the soft tissues of the body, including the kidneys, blood vessels, heart, and lungs. Hypercalcemia also seems to affect the central nervous system, causing a severe depressive illness as well as nausea, vomiting, and loss of appetite.

Excess vitamin D can also promote loss of bone mass as the increased levels of calcitriol help pull calcium from the bones into the bloodstream. In one report of 40 cases of vitamin D toxicity in adults 50 and older, four people who were taking more than 30 micrograms (1,200 IU) of supplemental vitamin D a day were losing three times as much calcium through their urine as people who were taking less vitamin D.[40]

Key Concepts: Because vitamin D's primary function is to regulate the level of calcium in the blood, which affects storage of calcium in bone, a deficiency of the nutrient affects the skeletal system. In children, vitamin D deficiency leads to rickets; in adults, lack of the nutrient causes osteomalacia and contributes to osteoporosis. Consumed in excess, vitamin D is toxic and should be taken only under a physician's supervision. Exposure to sun does not cause vitamin D toxicity.

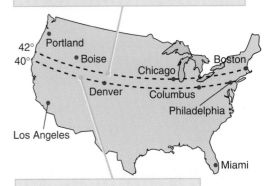

North of 42 degrees latitude, sunlight is too weak to synthesize vitamin D from late October through early March. The same effect occurs during the winter in the southern hemisphere south of 42 degrees latitude

At 40 degrees latitude, sunlight is too weak to synthesize vitamin D during January and February

Figure 9.17 **Mapping vitamin D synthesis.** Vitamin D synthesis halts for part of the winter if sunlight is too weak. In Los Angeles and Miami, the sunlight is strong enough to synthesize vitamin D year round, even in January.

rickets A bone disease in children that results from vitamin D deficiency.

osteomalacia A disease in adults that results from vitamin D deficiency; it is marked by softening of the bones, leading to bending of the spine, bowing of the legs, and increased risk for fractures.

osteoporosis A bone disease characterized by a decrease in bone mineral density and the appearance of small holes in bones due to loss of minerals.

hypercalcemia Excess calcium in the blood that causes the deposition of calcium in soft body tissues and affects the nervous system. It is caused by various conditions, including excess vitamin D intakes, but does not develop from a high calcium intake.

Quick Bites

Too Much Cover

Many Arab women are clothed so that only their eyes are exposed to sunlight. Even though these women live in sunny climates near the equator, many suffer from osteomalacia.

Vitamin E

Consumers have long embraced the practice of taking large amounts of vitamin E, once touted as being able to boost sexual prowess and to prevent gray hair, wrinkles, and other signs of aging. Although many of these rumored benefits of vitamin E have never been supported by science, a growing body of research suggests that the nutrient may, in fact, be an important protector against chronic diseases associated with aging.

Forms of Vitamin E

In 1922 researchers discovered that an unknown substance in vegetable oils was necessary for reproduction in rats. It was given the chemical name **tocopherol**, from the Greek word *tokos*, meaning "childbirth," added to the verb *phero*, meaning "to bring forth." The ending *ol* reflects the alcohol nature of the molecule. It was a full forty years after discovery, however, before scientists gathered evidence showing that humans also need this substance, which they labeled vitamin E. In 1968 the Food and Nutrition Board of the National Academy of Sciences officially recognized vitamin E as an essential nutrient.

Vitamin E is not a single compound. It is actually two sets of four compounds each: the tocopherols (alpha, beta, gamma, and delta) and the chemically related **tocotrienols** (alpha, beta, gamma, and delta). Although all of these can be absorbed, only alpha-tocopherol is considered to have vitamin E activity in the body. Alpha-tocopherol is the most common form of vitamin E in food.

As for all fat-soluble vitamins, absorption of vitamin E requires adequate absorption of dietary fat. Like the other fat-soluble vitamins, it travels via chylomicrons and other lipoproteins for distribution throughout the body. The GI tract absorbs 20 percent to 80 percent of dietary alpha-tocopherol, and the percentage declines as the amount of vitamin E consumed increases. Unabsorbed vitamin E is excreted in fecal matter. (See **Figure 9.18**.)

Unlike the fat-soluble vitamins A and D, vitamin E does not accumulate in the liver. Adipose tissue contains about 90 percent of the vitamin E in the body. The remaining vitamin E is found in virtually every cell membrane in every tissue. **Table 9.1** shows the amount of vitamin E in various tissues of the body.

Functions of Vitamin E

Vitamin E is an antioxidant and its activity is enhanced by other antioxidants such as vitamin C and selenium (a mineral). During normal metabolic processes, oxygen often reacts with other compounds to generate free radicals—highly unstable, toxic molecules that contain one unpaired electron. These unpaired electrons make free radicals highly reactive. Typically, a free radical attacks a nearby compound and steals an electron from it. While that stabilizes the original free radical "thief," it turns the "robbed" molecule into a free radical, sparking a chain reaction capable of instantly producing a flood of free radicals.

Under normal circumstances, your body generates free radicals to help eliminate unwanted molecules. If various enzymes and antioxidants fail to control free radical activity, these highly reactive compounds attack cell membranes and cell constituents, including DNA. This unleashing of free radicals sets the stage for chronic diseases such as cancer and atherosclerosis.

A form of free radical damage that promotes atherosclerosis is **lipid peroxidation**—the production of unstable lipid molecules that contain

Table 9.1 Vitamin E Content of Tissues

Tissue	Fresh Weight (µg/g)
Adipose	150
Adrenal	132
Pituitary	40
Testis	40
Platelets	30
Heart	20
Muscle	19
Liver	13
Ovary	11
Plasma	9.5
Uterus	9
Kidney	7
Erythrocytes	2.3

Source: *An Overview of Vitamin E Efficacy.* LaGrange, IL: VERIS; October 1998.

tocopherol The chemical name for vitamin E. There are four tocopherols (alpha, beta, gamma, delta), but only alpha-tocopherol is active in the body.

tocotrienols Four compounds (alpha, beta, gamma, delta) chemically related to tocopherols. The tocotrienols and tocopherols are collectively known as vitamin E.

lipid peroxidation Production of unstable, highly reactive lipid molecules that contain excess amounts of oxygen.

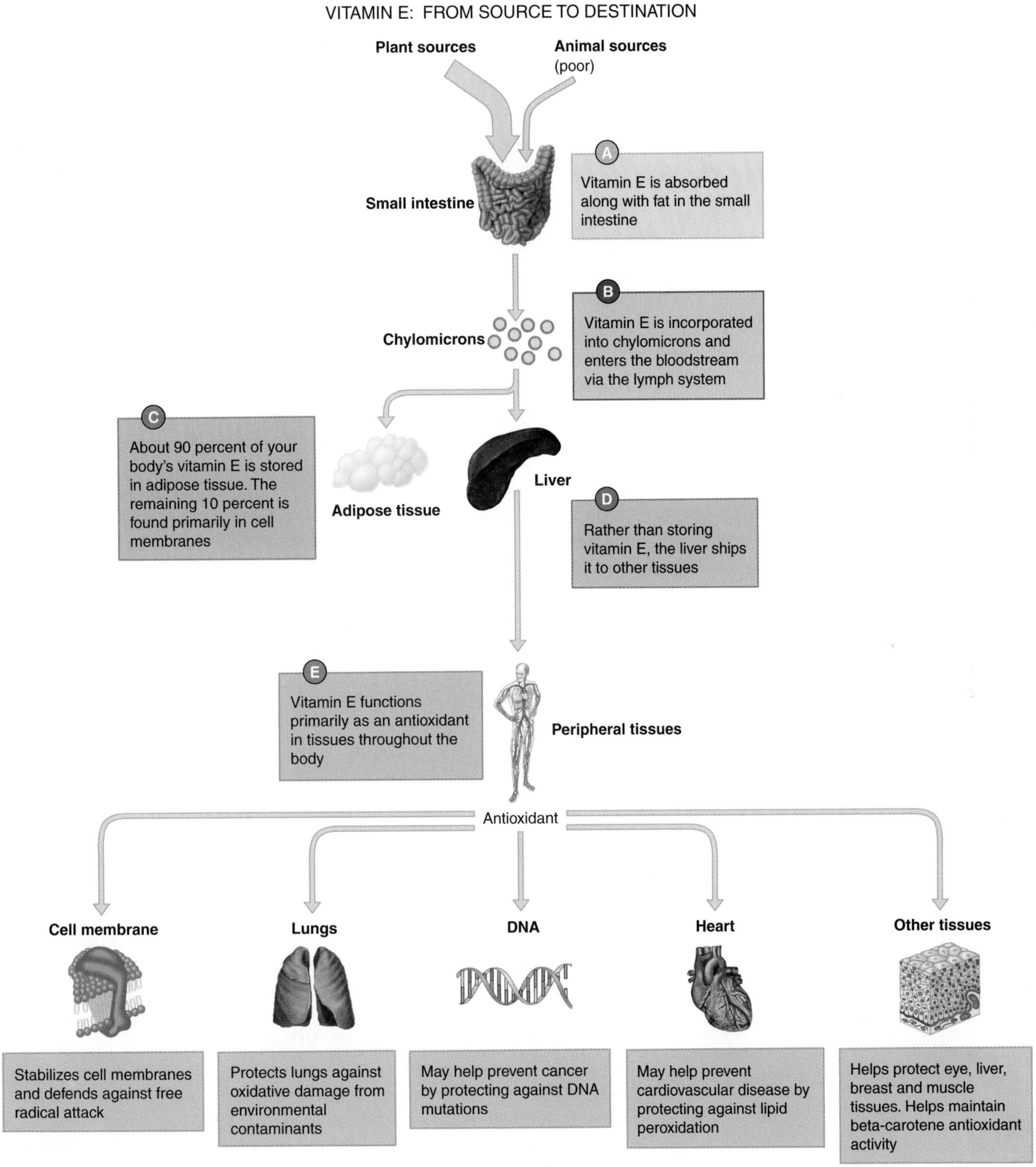

VITAMIN E: FROM SOURCE TO DESTINATION

Plant sources   **Animal sources**
(poor)

Small intestine

A Vitamin E is absorbed along with fat in the small intestine

Chylomicrons

B Vitamin E is incorporated into chylomicrons and enters the bloodstream via the lymph system

C About 90 percent of your body's vitamin E is stored in adipose tissue. The remaining 10 percent is found primarily in cell membranes

Adipose tissue

Liver

D Rather than storing vitamin E, the liver ships it to other tissues

E Vitamin E functions primarily as an antioxidant in tissues throughout the body

Peripheral tissues

Antioxidant

Cell membrane

Stabilizes cell membranes and defends against free radical attack

Lungs

Protects lungs against oxidative damage from environmental contaminants

DNA

May help prevent cancer by protecting against DNA mutations

Heart

May help prevent cardiovascular disease by protecting against lipid peroxidation

Other tissues

Helps protect eye, liver, breast and muscle tissues. Helps maintain beta-carotene antioxidant activity

Figure 9.18 **Vitamin E: from source to destination.** Vitamin E is absorbed in the small intestine and carried to the liver by chylomicrons. The antioxidant activity of vitamin E helps stabilize cell membranes, protects tissues from oxidative damage, and may reduce the risk of cancer and heart disease.

Key

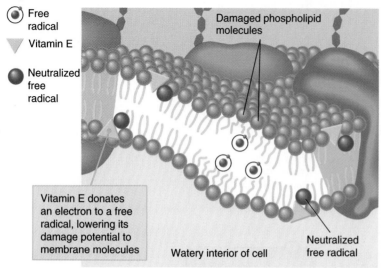

Figure 9.19 **Free radical damage.** Vitamin E helps prevent free radical damage to polyunsaturated fatty acids in cell membranes.

glutathione A tripeptide of glycine, cysteine, and glutamic acid that is involved in protection of cells from oxidative damage.

an excess of oxygen. In this process, the cleavage of a carbon-carbon double bond in a fatty acid yields an intermediate compound that reacts with oxygen to form peroxides or free radicals. To stop lipid peroxidation, vitamin E acts as a potent antioxidant and interrupts the cascade of free radical formation. Vitamin E donates an electron to the electron-seeking free radical, thus preventing the free radical from finding an electron somewhere else and causing more damage. This makes vitamin E itself a free radical, but not a very reactive one. The body excretes some of this altered vitamin E and recycles the rest by adding an electron from another antioxidant, such as vitamin C. This vitamin C radical can regain its antioxidant form by swiping an electron from **glutathione**. The enzyme glutathione reductase restores glutathione to its antioxidant form and depends on the mineral selenium.

The polyunsaturated fatty acids (PUFAs) in cell membranes are especially vulnerable to assault by free radicals. Vitamin E resides in cell membranes and other phospholipid-rich tissues, where it serves as one of the body's chief defenses against damage by free radicals. (See **Figure 9.19**.)

Laboratory evidence suggests that oxidative stress, which occurs when free radical formation overwhelms the body's counterbalancing mechanisms, leads to premature aging, cancer, atherosclerosis, cataracts, age-related macular degeneration, and an array of degenerative diseases. The current scientific evidence suggests that antioxidants like vitamin E have essential roles in slowing or preventing these disease processes.[41]

Thus, vitamin E functions as an antioxidant by

- stabilizing cell membranes and defending cells against free radical attack;
- protecting the lungs from oxidative damage due to environmental contaminants such as air pollution;
- helping to prevent cancer—cells damaged by free radicals are prone to mutation;
- protecting the tissues of the skin, eye, liver, breast, and calf muscle; and
- maintaining the effectiveness of the antioxidant beta-carotene.

Key Concepts: *Vitamin E is really a set of compounds called tocopherols and tocotrienols, but in the body, alpha-tocopherol is the only active vitamin E compound. Vitamin E functions as an antioxidant, protecting cell membranes in all parts of the body from the damaging effects of oxidation. Vitamin E has been connected to reduction of risk for many degenerative diseases such as heart disease and cancer.*

Dietary Recommendations for Vitamin E

To prevent vitamin E deficiency, the intake requirement must be related to body size and to polyunsaturated fatty acid (PUFA) intake. When PUFA intake is minimal, small amounts of vitamin E will prevent symptoms of deficiency. As PUFA intake increases, the concentration of PUFA in tissues also rises and more vitamin E is needed to prevent oxidation. Since the vitamin E content of oils tends to parallel the PUFA concentration, balancing the two is usually not a problem; but as more people limit fat intake, they may also limit vitamin E intake.

The RDA for vitamin E is 15 milligrams of alpha-tocopherol for men and women. The recommendations for pregnant and lactating women are 15 milligrams of alpha-tocopherol and 19 milligrams of alpha-tocopherol, respectively. A number of double-blind, placebo-controlled studies are looking at the effectiveness of vitamin E in preventing or slowing heart disease. If these studies yield positive results, recommendations for vitamin intake in adults older than 50 may increase.[42] Although officially discontinued, International Units (IU) are still found on supplement labels. If the vitamin E in the supplement is from natural sources, 1 IU = 0.67 mg alpha-tocopherol. If synthetic vitamin E is used, the conversion is 1 IU = 0.45 mg alpha-tocopherol.

Sources of Vitamin E

Vitamin E is found in many different foods from both plant and animal sources. Wheat germ oil contains the highest concentration of usable vitamin E. Vegetable and seed oils, such as safflower, cottonseed, and sunflower seed oils, are also rich sources. Although soybean and corn oils contain much vitamin E, only about 10 percent is alpha-tocopherol, the active form of vitamin E.[43] Foods made from vegetable oils, such as margarine and salad

---

 Are Megadoses of Vitamin E Appropriate?

FOR YOUR INFORMATION

Vitamin E is second only to vitamin C as the most popular single vitamin supplement in the United States.[1] Preliminary research shows that large doses of vitamin E may bolster immune function as well as help prevent such chronic conditions as heart disease, cancer, and Alzheimer's disease. These compelling studies have no doubt contributed to the ever-increasing sales of vitamin E supplements. Still, no major health organization endorses widespread use of vitamin E supplements because the research, though encouraging, is not definitive.

Vitamin E and Heart Disease

Vitamin E is a potent antioxidant that may help prevent heart disease, the number one killer of both men and women. Experiments suggest that vitamin E stymies the LDL-oxidation process, lending biological plausibility to a number of epidemiological studies that have shown an association between high intakes of vitamin E and reduced risk of heart disease.

LDL cholesterol appears to trigger plaque formation in the arteries of the heart when it undergoes oxidation—the chemical reaction sparked by free radicals. Oxidized LDL is more likely than unoxidized LDL to form foam cells, which are the foundation of atherosclerotic

plaques. In addition, oxidized LDL may destroy nearby cells and attract cell debris and other matter that clumps and forms fatty streaks that eventually narrow arteries.

Two major Harvard University studies of participants in the ongoing Health Professionals Follow-Up Study and the Nurses' Health Study support vitamin E's potential to prevent heart disease. Researchers monitored some 40,000 men for four years and nearly 90,000 women for eight years. Men taking at least 100 IU of vitamin E for a minimum of two years had a 37 percent lower risk of heart disease than those not taking a supplement. Similarly, women who took at least 100 IU of E had a 41 percent drop in risk.[2]

Although findings are promising, major health organizations await confirmation by clinical trials before recommending vitamin E supplements to the general public. In fact, a recent study of men and women at high-risk for heart attack because of pre-existing cardiovascular disease found no protective effect of 400 IU of vitamin E daily for an average of 4.5 years.[3] Randomized, placebo-controlled clinical trials are needed to determine whether long-term use of vitamin E supplements over the course of decades causes side effects that haven't been

seen in trials that lasted only a few years.

What's more, vitamin E can pose the risk of increased bleeding in people with heart disease who take warfarin (Coumadin), aspirin, and other anticoagulants to prevent blood clots. Vitamin E's anticlotting properties also raise a person's risk of hemorrhagic stroke—a type of stroke resulting from bleeding into the brain and the rest of the central nervous system. Hemorrhagic strokes are less frequent than the thrombotic type, in which a clot blocks blood flow in the brain. Still, hemorrhagic strokes are more often fatal. Until the benefits of taking megadoses of vitamin E clearly outweigh the risks, caution is in order. Before taking supplemental vitamin E, a person should consult a physician.

1 Richman A, Witkowski JP. Sixth Annual Dietary Supplement Survey. *Whole Foods.* June 1998:23–28.

2 Rimm EB, Stampfer MJ, Ascherio A, et al. Vitamin E consumption and the risk of coronary heart disease in men. *N Engl J Med.* 1993;328(20):1450–1456.

Stampfer MJ, Hennekens CH, Manson JE, et al. Vitamin E consumption and the risk of coronary heart disease in women. *N Engl J Med.* 1993;328(20):1444–1449.

3 Yusuf S, Dagenais G, Pogue J, et al. Vitamin E supplementation and cardiovascular events in high-risk patients. The Heart Outcomes Prevention Evaluation Study Investigators. *N Engl J Med.* 2000;342:154–160.

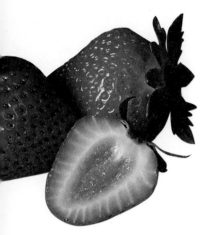

dressings, as well as nuts and seeds, also are good sources. Although substantial amounts of vitamin E are found in strawberries and some green leafy vegetables, most fruits and vegetables contribute only small amounts. Animal products are medium to poor sources of vitamin E and vary widely in their content depending on the fat composition of the given animal's diet.

In the typical U.S. diet, about 20 percent of vitamin E intake comes from salad oils, margarine, and shortening. Vegetables supply about 15 percent, and more than 12 percent comes from meat, poultry, and fish. Breakfast cereal supplies about 10 percent and fruit contributes about 9 percent of the dietary vitamin E.[44] NHANES III data suggest that American adults consume 8 to 12 milligrams of vitamin E per day from foods. However, this value is likely to be less than actual consumption due to typical underreporting of total fat and energy intake.[45] **Figure 9.20** shows foods that are good sources of vitamin E.

Cooking, processing, and storage can reduce the vitamin E content of foods substantially. (See **Table 9.2**.) During the milling of wheat to make white flour, for instance, vitamin E–rich wheat germ is removed, and if chloride dioxide is used for the bleaching process, all vitamin E is lost. Refining and purifying vegetable oils takes a substantial toll on their vitamin E content. In fact, the byproducts of the refining process contain so much vitamin E that they are used to make supplements. Oxygen is the destructive culprit that attacks vitamin E, and both light and heat accelerate oxidation. Safflower oils stored at room temperature for three months lose more than half of their vitamin E. Roasting destroys 80 percent of the vitamin E in almonds.

Key Concepts: *The RDA for vitamin E is 15 milligrams of alpha-tocopherol for both men and women. Vitamin E is found in wheat germ, vegetable and seed oils, and products made from these oils such as salad dressing and margarine. Processing foods can reduce their vitamin E content.*

Figure 9.20 **Foods sources of vitamin E.** Nuts and seeds, vegetable oil, and products made from vegetable oil, such as margarine, are among the best sources of vitamin E. Units are IU to be consistent with Daily Value definitions. **Note:** USDA tables list vitamin E in mg-alpha tocopherol equivalents. Conversion to IU was done using 1 mg-ATE=1.5 IU. USDA database is not complete for vitamin E. **Source:** U.S. Department of Agriculture, Agricultural Research Service, 1999. USDA Nutrient Database for Standard Reference, Release 13. Nutrient Data Laboratory Home Page, http://www.nal.usda.gov/fnic/foodcomp.

VITAMIN E

Daily Value = 30 IU

Exceptionally good sources		
Wheat germ oil	1 Tbsp.	39.3 IU
Total cereal	30 g (~3/4 cup)	35.2 IU
Product 19 cereal	30 g (~1 cup)	33.3 IU

High: 20% DV or more

Sunflower seeds	30 g	22.6 IU
Almonds	30 g	11.8 IU
Wheat bran flakes cereal	30 g (~3/4 cup)	8.3 IU
Cottonseed oil	1 Tbsp.	7.8 IU
Margarine, hard, soybean oil	1 Tbsp.	7.3 IU
Safflower oil	1 Tbsp.	7.0 IU
Hazelnuts	30 g	6.8 IU
Strawberries, fresh	140 g (~1 cup)	6.3 IU

Good: 10-19% DV

Italian dressing	30 g (~2 Tbsp.)	4.7 IU
Corn oil	1 Tbsp.	4.3 IU
French dressing	30 g (~2 Tbsp.)	3.8 IU
Soybean oil	1 Tbsp.	3.7 IU
Brazilnuts	30 g	3.4 IU
Peanuts	30 g	3.3 IU
Tomato juice, canned	240 ml (1 cup)	3.3 IU
Margarine, hard, corn oil	1 Tbsp	3.1 IU

Vitamin E Deficiency

Because of the widespread use of vegetable oils and other sources in the food supply, vitamin E deficiency is rare in North America. Most deficiencies occur in people with fat-malabsorption syndromes such as cystic fibrosis. One feature of vitamin E deficiency is premature **hemolysis**—the breakdown of red blood cells. Without vitamin E to protect the cells against oxidation, destruction of cell membranes is rampant, causing red blood cells to burst. Hemolysis, and the associated anemia (called hemolytic anemia) is most often seen in infants born prematurely, before vitamin E has been transferred from mother to fetus in the last weeks of pregnancy. Special formulas and supplemental vitamin E are administered to premature babies to help correct the problem.

In children and adults, fat malabsorption disorders and subsequent vitamin E deficiency usually cause neurological problems that affect the spinal cord and peripheral nerves. In adults, malabsorption must be prolonged, from 5 to 10 years, before signs of deficiency surface.

hemolysis The breakdown of red blood cells that usually occurs at the end of a red blood cell's normal life span. This process releases hemoglobin.

Vitamin E Toxicity

Vitamin E is relatively nontoxic, especially compared with fat-soluble vitamins A and D. One hazard of large doses of vitamin E, however, is that the dose counters vitamin K's blood-clotting mechanism, described in the next section. People who take anticoagulant medications such as warfarin (Coumadin) or aspirin to prevent blood clots should confer with a physician before they self-prescribe large doses of vitamin E.

A large and growing body of experimental evidence suggests high intakes of vitamin E may lower the risk of some chronic diseases, especially heart disease. Clinical trials, however, are limited and their results are inconsistent, so it is not yet appropriate to recommend high vitamin E intake to reduce risk of chronic disease. For adults, the UL is 1,000 milligrams per day of any form of supplemental alpha-tocopherol.[46]

Key Concepts: *Deficiencies of vitamin E are rare in adults, occurring primarily in people with fat-malabsorption syndromes. Preterm infants also run a high risk of vitamin E deficiency because they are delivered before the nutrient has a chance to move from the mother to the infant. Hemolysis is the hallmark of such a deficiency. Vitamin E toxicity is also rare, though large doses of the nutrient pose a hazard to people who take blood-thinning medications.*

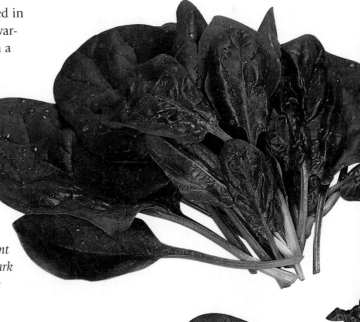

Table 9.2 **Reported Storage and Processing Losses of Vitamin E**

Food	Test Conditions	Vitamin E Loss
Peanut oil	Frying at 347°F, 175°C, 30 minutes	32%
Safflower oil	Stored at room temperature, 3 months	55%
Tortillas	Stored at room temperature, 12 months	95%
Almonds	Roasting	80%
Wheat germ	Storage at 39°F, 4°C, 6 months	10%
Wheat	Processing to white flour	92%
Bread	Baking	5–50%

Source: *Vitamin E Factbook,* LaGrange, IL: VERIS; 1999.

phylloquinone The form of vitamin K that comes from plant sources. Also known as vitamin K_1.

menaquinone The form of vitamin K that comes from animal sources. Also produced by intestinal bacteria, this form of vitamin K is known as vitamin K_2.

menadione A medicinal form of vitamin K that can be toxic to infants. Also known as vitamin K_3.

Vitamin K

In 1929 Danish researcher Henrik Dam discovered a nutrient that plays a crucial role in blood clotting. He named it vitamin "K" for "koagulation." Although most people give little thought to consuming enough of this nutrient, vitamin K stands between life and death. Without vitamin K to promote blood clotting, a single cut would eventually lead to death by blood loss.

Vitamin K refers to a family of compounds, known as quinones. It includes **phylloquinone** (K_1) from plant sources, **menaquinones** (collectively known as K_2) from animal sources and synthesized by our intestinal bacteria, and the synthetic substances **menadione**, Synkayvite, and Hykinone (collectively known as K_3). Phylloquinone is the most biologically active form. Menaquinone is only 70 percent as active and the synthetics drop to 20 percent. Phylloquinone, menaquinone, and the synthetic compound menadione are

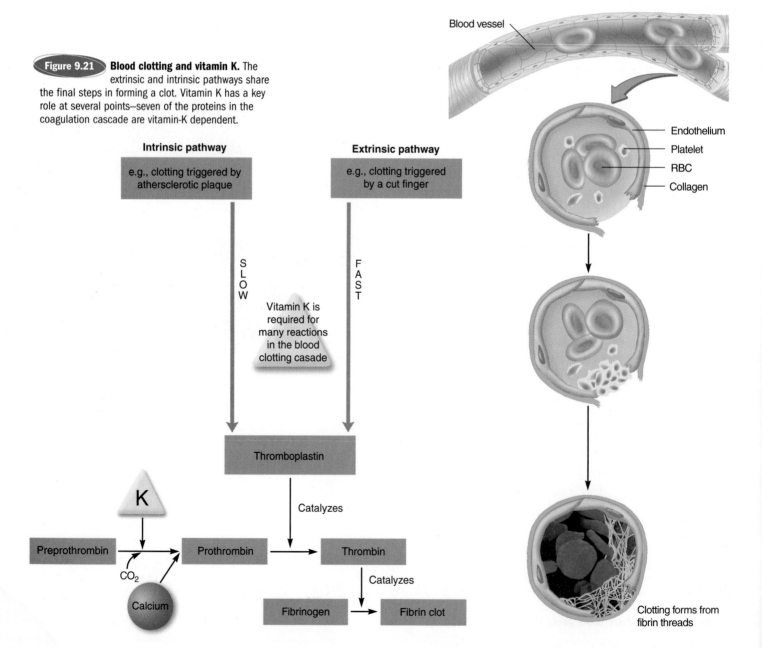

Figure 9.21 **Blood clotting and vitamin K.** The extrinsic and intrinsic pathways share the final steps in forming a clot. Vitamin K has a key role at several points—seven of the proteins in the coagulation cascade are vitamin-K dependent.

fat soluble and primarily stored in the liver. These stores are relatively small and used up rapidly.

The synthetic compounds Synkayvite and Hykinone are water soluble. These forms are well suited to the treatment of vitamin K deficiency caused by fat malabsorption disorders. Menadione is considered an unsafe supplemental form of vitamin K.

Functions of Vitamin K

When you get a cut, small or large, and start to bleed, a series of reactions forms a clot that stops the flow of blood. This cascade of reactions involves the production of a series of proteins, and ultimately the protein fibrin. Seven of the proteins in this coagulation cascade are vitamin K–dependent, and all require calcium for activation. For example, vitamin K converts the precursor protein preprothrombin to prothrombin by adding carbon dioxide to glutamic acid (an amino acid) in the protein. This change imparts a calcium-binding capacity, which allows prothrombin to be changed to thrombin. These reactions are integral to the formation of a blood clot.

In addition to promoting the formation of blood clots (**Figure 9.21**), vitamin K appears to assist in bone formation. The vitamin is thought to work by facilitating a process needed to allow the protein osteocalcin to strengthen the skeleton.

Vitamin K is important to the carboxylation of osteocalcin, which allows osteocalcin to become saturated with carboxyl groups. (See **Figure 9.22.**) Some research has shown a correlation between undercarboxylated osteocalcin and bone fractures; other evidence suggests an association between elevated risk of fractures and low levels of vitamin K in the blood.[47] At least two other bone proteins require vitamin K for carboxylation, underscoring the vitamin's importance to bone health.

Key Concepts: *Vitamin K was named for the Danish word koagulation because the nutrient works to promote the formation of blood clots. Vitamin K also is involved in bone health.*

Dietary Recommendations for Vitamin K

Dietary intake of vitamin K varies with age. In general, adults under age 45 have intakes that range from 60 to 110 micrograms of phylloquinone per day. In contrast, intakes for adults over age 55 range from 80 to 210 micrograms of phylloquinone per day. Experts attribute this difference to the greater vegetable consumption of older adults than that of younger adults.[48]

As with other fat-soluble vitamins, vitamin K absorption depends on normal consumption and digestion of dietary fat. Absorption is poor in people with fat-malabsorption syndromes. Even under normal conditions, absorption of dietary vitamin K may be as low as 40 percent.

Typical diets easily support vitamin K's role in blood clotting but researchers have found preliminary evidence that more than 400 micrograms per day of dietary vitamin K may be necessary to support its role in bone health.[49]

The AI for vitamin K for adult males (or males over the age of 19) is 120 micrograms. Recommendations for women are slightly lower: 90 micrograms per day. The AI doesn't change for pregnant and lactating women.

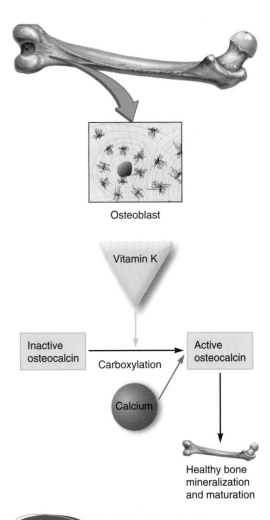

Osteoblast

Vitamin K

Inactive osteocalcin → Carboxylation → Active osteocalcin

Calcium

Healthy bone mineralization and maturation

Figure 9.22 **Vitamin K and bone health.** Osteocalcin is an abundant bone protein that is required for bone mineralization and maturation. Vitamin K helps in the carboxylation of osteocalcin, greatly enhancing its calcium binding properties.

Sources of Vitamin K

Scientists have long believed that intestinal bacteria synthesize about half of the body's vitamin K and dietary (mostly plant) sources supply the rest;

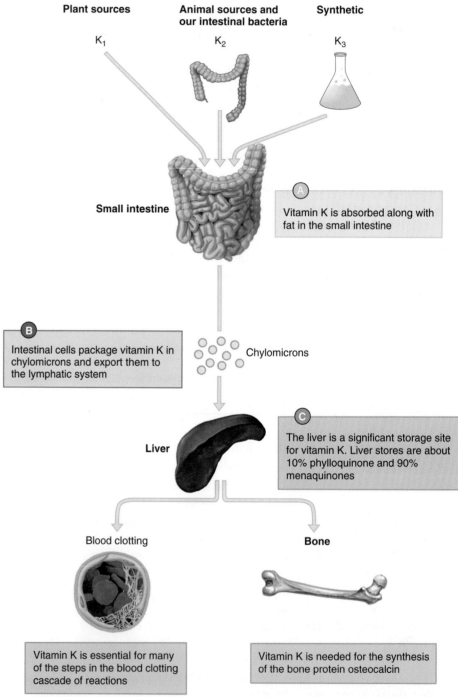

VITAMIN K: FROM SOURCE TO DESTINATION

Plant sources

Animal sources and our intestinal bacteria

Synthetic

K_1

K_2

K_3

Small intestine

A Vitamin K is absorbed along with fat in the small intestine

B Intestinal cells package vitamin K in chylomicrons and export them to the lymphatic system

Chylomicrons

Liver

C The liver is a significant storage site for vitamin K. Liver stores are about 10% phylloquinone and 90% menaquinones

Blood clotting

Bone

Vitamin K is essential for many of the steps in the blood clotting cascade of reactions

Vitamin K is needed for the synthesis of the bone protein osteocalcin

Figure 9.23 **Vitamin K: from source to destination.** Green leafy vegetables are rich sources of vitamin K. Intestinal bacteria produce 10–15 percent of our vitamin K, much less than previously believed. Vitamin K is important in both blood clotting and bone health.

however, current research indicates that intestinal bacteria produce only about 10 to 15 percent of the body's vitamin K.[50] (See **Figure 9.23**.)

Phylloquinone is the primary form of dietary vitamin K. Green leafy vegetables, especially spinach, turnip greens, broccoli, and Brussels sprouts, supply substantial amounts of phylloquinone. Certain vegetable oils (soybean, cottonseed, canola, and olive) also are good sources.[51] Exposure to light degrades vitamin K, so the phylloquinone content of oils varies not only with brand and batch but also with storage time if the oils are bottled in transparent containers. Therefore, vegetable oils may not be a reliable source of vitamin K.

In general, animal products contain limited amounts of vitamin K. Small amounts of menaquinones are found in egg yolks and butter, and various cheeses contain moderate amounts. Soybean products such as tofu contain substantial amounts of menaquinones. Liver contains moderate amounts of menaquinones, but because most people rarely eat liver it is unlikely to contribute much to the general consumption of vitamin K. The concentrations of menaquinones in other animal organs, such as kidney, heart, and muscle, are low and nutritionally insignificant.[52] **Figure 9.24** shows foods that contain vitamin K.

Key Concepts: *Dietary recommendations for vitamin K intake are small: the AI for adult men is 120 micrograms and for adult women it is 90 micrograms. Vitamin K*

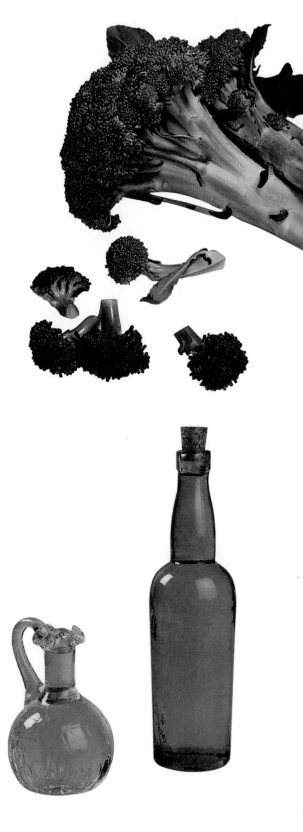

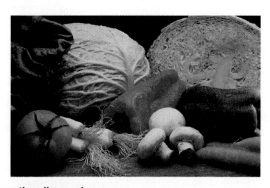

VITAMIN K

Daily Value = 80 µg

Exceptionally good sources

Turnip greens, raw	85 g (~3 cups)	552 µg
Spinach, raw	85 g (~3 cups)	225 µg
Cauliflower, raw	85 g (~3/4 cup)	163 µg
Cabbage, raw	85 g (~1 1/4 cups)	126 µg

High: 20% DV or more

Beef liver	85 g (3 oz)	88 µg
Soybean oil	1 Tbsp.	76 µg
Chicken liver	85 g (3 oz)	68 µg
Broccoli, cooked	85 g (~1/2 cup)	58 µg
Tomato, green, raw	85 g (1 small)	40 µg
Green beans, cooked	85 g (~2/3 cup)	28 µg
Egg	50 g (1 large)	25 µg
Asparagus, cooked	85 g (~1/2 cup)	23 µg
Strawberries, fresh	140 g (~1 cup)	20 µg
Tomato, red, raw	85 g (1 small)	19 µg

Good: 10-19% DV

Milk, nonfat	240 ml (1 cup)	10 µg
Milk, whole (3.25%)	240 ml (1 cup)	10 µg
Corn oil	1 Tbsp.	8 µg

Figure 9.24 **Food sources of vitamin K.** The best sources of vitamin K are vegetables, especially those in the cabbage family. Liver, eggs, and milk are good sources as well. **Note:** USDA Database does not include vitamin K.
Source: Pennington, JAT. Bowes and Church's Food Values of Portions Commonly Used, 17th ed, Philadelphia, PA: Lippincott-Raven Publishers, 1998.

Label [to] Table

I t is well known that milk is an excellent source of calcium, but did you know that milk also contains three of the four fat-soluble vitamins? Let's take a look at the Nutrition Facts from a carton of nonfat milk.

Skim milk

Calories	90
Total Fat	0
Cholesterol	less than 5mg
Sodium	130mg
Total Carbohydrate	13g
Dietary Fiber	0g
Sugars	12g
Protein	9g
Vitamin A	10% DV
Vitamin C	4% DV
Calcium	30% DV
Iron	0% DV
Vitamin D	25% DV

Milk contains the fat-soluble vitamins A, D, and K. Vitamin A is naturally in whole milk and is added to reduced-fat milks. All milks are fortified with vitamin D. Although it is true that fat-soluble vitamins can be toxic in large doses because they are stored in the body, the amounts added to milk are not of concern. Vitamin K is not listed on the label, but milk is a good source of this fat-soluble vitamin as well.

A one-cup serving of fortified milk provides 10 percent of the 5,000 IU Daily Value of vitamin A. If you drank three cups of milk per day, you would get about a third of your recommended amount of vitamin A. That's good news because dietary vitamin A is not always easy to obtain. One form, retinol, is found mainly in liver and fish liver oil, which are not always staples of the typical American. The provitamin forms of vitamin A, the carotenoids, are found in green leafy and dark orange vegetables.

Vitamin D is important because it helps with the absorption of calcium and phosphorus, both important for bone health. Fish liver oil, sardines, and some fortified cereals are also good sources of vitamin D. As shown in the nutrition label above, just one cup of milk gives you one-quarter of the vitamin D Daily Value. That's 25 percent of 10 µg, or 2.5 µg.

Keep in mind when selecting milk that nonfat (skim) milk contains vitamins A and D just like the higher fat 2% and whole milk. Don't let the large banner "Vitamin A and D" printed on containers of whole milk trick you into thinking it contains more. It doesn't!

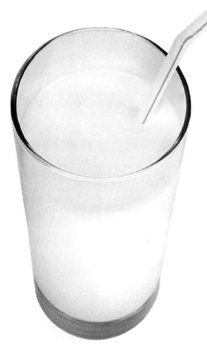

Nutrition Facts

Serving Size: 1 cup (240mL)
Servings Per Container about 8

Amount Per Serving

Calories 90   Calories from fat 0

	% Daily Value*
Total Fat 0g	0%
Saturated Fat 0g	0%
Cholesterol less than 5mg	1%
Sodium 130mg	5%
Total Carbohydrate 13g	4%
Dietary Fiber 0g	0%
Sugars 12g	
Protein 9g	18%

Vitamin A 10%	•	Vitamin C 4%
Calcium 30%	•	Iron 0%
Vitamin D 25%		

* Percent Daily Values are based on a 2,000 calorie diet. Your daily values may be higher or lower depending on your calorie needs:

		Calories:	2000	2,500
Total Fat	Less Than		65g	80g
Sat Fat	Less Than		20g	25g
Cholesterol	Less Than		300mg	300mg
Sodium	Less Than		2,400mg	2,400mg
Total Carbohydrate			300g	375g
Dietary Fiber			25g	30g
Protein			50g	65g

Calories per gram:
Fat 9 • Carbohydrate 4 • Protein 4

AMOUNTS PER 1 CUP SERVING:	FAT
WHOLE MILK	8g
FAT FREE MILK	0g

INGREDIENTS: GRADE A FAT FREE MILK, VITAMIN A PALMITATE, VITAMIN D₃.

is found primarily in green vegetables and in some vegetable oils. Animal foods, in general, contain limited amounts of vitamin K.

Vitamin K Deficiency

Although vitamin K has a crucial role in blood clotting, the body needs only small amounts. This makes vitamin K deficiency rare in healthy adults. On the other hand, preliminary research suggests that typical diets are supplying less than optimal amounts for bone health.

People who suffer fat-malabsorption syndromes, such as celiac disease, sprue, cystic fibrosis, ulcerative colitis, and Crohn's disease, however, can develop vitamin K deficiency. Prolonged use of antibiotics may cause a deficiency because the drugs can destroy the intestinal bacteria that produce vitamin K. Prior to surgery, a patient's vitamin K status is often tested to assess the risk for hemorrhaging and because antibiotics are frequently part of the treatment regimen.

Megadoses of vitamins A and E counteract the actions of vitamin K. Vitamin A appears to hamper intestinal absorption of vitamin K, and excess vitamin E seems to decrease the vitamin K–dependent clotting factor, thus promoting bleeding.

Physicians prescribe anticoagulant medications, such as warfarin (Coumadin) to reduce the risk of internal blood clotting that could block blood vessels leading to the heart or brain. People who take anticoagulants should maintain a consistent pattern of vitamin K consumption, because large fluctuations can interfere with the effectiveness of these drugs.[53]

Newborn babies, especially those who are breast-fed, also run a risk of vitamin K deficiency because at birth they lack the intestinal bacteria that produce the nutrient, and they don't receive much vitamin K via the diet. To prevent hemorrhaging, infants typically receive an injection of vitamin K at birth. This dose usually meets their needs for several weeks, when the vitamin K–producing bacteria begin to flourish.

Vitamin K Toxicity

Vitamin K is stored primarily in the liver and is also found in bone. Toxicity from food is rare because the body excretes vitamin K much more rapidly than the other fat-soluble vitamins. No UL has been set for vitamin K. A vitamin K overdose can cause hemolytic anemia. This condition has been seen in newborns who receive vitamin K in the form of menadione, rather than the recommended form, phylloquinone.

Key Concepts: *Vitamin K deficiencies are extremely rare. Because it takes several weeks before the intestinal bacteria that produce vitamin K begin to flourish in the intestine, newborns are routinely given injections of vitamin K at birth. Vitamin K toxicity is rare because from the body excretes the nutrient more readily than the other fat-soluble vitamins.*

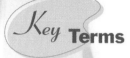

LEARNING *Portfolio* c h a p t e r 9

Key Terms

	page
antirachitic	344
bleaching process	334
calcitonin	346
calcitriol	344
carotenodermia	328
carotenoids	330
cone cells	332
cornea	332
dark adaptation	334
epithelial cells	336
epithelial tissues	336
free radical	341
glutathione	352
goblet cells	336
hemolysis	355
hypercalcemia	349
hyperkeratosis	339
international units (IU)	337
iodopsin	336
keratin	339
lipid peroxidation	350
megadose	330
menadione	356
menaquinone	356
night blindness	334
opsin	334
osteoblasts	346

	page
osteoclasts	346
osteomalacia	349
osteoporosis	349
parathyroid hormone	346
phylloquinone	356
preformed vitamin A	337
provitamin	330
provitamin A	330
retina	332
retinal	330
retinoic acid	330
retinoids	330
retinol	330
retinol-binding protein (RBP)	332
retinol activity equivalents (RAE)	337
retinyl esters	332
rhodopsin	334
rickets	349
rod cells	332
stem cells	336
teratogen	340
tocopherol	350
tocotrienols	350
vitamin precursor	330
xerophthalmia	338

Study Points

➤ Vitamins are organic substances the body needs in minuscule amounts.

➤ Two classes of vitamins exist: fat-soluble vitamins (A, D, E, K) and water-soluble vitamins (B vitamins and vitamin C).

➤ Vitamin A comes from preformed retinoids and the precursor carotenoids.

➤ Vitamin A functions in vision, cell differentiation, growth and development, and immune function.

➤ Sources of vitamin A include milk fat, liver, green leafy and yellow-orange vegetables, and yellow-orange fruits.

➤ Night blindness is an early symptom of vitamin A deficiency that, if not treated, can result in permanent blindness.

➤ Vitamin A is toxic when taken in large doses, causing liver damage and other problems.

➤ Vitamin D functions like a hormone and the body can synthesize it, but is still considered a vitamin.

➤ Vitamin D precursor is produced from cholesterol when UV light hits the skin. Reactions in the liver and kidney are needed to produce a fully active vitamin D molecule.

➤ Vitamin D in foods is available mainly from fortified milk and other fortified products.

➤ The primary function of vitamin D is the regulation of blood levels of calcium.

➤ Vitamin D deficiency contributes to skeletal problems.

➤ Toxicity of vitamin D can develop with doses just a few times larger than the AI level.

➤ Vitamin E is an important antioxidant in the body and may help reduce the risk of chronic diseases such as heart disease and cancer.

➤ Vitamin E is found in vegetable oils and foods made from those oils.

➤ Deficiency and toxicity of vitamin E are relatively rare.

➤ Vitamin K is an important factor in blood coagulation.

➤ Although synthesized by intestinal bacteria, most of the vitamin K in the body comes from dietary sources, especially green vegetables.

➤ Vitamin K deficiency is rare, but newborns are susceptible if not given an injection of vitamin K at birth.

➤ Because the body excretes vitamin K easily, toxicity is unlikely.

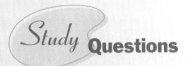

Study Questions

1. **List at least three characteristics of fat-soluble vitamins.**

2. **List the four fat-soluble vitamins by their general names and specific active forms.**

3. **What are the main roles of vitamin A in the body?**

4. **What vitamin deficiency is associated with night blindness?**

5. **What antioxidant is responsible for the yellow-orange color of cantaloupes?**

6. **Which fat-soluble vitamin is considered a hormone? What organs do this hormone affect?**

7. **From what precursor can vitamin D be synthesized?**

8. **What are the toxicity and deficiency symptoms of vitamin E?**

9. **How does a vitamin K deficiency lead to the inability to form a blood clot?**

10. **Which two fat-soluble vitamins are most toxic? Least toxic?**

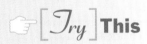

[Try] This

The PUFA Protection Challenge:
Vitamin E vs. Oxygen

The object of this experiment is to see if vitamin E protects polyunsaturated fats (PUFAs) from oxidation. You'll need two glasses, one bottle of either safflower or corn oil, and some liquid vitamin E gel caps (can be purchased at any pharmacy). Pour equal amounts of oil in each of the glasses. Bite a hole in 10 of the vitamin E gel caps and squeeze their contents into ONE of the glasses. Mark this glass with tape and write the letter E on it. Let the glasses sit uncovered on a countertop for several days or weeks. Check the freshness or rancidity of the oils by smelling them and noting whether they look clear or cloudy. Over time, one will become more rancid than the other. Which glass container won the challenge—the one with or without vitamin E? Why?

What About Bobbie?

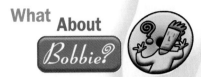

Let's check out Bobbie's intake of vitamin A. Refresh yourself with her day of eating by reviewing page 28. How do you think Bobbie did in terms of this fat-soluble vitamin? Her intake of 680 RAE is quite close to the RDA of 700 RAE, so Bobbie is likely meeting her needs for vitamin A. Here are her best vitamin A sources:

Food	Vitamin A (µg RAE)
Carrot (2 Tbsp)	193
Cream cheese (3 Tbsp)	97
Spaghetti sauce (3 oz)	83
Cheese pizza (1 slice)	83
Salsa (1/2 cup)	43

Bobbie's best sources of vitamin A were both preformed vitamin A sources (animal origin foods such as cream cheese and pizza cheese) and foods with vitamin A precursors (e.g., beta-carotene from carrots.)

Although Bobbie's intake of vitamin A was on target with her RDA, if this day's intake is typical of her usual eating pattern, she may want to try some of the following ideas to keep her vitamin A intake adequate:

- Use spinach greens as the base of her salad instead of iceberg lettuce.
- Continue adding shredded carrots to her salad and consider adding them to her sandwich too.
- Add a slice or two of tomato on top of the bagel with cream cheese.
- Alternate bagels (not high in vitamin A) and fortified cereals (high in vitamin A) for breakfast. This change would also add some milk to her diet, which would further increase her vitamin A intake (130 RAE per cup).

References

1 Mahan KL, Escott-Stump S, eds. *Krause's Food, Nutrition & Diet Therapy.* Philadelphia: WB Saunders, 2000.

2 Guyton AC, and Hall JE, *Textbook of Medical Physiology,* 9th ed., Philadelphia: WB Saunders, 1996.

3 McCollough FS, Northrop-Clewes CA, Thurnham DI. The effect of vitamin A on epithelial integrity. *Proc Nutr Soc,* 1999, May, 58:2,289–293.

4 Semba RD. The role of vitamin A and related retinoids in immune function. *Nutr Rev,* 1998;56:1 Pt 2:S38–48.

5 Institute of Medicine. Food and Nutrition Board. *Dietary Reference Intakes for Vitamin A, Vitamin K, Arsenic, Boron, Chromium, Copper, Iron, Manganese, Molybdenum, Nickel, Silicon, Vanadium, and Zinc.* Washington, DC: National Academy Press; 2001.

6 McCollough FS, Northrop-Clewes CA, Thurnham DI. Op. cit.

7 Semba RD. Op. cit.

8 Rothman KJ, Moore LL, Singer MR, et al. Teratogenicity of high vitamin A intake. *N Engl J Med* 1995; 333(21):1360–1373 and Oakley GP, Erickson JD. Vitamin A and birth defects, *N Engl J Med* 1995;333(21):1414–1415.

9 Koo, J. Acne: Psychological effects are more than skin deep. *Skin Care Today.* 1998;4:4–5.

10 Institute of Medicine (Food and Nutrition Board). *Dietary Reference Intakes for Vitamin C, Vitamin E, Selenium, and Carotenoids.* Washington, DC: National Academy Press; 2000

11 Olson JA, Krinsky NI. Introduction: the colorful, fascinating world of the carotenoids: important physiologic modulators. *The FASEB J.* 1995;9:1547.

12 Institute of Medicine. Op. cit.

13 Jacob RA, Burri BJ. Oxidative damage and defense. *Am J Clin Nutr.* 1996;63:985S–990S.

14 Rock CL, Jacob RA, Bowen PE. Update on the biological characteristics of the antioxidant micronutrients: vitamin C, vitamin E, and the carotenoids. *J Am Diet Assoc.* 1996;96:693–702.

15 Santos MS, Meydani SN, Leka L, et al. Natural killer cell activity in elderly men is enhanced by beta-carotene supplementation. *Am J Clin Nutr.* 1996;64:772777.

16 Hughes DA, Wright AJ, Finglas PM, et al. The effect of beta-carotene supplementation on the immune function of blood monocytes from healthy male nonsmokers. *J Lab Clin Med.* 1997;129:309–317.

17 Gollnick H, Hopfenmuller W, Hemmes C, et al. Systemic beta-carotene plus topical UV sunscreen are an optimal protection against harmful effects of natural UV sunlight: results of the Berlin-Eilath Study. *Eur J Dermatol.* 1996;6:200–205; and Fuller CJ, Faulkner H, Bendich A, et al. Effect of beta-carotene supplementation on photosuppression of delayed-type hyperactivity in normal young men. *Am J Clin Nutr.* 1992;56:684–690.

18 Rock CL, Jacob RA, Bowen PE. Op. cit.

19 Institute of Medicine. Op. cit.,

20 Rock CL, Jacob RA, Bowen PE. Op. cit.; and Zhang LX, Cooney RV, Bertram JS. Carotenoids up-regulate connexin43 gene expression independent of their provitamin A or antioxidant properties. *Cancer Res.* 1992;52:5707–5712.

21 Toma S, Losardo PL, Vinvent M, Palumb, R. Effectiveness of beta-carotene in cancer chemoprevention. *Eur J Cancer Prev.* 1995;4:213–224.

22 Rock CL, Jacob RA , Bowen PE. Op. cit.

23 Institute of Medicine, 2000. Op. cit.

24 Mangels AR, Holden JM, Beecher GR, et al. Carotenoid content of fruits and vegetables: an evaluation of analytic data. *J Am Diet Assoc.* 1993;93:284–296.

25 Rock CL, Lovalo JL, Emenhiser C, et al. Bioavailability of beta-carotene is lower in raw than in processed carrots and spinach in women. *J Nutr.* 1998;128:5, 913–916.

26 Hinds TS, West W L, Knight EM. Carotenoids and retinoids: a review of research, clinical, and public health applications. *J Clin Pharmacol.* 1997;37:551–558.

27 Institute of Medicine, 2000. Op. cit.

28 Utiger RD. The need for more vitamin D. *N Engl J Med.* 1998;328:828–829.

29 Eastell R, Riggs BL. Vitamin D and osteoporosis. In: Feldman D, Glorieux FH, Piek JW, eds. *Vitamin D.* San Diego: Academic Press; 1997:695–711.

30 Institute of Medicine. Food and Nutrition Board. *Dietary Reference Intakes for Calcium, Phosphorus, Magnesium, Vitamin D, and Fluoride.* Washington, DC: National Academy Press; 1997.

31 Vitamin D Deficiency Deemed Widespread. *Tufts University Health & Nutrition Letter.* May 1998;16(3):1.

32 The Sun and Your Skin. American Academy of Dermatology, 1994. www.aad.org/pamphlets/SunSkin.html. Accessed 6/11/00.

33 Vitamin D deficiency: the silent epidemic. *Nutr Action.* 1997;24(8):4.

34 Chen TC, Shao A, Heath H, Holick MF. An update on the vitamin D content of fortified milk from the United States and Canada. *N Engl J Med.* 1993;329:1507; and Holick MF, Shao Q, Liu WW, Chen TC. The vitamin D content of fortified milk and infant formula. *N Engl J Med.* 1992;326:1178–1181.

35 Gessner BD, de Schweinitz E, Petersen KM, Lewandowski C. Nutritional rickets among breast-fed black and Alaska Native children. *Alaska Med.* 1997;39:72–4, 87.

36 Eastell R, Riggs BL. Vitamin D and osteoporosis. In: Feldman D, Glorieux FH, Piek JW, eds. Op. cit. 695–711; and Chapuy M-C, Meunier PJ. Vitamin D insufficiency in adults and the elderly. In: Feldman D, Glorieux FH, Piek JW, eds. Op. cit., 679–693.

37 Chapuy MC, Arlot ME, Duboeuf F, et al. Vitamin D3 and calcium to prevent hip fractures in elderly women. *N Engl J Med.* 1992;327:1637–1642; Chapuy MC, Arlot ME, Delmas PD, Meunier PJ. Effect of calcium and cholecalciferol treatment for three years on hip fractures in elderly women. *BMJ.* 1994;308:1081–1082.

38 Thomas MK, Lloyd-Jones DM, Thadhani RF, et al. Hypovitaminosis D in medical inpatients. *N Engl J Med.* 1998;338:777–783.

39 Need AG, Morris HA, Horowitz M, Nordin C. Effects of skin thickness, age, body fat, and sunlight on serum 25-hydroxy-

vitamin D. *Am J Clin Nutr.* 1993;58:882–885; and Holick MF, Matsuoka LY, Wortsman J. Age, vitamin D, and solar ultraviolet. *Lancet.* Nov 4, 1989;2(8671):1104–1105. Letter.

40 Adams JS, Lee G. Gains in bone mineral density with resolution of vitamin D intoxication. *Ann Int Med.* 1997;127(3):203–206; and Marriott BM. Vitamin D supplementation: a word of caution. *Ann Int Med.* 1997;127(3):231–233.

41 Traber MG, Sies, H. Vitamin E in humans: demand and delivery, *Ann Rev Nutr.* 1996;16:321–347.

42 Institute of Medicine. Food and Nutrition Board. Dietary Reference Intakes for Vitamin C, Vitamin E, Selenium, and Carotenoids. Washington, DC: National Academy Press; 2000.

43 Ibid.

44 Ibid.

45 Ibid.

46 Institute of Medicine. *Dietary Reference Intakes for Vitamin C.*

47 Sokoll LJ, Booth SL, O'Brien ME, et al. Changes in serum osteocalcin, plasma phylloquinone, and urinary γ-carboxyglutamic acid in response to altered intakes of dietary phylloquinone in human subjects. *Am J Clin Nutr.* 1997;65:779–784.

48 Booth SL, Suttle JW. Dietary intake and adequacy of vitamin K. *J Nutr.* 1998;128(5):785–788.

49 "Special K" Takes on New Meaning. *Tufts University Health & Nutrition Letter.* 1997;15(5):1, 7.

50 Ibid.

51 Booth SL, Davidson KW, Lichtenstein AH, Sadowski JA. Plasma concentrations of dihydro-vitamin K_1 following dietary intake of a hydrogenated vitamin K_1-rich vegetable oil. *Lipids.* 1996; 31:709–713; and Fenton ST, Price RJ, Bolton-Smith C, Harrington D, Shearer MJ. Nutrient sources of phylloquinone (vitamin K_1) in Scottish men and women. *Proc Nutr Soc.* 1997;56:301. Abstract.

52 Shearer MJ, Bach A, Kohlmeier M. Chemistry, nutritional sources, tissue distribution and metabolism of vitamin K with special reference to bone health. *J Nutr.* 1996;126(suppl):1181S–1186S.

53 Booth SL, Charnley JM, Sadowski JA, et al. Dietary vitamin K_1 and stability of oral anticoagulation: proposal of a diet with constant vitamin K_1 content. *Thrombosis Haemostasis.* 1997;77:504–509.

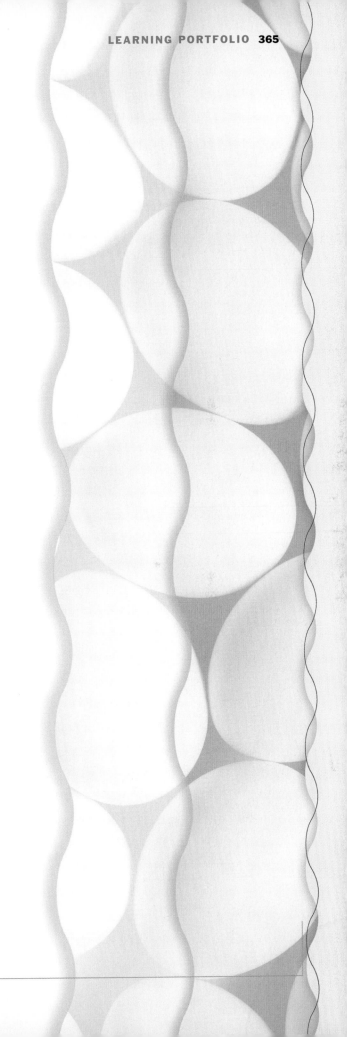

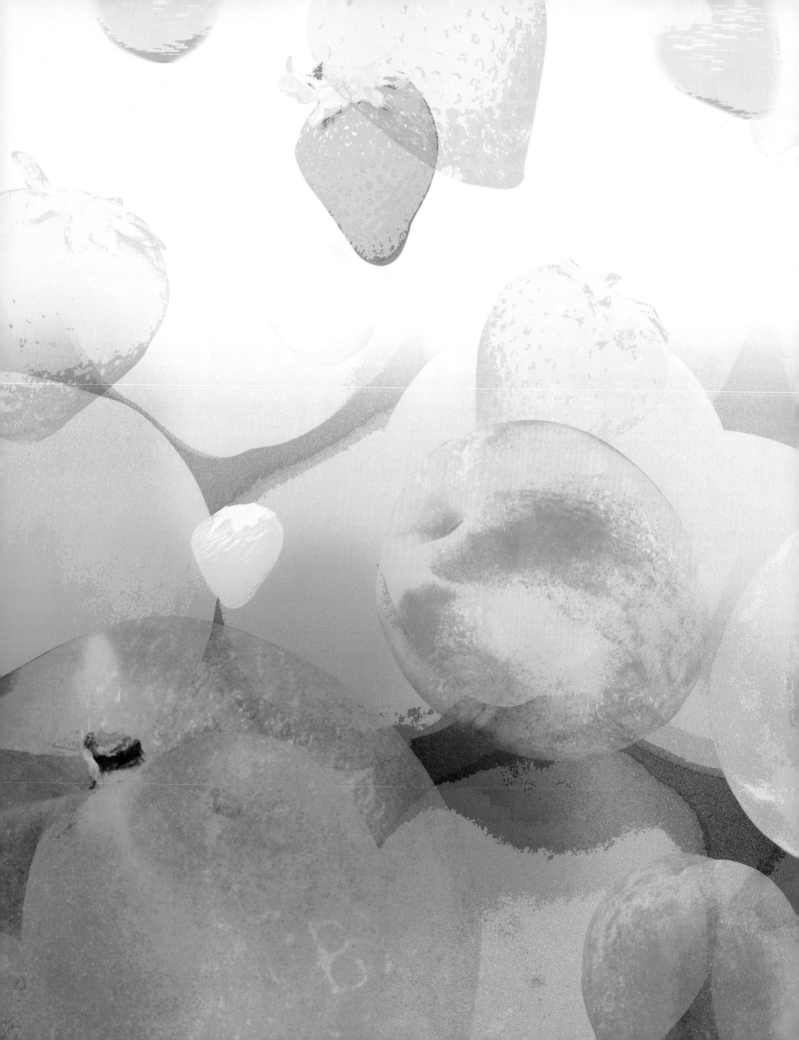

Chapter 10

Water-Soluble Vitamins

Think About It

1 When cooking vegetables, how often do you think about vitamin loss?

2 Because of a friend's suggestion you take a vitamin pill, and it causes intense flushing and itching. What has she probably given you and what does your reaction tell you?

3 You decide to follow a vegetarian lifestyle. What vitamin deficiency should you watch out for?

4 Do you know anyone who takes vitamin C to prevent colds? What do you think of this strategy?

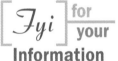

Fyi for your Information

This chapter's FYI boxes include practical information on the following topics:

- Fresh, Frozen, or Canned? Raw or Cooked?

- The B Vitamins and Heart Disease

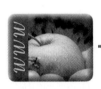

The web site for this book offers many useful tools and is a great source for additional nutrition information for both students and instructors. Visit the site at nutrition.jbpub.com for information on water-soluble vitamins. You'll find exercises that explore the following topics:

- Safe Supplements

- Exercise and Water-soluble Vitamins

- Overdosing on Niacin

Key to Illustrations

 Amino Acids

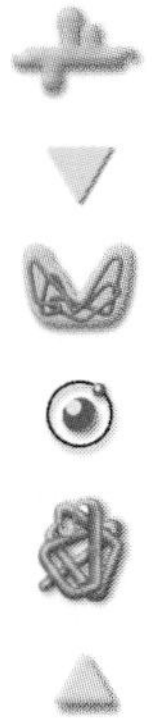

 Co-enzymes

 Enzymes

 Free Radical

 Proteins

 Water-Soluble Vitamins

What About Bobbie?

Track the choices Bobbie is making with the EatRight Analysis software.

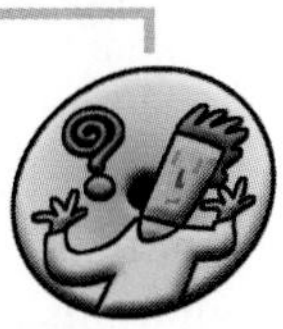

*F*eeling tired, run down, stressed out? Burning the candle at both ends? Too many workouts wearing you out? You must need a vitamin, right? Surely you've heard that vitamins give you energy, so a lack of energy must be a signal that you need more vitamins, right? Well, probably not.

First the facts: Because the body does not metabolize vitamins to yield ATP, they are not a source of energy. However, many of the B vitamins (water-soluble vitamins) facilitate the metabolic reactions that release energy from carbohydrate, fat, and protein. So in a sense, vitamins *help* you get energy by allowing carbohydrate, fat, and protein to become cellular fuel.

In times of stress, you need more energy and therefore more vitamins, so a supplement is in order, right? Well, not really. First we need to define *stress*. Certainly physical stress (e.g., injury and illness) increases the body's need for energy, protein, and many vitamins and minerals to aid healing. But emotional stress (e.g., anxiety, and fear) does not. It may seem that you expend a lot of *mental* energy studying for finals, but studying requires no more energy than sitting and chatting with your friends.

But surely if you do more physical exercise, you should take a vitamin, right? Again, not necessarily. Physical activity requires energy and therefore vitamins to help extract energy from food. But, the food you consume to meet your energy needs for physical activity contains vitamins, too, unless you meet your extra energy needs with chips and sodas! In most cases, healthful food choices—plenty of whole grains, fruits, vegetables, lean meats or meat alternatives, and low-fat dairy products—provide all the vitamins you need. So, check out your diet before you check out the vitamin supplements.

The Water-Soluble Vitamins: Eight Bs and a C

Water-soluble vitamins consist of the eight B vitamins and vitamin C. Scientists first viewed vitamin B as a single compound. However, the more they studied it, they discovered that "it" was actually several vitamins. To differentiate the various B vitamins, scientists initially added numbers to the letter *B*—vitamins B_6 and B_{12}, for example. Today, with the exception of B_6 and B_{12}, we usually refer to the B vitamins by their names: thiamin (B_1), riboflavin (B_2), niacin (B_3), pantothenic acid, biotin, and folate.

Although fat-soluble vitamins tend to accumulate in the body, the kidney readily removes and excretes excess water-soluble vitamins, with the exception of B_{12}. Also in contrast to fat-soluble vitamins, water-soluble vitamins are particularly susceptible to destruction by heat or alkalinity, which can break the chemical bonds between atoms. Some cooking practices are particularly harmful to vitamins in foods. Prolonged heat, such as that used to bake a vegetable casserole, tends to destroy the chemical bonds. Many cooks add baking soda, which is alkaline, to cooking water to reduce cooking time and intensify the vegetable's color. Vitamin C, thiamin, and riboflavin are especially vulnerable to heat and alkalinity. Water-soluble vitamins are hydrophilic by nature, and water will leach them from

Quick Bites

What do you believe?

*T*hirty-five percent of Americans surveyed in 1997 said that they believed vitamin supplements were necessary to ensure good health. Women were more likely than men to believe they needed supplements.

Quick Bites

Is it a fruit or vegetable?

*I*n the eighteenth century, botanists defined fruits as the organ surrounding the seeds. This definition considers cucumbers, eggplants, peppers, pea pods, and corn kernels as fruits. Legally though, these are all vegetables. In the late 1800s, the U.S. Supreme Court, while trying the case of a tomato importer, established a definition based on linguistic custom and usage. The importer had to pay the vegetable tax.

beriberi Thiamin-deficiency disease. Symptoms include muscle weakness, loss of appetite, nerve degeneration, and edema in some cases.

vegetables during cooking. Cooking only partially destroys the vitamin content of a food and some cooking methods are less destructive than others. The best cooking methods—steaming, stir-frying, and microwaving—use minimal amounts of water.

The B Vitamins

B vitamins act primarily as coenzymes, or as parts of coenzymes (compounds that enable specific enzymes to function). (See **Figure 10.1**.) The B vitamin part of a coenzyme helps catalyze the workings of metabolic pathways in cells. All B vitamins function in energy-producing metabolic reactions, and some also participate in other aspects of cellular metabolism.

Varied diets contain significant amounts of many vitamins, and vitamins often are added to foods like cereals and other grain products. In the 1940s, the U.S. government mandated enrichment of bread and cereal products made from milled grains. During the milling process, much of the B vitamin content is removed along with the germ, bran, and husk. (See **Figure 10.2**.) The addition of the B vitamins thiamin, riboflavin, and niacin helps restore the lost vitamins. Now, because of a 1998 FDA requirement, all enriched bread, flour, corn meal, pasta, rice, and other grains products must be fortified with folic acid.[1]

During the production of highly refined grain products, processing also removes vitamin B_6, magnesium, and zinc. Although current enrichment and fortification protect consumers from numerous deficiency diseases, they do not replace these nutrients. To ensure a good balance of nutrients, experts recommend that people regularly eat whole-grain products such as whole-wheat bread, brown rice, and oatmeal.

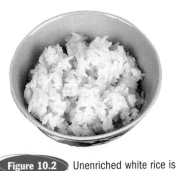

Figure 10.2 Unenriched white rice is low in thiamin.

Thiamin

Although mentioned in ancient Chinese writings from 2600 B.C.E., the thiamin-deficiency disease **beriberi** remained largely unknown until the nineteenth century when milling and refining grains became popular. In 1855 Dr. K. Takaki, Director General of the Japanese Naval Medical Services, demonstrated beriberi's dietary origins when he cured afflicted sailors by supplementing their diets with meat, milk, and whole grains. Some years later, Christian Eijkman, a Dutch medical officer, induced beriberi in birds by feeding them only white rice, and then cured them by adding bran to their diet. This led to the discovery of an "anti-beriberi" factor—thiamin.

Isolated in 1926, thiamin (also known as vitamin B_1) was named for *thio*, meaning "sulfur," and *amine*, the nitrogen-containing group in the vitamin. As **Figure 10.3** shows, thiamin consists of a sulfur-containing ring and a nitrogen-containing ring attached to a carbon atom. Heat easily breaks the bonds between the two rings and the carbon atom, so cooking reduces a food's thiamin content. Alkaline solutions (those with a pH of 8 or higher) also break these bonds.

Functions of Thiamin

Like the other B vitamins, thiamin is an important participant in many energy-yielding reactions. Specifically, thiamin is the vitamin portion of the

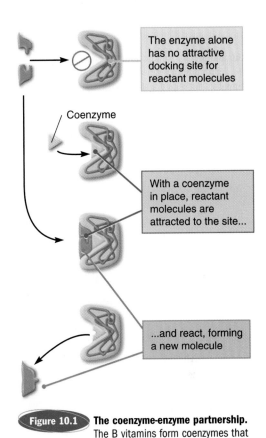

THIAMIN

Figure 10.3 **Thiamin structure and vulnerability.**
Water-soluble vitamins, especially thiamin, riboflavin, and vitamin C, are vulnerable to heat and alkalinity.

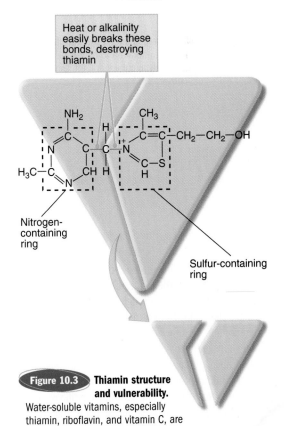

Figure 10.1 **The coenzyme-enzyme partnership.** The B vitamins form coenzymes that enable specific enzymes to catalyze reactions.

thiamin pyrophosphate (TPP) A coenzyme of which the vitamin thiamin is a part. It plays a key role in decarboxylation and helps drive the reaction that forms acetyl CoA from pyruvate during metabolism.

decarboxylation Removal of a carboxyl group (—COOH) from a molecule. The carboxyl group is then released as carbon dioxide (CO_2).

coenzyme **thiamin pyrophosphate (TPP)**, shown in **Figure 10.4**. TPP participates in a vital reaction known as **decarboxylation**, which removes a carboxyl group (—COOH) and releases it as carbon dioxide (CO_2). During glucose metabolism, for example, decarboxylation removes one carbon from the three-carbon substance pyruvate to form the two-carbon molecule acetyl CoA. (See **Figure 10.5**.) TPP is also involved in a decarboxylation step in the citric acid cycle.

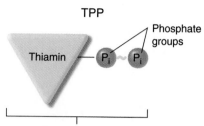

Thiamin pyrophosphate (TPP)

Figure 10.4 **Thiamin pyrophosphate (TPP).** Thiamin pyrophosphate (TPP) contains the B-vitamin thiamin and two phosphate groups.

Cells also use TPP in the pentose phosphate pathway, an alternative pathway to glycolysis. This series of reactions metabolizes glucose to make, among other products, the five-carbon monosaccharide deoxyribose for DNA synthesis, the five-carbon monosaccharide ribose for RNA synthesis, and the energy-rich molecule NADPH to help power biosynthesis.

Thiamin pyrophosphate also plays a role in nerve function, though the mechanism is still under investigation. Scientists suspect that TPP helps synthesize and regulate neurotransmitters—chemicals involved in the transmission of messages throughout the nervous system. TPP also may help produce energy to fuel nerve tissue.

Dietary Recommendations for Thiamin

The small difference in the RDA for adult men and women reflects the differences in their average size and energy use. The RDA for adult men aged 19 years and older is 1.2 milligrams; for adult women of the same age, the RDA is 1.1 milligrams per day. Pregnancy and lactation increase energy requirements so thiamin requirements rise during these life stages. Thiamin intake recommendations are 1.4 milligrams a day during pregnancy and 1.5 milligrams a day during lactation. If a person's diet supplies adequate energy and includes thiamin-rich foods, it generally contains adequate amounts of thiamin.

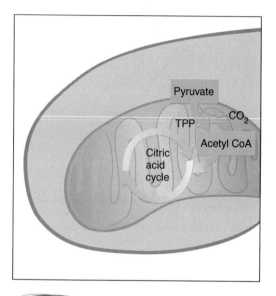

Figure 10.5 **TPP helps convert pyruvate to acetyl CoA.** In addition to coenzyme A and NAD⁺, three other catalytic cofactors—TPP, lipoamide, and FAD—help convert pyruvate to acetyl CoA.

[*Fyi*] Fresh, Frozen, or Canned? Raw or Cooked?

FOR YOUR INFORMATION

Selecting and Preparing Foods to Maximize Vitamin Content

A food's vitamin content depends first on the original amount in the plant or animal while it is alive and growing. Although grazing materials and feed may have a minor impact on vitamin content, animal products tend to have fairly consistent levels. This reflects the animal's ability to concentrate and store vitamins. The vitamin content of plants, however, depends more on soil and growing conditions such as available moisture and sunlight. The maturity of a fruit or vegetable at the time it is harvested also influences its vitamin content.

Light, heat, air, acid, alkali, and cooking fluids can attack vitamins, so proper storage, processing, and cooking are important. Ideally, you should shop for produce as the Europeans do: choose fresh fruits and vegetables daily to minimize nutrient losses associated with prolonged storage. Barring that, choose clean, undamaged produce at each of your regular shopping trips. When storing foods, avoid temperature extremes, and minimize exposure to light and air with refrigeration or covered storage. It's best to eat fruits and vegetables soon after purchase; normal storage can decrease their vitamin content. The vitamin C content of

fresh green beans, for example, drops by half after six days at home.

What about frozen and canned foods? The heat processing used in canning fruits and vegetables does deplete small amounts of vitamins. Researchers at the University of Illinois determined, however, that most of what is lost ends up in the liquid in which the food is packed.[1] In addition, the vitamin content of canned foods is shelf stable and remains constant even after two years. The thiamin content of canned meats and beans is comparable to home-prepared versions. Vegetable sources of folate, such as spinach,

Sources of Thiamin

Thiamin is found throughout the food supply, though most foods contain only small amounts. Pork and wheat germ are the richest food sources of thiamin. Sunflower seeds, legumes, watermelon, nuts, and organ meats such as liver, also rank as good thiamin sources. Most thiamin in the U.S. diet, however, comes from enriched or whole-grain products such as bread, pasta, rice, and ready-to-eat cereals.[2] **Figure 10.6** shows some foods that provide thiamin.

Meat (except pork and organ meats), dairy products, seafood, and most fruits contain very little thiamin. Eating a wide variety of foods is the best way to ensure adequate thiamin consumption.

There are few data from studies of humans on the bioavailability of thiamin from food.[3] See the section on thiamin toxicity for details about absorption of thiamin from supplements.

Thiamin Deficiency

In industrialized countries, thiamin deficiency usually is related to heavy alcohol consumption combined with limited food consumption. Alcoholics are at risk for thiamin deficiency for two reasons: (1) alcohol contributes calories without contributing nutrients, and (2) alcohol interferes with absorption of thiamin and many other vitamins. The poor and the elderly also may be at risk of deficiency due to inadequate energy intake or consumption of nutrient-poor foods. Eating mostly highly processed but unenriched foods and empty-calorie items such as alcohol, sugar, and fat can lead to a deficiency.

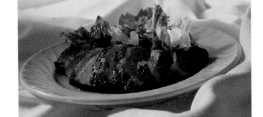

THIAMIN

Daily Value = 1.5 mg

High: 20% DV or more

Good: 10-19% DV

Exceptionally good source

Wheat germ	15 g	1.50 mg
Pork, loin chops, lean only, cooked	85 g (3 oz)	0.76 mg
Oatmeal, instant, fortified, cooked	1 cup	0.70 mg
Sunflower seeds	30 g	0.69 mg
Ham, extra lean, cooked	85 g (3 oz)	0.64 mg
Turkey, dark meat	85 g (3 oz)	0.54 mg
Soy milk	240 ml	0.39 mg
Corn flakes	30 g (1 cup)	0.39 mg
Cheerios cereal	30 g (1 cup)	0.39 mg
Fiber One cereal	30 g (1/2 cup)	0.39 mg
Rice, white, enriched	140 g (~3/4 cup)	0.35 mg
Brazilnuts	30 g	0.30 mg
Spaghetti, enriched, cooked	140 g (1 cup)	0.29 mg
Orange juice, chilled	240 ml (1 cup)	0.28 mg
Carrots, cooked	85 g (~1/2 cup)	0.26 mg
Grits, corn, enriched	1 cup	0.24 mg
Sesame seeds	30 g	0.24 mg
White bread, enriched	50 g (2 slices)	0.24 mg
Soybeans, cooked	90 g (~1/2 cup)	0.23 mg
Watermelon, fresh	280 g (1/16 melon)	0.22 mg
Black beans, cooked	90 g (~1/2 cup)	0.22 mg
Baked beans, canned	130 g (~1/2 cup)	0.20 mg
Pecans	30 g	0.20 mg
Salmon, cooked	85 g (3 oz)	0.18 mg
Navy beans, cooked	90 g (~1/2 cup)	0.18 mg
Whole wheat bread	50 g (2 slices)	0.18 mg
Oysters, cooked	85 g (3 oz)	0.16 mg
Lentils, cooked	90 g (~1/2 cup)	0.15 mg

Figure 10.6 **Food sources of thiamin.** Pork, whole and enriched grains, and fortified cereals are rich in thiamin. Most animal foods contain little thiamin.
Source: U.S. Department of Agriculture, Agricultural Research Service, 1999. USDA Nutrient Database for Standard Reference, Release 13. Nutrient Data Laboratory Home Page, http://www.nal.usda.gov/fnic/foodcomp.

---

retain most of their folate content when canned or frozen. The carotenes in vegetables and fruits are stable during the canning process. In fact, current research suggests the lycopene in tomatoes is a more effective antioxidant (it has been linked to reducing prostate cancer[2]) after tomatoes have been heated or canned.[3] During canning, fruits and vegetables lose some vitamin C to the surrounding fluid. You still get the benefit when you use liquids from canned vegetables in soups and stews.

Once fruits and vegetables are home and stored carefully, what is the best way to cook

them? To maximize the vitamin content, think minimal—minimal amounts of heat, minimal amounts of cooking water, and minimal exposure to air. Try to minimize handling the food before and during cooking. While dicing a food such as a potato reduces cooking time, it also exposes more surface area to vitamin-destroying influences. So, cut if you must, but not too small.

Steaming and microwaving are the best cooking methods for preserving vitamin content, because they minimize cooking time and water use. If you boil foods, try to use the cooking water for sauces, stews, or soups,

because it contains many of the water-soluble vitamins lost from the food during cooking.

To retain the most vitamins in your food, be gentle with storage and handling, and kind with cooking. Minimize (heat, water, air exposure) to maximize!

1 University of Illinois, Department of Food Science and Human Nutrition. *Nutrient Conservation in Canned, Frozen, and Fresh Foods.* Urbana, IL: Oct 1997.

2 Giovannucci E, Ascherio A, Rimm EB, et al. Intake of carotenoids and retinol in relation to risk of prostate cancer. *J Natl Cancer Inst.* 1995;87:1767–1779.

3 Tonucci LH, Holden JM, Beecher GR, et al. Carotenoid content of thermally processed tomato-based food products. *J Agr Food Chem.* 1995;43:579–583.

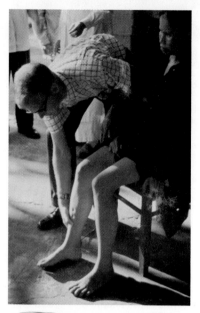

Figure 10.7 **Edema is a symptom of wet beriberi.**

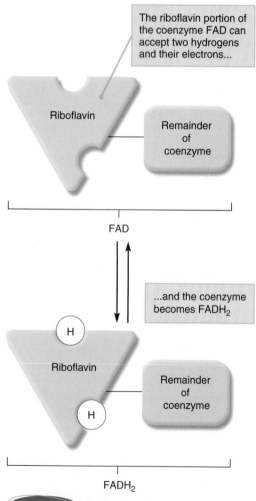

The riboflavin portion of the coenzyme FAD can accept two hydrogens and their electrons...

Riboflavin

Remainder of coenzyme

FAD

...and the coenzyme becomes FADH₂

H

Riboflavin

Remainder of coenzyme

H

FADH₂

Figure 10.8 **Riboflavin coenzymes easily transfer hydrogens.** The riboflavin coenzyme *flavin adenine dinucleotide* (FAD) accepts hydrogens and electrons to become FADH₂.

Beriberi

Beriberi is a term from the Singhalese language (spoken in Sri Lanka) that means "I can't, I can't." This is a perfect description of beriberi, the hallmarks of which include muscle weakness, loss of appetite, and nerve degeneration. This deficiency disease occurs in people whose major source of energy is polished rice, which is common in Southeast Asia. Polishing removes the rice hulls and thus their major source of thiamin.

An inadequate supply of this essential nutrient affects the cardiovascular, muscular, nervous, and gastrointestinal systems, which all rely on thiamin to help fuel their activities. The brain and nervous system rely on glucose for energy, and thiamin, as part of TPP, is crucial in glucose metabolism. The first signs of thiamin deficiency are weakness, irritability, headache, fatigue, and depression—functions associated with the brain and nervous system. These disturbances may appear after only 10 days on a thiamin-free diet.

As symptoms progress, "dry" beriberi (beriberi without edema) causes nerve degeneration, loss of nerve transmission leading to nervous tingling throughout the body, muscle wasting, poor arm and leg coordination, and deep pain in the calf muscles. "Wet" beriberi has additional symptoms, including an enlarged heart, heart failure, and severe edema (**Figure 10.7**). Because many B vitamins are in the same foods as thiamin, thiamin deficiency and other B vitamin deficiencies often go hand in hand.

Wernicke-Korsakoff Syndrome

Alcohol-induced malnutrition is the most common cause of Wernicke-Korsakoff syndrome, another thiamin deficiency disease. Symptoms include mental confusion, staggering, and constant rapid eye movements or paralysis of the eye muscles.

Thiamin Toxicity

To date, there are no reports of thiamin toxicity from either food or supplements. Supplements, which are cheap to produce, often include up to 200 times the Daily Value for thiamin. The Food and Nutrition Board has not set a Tolerable Upper Intake Level (UL) for this nutrient. Because thiamin absorption declines rapidly when a person consumes five or more milligrams at once, large doses of thiamin appear to be relatively innocuous. In addition, the kidneys rapidly excrete excess thiamin via urine.[4]

Riboflavin

Scientists discovered that heating the "anti-beriberi factor" destroyed its anti-beriberi properties but left its growth-promoting properties unscathed. The factor actually contained two active compounds—heat-vulnerable thiamin and a heat-stable component. In 1917, scientists identified the heat-stable component as another vitamin—called vitamin B₂ in England and vitamin G in the United States. This naming confusion ended when the new vitamin was finally dubbed riboflavin.

Riboflavin is named for its yellow color (*flavin* means "yellow" in Latin). The vitamin accepts and donates electrons with ease, so it participates in many oxidation-reduction reactions.

Functions of Riboflavin

Riboflavin is a part of two coenzymes: flavin mononucleotide (FMN) and flavin adenine dinucleotide (FAD). These coenzymes participate in numerous metabolic pathways, including the citric acid cycle and the beta-oxidation pathway that breaks down fatty acids. FMN and FAD act first as electron and hydrogen acceptors. In the citric acid cycle, for instance, FAD accepts hydrogen and electrons, forming the reduced form, $FADH_2$ (**Figure 10.8**). Later, this coenzyme delivers its high-energy electrons to the mitochondrial electron transport chain to produce ATP. Another riboflavin coenzyme, FMN, also accepts hydrogen and electrons, forming $FMNH_2$. FMN works in the electron transport chain to move electrons. Both coenzymes are crucial in energy metabolism.

Riboflavin-containing coenzymes also participate in reactions that remove ammonia during the deamination of some amino acids.[5] Riboflavin also is associated with the antioxidant performance of **glutathione peroxidase**.

Dietary Recommendations for Riboflavin

For adults aged 19 and older the RDA is 1.1 milligrams per day for women and 1.3 milligrams per day for men. Intake recommendations for riboflavin, like those for thiamin, reflect the higher energy needs of males. Pregnancy and lactation increase energy needs, so the RDA for women rises to 1.4 milligrams per day during pregnancy and to 1.6 milligrams per day during lactation.

Sources of Riboflavin

Although most plant and animal foods contain some riboflavin, milk, milk drinks, and yogurt supply about 15 percent of the riboflavin in the U.S. diet. Bread and bread products contribute approximately 10 percent, and ready-to-eat cereals add nearly as much.[6] Riboflavin is one of the four vitamins (thiamin, riboflavin, niacin, and folic acid) and one mineral (iron) that are added to enriched grain products. Organ meats such as liver and kidney are good sources of riboflavin, as are mushrooms and cottage cheese. **Figure 10.9** shows foods that provide riboflavin.

Riboflavin is more stable than thiamin and is resistant to acid, heat, and oxidation. On the other hand, light easily breaks it down. Riboflavin-rich foods should be stored in opaque packages. Milk, for example, usually is stored and sold in paper or plastic cartons rather than glass. (See **Figure 10.10**.)

About 95 percent of the riboflavin in food is bioavailable, and the body can absorb large amounts from a single meal or supplement.[7]

Riboflavin Deficiency

Riboflavin deficiencies are rare. Several large surveys suggest that in the United States men take in about 2 milligrams of riboflavin a day, and women consume about 1.5 milligrams a day. Some people, however, consume only marginal amounts. Because people with alcoholism tend to have poor diets, for example, they risk riboflavin deficiency. Long-term use of barbiturate drugs like phenobarbital also may lead to riboflavin deficiency. Repeated exposure to these drugs activates enzymes in the liver which accelerate the metabolism of riboflavin. Cancer, heart disease, and diabetes may also cause or worsen a riboflavin deficiency.[8]

RIBOFLAVIN

Daily Value = 1.7 mg

Exceptionally good source

Beef liver, cooked	85 g (3 oz)	3.52 mg

High: 20% DV or more

Chicken liver, cooked	85 g (3 oz)	1.49 mg
Yogurt, plain, nonfat	225 g (1 8-oz container)	0.53 mg
Yogurt, plain, lowfat	225 g (1 8-oz container)	0.48 mg
Wheat bran flakes cereal	30 g (3/4 cup)	0.45 mg
Cheerios cereal	30 g (1 cup)	0.43 mg
Fiber One cereal	30 g (1/2 cup)	0.43 mg
Corn flakes cereal	30 g (1 cup)	0.42 mg
Milk, 1%	240 ml (1 cup)	0.41 mg
Milk, 2%, whole (3.25%)	240 ml (1 cup)	0.40 mg
Squid, cooked	85 g (3 oz)	0.39 mg
Buttermilk, lowfat	240 ml (1 cup)	0.38 mg
Oatmeal, instant, fortified, cooked	1 cup	0.37 mg
Clams, cooked	85 g (3 oz)	0.36 mg
Milk, nonfat	240 ml (1 cup)	0.34 mg

Good: 10-19% DV

Pork, loin chops, lean only, cooked	85 g (3 oz)	0.28 mg
Egg, hardcooked	50 g (1 large)	0.26 mg
Mushrooms, cooked	85 g (~1/2 cup)	0.26 mg
Herring, cooked	85 g (3 oz)	0.25 mg
Almonds	30 g	0.24 mg
Beef, ground, extra lean, cooked	85 g (3 oz)	0.23 mg
Turkey, dark meat	85 g (3 oz)	0.21 mg
Cottage cheese, 2% milkfat	110 g (~1/2 cup)	0.20 mg
Chicken, dark meat, cooked	85 g (3 oz)	0.19 mg
Beef, porterhouse steak, cooked	85 g (3 oz)	0.19 mg
Ham, extra lean, cooked	85 g (3 oz)	0.17 mg
Soy milk	240 ml (1 cup)	0.17 mg
White bread, enriched	50 g (2 slices)	0.17 mg

Figure 10.9 **Food sources of riboflavin.** The best sources of riboflavin include milk, liver, whole and enriched grains, and fortified cereals.
Source: U.S. Department of Agriculture, Agricultural Research Service, 1999. USDA Nutrient Database for Standard Reference, Release 13. Nutrient Data Laboratory Home Page, http://www.nal.usda.gov/fnic/foodcomp.

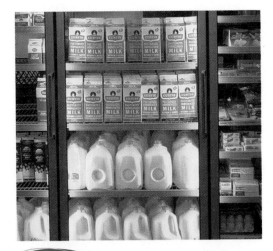

Figure 10.10 Packaging affects riboflavin content in milk.

glutathione peroxidase A selenium-containing enzyme that promotes the breakdown of fatty acids that have undergone peroxidation.

ariboflavinosis Riboflavin deficiency.

glossitis Inflammation of the tongue; a symptom of riboflavin deficiency.

stomatitis Inflammation of the mouth; a symptom of riboflavin deficiency.

cheilosis Cracking of the skin at the corners of the mouth and inflammation of the lips.

seborrheic dermatitis Disease of the oil-producing glands of the skin; a symptom of riboflavin deficiency.

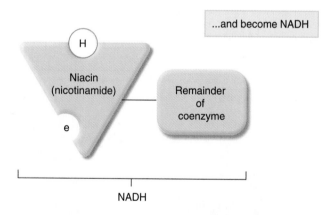

Figure 10.11 **Niacin is part of the coenzymes NAD+ and NADP+.** Niacin, as nicotinamide, is an integral part of coenzymes critical to several metabolic reactions. NAD+ is crucial to the formation of ATP and NADP+ is crucial to biosynthesis.

The niacin portion of the coenzyme NAD+ can accept one hydrogen and its electron as well as another electron...

...and become NADH

NADP+ is similar to NAD+ but it has a phosphate group

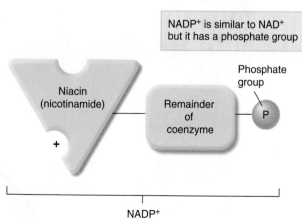

Riboflavin deficiency (**ariboflavinosis**) has characteristic symptoms that include sore throat, inflammation of the tongue (**glossitis**) and mouth (**stomatitis**), cracking of the membranes at the corners of the mouth (**cheilosis**), disease of the oil-producing glands of the skin (**seborrheic dermatitis**), and anemia. Riboflavin deficiency usually goes hand in hand with other nutrient deficiencies. In addition, riboflavin deficiency may lead to vitamin B_6 deficiency by interfering with vitamin B_6 metabolism.[9]

Riboflavin Toxicity

No cases of riboflavin toxicity have been reported. Because the body readily excretes excess riboflavin, even large doses appear to pose no risk of accumulating harmful levels. A UL has not been set for riboflavin.

Niacin

In 1867 scientists first produced a substance called nicotinic acid by oxidizing the nicotine from tobacco. Nicotinic acid is not, however, the same as or even closely related to the nicotine molecule. Seventy years later, Conrad Elvehjem at the University of Wisconsin demonstrated that nicotinic acid cured dogs of a canine version of the human niacin-deficiency disease, pellagra. In the early forties, the vitamin was renamed "niacin," an anagram of "nicotinic acid vitamin," so that people would not confuse it with nicotine.

Niacin actually is the name for two similarly functioning compounds: nicotinic acid and nicotinamide (also known as niacinamide). Like the other B vitamins, niacin is a coenzyme component (see **Figure 10.11**) and participates in at least 200 metabolic pathways.

Functions of Niacin

The niacin coenzymes, nicotinamide adenine dinucleotide (NAD+) and nicotinamide adenine dinucleotide phosphate (NADP+), play key roles in oxidation-reduction reactions. NAD+ accepts electrons and hydrogen (is reduced) to form NADH. Under aerobic conditions, NADH carries high-energy electrons to the electron transport chain to help produce ATP. When you need energy in anaerobic conditions (say, during vigorous activity that pushes the body beyond its aerobic capacity), NADH powers the conversion of pyruvate to lactate as it loses electrons and a hydrogen (is oxidized) to become NAD+. This regenerated NAD+ helps power the continued operation of glycolysis. Without it, glycolysis would halt, shutting off the supply of energy from glucose.

Many metabolic pathways that promote the synthesis of new compounds, such as fatty acids, rely on NADPH, the reduced form of NADP+. NADPH is concentrated in cells (such as liver cells) that make large amounts of fatty acids.

Dietary Recommendations for Niacin

Niacin is unique among the B vitamins because your body can make it from the amino acid **tryptophan** as well as obtain it from foods. Intake recommendations are expressed as **niacin equiva-**

lents (NE), a measure that includes both preformed dietary niacin and niacin derived from tryptophan. The RDA for adult men of all ages is 16 milligrams of NE per day, and the RDA for adult women of all ages is 14 milligrams of NE. It increases to 18 milligrams of NE for pregnancy and 17 milligrams of NE for lactation.

Sources of Niacin

Most of the preformed niacin in the U.S. diet comes from meat, poultry, fish, enriched and whole-grain breads and grain products, and fortified ready-to-eat cereals. In a typical U.S. diet, beef and processed meats are substantial contributors.[10] Other good sources of niacin include mushrooms, peanuts, liver, and seafood. **Figure 10.12** shows foods that provide niacin. Because the vitamin is stable when heated, little niacin is lost during cooking.

The niacin precursor, tryptophan, is found in protein-rich animal foods, with the exception of gelatin. To convert tryptophan to niacin, your body needs other nutrients: riboflavin, vitamin B₆, and iron. Sixty milligrams of

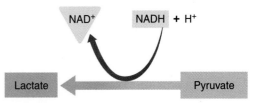

Niacin helps convert pyruvate to lactate. As a component of the coenzymes NAD⁺ and NADH, niacin participates in many metabolic reactions.

tryptophan An amino acid that serves as a niacin precursor in the body. In the body, 60 milligrams of tryptophan yield about one milligram of niacin, or one niacin equivalent (NE).

niacin equivalents (NE) A measure that includes preformed dietary niacin as well as niacin derived from tryptophan; 60 milligrams of tryptophan yield about one milligram of niacin.

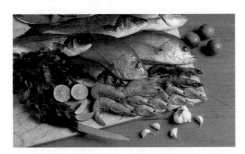

NIACIN

Daily Value = 20 mg

High: 20% DV or more	Beef liver, cooked	85 g (3 oz)	12.3 mg
	Chicken, light meat, cooked	85 g (3 oz)	10.6 mg
	Tuna, canned	55 g (2 oz)	7.3 mg
	Oatmeal, instant, fortified, cooked	1 cup	7.2 mg
	Halibut, cooked	85 g (3 oz)	6.1 mg
	Turkey, light meat, cooked	85 g (3 oz)	5.8 mg
	Salmon, cooked	85 g (3 oz)	5.7 mg
	Chicken, dark meat, cooked	85 g (3 oz)	5.6 mg
	All Bran cereal	30 g (1/2 cup)	5.2 mg
	Corn flakes, Cheerios cereals	30 g (1 cup)	5.0 mg
	Fiber One cereal	30 g (1/2 cup)	5.0 mg
	Pork, loin roast, lean only, cooked	85 g (3 oz)	4.6 mg
	Peanut butter	2 Tbsp.	4.3 mg
	Beef, ground, extra lean, cooked	85 g (3 oz)	4.2 mg
Good: 10–19% DV	Mushrooms, cooked	85 g (~1/2 cup)	3.8 mg
	Chicken liver, cooked	85 g (3 oz)	3.8 mg
	Salmon, canned, solids + bones	55 g (2 oz)	3.6 mg
	Beef, porterhouse steak, cooked	85 g (3 oz)	3.6 mg
	Ham, extra lean, cooked	85 g (3 oz)	3.4 mg
	Beef, T-bone steak, cooked	85 g (3 oz)	3.4 mg
	Turkey, dark meat, cooked	85 g (3 oz)	3.1 mg
	Barley, cooked	140 g (~1 cup)	2.9 mg
	Sardines, canned, solids + bones	55 g (2 oz)	2.9 mg
	Clams, cooked	85 g (3 oz)	2.9 mg
	Spaghetti, enriched, cooked	140 g (~1 cup)	2.3 mg
	Shrimp, cooked	85 g (3 oz)	2.2 mg
	Rice, brown, cooked	140 g (~3/4 cup)	2.1 mg
	Cod, cooked	85 g (3 oz)	2.1 mg
	White bread, enriched	50 g (2 slices)	2.0 mg
	Grits, corn, enriched, cooked	1 cup	2.0 mg
	Rice, white, enriched, cooked	140 g (~3/4 cup)	2.0 mg

Quick Bites

Are you smoking that bread?

In the 1940s, antitobacco forces were confused about the differences between niacin and nicotine. They mistakenly warned that niacin-enriched bread could cause an addiction to cigarettes!

Figure 10.12 **Food sources of niacin.** Niacin is found mainly in meats and grains. Enrichment adds niacin as well as thiamin, riboflavin, folic acid, and iron to processed grains. **Source:** U.S. Department of Agriculture, Agricultural Research Service, 1999. USDA Nutrient Database for Standard Reference, Release 13. Nutrient Data Laboratory Home Page, http://www.nal.usda.gov/fnic/foodcomp.

CALCULATION OF NE FOR AN 80-KG (176-LB) MAN

> His protein RDA is
>
> 80kg x 0.8g/kg = 64g protein

Let us assume his diet contains 94g of high-quality protein so that

> 94g dietary protein
> − 64g protein (his protein RDA)
> 30g protein in excess of needs

Tryptophan makes up about 1% of the protein so that

> 30g protein × .01 = 0.3g tryptophan
> (300mg tryptophan)

60 mg tryptophan ≐ 1mg niacin (1 NE) so that

> 300mg tryptophan ÷ 60 =
> 5mg niacin (5 NE)

> Shortcut Method
> 30g excess protein ÷ 6 = 5mg niacin (5 NE)

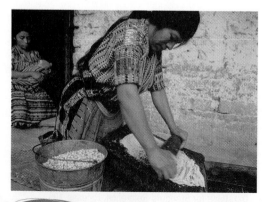

Figure 10.13 Soaking corn in lime water releases bound niacin.

tryptophan yield about one milligram of niacin, or one niacin equivalent (NE). To quickly determine the number of milligrams of niacin derived from tryptophan, divide the grams of high-quality dietary protein that exceed protein needs by six. For instance, 30 grams of excess protein, divided by six, yields five milligrams of niacin.

Because riboflavin, vitamin B_6, and iron affect the conversion of tryptophan to niacin, a deficiency of any one of these nutrients decreases tryptophan conversion. Certain rare metabolic disorders disrupt tryptophan conversion pathways. Pregnancy, on the other hand, increases the efficiency of converting tryptophan to niacin.

Tryptophan supplies about half of the average American's niacin intake. When estimating niacin consumption, remember that tables of food composition list only preformed niacin and therefore underestimate the amount of niacin some foods contribute via tryptophan.

Niacin Deficiency

First recorded in 1735 by a Spanish physician named Gaspar Casal, the niacin-deficiency disease pellagra was originally named *mal de la rosa*, or "red sickness," for the telltale redness that appears around the necks of people with the disease. Severely roughened skin is another hallmark and the condition was later dubbed pellagra for the Italian *pelle*, or "skin," and *agra*, or "rough." Because the niacin coenzymes NAD^+ and $NADP^+$ are involved in just about every metabolic pathway, niacin deficiency wreaks havoc throughout the body. The primary symptoms of pellagra are known as the three Ds: dementia, diarrhea, and dermatitis. In severe cases, a fourth *D*—death—is the final outcome. Deficiencies of iron and vitamin B_6 may also contribute to pellagra.

During the early 1900s, as corn became a staple in the southwestern United States, pellagra emerged in epidemic proportions. A protein in corn tightly binds niacin, so only about 30 percent is bioavailable.[11] We now know, however, that soaking corn in lime water releases that bound niacin, as **Figure 10.13** shows. This disease also was common among the rural poor in the southeast, who subsisted on a diet of corn (maize), molasses, and salt pork, which is mostly fat. Between the end of World War I and the end of World War II, pellagra afflicted some 200,000 Americans. The incidence of pellagra started to decline during World War II because of the mandatory enrichment of bread flour and other cereal grains with niacin. After World War II, the enrichment program combined with the post-war affluence that allowed people to purchase more protein-rich meat, poultry, and fish, finally curbed the disease. Sadly, pellagra continues to plague people living in Southeast Asia and Africa, whose diets lack sufficient niacin and protein.

Niacin Toxicity and Medicinal Uses of Niacin

Niacin has long been known to lower blood levels of LDL cholesterol while raising HDL cholesterol levels when taken in doses of 1,300 to 3,000 milligrams a day. However, adverse effects can be seen at much lower doses. Consuming as little as 250 milligrams of niacin at one time—about 15 to 17 times the RDA for adults—can cause flushing of the face, arms, and chest; itching; headaches; rash; nausea; glucose intolerance; and blurred vision.[12] Moreover, liver abnormalities sometimes show up within a week in people who take high-dose niacin supplements. Based on these complications, the established UL for niacin is 35 milligrams per day for adults.

Think About It

2

Sustained-release niacin supplements deliver the dose throughout the day rather than all at once. This may alleviate flushing and some of the other immediate side effects, but sustained-release supplements can be toxic to the liver when taken for months or years.[13] Niacin supplements containing more than the RDA should be taken only under medical supervision.

Researchers are currently studying nicotinamide in large doses as a possibility for prevention of type 1 diabetes. A recent study shows that nicotinamide protects insulin-secreting cells from inflammation and improves their function after the onset of diabetes.[14]

Key Concepts: *Thiamin, riboflavin, and niacin are all incorporated into coenzymes that catalyze energy-yielding reactions. All three B vitamins participate in pathways that metabolize carbohydrate, protein, and fat. Enriched grains are a major source of these B vitamins, with pork ranking as a good source of thiamin; milk as a major source of riboflavin; and high-protein foods as sources of niacin. Deficiencies of these vitamins are rare in the United States. People with alcoholism have the highest risk of deficiencies. High doses of thiamin and riboflavin appear to be harmless, but megadoses of niacin should be taken only under medical supervision.*

Pantothenic Acid

In the 1930s a chemist named Roger J. Williams discovered that yeast require a certain nutrient, which he called pantothenic acid. He suggested that if yeast needed this nutrient, humans might need it, too. First isolated in 1938, scientists identified the chemical structure of pantothenic acid in 1940.

The name pantothenic acid is derived from the Greek word *pantothen,* meaning "from every side." This B vitamin is widespread in the food supply, so it is well named.

Functions of Pantothenic Acid

Pantothenic acid is a component of coenzyme A (CoA), which in turn, is a component of acetyl CoA. (See **Figure 10.14.**) Acetyl CoA sits at the crossroads of a number of metabolic pathways—both energy-generating pathways and biosynthetic pathways. It starts the citric acid cycle, is a key building block of fatty acids, and is a precursor of ketone bodies.

Fatty acids also are known as acyl groups and pantothenic acid is a component of the acyl carrier protein. During fatty acid synthesis, the acyl carrier protein binds fatty acids and carries them through a series of reactions that increase their chain length. (See **Figure 10.15.**)

Dietary Recommendations for Pantothenic Acid

There are few data upon which to base dietary recommendations for pantothenic acid. As you learned in Chapter 2, when the data are insufficient to set an Estimated Average Requirement (EAR) for a nutrient, an RDA cannot be established. In these cases, and thus for pantothenic acid, an Adequate Intake level is set instead. For adults aged 19 to 50, the AI for pantothenic acid is 5 milligrams per day.

Sources of Pantothenic Acid

Pantothenic acid is widespread in the food supply. Although data on the specific pantothenic acid content of foods are sparse, food sources known to contain this vitamin are chicken, beef, potatoes, oats, tomato products,

PANTOTHENIC ACID AND COENZYME A

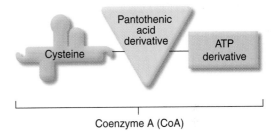

Coenzyme A (CoA)

Figure 10.14 **Pantothenic acid and coenzyme A.** Pantothenic acid forms part of coenzyme A, which in turn is a component of acetyl CoA. Through coenzyme A, pantothenic acid is involved in many metabolic reactions.

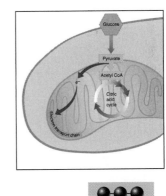

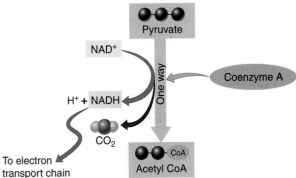

Figure 10.15 **Pantothenic acid helps convert pyruvate to acetyl CoA.** As part of coenzyme A, pantothenic acid helps form acetyl CoA from pyruvate. Niacin participates in this reaction as part of the coenzyme NAD^+.

PANTOTHENIC ACID

Daily Value = 10 mg

High: 20% DV or more	Beef liver, cooked	85 g (3 oz)	5.0 mg
	Chicken liver, cooked	85 g (3 oz)	4.6 mg
	Sunflower seeds	30 g	2.0 mg
Good: 10-19% DV	Mushrooms, cooked	85 g (~1/2 cup)	1.8 mg
	Yogurt, plain, nonfat	225 g (1 8-oz container)	1.4 mg
	Yogurt, plain, lowfat	225 g (1 8-oz container)	1.2 mg
	Turkey, dark meat, cooked	85 g (3 oz)	1.1 mg
	Chicken, dark meat, cooked	85 g (3 oz)	1.0 mg

Figure 10.16 **Food sources of pantothenic acid.** Pantothenic acid is found widely in foods, but is abundant in only a few sources such as liver.
Source: U.S. Department of Agriculture, Agricultural Research Service, 1999. USDA Nutrient Database for Standard Reference, Release 13. Nutrient Data Laboratory Home Page, http://www.nal.usda.gov/fnic/foodcomp.

liver, kidney, yeast, egg yolk, broccoli, and whole grains.[15] **Figure 10.16** shows foods that are good sources of pantothenic acid.

Pantothenic acid is damaged easily. Freezing and canning appear to decrease the pantothenic acid content of vegetables, meat, fish, and dairy products. Processing and refining grains can reduce their pantothenic acid content by nearly 75 percent.[16]

Scientists do not have clear information about the bioavailability of pantothenic acid. We assume that the nutrient is well absorbed.

Pantothenic Acid Deficiency

Pantothenic acid deficiencies are virtually nonexistent in the general population. The only observed cases of pantothenic acid deficiency are in people who were fed diets that completely lacked the nutrient or given a substance that prevents metabolism of pantothenic acid. These people suffered symptoms including irritability, restlessness, fatigue, apathy, malaise, sleep disturbances, nausea, vomiting, numbness, tingling, muscle cramps, staggering gait, and hypoglycemia.

Pantothenic Acid Toxicity

High intakes of pantothenic acid have not caused adverse effects. Risk of toxicity appears to be extremely low and therefore a UL has not been established.

Biotin

In 1924 three factors were identified as necessary for the growth of microorganisms. They were called "bios II," "vitamin H," and "coenzyme R." It soon became clear that all three were the same water-soluble, sulfur-containing vitamin—biotin.

In food, biotin is found both free and bound to protein. When proteins are digested, a biotin-lysine complex called **biocytin** is released.

Functions of Biotin

Biotin-containing enzymes mainly catalyze **carboxylation** reactions, in which carbon dioxide is added to a substrate. (See **Figure 10.17**.) Some of the reactions that rely on biotin-containing enzymes include

- adding carbon dioxide to three-carbon pyruvate to yield four-carbon oxaloacetate. This process is one of the first steps in gluconeogenesis.

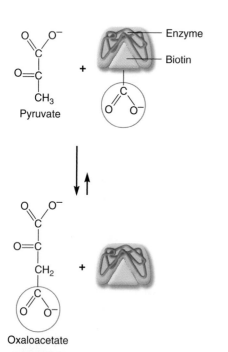

Pyruvate

Oxaloacetate

Figure 10.17 **Biotin aids carboxylation reactions.** Biotin is a coenzyme for several carboxylase enzymes. These enzymes transfer carboxyl groups such as in the conversion of pyruvate to oxaloacetate.

- entry of three-carbon fatty acids into the citric acid cycle to yield energy.
- elongating fatty acid chains during fatty acid synthesis.
- breaking down leucine to the ketone body acetoacetate.
- breaking down isoleucine, methionine, threonine, and valine for entry into the citric acid cycle.
- synthesizing DNA.

Dietary Recommendations for Biotin

Like pantothenic acid, there are not enough data on biotin to establish an EAR or an RDA. In fact, we know so little about human biotin requirements that the Adequate Intake value for adults is mathematically determined from the AI level for infants.[17] The infant value is based on the amount of biotin in human milk. The AI for biotin for adult men and women of all ages is 30 micrograms a day.

Sources of Biotin

Most tables of food composition do not list biotin content because it hasn't been determined for many foods. Good sources of biotin include cauliflower, liver, peanuts, and cheese. Most fruits and meats rank as poor sources. The enzyme **biotinidase** readily releases biotin from biocytin. Egg yolks are also a good source of biotin, but a protein called **avidin** in raw egg whites binds biotin and prevents its absorption from raw eggs. Heat destroys avidin, so it is unlikely to cause a biotin deficiency unless you eat a lot of raw eggs—at least a dozen daily. Of course, you should avoid eating anything that contains raw eggs because they might harbor Salmonella bacteria and cause food-borne illness.

Biotin Deficiency

Eating raw egg whites over a long period—months or years—can cause biotin deficiency. Because some anticonvulsant drugs break down biotin, people who take them for long periods also risk a deficiency. Infants born with biotinidase deficiency suffer from a rare genetic defect that leads to biotin depletion. Symptoms progress from initial hair loss and rash to convulsions and other neurologic disorders. The deficiency also can delay growth and development. Early diagnosis and daily high doses of biotin (e.g., 10 milligrams per day) usually clear up symptoms. If not treated, biotin deficiency causes changes in blood pH that can lead to coma and death.

Biotin Toxicity

Biotin does not appear to be toxic at high doses. Children with biotinidase deficiency have been given as much as 200 milligrams of biotin daily without adverse side effects. A UL for biotin has not been established.

Vitamin B$_6$

Vitamin B$_6$ is a group of six compounds: pyridoxal (PL), pyridoxine (PN), pyridoxamine (PM), and their phosphorylated forms PLP, PNP, and PMP where a phosphate group has been added (see **Figure 10.18**). While food contains the phosphated forms, PLP, PNP, and PMP, digestion strips the phosphate groups. PL, PN, and PM travel to the liver, which converts them to PLP (pyridoxal phosphate), the primary active coenzyme form.[18]

biocytin A biotin-lysine complex released from digested protein.

carboxylation A reaction that adds a carboxyl group (—COOH) to a substrate, replacing a hydrogen atom.

biotinidase An enzyme in the small intestine that releases biotin from biocytin.

avidin A protein in raw egg whites that binds biotin, preventing its absorption. Avidin is destroyed by heat.

Quick Bites

Busy Bacteria

You may be aware that bacteria in the colon synthesize vitamin K, but did you know that colonic bacteria also make some biotin? Then again, when synthesizing this B vitamin these busy microbes may be pursuing a futile effort. Since the colon is downstream from the small intestine, the site of most biotin absorption, the bacteria's biotin may not be absorbed efficiently. Bacterial synthesis of biotin probably does not make an important contribution to your body's supply of biotin.

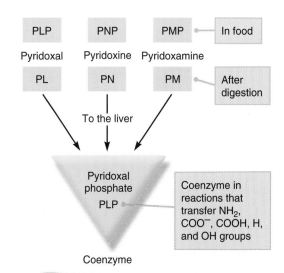

Figure 10.18 **The vitamin B$_6$ family and coenzyme form.** Vitamin B$_6$ is a group of six compounds: pyridoxal (PL), pyridoxine (PN), pyridoxamine (PM), and their phosphorylated forms PLP, PNP, and PMP. Digestion removes the phosphate groups and the liver converts PL, PN, and PM to PLP (pyridoxal phosphate), the active coenzyme form.

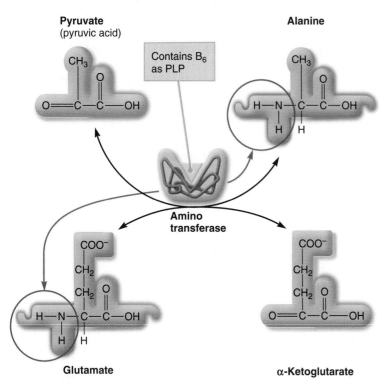

Pyruvate
(pyruvic acid)

Contains B₆ as PLP

Alanine

Amino transferase

Glutamate

α-Ketoglutarate

Figure 10.19 **Vitamin B₆ aids transamination reactions.** Vitamin B₆, as part of PLP, helps transfer an amino group from an amino acid to a keto acid, thus producing a new amino acid.

Functions of Vitamin B₆

The vitamin B₆ coenzyme PLP supports more than 100 different enzymes involved in reactions that include the transfer of amino groups (NH_2), carboxyl groups (COO^- or $COOH$), or water (as H and OH). These enzymes support protein metabolism, blood cell synthesis, carbohydrate metabolism, and neurotransmitter synthesis.

Protein Metabolism

One of the primary tasks of PLP is to help metabolize amino acids and other nitrogen-containing compounds. As **Figure 10.19** shows, PLP plays a key role in transamination reactions, helping transfer an amino group from an amino acid to a keto acid, thus producing a new amino acid. Transamination, catalyzed by PLP, enables the body to make the 11 nonessential amino acids. Without adequate supplies of vitamin B₆, all amino acids become "essential," meaning the body cannot synthesize them and must obtain them from the diet (see discussion of amino acids in Chapter 6, "Proteins"). Over time, vitamin B₆ deficiency impairs protein synthesis and cell metabolism.

Blood Cell Synthesis

PLP supports the synthesis of the white blood cells of the immune system and is crucial for the synthesis of the red blood cells' hemoglobin rings, which carry oxygen. PLP also helps bind oxygen to hemoglobin. Inadequate vitamin B₆ disturbs this binding process, causing **microcytic hypochromic anemia**. In this type of **anemia**, red blood cells are smaller than normal and also lack sufficient hemoglobin to carry oxygen. Iron deficiency also can cause microcytic hypochromic anemia.

Vitamin B₆, Folate, and Heart Disease

Moderately high blood levels of the amino acid homocysteine are associated with fatal cardiovascular events. Homocysteine blood levels are influenced by dietary intake of B₆, folate, and vitamin B₁₂. Low intake of B₆ or folate can result in high homocysteine levels. Because the body accumulates large vitamin B₁₂ stores to draw on when needed, variations in B₁₂ intake seldom affect homocysteine levels. The body lowers homocysteine levels in one of two ways: (1) two PLP-dependent enzymes help convert homocysteine to cysteine, or (2) folate and vitamin B₁₂-dependent enzymes help convert homocysteine to methionine. An increase in fruit and vegetable intake also can affect homocysteine levels. In a Dutch study, subjects who consumed a "high" fruit and vegetable diet (500 g fruits and vegetables plus 200 mL of juice per day; ~ 1.6 mg B₆ and 170 μg folate per 2,000 kcal) had significantly lower plasma homocysteine concentrations that those who consumed a "low" fruit and vegetable diet (100 g of fruits and vegetables per day; ~ 1.2 mg B₆, and 100 mg folate per 2,000 kcal).[19] Because the differences in vitamin B₆ and folate content between the diets were so small, the authors suggest that other components in fruits and vegetables also may influence homocysteine.

A recent study found that women with the highest intakes of B₆ and folate have about half the risk of a heart attack as women with the lowest intakes. Furthermore, when intakes were considered separately, B₆ and folate had similar disease-reduction effects.[20]

microcytic hypochromic anemia Anemia characterized by small, pale red blood cells that lack adequate hemoglobin to carry oxygen; can be caused by deficiency of iron or vitamin B₆.

anemia Abnormally low concentration of hemoglobin in the bloodstream; can be caused by impaired synthesis of red blood cells, increased destruction of red cells, or significant loss of blood.

Carbohydrate Metabolism

Through its role in transamination reactions, PLP participates in gluconeo-genesis—producing glucose from amino acids. In addition, PLP facilitates glycogen breakdown.

Neurotransmitter Synthesis

PLP helps produce a number of neurotransmitters including serotonin, gamma-amino butyric acid (GABA), dopamine, and norepinephrine. A vitamin B₆ deficiency can cause neurologic symptoms—depression, headaches, confusion, and convulsions.

Other Functions

The vitamin B₆ coenzyme also helps convert tryptophan to the B vitamin niacin, as described earlier.

Dietary Recommendations for Vitamin B₆

The RDA for vitamin B₆ for men and women aged 19 to 50 is 1.3 milli-grams per day. For men 51 years and older, the RDA is 1.7 milligrams per day, and for women 51 years and older, the RDA is 1.5 milligrams per day. Due to the role of vitamin B₆ in amino acid metabolism, people on very high protein diets may need higher intakes.[21]

Sources of Vitamin B₆

In the United States, the primary sources of vitamin B₆ are fortified, ready-to-eat cereals; mixed foods (including sandwiches) that contain primarily meat, fish, or poul-try; white potatoes and other starchy vegetables; and noncitrus fruits.[22] Highly fortified cereals, beef liver and other organ meats, and fortified soy-based meat substi-tutes are especially rich sources. Other good sources of vitamin B₆ include bananas, watermelon, potatoes, and sunflower seeds. Although whole grains contain vitamin B₆, refining removes B₆ and enrichment does not replace it. **Figure 10.20** shows foods that provide vitamin B₆.

Vitamin B₆ is not particularly stable and is especially sensitive to temperature. Heat can destroy as much as 50 percent of a food's vitamin B₆ content. About 75 percent of the vitamin B₆ in a varied diet is bioavailable, and vitamin B₆ taken without food is almost completely absorbed, even when taken in megadoses.[23]

Vitamin B₆ Deficiency

Vitamin B₆ deficiencies are rare. When one does occur, the deficiency leads to microcytic hypochromic anemia, seborrheic dermati-tis, and neurologic symptoms such as depression, confusion, and convul-sions.

Alcoholism boosts the risk of vitamin B₆ deficiency because alcohol decreas-es absorption of the nutrient and hampers synthesis of the coenzyme PLP. A breakdown product of alcohol metabolism also interferes with the functioning of vitamin B₆ coenzymes. In addition, two conditions frequently suffered by

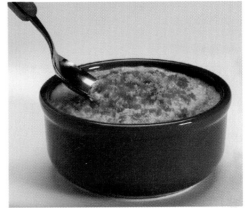

VITAMIN B₆

Daily Value = 2 mg

Food	Amount	Vitamin B₆
High: 20% DV or more		
Beef liver, cooked	85 g (3 oz)	1.22 mg
Oatmeal, instant, fortified, cooked	1 cup	0.98 mg
Banana, fresh	140 g (1 9" banana)	0.81 mg
Garbanzo beans, canned	130 g (~1/2 cup)	0.61 mg
Chicken, light meat, cooked	85 g (3 oz)	0.51 mg
All Bran cereal	30 g (1/2 cup)	0.51 mg
Wheat bran flakes cereal	30 g (3/4 cup)	0.51 mg
Corn flakes cereal	30 g (1 cup)	0.51 mg
Fiber One cereal	30 g (1/2 cup)	0.50 mg
Cheerios cereal	30 g (1 cup)	0.50 mg
Chicken liver, cooked	85 g (3 oz)	0.49 mg
Turkey, light meat, cooked	85 g (3 oz)	0.46 mg
Watermelon, fresh	280 g (1/16 melon)	0.40 mg
Good: 10-19% DV		
Pork, loin chops, roast, lean only, cooked	85 g (3 oz)	0.34 mg
Ham, extra lean, cooked	85 g (3 oz)	0.34 mg
Halibut, cooked	85 g (3 oz)	0.34 mg
Potato, baked	110 g (1 small)	0.33 mg
Turkey, dark meat, cooked	85 g (3 oz)	0.31 mg
Chicken, dark meat, cooked	85 g (3 oz)	0.31 mg
Beef, porterhouse steak, cooked	85 g (3 oz)	0.31 mg
Herring, cooked	85 g (3 oz)	0.30 mg
Tomato juice, canned	240 ml (1 cup)	0.27 mg
Sweet potato, cooked	110 g (1 small)	0.27 mg
Sesame seeds	30 g	0.24 mg
Sunflower seeds	30 g	0.23 mg
Beef, ground, extra lean, cooked	85 g (3 oz)	0.23 mg
Carrots, cooked	85 g (~1/2 cup)	0.21 mg
Rice, brown, cooked	85 g (~3/4 cup)	0.20 mg

Figure 10.20 **Food sources of vitamin B₆.** Meats are generally good sources of vitamin B₆ along with certain fruits (e.g., bananas, watermelon) and vegetables (e.g., potatoes, carrots).
Source: U.S. Department of Agriculture, Agricul-tural Research Service, 1999. USDA Nutrient Database for Standard Reference, Release 13. Nutrient Data Laboratory Home Page, http://www.nal.usda.gov/fnic/foodcomp.

people with alcoholism—cirrhosis and hepatitis—damage liver tissue, preventing the liver from metabolizing vitamin B_6 to its coenzyme form.

Vitamin B_6 Toxicity and Medicinal Uses of Vitamin B_6

Megadoses of supplemental vitamin B_6—2,000 milligrams or more a day—can cause irreversible nerve damage that affects the ability to walk and causes numbness in the extremities.[24] Side effects have been noted at levels of 1,000 milligrams a day as well.

Some women self-prescribe large doses of vitamin B_6 to treat premenstrual syndrome (PMS)—the headache, bloating, irritability, and depression that may occur during the week or so before the onset of menstruation. Although vitamin B_6 has long been reputed to be an antidote for PMS, research has failed to prove its effectiveness.[25]

Despite the risk of toxicity, some people have recommended high doses of vitamin B_6 as a treatment for carpal tunnel syndrome—a repetitive strain injury characterized by painful tingling in the wrist and fingers. Most well-designed scientific studies carried out in recent years, however, have failed to find a link between vitamin B_6 and improvement of carpal tunnel syndrome.[26]

The reasons for the nerve damage associated with B_6 excess are unclear, but modification of proteins by PLP may be involved. The UL for vitamin B_6 intake is 100 milligrams per day, a common amount in over-the-counter vitamin supplements. Because of the hazards of vitamin B_6 megadoses, high doses should be taken only under medical supervision.

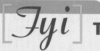

The B Vitamins and Heart Disease

FOR YOUR INFORMATION

In 1968 a young pathologist named Kilmer McCully examined the body of a 2-month-old boy who had died of the rare genetic disease homocystinuria—a condition with sky-high levels of the amino acid homocysteine in the urine. The child's arteries were so hardened and clogged that they resembled those of an adult with severe heart disease. This incident was reminiscent of a similar case that involved an 8-year-old child.

These two cases led Dr. McCully to postulate that high blood levels of homocysteine may be linked to increased risk of heart disease. For the next decade, Dr. McCully held fast to his controversial theory despite the skepticism of his colleagues who found only scant and largely unsubstantiated supporting evidence. In 1978, his outspoken defense of homocysteine as a risk factor for heart disease cost him his job.[1]

In the 1990s, a landmark report from the Physicians' Health Study sparked renewed interest in Dr. McCully's theory linking homocysteine and heart disease. In this ongoing study of a large group of physicians, Harvard University researchers found that those with the highest blood levels of homocysteine had more than triple the heart disease risk of their counterparts with lower homocysteine blood levels.[2] This suggests that homocysteine is an independent risk factor for cardiovascular disease that may be on a par with high blood cholesterol and smoking.

In 1993 a research team from the Jean Mayer USDA Human Nutrition Research Center on Aging at Tufts University showed that high homocysteine levels go hand in hand with low blood levels of vitamins B_6, B_{12}, and especially folate.[3] This association makes sense, since these three nutrients participate in metabolic

pathways that break down homocysteine in the body. When one or more of these vitamins is lacking, homocysteine builds up in the blood over time. Based on the Tufts study, one in five older adults may have homocysteine levels high enough to put them at risk.

During the 1990s scores of studies clearly linked elevated homocysteine to heart attacks, as well as to strokes, blood clots in the legs, and damage to arteries throughout the rest of the body.[4] Homocysteine may contribute to clogged arteries by triggering the proliferation of smooth muscle cells just beneath the innermost layer of the artery wall. These excess cells add to the plaque and other debris that line the arteries and promote blood clots.

Should people take B vitamin supplements to reduce their risk of heart disease? Most research suggests that the RDA levels for folate, vitamin B_6, and vitamin B_{12} may be

Key Concepts: *Pantothenic acid and biotin are widespread in the food supply. Deficiencies of these B vitamins are rare because most people consume adequate amounts. Like the other B vitamins, pantothenic acid and biotin are parts of coenzymes involved in the metabolism of fat, carbohydrate, and protein. Vitamin B$_6$ is found in animal and plant foods and participates in protein metabolism, synthesis of neurotransmitters, and other metabolic pathways. Prolonged megadoses of vitamin B$_6$ can cause nerve damage.*

Folate

Eating raw liver, unappetizing though that may be, has long been known to cure a degenerative type of anemia. In 1945 a search for liver's curative component led to the discoveries of folate and vitamin B$_{12}$. Because folate and B$_{12}$ work together to perform a number of biochemical functions, a deficiency of either one produces the same abnormalities in red blood cells.

As **Figure 10.21** shows, folate has three parts: pteridine, *para*-aminobenzoic acid (PABA), and at least one molecule of glutamic acid (glutamate). About 90 percent of the folate molecules in foods contain 3 to 11 glutamates. All but one of these glutamates is removed in the small intestine prior to absorption. The folic acid form of folate has only one glutamate. Folic acid is the most stable form of folate and is the form used for supplementation and fortification.

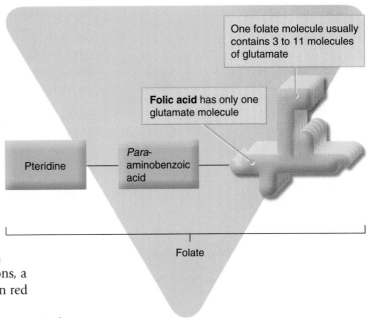

Figure 10.21 **Folate and its major components.** Folate is made up of pteridine, *para*-aminobenzoic acid (PABA), and at least one molecule of glutamic acid (glutamate).

---

sufficient to keep homocysteine levels down. In 1998 a report from the Nurses' Health Study examined whether B vitamin intake affects heart disease risk. In this ongoing study, Harvard researchers have been monitoring the health and eating habits of more than 80,000 female nurses since 1980. They found that women who took in the most folate—from either foods or supplements—were 31 percent less likely to suffer a heart attack than the women who consumed the least folate. The same held true for vitamin B$_6$.[5] More research is under way to determine whether the results hold up in different populations, such as men, and under different circumstances.

At this time, no major health organization recommends across-the-board testing for homocysteine. Some physicians, however, do advise testing for people with a strong family history of heart disease and those who have suffered a heart attack or other coronary event in the absence of high blood cholesterol or other risk factors. A simple blood test can measure homocysteine levels at a cost between $50 and $120. When ordered by a physician, many insurers, including Medicare, will cover the expense.

1 McCully KS. *The Homocysteine Revolution.* New Canaan, CT: Keats Publishing; 1997.

2 Stampfer MJ, Malinow MR, Willett WC, et al. A prospective study of plasma homocyst(e)ine and risk of myocardial infarction in US physicians. *JAMA.* 1992;268:877–881.

3 Selhub J, Jacques PF, Wilson PW, et al. Vitamin status and intake as primary determinants of homocysteinemia in an elderly population. *JAMA.* 1993;270:2693–2698.

4 McCully KS. Homocysteine, folate, vitamin B$_6$, and cardiovascular disease. *JAMA.* 1998;279:392–393.

5 Rimm E, Willett WC, Hu FB, et al. Folate and vitamin B$_6$ from diet and supplements in relation to risk of coronary heart disease among women. *JAMA.* 1998;279:359–364.

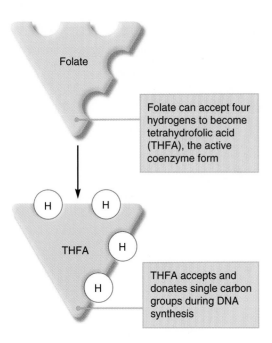

Figure 10.22 **Folate, THFA, and DNA.** Five forms of tetrahydrofolic acid (THFA) are the active coenzyme forms of folate.

Folate can accept four hydrogens to become tetrahydrofolic acid (THFA), the active coenzyme form

THFA accepts and donates single carbon groups during DNA synthesis

dietary folate equivalents (DFE) A measure of folate intake used to account for the high bioavailability of folic acid taken as a supplement compared with the lower bioavailability of the folate found in foods.

DRI Values and Bioavailability of Folate

1 μg DFE = 1 μg food folate

= 0.5 μg folic acid taken on an empty stomach

= 0.6 μg folic acid consumed with meals

Functions of Folate

The body converts folate to a coenzyme called tetrahydrofolic acid (THFA). THFA has five active forms, all of which accept and donate one-carbon units during DNA synthesis, amino acid metabolism, cell division, and the maturation of red blood cells and other cells. (See **Figure 10.22**.)

Dietary Recommendations for Folate

The bioavailability of folate varies depending on stomach contents and the folate source. The body absorbs nearly 100 percent of folic acid in supplements taken on an empty stomach. Some research suggests, however, that the presence of even a small portion of food reduces the absorption of supplemental folic acid to about 85 percent—the same as the bioavailability of folic acid in fortified breads and cereals.[27] The bioavailability of folate naturally present in food is lower—about 50 to 67 percent of intake.[28] To account for these differences, DRI values are expressed as **dietary folate equivalents (DFE)**.

The RDA for folate for males and females age 19 years and older is 400 micrograms of DFE per day. The folate RDA for women increases significantly during pregnancy and lactation: 600 micrograms of DFE per day for pregnant women and 500 micrograms DFE per day while a woman is breastfeeding. To reduce the risk of bearing a child with certain birth defects, especially neural tube defects, the Institute of Medicine and the U.S. Public Health Service advise women of childbearing age to take in 400 micrograms of synthetic folic acid daily, from fortified foods or supplements, as well as to eat folate-containing foods.[29]

Sources of Folate

Most folate in the U.S. diet comes from fortified ready-to-eat cereals and various vegetables. Spinach and other dark green leafy vegetables, asparagus, broccoli, orange juice, wheat germ, liver, sunflower seeds, and legumes are particularly good sources. Although vegetables other than dark green leafy ones are less rich in folate, we eat foods such as green beans and vegetable soup so often that they make major contributions to our total folate intake.[30] **Figure 10.23** shows foods that provide folate.

Folate status during the early stages of pregnancy is strongly linked with birth defects, specifically neural tube defects. Studies consistently show that folic acid supplementation around the time of conception reduces risk of these birth defects by nearly 70 percent. This link prompted the U.S. government to mandate folate fortification of enriched cereal grains, including bread, pasta, flour, breakfast cereal, and rice.[31] This 1998 mandate called for a fortification level of 1.4 milligrams of folic acid per kilogram of grain. Scientists estimate that folate fortification increases folic acid intake by about 100 micrograms per day (an amount provided by slightly more than $\frac{1}{2}$ cup of pasta or one slice of bread) and boosts daily consumption by women of childbearing age to 400 micrograms of folic acid. When food survey data was adjusted to reflect folic acid supplementation and correct for differences in bioavailability, folate intakes met or surpassed the EAR in 67 percent to 95 percent of the population groups. However, 68 percent to 87 percent of women of childbearing age had synthetic folic acid intakes less than 400 micrograms per day.[32]

Folate is extremely vulnerable to heat, ultraviolet light, and exposure to oxygen. Cooking and other food-processing and preparation techniques can destroy 50 percent to 90 percent of a food's folate. Experts recommend eating folate-rich fruits and vegetables raw, or cooking them quickly in minimal amounts of water via steaming, stir-frying, or microwaving. Vitamin C in foods also helps protect folate from oxidation.

Folate Deficiency

Many scientists believe that folate deficiency is the most prevalent of all vitamin deficiencies. Studies suggest that up to 10 percent of the U.S. population have insufficient folate stores. Deficiency may stem from the following conditions:

- *Inadequate folate consumption.* General malnutrition, often due to famine or poverty, causes folate deficiency. Cultural cooking habits that destroy folate, eating habits that avoid raw folate-rich vegetables, alcoholism, excessive dieting, and anorexia nervosa and bulimia nervosa can severely limit folate intake. The infirm or neglected elderly and institutionalized psychiatric patients also are at risk.

Quick Bites

Can Folate Prevent Cancer?

When women took multivitamins containing folate for at least 15 years, they had a 75 percent reduction in colon cancer risk, according to the Harvard Nurses' Health Study. Folate intakes of more than 600 micrograms per day reduced breast cancer risk by 50 percent.

FOLATE

Daily Value = 400 μg

High: 20% DV or more

Exceptionally good source

Food	Amount	Folate
Chicken liver, cooked	85 g (3 oz)	655 μg
Beef liver, cooked	85 g (3 oz)	187 μg
Spinach, raw	85 g (~3 cups)	165 μg
Lentils, cooked	90 g (~1/2 cup)	163 μg
Pinto beans, cooked	90 g (~1/2 cup)	155 μg
Black beans, cooked	90 g (~1/2 cup)	134 μg
Oatmeal, instant, fortified, cooked	1 cup	129 μg
Asparagus, cooked	85 g (~1/2 cup)	124 μg
Okra, cooked	85 g (~1/2 cup)	124 μg
Romaine lettuce, raw	85 g (~1 1/2 cups)	115 μg
Blackeyed peas, cooked	90 g (~1/2 cup)	114 μg
Corn flakes cereal	30 g (1 cup)	106 μg
Artichokes, cooked	85 g (~1/2 cup)	101 μg
Turnip greens, cooked	85 g (~2/3 cup)	101 μg
Cheerios cereal	30 g (1 cup)	100 μg
Soybeans, cooked	90 g (~1/2 cup)	100 μg
Spaghetti, enriched, cooked	140 g (1 cup)	98 μg
Spinach, cooked	85 g (~1/2 cup)	91 μg
All Bran cereal	30 g (1/2 cup)	90 μg

Good: 10-19% DV

Food	Amount	Folate
Collards, cooked	85 g (~1/2 cup)	79 μg
Grits, corn, enriched, cooked	85 g (~1/2 cup)	75 μg
Rice, white, enriched, cooked	140 g (~3/4 cup)	70 μg
Sunflower seeds	30 g	68 μg
Beets, cooked	85 g (~1/2 cup)	68 μg
Kidney beans, canned	85 g (~1/2 cup)	66 μg
Mustard greens, cooked	85 g (~2/3 cup)	62 μg
Wheat germ	15 g	53 μg
Tomato juice, canned	240 ml	48 μg
Broccoli, cooked	85 g (~1/2 cup)	48 μg
White bread, enriched	50 g (2 slices)	48 μg
Orange juice, chilled	240 ml (1 cup)	45 μg
Crab, Alaska king, cooked	85 g (3 oz)	43 μg
Orange, fresh	140 g (1 medium)	42 μg

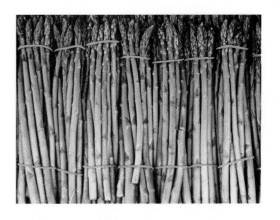

Figure 10.23 **Food sources of folate.** Good sources of folate are a diverse collection of foods: liver, legumes, leafy greens, and orange juice. Enriched grains and fortified cereals are other ways to include folic acid in the diet.
Source: U.S. Department of Agriculture, Agricultural Research Service, 1999. USDA Nutrient Database for Standard Reference, Release 13. Nutrient Data Laboratory Home Page, http://www.nal.usda.gov/fnic/foodcomp.

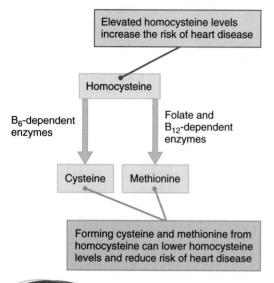

Figure 10.24 **Homocysteine and heart disease.** Elevated homocysteine levels are linked to an increased risk of heart disease. B_6-, B_{12}-, and folate-dependent enzymes help lower the amount of homocysteine by converting it to cysteine and methionine.

Normal red blood precursor

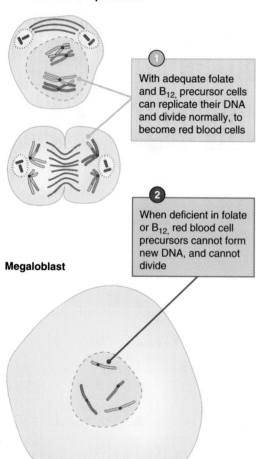

① With adequate folate and B_{12}, precursor cells can replicate their DNA and divide normally, to become red blood cells

② When deficient in folate or B_{12}, red blood cell precursors cannot form new DNA, and cannot divide

Megaloblast

- *Inadequate folate absorption* due to abnormalities in the mucosal cells lining the GI tract.
- *Increased folate requirements* due to pregnancy and lactation, or other conditions. Certain diseases such as blood disorders, leukemia, lymphoma, and psoriasis can increase folate needs.
- *Impaired folate utilization* typically associated with a vitamin B_6 deficiency.
- *Altered folate metabolism* arising from use of alcohol or certain prescription drugs such as barbiturates. Sulfa drugs and anticonvulsants probably impair folate absorption.
- *Excessive folate excretion* due to prolonged diarrhea.

Folate and Heart Disease

Recent research suggests that folate has an important role in preventing heart disease. Folate works with vitamin B_{12} and vitamin B_6 to reduce elevated homocysteine, which is a risk factor for heart attacks.[33] (See **Figure 10.24.**) When folate intake is inadequate, homocysteine levels rise; during a folate deficiency, homocysteine levels are markedly elevated. As folate intake increases, homocysteine levels drop. The Food and Nutrition Board used homocysteine levels as a primary factor in estimating the folate RDA and the recommended folate intakes help maintain homocysteine at reduced levels.

Megaloblastic Anemia

A cellular deficiency of either folate or vitamin B_{12} can impair DNA synthesis in proliferating cells without significant alterations in RNA and protein synthesis. The lack of DNA first affects red blood cells, which are rapidly dividing cells that typically turn over every 120 days. When red blood cell precursors in the bone marrow cannot form new DNA, they cannot divide normally to become red blood cells. As these precursor cells continue to synthesize protein and other cell components, they grow into large bizarre shapes. These large, fragile, immature cells, called **megaloblasts**, displace red blood cells and are a hallmark of megaloblastic anemia, which is shown in **Figure 10.25**.

Megaloblasts may mature into **macrocytes**—abnormally large red blood cells with short life spans. As megaloblasts and macrocytes proliferate and the number of normal red blood cells diminishes, the blood's ability to carry oxygen drops, causing weakness and fatigue. Folate-deficiency anemia commonly causes depression, irritability, forgetfulness, and disturbed sleep.

Impaired DNA synthesis also affects the rapidly dividing cells lining the gastrointestinal tract. As a result, large, immature GI cells multiply and accumulate along the absorptive surface of the digestive tract where they interfere with absorption, causing chronic diarrhea. In the mouth, these defective cells cause the tongue to appear beefy red. A lack of folate also impairs the synthesis of white blood cells, which are vital to the immune response.

Depending on their magnitude, the body's folate stores can sustain normal functioning for two to four months after folate intake stops. Appropriate vitamin replacement restores normal cell reproduction within 24 hours.

Figure 10.25 **Megaloblastic anemia.** When red blood cell precursors in the bone marrow cannot form new DNA, they cannot divide normally. These precursor cells continue to grow and become large, fragile, immature cells called megaloblasts. Megaloblasts displace red blood cells, resulting in megaloblastic anemia.

Neural Tube Defects

A large body of evidence links poor folate status during the early stages of pregnancy to an increased risk of a birth defect known as a **neural tube defect (NTD)**. In this type of birth defect, the neural tube fails to encase the spinal cord during early fetal development. This causes a number of disorders such as **spina bifida** and **anencephaly** (See **Figure 10.26.**). Worldwide, NTDs afflict one to nine of every 1,000 infants born. The FDA's mandate to fortify foods with folic acid should help reduce the rate of NTD. Interestingly, a recent study suggests that both Down syndrome and spina bifida may result from the same genetic abnormality in folate metabolism.[34]

Folate Toxicity

Because folate works so closely with vitamin B$_{12}$, it can mask a vitamin B$_{12}$ deficiency. Consuming excess folate can prevent the formation of altered red blood cells that signals a lack of B$_{12}$. Some evidence also suggests that high intakes of folic acid may prompt or exacerbate the neurological problems associated with vitamin B$_{12}$ deficiency.

Although rare, when hypersensitive people take folic acid supplements, they may suffer hives or respiratory distress. The UL for adults is 1,000 micrograms per day of folic acid from supplements and fortified foods. Researchers have found that folate intake in elders did not generally exceed the UL: however, 20 percent to 30 percent of children exceed the UL for their age groups (UL for ages 1–3 yr. = 300 mg/d; UL for ages 4–6 yr. = 400 mg/d).[35]

Vitamin B$_{12}$

Vitamin B$_{12}$ is also called cobalamin, a generic term that describes a group of cobalt-containing compounds. Scientists usually use the term *vitamin B$_{12}$* to refer to the free vitamin compound called cyanocobalamin. In the United States, this is the only form of vitamin B$_{12}$ commercially available in supplements.

Functions of Vitamin B$_{12}$

Vitamin B$_{12}$ plays a key role in folate metabolism, by transferring a methyl group (—CH3) from the folate coenzyme THFA, as **Figure 10.27** shows. Without vitamin B$_{12}$, THFA cannot change into its methylene form—the

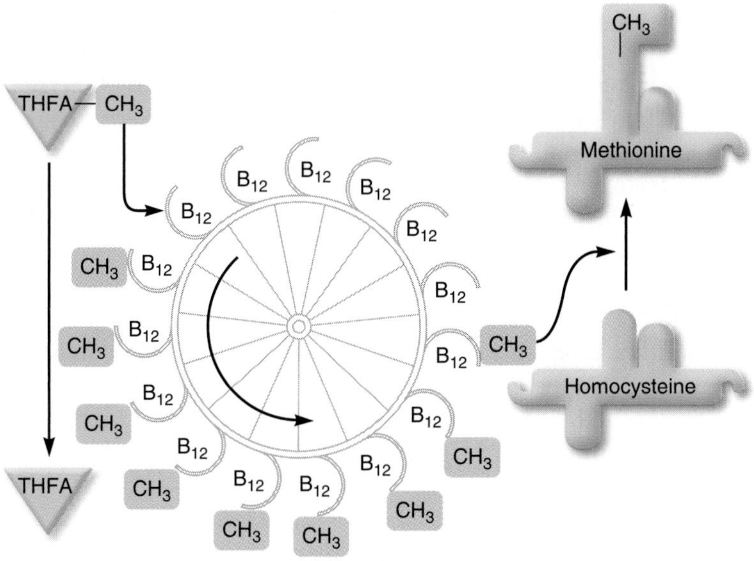

megaloblasts Large, immature red blood cells produced when precursor cells fail to divide normally due to impaired DNA synthesis.

megaloblastic anemia Excess amounts of megaloblasts in the blood caused by deficiency of folate or vitamin B$_{12}$.

macrocytes Abnormally large red blood cells with short life spans.

neural tube defect (NTD) A birth defect resulting from failure of the neural tube to develop properly during early fetal development.

spina bifida A type of neural tube birth defect.

anencephaly A type of neural tube birth defect in which part or all of the brain is missing.

SPINE AFFECTED BY SPINA BIFIDA

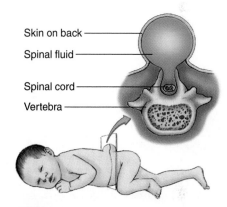

Skin on back
Spinal fluid
Spinal cord
Vertebra

Figure 10.26 **Neural tube defects.** Poor folate status during the early stages of pregnancy, even before a woman may realize she is pregnant, increases the risk of a neural tube defect.

Figure 10.27 **Vitamin B$_{12}$ helps transfer methyl groups (—CH$_3$).** Vitamin B$_{12}$ helps transfer a methyl group (—CH$_3$) from the folate coenzyme THFA. One destination for the methyl group is the reaction that converts homocysteine to methionine. This conversion reduces homocysteine blood levels thereby lowering the risk of heart disease.

myelin sheath The protective coating that surrounds nerve fibers.

R-protein A protein produced by the salivary glands that may protect vitamin B_{12} as it travels through the stomach and into the small intestine.

atrophic gastritis An age-related condition in which the stomach loses its ability to secrete acid. In severe cases, ability to make intrinsic factor is also impaired.

active form in many important metabolic pathways. For instance, a deficiency of the methylene form of THFA inhibits DNA synthesis. The partnership between B_{12} and folate coenzyme THFA means that a vitamin B_{12} deficiency can lead to a folate deficiency, and a lack of either B_{12} or folate can precipitate megaloblastic anemia. Vitamin B_{12}–dependent enzymes also work with THFA to convert homocysteine to methionine, thereby reducing homocysteine blood levels and lowering the risk of heart disease.

Vitamin B_{12} also helps maintain the **myelin sheath**, the protective coating that surrounds nerve fibers. In addition, by helping to rearrange carbon atoms in fatty acid chains, vitamin B_{12} helps prepare them to enter the citric acid cycle.

Absorption of Vitamin B_{12}

The absorption of vitamin B_{12} is a complex process that requires several factors. (See **Figure 10.28.**) In the stomach, vitamin B_{12} binds with **R-protein**, a protein produced by the salivary glands that may protect vitamin B_{12} as it travels through the stomach and into the small intestine. Once there, pancreatic proteases such as trypsin cleave vitamin B_{12} from R-protein. Vitamin B_{12} then binds to intrinsic factor, a substance produced by the parietal cells of the stomach, the same cells that produce hydrochloric acid. Together, the two substances journey to the ileum of the small intestine and attach to receptor cells on the organ's brush border. The receptor cells absorb vitamin B_{12} and transfer it to transcobalamin II, a protein carrier in the blood. Transcobalamin II enters the bloodstream and delivers vitamin B_{12} to the liver, bone marrow, and developing blood cells.

A defect at any point in this process can cause a vitamin B_{12} deficiency. Factors that can impair vitamin B_{12} absorption include

- lack of R-protein, pancreatic enzymes, or intrinsic factor;
- absence or removal of the ileum or stomach;
- overgrowth of bacteria in the stomach;
- tapeworm; and
- reduction of gastric acid production due to prolonged use of acid-inhibiting medications or an age-related condition called **atrophic gastritis**.

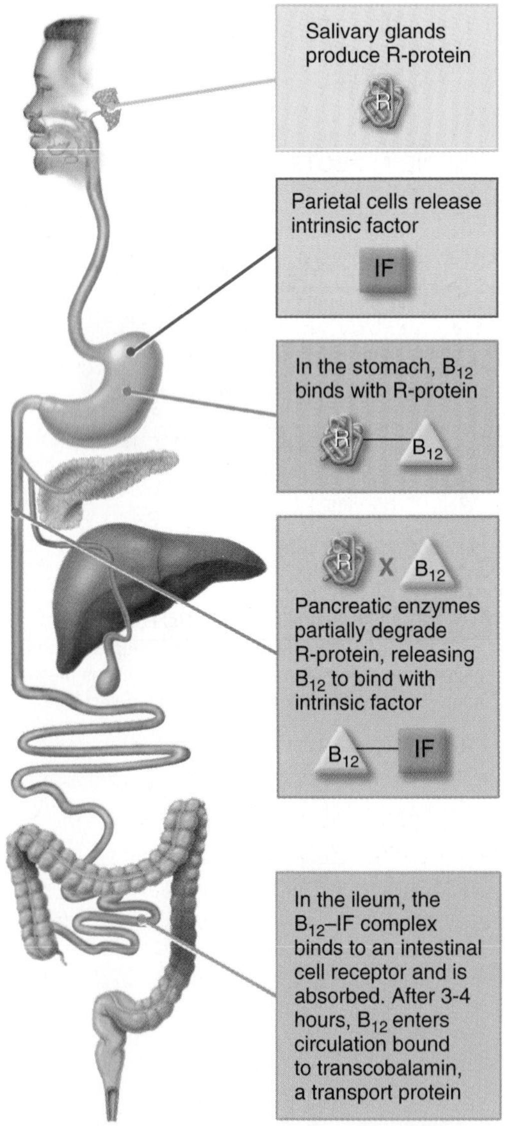

Dietary Recommendations for Vitamin B_{12}

The RDA for men and women aged 19 to 50 is 2.4 micrograms per day. Although the value for adults 51 and older is the same, up to 30 percent of these older adults have atrophic gastritis, which decreases the bioavailability of vitamin B_{12} naturally found in animal foods. People with atrophic gastritis should focus on fortified foods and dietary supplements for most of their B_{12} intake. The form of vitamin B_{12} in these sources is well absorbed—even by people with atrophic gastritis.[36]

Sources of Vitamin B_{12}

Except for fortified foods such as ready-to-eat cereals or some soy milks, animal-derived foods are the only good sources of vitamin B_{12}. Bacteria in animal stomachs synthesize B_{12}, and B_{12} is in the soil that animals consume when eating and grazing. Animals store excess B_{12} in their tissues, especially their livers. Unlike the other B vitamins, B_{12} is not normally present in plant foods. While products made from soy paste and sea algae list vitamin B_{12} as an ingredient, they only contain an inactive and biologically unavailable form.

Salivary glands produce R-protein

Parietal cells release intrinsic factor

IF

In the stomach, B_{12} binds with R-protein

B_{12}

X B_{12}

Pancreatic enzymes partially degrade R-protein, releasing B_{12} to bind with intrinsic factor

B_{12} — IF

In the ileum, the B_{12}–IF complex binds to an intestinal cell receptor and is absorbed. After 3-4 hours, B_{12} enters circulation bound to transcobalamin, a transport protein

Figure 10.28 **Absorption of vitamin B_{12}.** Absorption of B_{12} is a complex process that involves many factors and sites in the GI tract. Defects in this process, especially a lack of intrinsic factor, impair B_{12} absorption and can result in pernicious anemia.

Mixed foods, including sandwiches whose main ingredient is meat, fish, or poultry, contribute most of our dietary B$_{12}$. The next most important sources are milk and milk products for women and beef for men. Although shellfish, liver and other organ meats, some game meat, and some kinds of fish are the richest sources of B$_{12}$, few people regularly eat these foods.[37] **Figure 10.29** shows foods that provide vitamin B$_{12}$.

Although definitive data are lacking, scientists conservatively estimate that about 50 percent of dietary B$_{12}$ is bioavailable. That percentage may drop when a person consumes foods particularly high in vitamin B$_{12}$.

Vitamin B$_{12}$ Deficiency

While a folate deficiency has several causes, often in combination, a vitamin B$_{12}$ deficiency is almost always due to impaired absorption. To circumvent malabsorption, vitamin B$_{12}$ injections deliver the vitamin directly to the bloodstream. Because the liver stores a substantial amount of B$_{12}$, monthly shots usually are sufficient. Other treatments include taking megadoses of vitamin B$_{12}$ supplements (300 times the RDA) that overwhelm impaired absorption, and using a vitamin B$_{12}$-containing nasal gel.

Vegetarians who eat neither meat nor dairy products are at risk of vitamin B$_{12}$ deficiency unless they take vitamin B$_{12}$ supplements or regularly eat fortified cereals. Adult livers store large amounts of vitamin B$_{12}$, so deficiencies develop slowly—over 3 to 12 years. Strict vegetarian (vegan) mothers who breastfeed may put their infants at risk of long-term neurologic problems unless they include supplemental vitamin B$_{12}$ in their diets.

Think About It 3

Pernicious Anemia

The major outcome of impaired vitamin B$_{12}$ absorption is vitamin B$_{12}$-deficiency anemia, or **pernicious anemia**. Like folate-deficiency anemia, pernicious anemia causes the formation of megaloblasts and macrocytes rather than normal red blood cells. But there are important differences. Folate deficiency may lead to cognitive defects and depression, but B$_{12}$ deficiency causes the myelin sheath to swell and break down, leading to brain abnormalities and spinal cord degeneration. If pernicious anemia is not treated, nerve degeneration becomes irreversible and ultimately fatal. Indeed, pernicious means "leading to death." Fortunately, timely vitamin B$_{12}$ injections usually reverse the blood abnormalities and some other signs of pernicious anemia within a matter of days.

Pernicious anemia also attacks the stomach's parietal cells, diminishing their ability to produce intrinsic factor and stomach acid. Pernicious anemia can affect people of all ages, races, and ethnic origins. It runs in families and is associated with several autoimmune disorders, such as Graves' disease.

Vitamin B$_{12}$ Toxicity

High levels of vitamin B$_{12}$ from food or supplements have not been shown to cause harmful side effects in healthy people. Doses of 1 milligram are

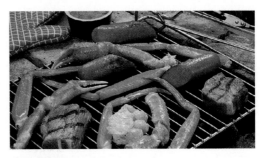

VITAMIN B$_{12}$

Daily Value = 6 µg

Exceptionally good sources

Beef liver, cooked	85 g (3 oz)	95.0 µg
Clams, cooked	85 g (3 oz)	84.1 µg
Oysters, cooked	85 g (3 oz)	29.8 µg
Chicken liver, cooked	85 g (3 oz)	16.5 µg
Herring, cooked	85 g (3 oz)	11.1 µg
Crab, Alaska king, cooked	85 g (3 oz)	9.8 µg
Crab, blue, cooked	85 g (3 oz)	6.2 µg
Salmon, cooked	85 g (3 oz)	4.9 µg
Sardines, canned, solids + bones	55 g (2 oz)	4.9 µg
Lobster, cooked	85 g (3 oz)	2.6 µg
Beef, ground, extra lean, cooked	85 g (3 oz)	1.8 µg
Beef, T-bone steak, cooked	85 g (3 oz)	1.8 µg
Tuna, canned	55 g (2 oz)	1.6 µg
Wheat bran flakes cereal	30 g (3/4 cup)	1.5 µg
All Bran cereal	30 g (1/2 cup)	1.5 µg
Yogurt, plain, nonfat	225 g (8-oz container)	1.4 µg
Shrimp, cooked	85 g (3 oz)	1.3 µg
Yogurt, plain, lowfat	225 g (8-oz container)	1.3 µg
Halibut, cooked	85 g (3 oz)	1.2 µg
Squid, cooked	85 g (3 oz)	1.0 µg
Milk, nonfat	240 ml (1 cup)	0.9 µg
Milk, 1%	240 ml (1 cup)	0.9 µg
Cod, cooked	85 g (3 oz)	0.9 µg
Milk, 2%	240 ml (1 cup)	0.9 µg
Milk, whole (3.25%)	240 ml (1 cup)	0.9 µg
Cottage cheese, 2% milkfat	110 g (~1/2 cup)	0.8 µg
Bologna, beef	55 g (2 slices)	0.8 µg
Frankfurter, beef	55 g (1 each)	0.7 µg
Pork, loin chops, lean only, cooked	85 g (3 oz)	0.6 µg

High: 20% DV or more

Good: 10-19% DV

Figure 10.29 **Food sources of vitamin B$_{12}$.** Vitamin B$_{12}$ is found naturally only in foods of animal origin such as liver, meats, and milk. Some cereals are fortified with vitamin B$_{12}$. **Note:** The DV for vitamin B$_{12}$ is substantially higher than the current (1998) RDA of 2.4 micrograms for those age 14 and older. **Source:** U.S. Department of Agriculture, Agricultural Research Service, 1999. USDA Nutrient Database for Standard Reference, Release 13. Nutrient Data Laboratory Home Page, http://www.nal.usda.gov/fnic/foodcomp.

pernicious anemia Result of the inability to absorb vitamin B$_{12}$. Hallmarks of the condition are excess megaloblasts and nerve degeneration that can result in paralysis and death.

reducing agent A compound that donates electrons or hydrogen atoms to another compound.

connective tissues Tissue composed primarily of fibrous proteins such as collagen, and which contains few cells. Its primary function is to bind together and support various body structures.

Quick Bites

Chili Peppers Are Hot Stuff

*A*n estimated one-quarter of the world's adults eat chili peppers every day. By weight, chili peppers are one of the richest sources of vitamins A and C. In addition, capsaicin, the substance that causes your mouth to burn, jump-starts the digestive process by stimulating salivation, gastric secretions, and gut motility.

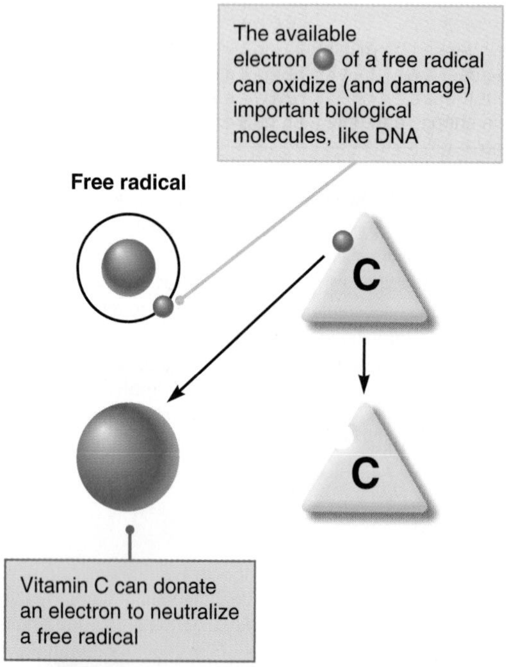

The available electron ● of a free radical can oxidize (and damage) important biological molecules, like DNA

Free radical

Vitamin C can donate an electron to neutralize a free radical

Figure 10.30 **Vitamin C is an antioxidant.** Vitamin C minimizes free radical damage by donating an electron. Vitamin C also indirectly activates many enzymes. Although essential to enzyme activity, unlike the B vitamins, vitamin C is not a coenzyme.

routinely used to treat pernicious anemia with no ill effects. A UL for vitamin B_{12} has not been determined.

Key Concepts: *Folate and vitamin B_{12} work closely together. Fruits, vegetables, enriched grains, and fortified cereals contain folate, but only animal foods and fortified cereals contain bioavailable vitamin B_{12}. A deficiency of folate causes megaloblastic anemia and has been associated with neural tube defects. Deficiency of B_{12} can cause pernicious anemia, a form of megaloblastic anemia, and irreversible nerve damage. Because vitamin B_{12} is found only in animal foods, strict vegetarians must find an alternative source. Folate, vitamin B_{12}, and vitamin B_6 all play roles in the metabolism of the amino acid homocysteine, which has been implicated in heart disease.*

Vitamin C

For centuries, the insidious disease scurvy dogged mankind. Explorers and seafaring men especially feared this mysterious ailment that inflicted aching pain and made each journey a gamble with death. Writings that date back as far as 1500 B.C.E. describe their suffering in detail.

Though they did not know why, some travelers avoided this scourge. Unknowingly, they had eaten foods that contained vitamin C. The mystery began to be solved in 1747 by James Lind, a Scottish physician. In a controlled human nutrition experiment (see Figure 1.12 in Chapter 1), he discovered that eating lemons and oranges cured the disease. But not until 1930 did scientists isolate the substance responsible for curing scurvy and name it vitamin C.

Vitamin C comes in two interchangeable biologically active forms: a reduced form called ascorbic acid and an oxidized form called dehydroascorbic acid. Although most animals can synthesize the nutrient, humans cannot make their own vitamin C. For some unknown reason, humans also appear to require much less than other animals.

Functions of Vitamin C

Vitamin C is an antioxidant—it acts as a **reducing agent** and participates in many reactions by donating electrons or hydrogen ions. It also is essential to the activity of many enzymes. But unlike the B vitamins, it is not a coenzyme, and only indirectly activates enzymes.

Collagen Synthesis

Vitamin C plays an important role in the formation of collagen, a fibrous protein that helps reinforce the **connective tissues** that hold together the structures of the body. Collagen is the most abundant protein in our bodies and the main fibrous component of skin, bone, tendons, cartilage, and teeth. It also is the major protein in connective tissue, which binds cells and tissues together, and in scar tissue.

Antioxidant Activity

Like vitamin E and beta-carotene (see Chapter 9), vitamin C works as an antioxidant and minimizes free radical damage in cells. In its antioxidant role, vitamin C may reduce the risk of chronic diseases such as heart disease, certain forms of cancer, and cataracts. Research results are contradictory, however, and scientists continue to explore the impact of vitamin C on chronic disease. In addition to working independently as an antioxidant (**Figure 10.30**), vitamin C helps recycle oxidized vitamin E for reuse in the cells.[38] Finally, vitamin C stabilizes the reduced form of the folate coenzyme.

Iron Absorption

As a reducing agent, vitamin C enhances the absorption of nonheme iron, which comes mainly from plant foods (the small intestine absorbs nonheme iron better when it is reduced).

Synthesis of Vital Cell Compounds

Vitamin C helps synthesize carnitine, a compound that carries fatty acids from the cytosol to the mitochondria for energy production. Vitamin C also helps synthesize norepinephrine, epinephrine, the neurotransmitter serotonin, the thyroid hormone thyroxine, bile acids, steroid hormones, and purine bases used in DNA synthesis.

Immune Function

Vitamin C enables lymphocytes and other cells of the immune system to function properly. This explains why people may need more vitamin C during an illness. Because chemical-detoxifying systems in cells use vitamin C, drug use also can boost vitamin C requirements.

Dietary Recommendations for Vitamin C

For adults age 19 and older, the RDA for vitamin C is 90 milligrams per day for men and 75 milligrams per day for women. For women, the RDA rises to 85 milligrams per day during pregnancy and 120 milligrams per day during lactation. Because smoking increases the metabolic turnover of vitamin C, the Food and Nutrition Board estimates that smokers require 35 milligrams per day more than nonsmokers.[39]

Sources of Vitamin C

Particularly good sources of vitamin C include potatoes, citrus fruits, tomatoes, fortified juice drinks, broccoli, strawberries, kiwi fruit, cabbage, spinach and other leafy greens, and green peppers. Because vitamin C is highly vulnerable to heat and oxygen, *fresh* fruits and vegetables are the optimal sources. **Figure 10.31** shows some foods that provide vitamin C.

When people take in 30 milligrams to 120 milligrams daily, the intestine absorbs about 80 percent to 90 percent of vitamin C. However, when vitamin C consumption exceeds 6,000 milligrams daily, absorption drops to about 20 percent. Most of the residual vitamin C is excreted in the urine.

Vitamin C Deficiency

Scurvy is the well-known vitamin C deficiency disease. Its first symptoms surface after about a month on a vitamin C–free diet. As the body loses its ability to synthesize collagen, connective tissue starts breaking down and gums and joints begin to bleed. Weakness develops and small hemorrhages appear around the hair follicles on the arms and legs. As the disease progresses, previously healed wounds reopen and bone pain, fractures, diarrhea, and psychological problems such as depression, commonly emerge. Scurvy is rare in developed countries, but possible among those who eat few fruits and

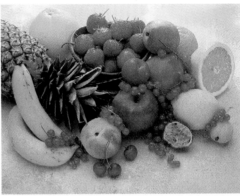

VITAMIN C

Daily Value = 60 mg

Exceptionally good sources

Orange juice, chilled	240 ml (1 cup)	81.9 mg
Strawberries, fresh	140 g (~1 cup)	79.4 mg
Orange, fresh	140 g (1 medium)	74.5 mg
Cantaloupe, fresh	140 g (1/4 medium melon)	59.1 mg
Tomato juice, canned	240 ml (1 cup)	44.5 mg
Mango, fresh	140 g (~3/4 cup)	38.8 mg
Cauliflower, cooked	85 g (~3/4 cup)	37.7 mg
Broccoli, cooked	85 g (~1/2 cup)	34.1 mg
Watermelon, fresh	280 g (1/16 melon)	26.9 mg
Spinach, raw	85 g (~3 cups)	23.9 mg
Pineapple, fresh	140 g (~1 cup)	21.6 mg
Mustard greens, cooked	85 g (~2/3 cup)	21.5 mg
Romaine lettuce, raw	85 g (~1 1/2 cups)	20.4 mg
Beef liver, cooked	85 g (3 oz)	19.6 mg
Sweet potato, cooked	110 g (1 small)	18.8 mg
Clams, cooked	85 g (3 oz)	18.8 mg
Blueberries, fresh	140 g (~3/4 cup)	18.2 mg
Cabbage, cooked	85 g (~1/2 cup)	17.0 mg
Wheat bran flakes	30 g (3/4 cup)	15.5 mg
Collards, cooked	85 g (~1/2 cup)	15.5 mg
Soybeans, cooked	90 g (~1/2 cup)	15.3 mg
Swiss chard, cooked	85 g (~1/2 cup)	15.3 mg
Cheerios cereal	30 g (1 cup)	15.0 mg
Corn flakes cereal	30 g (1 cup)	15.0 mg
Potato, baked	110 g (1 small)	14.1 mg
Banana, fresh	140 g (1 9" banana)	12.7 mg

High: 20% DV or more

- -

Spinach, cooked	85 g (~1/2 cup)	10.5 mg
Okra, cooked	85 g (~1/2 cup)	10.4 mg
Peach, fresh	140 g (2 small)	9.2 mg
Acorn squash, cooked	85 g (~1/2 cup)	9.2 mg
Asparagus, cooked	85 g (~1/2 cup)	9.2 mg
Green beans, cooked	85 g (~3/4 cup)	8.2 mg

Good: 10-19% DV

Figure 10.31 **Food sources of vitamin C.** Vitamin C is found mainly in fruits and vegetables. Although citrus fruits are notoriously good sources, many other popular fruits and vegetables are rich in vitamin C. **Source:** U.S. Department of Agriculture, Agricultural Research Service, 1999. USDA Nutrient Database for Standard Reference, Release 13. Nutrient Data Laboratory Home Page, http://www.nal.usda.gov/fnic/foodcomp.

vegetables, follow extremely restricted diets, or abuse alcohol or drugs.[40] Less severe vitamin C deficiency can impair cellular functions without causing overt scurvy. The most common symptoms are inflammation of the gums and fatigue.

Vitamin C Toxicity

Although megadoses of vitamin C do not appear to be acutely toxic to most healthy people, taking more than 2,000 milligrams daily for a prolonged period may lead to nausea, abdominal cramps, diarrhea, and nosebleeds.[41] The UL for vitamin C is 2,000 milligrams per day. In people with kidney disease, excess vitamin C also may contribute to oxalate-containing kidney stones. In healthy people, epidemiological studies do not support an association between excess vitamin C intake and kidney stones.[42] High vitamin C intakes also may bolster iron absorption—useful for some, but problematic for people with **hemochromatosis**, a metabolic disease that causes excess iron accumulation.

Finally, some experts suspect that large amounts of vitamin C may stimulate free radical damage by enhancing oxidation (a pro-oxidant effect), the opposite of its usual antioxidant activity. This suspicion is based on test-tube experiments that show vitamin C acting as a pro-oxidant when it comes into contact with iron or another metal.[43]

As for vitamin C's notoriety as a purported cure for the common cold, reviews of relevant research show no significant effect on the incidence of colds. At best, in some people, high doses may reduce the severity and duration of cold symptoms.[44]

Think About It 4

Key Concepts: *Vitamin C, which is found in many fruits and vegetables, functions mainly in collagen synthesis. It also acts as an antioxidant. Vitamin C helps boost iron absorption and plays a part in hormone and neurotransmitter synthesis. A deficiency of vitamin C leads to scurvy, although this is rare today. Megadoses of vitamin C can cause gastrointestinal disturbances.*

Vitamin-Like Compounds

The body synthesizes a number of vitamin-like compounds that play essential roles in maintaining metabolism. These include choline, carnitine, inositol, taurine, and lipoic acid. Although the risk of a deficiency is minimal in healthy people, it is unclear whether certain diseases cause deficiencies of these compounds and whether they should be added to infant formulas. Currently, many manufacturers of infant formula do add some of these compounds to their products.

Choline

Choline helps maintain the structural integrity of cell membranes and it accelerates the production of acetylcholine, an important neurotransmitter involved in memory, muscle control, and other functions. Choline also is a component of lecithins and bile (choline was named after the French word for bile, *chole*).

With the help of vitamin B_{12} and folate, the liver forms choline from the amino acids serine and methionine. If you eat enough protein to provide the essential amino acid methionine, your body can manufacture choline. Insufficient data are available to determine if choline is essential in the human diet. The research that exists suggests that people on diets devoid of choline develop fatty liver and liver damage.

hemochromatosis A metabolic disorder that results in excess iron deposits in the body.

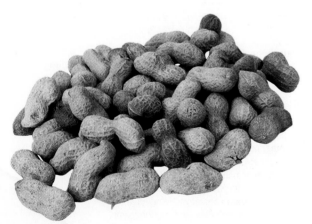

Because choline is widespread in the food supply, the risk of a deficiency is minimal in healthy people. Milk, liver, eggs, and peanuts are especially rich in choline. An AI for choline has been set at 550 milligrams per day for adult men, and 425 milligrams a day for adult women.

High doses of choline can cause hypotension (low blood pressure), sweating, diarrhea, and fishy body odor. The UL for adults is 3,500 milligrams of choline per day.

Carnitine

Carnitine carries fatty acids from the cytosol into the mitochondria for entry into the citric acid cycle. In the mitochondria, carnitine also helps dispose of excess organic acids produced via metabolic pathways. The liver synthesizes carnitine from the amino acids lysine and methionine.

Meat and dairy products are the major dietary sources of carnitine. Carnitine does not appear to be an essential compound for healthy people, because strict vegetarians often eat diets virtually lacking carnitine without suffering ill effects. Low blood levels of carnitine have been observed in malnourished children and adults. Diets deficient in the amino acids needed to make carnitine may cause abnormal fatty acid metabolism.

Carnitine in large doses has been helpful in removing toxic compounds in people with certain inborn errors of metabolism. In addition, high doses of carnitine have been successful in treating progressive muscle disease and deterioration of the heart muscle.

Inositol

Inositol is part of cell membrane phospholipids. Inositol phospholipids, a family of lipids containing inositol derivatives, are precursors of eicosa-noids, substances that work like hormones in the body (for more on eicosanoids, see Chapter 5, "Lipids"). Inositol participates in a chain of reactions that ultimately increases the concentration of intracellular calcium, which in turn elicits a number of cell responses such as the relaying of messages by nerve cells. This may explain why inositol phospholipids are concentrated in brain tissue.

The body synthesizes inositol from glucose and these two molecules have similar structures. Although there are nine forms of inositol, myo-inositol is the only one involved in human nutrition.

While some plant foods contain inositol, animal-derived foods supply most dietary inositol. There is no reason to suspect inositol deficiency in the general population and the Food and Nutrition Board has not set recommended intake levels. Inositol seems to become essential only for people with impaired inositol metabolism. Abnormal inositol metabolism appears to be associated with certain medical conditions such as diabetes, multiple sclerosis, kidney failure, and some cancers.

Taurine

Taurine seems to play a role in photoreceptor activity in the eye, antioxidant activity in white blood cells and pulmonary tissue, central nervous system function, platelet aggregation, heart muscle contraction, insulin activity, and cell growth and differentiation. Derived from the amino acids methionine and cysteine, taurine is concentrated in muscle, platelets, and nerve tissue and is attached to bile acids.

There is no evidence of taurine deficiency in the general population. Although it is found only in foods from animal sources, strict vegetarians are not deficient. Apparently, people are able to synthesize all the taurine they need.

Taurine supplements may be useful for children with cystic fibrosis and preterm infants who absorb fat poorly. In these children, the taurine attached to bile acids may help increase fat absorption. Taurine is one of several amino acids that have become popular additives to so-called smart drinks designed to assist in mental activities. However, no solid scientific evidence links taurine to improved mental abilities.

Lipoic Acid

Lipoic acid is a necessary cofactor in energy-producing reactions in mitochondria. For instance, lipoic acid helps convert pyruvate to acetyl CoA, the major linking step between glycolysis and the citric acid cycle. It is a potent antioxidant and is unique because it can neutralize both fat-soluble and water-soluble free radicals. Although health food stores sell lipoic acid supplements, no evidence supports their use by healthy people.

Bogus Vitamins

Many dietary supplements contain unnecessary substances. Yet hucksters often call these substances vitamins and tout their supposed benefits as health enhancers and disease treatments. Despite ample scientific evidence to the contrary, quacks still hawk laetrile ("vitamin B_{17}") as a cancer cure. Some supplements contain hesperidin, *para*-aminobenzoic acid (PABA), pangamic acid, or rutin even though these substances are not essential for human health. Think twice before you pay a premium price for supplements that contain these bogus vitamins.

Key Concepts: *The body contains a number of vitamin-like compounds synthesized from glucose and amino acids and found in the food supply. Although deficiencies of these substances are unlikely, some people with certain medical conditions may benefit from supplemental amounts of some of these compounds. Of course, supplements should be taken only with a physician's recommendation. Researchers are examining the needs for these substances and their effects on the body.*

Label [to] **Table**

As of January 1998, the FDA requires all manufacturers to add folic acid to enriched grain products such as bread, flour, rice, and pasta. Folic acid, the synthetic form of folate, has been shown to decrease risk of neural tube defects. Folate or folic acid may also be important in reducing risk of heart disease and colon cancer. Prior to the fortification of enriched grains, it was difficult for some people to get enough of this B vitamin, in part because it is destroyed easily during cooking and storage. The purpose of folic acid fortification is to ensure most people, especially women of childbearing age, can meet their needs for this B vitamin. Look at the Nutrition Facts label on a pasta package. Note how much folic acid is in a serving of pasta!

Nutrition Facts

Serving Size: 1/2 cup (56g)
Servings Per Container: 8

Amount Per Serving

Calories 200   Calories from fat 10

	% Daily Value*
Total Fat 1g	2%
Saturated Fat 0g	0%
Cholesterol 0mg	0%
Sodium 0mg	0%
Total Carbohydrate 41g	14%
Dietary Fiber 2g	8%
Sugars 1g	
Protein 7g	

Vitamin A 0%	•	Vitamin C 0%
Calcium 0%	•	Iron 10%
Thiamin 35%	•	Riboflavin 15%
Niacin 20%	•	Folic acid 30%

* Percent Daily Values are based on a 2,000 calorie diet. Your daily values may be higher or lower depending on your calorie needs:

		Calories:	2000	2,500
Total Fat	Less Than		65g	80g
Sat Fat	Less Than		20g	25g
Cholesterol	Less Than		300mg	300mg
Sodium	Less Than		2,400mg	2,400mg
Total Carbohydrate			300g	375g
Dietary Fiber			25g	30g

Calories per gram:
Fat 9   Carbohydrate 4   Protein 4

Calories	200
Total fat	2% (1g)
Saturated fat	0%
Cholesterol	0%
Sodium	0%
Total carbohydrate	14%
Vitamin A	0%
Vitamin C	0%
Calcium	0%
Iron	10%
Folic acid	30%
Thiamin	35%
Niacin	20%
Riboflavin	15%

Some vegetables and legumes also contain folate, so combining pasta with vegetables, or enriched rice with black beans, would provide substantial amounts of folate. The next time you are at the grocery store, pay close attention to the food labels on grain products to see just how much folate you could consume from different grain products.

Looking again at this food label, what other water-soluble vitamins do you see? In addition to folic acid, this pasta also contains thiamin, niacin, and riboflavin. These are the "enrichment" vitamins and one serving of pasta provides 15 to 30 percent of the Daily Value of each.

LEARNING *Portfolio* chapter 10

Key Terms

	page		page
anemia	380	macrocytes	386
anencephaly	387	megaloblastic anemia	386
ariboflavinosis	374	megaloblasts	386
atrophic gastritis	388	microcytic hypochromic	
avidin	379	anemia	380
beriberi	368	myelin sheath	388
biocytin	379	niacin equivalents (NE)	375
biotinidase	379	neural tube defect	386
carboxylation	379	pernicious anemia	389
cheilosis	374	R-protein	388
connective tissues	390	reducing agent	390
decarboxylation	370	seborrheic dermatitis	374
dietary folate equivalents		spina bifida	386
(DFE)	384	stomatitis	374
glossitis	374	thiamin pyrophosphate	
glutathione peroxidase	373	(TPP)	370
hemochromatosis	392	tryptophan	375

Study Points

➤ The water-soluble vitamins include the eight B vitamins and vitamin C.

➤ Thiamin (vitamin B₁) functions as the coenzyme thiamin pyrophosphate (TPP) in energy metabolism.

➤ Thiamin deficiency results in the classic disease beriberi. In industrialized countries, thiamin deficiency most often is associated with alcoholism. There is no known danger of toxicity related to high intakes of thiamin.

➤ Riboflavin (vitamin B₂) forms part of the coenzymes FAD and FMN, which function in energy metabolism as hydrogen and electron carriers.

➤ Ariboflavinosis (riboflavin deficiency) is characterized by inflammation of the mouth and tongue.

➤ Niacin (vitamin B₃) participates in energy metabolism as part of the coenzymes NAD⁺ and NADP⁺.

➤ Niacin deficiency results in pellagra, a disease characterized by diarrhea, dermatitis, dementia, and death.

➤ High doses of niacin, such as in the treatment of high blood cholesterol, can have toxic side effects including liver damage.

➤ Pantothenic acid is a part of coenzyme A, a critical player in energy metabolism.

➤ The active coenzyme form of biotin is biocytin, and it is involved in many reactions involving energy-yielding nutrients.

➤ Biotin deficiency is rare, but may be induced by regularly consuming large quantities of raw egg whites.

➤ The coenzyme form of vitamin B₆ (pyridoxine) is called pyridoxal phosphate (PLP); it participates in a variety of reactions, primarily involving amino acid metabolism.

➤ Megadoses of vitamin B₆ can cause permanent nerve damage.

➤ Folate and vitamin B₁₂ work closely together in a number of metabolic pathways including reactions in cell division and DNA synthesis.

➤ Deficiency of either folate or vitamin B₁₂ will result in megaloblastic anemia, but vitamin B₁₂ deficiency (pernicious anemia) also causes irreversible nerve damage.

➤ Poor folate status is associated with development of neural tube defects during pregnancy. Therefore, women of childbearing age are advised to take in 400 micrograms of folic acid each day from fortified foods or supplements in addition to other dietary folate.

➤ Vitamin C (ascorbic acid) functions in the synthesis of collagen and other vital compounds, and also works as an antioxidant.

➤ Vitamin C deficiency can cause scurvy, which is characterized by bleeding gums and small hemorrhages on the skin.

➤ A number of vitamin-like compounds have been identified including choline, inositol, and taurine. These compounds are synthesized by the body, and are not dietary essentials.

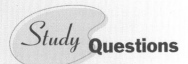

Study Questions

1. **List the nine water-soluble vitamins and one main function for each.**

2. **Which water-soluble vitamin can be made from an amino acid?**

3 **Name the diseases and/or characteristic symptoms of deficiency of each water-soluble vitamin.**

4. **A lack of which three B vitamins can cause anemia? Describe the differences among these anemias.**

5. **List the water-soluble vitamins demonstrated to be toxic in large doses. What signs indicate toxic levels of each vitamin?**

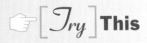

Try This

The Antioxidant and the Apple

This experiment will help you see how vitamin C acts as an antioxidant. You will need an apple and a lemon. Slice the apple into eight pieces. Put four on one plate and four on another. Slice open the lemon and squeeze its juices over the apple slices on one plate. Leave the lemon on this plate to remind you which apple slices have been sprayed with lemon juice. Let both plates sit for 30 minutes. Do the apple slices look any different after 30 minutes? What is the difference? Why?

Supplemental Income

The object of this exercise is to critically review vitamin supplements. Go to the drug store and look at a few multivitamin supplements and "stress" formulas. Look at the %DV for the water-soluble vitamins. Do you see any that have more than 1000% of the DV? Compare prices. Is it more expensive to buy supplements with more of these vitamins? Considering what you learned in this chapter, would it benefit you to take supplements that contain such a high amount of these vitamins? Why do you think supplements contain such large quantities of these vitamins?

What About Bobbie?

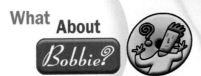

Let's take a look at Bobbie's intake of five water-soluble vitamins: thiamin, riboflavin, niacin, vitamin B_{12}, and vitamin C. Let's examine her day of eating (see Chapter 1) using the guidelines you've learned in this chapter. How did Bobbie do in terms of these water-soluble vitamins? She did well; she consumed ample amounts of most due to her varied food choices. Here is a summary of each of the vitamins.

Thiamin

Bobbie consumed 1.8 milligrams of thiamin, which is 164 percent of the RDA of 1.1 milligrams. Most of the foods Bobbie ate this day contributed to her thiamin intake, but the ones that contributed the most were the enriched grains from the bread, bagel, and spaghetti.

Riboflavin

Bobbie consumed 1.9 milligrams of riboflavin on this day or 171 percent of the RDA of 1.1 milligrams. As with thiamin, it was a variety of foods that contributed to her riboflavin intake but the enriched grains (bread, bagel, and pasta) were among the best contributors. The meatballs Bobbie ate at dinner also contributed riboflavin.

Niacin

Bobbie's intake of niacin was also above her RDA. She consumed 21.7 milligrams this day compared to her RDA of 14 milligrams. If you remember from the protein chapter that Bobbie's intake of protein was quite high, it shouldn't surprise you that her niacin intake is high, too. Meat, poultry, fish, and other protein-containing foods are some of the best sources of niacin. In this case, Bobbie's turkey sandwich, meatballs, and cheese pizza contributed niacin.

Vitamin B_{12}

Bobbie's intake of vitamin B_{12} (3.6 µg), like her intake of the other B vitamins, was above the RDA (2.4 µg). The foods that contributed to Bobbie's vitamin B_{12} intake were the animal products (turkey, egg, meatballs, parmesan cheese, and cheese pizza).

Vitamin C

Although Bobbie enjoys tomato products like salsa, spaghetti sauce, and pizza sauce, her intake of vitamin C (61 milligrams) was less than the RDA of 75 milligrams. Here are some other ways Bobbie could have included more vitamin C in her diet:
- Have some orange or grapefruit juice with breakfast.
- Choose spinach, broccoli, or Brussels sprouts instead of green beans for dinner.
- Use spinach as the base of her salad instead of iceberg lettuce.
- Add some sliced red pepper to her salad at lunch.
- Have an orange as a snack instead of the tortilla chips.

References

1 US Department of Health and Human Services. FDA Announces Name Changes for Lower-Fat Milks and Folic Acid Fortification for Bakery Products. *HHS News*; Dec 31, 1997.

2 Institute of Medicine. Food and Nutrition Board. *Dietary Reference Intakes for Thiamin, Riboflavin, Niacin, Vitamin B₆, Folate, Vitamin B₁₂, Pantothenic Acid, Biotin, and Choline.* Washington, DC: National Academy Press; 1998.

3 Ibid.

4 Ibid.

5 Murray RK, Granner DK, Mayes PA, Rodwell VW. *Harper's Biochemistry.* 24th ed. Stamford, CT: Appleton & Lange; 1996.

6 Institute of Medicine. Food and Nutrition Board. Op. cit.

7 Zempleni J, Galloway JR, McCormick DB. Pharmacokinetics or orally and intravenously administered riboflavin in healthy humans. *Am J Clin Nutr.* 1996;63:54–66.

8 Institute of Medicine. Food and Nutrition Board. Op. cit.

9 McCormick DB. Two interconnected B vitamins: riboflavin and pyridoxine. *Physiol Rev.* 1989;69:1170–1198.

10 Institute of Medicine. Food and Nutrition Board. Op. cit.

11 Carpenter KJ, Lewin WJ. A reexamination of the composition of diets associated with pellagra. *J Nutr.* 1985;115:543–552.

12 McKenney JM, Proctor JD, Harris S, Chinchili VM. A comparison of the efficacy and toxic effects of sustained- vs. immediate-release niacin in hypercholesterolemic patients. *JAMA.* 1994;271:672–677.

13 Ibid.; and Gibbons LW, Gonzalez V, Gordon N, Grundy S. The prevalence of side effects with regular and sustained-release nicotinic acid. *Am J Med.* 1995;99:378–385.

14 Visalli N, Cavallo MG, Signore A, et al. A multi-centre randomized trial of two different doses of nicotinamide in patients with recent-onset type 1 diabetes (the IMDIAB VI). *Diabetes Metab Res Rev.* 1999; 15:181–185.

15 Plesofsky-Vig N. Pantothenic acid. In: Ziegler EE, Filer LJ, eds. *Present Knowledge in Nutrition.* 7th ed. Washington, DC: ILSI Press; 1996.

16 Institute of Medicine. Food and Nutrition Board. Op. cit.

17 Ibid.

18 Ibid.

19 Broekmans WMR, Klöpping-Ketelaars IAA, Schuurman CRWC, et al. Fruits and vegetables increase plasma carotenoids and vitamins and decrease homocysteine in humans. *J Nutr.* 2000;130:1578–1583.

20 Rimm EB, Willett WC, Hu FB, et al. Folate and vitamin B6 form diet and supplements in relation to risk of coronary heart disease among women. *JAMA.* 1998;279:359–364.

21 Institute of Medicine. Food and Nutrition Board. Op. cit.

22 Ibid.

23 Gregory JF. Bioavailability of vitamin B₆. *Eur J Clin Nutr.* 1997;51:S54–S59.

24 Schaumberg H, Kaplan J, Windebank A, et al. Sensory neuropathy from pyridoxine abuse. *N Engl J Med.* 1983;309:445–448.

25 Kurzer MS. Women, food and mood. *Nutr Rev.* 1997;55:268.

26 Franzblau A. The relationship of vitamin B6 status to median nerve function and carpal tunnel syndrome among active industrial workers. *J Occupation Environment Med.* 1996;38:485–491.

27 Pfeiffer CM, Rogers LM, Bailey LB, et al. Absorption of folate from fortified cereal-grain products and of supplemental folate consumed with or without food determined by using a dual-label stable-isotope protocol. *Am J Clin Nutr.* 1997;66:1388–1397.

28 Institute of Medicine. Food and Nutrition Board. Op. cit., 8–11; and Suitor CW, Bailey LB. Dietary folate equivalents: interpretation and application. *J Am Diet Assoc.* 2000;100:88–94.

29 Mills JL. Fortification of foods with folic acid: how much is enough? *N Engl J Med.* 2000;342:1442–1445

30 Institute of Medicine. Food and Nutrition Board. Op. cit.

31 US Department of Health and Human Services. Op. cit.

32 Lewis CJ, Crane NT, Wilson DB, Yetley EA. Estimated folate intakes: data updated to reflect food fortification, increased bioavailability, and dietary supplement use. *Am J Clin Nutr.* 1999;70:198–207.

33 Institute of Medicine. Food and Nutrition Board. Op. cit., 260–264; and Jacques PF, Sselhub J, Bostom AG, et al. The effect of folic acid fortification on plasma folate and total homocysteine concentrations. *N Engl J Med.* 1999;340:1449–1454.

34 James SJ, Pogribna M, Pogribny IP, et al. Abnormal folate metabolism and mutation in the methyelenetetrahydrofolate reductase gene may be maternal risk factor for Down syndrome. *Am J Clin Nutr*. 1999;70:495–501.

35 Lewis CJ, et al. Op. cit.

36 Hurwitz A, Brady DA, Schaal SE, et al. Gastric acidity in older adults. *JAMA*. 1997;278: 659–662.

37 Institute of Medicine. Food and Nutrition Board. Op. cit.

38 Sauberlich HE. Pharmacology of vitamin C. *Ann Rev Nutr*. 1994;14:371.

39 Institute of Medicine. Food and Nutrition Board. *Dietary Reference Intakes for Vitamin C, Vitamin E, Selenium, and Carotenoids*. Washington, DC: National Academy Press; 2000.

40 Ibid.

41 Johnston CS, Retrum KR, Srilakshmi JC. Antihistamine effects and complications of supplemental vitamin C. *J Am Diet Assoc*. 1992;8:988–989.

42 Institute of Medicine. Food and Nutrition Board. Op. cit.

43 Halliwell B. Antioxidants: sense or speculation? *Nutr Today*. 1994;29:15–19.

44 Institute of Medicine. Food and Nutrition Board. Op. cit.

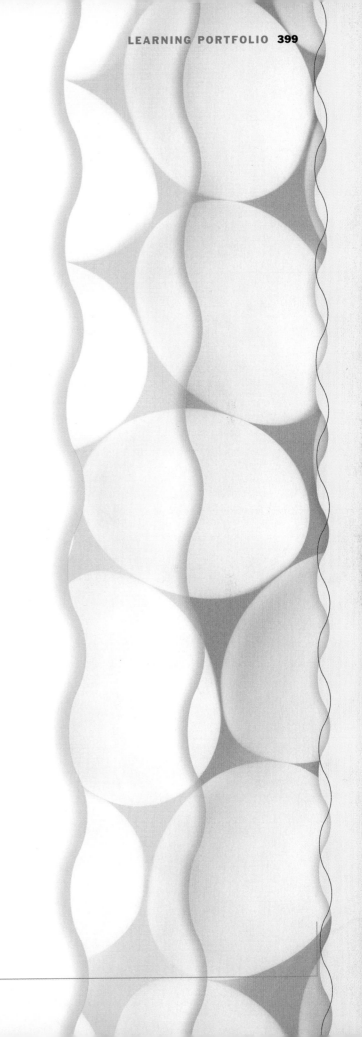

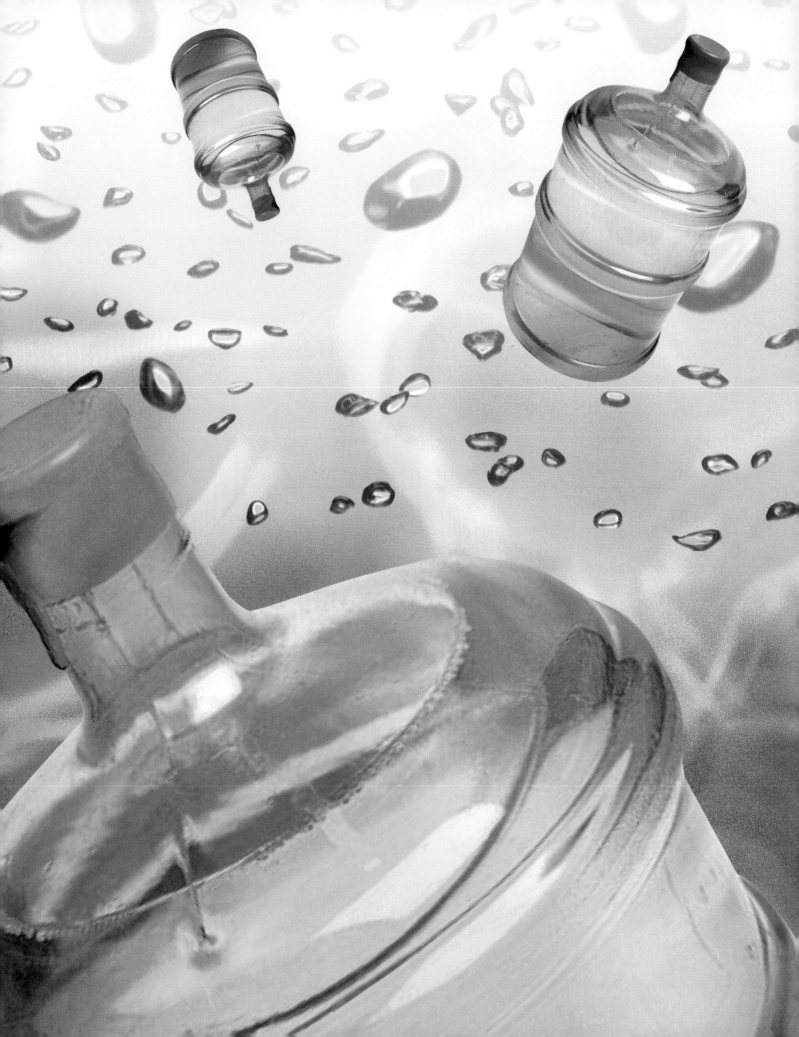

Chapter 11

Water and Major Minerals

FYI for your Information

This chapter's FYI boxes include practical information on the following topics:

• Tap, Filtered, or Bottled: Which Water Is Best

• Calcium Supplements: Are They Right for You?

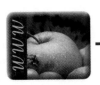

The web site for this book offers many useful tools and is a great source for additional nutrition information for both students and instructors. Visit the site at **nutrition.jbpub.com** for information on water and major minerals. You'll find exercises that explore the following topics:

• The Water in Your State

• The DASH Diet

• Calcium

• Making Hard Water Soft

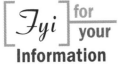
Key to Illustrations

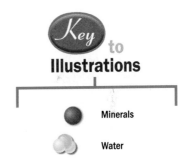

Minerals

Water

What About Bobbie?

Track the choices Bobbie is making with the EatRight Analysis software.

electrolyte [ih-LEK-tro-lite] Substances that dissociate into charged particles (ions) when dissolved in water or other solvents and thus become capable of conducting an electrical current. The terms *electrolyte* and *ion* often are used interchangeably.

hydrogen bond Noncovalent bond between hydrogen and an atom, usually oxygen, in another molecule.

heat capacity The amount of energy required to raise the temperature of a substance 1°C.

You take a coast-to-coast flight with your father and your brother. You watch as your father drinks water frequently throughout the flight, while your brother alternates between Coke and beer. When you arrive at your destination, your brother complains of feeling utterly exhausted. In contrast, your father is lively and ready for a "night on the town!" How do you explain this?

First, it's important to know that the familiar airline beverage cart is not just a kind gesture by the airline; regular fluid intake on flights is necessary! Although you are unaware of it, water evaporates from the skin at an accelerated rate in the low-humidity, high-altitude, pressurized cabin of an airplane. So, drinking fluids during the flight helps prevent dehydration. But, you must choose the fluids carefully. Alcoholic and caffeinated beverages are diuretics. This means that they increase fluid loss as urine, and therefore do not replace fluid losses as effectively as water, juice, and caffeine-free beverages.

Your brother's lack of energy may be a symptom of mild dehydration. Although he has been drinking fluids, the diuretic effect of alcohol and caffeine limits replacement of fluid. Dad, however, had the right idea—plenty of water along the way—and he's ready for action!

This chapter focuses first on water, the most essential nutrient; then it turns to the minerals sodium, potassium, and chloride, which the body needs to maintain normal fluid balance; and finally, it discusses other major minerals, along with their functions and food sources.

Water: The Essential Ingredient for Life

Water in your body contains numerous dissolved minerals, called **electrolytes**, that are kept in constant balance. To live, each cell must have just the right mix of water and electrolytes. Although intracellular and extracellular fluids have different mixes, the proportions in each must stay within a narrow range. Despite a continuous flow of molecules between intracellular fluid, extracellular fluid, and the outside environment, the body maintains its electrolyte balances through the intake and excretion of water and the movement of ions.

Humans can survive for weeks without food, but can live only a few days without water. The body has no capacity to store "spare" water, so it must quickly replace lost fluid. Overall, water makes up between 50 and 75 percent of your weight. (See **Figure 11.1**.) Leaner people have proportionately more water, because muscle tissue is nearly three-fourths water by weight, while adipose tissue is only about 10 percent water.

The one bit of chemistry that almost everyone can rattle off is the chemical formula for water: H_2O. Water is such a simple molecule (see **Figure 11.2**) that people often do not appreciate its extraordinary physical and chemical properties. Water's strong surface tension, high heat capacity, and ability to dissolve many substances result from **hydrogen bonds** between a hydrogen atom of one water molecule and the oxygen atom of another water molecule.

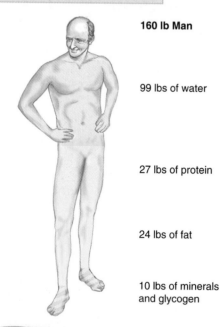

An adult male is approximately 62% water, 17% protein, 15% fat, and 6% minerals and glycogen

160 lb Man

99 lbs of water

27 lbs of protein

24 lbs of fat

10 lbs of minerals and glycogen

Figure 11.1 **Body composition.** The main constituent of the body is water. Adult males have more lean tissue and less fat than adult females.

Functions of Water

Water performs a wide variety of tasks in the body (see **Figure 11.3**). Water is the highway that moves nutrients and wastes between cells and organs. In the intestines, water solubilizes and moves nutrients to your cells and tissues, and it also carries waste out of your body in urine. What about nutrients and wastes that are not water soluble? Your body either modifies them chemically so they dissolve in water or packages them with proteins (e.g., lipoproteins). Your body's watery fluids, such as the bloodstream, can easily transport these protein packages throughout the body.

Heat Capacity

The **heat capacity** of a substance is the amount of energy required to raise its temperature 1°C. Raising the temperature of a substance with a high heat capacity requires more energy than raising the temperature of a substance with a low one. Water, for instance, has about three times the heat capacity of iron. Warming or cooling a substance with a high heat capacity requires a relatively large amount of energy. You may have noticed this property when heating items in a microwave oven. Watery foods like soup take much longer to heat than foods that contain little water, such as pizza and butter. Because of water's high heat capacity, it takes a lot of heat to change the temperature of the body; body water dampens the effects of extreme environmental temperatures on conditions in cells.

Cooling Ability

A rise in body temperature, whether due to exercise, environmental conditions, or illness, triggers the body's cooling system. If you get too warm, blood vessels dilate and you begin to sweat. The perspiration evaporates on the skin, thereby cooling your body. Moisture readily evaporates in dry air, so perspiring is most effective for cooling when the humidity is low. When the humidity is high, such as in humid, tropical environments, sweat does not evaporate readily so even profuse sweating may not cool the body effectively.

Participation in Metabolism

Nearly all the chemical reactions of metabolism involve water. Water is the solvent for many biologically essential molecules (e.g., glucose, vitamins, minerals, and amino acids), and it is a product or reactant in many biochemical reactions.

pH Balance

Water is also an essential component of the body's mechanisms to maintain pH (acid-base) balance in the narrow range necessary for life. One of the major buffer systems involves carbonic acid and bicarbonate. Carbonic acid forms when dissolved carbon dioxide reacts with water ($CO_2 + H_2O \rightarrow H_2CO_3$). Carbonic acid can then dissociate to form H^+ and HCO_3^- (bicarbonate). The resulting H^+ helps increase acidity, lowering pH.

Body Fluids

Water is the major component of all body fluids. These fluids also serve essential mechanical functions such as shock absorption, lubrication, cleansing, and protection. For example, amniotic fluid provides a gentle cushion that protects the fetus, synovial fluid allows joints to move smoothly, tears lubricate and cleanse the eyes, and saliva moistens food and makes swallowing possible.

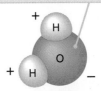

Water is a polar molecule. Although its net charge is zero, oxygen's strong attraction of the hydrogens' electrons makes it positive at one end and negative at the other

The more positive end of each water molecule is attracted to the more negative end of another – these weak attractions are called hydrogen bonds

The millions of weak hydrogen bonds between water molecules are strong enough to support this water strider

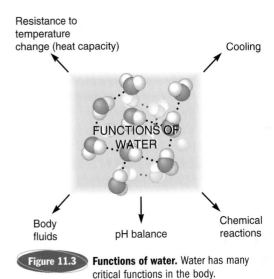

Figure 11.2 **Water—a simple, yet powerful, molecule.** Water has a strong surface tension and high heat capacity. Because dissolved molecules are more likely to come together and react with one another, water's ability to dissolve substances makes chemical reactions more efficient.

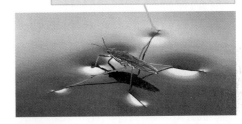

Resistance to temperature change (heat capacity)

Cooling

FUNCTIONS OF WATER

Body fluids

pH balance

Chemical reactions

Figure 11.3 **Functions of water.** Water has many critical functions in the body.

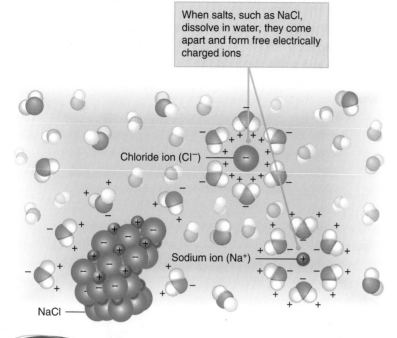

When salts, such as NaCl, dissolve in water, they come apart and form free electrically charged ions

Chloride ion (Cl⁻)

Sodium ion (Na⁺)

NaCl

Figure 11.4 **Dissolving salt in water.** When dissolving salt, the oxygen atoms of the water molecules are attracted to the negatively charged chloride ions. Water's hydrogen atoms are attracted to the positively charged sodium ions.

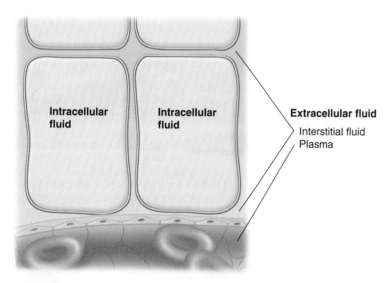

Intracellular fluid

Intracellular fluid

Extracellular fluid
Interstitial fluid
Plasma

Figure 11.5 **Intracellular and extracellular fluid.** Extracellular fluids and their solutes (except for proteins) move across capillary membranes easily. Plasma (the fluid portion of the blood) has a higher concentration of proteins than interstitial fluid. Excluding protein, their compositions are roughly the same.

Electrolytes and Water: A Delicate Equilibrium

Your body precisely controls and balances the concentration of electrolytes dissolved in its watery fluids. When **salts**, such as sodium chloride, dissolve in water (see **Figure 11.4**) they come apart and form free **ions**, which are positively (e.g., Na⁺) and negatively (e.g., Cl⁻) charged particles. In an electrolyte solution the number of positive charges always equals the number of negative charges. The main positively charged ions (**cations**) in the body are sodium and potassium, and the main negatively charged ions (**anions**) are chloride and phosphate.

There are two major fluid compartments in the body. About two-thirds of body water is in intracellular fluid and one-third is in extracellular fluid. The major components of extracellular fluid are interstitial fluid (the fluid between cells) and blood **plasma** (the fluid portion of blood). (See **Figure 11.5**.)

Sodium is the main cation in extracellular fluid, whereas potassium is the predominant cation of intracellular fluid. To maintain the balance of sodium and potassium, all cell membranes incorporate **sodium-potassium pumps (Figure 11.6)** that actively pump sodium out of the cell while allowing potassium back in. If solutes are more concentrated on one side of a **semipermeable membrane** (through which water, but not **solutes**, can pass easily), water flows to the side of higher concentration until the concentrations on both sides are the same. This movement is called **osmosis**; **osmotic pressure** is the force that causes water to flow across a membrane to the side with a higher concentration of ions (**Figure 11.7**).

Key Concepts: *Water is the most essential nutrient; we can survive much longer without food than without water. Water's functions in the body include temperature regulation, metabolism, acid-base regulation, lubrication, and protection. The balance of body fluids and the amount of electrolytes dissolved in the body's water are controlled precisely. Potassium is the main intracellular cation, and sodium is the main extracellular cation.*

salts Compounds that result from the replacement of the hydrogen of an acid with a metal or a group that acts like a metal.

ion An atom or group of atoms with an electrical charge resulting from the loss or gain of one or more electrons.

cation Ion that carries a positive charge

anion Ion that carries a negative charge.

plasma The fluid portion of the blood that contains blood cells and other components.

sodium-potassium pump Mechanism that pumps sodium ions out of a cell, allowing potassium ions to enter the cell.

semipermeable membrane Membrane that allows passage of some substances but blocks others.

solute A substance that is dissolved in a solvent.

osmosis The movement of a solvent, such as water, through a semipermeable membrane from the low-solute to the high-solute solution until the concentrations on both sides of the membrane are equal.

osmotic pressure The pressure exerted on a semipermeable membrane by a solvent, usually water, moving from the side of low-solute to the side of high-solute concentration.

Key

Na⁺ Sodium

K⁺ Potassium

P Phosphate molecule

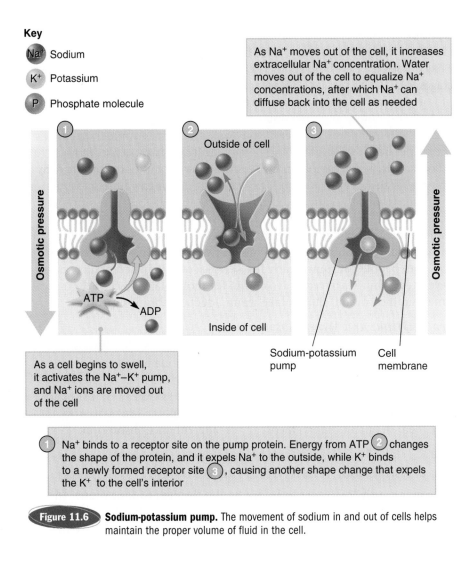

As Na⁺ moves out of the cell, it increases extracellular Na⁺ concentration. Water moves out of the cell to equalize Na⁺ concentrations, after which Na⁺ can diffuse back into the cell as needed

Outside of cell

Inside of cell

Sodium-potassium pump

Cell membrane

As a cell begins to swell, it activates the Na⁺–K⁺ pump, and Na⁺ ions are moved out of the cell

① Na⁺ binds to a receptor site on the pump protein. Energy from ATP ② changes the shape of the protein, and it expels Na⁺ to the outside, while K⁺ binds to a newly formed receptor site ③, causing another shape change that expels the K⁺ to the cell's interior

Figure 11.6 **Sodium-potassium pump.** The movement of sodium in and out of cells helps maintain the proper volume of fluid in the cell.

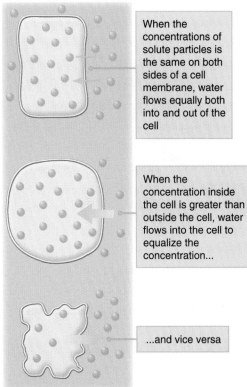

When the concentrations of solute particles is the same on both sides of a cell membrane, water flows equally both into and out of the cell

When the concentration inside the cell is greater than outside the cell, water flows into the cell to equalize the concentration...

...and vice versa

Figure 11.7 **Osmosis and osmotic pressure.** Relatively small changes in the concentration of extracellular solutes can result in large osmotic pressures across the cell membrane.

Intake Recommendations: How Much Water Is Enough?

There is no single answer to this question. Each individual needs a different amount of water depending on body size and composition, activity level, and the temperature and humidity of the environment. An "average" adult who expends 2,400 kilocalories daily loses approximately 2.4 liters (about 10 cups) of water each day. Because we cannot store water, the average adult needs to replace at least 2.4 liters of water a day. Although there is no RDA for water, the Food and Nutrition Board recommends a fluid intake for adults of 1.0 milliliters to 1.5 milliliters per kilocalories expended.[1] Athletes and very active people need much more than this, especially if they work and train in warm, humid climates.

Beverages, foods, and water produced by metabolic reactions supply the water that the body needs (remember that the electron transport chain produces water along with ATP). **Figure 11.8** shows the water content of various foods. You may have heard that you should drink 8 to 10 glasses of water every day. Let's take a closer look at this recommendation.

With an energy expenditure of 2,000 kilocalories per day, the body would need 2,000 milliliters to 3,000 milliliters of water. Metabolism

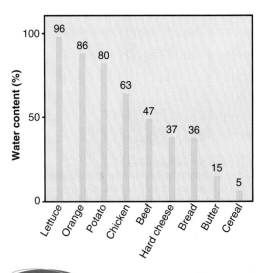

Figure 11.8 **Water content of various foods.**

typically provides about 400 milliliters to 500 milliliters, so the remainder (1,500 ml to 2,500 ml) must come from beverages and foods. You could expect foods to contribute about 1,000 milliliters of water, which leaves beverages to make up the rest. So, what is the milliliter equivalent of 8 glasses of water? If each glass is 8 fluid ounces (~ 240 ml), then 8 glasses would be 1,920 milliliters, and this combined with just metabolic water provides 2,320–2,420 milliliters. So even if you don't drink the recommended 8 glasses per day, it's not difficult to obtain adequate water for the body.

Some experts suggest that many Americans suffer mild but chronic dehydration because they drink too little water and too many diuretic-containing fluids (especially caffeinated and alcoholic beverages).[2] A recent survey does not bear this out, however. It shows that the average American consumes nearly 8 servings of a combination of water, juice, milk, and soda without caffeine.[3] This would provide nearly 2,000 milliliters of fluid. In addition, people consume nearly five servings of caffeinated or alcoholic beverages. While there certainly is room for more plain water in the typical American diet, overall fluid intake seems adequate for most people.

Think About It **1**

Sports Drinks and Water Absorption

Drinking plenty of plain water and eating a healthful diet easily replaces the fluid and electrolytes a person loses during moderate exercise in pleasant weather. But if you are involved in endurance activities or strenuous exercise in hot weather, consider using sports drinks instead of just plain water. The glucose and mineral content of good sports drinks improve the taste, help maintain blood glucose levels, and enhance absorption.[4] (See Chapter 13, "Sports Nutrition.")

Water Excretion: Where Does the Water Go?

We continuously lose water from our bodies through various routes. In the lungs, water evaporates and exits in exhaled air. Water also departs through the skin by evaporation and perspiration. In the GI tract, feces carry water out of the body. The kidneys excrete water in urine. **Figure 11.9** summarizes sources and amounts of fluid output and shows how these balance with fluid intake.

Depending on the amount of water, protein, and sodium consumed, the body loses about 1 to 2 liters of water each day through urine. During exercise, urine production declines and fluid losses from the skin and lungs increase. **Insensible water loss**—the continuous evaporation of water from the lungs and skin—typically accounts for about one-quarter to one-half of daily fluid loss. High altitude, low humidity, and high temperatures increase these losses. During a coast-to-coast airplane flight, the low cabin humidity can cause fluid losses of 4 to 6 cups (about 1,000 ml to 1,500 ml)![5]

Insensible losses rise, sometimes dramatically, during illness. Fever, coughing, rapid breathing, and watery nasal secretions all significantly increase water loss. This is one of the reasons that doctors recommend increasing your fluid intake when you are ill.

Water plays a critical role in the elimination of wastes. Urea, a breakdown product of protein metabolism, is a major component of urine. If we overconsume protein and salt (a common situation with the typical American diet), the kidneys have to work harder to eliminate excess urea and sodium from the body. This task requires water, so unless kidney function is impaired, the more protein and sodium you consume, the more fluid you need to consume and the more urine you are likely to produce.

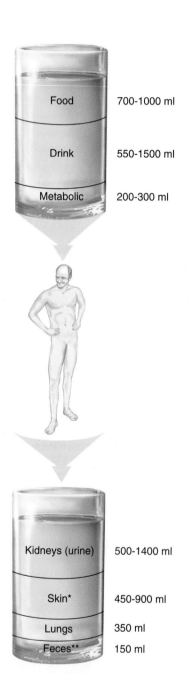

Food	700-1000 ml
Drink	550-1500 ml
Metabolic	200-300 ml

Kidneys (urine)	500-1400 ml
Skin*	450-900 ml
Lungs	350 ml
Feces**	150 ml

* (Insensible and perspiration)
The volume of perspiration is normally about 100 ml per day. In very hot weather or during heavy exercise, a person may lose 10 to 20 times this amount (1 to 2 liters) per hour.

**People with severe diarrhea can lose several liters of water per day in feces.

Figure 11.9 **Typical daily water intake and output.**

Key Concepts: A typical adult needs 1.0 milliliter to 1.5 milliliters of fluid per kilo-calorie expended. Water intake comes from a combination of foods, fluids, and water produced in normal metabolism. The main method of water excretion is in urine. In addition, fluid is lost through the skin and lungs, and with feces. Losses are higher when a person perspires heavily or is ill. Water is critical in eliminating the body's waste products.

Water Balance

Our bodies maintain water balance by mechanisms that control water intake (e.g., thirst) and water excretion. Because of water's critical roles, the body works not only to balance fluid between compartments, but to closely regulate total body water.

Regulation of Fluid Excretion

Our kidneys adjust the amount and concentration of urine in response to the body's hydration status. The kidneys can excrete a small volume of concentrated urine or a large volume of dilute urine while maintaining a relatively constant excretion of solutes such as sodium and potassium. This ability to regulate water excretion without major changes in solute excretion is an important survival mechanism, especially when water is in short supply.

When water intake is low, the kidneys conserve water. While continuing to excrete solutes, they reabsorb water, thus decreasing urine volume and concentrating the urine. When the body has an excess of water, the kidneys form and excrete a large volume of dilute urine.

How do the kidneys know when to conserve water? **Osmoreceptors**, special cells in the hypothalamus of the brain, are exquisitely sensitive to very small increases in extracellular sodium concentration and thus sense the body's need for water. If the sodium concentration rises, these receptors signal the pituitary gland to release **antidiuretic hormone (ADH)**. ADH decreases water loss by causing the kidneys to reabsorb water rather than excrete it in the urine (**Figure 11.10**).

In minute concentrations, ADH signals the kidney to conserve water. In higher concentrations ADH is a potent **vasoconstrictor**, which is why it also is called **vasopressin**. Although ADH is far less sensitive to blood volume than to plasma **osmolarity** (concentration of electrolytes), a severe loss of blood also triggers its release. A loss of 15 to 25 percent of blood volume will cause up to a 50-fold increase in ADH levels. Nausea is a potent trigger. ADH levels increase 100-fold after vomiting. Some drugs (e.g., nicotine and morphine) stimulate the release of ADH, but others (e.g., alcohol and caffeine) inhibit it.[6]

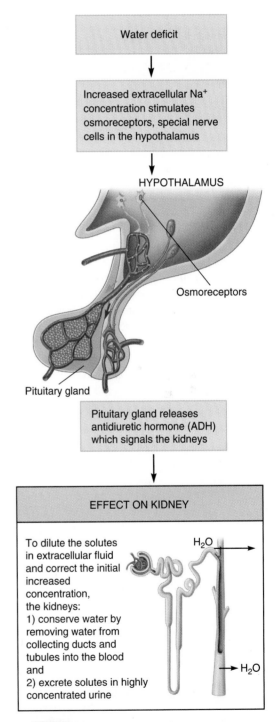

Figure 11.10 **Antidiuretic hormone regulates excretion.** In response to a water deficit, the osmoreceptor-ADH feedback system regulates solute concentrations in extracellular fluid.

insensible water loss The continual loss of body water by evaporation from the respiratory tract and diffusion through the skin.

osmoreceptors Neurons in the hypothalamus that detect changes in the fluid concentration in blood and regulate the release of antidiuretic hormone.

antidiuretic hormone (ADH) A peptide hormone secreted by the pituitary gland, it increases blood pressure and prevents fluid excretion by the kidneys. Also called vasopressin.

vasoconstrictor A substance that causes blood vessels to constrict.

vasopressin See antidiuretic hormone.

osmolarity The concentration of dissolved particles (e.g., electrolytes) in a solution expressed per unit of volume.

renin An enzyme, produced by the kidney, that affects blood pressure by catalyzing the conversion of angiotensinogen to angiotensin I.

angiotensin I [an-jee-oh-TEN-sin one] A 10-amino-acid peptide that is a precursor of angiotensin II.

angiotensinogen A circulating protein produced by the liver from which angiotensin I is cleaved by the action of renin.

angiotensin II In the lungs, the 8-amino-acid peptide angiotensin II is formed from angiotensin I. Angiotensin II is a powerful vasoconstrictor that rapidly raises blood pressure.

Quick Bites

How do desert-dwelling animals avoid dehydration?

Some desert animals can concentrate their urine to nearly 100 times the maximum concentration of human urine. This allows such animals to survive on water obtained from food and their own metabolic reactions. Aquatic animals, on the other hand, minimally concentrate their urine. Beavers concentrate their urine to only about half that of humans.

Regulation of Blood Volume and Pressure

The kidneys themselves have sensors that detect falling blood pressure. (See **Figure 11.11**.) In response, the kidneys release **renin**, an enzyme that splits off a small protein, **angiotensin I**, from the blood protein **angiotensinogen**. Within seconds, enzymes in the small blood vessels of the lungs convert nearly all angiotensin I to **angiotensin II**. While angiotensin II is a powerful vasoconstrictor, it also acts directly on the kidneys to decrease excretion of sodium and water. In addition, this protein causes the release

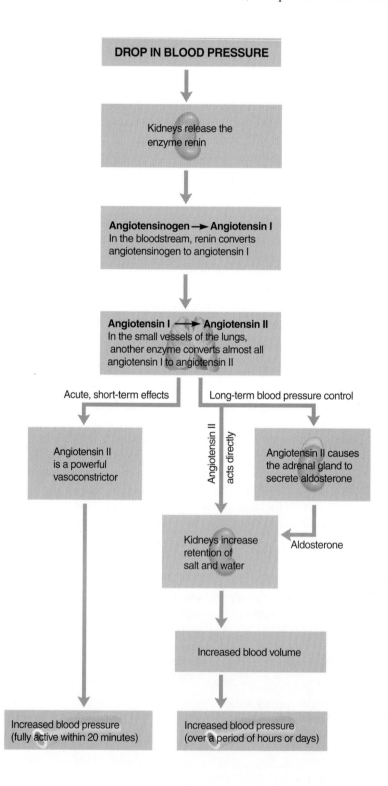

Figure 11.11 **Regulating blood volume and pressure.** Within minutes after severe hemorrhage, the renin-angiotensin-vasoconstrictor mechanism is powerful enough to cause a lifesaving rise in blood pressure. Malfunctions in the long-term blood pressure control mechanism can cause persistently high blood pressure (hypertension).

of **aldosterone**, a hormone from the adrenal glands. Aldosterone also causes the kidneys to retain sodium, and since water follows sodium, water retention increases as well. All of these processes work to restore blood pressure and volume.

The ability of angiotensin II to act as a vasoconstrictor and increase blood pressure is a life-saving measure. This acute short-term action helps compensate for a severe loss of blood, such as occurs during a hemorrhage. Angiotensin II's effect on the kidney increases extracellular fluid volume and arterial blood pressure over a period of hours or days. Although slower, this long-term action is more powerful than acute vasoconstriction in returning blood pressure to normal.

Perhaps the most important role of the renin-angiotensin system is its response to dietary sodium. It allows a person to consume either very small or very large amounts of sodium without causing major changes in extracellular fluid volume or blood pressure. Since water follows sodium, increased sodium intake increases extracellular fluid volume and blood pressure. This reduces the secretion of renin and production of angiotensin, leading to decreased retention of sodium and water by the kidneys. The resulting excretion of water and sodium returns extracellular volume and blood pressure to normal. A low sodium intake triggers the opposite effects.

Thirst

While taste, availability, cultural patterns, and personal habits affect the amount of fluids we consume, thirst is our most important stimulus for drinking. Why do we become thirsty? The four major stimuli for thirst are

1. increased osmolarity of the fluid surrounding the osmoreceptors in the hypothalamus,

2. reduced blood volume and blood pressure,

3. increased angiotensin II, and

4. dryness of the mouth and mucous membranes lining the esophagus.[7]

Drinking fluids temporarily alleviates thirst, so we do not drink to the point of overhydration and dilution of body fluids. Remarkably, studies show that animals drink almost precisely the amount of water necessary to return their blood volume and electrolyte concentrations to normal.[8]

Nevertheless, thirst is not always a reliable guide to avoiding dehydration. Hot weather or heavy exercise can cause fluid losses of up to 1 to 2 liters per hour[9] and deplete our fluids before we feel thirsty. After you drink water, your body can take 30 to 60 minutes to absorb and distribute it throughout the body. For example, imagine you are roller blading in the hot sun and after an hour you pause momentarily to quench your thirst with a $1/_2$-liter bottle of water. That's not enough—you still have a deficit of $1/_2$ to $1 \, 1/_2$ liters of water, and you'll continue to lose water while your body absorbs and distributes the water you just drank. To avoid dehydration in hot weather or when exercising, you need to drink fluids early and often.

Because heavy activity easily can cause dehydration, athletes also must be careful to drink adequate amounts of fluid. Athletic performance improves if athletes anticipate their water needs well before they begin to feel thirst. (See Chapter 13, "Sports Nutrition," for more on water recommendations for athletes.)

aldosterone [al-DOS-ter-own] A steroid hormone secreted from the adrenal glands that acts on the kidneys to regulate electrolyte and water balance. It raises blood pressure by promoting retention of sodium (and thus water) and excretion of potassium.

Quick Bites

Water, Water Everywhere and Not a Drop to Drink!

When shipwrecked sailors drink seawater, they quickly become severely dehydrated. This is because the concentration of salt in seawater is about double the maximum concentration of salt in urine. Thus, it takes 2 liters of urine to rid the body of the solutes ingested by drinking 1 liter of seawater.

Think About It 2

Older people and infants are particularly vulnerable to dehydration. The sensitivity of the thirst response declines with age, putting the elderly at high risk. Infants need to take in a large amount of water relative to their size because a large proportion of their body weight is water. Breast milk or infant formula provides an appropriate amount of fluid for infants. People who care for children and elders must remember to give them fluids often.

Water Reabsorption in the Gastrointestinal Tract

The operation of the gastrointestinal tract requires many liters of fluid each day. If all the secretions from the salivary glands, stomach, small intestine, pancreas, and gallbladder passed through the GI tract and out in the feces, we would dehydrate very rapidly! Fortunately, the small and large intestines reabsorb almost all of the water that enters them, so little water actually is lost in feces.

Key Concepts: *The body has mechanisms that balance water among compartments and regulate total body water. Antidiuretic hormone (ADH) stimulates water reabsorption in the kidneys, while aldosterone stimulates the kidneys to reabsorb sodium. Thirst is not a reliable indicator to avoid dehydration when fluid losses are high, such as during hot weather or heavy exercise.*

Quick Bites

Why do salty foods make you thirsty?

The thirst mechanism is highly sensitive to extra-cellular sodium concentration. Even a tiny rise in sodium crosses the thirst threshold and triggers the desire to drink.

Fyi Tap, Filtered, or Bottled: Which Water Is Best?

FOR YOUR INFORMATION

Everywhere you look, it seems like more and more people are carrying and sipping on bottles of water. Theme parks even sell shoulder holsters for you to carry your bottle around with you. What's with the water craze? And what's wrong with the good old water fountain?

During the mid to late 1980s, the growth in use of bottled water began. Initially, bottled mineral waters, like Perrier, were associated with wealth and glamour. But like many trends adopted by the wealthy (white bread, for instance), bottled water soon became desirable to a wider range of people. It is now estimated that Americans drink 2.5 billion gallons of bottled water each year![1] In 1997 U.S. sales of fruit beverages grew 2.5 percent, beer 0.8 percent, and soft drinks 3.3 percent, while bottled water sales grew 9.6 percent.[2] Even the major soft drink companies Coca-Cola and Pepsico have gotten into the act, and now sell their own brands of bottled water.

There are probably several factors fueling the growth of the bottled-water industry.

Baby boomers are seeking natural, low-calorie beverages, and fitness consciousness has re-emphasized the importance of hydration. Media reports of contamination of tap water in major metropolitan areas spark concerns about the safety and quality of tap water. Most Americans choose bottled water for what they think is *not* in it, rather than for what it contains.

From a nutritional perspective, it's important to drink plenty of fluids, and water is one of the best ways to replace lost fluids. And so, at the simplest level, the source of water doesn't really matter. Standards for municipal water systems are enforced by the Environmental Protection Agency (EPA), which requires regular testing and monitoring. Tap water can be considered a safe, clean source of water. Many municipal water systems add fluoride to tap water, an important weapon in the prevention of tooth decay. However, home-installed filtration systems for removing chlorine may also remove added fluoride, and most bottled waters do not contain fluoride.

Some people don't like the taste of their local water supply, and don't want to bother with maintaining a filtration system. In this case, or if you want your water "to go," bottled water may be the choice. The bottled-water industry offers

- high-volume, returnable containers from suppliers who stock the "water coolers" for offices or supermarkets;
- the familiar brands (e.g., Evian, Zephyrhills, Dannon, Nala) that are sold as alternatives to soft drink; and
- bottled-water in vending machines.

The bottled-water industry is regulated by the Food and Drug Administration (FDA) which, in 1995, published Standards of Identity for bottled water, set maximum allowable standards for contaminants, and established Current Good Manufacturing Practices (CGMP) for bottling plants. Keep in mind that FDA regulates bottled waters that are sold interstate, and not those sold only in a particular area or state. Individual states may have their own quality standards for locally distributed waters.

Substances That Affect Fluid Balance

Alcohol

Anyone who has experience with alcohol probably realizes that it is a diuretic—a drug that increases fluid loss through increased urination. Alcohol increases fluid loss by suppressing ADH production, and excessive alcohol consumption can cause dehydration. Symptoms of mild to moderate dehydration include thirst, weakness, dryness of mucous membranes, dizziness, and lightheadedness—all common effects of a hangover. Drinking a few glasses of water before bed often can prevent some of the morning regret. It is also an excellent idea for people who drink alcohol to combine it with a meal that includes water. Better yet, keep alcohol consumption low—less than one drink per day for women and fewer than two for men.

Caffeine

Commonly known as a stimulant, caffeine also is a strong diuretic. Like alcohol, it inhibits ADH activity. A study of 12 healthy volunteers demonstrates the power of caffeine's dehydrating effects. The subjects abstained from caffeine for five days, then drank mineral water as their only fluid for one day. On the following day they drank the same amount of fluid, but substituted six cups of coffee for some of the mineral water.

Look beyond the terms like *artesian, mineral, spring,* or *purified* (see Table A). The labels on most bottled water list the source of the water. Some consumers may be surprised to find that their favorite brand of water is really from a municipal source, not an underground spring! Nutrition Facts labels are required if the manufacturer makes a claim (e.g., sodium-free) or adds minerals. These labels often do not show the natural mineral content of the water, which is really the only other nutritional aspect that could be expected.

Once again, the choice is up to the consumer—there is no clearly best choice of water. Cost, taste, convenience, and safety are all issues to consider.

[1] Tip of the Day! Water to tap. American Dietetic Association Web site: www.eatright.org/erm/erm 070798.html. Accessed 7/29/99.

[2] BottledWaterWeb: www.bottledwaterweb.com/indus.html; Accessed 8/1/99.

Table A **Definitions of Bottled Water Terms**

- *Mineral water* must contain at least 250 parts per million (ppm) of dissolved minerals and come from a geologically and physically protected underground water source.
- *Purified water* is tap or ground water that has been treated by distillation, deionization, or reverse osmosis. This may be labeled "distilled water" if produced by steam distillation and condensation.
- *Spring water* comes from an underground formation from which water flows naturally to the surface; it is collected either at the spring or from a bore hole to the underground formation.
- *Artesian water* comes from tapping a confined underground aquifer that is below the natural water table. Generally the artesian well is located in a depression where the water table of the surrounding hills is higher. The "head" of pressure from the water table forces the water up through the tap line.
- *Ground water* comes from a subsurface saturated zone and is not under the direct influence of surface water.
- *Well water* comes from a drilled hole that taps the water of an aquifer, and is pumped to the surface.

Source: Bottled Water Industry Facts. www.bottledwaterweb.com/indus.html; Accessed 8/1/99; and from FDA regulations 21CFR165.110. frwebgate5.access.gpo.gov/cgibin/...docID=374908008+2+2+0&WAISaction=retrive. Accessed 8/1/99.

Excess water intake and diuretics such as alcohol and caffeine decrease the secretion of antidiuretic hormone (ADH)

↓

A fall in ADH levels signals the kidney to concentrate solutes in extracellular fluid by excreting water

↓

EFFECT ON KIDNEY

To concentrate solutes in extracellular fluid and correct the initial decreased concentration, the kidneys:

1) decrease permeability so collecting ducts and tubules retain water for excretion
2) excrete large volumes of dilute urine

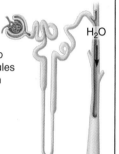

H_2O

Figure 11.12 **Effects of decreased ADH level on kidney output.** Alcohol and caffeine increase water excretion by slowing the release of antidiuretic hormone (ADH).

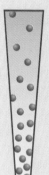

% Body weight loss

0
1 Thirst
2 Increased thirst, loss of appetite, discomfort
3 Impatience, decreased blood volume
4 Nausea, slowing of physical work
5 Difficulty concentrating, apathy, tingling extremities
6 Increasing body temperature, pulse and respiration rate
7 Stumbling, headache
8 Dizziness, labored breathing
9 Weakness, mental confusion
10 Muscle spasms, indistinct speech
11 Kidney failure, poor circulation due to decreased blood volume

Figure 11.13 **Effects of progressive dehydration.**

During the coffee-drinking day, urine output exceeded fluid intake and the subjects lost, on average, 2.7 percent of their body water. The subjects were not aware that they were dehydrated and only 2 of the 12 felt thirsty.[10] **Figure 11.12** shows the effects of decreased ADH on the amount of urine the kidneys process.

Many Americans rely primarily on caffeinated beverages for their daily fluid intake. A few cups of coffee in the morning, a caffeinated soda with lunch, another in the afternoon, and maybe a glass of wine or a beer with dinner—this pattern is typical for many busy Americans. Although some suggest that a fondness for caffeinated beverages can cause chronic mild dehydration, Americans seem to consume a sufficient quantity and variety of beverages to maintain fluid balance.[11]

Diuretic Medications

Diuretics are some of the most common medications. They can help lower blood pressure, decrease high intracranial pressure, or reduce excess pressure in the eye. On the other hand, diuretics can significantly disrupt sodium and potassium balance. Typically, a physician monitors the blood electrolyte levels of a patient taking diuretics. To prevent a low blood potassium level, patients on certain diuretics may require potassium supplementation.

Dehydration

Dehydration, or too little water, is a major killer worldwide—infants and the frail elderly are especially vulnerable. (See **Figure 11.13**.) Gastrointestinal infections are primarily responsible. These infections cause diarrhea and prolonged vomiting, leading to excessive water loss. Unless treated rapidly, a person who loses an amount of water equal to 20 percent of body weight is likely to become comatose and die. Burns also can cause deadly dehydration. Extensively damaged skin cannot protect the body and prevent excessive fluid loss.

Dehydration diminishes physical and mental performance. Early signs of dehydration include fatigue, dry mouth, headache, and dark urine with a strong odor. Change in urine color reflects the body's attempt to conserve water by increasing water reabsorption in the kidney. You probably have noticed that your urine becomes darker when you haven't had much to drink, whereas your urine is almost colorless when you've had plenty to drink. Low fluid intake increases the risk of kidney stones, and some experts believe it also increases the risk of urinary tract, breast, and colon cancers.[12]

Water consumption, of course, is the primary treatment for dehydration. Oral-rehydration solutions also can be used; typically these consist of simple ingredients including clean water, sugar, and table salt. Oral rehydration may be sufficient for mild dehydration, but intravenous fluids and hospitalization may be necessary for moderate to severe dehydration. Diarrhea and prolonged vomiting, which cause heavy fluid and electrolyte losses, can be fatal unless the person is rapidly rehydrated with electrolyte solutions.

Water Intoxication

Overhydration is a much less common problem than dehydration, but does occur occasionally. In certain disorders, excessive secretion of ADH causes the kidney to reabsorb too much water, leading to overhydration and dilution of sodium in extracellular fluid. People with certain mental disorders have a compulsion to drink huge quantities of water, but their kidneys usually are able to keep up, since normal kidneys can excrete 15 to 20 liters of urine per day.

Key Concepts: Alcohol, caffeine, and diuretic medications increase urinary fluid losses. Chronic ingestion of these substances may contribute to dehydration. Dehydration occurs when fluid loss exceeds fluid intake; it is a potential consequence of gastrointestinal disease, burns, and heavy sweating. Treatment involves replacing fluids, along with electrolytes if the condition is severe. Water intoxication is rare; normal kidneys can excrete many liters of fluid each day.

Major Minerals

Unlike the nutrient molecules you have studied so far, minerals are inorganic elemental atoms or ions. Unlike carbohydrate, protein, and fat, minerals are not changed during digestion or when the body uses them. Unlike many vitamins, minerals are not destroyed by heat, light, or alkalinity. Calcium remains calcium, be it in seashells, milk, or bones. Iron remains iron, whether it is part of a cast-iron skillet or carried in the bloodstream as part of hemoglobin. This is true for all minerals.

Minerals play many essential roles in the body. Some minerals, such as magnesium, participate in the catalytic activity of enzymes. Others serve a structural function; for example, calcium and phosphorus are among the minerals that make our bones hard. Minerals are categorized as major or trace minerals, based on the amount needed in the diet and the amount of the mineral in the body. The body requires more than 100 milligrams per day of each **major mineral**, while the dietary need for each **trace mineral** is less than 100 milligrams daily. **Figure 11.14** lists the major and trace minerals and shows the relative amounts of each in the body. This classification of minerals is unrelated to the mineral's biological importance. For example, iron is a trace mineral but it plays a critical role in many major metabolic reactions. The trace minerals are discussed in Chapter 12.

Minerals in Foods

Although we often associate minerals with animal foods (e.g., calcium in dairy products, iron in meats), minerals are found throughout the groups that make up the Food Guide Pyramid. Generally speaking, animal foods are more reliable sources of minerals than plants are, because animal tissues contain minerals in the proportions that animal tissues need. Drinking water can sometimes be a significant source of several minerals such as sodium, magnesium, and fluoride. The specific sources of each major mineral are discussed later in the chapter.

Bioavailability of Minerals

A variety of factors affect the bioavailability (the amount available to the body) of minerals from foods. The body absorbs many minerals in proportion to its needs. For example, a calcium-deficient person more readily absorbs calcium than does a person with normal calcium levels. Overloading one mineral by taking supplements can hamper the absorption of other minerals. Minerals like calcium, iron, and magnesium (which all have similar chemical properties, including a 2+ charge) compete for absorption. Fiber content of food also can affect mineral bioavailability. High-fiber diets can reduce the absorption of iron, calcium, zinc, and magnesium. **Phytate** in grain fibers binds minerals, sequestering them and carrying them out of the intestine unabsorbed. **Oxalate**, found in spinach and rhubarb, binds calcium and prevents absorption of all but about 5 percent of the plant's calcium.

major minerals Major minerals are required in the diet and present in the body in large amounts compared to trace minerals.

trace minerals Minerals required in the diet and present in the body in very small quantities, less than 100 mg each.

phytate (phytic acid) A phosphorus-containing compound in the outer husks of cereal grains that binds with minerals and inhibits their absorption.

oxalate (oxalic acid) An organic acid in some leafy green vegetables, such as spinach, that binds to calcium to form calcium oxalate, an insoluble compound the body cannot absorb.

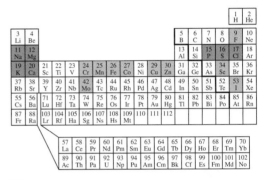

Key

■ Major minerals
■ Trace minerals

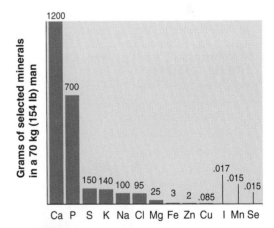

Figure 11.14 **Minerals in the human body.** Dietary minerals also are elements in the periodic table. Based on the amount of a mineral needed in the diet and the amount in the body, nutritionists categorize a mineral as major or trace. Other minerals are found in minute quantities in the body, and may or may not be essential nutrients.

Source: Groff JL and Gropper SS, *Advanced Nutrition and Human Metabolism*, 3rd ed., Belmont CA: Wadsworth/Thomson Learning, 2000 and Stipanuk MH, *Biochemical and Physiological Aspects of Human Nutrition*, Philadelphia: WB Saunders Co, 2000.

Key Concepts: Minerals are essential inorganic elements. Those that we need and store in larger amounts are called major minerals, and those we need in very small quantities are the trace minerals. A wide variety of foods contain minerals. Physiological needs, competition with minerals, and fiber content of food all affect mineral bioavailability.

Electrolytes	Extracellular* fluid concentration	Intracellular** fluid concentration
	meq/L	meq/L
Cations		
Sodium (Na^+)	140	13
Potassium (K^+)	5	140
Calcium (Ca^{2+})	5	Minimal
Magnesium (Mg^{2+})	2	7
Total	**151**	**160**
Anions		
Chloride (Cl^-)	104	3
Bicarbonate (HCO_3^-)	24	10
Sulfate (SO_4^{2-})	1	---
Phosphate (HPO_4^{2-})	2	107
Proteins	15	40
Organic anions	5	---
Total	**151**	**160**

* Values are for plasma. Interstitial fluid concentrations vary slightly (about 4 percent)

** Values are for cell water in muscle

Figure 11.15 **Cations and anions in intracellular and extracellular fluid.** Potassium, magnesium, phosphate, and proteins are the main solutes inside a cell. Sodium, chloride, and bicarbonate are the main solutes outside the cell.
Source: Oh MS, Uribarri J. Electrolytes, water, and acid-base balance. In: Shils ME, Olson JA, Shike M, Ross AC, eds. *Modern Nutrition in Health and Disease,* 9th ed. Philadelphia: Lippincott Williams & Wilkins, 1999:222, 105–139.

Quick Bites

Sacred Salt

The physiological need for salt played an important role in shaping human history. Population groups tended to congregate where salt can be found, and civilizations in Africa, India, the Middle East, and China developed around rich salt deposits. At times, salt was traded at a value twice that of gold.

Sodium

Many people do not realize that sodium (Na) is an essential nutrient. We know sodium best as a component of sodium chloride (table salt); and we have heard for years that we shouldn't eat too much salt. The *Dietary Guidelines* suggest that Americans "choose and prepare foods with less salt."[13] But, some sodium in the diet is essential for normal body function.

Functions of Sodium

Sodium is the major cation in extracellular fluid and a critical electrolyte in the regulation of body fluids. It acts in concert with potassium, the major cation in intracellular fluid, and chloride, the major anion in extracellular fluid, to maintain proper body water distribution and blood pressure. (See **Figure 11.15**.) Nerve transmission and muscle function require sodium. Sodium also helps control the body's acidity, and aids the absorption of some nutrients such as glucose.

Dietary Recommendations for Sodium

There is no RDA for sodium. Diets rarely are too low in sodium, and the body needs substantially less than the amount in a typical diet. Instead, the Food and Nutrition Board estimates that healthy adults require a minimum of 500 milligrams per day, an amount vastly exceeded by most people.[14] The American Heart Association recommends that individuals avoid taking in more than 2,400 milligrams of sodium per day, the level adopted by the FDA as the Daily Value for food labels. This amounts to about 1 teaspoon of table salt, or about 2 teaspoons of baking soda. Even when the body loses considerable sodium, for example when sweating heavily, dietary sources easily replenish it. In extreme cases, such as severe diarrhea, a balanced electrolyte solution is the best source of replacement sodium.

Sources of Sodium

A typical American diet contains between 3,000 milligrams and 6,000 milligrams of sodium. Of our total sodium intake, sodium added during food processing supplies about 75 percent, naturally occurring sodium in foods provides another 10 percent, and salt added during cooking and at the table contributes the remaining 15 percent. Table salt and soy sauce are high in sodium, as are foods in brine (e.g., pickles, olives, and sauerkraut). Other foods with significant levels of sodium include salty or smoked meats and fish, salted snack foods, bouillon cubes, bottled sauces, processed cheeses, and canned and instant soups. A diet based on Asian foods, which includes liberal amounts of soy sauce and monosodium glutamate (a flavor enhancer), may contain 12,000 milligrams to 16,000 milligrams of sodium per day. **Table 11.1** lists the sodium content of some common foods.

Your intestinal tract absorbs nearly all dietary sodium, which then travels throughout the body in the bloodstream. Your kidneys, those remarkable organs, retain the exact amount of sodium the body needs and excrete the excess sodium in the urine along with water.

Because excreting excess sodium wastes water, taking in too much sodium and not enough water can worsen dehydration. The old practice of giving athletes salt tablets before or after exercise is unnecessary and possibly harmful. On the other hand, radical sodium restriction is not a good idea, either. Even though most Americans consume too much sodium, severe sodium restriction can limit the availability of other essential nutrients like vitamin B$_6$, calcium, iron, and magnesium.[15]

Hyponatremia

Blood sodium concentration sometimes can drop too low, usually as a result of severe diarrhea, vomiting, or intense prolonged sweating. Consuming only water without food or other mineral sources also can depress blood sodium levels. The primary symptoms of low blood sodium, **hyponatremia**, resemble dehydration symptoms and the treatment is similar—replacement of fluid and minerals through liquids and foods or intravenous solutions if necessary. If severe hyponatremia is not treated, extracellular fluid moves into cells, causing them to swell. As brain cells swell and malfunction, the afflicted person can experience headache, confusion, seizures, or coma. Many illnesses, including cancer, kidney disease, and heart disease, can cause low blood sodium concentration. In these situations, treatment usually targets the underlying condition that caused the electrolyte imbalance.[16]

Hypernatremia

Rapid intake of large amounts of sodium (e.g., drinking seawater) can cause the retention of sodium and water in the blood. This causes **hypernatremia**, abnormally high concentration of sodium in the blood, and **hypervolemia**, an abnormal increase in blood volume. This results in edema (swelling) and a rise in blood pressure. A healthy person with normal kidneys and ample water intake rapidly excretes excess sodium, so hypernatremia usually is

hyponatremia Abnormally low sodium concentrations in the blood due to excessive excretion of sodium (by the kidney), prolonged vomiting, or diarrhea.

hypernatremia Abnormally high sodium concentrations in the blood due to increased kidney retention of sodium or rapid ingestion of large amounts of salt.

hypervolemia An abnormal increase in the circulating blood volume.

Table 11.1 **Sodium Content of Various Foods**

Food	Serving Size	Sodium (mg)
Dill pickle	1 large (4")	1730
Ham, cured	3 oz. (85 g)	1180
Biscuit from mix	1	540
Spaghetti sauce, jar	½ C	520
American cheese	1 oz.	400
Potato chips	1 oz.	170
Whole-wheat bread	1 slice	150
Two-percent milk	1 C (240 ml)	120
Roast pork	3 oz. (85 g)	50
Fresh tomato	1 medium	10
Baked potato	1 medium	8
Cucumber, fresh	1 large (8 ¼")	6

Source: US Department of Agriculture. Agricultural Research Service. 1999. USDA Nutrient Database for Standard Reference, Release 13. Nutrient Data Laboratory Home Page, http://www.nal.usda.gov/fnic/foodcomp. Accessed 7/26/00.

seen only in patients with congestive heart failure or kidney disease. Eating too much sodium over a long period of time can contribute to high blood pressure in some people (see this chapter's section on hypertension). Excess dietary sodium can also contribute to osteoporosis by increasing calcium loss in the urine.

Key Concepts: *Sodium is the major cation in the extracellular fluid; it plays a critical role in regulating proper water distribution and blood pressure. Nearly all of the sodium that people ingest is absorbed. Control of serum sodium is regulated by excretion. There is no RDA for sodium, and our diets contain an overabundance of sodium, largely from processed foods. The American Heart Association recommends limiting sodium intake to less than 2,400 milligrams per day. A typical American diet contains between 3,000 and 6,000 milligrams of sodium per day. Abnormally low or high levels of sodium in the blood usually are associated with heart or kidney disease, rather than dietary deficiency or excess.*

Potassium

Just as sodium is the major extracellular cation, potassium (K) is the key cation in cells. Potassium also can affect hypertension, but in a different way. If people with hypertension eat a diet rich in potassium-containing foods (like fruits and vegetables), their blood pressure often improves.[17]

Functions of Potassium

Intracellular fluid contains about 95 percent of the body's potassium, with the highest amount in skeletal muscle cells. The flow of sodium and potassium in and out of cells is an important component of muscle contractions and the transmission of nerve impulses. The central nervous system (CNS) zealously protects its potassium—CNS potassium levels remain constant even in the face of falling levels in the muscle and blood. Potassium also helps regulate blood pressure.

Dietary Recommendations for Potassium

Although food manufacturers often add sodium to processed foods, they do not routinely add potassium. So if a person's diet includes a lot of processed foods, it may fail to meet the minimum potassium recommendations. For healthy adults, the Food and Nutrition Board estimates the minimum requirement to be 2,000 milligrams per day, and 3,500 milligrams is the Daily Value used for food labels. A balanced healthy diet supplies between 2,000 and 4,000 milligrams of potassium per day. **Figure 11.16** shows the effects that food processing has on the sodium and potassium levels in foods.

Sources of Potassium

Fresh vegetables and fruits, especially potatoes, spinach, melons, and bananas, are major dietary sources of potassium. Fresh meat, milk, coffee, and tea also contain significant potassium. (See **Figure 11.7**.) Some salt substitutes contain potassium chloride, but check the label to be sure.

Hypokalemia

Hypokalemia, low blood potassium, results from potassium depletion, most commonly caused by vomiting, diarrhea, or diuretics. In many cases of hypokalemia, insufficient dietary potassium intake magnifies the effects of excess potassium loss. Symptoms include muscle weakness, loss of appetite, and confusion. Severe or rapid potassium depletion can disrupt heart rhythms—a potentially fatal problem.

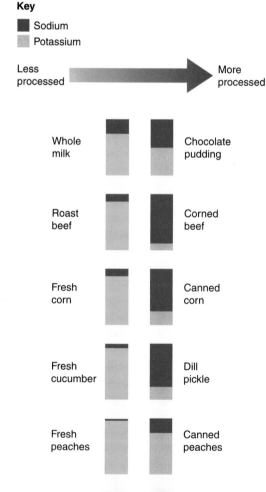

Key

■ Sodium
■ Potassium

Less processed → More processed

Whole milk / Chocolate pudding

Roast beef / Corned beef

Fresh corn / Canned corn

Fresh cucumber / Dill pickle

Fresh peaches / Canned peaches

Wheat flour / Whole wheat bread

Figure 11.16 **Effects of food processing on sodium and potassium content.**
Food processing tends to remove potassium and add sodium. Even when potassium is not removed, adding sodium reduces the ratio of potassium to sodium.

People with poor diets, such as alcoholics and individuals who suffer from anorexia nervosa or bulimia nervosa, are at highest risk of potassium deficiency. Hypokalemia also is possible in people who overuse strong laxatives. Some diuretics prescribed for hypertension cause increased excretion of both water and potassium. People taking these diuretics are at increased risk for hypokalemia and must pay special attention to their potassium intake. Their doctors may prescribe potassium supplements to counter losses. Athletes and people doing physical labor in high temperatures have high water losses, so they also risk potassium deficiency.

Hyperkalemia

The kidneys effectively remove excess potassium, so the risk of toxicity from dietary intake is usually low. However, malfunctioning kidneys or an excess of intravenous potassium can cause **hyperkalemia**, or a high concentration of potassium in the blood. Because severe hyperkalemia can slow and eventually stop the heart, people who suffer from kidney failure must monitor their potassium intake carefully. The "cocktail" of drugs administered during execution by lethal injection sometimes includes potassium.

Key Concepts: *Potassium is the major cation in the intracellular fluid. With sodium, it regulates muscle contractions and nerve impulse transmissions. For healthy adults, the minimum potassium requirement is 2,000 milligrams per day. A healthy diet has an average of 2,000 to 4,000 milligrams of potassium per day. The major sources of dietary potassium are vegetables and fruits. The symptoms of hypokalemia are loss of appetite, muscle cramps, and confusion. Severe hyperkalemia can cause cardiac arrest and death.*

Quick Bites

Versatile Potassium

During the Middle Ages, saltpeter (potassium nitrate) was discovered to be a useful substance. It was used to extract other minerals from rock, as a fertilizer, and as an ingredient in gunpowder. It wasn't used to cure meat until the sixteenth or seventeenth century. Saltpeter was a major ingredient in the curing mixture until 1940, about the time that refrigeration emerged. Today, food manufacturers use small amounts of nitrites rather than saltpeter to preserve foods such as bacon, ham, and some sausages.

hypokalemia Inadequate levels of potassium in the blood.

hyperkalemia Abnormally high potassium concentrations in the blood.

POTASSIUM

Daily Value = 3500 mg

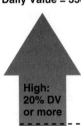
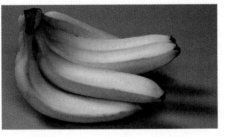

High: 20% DV or more

Good: 10-19% DV

Food	Serving	Potassium
Yogurt, plain, nonfat	225 g (1 8-oz container)	574 mg
Banana	One 9"	554 mg
Tomato juice	240 ml (1 cup)	535 mg
Clams, cooked	85 g (3 oz)	534 mg
Lima beans, cooked	90 g (~1/2 cup)	513 mg
Halibut, cooked	85 g (3 oz)	490 mg
Spinach, raw	85 g (~3 cups)	474 mg
Orange juice, chilled	240 ml (1 cup)	473 mg
Cantaloupe	140 g (1/4 medium melon)	433 mg
Potato, baked	110 g (1 small)	430 mg
Apricot, fresh	140 g (~ 4 apricots)	414 mg
Baked beans, canned	130 g (~1/2 cup)	385 mg
Milk, 1% milkfat	240 ml (1 cup)	381 mg
Acorn squash, cooked	85 g (~1/3 cup)	371 mg
Milk, whole (3.25% fat)	240 ml (1 cup)	370 mg

Figure 11.17 **Food sources of potassium.** The best food sources of potassium are fresh fruits and vegetables, and certain dairy products and fish.
Source: U.S. Department of Agriculture, Agricultural Research Service. 1999. USDA Nutrient Database for Standard Reference, Release 13. Nutrient Data Laboratory Home Page, http://www.nal.usda.gov/fnic/foodcomp.

Quick Bites

Banana Facts

You may know that bananas are high in potassium, but did you also know that they have an unusually high carbohydrate content? Before ripening, a banana is almost entirely starch. After ripening, the dessert varieties are almost entirely sugar—as much as 20 percent by weight.

chloride shift The movement of chloride ions in and out of red blood cells to maintain a lower level of chloride in red blood cells in the arteries than in the veins.

Chloride

Chloride (Cl^-) and chlorine (Cl_2) are not the same. Chloride is a single negatively charged atom that people commonly eat as a component of table salt (NaCl). Chlorine, a highly reactive molecule composed of two atoms, is a poisonous gas. Water treatment facilities commonly use chlorine to kill bacteria and other germs.

Functions of Chloride

Chloride is the major extracellular anion in the body. Although mostly found outside cells, chloride readily moves in and out of red blood cells. As these cells transport oxygen to body tissues or carbon dioxide to the lungs, the concentration of chloride ions shifts to sustain a neutral charge in the cell. This **chloride shift** maintains lower levels of chloride ions in arterial red blood cells than in venous red blood cells.

You have probably noticed the salty taste that sodium chloride (NaCl) imparts to blood, sweat, and tears. Both sodium and chloride help maintain the body's fluid balance. Chloride also readily combines with hydrogen ions (H^+) to form hydrochloric acid (HCl). In the stomach, hydrochloric acid kills many disease-causing bacteria that have been ingested and helps prepare protein for enzymatic digestion. In the large intestine, bacterial activity forms acid products. To neutralize these acid products, the cells lining the large intestine absorb chloride ions and secrete alkaline bicarbonate ions.[18] During an immune response, white blood cells use chloride ions to form a powerful chemical weapon to kill invading bacteria. In neurons, the coordinated movements of chloride, and the cations sodium, potassium, and calcium, help transmit nerve impulses.

Dietary Recommendations for Chloride

Most of us consume much more chloride than 750 milligrams per day, the adult minimum requirement estimated by the Food and Nutrition Board. Consumption of excess sodium and chloride may aggravate hypertension in salt-sensitive people, so the American Heart Association recommends that healthy adults limit their consumption of salt (NaCl) to no more than 6,000 milligrams per day; about 2,400 milligrams sodium and 3,600 milligrams chloride. The Daily Value for chloride is 3,400 milligrams.

Sources of Chloride

Although some fruits and vegetables naturally contain chloride, most of our chloride intake comes from salt (for dietary sources of salt see the "Sodium" section earlier in this chapter). You usually can estimate the chloride content of processed foods from the sodium content by using this simple formula:

$$\text{chloride content} = 1.5 \times \text{sodium content.}$$

The average intake of chloride from salt is 4,500 milligrams per day (7.5 g of salt), which is much more than adequate. The kidneys excrete excess chloride, and some chloride also is lost in sweat. The only known cause of high blood chloride levels is severe dehydration.

Hypochloremia

Because vomiting removes hydrochloric acid along with other stomach contents, frequent vomiting can cause a chloride deficiency. People with bulimia nervosa compulsively gorge and purge, so they often suffer from

---

Quick Bites

Low-Calorie Chlorine?

Sucralose is a low-calorie sweetener made from sugar. During manufacture, a multistep process substitutes three chlorine atoms for three hydrogen-oxygen groups on the sugar molecule. This creates an exceptionally stable molecular structure that is 600 times sweeter than sugar. The sucralose molecule is chemically and biologically inert so it passes through the body without being digested and is eliminated after consumption.

Quick Bites

Discouraging Discoloration

Cutting or bruising causes discoloration of many fruits and vegetables such as apples, bananas, pears, eggplants, avocados, and raw potatoes. Chloride ions inhibit the responsible enzyme, so salt will retard discoloration although it changes the flavor.

low chloride, as well as low levels of other critical electrolytes, such as potassium. A person who combines repeated vomiting with inadequate consumption of fluid and minerals can suffer dehydration and **metabolic alkalosis** (high blood pH). Small variations in blood pH can have profound consequences—a 5 percent rise in pH can be fatal. Alkalosis can cause abnormal heart rhythm, a substantial drop in blood flow to the brain, decreased oxygen delivery to tissues, and abnormal metabolic activity. To treat this problem, doctors administer oral or intravenous fluids containing the deficient minerals. This replenishment of minerals and fluids restores pH balance.[19]

Key Concepts: *Chloride is involved in many important metabolic functions. It is used to form the hydrochloric acid secreted in the stomach, and is important in the generation of nerve impulses, as well as in immune function. The minimum chloride requirement for a healthy adult is 750 milligrams per day; average chloride intake from salt is 4,500 milligrams per day. People with bulimia nervosa may develop chloride deficiency as a result of self-induced vomiting.*

Calcium

Our bodies contain more calcium (Ca) than any other mineral, about 1.5 to 2 percent of our total weight. Adequate calcium intake over one's lifetime is essential for healthy bones and teeth that will remain strong into old age. While we associate calcium primarily with bones, it plays many important roles in the body. Getting enough calcium in your diet not only maintains healthy bones, but also may help prevent hypertension, decrease your odds of getting colon or breast cancer, and reduce the risk of developing kidney stones.

Functions of Calcium

Bones and teeth contain more than 99 percent of the body's calcium. This mineral makes bones hard and strong, able to withstand tremendous force without breaking—most of the time. The other 1 percent of body calcium is in blood and soft tissues, where it plays many equally crucial roles in such vital functions as muscle contraction, nerve impulse transmission, blood clotting, and cell metabolism. **Figure 11.18** shows the functions of calcium.

Bone Structure

Most of us think of bone as a simple structural framework for our bodies. We forget that bone is living tissue that changes in response to physical stresses. Bone also encases the marrow, the source of many types of blood and immune cells, and it also serves as the reserve site for minerals such as calcium and phosphorus.

Bone is made up of cells and an extracellular matrix. Two types of cells, **osteoblasts** and **osteoclasts**, continually remodel our bones—building them up and tearing them down. Osteoblasts are the construction team and osteoclasts are the demolition team. Osteoblasts first secrete the collagen protein matrix that forms the initial framework for new bone. Then these bone builders help move minerals from the extracellular fluid to the bone surface, where the minerals become a hard crystalline material that surrounds the collagen fibers. Most of the calcium in bone is in the form of **hydroxyapatite**—a crystalline mineral complex of calcium and phosphorus. By weight, bone is two-thirds mineral and one-third water and protein, primarily collagen. While osteoblasts continually deposit bone, osteoclasts perform the opposite function by resorbing bone. As they break down bone, they release calcium and phosphate, which enter the bloodstream.

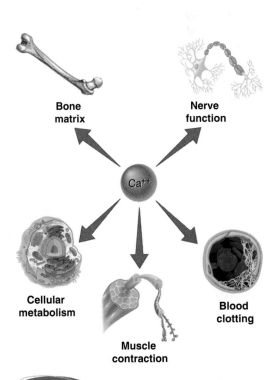

Figure 11.18 Functions of calcium. Calcium is important for many cellular processes in addition to its key role in bone mineralization.

linear growth Increase in body length/height.

fibrin A stringy, insoluble protein that is the final product of the blood-clotting process.

calmodulin A calcium-binding protein that regulates a variety of chemical reactions and physiological activities, such as muscle contractions and norepinephrine release.

ciliary action Wavelike motion of small hairlike projections on some cells.

The activities of osteoblasts and osteoclasts determine how bones grow and change over time. Mineralization of bone is favored during **linear growth** (growth in height) and for 5 to 10 years thereafter. It is thought that we achieve peak bone mass sometime around age 30.

Throughout life, our bones change in response to our activities. The dynamic nature of bone allows it to be strengthened and rebuilt in areas under repeated stress—bone thickens when repeatedly subjected to loads. Even elderly adults can strengthen and rebuild their bones by performing weight-bearing exercise such as walking or weight lifting.[20]

The calcium in bones serves as a reservoir for calcium that is needed throughout the body. The body maintains a constant calcium blood level at all costs—at the expense of bone strength if necessary. Even if calcium intake is very low, the calcium concentration in the bloodstream remains steady because the body removes calcium from bone to sustain an adequate supply to other tissues. In the absence of kidney disease or hormonal abnormalities, your blood calcium level remains normal, even if your diet is extremely deficient in calcium.

Nerve Function

Calcium is a key factor in normal transmission of nerve impulses. The movement of calcium into nerve cells triggers the release of neurotransmitters at the junction between nerves. The neuron releases neurotransmitters in direct proportion to the number of calcium ions that flow through the cell's calcium channels. Insufficient calcium can inhibit nerve transmissions.

Blood Clotting

Calcium is essential for the formation of **fibrin**, the fibrous protein that makes up the structure of blood clots. Calcium participates in nearly every step of the blood-clotting cascade. Blood will not clot in the absence of calcium, but calcium levels in the body seldom fall low enough to significantly impair blood clotting.

Muscle Contraction

The flow of sodium and calcium is crucial for mechanical contraction of muscle. Calcium sits at a critical location on the muscle fiber, facilitating the interaction of the muscle proteins myosin and actin. Stimulation of muscle fibers by nerve impulses, hormones, or stretch in the fiber increases the amount of calcium in the muscle cells and causes the muscle to contract. As the cells pump calcium ions back outside, the muscle relaxes.

Cellular Metabolism

Calcium is also a key player in regulation of cellular metabolism. When calcium enters a cell, it can bind **calmodulin**, a regulatory protein. This activates calmodulin so it can regulate a variety of enzymatic processes that affect cell secretions, **ciliary action**, cell division, and cell proliferation.

Regulation of Blood Calcium

Circulating calcium performs a myriad of functions that are so critical the body will demineralize bone to prevent even minor dips in blood calcium levels. Three hormones, calcitriol (the active form of vitamin D), parathyroid hormone, and calcitonin, regulate calcium status. They control intestinal absorption of calcium, bone calcium release, and calcium excretion by the kidneys. (See **Figure 11.19.**) In people with inadequate calcium intakes, high sodium intake, excess caffeine, and other diuretics can affect calcium balance by increasing the rate of calcium excretion in the urine.[21]

Vitamin D

Vitamin D increases calcium absorption by the intestine. Calcitriol, the active form of vitamin D, increases the production of calcium-binding proteins in the lining of the small intestine. The rate of calcium absorption seems to be directly proportional to the quantity of calcium-binding proteins.

Parathyroid Hormone

When plasma calcium levels are too low, the parathyroid gland secretes parathyroid hormone (PTH). PTH activates bone-resorbing osteoclasts that break down bone and release calcium and phosphorus into the blood. It also increases kidney reabsorption of calcium and stimulates calcitriol production, which then enhances intestinal calcium absorption. PTH greatly increases

LOW BLOOD CALCIUM		HIGH BLOOD CALCIUM	
Increase PTH secretion and calcitriol formation	**Thyroid/Parathyroid**	**Secrete calcitonin**	**Decrease PTH secretion and calcitriol formation**
Parathyroid gland secretes parathormone (PTH). Increased PTH levels stimulate calcitriol (vitamin D₃) production in the kidney	Thyroid — Parathyroid (embedded in the thyroid)	Thyroid gland secretes calcitonin	Parathormone formation slows and PTH levels drop. Decreased PTH levels slow calcitriol formation
Absorb more dietary calcium	**Small intestine**	**Absorb less dietary calcium**	
Calcitriol increases intestinal absorbtion of calcium and phosphorus		No major effect – calcitonin slightly inhibits calcium absorption	Decreased calcitriol slows intestinal absorption of calcium and phosphorus
Retain calcium	**Kidney**	**Excrete calcium**	
PTH and calcitriol increase calcium reabsorption in the kidney, thus decreasing calcium excretion		No major effect – calcitonin slightly increases calcium excretion	Decreased PTH and calcitriol levels increase calcium excretion
Move calcium from bone to bloodstream	**Bone**	**Move calcium from bloodstream to bone**	
PTH and calcitriol work together to stimulate osteoclast activity. The osteoclasts gobble up bone, releasing calcium into the bloodstream	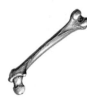	Calcitonin inhibits the activity of osteoclasts, shifting the balance toward the deposition of calcium in bone	Decreased PTH and calcitriol levels slow osteoclast activity and breakdown of bone
RAISE BLOOD CALCIUM		**LOWER BLOOD CALCIUM**	

Figure 11.19 **Regulating blood calcium levels.** Calcitonin has only a weak effect on calcium ion concentration. It is fast acting, but any decrease in calcium ion concentration triggers the release of PTH, which almost completely overrides the calcitonin effect. In prolonged calcium excess or deficiency, the parathyroid mechanism is the most powerful hormonal mechanism for maintaining normal blood calcium levels.

phosphorus excretion, so phosphorus blood levels actually drop in response to PTH despite an initial increase in supply from the breakdown of bone.

Calcitonin

When plasma calcium is too high, the thyroid gland secretes calcitonin. Calcitonin has weak effects on plasma calcium levels and acts in opposition to parathyroid hormone. While it has no major effects in the small intestine and kidney, it inhibits the formation and activity of osteoclasts. This shifts the osteoclast-osteoblast balance toward bone deposition. High concentrations of calcium in the blood decrease parathyroid hormone production, and thus calcitriol production, slowing processes that move calcium into the bloodstream.

Dietary Recommendations for Calcium

Optimal calcium intake throughout life is extremely important. Bones become stronger and denser as children and young adults develop. Later in life, bones gradually become less dense. If children and young adults fail to take in enough calcium, they are more likely to develop osteoporosis (fragile, porous bones that easily break) later in life. The Adequate Intake level for calcium is 1,000 milligrams per day for adults aged 19 to 50, although calcium intake recommendations vary slightly among public health organizations. Adolescents need more calcium to maximize peak bone mass (AI for ages 9 to 18 is 1,300 mg per day). The AI for adults aged 51 and older increases to 1,200 milligrams per day.

Unfortunately, many of us fall far short of these recommended calcium intakes. Although average calcium intake has increased slightly (from 743 milligrams per day in 1977-1978 to 813 milligrams per day in 1995),[22]

Figure 11.20 **Food sources of calcium.** Calcium is found in milk and dairy products, certain green leafy vegetables, and canned fish with bones.
Source: U.S. Department of Agriculture, Agricultural Research Service. 1999. USDA Nutrient Database for Standard Reference, Release 13. Nutrient Data Laboratory Home Page, http://www.nal.usda.gov/fnic/foodcomp

CALCIUM

Daily Value = 1000 mg

High: 20% DV or more

Food	Serving	Amount
Tofu, calcium processed	85 g (~1/3 cup)	581 mg
Yogurt, plain, lowfat	225 g (1 8-oz container)	411 mg
Milk, skim	240 ml (1 cup)	302 mg
Milk, 1% milkfat	240 ml (1 cup)	300 mg
Milk, 2% milkfat	240 ml (1 cup)	297 mg
Sesame seeds, whole roasted, toasted	30 g (1 oz)	297 mg
Cheese, swiss	30 g (1 oz)	288 mg
Cheese, cheddar	30 g (1 oz)	216 mg
Sardines, canned	55 g (2 oz)	210 mg

Good: 10-19% DV

Food	Serving	Amount
Cheese, mozzarella	30 g (1 oz)	194 mg
Molasses, blackstrap	1 Tbsp.	172 mg
Soybeans, cooked	90 g (~1/2 cup)	131 mg
Spinach, cooked*	85 g (~1/2 cup)	124 mg
Salmon, canned, + bones	55 g (2 oz)	117 mg
Turnip greens, cooked	85 g (~1/2 cup)	116 mg
Blackeyed peas, cooked	90 g (~1/2 cup)	115 mg
All Bran cereal	30 g (~1/2 cup)	106 mg
Collards, cooked	85 g (~1/2 cup)	101 mg

*In spinach, oxalate binds calcium and prevents absorption of all but about 5 percent of the plant's calcium.

most Americans still fail to meet current recommendations. Population surveys of girls and young women 12 to 19 years old show their average calcium intake to be less than 900 milligrams per day, which is well below recommended intake levels.[23] Many of these young women will attain a suboptimal peak bone mass and will be prone to osteoporosis as they age.

Sources of Calcium

Dairy products provide more than half of the calcium in the typical American diet. Of all the dairy products, nonfat milk is the most nutrient dense because of its high calcium content and low fat and calorie content. Nonfat yogurt is another excellent source of calcium. Cottage cheese has the least calcium of the dairy foods because processing removes much of its calcium. Ice cream and cheese are good sources of calcium, but they should be eaten only in moderation because of their high fat content. Green leafy vegetables such as spinach, have high levels of calcium, but most of the calcium is bound to oxalate and therefore cannot be absorbed. Chinese cabbage, kale, turnip greens, and calcium-processed tofu contain significant amounts of bioavailable calcium. Canned fish with bones such as sardines provide lots of calcium as long as you eat the bones. **Figure 11.20** shows food sources of calcium. Some brands of orange juice, cereal, bread, and yogurt products are now fortified with calcium, making them good sources. Check labels carefully because only a few of the many products on grocery shelves are fortified with calcium. **Figure 11.21** shows the variation in bioavailability among various sources of calcium.

While eating a variety of healthful foods is always the best way to obtain nutrients, some people, especially those with limited dairy intake, may need to take supplements to ensure adequate calcium intake. Flavored,

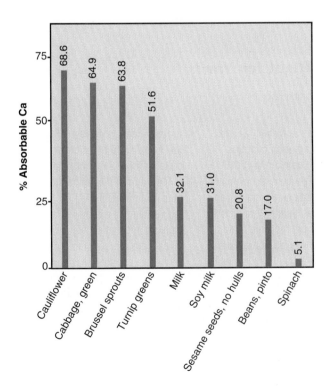

Figure 11.21 Bioavailability of calcium from different sources.

Source: Adapted from Weaver CM, Plawecki KL. Dietary calcium: Adequacy of a vegetarian diet. *Am J Clin Nutr.* 1994; 59(suppl):1238S–1241S.

chewable, calcium-containing antacids are an inexpensive and easy-to-take source of extra calcium. For more information, see the FYI feature "Calcium Supplements: Are They Right for You?"

Calcium Absorption

The body normally absorbs 25 to 75 percent of dietary calcium, depending on a variety of factors including age, presence of adequate vitamin D, the body's need for calcium, and calcium intake. For example, if a child and a healthy elderly person eat exactly the same meal, the child may absorb 75 percent of the calcium in the food, whereas the elderly person might absorb only 25 percent. Calcium absorption is particularly high during pregnancy and infancy, and is at its lowest in old age.

Calcium absorption is inversely related to calcium intake. The body adjusts the percentage it absorbs based on the amount in the diet—an increase in dietary calcium reduces absorption and a decrease in dietary calcium enhances absorption.[24] In the absence of vitamin D, calcium absorption can drop to less than 10 percent of dietary calcium.[25] Phytates (in nuts, seeds, and grains) depress calcium absorption, as do high levels of phosphorus and magnesium from supplements. Dietary fiber, except for wheat bran, has little effect on calcium absorption. High intakes of wheat bran have been found to depress calcium absorption from milk. Low estrogen levels, as seen in postmenopausal women, can lower calcium absorption to about 20 percent. Many women take estrogen supplements after menopause to maintain calcium absorption and lower the risk of osteoporosis. Calcium from supplements is absorbed most efficiently when taken between meals at individual doses of 500 milligrams or less.[26]

[Fyi] Calcium Supplements: Are They Right for You?

FOR YOUR INFORMATION

After reading the section on calcium, you may be wondering whether you need a calcium supplement. After all, calcium is critical for so many bodily functions, and getting enough calcium reduces the risk of osteoporosis later in life.

Before you head to the supplement aisle at the grocery store, take a critical look at your diet, especially your intake of milk and other dairy products. In the United States dairy foods are the major sources of dietary calcium; without them, it may be difficult to reach the AI for calcium. People who exclude dairy products, such as vegans and those with milk allergy, must choose foods carefully to find rich calcium sources.

Calcium sources vary widely in their bioavailability. While labels are required to list the %DV for calcium, they don't indicate how much of that calcium the body will absorb. For example, 1/2 cup of spinach contains about 120 milligrams of calcium, but the body will absorb only 5 percent of that calcium! Intake recommendations are based on the mix of sources in the typical American diet. Other cultures manage on much lower intakes in part because they do not consume the many food constituents that deplete calcium or reduce its absorption. Vegetarians may, in fact, need less calcium than meat eaters. If you are considering spinach as your sole source of calcium, however, check out **Table A.** It shows the amount of certain foods needed to equal the calcium available from 1 cup of milk (about 30 percent of the 300 milligrams of calcium in 1 cup of milk is bioavailable).

You can see from Table A that the amount of bioavailable calcium varies quite a bit among green leafy vegetables! If your diet is low in calcium, try adding some of the higher calcium foods. Incorporating calcium-rich foods into the diet adds other important vitamins and minerals.

Even armed with more information about calcium in the diet, you may still decide to investigate the supplement market. Again, there are a variety of choices: calcium carbonate, calcium citrate, calcium lactate, calcium phosphate...how to decide? First, it's important to know that the absorption of calcium from most supplements is about equal—roughly 30 percent. The calcium citrate malate that is used in some brands of fortified juice, and a limited number of supplements, is absorbed better, 35 percent. However, a typical calcium citrate malate tablet has less calcium than a tablet of

Hypocalcemia

A lower than normal level of calcium in the blood is called **hypocalcemia**. Because the body uses bone calcium to maintain normal blood calcium levels, hypocalcemia is relatively uncommon. The causes of hypocalcemia include kidney failure, parathyroid disorders, and vitamin D deficiency. Significant hypocalcemia can cause muscle spasms, facial grimacing, and convulsions.

A chronic dietary calcium deficiency can result in osteoporosis either by sub-optimal bone growth in childhood and adolescence or increased rate of bone loss after menopause (see the section "Osteoporosis" later in this chapter). Studies also link low calcium intake to an increased risk of hypertension, colon cancer, and preeclampsia (a complication of pregnancy marked by high blood pressure, edema, and protein in the urine).[27]

Hypercalcemia

The two major causes of **hypercalcemia** are cancer and the overproduction of PTH by the parathyroid gland. Hypercalcemia can result in fatigue, confusion, loss of appetite, and constipation. Calcium may be deposited in the soft tissues where it can impair organ function. Very high levels of blood calcium can lead to coma and cardiac arrest.

Excess calcium supplementation usually does not result in hypercalcemia, but may cause mineral imbalances by interfering with the absorption of other minerals, such as iron, magnesium, and zinc. Calcium supplements that contain citrate and ascorbic acid enhance iron absorption, but other forms can cut iron absorption in half. Calcium also may interfere with absorption of some medications, such as tetracycline.[28] The Food and Nutrition Board has established a UL for calcium of 2,500 milligrams per day.

hypocalcemia A deficiency of calcium in the blood.
hypercalcemia Abnormally high concentrations of calcium in the blood.

---

another type such as calcium carbonate. Calcium carbonate is usually the most concentrated per tablet, so taking fewer pills per day will supply enough; also, this type of supplement tends to be less expensive. Chelated calcium supplements can improve absorption a bit, but the extra expense is probably not worth it.

Other factors to consider are that calcium supplements may be absorbed better if taken between meals. Also, you need to get plenty of vitamin D, either through casual exposure to the sun, in fortified milk, or as part of a supplement (many calcium supplements have added vitamin D). Vitamin D is important for the absorption of calcium. In addition, bones get stronger with regular, weight-bearing exercise, so make sure to include that in your healthful lifestyle.

Table A **Foods That Provide the Calcium Equivalent of 1 Cup (8 fl oz) of Milk**

Food	Amount	Food	Amount
Almonds, dry roasted	6 oz	Mustard greens	1 1/3 C
Beans, pinto	6 1/3 C	Radish	4 1/2 C
Beans, red	7 C	Rutabaga	2 1/4 C
Beans, white	2 1/2 C	Sesame seeds, no hulls	12 oz
Broccoli	2 1/2 C	Soy milk, unfortified	30 C
Brussels sprouts	4 C	Spinach	7 3/4 C
Cabbage, Chinese	1 C	Tofu, calcium set	1/2 C
Cabbage, green	3 C	Turnip greens	1 C
Calcium-fortified juices*	5 fl oz	Watercress	3 1/2 C
Cauliflower	4 C		
Kale	1 3/4 C		
Kohlrabi	3 1/2 C		

*Fortified with calcium as calcium citrate malate.
Source: Adapted from Weaver CM, Plawecki KL. Dietary calcium: Adequacy of a vegetarian diet. *Am J Clin Nutr.* 1994;59(suppl):1238S–1241S.

phosphorylation The addition of phosphate to an organic (carbon-containing) compound. Oxidative phosphorylation is the formation of high-energy phosphate bonds (ADP + Pi → ATP) from the energy released by oxidation of energy-yielding nutrients.

Key Concepts: *Calcium is a major component of bones and teeth. In addition, calcium is required for muscle contraction, nerve impulse transmission, blood clotting, and regulation of cell metabolism. For adults, 1,000 milligrams per day is recommended, and more is suggested for adolescents and older adults. Dairy foods and fortified foods are major dietary sources of calcium. Calcium status is regulated by three hormones that control intestinal absorption, bone calcium release, and kidney excretion: calcitriol, parathyroid hormone, and calcitonin. Lack of dietary calcium contributes to the development of osteoporosis.*

Phosphorus

Phosphorus (P), like calcium, serves many roles in the biochemical reactions of cells and it has a critical role in bone as part of the mineral complex hydroxyapatite. Phosphorus intake typically exceeds that of calcium because it is so widespread in the food supply. Most phosphorus in the body is in the form of the phosphate ion (PO_4^{3-}). In fact, phosphate is the most abundant intracellular anion.

Functions of Phosphorus

Bones are the major storehouse of phosphorus, with nearly 85 percent of the body's supply. The remaining phosphorus is found in cells of soft tissues (~15 percent) and extracellular fluid (~0.1 percent). It helps activate and deactivate enzymes in a process called **phosphorylation**. Phosphorus is an essential component of ATP, the universal energy source for all cells. Phosphorus also is a component of DNA, RNA, and phospholipids in cell membranes and lipoproteins.

Dietary Recommendations for Phosphorus

The phosphorus RDA for adults is 700 milligrams per day. Adolescents need more, about 1,250 milligrams per day, to support growth. The average adult intake is between 1,000 and 1,500 milligrams per day, so phosphorus deficiencies due to dietary insufficiency are rarely seen.

Sources of Phosphorus

Phosphorus is abundant in our food supply. In general, foods rich in protein (milk, meat, and eggs) also are rich in phosphorus. Food additives, especially those in processed meat and soft drinks, supply up to 30 percent of our phosphorus. **Figure 11.22** shows selected food sources of phosphorus. Food manufacturers often add phosphate salts to processed foods to improve moisture retention and smoothness.

Since phosphorus density is higher in cow's milk than in most other foods, people with high dairy-product intakes have high phosphorus diets. This is also true for people who drink several colas daily or the few other soft drinks that contain phosphoric acid. One 12-ounce cola contains about 50 milligrams of phosphorus—only 5 percent of an adult woman's typical intake. However, when five or more are consumed daily, colas may contribute substantial amounts of phosphorus to the diet.[29]

Our bodies directly absorb phosphorus from most food sources, with one major exception—plant seeds. All plant seeds (beans, peas, cereals, and nuts) contain phosphorus in a storage form, phytic acid. Our bodies do not produce the enzymes necessary to break down phytic acid. Still, we can absorb up to 50 percent of this phosphorus because other foods and bacteria in our large intestines contain the necessary enzymes. Yeasts also can

Quick Bites

The Double Helix Depends on Phosphorus

The backbone of DNA's twisting ladderlike structure contains alternating molecules of phosphoric acid and deoxyribose.

break down phytic acid, so our bodies absorb more phosphorus from whole-grains when part of leavened bread, for example, than from grains in unleavened bread and breakfast cereals. While excess calcium interferes with phosphorus absorption—possibly because unabsorbed calcium binds with phytic acid and prevents bacterial breakdown—typical dietary calcium levels have no effect.

Generally, we absorb between 55 and 70 percent of dietary phosphorus and the kidneys excrete any excess in the urine. Unlike calcium absorption, phosphorus absorption does not increase as dietary intake decreases.[30] On the other hand, the body's phosphorus needs can drive phosphorus absorption efficiency. While the efficiency of phosphorus absorption, unlike calcium absorption, does not vary with increased dietary intake, it rises dramatically when the body has low phosphorus levels. In the intestines, calcitriol enhances both calcium and phosphorus absorption. Parathyroid hormone, on the other hand, has opposite effects on calcium and phosphorus levels. PTH not only maintains calcium levels by stimulating the kidneys to reabsorb calcium, but also causes rapid loss of phosphorus in the urine. The two most important regulators of urinary phosphorus excretion are PTH and the amount of phosphorus in the diet.[31]

Hypophosphatemia

Phosphorus is so common in foods that only near total starvation will cause a dietary phosphorus deficiency. Rather, an underlying disorder typically causes **hypophosphatemia**, low blood phosphate, either by restricting absorption or enhancing excretion. Physicians commonly encounter hypophosphatemia, and about 2 percent of patients admitted to general hospitals suffer from it.[32] Some of its more common causes include **hyperparathyroidism** (excessive secretion of PTH, often because of a parathyroid tumor), vitamin D deficiency, and overuse of aluminum-, magnesium-, or calcium-containing antacids that bind phosphate. Common symptoms of hypophosphatemia include anorexia, dizziness,

hypophosphatemia Abnormally low phosphate concentration in the blood.

hyperparathyroidism Excessive secretion of parathyroid hormone, which alters calcium metabolism.

PHOSPHORUS

Daily Value = 1000 mg

High: 20% DV or more

Beef liver, cooked	85 g (3 oz)	392 mg
Yogurt, plain, nonfat	225 g (8 oz)	352 mg
Sunflower seeds	30 g (1 oz)	347 mg
All Bran cereal	30 g (~1/2 cup)	294 mg
Herring, cooked	85 g (3 oz)	258 mg
Milk, skim	240 ml (1 cup)	247 mg
Milk, 1% milkfat	240 ml (1 cup)	235 mg
Milk, 2% milkfat	240 ml (1 cup)	232 mg
Cheese, provolone	85 g (3 oz)	227 mg
Chicken, dark meat, cooked	85 g (3 oz)	204 mg

Good: 10-19% DV

Chicken, white meat, cooked	85 g (3 oz)	184 mg
Oysters, cooked	85 g (3 oz)	173 mg
Lentils, cooked	90 g (~1/2 cup)	162 mg
Tofu, calcium processed	85 g (~1/3 cup)	162 mg
Almonds	30 g (1 oz)	140 mg
Beef, ground, extra lean	85 g (3 oz)	136 mg
Black beans, cooked	90 g (~1/2 cup)	126 mg
Soy milk	240 ml (1 cup)	120 mg
Peanut butter	2 Tbsp.	118 mg

Figure 11.22 **Food sources of phosphorus.**
Phosphorus is abundant in the food supply. Meats, legumes, nuts, dairy products, and grains tend to have more phosphorus than fruits and vegetables.
Source: U.S. Department of Agriculture, Agricultural Research Service. 1999. USDA Nutrient Database for Standard Reference, Release 13. Nutrient Data Laboratory Home Page, http://www.nal.usda.gov/fnic/foodcomp.

hyperphosphatemia Abnormally high phosphate concentration in the blood.

bone pain, muscle weakness, and a waddling gait. Chronic hypophosphatemia affects primarily the musculoskeletal system, causing muscle weakness and damage, including respiratory problems due to poor diaphragm function. Long-standing hypophosphatemia can cause rickets and osteomalacia.

Hyperphosphatemia

Physicians also frequently see **hyperphosphatemia**, high blood phosphate, which most commonly is a consequence of kidney disease. Other causes include an underactive parathyroid gland, taking too many vitamin D supplements, and overuse of phosphate-containing laxatives. Excess phosphorus can bind calcium, and since low calcium concentrations can cause nerve fibers to discharge repeatedly without provocation, this can lead to severe muscle spasms and convulsions. If your diet contains excessive phosphorus and not enough calcium, you may be at risk for increased bone loss. However, a high phosphorus intake alone is unlikely to have an adverse affect on bone health.[33] Replacing milk as a beverage with cola, a common practice among adolescents and Americans of all ages, increases phosphates in the diet (from cola), while reducing calcium intake. Some experts believe that this practice may be a significant factor in the development of osteoporosis later in life. The UL for phosphorus is 4,000 milligrams per day for people aged 9 to 70.

Key Concept: *Phosphorus is common in many crucial metabolic systems. It is used to activate and deactivate enzymes, and is an essential component of ATP, the energy source of the cell. Phosphorus is found in the phospholipids of cell membranes and is part of the hydroxyapatite in bone. About 85 percent of phosphorus is found in bone. Milk and meat are major sources of dietary phosphorus, and up to 30 percent of dietary intake comes from food additives. The RDA for adults is 700 milligrams per day, increasing to 1,250 milligrams per day for teens. Diets high in phosphorus and low in calcium can contribute to bone loss.*

Magnesium

Magnesium (Mg) is the fourth most abundant cation in the body, and is about one-sixth as plentiful in cells as potassium. About 50 to 60 percent of the body's magnesium is in bone, with the remainder distributed equally between muscle and other soft tissue. The magnesium in bone provides a large reservoir in case deficiencies in soft tissue magnesium occur. Most magnesium resides in cells, with only 1 percent in extracellular fluid.

Functions of Magnesium

Magnesium participates in more than 300 types of enzyme-mediated reactions in the body including those in DNA and protein synthesis. In the mitochondria, magnesium is essential for the production of ATP via the electron transport chain. Since ATP is the universal energy source for all cells, an absence of magnesium would quickly halt cellular activity. In the glycolysis pathway alone, seven key enzymes require magnesium. Magnesium also participates in muscle contraction and blood clotting.

Dietary Recommendations for Magnesium

Because of the large amount of magnesium in bone, blood magnesium levels may not be indicative of total body status. Therefore assessing deficiency and setting intake recommendations is difficult. The RDA for magnesium in adults (aged 19 to 30 years) is 400 milligrams per day for men and 310

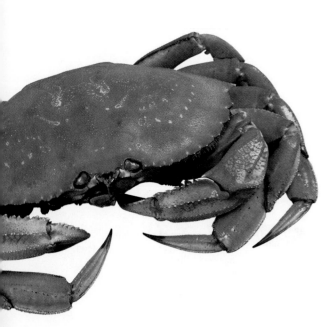

milligrams per day for women. This value rises slightly, in adults aged 31 to 70, to 420 milligrams for men and 320 milligrams for women. The average adult diet in the United States contains only about three-fourths of the magnesium RDA, and slightly less than the EAR (Estimated Average Requirement) for magnesium. Despite this, symptoms due to low magnesium are relatively uncommon in healthy people. This is because so much magnesium is stored in bone that levels in cells and body fluids remain constant even if intake is somewhat less than optimal.

Sources of Magnesium

Magnesium is ubiquitous in foods, but the amount varies widely depending on the food source. This mineral enters our diet mostly from plants. Whole grains and vegetables such as spinach and potatoes are good sources of magnesium, as are legumes, tofu, and some types of seafood. **Figure 11.23** shows food sources or magnesium. Refined foods are low in magnesium content. Processed grains lose up to 80 percent of their magnesium and enrichment does not replace it. Chocolate contains modest amounts of magnesium—but unfortunately not enough to compensate for its high fat and calorie content. Tap water can also be a significant source of the mineral in some communities with "hard" water. Total magnesium intake usually is proportional to calorie intake, so young people and adult men have higher intakes than women and the elderly.

We generally absorb about 50 percent of dietary magnesium. High-fiber diets can decrease absorption, as does a high-phosphorus diet. High calcium intake, usually in the form of supplements, also can interfere with magnesium absorption. This is another reason why food is a better source of nutrients than supplements. People who must take calcium supplements should be sure to regularly eat foods with high magnesium content.

Hypomagnesemia

Deficiency in any of the three major intracellular minerals—magnesium, potassium, and phosphorus—usually is associated with deficiencies in the other two. It is uncommon to see an isolated deficiency of any of the intracellular minerals.[34] **Hypomagnesemia**, or magnesium deficiency, occurs with a variety of diseases, including kidney disease, and is associated with alcoholism and some types of diuretic drugs. People who have prolonged diarrhea can be at risk for magnesium deficiency. People who have chronically poor diets are also at risk, especially if they abuse alcohol. Nearly all chronic alcoholics have symptoms of hypomagnesemia because they often have poor diets and because alcohol increases urinary excretion of magnesium.

In research studies, healthy people whose diets are deficient in magnesium usually have no symptoms for a few weeks, because of the large supply of magnesium stored in bone. Gradually, loss of appetite, nausea, and weakness develop. After more time, muscle cramps, irritability, and confusion occur. The heart rhythm may become disturbed. If hypomagnesemia becomes extreme, death can result, usually due to heart rhythm problems.

hypomagnesemia An abnormally low concentration of magnesium in the blood.

MAGNESIUM

Daily Value = 400 mg

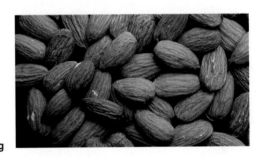

Cheese, provolone		149 mg
All Bran cereal		129 mg
Sesame seeds		107 mg
Halibut, cooked		91 mg
Almonds		82 mg
Oysters, cooked		81 mg
Cashews		78 mg
Spinach, raw		67 mg
Lima beans, cooked		67 mg
Black beans, cooked		63 mg
Rice, brown, cooked		60 mg
Wheat bran flakes cereal		60 mg
Crab, Alaska King, cooked		54 mg
Peanut butter		51 mg
Tofu, calcium processed	85 g (~1/3 cup)	49 mg
Blackeyed peas, cooked	90 g (~1/2 cup)	47 mg
Yogurt, plain, nonfat	225 g (1-8 oz container)	43 mg
Whole wheat bread	50 g (2 slices)	43 mg
Molasses, blackstrap	1 Tbsp.	43 mg
Banana	One 9"	41 mg

High: 20% DV or more

Good: 10-19% DV

Figure 11.23 **Food sources of magnesium.** Most of the magnesium in the diet comes from plant foods such as grains, vegetables, and legumes.
Source: U.S. Department of Agriculture, Agricultural Research Service. 1999. USDA Nutrient Database for Standard Reference, Release 13. Nutrient Data Laboratory Home Page, http://www.nal.usda.gov/fnic/foodcomp.

hypermagnesemia An abnormally high concentration of magnesium in the blood.

hypertension When resting blood pressure persistently exceeds 140 mm Hg systolic or 90 mm Hg diastolic.

systolic Pertaining to a heart contraction. Systolic blood pressure is measured during a heart contraction, a time period known as systole.

diastolic Pertaining to the time between heart contractions. Diastolic blood pressure is measured at the point of maximum cardiac relaxation.

essential hypertension Hypertension for which no specific cause can be identified. Ninety to 95 percent of people with hypertension have essential hypertension.

Quick Bites

Do onions make you cry?

The cabbage and onion families have sulfur-based compounds that are transformed into odiferous compounds when their tissues are broken. Cutting into a raw onion mixes the contents of its cells, bringing enzymes into contact with an odorless precursor substance apparently derived from the sulfur-containing amino acid cysteine. The volatile result, a powerful sulfur-containing irritant, causes most people's eyes to water, apparently by dissolving in fluids that surround the eye and forming sulfuric acid.

Hypermagnesemia

Hypermagnesemia, an abnormally high concentration of magnesium in the blood, is uncommon in the absence of kidney disease. People with kidney failure, especially if they use magnesium-containing antacids or laxatives, are most likely to suffer hypermagnesemia. High blood magnesium leads to nausea and general weakness. The UL established by the Food and Nutrition Board recommends that healthy people not take more than 350 milligrams of magnesium per day as a supplement or in medicines. Physicians sometimes intentionally administer high doses of magnesium during pregnancy to stop premature labor. This requires frequent monitoring to avoid toxicity that can lead to respiratory paralysis and death.

Key Concepts: *Magnesium is a cofactor for more than 300 enzymes. Magnesium is required for cardiac and nerve function and it helps form ATP. Sixty percent of magnesium is stored in bone. The RDA for magnesium in adults is 400 milligrams per day for men and 310 milligrams per day for women. Whole grains and vegetables are good sources of magnesium. People who suffer from chronic diarrhea or vomiting can be at risk for magnesium deficiency. Alcoholism is associated with magnesium deficiency because alcoholics are often malnourished and because alcohol stimulates urinary loss of magnesium.*

Sulfur

Sulfur (S) is different from the other minerals discussed in this chapter because it is not used alone as a nutrient. In the body, sulfur primarily is a component of organic compounds, such as the vitamins biotin and thiamin and the amino acids methionine and cysteine. Sulfur in these amino acids is especially important to protein structure. Disulfide bridges that form when sulfur atoms bind to each other cause proteins to fold in specific ways as sulfur atoms along the protein are pulled together. A protein's folding and shape is critical for its function. Sulfur is also important in some of the liver's drug detoxifying pathways. In its ionic form, sulfate (SO_4^{2-}), sulfur helps maintain acid-base balance.

Sulfur-containing amino acids provide ample sulfur for anyone who consumes adequate amounts of protein. Deficiency of sulfur is unknown in humans.

Key Concepts: *Sulfur is a component of the amino acids methionine and cysteine, as well as of the vitamins biotin and thiamin. Sulfur is important in drug detoxification and in maintaining acid-base balance. Since sulfur is a component of all proteins, a diet sufficient in protein contains adequate sulfur.*

Major Minerals and Health

Hypertension

Hypertension, or high blood pressure, affects nearly 25 percent of adult Americans. Hypertension is defined as a persistent **systolic** blood pressure of 140 or higher, or a **diastolic** blood pressure of 90 or higher, or both. The systolic blood pressure is the arterial pressure exerted when the heart beats and sends blood into the body. The diastolic blood pressure is the arterial pressure when the heart relaxes between beats. Normal blood pressure is about 120/80 or lower. The majority of people with high blood pressure have **essential hypertension**, meaning that the cause of their hypertension is unknown.

When hypertension is left untreated or is treated ineffectively, the heart can become enlarged, making it work much less efficiently. Hypertension accelerates atherosclerosis (see Chapter 5, "Lipids," for more on atherosclerosis) by scarring, narrowing, and reducing the elasticity of the arteries and arterioles. This may limit the heart's ability to supply nutrients and oxygen, and limit the functional capacity of the organs and tissues. A narrowed and less elastic artery is also at risk for blockage by a blood clot, which could result in a heart attack or stroke. The brain, kidneys, and heart are especially sensitive to the effects of high blood pressure.

Blood pressure tends to increase with age in Western societies. In the United States more than half the people older than 65 have hypertension. Risk varies among ethnic groups. African Americans are at highest risk for hypertension. They face high blood pressure at a greater rate and usually at a much earlier age than Caucasians.[35]

Sodium and Hypertension

Many experts believe that a major cause of essential hypertension in many cases is a high-sodium diet combined with a genetic predisposition to hypertension. In population studies, people from high sodium-consuming countries have a higher incidence of hypertension than people from countries with lower sodium intakes. Researchers have studied primitive people from different parts of the world whose diets contain very little sodium. These people have no hypertension, and their blood pressure does not rise with age as long as they continue to eat their traditional diets. However, if they adopt "modern" diets, their blood pressure rises and some develop hypertension.[36]

The consumption of large amounts of sodium is a relatively recent phenomenon. Our distant ancestors ate very limited amounts of sodium, and much higher levels of potassium than we now typically consume. Our bodies appear to be poorly adapted to handle our modern high-sodium, low-potassium diets.[37]

The treatment of hypertension with sodium restriction remains controversial, as does the recommendation that *all* Americans limit their sodium intake to no more than 2,400 milligrams per day.[38] About 10 to 15 percent of people with hypertension are particularly sensitive to salt. If these people decrease their salt intake, their blood pressure improves significantly. For non-salt-sensitive hypertensive individuals, reducing salt intake has only a minimal effect on blood pressure. However, a review of clinical trials on the effects of sodium reduction concluded that (1) there is no evidence that moderate sodium reduction presents any hazards and (2) the blood pressure reduction that would result from a substantial lowering of dietary sodium in the U.S. population could reduce cardiovascular morbidity and mortality.[39] Further, the National Heart, Lung and Blood Institute (NHLBI) continues to support reduction of sodium intake to 2,400 milligrams per day as recommended by the National High Blood Pressure Education Program, the American Heart Association, and the *Dietary Guidelines for Americans.*[40]

Other Dietary Factors

Sodium is not the only dietary factor associated with hypertension. Excess weight tends to raise blood pressure; regular exercise and weight loss help to reduce blood pressure. Reducing consumption of alcohol also tends to reduce blood pressure, and improves the effectiveness of antihypertensive medications. Diets rich in calcium, magnesium, and potassium reduce blood pressure as well.[41] The mechanism for the impact of these minerals

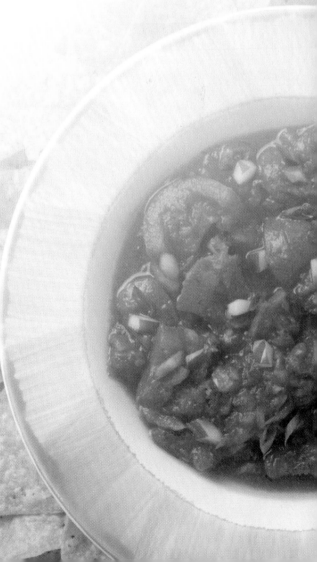

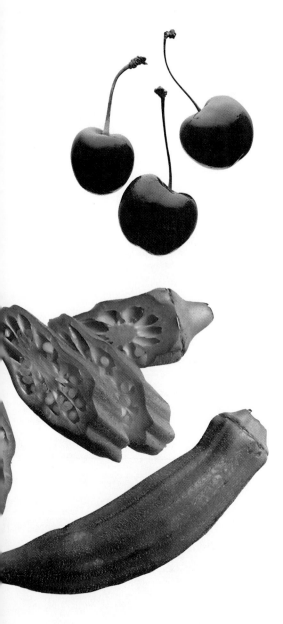

on hypertension may be due in part to their interrelationship with sodium metabolism.

The DASH (Dietary Approaches to Stop Hypertension) study, a multicenter NHLBI-sponsored trial, tested the effects of different dietary patterns on blood pressure. After a control period, the 459 subjects in this study received one of three diets for an eight-week period:

1. *Control Diet:* macronutrient and fiber content equal to U.S. average; 4 servings of fruits and vegetables per day; $1/2$ serving of dairy products per day; potassium, magnesium, and calcium levels close to the 25th percentile of U.S. consumption

2. *Fruit and Vegetable Diet:* 8.5 servings of fruits and vegetables per day; potassium and magnesium levels at the 75th percentile of U.S. consumption; other nutrients similar to control diet

3. *Combination Diet:* 10 servings of fruits and vegetables per day; 2.7 servings of low-fat dairy products per day; less fat, saturated fat, and cholesterol than control diet; potassium, magnesium and calcium levels at the 75th percentile of U.S. consumption[42]

The sodium content of the diets averaged about 3,000 milligrams per day. The study excluded subjects who were taking antihypertensive medications, unless their physicians had given them permission to discontinue their medication for the course of the study.[43]

Both the fruit and vegetable diet and the combination diet significantly lowered the systolic and diastolic blood pressure in all subjects and in subgroups analyzed by sex, ethnicity, and hypertensive/normotensive states. For hypertensive individuals, the DASH combination diet lowered blood pressure comparably to antihypertensive drugs. It is believed that adoption of the DASH combination diet could result in a downward shift in the incidence and severity of the disease.[44] Because recent data indicate a slight rise in the incidence of stroke, increased kidney disease, and heart failure, and a leveling of the heart disease death rate among U.S. adults, the NHLBI recommends that all Americans, not just those with hypertension, follow the DASH combination diet.[45] **Table 11.2** shows sample meals from the three DASH diets used in the study.

Preliminary results from a follow-up study, the DASH-Sodium trial, support both the DASH-style dietary changes and lower sodium intake. This study used different levels of sodium restriction (3,300 mg/d, 2,400 mg/d, and 1,500 mg/d) and two diet plans (a "typical" American diet and the DASH diet). About 41 percent of the participants had hypertension. Reducing sodium intake lowered blood pressure for both dietary treatments; lower sodium intake resulted in lower blood pressure. The DASH diet in combination with sodium restriction was more effective than the low-sodium control diet.[46]

Key Concepts: *Hypertension is a risk factor for atherosclerosis, kidney disease, and stroke. Blood pressure tends to rise with age, and rates of hypertension are higher among African Americans. Sodium intake has an impact on blood pressure, especially in those who are salt sensitive. There is also evidence that low intake of potassium, calcium, and possibly magnesium may also contribute to the development of hypertension. Eating a diet with lots of fresh foods and avoiding processed foods will not only improve the balance of minerals in our diet, but may also reduce risk of disease.*

Osteoporosis

Osteoporosis (literally, "porous bone") is a disease characterized by low-density bone mass and structural deterioration of bone tissue, leading to bone fragility and an increased susceptibility to fractures especially of the hip, spine, and wrist. Osteoporosis is often called a "silent disease" because bone loss occurs over many years without symptoms. It may remain undiagnosed until the bones become so weak that a sudden strain, bump, or fall causes a fracture. Sometimes the fracture occurs first, such as in a hip, and causes the fall! Osteoporosis is the major cause of bone fractures in older adults, primarily postmenopausal women.

More than 25 million Americans are affected by osteoporosis, which makes it a major public health problem. Eighty percent of those afflicted are women, but one-third of all men will also be affected by age 75. One half of all women and one in five men will have an osteoporosis-related fracture in their lifetime. Osteoporosis is responsible for 1.5 million fractures annually, including more than 300,000 hip fractures, 500,000 vertebral fractures, and 200,000 wrist fractures. The estimated annual cost for treatment of osteoporotic fractures is $10 to $15 billion.[47] Risk factors for osteoporosis are listed in **Table 11.3**.

Table 11.2 Sample DASH Menus

Meal	Control Diet	Fruit and Vegetable Diet	Combination Diet
Breakfast	Apple juice Sugar-frosted flakes White toast Butter Jelly Whole milk	Orange juice Oat bran muffin Raisins Dried apricots Butter	Orange juice Granola bar Fat-free yogurt 1% low-fat milk Banana
Lunch	Ham-and-chicken sandwich on white bread, with lettuce, pickles, mustard, and mayonnaise Fruit cocktail	Ham-and-Swiss cheese sandwich on whole-wheat bread Banana	Smoked turkey sandwich on whole-wheat bread with lettuce and mayonnaise Fresh orange
Dinner	Spiced cod Scallion rice Carrots Butter French rolls	Spiced cod Scallion rice Lima beans Butter Dinner rolls Melon balls	Spiced cod Scallion rice Spinach Margarine Dinner rolls Melon balls 1% low-fat milk
Snack	Graham crackers Vanilla frosting Tropical fruit punch	Peanuts	Peanuts Dried apricots Melon balls

Source: Karanja NM, Obarzanek E, Lin P-H, McCullough ML, Phillips KM, Swain JF, Champagne CM, Hoben KP. Descriptive characteristics of the dietary patterns used in the Dietary Approaches to Stop Hypertension trial. *J Am Diet Assoc.* 1999;99(8):S19.

Table 11.3 Risk Factors for Osteoporosis

Advanced age
Female
Thin and/or small frame
Family history of osteoporosis
Early menopause, whether natural or surgically-induced
Low testosterone levels in men
Abnormal absence of menstrual periods (amenorrhea)
Anorexia nervosa or bulimia nervosa
Medical conditions, such as thyroid disease, rheumatoid arthritis, and problems that block intestinal absorption of calcium
Use of certain medications, such as corticosteroids and anticonvulsants
Insufficient dietary calcium
Lack of weight-bearing exercise
Cigarette smoking
Excessive use of alcohol or caffeine

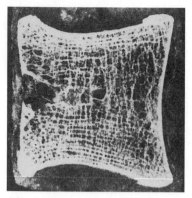

(a)

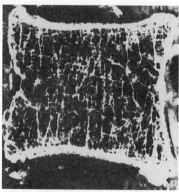

(b)

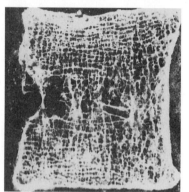

(c)

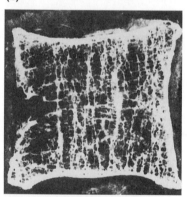

(d)

Figure 11.24 **Healthy and osteoporotic bone in women.** The photos above show the progression of Osteoporosis in the lumbar vertebra of (a) a 29-year-old woman, (b) a 40-year-old woman, (c) a 84-year-old woman, (d) a 92-year-old woman.

Development of Osteoporosis

Normal maintenance of bone tissue relies on the balance of activity between osteoblasts and osteoclasts. Bone mass typically peaks sometime around age 30. At about age 40, bone breakdown begins to exceed formation, and the progressive loss of bone begins. Adequate intake of calcium and vitamin D in the early years help to maximize bone mass, so that even when bone loss begins, an individual is a long way from reaching a lowered bone mineral density that is associated with fractures. Women are at highest risk for osteoporosis because the decline of estrogen secretion that occurs with menopause accelerates the rate of bone loss. By age 65, some women have lost half their skeletal mass. Women who reach menopause with low bone mass are at risk for later fractures. **Figure 11.24** shows typical changes in bone density in women that are associated with aging.

The only way to detect osteoporosis before a fracture occurs is to measure bone density. Typically bone-density measurement requires a high-tech bone-scanning device called dual energy x-ray absorptiometer (DEXA or DXA). Testing is expensive and access may be limited. Newer screening methods such as a portable scanning device called the Sahara, and a urine test that helps identify fast losers of bone, may improve early identification of osteoporosis so that measures can be taken to reduce or perhaps even reverse bone loss.

Calcium and Osteoporosis

Most people link the mineral calcium with osteoporosis. Calcium is certainly an important nutrient in bone formation, but it is not the only one. Normal development and mineralization of bone requires calcium, phosphorus, fluoride, magnesium, vitamin D, vitamin A, vitamin K, and protein.

Experts agree that adequate calcium intake throughout life can help prevent osteoporosis. Increasing calcium intake during childhood and adolescence helps to maximize peak bone mass. Even in adulthood, adequate calcium intake will slow bone loss, and in postmenopausal women, measures to ensure adequate calcium intake have been shown to reduce fracture rates.

Other Dietary and Lifestyle Factors

Vitamin D is important for calcium absorption and bone maintenance. Aging decreases our ability to produce the active form of vitamin D.[48] To prevent deficiency, milk and some cereals are fortified with vitamin D. Some older adults who do not include milk in the diet may need supplements. Diets that are very high in sodium can increase calcium excretion and may increase risk for osteoporosis. Also, phytates and oxalates, caffeine, and smoking can reduce calcium absorption and increase excretion rates. Regular weight-bearing exercise enhances bone remodeling and strength, and is important in preventing loss of bone mass. A recent study of postmenopausal women shows that higher protein intake is associated with a reduced rate of hip fractures.[49] Osteoporosis can be prevented to a significant extent by maintaining adequate calcium and vitamin D intake throughout life, performing weight-bearing exercise, and in the case of postmenopausal women, taking estrogen supplements.[50]

Key Concepts: *Osteoporosis is the progressive loss of bone mass, resulting in fragile bones that are susceptible to fracture. Osteoporosis primarily affects post-menopausal women who, as a result of reduced estrogen secretion, experience an accelerated rate of bone loss with aging. Adequate calcium intake early in life helps maximize peak bone mass and reduce the risk of osteoporosis. Adequate amounts of vitamin D and regular exercise are also important to maintain bone health.*

Label [to] **Table**

After reading this chapter you should have a greater appreciation of the importance of calcium in your diet. If you don't consume dairy products, or consume them infrequently, getting enough of it can be difficult. Today, soft drinks have become more popular than milk. To combat your potential lack of calcium, more and more food products are being fortified with this mineral. Did you know that many brands of orange juice now provide as much calcium per serving as a glass of milk? Check out the following Nutrition Facts label from a calcium-fortified orange juice.

This orange juice contains 35% of the Daily Value for calcium (1,000 mg). That's 350 milligrams of the 1,000 milligrams you need. That's a pretty good hit of calcium for just one 8-ounce glass of OJ. Surprisingly, it's slightly more than an 8-ounce cup of milk. You can see from the comparison at the bottom of the label that this fortified juice increases the calcium %DV from 2% (in regular orange juice) to 35%.

Look at the label again. How much fiber can you get from this juice? That's right; fiber isn't listed on the label because most juices don't contain fiber. Since the majority of Americans need more fiber in their diets, it's a good idea not to go overboard on juices and choose whole pieces of fruit as well.

In addition to being a great source of calcium, this orange juice contains folate (another hard-to-get nutrient), lots of vitamin C, other B vitamins, and potassium. As part of a breakfast or even with a snack, this juice packs a lot of nutrients in its 110 calories.

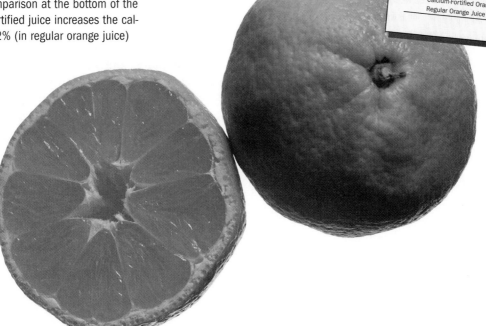

Nutrition Facts

Serving Size: 8 fl oz (240 mL)
Servings Per Container: 8

Amount Per Serving

Calories 110   Calories from fat 0

	% Daily Value*
Total Fat 0g	
Sodium 0mg	0%
Potassium 450mg	13%
Total Carbohydrate 26g	9%
Sugars 22g	
Protein 2g	

Vitamin C 180%	•	Calcium 35%
Thiamin 10%	•	Niacin 4%
Vitamin B 6%	•	Folate 15%

Not a significant source or saturated fat, cholesterol, dietary fiber, vitamin A, and iron.

* Percent Daily Values are based on a 2,000 calorie diet.

% of Daily Value of Calcium:	
Calcium-Fortified Orange Juice	35%
Regular Orange Juice	2%
% of Daily Value of Viatmin C:	
Calcium-Fortified Orange Juice	180%
Regular Orange Juice	120%

LEARNING *Portfolio* chapter 11

Key Terms

	page		page
aldosterone		hypomagnesemia	429
[al-DOS-ter-own]	409	hyponatremia	415
angiotensin I		hypophosphatemia	427
[an-jee-oh-TEN-sin one]	408	insensible water loss	407
angiotensin II	408	ion	404
angiotensinogen	408	linear growth	420
anion	404	major minerals	413
antidiuretic hormone (ADH)	407	metabolic alkalosis	419
calmodulin	420	osmolarity	407
cation	404	osmoreceptors	407
chloride shift	418	osmosis	404
ciliary action	420	osmotic pressure	404
diastolic	430	osteoblasts	419
electrolyte [ih-LEK-tro-lite]	403	osteoclasts	419
essential hypertension	430	oxalate [oxalic acid]	413
fibrin	420	phosphorylation	426
heat capacity	403	phytate [phytic acid]	413
hydrogen bond	403	plasma	404
hydroxyapatite	419	renin	408
hypercalcemia	425	salts	404
hyperkalemia	417	semipermeable membrane	404
hypermagnesemia	430	sodium-potassium pump	404
hypernatremia	415	solute	404
hyperparathyroidism	427	systolic	430
hyperphosphatemia	428	trace minerals	413
hypertension	430	vasoconstrictor	407
hypervolemia	415	vasopressin	407
hypocalcemia	425		
hypokalemia	417		

Study Points

➤ Water is the most essential nutrient; we can live much longer without food than without water. Recommended water intake is 1.0 milliliter to 1.5 milliliter per kilocalorie expended.

➤ Water is important for the movement of nutrients and waste, cellular reactions, temperature regulation, and acid-base balance. Moreover, fluids in the body lubricate and cushion joints, cleanse the eyes, and moisten the food we eat.

➤ Dissolved ions, or electrolytes, help to maintain normal fluid balance.

➤ Fluid is lost from the body via the urine, skin, feces, and lungs. The hormones ADH and aldosterone regulate fluid excretion from the kidneys.

➤ The thirst response stimulates fluid intake. Caffeine, alcohol, and diuretic medications increase fluid excretion. Dehydration results when fluid intake is less than losses; it can seriously impair physical and mental performance.

➤ Minerals are inorganic elements, and are categorized as major or trace depending on the amount in the body and the amount needed in the diet.

➤ The bioavailability of minerals may be affected by excess intake of single mineral supplements, phytate, oxalate, and fiber in plant foods, and mineral status in the body.

➤ Sodium, the major extracellular cation, helps regulate water distribution and blood pressure. Sodium needs (500 mg per day) are well below average intakes (3,000 mg to 6,000 mg per day).

➤ Potassium, the major cation in the intracellular fluid, is necessary for nerve and muscle function. It is provided in the diet mainly from unprocessed foods including fruits and vegetables.

➤ Chloride is the major extracellular anion, and a component of stomach acid. Chloride deficiency is most often associated with prolonged vomiting.

➤ **Calcium**, the most abundant mineral in the body, is found in bones. It also functions in blood clotting, nerve and muscle function, and cellular metabolism. Major dietary sources of calcium are dairy products, calcium-fortified foods, and certain vegetables.

➤ **Phosphorus** is a key component of ATP, DNA, RNA, phospholipids, and lipoproteins. Because phosphorus is widespread in foods, dietary phosphorus intake is rarely inadequate.

➤ **Plant foods** like whole grains and vegetables are important sources of magnesium, which is a cofactor for hundreds of enzymes. Low levels of magnesium are associated with kidney disease, alcoholism, and use of diuretics.

➤ **Sulfur** does not function alone as a nutrient, but as a component of certain amino acids, and the vitamins biotin and thiamin.

➤ **Hypertension** increases risk for heart disease, stroke, and kidney disease. Sodium has long been linked to hypertension, but only some individuals are salt sensitive. Other dietary factors linked to hypertension include high chloride intake and low potassium, calcium, and magnesium intake.

➤ **Osteoporosis** results from excessive bone loss. Postmenopausal women are at highest risk for osteoporosis. Adequate dietary calcium, vitamin D, and physical activity throughout the life span reduces the risk for osteoporosis.

Study **Questions**

1. **What are the two main factors that affect absorption of a mineral?**

2. **What functions does chloride perform in the human body?**

3. **What is the role of aldosterone in the body, and how is it released?**

4. **Name four of the main biological functions of water?**

5. **What is the recommended intake level for sodium?**

6. **What three major minerals affect bone health?**

7. **What are the major functions of calcium, other than its relation to bone health?**

8. **How does the body compensate for low calcium intake?**

9. **Which people have a high risk of hypomagnesemia?**

10. **How does the body use sulfur? What is its role in protein function?**

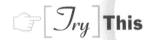

☞ [*Try*] **This**

Calcium Food Diary

The purpose of this exercise is to see how much calcium you consume in a typical day. Start by keeping a food diary for three days (two weekdays and one weekend day). While keeping the diary, try not to change your eating habits. (Altering the way you eat would reduce the accuracy of your project.) After completing the diary, add up the amounts of calcium you consume using Appendix A in the back of your textbook or using the EatRight Analysis software. The calcium AI value for adults between the ages of 19 and 50 is 1,000 milligrams. How does your average calcium intake compare? If your calcium intake is not meeting the AI, how can you include more calcium in your diet?

Osmosis Experiment

Purchase some celery and let it sit for a week or two until it becomes limp. When the celery looks limp and lifeless, fill your sink with cold water and soak the celery. When it has soaked for several hours, take the celery out and examine its appearance. Notice anything different? Since the crispness of celery is due to osmotic pressure, when you soaked the limp celery, it absorbed water into its cells and became crisp again.

What About Bobbie?

Let's take a look at Bobbie's intake of water and the major minerals calcium, magnesium, and sodium. Refer to Chapter 1 to refresh yourself with Bobbie's one-day intake. How do you think she did?

Water

Bobbie's fluid intake is on the low side. She consumed 10 ounces of coffee with breakfast, a 12-ounce soda with lunch, 16 ounces of water with her afternoon snack, and another 12-ounce diet soda with dinner. Caffeinated beverages (coffee, and possibly the sodas) are diuretics, and therefore, are not the best hydrators. Her fluid intake is about 1.5 liters from beverages and 1.0 liter from food. This is at the low end of the recommended fluid intake of 2.4 to 3.6 liters for someone consuming approximately 2,400 kilocalories per day (1–1.5 ml/kcal consumed). What could Bobbie do differently? The following tips could help her increase her fluid consumption:

* Leave for class with a water bottle in her backpack so she can sip on it throughout the day.
* Drink a glass of water with every caffeine-containing fluid to off-set the diuretic effect—this means water before her coffee and diet soda.
* Include fluids like water, juices, or milk with every meal and snack. She didn't drink anything with her evening snack.
* Mix fruit juice with sparkling water for a change of pace.

Calcium

Bobbie's calcium intake was quite low on the day she recorded her food intake. She consumed 745 milligrams but the Adequate Intake (AI) for a 20-year-old woman is 1,000 milligrams. If this day reflects her usual intake, then she is at risk of poor bone mineralization and a lower than average peak bone mass. This increases her risk of osteoporosis.

Magnesium

Bobbie's intake of magnesium was 330 milligrams and the Recommended Dietary Allowance (RDA) for a woman her age is 320 milligrams. If this one-day record reflects her usual eating, she is consuming an adequate amount of magnesium and does not need to increase her intake of this mineral. Some of the best sources of magnesium in her diet were the banana, pizza, and spaghetti noodles.

Sodium

Bobbie's intake of 4,659 milligrams of sodium was much higher than the recommended amount (2,400 mg) and close to the average American's intake. This should not be a surprise since most of Bobbie's meals are either convenience items or prepared by someone else (e.g., the school's cafeteria), which makes it hard to control sodium content. The biggest contributors to her high intake of sodium were the sourdough bread, turkey lunchmeat, pickle (on sandwich), salsa, spaghetti sauce, and pizza. Bobbie would benefit from drinking the extra water discussed above since her intake of sodium is so high.

References

1 Institute of Medicine, Food and Nutrition Board, Commission on Life Sciences, National Research Council. *Recommended Dietary Allowances.* 10th ed. Washington, DC: National Academy Press; 1989.

2 Kleiner SM. Water: an essential but overlooked nutrient. *J Am Diet Assoc.* 1999;2:200–206.

3 Levine B. Water: the elixir of life. *Current Concepts and Perspectives in Nutrition.* 1999;9(1). (publication of the Nutrition Information Center, Clinical Nutrition Research Unit of Weill Medical College of Cornell University, Ithaca, NY.)

4 Davis JM, Burgess WA, Slentz CA, Bartoli WP. Fluid availability of sports drinks differing in carbohydrate type and concentration. *Am J Clin Nutr.* 1990;51(6):1054–1057; and Millard-Stafford M, Rosskopf LB, Snow TK, Hinson BT. Water versus carbohydrate-electrolyte ingestion before and during a 15-km run in the heat. *Int J Sport Nutr.* 1997;7(1):26–38.

5 Johnson R, Tulin B. *Travel fitness.* Champaign, IL: Human Kinetics; 1995.

6 Guyton AC, Hall JE, *Textbook of Medical Physiology.* 9th ed. Philadelphia: WB Saunders; 1996.

7 Ibid.

8 Ibid.

9 Ibid.

10 Neuhauser-Berthold M, Beine S, Verwied SC, Luhrmann RM. Coffee consumption and total body water homeostasis as measured by fluid balance and bioelectrical impedance analysis. *Ann Nutr Metab.* 1997;41:29–36.

11 Kleiner SM. Op. cit.

12 Ibid.

13 *Nutrition and Your Health: Dietary Guidelines for Americans.* 5th ed. US Department of Agriculture, US Department of Health and Human Services; 2000. Home and Garden Bulletin 232.

14 Food and Nutrition Board. Op. cit.

15 Morris CD. Effect of dietary sodium restriction on overall nutrient intake. *Am J Clin Nutr.* 1997;65(2 suppl):687S–691S.

16 Cogan MG. *Fluid and Electrolytes.* Englewood Cliffs, NJ: Appleton & Lange; 1991.

17 Kaplan NM. *Clinical Hypertension.* Baltimore, MD: Williams & Wilkins. 1998;48–51.

18 Guyton AC, Hall JE. Op. cit.

19 Fauci AS, Braunwald E, Isselbacher KJ, Wilson JD, Martin JB, Kasper D, Hauser SL, Longo DL. *Harrison's Principles of Internal Medicine.* 14th ed. New York: McGraw-Hill; 1997.

20 Waltzer KB. Simple, sensible preventive measures for managed care settings. *Geriatrics.* 1998;53(10):65–68, 75–77, 81; quiz 82.

21 National Institutes of Health (NIH). Osteoporosis Prevention, Diagnosis, and Therapy. NIH Consensus Statement; 2000, March 27–29;17(2):1–34.

22 Frazão E, ed. *America's Eating Habits: Changes and Consequences.* Washington, DC: US Department of Agriculture. Food and Rural Economics Division. Economic Research Service; April 1999. Agriculture Information Bulletin 750 (AIB-750).

23 National Institutes of Health (NIH). Optimal Calcium Intake. NIH Consensus Statement 1994, June 6–8; 12(4):1–31.

24 Institute of Medicine, Food and Nutrition Board. *Dietary Reference Intakes for Calcium, Phosphorus, Magnesium, Vitamin D, and Fluoride.* Washington, DC: National Academy Press; 1999

25 National Institutes of Health (NIH). Op. cit.

26 Ibid.

27 Ibid.

28 Ibid.

29 Institute of Medicine, Food and Nutrition Board. Op. cit.

30 Ibid.

31 Ibid.

32 Stein JH. *Internal Medicine.* St. Louis: Mosby-Year Book: 1994.

33 Institute of Medicine, Food and Nutrition Board. Op. cit.

34 Fauci AS, et al. Op. cit.

35 Zemel MB. Dietary pattern and hypertension: the DASH study. *Nutr Rev.* 1997;55:303–308.

36 Ibid.

37 Kaplan NM. Op. cit.

38 Kaplan NM. The dietary guideline for sodium: should we shake it up? No. *Am J Clin Nutr.* 2000;71:1020–1026; and McCarron DA. The dietary guideline for sodium: should we shake it up? Yes! *Am J Clin Nutr.* 2000;71:1013–1019.

39 USDA Center for Nutrition Policy and Promotion. Dietary guidance on sodium: should we take it with a grain of salt? *Nutrition Insights;* May 1997.

40 National Institutes of Health, National Heart, Lung, and Blood Institute. Statement on Sodium Intake and High Blood Pressure.www.nih.gov/news/pr/aug98/nhlbi-17.htm. Accessed 8/1/00; Krauss RM, Eckel RH, Howard B, et al. AHA Dietary Guidelines Revision 2000: A statement for healthcare professionals from the Nutrition Committee of the American Heart Association. *Circulation,* 2000; 102:2296–2311; and *Nutrition and Your Health: Dietary Guidelines for Americans.* US Department of Agriculture, US Department of Health and Human Services; 2000. Home and Garden Bulletin 232.

41 Kotchen TA, McCarron DA. Dietary electrolytes and blood pressure: a statement for healthcare professionals from the American Heart Association Nutrition Committee. *Circulation.* 1998;6:613–617.

42 Harsha DW, Lin PW, Obarzanek E et al. Dietary approaches to stop hypertension: a summary of study results. *J Am Diet Assoc.* 1999;99(8 suppl):S35–S39

43 Vogt TM, Appel LJ, Obarzanek E, et al. Dietary approaches to stop hypertension: rationale, design, and methods. *J Am Diet Assoc.* 1999;99(8 suppl):S12–S18.

44 The DASH Study. Research and results. http://dash.bwh.harvard.edu/research.html. (1999;99(8 suppl):S12–S18. 10/25/00; and Harsha DW, et al. Op. cit.

45 Recommendations updated for hypertension. *Harvard Health Letter.* 1998;1:6–7.

46 Svetkey LP, Sacks FM, Obarzanek E, et al. The DASH Diet, Sodium Intake and Blood Pressure Trial (DASH-Sodium): rationale and design. DASH-Sodium Collaborative Research Group. *J Am Diet Assoc.* 1999;99:S96–S104; and "NHLBI Study Shows Large Blood Pressure Benefit From Reduced Dietary Sodium." NIH News Release, 5-17-00. http://www.nhlbi.nih.gov/press/may17-00.htm. Accessed 7/26/00.

47 National Institutes of Health (NIH). Osteoporosis Prevention, Diagnosis, and Therapy. Op. cit.

48 Fauci AS, et al. Op. cit.

49 Munger RG, Cerhan JR, Chiu BC-H. Prospective study of dietary protein intake and risk of hip fracture in post-menopausal women. *Am J Clin Nutr.* 1999;69:147–152.

50 New SA, Bolton-Smith C, Grubb DA, Reid DM. Nutritional influences on bone mineral density: a cross-sectional study in premenopausal women. *Am J Clin Nutr.* 1997;65(6): 1831–1839.

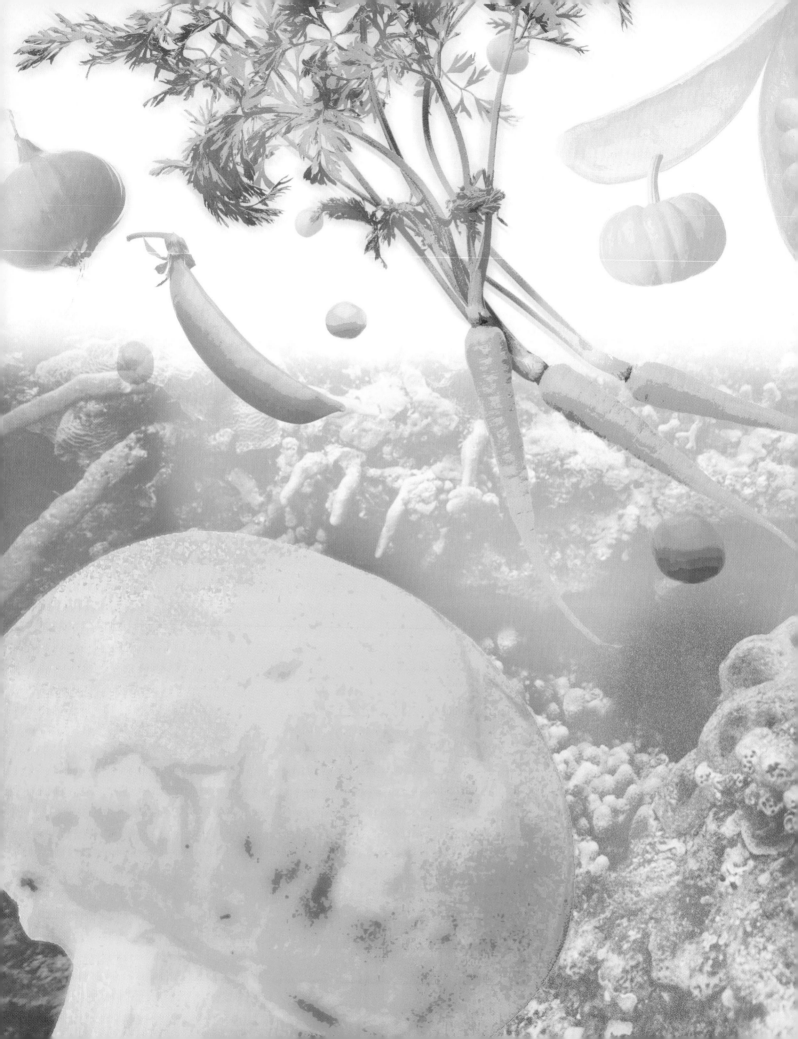

Chapter 12

Trace Minerals

Think About It

1 Do you think a person with an infection should take iron supplements?

2 You disclose to a friend that you tend to be low in iron. She knows you are a vegetarian and suggests you drink milk. What false assumption might she be making?

3 You know that a number of people in your family have had goiter or take thyroxine. You also notice that none of these people like fish. Any relationship?

4 Some people argue that fluoridation is overdone. What is your position? Would you vote for fluoridating all water supplies?

Fyi for your Information

This chapter's FYI boxes include practical information on the following topics:

• Zinc and the Common Cold

• Selenium and Cancer

• Chromium, Exercise, and Body Composition

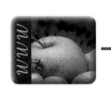

The web site for this book offers many useful tools and is a great source for additional nutrition information for both students and instructors. Visit the site at **nutrition.jbpub.com** for information on trace minerals. You'll find exercises that explore the following topics:

• Highlighting Heme

• The ADA's Stand on Supplements

• What Food Labels Can Claim

• Glowing Thyriods!

Key to Illustrations

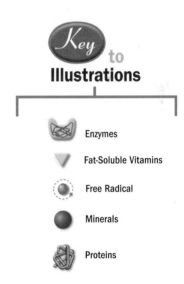

Enzymes

Fat-Soluble Vitamins

Free Radical

Minerals

Proteins

What About Bobbie?

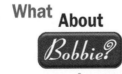

Track the choices Bobbie is making with the EatRight Analysis software.

One of your "meat-and-potatoes" friends argues that animal foods are the best sources of minerals because animals concentrate the minerals they eat from plants. Your vegetarian friend disagrees, saying that minerals are plentiful in plant foods, but processing removes them. Another friend contends that American agricultural practices have stripped the mineral content from the soil, and so supplements are really the only way to get adequate mineral intake. Who's right?

As you saw in the previous chapter, protein-rich animal foods are good sources of some minerals like calcium, phosphorus, and sulfur. Other major minerals (e.g., potassium and magnesium) are plentiful in plant foods.

This chapter focuses on trace minerals, that is, minerals present in the body in small quantities, and therefore needed by the body in small amounts. Meats are the best food sources for some of these minerals—iron and zinc, for instance. Whole grains are also good sources of several minerals, including iron, copper, selenium, and manganese. And water is a major source of fluoride, a mineral that often occurs naturally in water or is added during municipal water treatment.

But what about the mineral content of soil? (See **Figure 12.1**.) The mineral content of soil certainly influences the nutrient value of the plants that grow in it. This is especially true for the trace minerals selenium and iodine. How important is this to our dietary intake? Is the soil's mineral content depleted, as some supplement suppliers claim? Adequate nutrition is as important for healthy plants as it is for healthy livestock and people. If soil lacks a nutrient the plant needs, the plant will not grow. Fertilization adds nutrients to the soil and so does the natural degradation of rocks, plants, and animals. There is little evidence for specific nutritional claims based on the mineral content of the soil. In addition, few people consume only foods grown locally. A varied diet typically includes foods from many different locales and thus from a wide variety of soils.

What Are Trace Elements?

Trace elements are essential minerals found in a large variety of animal and plant foods; these nutrients have both regulatory and structural functions in the body. Trace elements differ from the major minerals (calcium, phosphorus, magnesium, etc.) in two ways. First, the dietary requirements for each of the trace elements are less than 100 milligrams per day. For example, iron and zinc intake recommendations for adults range from 12 milligrams to 15 milligrams per day, while the adult daily calcium recommendation is 1,000 milligrams per day. Second, the total amount of each trace element found in the body is small, less than 5 grams. For example, the total amount of iron in the body is 2 to 4 grams, or about the

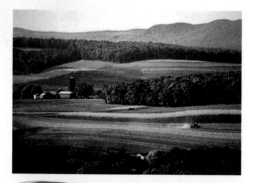

Figure 12.1 Mineral content of soil influences the nutrient value of plants.

amount of iron in a small nail. In contrast, a typical adult body contains more than *1,000* grams of calcium. **Figure 12.2** shows the trace elements on the periodic table.

Why Are Trace Elements Important?

Despite the minuscule amounts in the body, trace elements are crucial to many body functions including metabolic pathways. Trace elements serve as cofactors for enzymes, components of hormones, and participants in oxidation-reduction reactions. They are essential for growth and for normal functioning of the immune system. Deficiencies may cause delayed sexual maturation, poor growth, mediocre work performance, faulty immune function, tooth decay, and altered hormonal function.

Technological advances in recent years have triggered an explosion of exciting new research because scientists can now track trace elements throughout the body more effectively. Working together, nutritionists, biochemists, biologists, immunologists, geneticists, and epidemiologists are uncovering the mysteries behind many of these fascinating elements and finding new links between trace elements and a variety of diseases and genetic disorders.

Other Characteristics of Trace Elements

Foods from animal sources, particularly liver, are good sources of many trace minerals. Amounts in plant foods can differ dramatically from region to region, depending on the soil's mineral content. Even the maturity of a vegetable, fruit, or grain can influence its mineral content. Since actual mineral content is so variable, the values published in food composition tables can be misleading. Food tables, especially many of the popular

Quick Bites

Hair Analysis Is a Misguided Measure

Although discredited as a measure of trace mineral status in individuals, hair analysis is promoted with the claim that it can reveal mineral deficiencies. This measure lacks sensitivity and is unreliable. The color, diameter, and rate of growth of a person's hair, the season of the year, the geographic location, and the person's age and sex can affect the levels of minerals in hair. It is possible for hair concentration of an element (zinc, for example) to be high even though deficiency exists in the body. Hair dyes, colors, perming agents, and certain shampoos also alter the mineral content of hair.

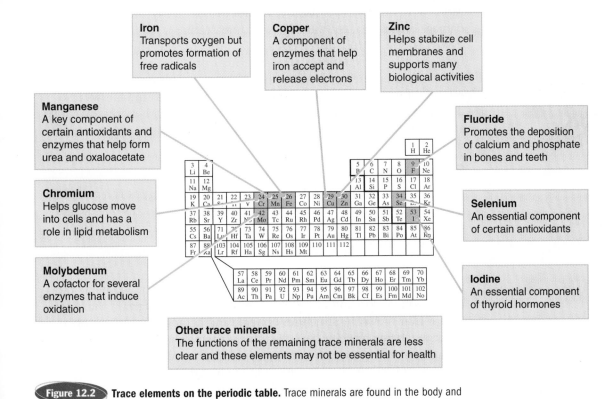

Figure 12.2 **Trace elements on the periodic table.** Trace minerals are found in the body and required in the diet in small amounts, but they play important roles in the body.

hemochromatosis A hereditary disorder whereby excessive absorption of iron results in abnormal iron deposits in the liver and other tissues.

ferrous iron (2+) The reduced form of iron most commonly found in food.

ferric iron (3+) The oxidized form of iron able to be bound to transferrin for transport.

heme A chemical complex with a central iron atom (ferric iron Fe^{3+}) that forms the oxygen-binding part of hemoglobin and myoglobin.

myoglobin The oxygen-transporting protein of muscle that resembles blood hemoglobin in function.

computerized nutrient databases, often have incomplete information about trace mineral content.

Even if we are fairly sure of the amount of a particular mineral in a food, other components of the diet can affect the mineral's bioavailability. Trace minerals are affected by the same factors that affect bioavailability of the major minerals (see **Figure 12.3**), including fiber, phytate, polyphenols, oxalate, the acidity of the intestinal environment, and the person's need for that mineral. High doses of other minerals can compete with trace minerals and inhibit their absorption. Treatment for mineral toxicity sometimes exploits these antagonistic interactions between minerals. For example, high doses of zinc may be given to patients with a genetic disorder of copper overload (Wilson's disease) because zinc inhibits copper absorption.

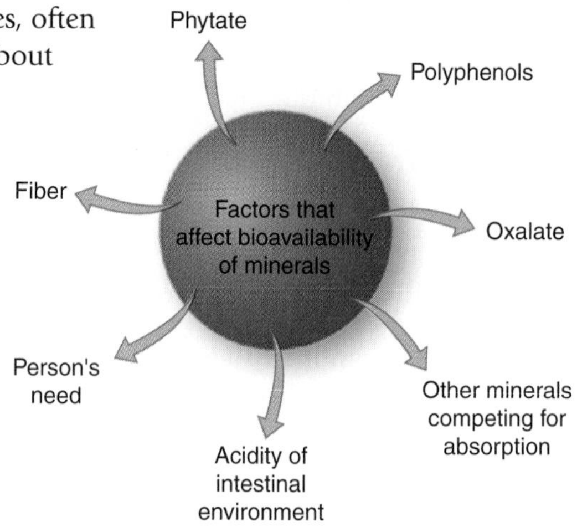

Figure 12.3 **Factors that affect the bioavailability of minerals.**

(Diagram labels: Phytate, Polyphenols, Fiber, Factors that affect bioavailability of minerals, Oxalate, Person's need, Acidity of intestinal environment, Other minerals competing for absorption)

Iron

Iron (Fe) is the fourth most abundant mineral in the earth's crust, yet iron deficiency is the most common nutrient deficiency in the world; from 500 to 600 million people suffer from iron-deficiency anemia.[1] On the other hand, **hemochromatosis**, a disease of excess iron absorption, is one of the most common inherited disorders. If not detected early, this disorder can damage organs severely, causing premature death.

Why is iron useful? Iron has a special property. It easily changes between its two oxidation states—**ferrous iron** (Fe^{2+}) and **ferric iron** (Fe^{3+})—by transferring electrons to other atoms. This property makes iron essential for numerous oxidation-reduction reactions, and allows it to bind reversibly with oxygen. The ability to shift easily between oxidative states also endows iron with its "dark side"—the ability to promote formation of destructive free radicals.

Functions of Iron

Iron is well known for its role in the body's use of energy; it is required for oxygen transport and is an essential component of hundreds of enzymes, many of which are involved in energy metabolism. In addition, iron plays a role in brain development and in the immune system.

Oxygen Transport

Iron's ability to carry oxygen is crucial. As a component of two **heme** proteins—hemoglobin and **myoglobin**—iron transports oxygen in the body. **Figure 12.4** shows the structures of heme and hemoglobin. With iron at the center, heme proteins have the unique chemical property of easily loading and unloading oxygen, and they give blood its red color. Hemoglobin in red blood cells transports oxygen in the blood, delivering it through the capillary beds to the tissues. Myoglobin in muscle facilitates the movement of oxygen into muscle cells.

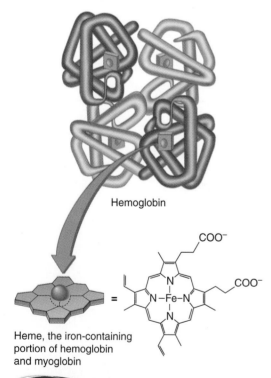

Hemoglobin

Heme, the iron-containing portion of hemoglobin and myoglobin

Figure 12.4 **Hemoglobin heme.** Iron in the heme portion of hemoglobin and myoglobin binds and releases oxygen easily. Hemoglobin in red blood cells transports oxygen in the blood and gives blood its red color.

Enzymes

Hundreds of enzymes have iron as a constituent or need it as a cofactor in reactions. One of iron's best-known roles is as a component of enzymes involved in energy metabolism. **Cytochromes**, for example, are heme-containing compounds critical to the electron transport chain.

The rate-limiting enzyme in gluconeogenesis requires iron. Iron also is a cofactor for antioxidant enzymes that protect against damaging free radicals. Interestingly, excess iron can also catalyze the formation of these highly reactive and potentially destructive substances.

Immune Function

Although iron is necessary for optimal immune function, it also serves as a nutrient for bacteria. Because iron supplementation can worsen an infection, this poses a dilemma for treating iron deficiencies in areas of the world with rampant infectious diseases. In the absence of an infection, however, current research indicates that iron supplementation is safe.[2]

Brain Function

Iron is essential for synthesizing neurotransmitters and for optimal brain growth.[3] Evidence also supports a role for iron in **myelinization**—the development of the myelin sheath around nerve fibers.[4] Iron's participation in brain development is an active area of research, since numerous studies report an association between iron-deficiency anemia in children and deficits in their behavioral and cognitive development. **Figure 12.5** shows the roles of iron.

Regulation of Iron in the Body

Total body iron averages approximately 3.8 grams in men and 2.3 grams in women. When the body has sufficient iron to meet its needs, most iron (greater than 70 percent) can be classified as functional iron; the remainder is storage or transport iron. More than 80 percent of the body's functional iron is found in the red blood cells as hemoglobin, and the rest is found in myoglobin and enzymes (e.g., cytochromes).[5] The body regulates its iron status by balancing absorption, transport, storage, and losses.[6] **Table 12.1** shows the normal distribution of iron in men and women.

cytochromes Heme proteins that transfer electrons in the electron transport chain through the alternate oxidation and reduction of iron.

myelinization Development of the myelin sheath, a substance that surrounds nerve fibers.

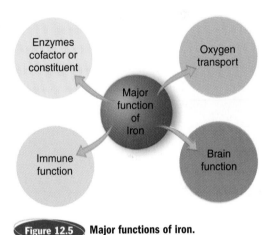

Figure 12.5 **Major functions of iron.**

Table 12.1 Normal Distribution of Iron-Containing Compounds (mg iron per kg body weight)

Compound	Men	Women
Storage Complexes		
Ferritin	9	4
Hemosiderin	4	1
Transport Protein		
Transferrin	<1	<1
Functional Compounds		
Hemoglobin	31	31
Myoglobin	4	4
Enzymes	2	2
TOTAL	50	42

Source: Recommendations to Report and Control Iron Deficiency in the United States. MMWR. 1998;(RR–3):7.

Quick Bites

But It Worked in the Lab...

The evidence is clear from carefully conducted clinical trials that supplements reduce iron deficiency during pregnancy. However, public health supplementation programs in communities often are unsuccessful. Why the discrepancy? Although the clinical trials support the distribution and consumption of iron pills, programs in the "real world" have several limiting factors: inadequate supply of iron tablets, limited access to care, poor or nonexistent nutrition counseling, lack of knowledge, and the uncomfortable side effects experienced by some women. These factors are important causes of noncompliance.

transferrin A protein synthesized in the liver that transports iron in the blood to the erythroblasts for use in heme synthesis.

ferritin A complex of iron and apoferritin that is a major storage form of iron.

heme iron The iron found in the hemoglobin and myoglobin of animal foods.

non-heme iron The iron in plants and the iron in animal foods that is not part of hemoglobin or myoglobin.

Iron Absorption

Iron absorption in the gastrointestinal tract is the primary regulator of iron levels. When the absorptive mechanism operates normally, a person maintains functional iron and tends to establish iron stores. The body's capacity to absorb dietary iron depends on the body's iron status and need, normal GI function, the amount and type of iron in the diet, and dietary factors that enhance or inhibit iron absorption.

Process of Iron Absorption. To avoid iron toxicity, the body regulates its absorption of iron (see **Figure 12.6**). Intestinal cells act as gatekeepers, forming an initial barrier that turns away excess (and potentially harmful) iron. Once admitted into the intestinal cell, iron has three potential fates:

- It can be used by the cell itself.
- It can be released into the blood and carried to other tissues by **transferrin**, the major iron-transporting protein in the body.
- It can be stored as **ferritin**.

The body's need for iron determines its fate: the greater the need, particularly for synthesis of red blood cells, the more transferrin binds iron and transports it to bone marrow and other tissues. If iron stores are high, the extra iron remains in the cell and is excreted along with mucosal cells that are sloughed off at the end of their life cycle. Some scientists propose that intestinal ferritin acts as an "iron sink," which prevents the accumulation of iron to toxic levels.[7]

Effect of the Body's Iron Status on Iron Absorption. Depending on the size of the body's iron stores, absorption of dietary iron (i.e., iron bioavailability)

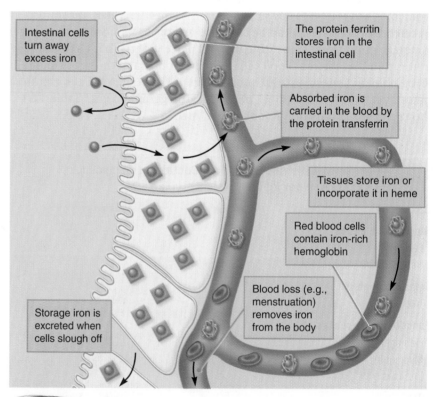

Figure 12.6 **Iron absorption.** The amount of iron absorbed depends on several factors— normal GI function, need for iron, the amount and kind of iron consumed, and dietary factors that enhance or inhibit iron absorption.

can vary from less than 1 percent to greater than 50 percent. The GI tract increases iron absorption when the body's iron stores are low and decreases absorption when stores are sufficient. The body also gives priority to red blood cell production; an increased production rate, such as during pregnancy or after blood loss, can trigger a several-fold increase in iron uptake.[8]

Among adults, men absorb approximately 6 percent of dietary iron and nonpregnant women of childbearing age absorb approximately 13 percent. The women's higher absorption rate primarily reflects their lower iron intake, and higher iron losses as a result of menstruation. Iron absorption also is high among iron-deficient persons.

Effect of GI Function on Iron Absorption. Although most iron absorption occurs in the duodenum and jejunum of the small intestine, the stomach also has an important role. To be absorbed, dietary iron must be dissolved in chyme, and gastric acid solubilizes iron in food. Acidity also promotes the conversion of ferric iron (Fe^{3+}) to ferrous iron (Fe^{2+}), the form that most easily enters the absorptive intestinal cells. The stomach's retention and mechanical mixing of food also maximizes iron's bioavailability. Gastric acid production generally declines with aging, reducing iron absorption in the elderly.

Effect of the Amount and Form of Iron in Food. Food contains two types of iron—**heme iron** and **non-heme iron**. Most heme iron is a part of hemoglobin and myoglobin, so it is found only in animal tissue. This association makes heme iron much more absorbable than non-heme iron, which usually is part of iron-containing salts. While meat, fish, and poultry contain various amounts of heme iron and non-heme iron, the mix averages about 40 percent heme iron and 60 percent non-heme iron.[9] In contrast, plant-based and iron-fortified foods contain only non-heme iron. (See **Figure 12.7**.) Vegetarian diets, by definition, contain little to no heme iron, so iron-deficiency anemia is a concern.

Heme iron is two to three times more absorbable than non-heme iron. Depending on the body's iron stores, heme iron absorption ranges from 15 to 35 percent of the amount ingested.[10] As the amount of iron ingested increases, the proportion absorbed decreases.

Dietary Factors That Enhance Iron Absorption. Heme iron absorption is relatively independent of meal composition. On the other hand, meal composition strongly influences non-heme iron absorption. **Table 12.2** lists factors that inhibit or enhance absorption of iron. The two most important dietary factors that boost absorption of non-heme iron are organic acids, especially vitamin C (ascorbic acid) and meat, including fish and poultry. Organic acids maintain the iron in a soluble, bioavailable form as the stomach contents enter the duodenum. To exert this effect, ascorbic acid must be present in the same meal as the non-heme iron. Other organic

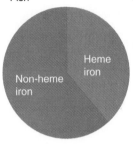

About 40% heme and 60% non-heme iron
Heme iron is supplied by animal foods which also contain non-heme iron

Beef
Chicken
Fish

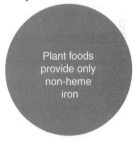

100% non-heme iron
Beans
Fortified cereals
Green leafy vegetables
Soy

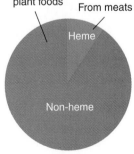

Average daily heme/non-heme iron

Table 12.2 **Factors That Affect Iron Absorption**

Inhibitors	Enhancers
Fiber and phytate	Vitamin C/ascorbic acid
Calcium and phosphorus (milk/dairy)	Meat factor in meat and poultry
Tannins, found in tea	HCl secreted in the stomach
Polyphenols	Citric, malic, and lactic acid
Oxalate	

Figure 12.7 **Sources of heme and non-heme iron.** Heme iron is found only in meats. Non-heme iron is found in both plant and animal foods.

polyphenols Organic compounds that include an unsaturated ring containing more than one —OH group as part of their chemical structures; may produce bitterness in coffee and tea.

acids (e.g., citric, malic, and tartaric acids) appear to have effects comparable to those of ascorbic acid. It is unclear exactly how meat enhances absorption of non-heme iron, but the presence of meat increases absorption efficiency. In fact, a recent study found that non-heme iron absorption in nonvegetarians was more than double that of lacto-ovo-vegetarians.[11] Despite this difference in absorption, this same study did not find evidence of iron deficiency in the vegetarians.[12]

Dietary Factors That Inhibit Iron Absorption. The most significant inhibitors of iron absorption are phytic acid (phytate), which is found in whole grains, and **polyphenols**, which are found in tea, coffee, other beverages, and many plants. (See **Figure 12.8**.) Even though minute amounts of these substances can reduce iron absorption, eating foods rich in vitamin C at the same meal counteracts this effect. The benefits of eating whole grains, which are nutrient dense and rich in fiber, outweigh the negative impact on iron absorption. Rather than cut back on whole grains, a person should include small amounts of meat and/or generous amounts of vitamin C–rich fruits and vegetables with meals to improve iron absorption.

Other inhibitors of non-heme iron absorption include soy, calcium, zinc, oxalates, and fiber. The long-term significance of these inhibitory factors on iron status is unclear. Since many women take calcium supplements to prevent osteoporosis, calcium's inhibition of iron absorption has come under scrutiny. A recent study found that 6 months of calcium supplementation (1,200 milligrams per day) reduces short-term iron absorption, yet overall iron status was unaffected.[13] To be safe, some experts recommend taking calcium supplements alone at bedtime rather than with meals.[14]

Zinc competes with iron for absorption. When they are taken together, large amounts of either mineral can inhibit the absorption of the other. Deficiency of both nutrients is common, so some developing countries promote enrichment of foods with balanced amounts of both iron and zinc.

Figure 12.8 Iron absorption from foods.

Source: Courtesy of Laurie Grace. From Scrimshaw NS. Iron deficiency. *Scientific American.* October 1991:48.

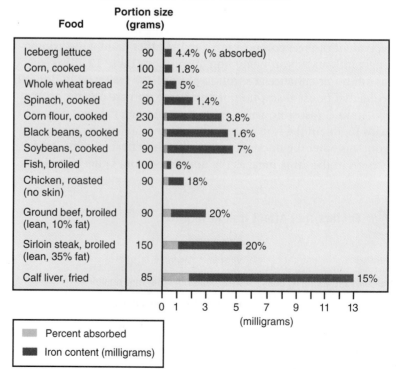

IRON ABSORPTION FROM FOODS

Food	Portion size (grams)	% absorbed
Iceberg lettuce	90	4.4% (% absorbed)
Corn, cooked	100	1.8%
Whole wheat bread	25	5%
Spinach, cooked	90	1.4%
Corn flour, cooked	230	3.8%
Black beans, cooked	90	1.6%
Soybeans, cooked	90	7%
Fish, broiled	100	6%
Chicken, roasted (no skin)	90	18%
Ground beef, broiled (lean, 10% fat)	90	20%
Sirloin steak, broiled (lean, 35% fat)	150	20%
Calf liver, fried	85	15%

0 1 3 5 7 9 11 13
(milligrams)

Percent absorbed
Iron content (milligrams)

Iron Transport and Storage

Transferrin delivers iron from the intestines to the tissues and redistributes iron from storage sites to various body compartments. Individual cells take up the iron transported on transferrin via **transferrin receptors** on the cell membranes.[15] The number of transferrin receptors varies with the cell's need for iron; tissues with the highest iron need (e.g., bone marrow, liver, and placenta) have the highest concentration of transferrin receptors. **Figure 12.9** shows iron in the body.

The body stores surplus iron either as part of the soluble protein complex ferritin or as the insoluble protein complex **hemosiderin**.[16] The liver, bone marrow, spleen, and skeletal muscle harbor most of the body's ferritin and hemosiderin, and small amounts of ferritin circulate in the bloodstream. In healthy people, ferritin contains most of the stored iron.[17] When long-term negative iron balance depletes iron stores, iron deficiency begins.

Iron Turnover and Loss

While protecting against toxicity, the body tightly regulates its iron content to ensure adequate stores. It recycles iron, and adjusts absorption and excretion as needed.

Red blood cell formation and destruction are responsible for most iron turnover. In adult men, for example, the breakdown of older red blood cells supplies approximately 95 percent of the iron required to produce

transferrin receptor Specialized receptor on the cell membrane that binds transferrin.

hemosiderin An insoluble form of storage iron.

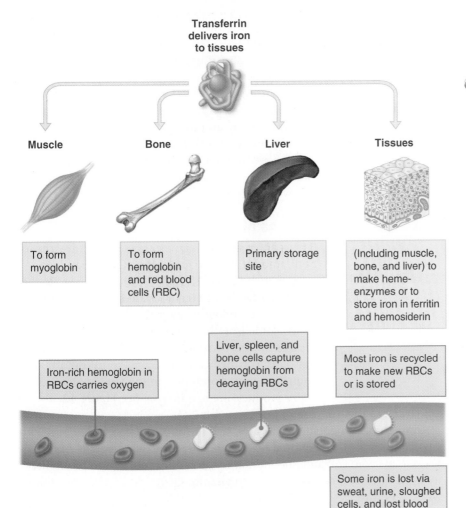

Transferrin delivers iron to tissues

Figure 12.9 **Iron in the body.** Transferrin transports iron to tissues for the synthesis of heme or storage in ferritin and hemosiderin.

Muscle — To form myoglobin

Bone — To form hemoglobin and red blood cells (RBC)

Liver — Primary storage site

Tissues — (Including muscle, bone, and liver) to make heme-enzymes or to store iron in ferritin and hemosiderin

Iron-rich hemoglobin in RBCs carries oxygen

Liver, spleen, and bone cells capture hemoglobin from decaying RBCs

Most iron is recycled to make new RBCs or is stored

Some iron is lost via sweat, urine, sloughed cells, and lost blood

new red blood cells. Dietary sources supply only 5 percent. In contrast, this balance is 70/30 in infants, whose growth needs tend to outstrip the recycled supply.

Adults lose about 1 milligram of iron daily in feces and sloughed-off mucosal and skin cells. Women of childbearing age require additional iron (an average of 0.3 to 0.5 mg of iron absorbed daily) to compensate for blood loss during menstruation. Support of tissue growth during pregnancy requires absorption of an average of 3 milligrams of additional iron daily over the 280 days of gestation.

All people lose tiny amounts of iron daily in normal gastrointestinal blood loss, but gastrointestinal problems can cause significant iron loss. Peptic ulcer, inflammatory bowel disease, and bowel cancer can cause gastrointestinal bleeding. Hookworm infections, although uncommon in the United States, also are associated with gastrointestinal blood loss and iron depletion.[18]

Dietary Recommendations for Iron

Scientists base recommendations for iron intake on the replacement of daily iron losses and the bioavailability of dietary iron. The primary routes of loss are bleeding, gastrointestinal losses (mainly exfoliation of the intestinal mucosa), sloughing of skin, and sweat. The RDA for iron is based on average losses of 1 milligram per day for adult men, and 1.4 milligrams per day for premenopausal women, combined with an absorption percentage of 18 percent from a mixed diet. The RDAs for adults are 8 milligrams per day for men and postmenopausal women and 18 milligrams per day for women of childbearing age. Dietary intakes of most men actually exceed their RDA, while women's intakes are well below the RDA for most age ranges, according to NHANES III. Researchers attribute the women's lower intake to lower energy intake, since women consume on average 1,800 kilocalories per day and the American diet contains about 6 milligrams iron per 1,000 kilocalories.[19] The average premenopausal woman therefore consumes less than 11 milligrams of iron daily, substantially below the recommended 18 milligrams.

Sources of Iron

Beef is an excellent dietary source of iron, in terms of both amount and bioavailability. Other excellent sources include clams, oysters, tofu, and liver. Poultry, fish, pork, lamb, and legumes are also good sources. Whole-grain and enriched-grain products contain less bioavailable iron than meat, but are significant sources of iron because they comprise a major part of our diets. Fortified cereals also make an important contribution to iron intake in the United States. Dairy products are low in iron. See **Figure 12.10**, which shows the iron content of some foods.

A varied diet (adequate in calories, rich in fruits and vegetables, and with small amounts of lean animal flesh) generally provides adequate iron. Vegetarians who consume no animal tissue can maximize iron bioavailability from other sources by consuming vitamin C–rich fruits and vegetables with every meal.

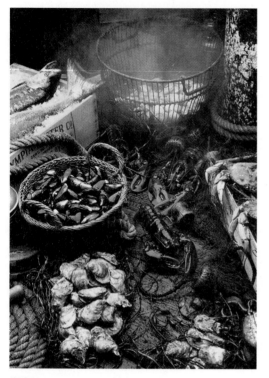

IRON

Daily Value = 18 mg

	Exceptionally good source		
High: 20% DV or more	Clams, cooked	85 g (3 oz)	24 mg
	Oysters	85 g (3 oz)	10 mg
	Corn flakes cereal	30 g (~1 cup)	9.3 mg
	Tofu, calcium processed	85 g (~1/3 cup)	8.9 mg
	Cheerios cereal	30 g (1 cup)	8.1 mg
	Beef liver	85 g (3 oz)	5.3 mg
	All Bran cereal	30 g (~1/2 cup)	4.5 mg
Good: 10-19% DV	Lentils, cooked	90 g (~1/2 cup)	3 mg
	Shrimp, cooked	85 g (3 oz)	2.6 mg
	Steak, porterhouse	85 g (3 oz)	2.4 mg
	Spinach, raw	90 g (~1/2 cup)	2.3 mg
	Lima beans, cooked	90 g (~1/2 cup)	2.2 mg
	Sunflower seeds	30 g (1 oz)	2 mg
	Turkey, roasted, dark meat	85 g (3 oz)	2 mg
	Spaghetti, enriched, cooked	140 g (~1 cup)	2 mg

Figure 12.10 **Food sources of iron.** Iron is found in red meats, certain seafood, vegetables and legumes, and is added to enriched grains and breakfast cereals.
Source: U.S. Department of Agriculture, Agricultural Research Service. 1999. USDA Nutrient Database for Standard Reference, Release 13. Nutrient Data Laboratory Home Page, http://www.nal.usda.gov/fnic/foodcomp.

Think About It

2

Iron Deficiency and Measurement of Iron Status

Iron deficiency is the most common nutritional deficiency worldwide. Although significantly more prevalent in developing countries than in the rest of the world, it is still a public health concern in the United States. Infants and toddlers, adolescent girls, women of childbearing age, and pregnant women are particularly vulnerable.

Iron deficiency is most prevalent in 6- to 24-month-old children, the period of rapid brain growth and development of cognitive and motor skills. If iron stores are not replaced before the child passes critical developmental milestones, developmental deficits from iron deficiency may be irreversible.

Studies of infants and children show a link between iron deficiency and delays in behavioral and cognitive development, but we do not yet understand how iron affects the brain.[20] Research in this area is complicated by the difficulty of separating the roles of iron deficiency and other environmental factors (e.g., generalized malnutrition, poverty, and low parental education) that also impair psychomotor and mental development.

Progression of Iron Deficiency

Iron deficiency is not the same as iron-deficiency anemia. Iron deficiency progresses through three distinct stages, which **Table 12.3** shows. The third stage is iron-deficiency anemia, a severe form of iron deficiency that is defined by low hemoglobin levels.

Depletion of iron stores is the first stage of iron deficiency, which causes no physiological impairments. Because serum ferritin is proportional to the body's total iron stores, a test of serum ferritin is a good way to assess iron deficiency.

Depletion of functional and transport iron is the second stage of iron deficiency—the stage between iron depletion and actual anemia. The newest and most sensitive measure of this intermediate stage is the serum level of transferrin receptors (TfRs). As the body's iron status falls, TfR levels increase in proportion to the iron deficit. Other blood values used to detect this stage are **transferrin saturation** and **protoporphyrin** levels. Transferrin saturation is a measure of the residual binding capacity for iron, which increases when a lack of iron does not saturate transferrin. Protoporphyrin and iron combine to make heme, the iron-containing portion of hemoglobin. When the supply of iron is inadequate for heme synthesis, blood levels of protoporphyrin rise.

Because second-stage iron depletion impairs the function of iron-requiring enzymes needed for aerobic energy production, an iron-depleted person may be unable to work at full capacity. Animal research shows a decreased exercise capacity among iron-deficient animals without anemia.

transferrin saturation The extent to which transferrin has vacant iron-binding sites (e.g., low transferrin saturation indicates a high proportion of vacant iron-binding sites).

protoporphyrin A chemical complex that combines with iron to form heme.

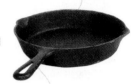

Quick Bites

Grandma's Cast-Iron Skillet Helped Her Avoid Iron Deficiency

Iron deficiency is the most common form of malnutrition in the United States. However, this is a relatively recent phenomenon. Americans used to cook using cast-iron pots and pans. A study showed that using these utensils to cook acidic foods like spaghetti sauce and apple butter increases the iron content of such foods by a factor of 30- to 100-fold. Our preference for stainless steel, aluminum, and enamelware does not allow us this fortification.

Table 12.3 Stages of Iron Deficiency

Stage	Biochemical Sign	Functional Implications
Depletion of iron stores	Decreased ferritin	None
Depletion of functional iron	Decreased transferrin receptors Decreased erythrocyte protoporphyrin	Decreased physical performance
Iron-deficiency anemia	Decreased hemoglobin Decreased hematocrit Decreased red cell size	Cognitive impairment, poor growth, decreased performance, and decreased exercise tolerance

hematocrit Percentage volume occupied by packed red blood cells in a centrifuged sample of whole blood.

microcytic anemia Anemia characterized by smaller than normal red blood cells, decreased mean corpuscular (RBC) volume, and mean corpuscular hemoglobin.

iron overload Toxicity from excess iron.

Quick Bites

Oceans Can Get Anemia, Too

Stretching from South America to New Zealand, a large region of the South Pacific Ocean that suffers from an iron deficiency. Phytoplankton and plant life are not growing properly in this area. Researchers have identified iron deficiency as the reason.

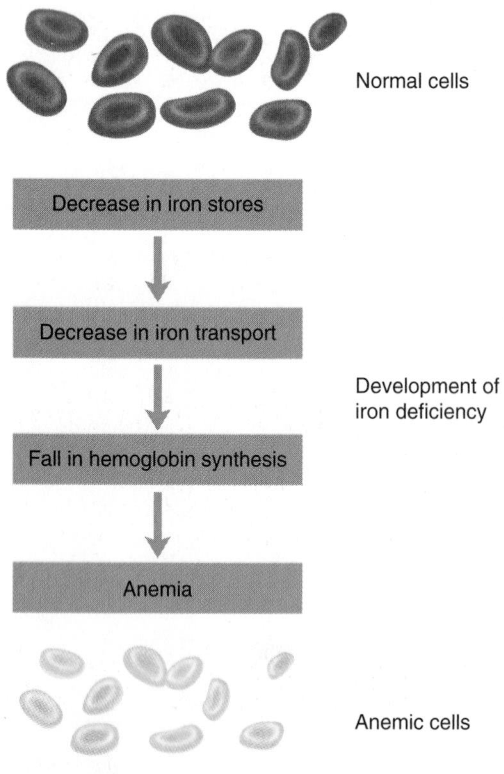

Normal cells

Decrease in iron stores

Decrease in iron transport

Development of iron deficiency

Fall in hemoglobin synthesis

Anemia

Anemic cells

Figure 12.11 **Normal and anemic red blood cells.** Iron deficiency can progress to iron-deficiency anemia, a severe form of iron deficiency that is accompanied by low hemoglobin levels.

Recent research in young women with iron deficiency but without anemia shows a similar decrease in their physical performance.[21] More human studies are required to determine if iron depletion affects other physiological processes.

The third and most severe stage of iron deficiency is anemia—a disease characterized by insufficient and/or defective red blood cells. A lack of iron inhibits production of normal red blood cells, while normal cell turnover continues to deplete the red blood cell population. Red blood cell production falters, producing red blood cells that are pale and smaller than normal. Hemoglobin and **hematocrit** (concentration of red blood cells in the blood) levels also are low. This type of anemia, known for its small, pale red blood cells, is called microcytic hypochromic anemia. Inadequate vitamin B_6 also can cause microcytic hypochromic anemia. Another type of anemia, megaloblastic anemia, is known for its abnormally large, immature red blood cells and is caused by inadequate folate or vitamin B_{12}. (See Chapter 10 for more details.) **Figure 12.11** shows normal and anemic blood cells.

The symptoms of **microcytic anemia** vary according to its severity, and the speed of its development. They include fatigue, pallor, breathlessness with exertion, decreased tolerance of cold, behavioral changes, deficits in immune function, cognitive impairment, decreased work performance, and impaired growth. In children, iron deficiency is associated with apathy, short attention span, irritability, and reduced ability to learn.[22]

Iron Toxicity

Iron Poisoning in Children

Accidental iron overdose is a leading cause of poisoning deaths in children younger than 6 years old in the United States.[23] The iron products involved range from nonprescription daily multivitamin/mineral supplements for children to high-potency prescription iron supplements for pregnant women. Parents who are cautious about keeping other medications out of reach often do not realize that over-the-counter iron tablets and iron-containing multivitamin/mineral supplements can be toxic to children. Even a few pills can cause the death of a small child. Symptoms of iron intoxication include nausea, vomiting, diarrhea, rapid heartbeat, dizziness, and confusion. Death can occur within hours of ingestion. If iron poisoning is suspected, the child should receive immediate emergency medical care.

Hereditary Hemochromatosis

Hereditary hemochromatosis, a form of chronic iron overload, was once thought to be rare but now is known to be quite common. A genetic defect causes excessive iron absorption. Over the years, iron can build up in many parts of the body, leading to severe organ damage and even death. Diabetes, heart disease, cirrhosis, liver cancer, and arthritis can all be consequences of hemochromatosis.

Serious complications of hemochromatosis are five to ten times more common in men than women, primarily because of women's blood loss associated with menstruation and pregnancy. Treatment of hemochromatosis includes minimizing iron intake and frequent phlebotomy (removal of blood) to withdraw some of the iron it carries in cells. With early diagnosis and treatment, a person with hemochromatosis can avoid organ damage and other complications, and have a normal life span.

Iron overload is highly prevalent in some African communities. Researchers originally thought the custom of consuming beer brewed in steel drums was entirely responsible. These beverages have a large amount of highly bioavailable iron and alcohol enhances the absorption of iron. However, researchers have found strong evidence for a gene, distinct from the hemochromatosis gene in Caucasians, that may predispose individuals to this disorder.[24] The UL for iron is 45 milligrams per day.

Key Concepts: Iron is essential for life but highly toxic in excess. Iron is a key component of the oxygen transporters hemoglobin and myoglobin, and of many enzymes involved in energy metabolism. Heme iron is absorbed more efficiently than non-heme iron. The body carefully regulates iron absorption; iron can be bound to transferrin for transport, or stored as ferritin or hemosiderin. The best dietary source of iron is red meat. Iron deficiency develops gradually, with anemia being the most severe manifestation of deficiency. Iron poisoning is potentially deadly, especially for young children. Hereditary hemochromatosis is a common genetic disease that causes iron overload.

Zinc

It's hard to believe that a nutrient so important to health could go unnoticed until as recently as 40 years ago, but that is the case with zinc (Zn). Some people may think of zinc only in connection with the "zinc oxide" cream used topically as a sunscreen or with zinc lozenges promoted as a treatment for colds; few consumers realize that dietary zinc is absolutely essential for health.

Scientists first recognized human zinc deficiency in 1961.[25] They found severe zinc deficiencies in young, severely growth-retarded, Iranian men. In addition to suffering from dwarfism, these men were anemic and extremely lethargic, had **hypogonadism** (poorly developed genitals), and some couldn't see well in the dark. Their diets consisted mainly of wheat bread, and was almost devoid of animal protein. These men also were known to eat clay (**geophagia**). Scientists hypothesized that the high phytate content of their diet, along with the geophagia, impaired absorption of both zinc and iron. Six years later, a study in Egypt confirmed zinc's role; zinc supplementation improved growth and genital development.[26]

Functions of Zinc

The body contains a small amount of zinc—between 1.5 and 2.5 grams, or about the same amount of zinc as is in a **galvanized** nail, which has a thin layer of zinc to protect it from corrosion. Zinc is a component of every living cell. Zinc is best known for its participation in enzyme structure and function, but it also supports many other diverse biological activities through a role in controlling gene regulation. **Figure 12.12** illustrates the functions of zinc in the body.

Zinc and Enzymes

Zinc is critical to the proper function of more than 80 enzymes and other **metalloproteins**, which are proteins that have a mineral as an essential part of their structures.[27] It is essential for their structural integrity and function, regulation of their activities, and their ability to catalyze reactions. In the cytoplasm, zinc and copper are key components of superoxide dismutase, an enzyme that speeds antioxidant reactions and helps protect cells from free radical damage.

hypogonadism Decreased functional activity of the gonads (ovaries or testes) with retardation of growth and sexual development.

geophagia Ingestion of clay or dirt.

galvanized Iron or steel with a thin layer of zinc plated onto it to protect against corrosion.

metalloprotein A protein with a mineral element as an essential part of its structure.

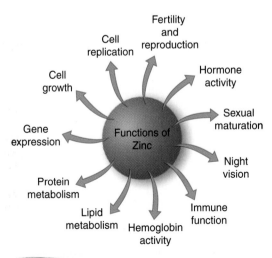

Figure 12.12 Functions of zinc in the body.

Zinc's Role in Nucleic Acid Metabolism

Zinc also is inextricably linked to gene expression. In severe zinc deficiency, cells fail to replicate. This may be why zinc is so important for normal growth of children and sexual maturation of adolescents. Furthermore, certain tissues with high turnover rates, such as cells lining the GI tract, skin cells, immune cells, and blood cells, are particularly vulnerable to a zinc deficiency. As a result, zinc-deficient people often have diarrhea, dermatitis, and depressed immunity.

Zinc and the Immune System

Zinc is vital to a vigorous immune response and is essential to the proper development and maintenance of the immune system. Without zinc, your body could not fight off invading viruses, bacteria, and fungi. Even mild deficiency may increase the risk of infection.

Zinc and Vision

Zinc-deficient people may show signs of night blindness, or other classic signs of vitamin A deficiency. Zinc is a key component of the enzyme that activates vitamin A in the retina. Thus, a lack of zinc interferes with vitamin A activity in the eye.

Zinc and Gene Regulation

Zinc enables certain small proteins to fold and form a stable "zinc-finger" structure. This structure interacts with a region of DNA. Without zinc, that area of a gene won't function. This function of zinc may explain how it influences the immune system. Discovery and characterization of zinc-finger protein families is an active area of nutrition research.[28]

Other Zinc Functions

Zinc is essential for a number of other diverse biological functions:

- *Hormonal:* Zinc interacts with a number of hormones including insulin.
- *Growth and Reproduction:* Zinc plays an important role in pregnancy outcome, fetal development, and bone health.
- *Hemoglobin Activity:* Zinc increases the affinity of hemoglobin for oxygen and indirectly influences hemoglobin synthesis.
- *Taste:* Some studies show that zinc participates in taste perception and appetite regulation.
- *Cell Death:* Zinc can induce as well as inhibit the process of apoptosis, also known as programmed cell death.[29]

Regulation of Zinc in the Body

Zinc Absorption

The body absorbs small amounts of zinc more effectively than large doses, and absorption ranges between 10 and 35 percent, a range similar to heme iron absorption. The degree of zinc absorption depends on the person's zinc status, zinc needs, and zinc content of the meal, and the presence of competing minerals. People with zinc deficiency absorb zinc more thoroughly than those with optimal zinc status. Absorption increases during times of increased need, such as growth spurts, pregnancy, and lactation. On the other hand, certain dietary factors such as phytate and fiber can impair absorption of zinc. See **Figure 12.13**, which shows zinc absorption.

metallothionein An abundant, nonenzymatic, zinc-containing protein.

Dietary Factors That Inhibit Zinc Absorption

Because of phytate and fiber, the body absorbs zinc poorly from whole grains—less than 15 percent on average.[30] Phytate can bind zinc in insoluble complexes, thus inhibiting zinc's absorption. Dietary fiber may also reduce zinc absorption but to a lesser extent than phytate. Calcium in a meal does not appear to affect zinc absorption, but supplemental calcium taken with meals high in phytate may increase phytate's ability to bind zinc and may decrease zinc's bioavailability.[31] However, American diets typically do not contain enough phytate and fiber to depress zinc absorption significantly. Exceptions are vegetarian diets that are high in phytate and fiber.[32]

The negative effect of high-dose non-heme iron supplementation (such as during pregnancy) on zinc absorption is well documented.[33] On the other hand, your body absorbs heme iron (from meat) differently, so heme iron has no effect on zinc absorption. Also, iron only inhibits zinc absorption when there is a high iron-to-zinc ratio.[34] Eating iron-fortified foods is unlikely to inhibit zinc absorption.

Zinc Transport and Distribution

Zinc circulates in the bloodstream loosely bound to albumin and more tightly bound to another protein, alpha$_2$macroglobulin. Zinc travels to the liver and to the tissues where it is most needed. Muscle and bone contain 90 percent of the body's zinc and the remainder is divided primarily among the liver, kidney, pancreas, brain, skin, and prostate. **Figure 12.14** shows zinc in the body.

Zinc Homeostasis and Excretion

The body has no long-term storehouse of zinc to draw upon when dietary zinc is low. Despite the lack of zinc storage, the body balances zinc absorption and excretion, thus maintaining zinc homeostasis even when confronted with varying needs and dietary conditions.

Intestinal cells act as temporary buffers that help regulate zinc absorption. The protein **metallothionein** binds zinc in the intestinal mucosal cells and impedes its movement into the bloodstream. When zinc intake is high, the body makes more metallothionein to retain more zinc in the intestinal cells. Intestinal cells and other cells produce zinc transporter proteins, which help to maintain body homeostasis.[35]

During digestion, the pancreas secretes as much as 4.0 milligrams of zinc per day in the pancreatic juice. When the body needs zinc, intestinal cells reabsorb most of this secreted zinc. Otherwise, the body excretes it in the feces along with unabsorbed dietary zinc and sloughed, zinc-containing intestinal cells. The body also excretes zinc in minor amounts via urine, sweat, skin, hair, semen, and menstrual fluids.

Key

● Zinc

● Non-heme iron

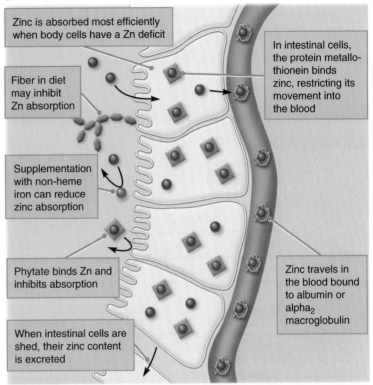

Zinc is absorbed most efficiently when body cells have a Zn deficit

Fiber in diet may inhibit Zn absorption

Supplementation with non-heme iron can reduce zinc absorption

Phytate binds Zn and inhibits absorption

When intestinal cells are shed, their zinc content is excreted

In intestinal cells, the protein metallothionein binds zinc, restricting its movement into the blood

Zinc travels in the blood bound to albumin or alpha$_2$ macroglobulin

Figure 12.13 **Zinc absorption.** Intestinal cells act as temporary buffers that help regulate zinc absorption.

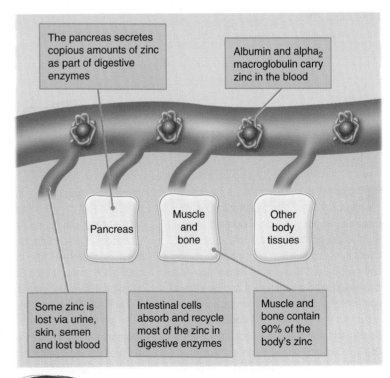

The pancreas secretes copious amounts of zinc as part of digestive enzymes

Albumin and alpha$_2$ macroglobulin carry zinc in the blood

Pancreas

Muscle and bone

Other body tissues

Some zinc is lost via urine, skin, semen and lost blood

Intestinal cells absorb and recycle most of the zinc in digestive enzymes

Muscle and bone contain 90% of the body's zinc

Figure 12.14 **Zinc in the body.** Zinc is a component of every living cell and helps stabilize cell membranes. More than 80 enzymes contain zinc.

Dietary Recommendations for Zinc

The RDA for adult males is 11 milligrams per day, and for females it is 8 milligrams per day. Experts recommend increasing zinc intake to 11 milligrams per day during pregnancy to provide for the growing fetus, and to 12 milligrams per day during the first 6 months of lactation.

Average zinc intake in the United States is generally below the RDA.[36] These dietary data raise the important question of whether marginal zinc deficiency is common or the RDA is set too high. Since RDA levels are set higher than the assumed *average* requirement, *average* population intakes that are lower than the RDA may not be of concern.

Sources of Zinc

Zinc usually is abundant in foods that are good sources of protein, especially red meat, seafood, oysters, and clams. Dark meat is a richer source than white meat, and unrefined whole grains have more zinc than processed grains. However, the bioavailability of zinc is just as important as the amount present. Although wheat-bran bread has a relatively high amount of zinc (2.4 milligrams), much of it is unavailable due to poor absorption (7 percent).[37] The bioavailability of zinc is highest from red meats, liver, eggs, and seafood. Fruits and vegetables generally are poor sources of dietary zinc.

In the United States, 44 percent of dietary zinc comes from meat, poultry, and seafood, 19 percent from dairy sources, and 17 percent from grains.[38] Adequate zinc intake is of special concern for vegetarians because they do not eat many of the foods that are the best sources of this mineral. **Figure 12.15** shows the zinc content of some foods.

ZINC

Daily Value = 15 mg

Exceptionally good source

Oysters, cooked	85 g (3 oz)	154 mg
Crab, Alaska King, cooked	85 g (3 oz)	6.5 mg
Beef liver	85 g (3 oz)	4.6 mg
Ground beef, extra lean	85 g (3 oz)	4.6 mg
Steak, porterhouse, cooked	85 g (3 oz)	4.0 mg
All Bran cereal	30 g (~1/2 cup)	3.8 mg
Turkey, roasted, dark meat	85 g (3 oz)	3.8 mg
Wheat bran flakes cereal	30 g (~3/4 cup)	3.8 mg
Cheerios cereal	30 g (~1 cup)	3.8 mg
Wheat germ	15 g	2.5 mg
Lobster, cooked	85 g (3 oz)	2.5 mg
Ham, extra lean, cooked	85 g (3 oz)	2.4 mg
Chicken, cooked, dark meat	85 g (~3 oz)	2.4 mg
Clams, cooked	85 g (3 oz)	2.3 mg
Yogurt, plain, nonfat	225 g (1 8-oz container)	2.2 mg
Refried beans, canned	130 g (~1/2 cup)	1.5 mg

High: 20% DV or more

Good: 10-19% DV

Figure 12.15 **Food sources of zinc.** Meat, organ meats, and seafood are the best sources of zinc.
Source: U.S. Department of Agriculture, Agricultural Research Service. 1999. USDA Nutrient Database for Standard Reference, Release 13. Nutrient Data Laboratory Home Page, http://www.nal.usda.gov/fnic/foodcomp.

Fyi Zinc and the Common Cold

FOR YOUR INFORMATION

The common cold, one of our most common illnesses, affects American adults 2 to 4 times per year and children 6 to 8 times per year.[1] Colds are even more frequent in young children in day-care settings and preschools. Because of missed work and decreased productivity, colds can be an economic stressor as well as a physical nuisance. A cure for the common cold would be of great benefit and scientists have long pursued this goal. Because of zinc's role in immune function, 11 placebo-controlled studies between 1984 and 1998 investigated the effect of zinc lozenges on the common cold. Roughly half of the studies produced positive results and the other half had negative findings.

One study with positive results gained considerable attention from the press. As a result, zinc lozenges are on nearly every pharmacy shelf in the United States. This study recruited 100 people during the winter of 1994. Researchers enrolled subjects within 24 hours of the onset of their common cold symptoms. Every 2 hours while awake, half the subjects took placebo lozenges and half took lozenges containing 13 milligrams of zinc, an average of 6 lozenges per day. They could take acetaminophen, but they were asked to refrain from taking other cold medicines or antibiotics during the trial. In the zinc group, colds resolved in an average of 4 days. In comparison, cold symptoms in the placebo group persisted for 7 days.[2]

Though scientists have suggested several hypotheses, the mechanism for the effect is unclear. Zinc deficiency is known to impair immune function, but could all these people have been zinc deficient? This is doubtful. Some speculate that zinc may inhibit viral replication.

During the trial, many of the experimental subjects experienced side effects including

Zinc Deficiency

Zinc deficiency is most prevalent in populations that subsist on cereal proteins, which have poorly available zinc.[39] Diarrhea and chronic infections like pneumonia can cause excessive zinc excretion. These diseases are commonplace in developing countries where zinc deficiency may be widespread. In some of these areas, zinc supplementation has decreased the incidence of acute lower respiratory infection, diarrhea, and attacks of malaria in children.

As **Table 12.4** shows, the primary culprits in marginal zinc deficiency are increased needs, poor intake, poor absorption, and excessive losses. During pregnancy, zinc deficiency may contribute to complications and low birth weight.[40] Zinc-deficient preschool-age children and patients on **hemodialysis** may have a poor appetite and a diminished sense of taste.[41] Malabsorption syndromes such as cystic fibrosis and **Crohn's disease** impair zinc absorption. Symptoms of moderate to severe zinc deficiency include poor growth, impaired immune response, and other conditions that may include

hemodialysis Technique for removing waste products by filtering blood, usually performed on patients with kidney failure.

Crohn's disease A disease that causes inflammation and ulceration along sections of the intestinal tract.

Table 12.4   Risks Factors for Zinc Deficiency

Dietary Deficiency	Protein calorie malnutrition	Vegan diets
	Poor food choices	IV feeding without zinc
Increased Requirements	Burn patients	Pregnancy and lactation
	Growth spurts	Chronic infection
Malabsorption	Acrodermatitis enteropathica	Geophagia or pica
	Celiac disease, Crohn's disease	High phytate diets
	Cystic fibrosis	Chronic iron supplementation
Increased Losses	Sickle cell disease	Burns and surgery
	Diabetes	Chronic diarrhea
	Renal disease	

nausea, bad taste, and sore mouths. In addition to the mild side effects and the cost of the lozenges, such high doses of zinc could have harmful effects. Long-term use of high doses of zinc induces copper deficiency. On average, those in the experimental group took close to 480 milligrams zinc during the week of their cold. If children have 8 colds per year and take nearly 500 milligrams of zinc per cold, could that be enough to induce widespread copper deficiency?

The same research group studied 249 randomly selected children in a double-blind, placebo-controlled trial. The experimental group took zinc gluconate lozenges at the first sign of cold symptoms. Depending on age, each child received 50 to 60 milligrams of zinc per day. There was no difference between groups in the time for all cold symptoms to resolve—a median of 9 days. Although the researchers noted several limitations of their study, they concluded that we still need additional studies to determine what role, if any, zinc has in treatment of the common cold.[3]

Since only half of the studies produced positive effects and excess zinc intake can cause deficiencies of other minerals, we should think twice before routinely giving children (and ourselves) zinc lozenges every time a cold strikes.

1 Gwaltney JM, Hendley JO, Simon G, Jordan WS. Rhinovirus infections in an industrial population. *N Engl J Med.* 1966;275:1261–1268.

2 Mossad SB, Macknin ML, Medendorp SV, Mason P. Zinc gluconate lozenges for treating the common cold: a randomized, double-blind placebo-controlled study. *Ann Intern Med.* 1996;125:81–88.

3 Macknin ML, Piedmonte M, Calendine C, et al. Zinc gluconate lozenges for treating the common cold in children: a randomized controlled trial. *JAMA.* 1998;279:1962–1967

acrodermatitis enteropathica *A genetic disorder that results in a deficiency in the absorption of zinc.*

Wilson's disease *Genetic disorder of increased copper absorption, which leads to toxic levels in the liver and heart.*

Keshan disease *Selenium deficiency disease that impairs the structure and function of the heart.*

selenomethionine *A selenium-containing amino acid derived from methionine that is the storage form of selenium.*

Table 12.5 **Effects of Zinc Deficiency**

Severe Deficiency	Moderate Deficiency
Hypogonadism	Delayed sexual maturation
Cessation of growth	
Patchy loss of hair	Growth retardation
Skin lesions and rashes	Pregnancy complications
Impaired taste (hypogeusia)	
	Acne
Loss of appetite/anorexia	Increased infections
Diarrhea	
Decreased thyroid hormone synthesis	
Night blindness	
Recurrent infections	

Quick Bites

On your next moonlit stroll, think selenium!

Selenium takes its name from the Greek word Selênê, "moon," because it has a pasty white color. In mythology, Selene is the Greek goddess of the moon. Ancient Greeks often blamed Selene and her brother Helios (god of the sun) for pestilent diseases and death.

impaired taste acuity. **Table 12.5** lists these and other characteristics of moderate and severe zinc deficiency.

Although severe zinc deficiency is uncommon, it can be caused by **acrodermatitis enteropathica**, a rare genetic disorder that impairs zinc absorption and produces skin problems and infections. In the past, long-term intravenous feeding severely depleted zinc in patients who could not eat normally. Today, trace minerals are added to intravenous solutions.

Zinc Toxicity

Because the body efficiently rids itself of excess zinc, toxicity from high dietary zinc intake is rare. Yet there have been isolated accounts of acute zinc toxicity in people who consumed large amounts of acidic foods or beverages that had been stored in galvanized containers. High doses of zinc (2 to 4 grams) may cause acute gastrointestinal distress, nausea, vomiting, and cramping.

Chronic intake of moderately elevated amounts of zinc is a more common cause of zinc toxicity. Usually, excessive zinc supplementation is at fault. In elderly patients, intakes of 100 to 150 milligrams of zinc per day for several weeks decreased immune function.[42] Higher doses can cause vomiting.[43] Excess zinc intake also affects blood lipids by elevating LDL and depressing HDL levels.[44] The UL for zinc is 40 milligrams per day.

Chronic high intakes of zinc relative to copper can inhibit copper absorption and with time may induce a copper deficiency. Doctors use the interaction of zinc and copper to treat patients with **Wilson's disease**, a genetic disorder of hyperabsorption and accumulation of copper in such patients. Daily doses between 100 and 150 milligrams of zinc effectively inhibit the harmful accumulation of copper in the liver.[45]

Key Concepts: *Zinc is important for normal growth and development, immune function, and the function of many enzymes. Zinc homeostasis is maintained by regulating intestinal absorption. Iron, zinc, and copper all compete for absorption, but problems don't usually occur if these minerals are coming from balanced dietary rather than supplemental sources. The best food sources for zinc are beef, oysters, crab, legumes, and unrefined whole grains. Zinc deficiency is most prevalent in populations that subsist on cereal protein.*

Selenium

The story of selenium (Se) is a recent one and becomes more complex as scientists explore its role at the molecular level. Historically, since animals grazing on selenium-rich soils suffered selenium poisoning, scientists focused on its toxicity. This changed in 1957, when researchers first demonstrated selenium's nutritional benefits in vitamin E-deficient animals. But not until 1979 did evidence emerge that selenium is essential for humans. Chinese scientists reported an association between low selenium status and **Keshan disease**, a heart disorder that strikes children in the Keshan province of China. The Chinese scientists demonstrated that selenium supplements could prevent the disease. Although selenium deficiency does not cause the disease, it predisposes a child to heart damage after a particular type of viral infection. When selenium intake is adequate, the virus apparently does not cause Keshan disease.

Functions of Selenium

Although scientists have identified nearly 50 selenium-containing proteins, two amino acid derivatives—**selenomethionine**, a methionine derivative, and **selenocysteine**, a cysteine derivative—contain most of the body's selenium. Selenomethionine is a selenium "storage compartment," and selenocysteine is selenium's biologically active form. As selenocysteine, selenium is a component of enzymes involved in antioxidant protection and thyroid hormone metabolism.

Selenium is best known as a component of glutathione peroxidases, a family of antioxidant enzymes. (See **Figure 12.16A**) The discovery of these enzymes resolved a puzzling overlap in the functions of selenium and vitamin E. Both nutrients play a role in preventing lipid peroxidation and membrane damage. Glutathione peroxidases promote the breakdown of fatty acids that have undergone peroxidation, thus eliminating highly reactive free radicals. This reduction in free radicals spares vitamin E, making it available to stop other chain reactions of free radicals (see **Figure 12.16B**). Since glutathione peroxidases require selenium, dietary selenium indirectly spares vitamin E.

In recent years, scientists identified selenium as a component of enzymes involved in the metabolism of iodine and thyroid hormone. Iodine deficiency alone causes **hypothyroidism**, and a combined deficiency of selenium and iodine increases the severity of the disease. There also is some evidence that a combined deficiency of both minerals during pregnancy is involved in some forms of **cretinism** in newborns.

Selenium is important in the immune system and its response to infections. Recent research also tentatively links low selenium status to increased cancer risk;[46] however, because small increases in selenium intake can be

selenocysteine A selenium-containing amino acid that is the biologically active form of selenium

hypothyroidism The result of a lowered level of circulating thyroid hormone with slowing of mental and physical functions.

cretinism A congenital condition often caused by severe iodine deficiency during gestation, which is characterized by arrested physical and mental development.

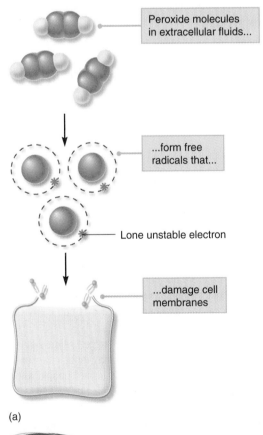

Peroxide molecules in extracellular fluids...

...form free radicals that...

Lone unstable electron

...damage cell membranes

(a)

Figure 12.16 **Peroxides form free radicals.** Free radicals damage cell membranes and have been implicated in heart disease.

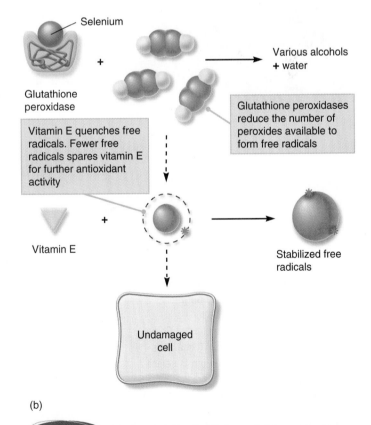

Selenium

Glutathione peroxidase

Various alcohols + water

Glutathione peroxidases reduce the number of peroxides available to form free radicals

Vitamin E quenches free radicals. Fewer free radicals spares vitamin E for further antioxidant activity

Vitamin E

Stabilized free radicals

Undamaged cell

(b)

Figure 12.16 **Selenium and vitamin E help combat free radicals.** Since glutathione peroxidases require selenium, dietary selenium indirectly spares vitamin E.

toxic, selenium supplements are not recommended for cancer prevention. Much more research and large-scale trials are needed to clarify selenium's relationship to cancer.

Regulation of Selenium in the Body

Selenomethionine and selenocysteine are the principal dietary forms of selenium. The body efficiently absorbs these selenoamino acids, with estimates ranging from 50 to 90 percent.[47] The presence of vitamins A, C, and E and reduced glutathione enhance selenium absorption, but phytates and heavy metals such as mercury interfere with its bioavailability.

The selenium regulatory process maintains a low concentration of highly reactive free selenocysteine, and achieves homeostasis through excretion of excess mineral. The major routes of selenium excretion are the urine and the feces. When intake is excessive, the skin and lungs serve as additional excretory routes.

Selenium status, like that of many trace minerals, is difficult to evaluate. There are no sensitive tests that can readily distinguish between adequate and suboptimal levels of selenium.

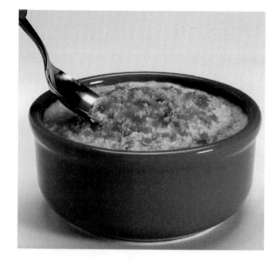

Dietary Recommendations for Selenium

Selenium is one of the "youngest" nutrients for which an RDA exists. The first RDA for selenium was established in 1989. The RDA was based on data from Chinese scientists who conducted repletion experiments in selenium-depleted subjects living in areas where Keshan disease was endemic. The RDA for selenium was revised in 2000. For both men and women the selenium RDA is 55 micrograms per day. [48]

Sources of Selenium

Since animals accumulate selenium in their tissues, the selenium content of food from animal sources generally is more consistent than the selenium content of plants. Organ meats and seafood are consistently good selenium sources. Other meats contain somewhat lower amounts of the mineral. The

---

[*Fyi*] Selenium and Cancer

FOR YOUR INFORMATION

Studies of animals indicate that high doses of selenium protect against cancer. In humans, the relationship between selenium and cancer is less clear.

Dietary intervention trials in Linxian, China, have yielded interesting results. These trials indicate that replenishing selenium in selenium-deficient individuals may decrease their risk of cancer. The Linxian region has one of the highest rates of esophageal and gastric cancer in the world. The population studied had multiple micronutrient deficiencies, which were thought to play a role in risk for

these cancers.[1] The study subjects took daily micronutrient supplements, with one group taking a combination of beta-carotene, selenium (50 micrograms per day), and alpha-tocopherol. The results indicate that supplements containing selenium might play a role in reducing cancer risk. Since the study design did not include evaluation of single nutrients, researchers could not draw conclusions about the role of selenium relative to the other nutrients. It is possible that the combination of nutrients or their interactions caused the improvements. Although the

data are not applicable to well-nourished populations, they do support the hypothesis that micronutrient deficiencies can increase cancer risk.

A more recent study suggests that dietary selenium supplements may reduce cancer risk in otherwise well-nourished people who live in areas where soil selenium is low.[2] Researchers found that people who lived in these regions and consumed supplemental selenium had significantly reduced cancer mortality, reduced incidence of all cancers, and reduced incidence of cancer at specific

American diet generally provides adequate selenium. **Figure 12.17** shows some sources of selenium.

Selenium Deficiency

Selenium deficiency predisposes a person to Keshan disease. Until recently, this disease was a major public health problem in China's Keshan province. Doctors have found selenium deficiency in people who receive long-term **total parenteral nutrition (TPN)**. Although after several years of TPN these patients may suffer heart problems and muscle weakness, no specific visible symptoms have been defined for selenium deficiency.

Selenium Toxicity

Chronic consumption of excess selenium can cause brittle hair and nails, and their eventual loss. While typical dietary intakes are unlikely to exceed safe amounts, selenium supplements can cause problems. Overenthusiastic media reports of research on selenium and cancer, coupled with easy access to selenium supplements, may cause some people to consume unhealthful quantities. The Tolerable Upper Level (UL) is set at 400 micrograms per day for adults.[49]

Key Concepts: *Selenium is best known for its role as an essential component of the antioxidant enzymes glutathione peroxidases. Selenium interacts with vitamin E in antioxidant systems and with iodine in thyroid hormone metabolism. It also is important for good immune function. Good dietary sources for selenium are organ meats and seafood. A deficiency of selenium may predispose a child to Keshan disease, a rare heart disease caused by a virus. New research also links marginal selenium status to cancer risk.*

total parenteral nutrition (TPN) Feeding a person by giving all essential nutrients intravenously.

SELENIUM

Daily Value = 70 μg

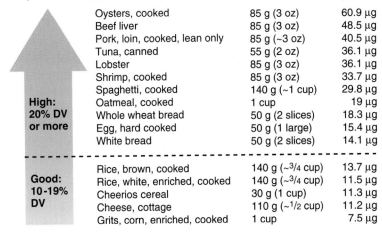

High: 20% DV or more		
Oysters, cooked	85 g (3 oz)	60.9 μg
Beef liver	85 g (3 oz)	48.5 μg
Pork, loin, cooked, lean only	85 g (~3 oz)	40.5 μg
Tuna, canned	55 g (2 oz)	36.1 μg
Lobster	85 g (3 oz)	36.1 μg
Shrimp, cooked	85 g (3 oz)	33.7 μg
Spaghetti, cooked	140 g (~1 cup)	29.8 μg
Oatmeal, cooked	1 cup	19 μg
Whole wheat bread	50 g (2 slices)	18.3 μg
Egg, hard cooked	50 g (1 large)	15.4 μg
White bread	50 g (2 slices)	14.1 μg
Good: 10-19% DV		
Rice, brown, cooked	140 g (~3/4 cup)	13.7 μg
Rice, white, enriched, cooked	140 g (~3/4 cup)	11.5 μg
Cheerios cereal	30 g (1 cup)	11.3 μg
Cheese, cottage	110 g (~1/2 cup)	11.2 μg
Grits, corn, enriched, cooked	1 cup	7.5 μg

Figure 12.17 **Food sources of selenium.** Selenium is found mainly in meats, organ meats, seafood, and grains.
Source: U.S. Department of Agriculture, Agricultural Research Service. 1999. USDA Nutrient Database for Standard Reference, Release 13. Nutrient Data Laboratory Home Page, http://www.nal.usda.gov/fnic/foodcomp

sites (lung, colorectal, and prostate). They concluded that although the findings support the hypothesis that supplemental selenium (within the range of normal dietary intakes) can reduce cancer incidence and mortality, the results are preliminary and confirmation is required from further research before public health recommendations can be made. The protective effect of selenium in this study was likely due to normalization of selenium status in previously selenium-deficient people. The results, then, may confirm those of the Linxian trial, which showed that dietary deficiency may contribute to development of certain types of cancers.

In 1984 a program was initiated in Finland to supplement fertilizer with selenium, since soil in that country is low in this mineral. This effort raised selenium intake from 30 to 40 micrograms per day to almost 100 micrograms per day. A rise in plasma selenium reflected this increased dietary intake. No dramatic change in cancer mortality or incidence attributable to selenium was seen in the 8 years from 1984 to 1992. Perhaps a higher intake (200 micrograms) would change cancer incidence, or perhaps an effect will be seen after a longer period. This area remains wide open for further research.

1 Mobarhan S. Micronutrient supplementation trials and the reduction of cancer and cerebrovascular incidence and mortality. *Nutr Rev.* 1994:52(3):102–105.

2 Fleet JC. Dietary selenium repletion may reduce cancer incidence in people at high risk who live in areas with low soil selenium. *Nutr Rev.* 1997;55(7):277–229.

goiter A chronic enlargement of the thyroid gland, visible as a swelling at the front of the neck; usually associated with iodine deficiency.

triiodothyronine (T3) An iodine-containing thyroid hormone with several times the biologic activity of thyroxine (T4).

thyroxine (T4) An iodine-containing hormone secreted by the thyroid gland to regulate the rate of cell metabolism; known chemically as tetraiodothyronine.

thyroglobulin The storage form of thyroid hormone in the thyroid gland

thyroid-stimulating hormone (TSH) Secreted from the pituitary gland at the base of the brain, this hormone regulates synthesis of thyroid hormones.

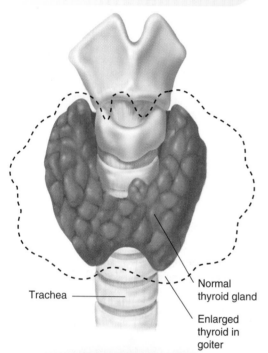

Trachea

Normal thyroid gland

Enlarged thyroid in goiter

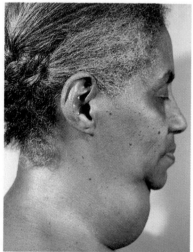

Figure 12.18 **Enlargement of the thyroid gland in goiter.** The finding that the use of iodized salt dramatically reduced goiter rates led to the widespread fortification of table salt with iodine.

Iodine

Ancient Chinese writings first recorded descriptions of what we now know to be the iodine-deficiency diseases cretinism and **goiter** (see **Figure 12.18**). Cretins were described as feeble-minded dwarfs with puffy facial features and a stumbling gait. In the Middle Ages, European paintings commonly depicted cretins as angels or demons.[50] As late as the early 1900s, goiter was common in certain parts of the United States, particularly the upper Midwest. In 1922 scientists demonstrated that the use of iodized salt by 50,000 school children dramatically reduced goiter rates. These findings led to the widespread fortification of table salt with of iodine (I). Although iodine deficiency remains a problem in many parts of the world, the World Health Organization plans to eradicate iodine deficiency disorders within the next decade through the use of iodized salt programs.[51]

Function of Iodine

Much of iodine is an essential component of the two thyroid hormones: **triiodothyronine (T3)** and **thyroxine (T4)**. Thyroid hormones control the regulation of body temperature, basal metabolic rate, reproduction, and growth. Although the thyroid hormones released by the thyroid gland are about 93 percent thyroxine and only 7 percent triiodothyronine, triiodothyronine is about four times more potent than thyroxine.[52] Within a few days of secretion, the body converts most of the thyroxine to the more active triiodothyronine.

Iodine Absorption and Metabolism

Much of the iodine in food is in the form of iodide (the reduced form), and iodates. The intestine absorbs nearly all of it, from 95 to 100 percent. The entire body contains between 15 and 20 milligrams, 70 to 80 percent of which resides in the thyroid gland. Each day the thyroid gland "traps" between 60 and 120 micrograms of iodide for eventual incorporation into the thyroid hormones. Enzymes oxidize the iodide, then other enzymes bind it to **thyroglobulin**, the storage form of thyroid hormones.

Thyroid stimulating hormone (TSH) signals the thyroid gland to cleave T3 and T4 from thyroglobulin and release them into the bloodstream. In various body organs, three different enzymes convert most of the T4 to the more active form, T3. Recent research reveals that all three of these converting enzymes are selenium dependent. Therefore, a deficiency in selenium may lead to inefficient use of iodine in thyroid hormones.

The kidneys excrete most excess iodine in urine, but some is lost in sweat, especially in hot, humid climates.

Dietary Recommendations for Iodine

To replace losses and prevent deficiency of iodine, the thyroid gland needs at least 60 micrograms daily. Because iodine absorption is so efficient, intakes of 75 micrograms per day should be sufficient for adults. To provide a margin of safety, however, the RDA is set at 150 micrograms per day for both men and women.

Sources of Iodine

Because the ocean is the best source of iodine, the best food sources are seafoods. Saltwater fish have higher concentrations of iodine than fresh water fish. The dairy industry adds iodide to cattle feed and uses sanitizing solutions that contain iodide. These measures add substantial amounts of

3

iodine to milk and dairy products. Natural iodine levels in plants reflect soil levels. For many people, iodized salt used in cooking and at the table is their primary source. In the United States, iodized salt contains an average of 76 micrograms of iodine per gram of salt.

Excluding iodized salt, the average U.S. diet contains between 230 and 400 micrograms of iodine per day. After salt, dairy products supply most of our dietary iodine, followed by 10 to 15 percent from meat, fish, and poultry and 5 to 15 percent from grains and cereals. Salt added during cooking and at the table contributes 35 to 70 micrograms of iodide to the average adult's daily diet. **Figure 12.19** shows the iodine content of some foods.

Iodine Deficiency

As early as 1830, iodine deficiency was linked to the presence of goiter. We now understand that a deficiency of iodine inhibits the synthesis of thyroid hormones. As the body senses the lack of thyroid hormones, it produces more and more TSH. TSH causes the thyroid gland to grow, eventually resulting in a goiter. Goiter in children has been linked to depressed IQ[53] in addition to the usual symptoms of hypothyroidism—cold intolerance, weight gain, sluggishness, and a decreased body temperature.

Severe iodine deficiency during early pregnancy causes cretinism. Most cretins have stunted growth and are deaf, mute, and mentally retarded. A selenium deficiency may be partly responsible for a form of cretinism commonly seen in Africa.

Raw cabbage, turnips, rutabagas, and cassava contain compounds known as **goitrogens**, which are compounds that block the body's absorption and use of iodine. Consuming large amounts of these foods in their raw form can cause problems; cooking inactivates the goitrogens. Iodine-deficiency disorders are common in developing countries where iodide consumption is low and raw cassava and similar vegetables are a major part of the diet.

Iodine Toxicity

Because high amounts of iodine inhibit synthesis of thyroid hormone and stimulate growth of the thyroid gland, iodine toxicity also can cause goiter. Overzealous supplementation is the most common cause of iodine toxicity. A successful program of iodine fortification must be balanced against the risk of iodine-induced hyperthyroidism, especially in areas of severe iodine deficiency. The UL for iodine is 1,100 micrograms per day.

Key Concepts: *Iodine is an essential component of thyroid hormones. Iodine deficiency causes overstimulation of the thyroid gland and eventual goiter. The best food source of iodine is seafood. Many people around the world are still at risk for iodine deficiency, but iodization of salt is a powerful preventive measure.*

IODINE

Daily Value = 150 µg

	Food	Portion	Iodine
High: 20% DV or more	Cod, cooked	85 g (~3 oz)	98.6 µg
	Corn grits, enriched, cooked	1 cup	67.8 µg
	Milk, 2% fat	240 ml (1 cup)	56.1 µg
	Milk, skim	240 ml (1 cup)	51 µg
	White bread	50 g (~2 slices)	45.5 µg
	Tortilla, flour	55 g	41.3 µg
	Beef liver, cooked	85 g (3 oz)	35.7 µg
	Navy beans, cooked	90 g (~1/2 cup)	35.1 µg
	Shrimp, cooked	85 g (3 oz)	34.9 µg
	Potato, baked	110 g (1 small)	34.1 µg
	Whole wheat bread	50 g (~2 slices)	31.5 µg
Good: 10-19% DV	Egg, cooked	50 g (1 large)	23.5 µg
	Turkey breast, cooked	85 g (~3 oz)	22 µg
	Oatmeal, cooked	1 cup	16.4 µg

Figure 12.19 **Food sources of iodine.** Few foods are rich in iodine; it is found mainly in milk, seafood, and some grain products.
Source: Pennington, JAT. *Bowes and Church's Food Values of Portions Commonly Used.* 17th ed. Philadelphia, PA: Lippincott-Raven Publishers, 1998.

Quick Bites

Iodine or Iodide: What's in a name?

Iodine (I_2) is a bluish-black solid that gives off a purple vapor, which gives the element its name. Iodine stems from the Greek word iôdêdes, meaning "violet-colored."

Iodide (I^-) is the colorless negative ion of iodine. Iodine circulates in the body either protein-bound or as free iodide ions. Sodium iodide and potassium iodide are iodide salts commonly used in medicines.

goitrogens Compounds that can induce goiter.

Menkes' syndrome A genetic disorder that results in copper deficiency.

ceruloplasmin A copper-dependent enzyme responsible for the oxidation of ferrous ion (Fe^{2+}) to ferric ion (Fe^{3+}), enabling iron to bind to transferrin. Also known as ferroxidase I.

Copper

In 1928 researchers recognized the essential nature of copper (Cu) for experimental animals. But not until the 1960s did evidence emerge that copper deficiency occurs in humans. Recent cloning of the genes for two genetic disorders of copper metabolism—Wilson's disease (copper toxicity) and **Menkes' syndrome** (copper deficiency)—has fueled interest in copper and led to exciting new discoveries about its metabolism and physiological role. Although simple dietary copper deficiency is not a significant public health concern, excessive supplementation of other trace minerals can cause a secondary copper deficiency.

Functions of Copper

Copper-containing enzymes have many functions including acting as an antioxidant, participating in the electron transport chain, as well as in the biosynthesis of the pigment melanin and the connective tissue proteins collagen and elastin. Perhaps the most important function of copper is as a component of **ceruloplasmin**, the enzyme that catalyzes the oxidation of ferrous (Fe^{2+}) to ferric (Fe^{3+}) iron for incorporation into transferrin. The absence of ceruloplasmin leads to accumulation of iron in the liver, similar to what is seen in iron overload or hemochromatosis. Copper is an important component of the superoxide dismutases, enzymes involved in antioxidant reactions. Copper also plays a role in various other activities including the myelinization of the nervous tissue, immune function, and cardiovascular function.

Copper Absorption, Use, and Metabolism

Depending on the amount of copper in the meal and other dietary factors, the intestine absorbs approximately 50 percent of dietary copper. Amino acids, particularly histidine, enhance copper absorption. On the other hand, a number of minerals, most notably iron and zinc, may interfere with copper absorption. Because high-dose iron supplementation is more common than zinc supplementation, the iron-copper interaction is of greater concern. Dietary phytates do not appear to inhibit copper absorption. Because copper is best absorbed in an acidic environment, antacids can reduce copper absorption.

Albumin transports copper from the intestinal cell to the liver, where about two-thirds is incorporated into ceruloplasmin. The average healthy adult body contains approximately 100 milligrams of copper at any time, mainly distributed among the liver, brain, blood, and bone marrow. The body stores relatively little copper, and excretes nearly all excess copper in feces and a minor amount in the urine. Copper excreted in the feces includes unabsorbed dietary copper, copper released in bile, and copper in cells sloughed from the intestinal wall.

Dietary Recommendations and Food Sources for Copper

There is no single reliable index of copper status. Balance studies have been previously used to estimate copper needs. However, balance studies in humans are problematic, and so a combination of plasma, serum, and blood cell measures were used to develop the copper RDA.[54] The RDA for both men and women is 900 micrograms per day.

Copper is widely distributed in foods. The richest food sources for copper include organ meats (e.g., liver), shellfish, nuts and seeds, legumes, peanut butter, and chocolate. (See **Figure 12.20**.) Although information

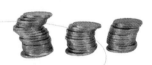

Quick Bites

A Penny for Your …

How do the amounts of zinc and copper in a U.S. penny compare to the amounts in your body? Today's penny is mostly zinc (2.4 grams), covered with some copper plating (62.5 mg). A penny's zinc is in the upper range of the body's zinc content, but the amount of copper falls short. It takes the copper in about $1\frac{1}{2}$ pennies to equal the amount of copper in your body.

about the copper content of foods is incomplete, dietary surveys in the United States suggest that adults consume an average of about 1,000 to 1,600 micrograms of copper per day.

Copper Deficiency

Overt copper deficiency is relatively rare in humans. Copper deficiency occurs most commonly in preterm infants. These babies have low copper stores at birth and a rapid growth rate, which elevates needs. Because cow's milk has little copper and it is poorly bioavailable, infants who are inappropriately fed unmodified cow's milk are more likely to develop a deficiency than breast-fed infants. Doctors have also observed copper deficiency, albeit less frequently than zinc deficiency, in people with malabsorption syndromes.[56]

Copper deficiency most commonly causes anemia, decreased numbers of white blood cells, and bone abnormalities. In copper-deficiency anemia, low ceruloplasmin activity causes defective iron mobilization. Copper-deficient young children are most likely to suffer bone abnormalities. Probably caused by poor synthesis of connective tissue, these abnormalities mimic the changes observed in scurvy. In experimental settings, copper deficiency causes elevated blood cholesterol, impaired glucose tolerance, and heart-related abnormalities. Some scientists suggest that copper deficiency during pregnancy may cause numerous gross structural and biochemical birth defects.[57]

Menkes' syndrome is an extremely rare (~1 in 100,000 live births) genetic copper disorder in which there is a failure to absorb copper into the bloodstream and therefore a lack of functional copper-containing proteins such as ceruloplasmin. Serum copper and ceruloplasmin levels are low, but copper accumulates in the intestinal mucosal cells, and in the muscle, spleen, and kidney.[58] Menkes' syndrome causes neurological degeneration,

Quick Bites

Egg whites? Please stand up!

Although cooking food in a copper pot is inadvisable, copper mixing bowls can be a plus. Meringues made in ceramic or steel bowls tend to be snowy white and drier than those made in copper bowls. Making meringue in a copper bowl leads to a creamier, yellowish foam that is harder to overbeat into a lumpy liquid. The copper bowl contributes copper ions to conalbumin, a metal-binding protein, thus stabilizing the whipped egg whites.

COPPER

Daily Value = 2 mg

Exceptionally good sources

Oysters, cooked	85 g (3 oz)	6.4 mg
Beef liver, cooked	85 g (3 oz)	3.8 mg
Lobster, cooked	85 g (3 oz)	1.6 mg
Crab, Alaska King, cooked	85 g (3 oz)	1.0 mg
Clams, cooked	85 g (3 oz)	0.6 mg
Sunflower seeds	30 g (~1 oz)	0.5 mg
Hazelnuts	30 g (~1 oz)	0.5 mg
Mushrooms, cooked	85 g (~1/2 cup)	0.4 mg
Peanuts	30 g (1 oz)	0.4 mg
All Bran cereal	30 g (~1/2 cup)	0.4 mg
Tofu, calcium processed	85 g (~1/3 cup)	0.3 mg
Baked beans, canned	130 g (~1/2 cup)	0.3 mg
Navy beans, cooked	90 g (~1/2 cup)	0.3 mg
Soy milk	240 ml (1 cup)	0.3 mg
Refried beans, canned	130 g (~1/2 cup)	0.2 mg
Cocoa	1 Tbsp.	0.2 mg

High: 20% DV or more

Good: 10-19% DV

Figure 12.20 **Food sources of copper.** Copper is found in a limited variety of foods. The best sources are seafood, legumes, and nuts. Source: U.S. Department of Agriculture, Agricultural Research Service. 1999. USDA Nutrient Database for Standard Reference, Release 13. Nutrient Data Laboratory Home Page, http://www.nal.usda.gov/fnic/foodcomp.

chelation therapy Use of a chelator (e.g., EDTA) to bind metal ions to remove them from the body.

peculiar kinky hair, abnormal connective tissue development, osteoporosis, and poor growth. Although this syndrome is usually fatal in infancy or early childhood, copper-histidine treatment within the first few days of life may prevent irreversible damage.[59]

Copper Toxicity

Compared to other trace elements, copper is relatively nontoxic. The UL for copper is 10,000 micrograms per day. Wilson's disease is a rare (1 in 200,000) genetic copper toxicity disorder that impairs copper excretion in bile, causing toxic accumulation in the liver, brain, kidney, and eye. As copper accumulates in red blood cells, it causes anemia. Without treatment, people with Wilson's disease develop serious liver and neurologic problems. Copper toxicity may be treated either by **chelation therapy** to bind and remove copper or with zinc supplementation to decrease copper absorption. Lifelong treatment can prevent many complications of Wilson's disease.

Key Concepts: *The most important function of copper is as a component of ceruloplasmin, the enzyme that catalyzes the oxidation of iron for transport in transferrin. Food sources for copper include organ meats, shellfish, nuts and seeds, legumes, peanut butter, chocolate, and dried fruits. Copper deficiency is relatively rare in humans. Usual copper intakes fall below the current safe and adequate level.*

Manganese

Recognized for centuries, manganese (Mn) derives its name from a Greek term for magic. While its many functions are not magical, they are unique. Manganese is essential not only in biological systems, but also in iron and steel production. It has many industrial uses in such diverse products as dry-cell batteries, glass, ceramics, paints, varnishes, inks, dyes, and fertilizers. Industrial exposure, rather than food intake, is the more frequent cause of manganese toxicity.

Functions of Manganese

The body contains between 10 and 20 milligrams of manganese, which is concentrated primarily in the bone, liver, pancreas, and brain. Despite this limited quantity, manganese is a key component of several enzymes:

- *Mn-superoxide dismutase,* located in the mitochondria of cells, is an antioxidant that prevents tissue damage due to lipid oxidation.
- *Arginase* helps form urea in the urea cycle.
- *Pyruvate carboxylase* helps convert pyruvate to oxaloacetate.

Manganese also activates numerous enzymes involved in the formation of cartilage in bone and skin.

Manganese Absorption, Use, and Homeostasis

Absorption of manganese is poor, only 1 to 15 percent. This low absorption rate may protect against toxicity. Some research suggests that high levels of iron, calcium, and phosphorus may inhibit absorption. Fiber and phytate also may limit manganese absorption, but to a lesser degree than they affect the absorption of most other trace minerals. Following absorption, transferrin binds manganese and transports it in the bloodstream.

Excretion, rather than absorption, regulates the body's manganese. Bile is the main excretory route. Should the intestine absorb excess manganese, the body may quickly dump this excess back into the intestine as part of

---

Quick Bites

Cooking in Copper

Because the copper imparted a bright green color to cooked green vegetables, cooking vegetables in uncoated copper pans was once encouraged. This practice often led to decreased liver and brain function. The Swedish military recognized copper toxicity and banned copper cooking utensils in 1753.

bile. There is no storage form of manganese. As with zinc, there does not appear to be a reliable indicator of manganese status in adults.

Dietary Recommendations and Food Sources for Manganese

The Adequate Intake (AI) level for manganese is 2.3 milligrams per day for men and 1.8 milligrams per day for women. Previous to 2001, manganese recommendations were higher: 2.0 to 5.0 milligrams per day, but these recommendations were questioned because they were close to the toxic levels suggested by the Environmental Protection Agency: more than 10 milligrams manganese per day from food or more than 4.2 milligrams from water.[60]

Tea, coffee, nuts, cereals, and some fruits are the best food sources of manganese. Some estimates suggest that coffee or tea supplies as much as 20 to 30 percent of our daily manganese intake. Meat, dairy products, poultry, fish, and refined foods are poor sources; they contain little manganese. **Figure 12.21** shows the manganese content of some foods.

Manganese Deficiency

Although people who consume normal varied diets do not appear to be at risk for manganese deficiency, certain disorders may cause suboptimal status. Studies report low manganese or altered manganese metabolism in some patients with nontrauma epilepsy, phenylketonuria (PKU),[61] **amyotrophic lateral sclerosis**,[62] and **multiple sclerosis**. In animal studies, manganese deficiency has dramatic effects—impaired growth, skeletal abnormalities, a staggering gait, and impaired fat and carbohydrate metabolism.

amyotrophic lateral sclerosis (ALS) A syndrome marked by muscular weakness and atrophy due to a degeneration of motor neurons of the spinal cord.

multiple sclerosis A progressive disease that destroys the myelin sheath surrounding nerve fibers of the brain and spinal cord.

Quick Bites

Highway Harvest

Oil companies often add a type of manganese to modern gasoline as an antiknock compound to increase the octane rating for high-compression engines. It is now evident that plants along highways accumulate manganese from passing cars.

MANGANESE

Daily Value = 2 mg

Exceptionally good sources

Wheat germ	15 g	3 mg
All Bran cereal	30 g (~1/2 cup)	2.7 mg
Pineapple, fresh	140 g (~1 cup)	2.3 mg
Blackberries, fresh	140 g (~1 cup)	2 mg
Hazelnuts	30 g (1 oz)	1.7 mg
Oatmeal, cooked	1 cup	1.4 mg
Whole wheat bread	50 g (2 slices)	1.2 mg
Okra, cooked	85 g (~1/2 cup)	0.9 mg
Spinach, cooked	85 g (~1/2 cup)	0.8 mg
Cantaloupe, fresh	140 g (~1/4 med. melon)	0.7 mg
Carrots, cooked	85 g (~1/2 cup)	0.6 mg
Tea, brewed	240 ml (1 cup)	0.5 mg
Baked beans, canned	130 g (~1/2 cup)	0.4 mg
Sweet potato, cooked	110 g (1 small)	0.4 mg
Turnip greens, cooked	85 g (~1/2 cup)	0.3 mg
Beets, cooked	85 g (~1/2 cup)	0.3 mg
Broccoli, cooked	85 g (~1/2 cup)	0.3 mg
Cocoa	1 Tbsp.	0.2 mg

High: 20% DV or more

Good: 10–19% DV

Figure 12.21 **Food sources of manganese.** Manganese is found mainly in plant foods such as grains, legumes, vegetables, and some fruits.
Source: U.S. Department of Agriculture, Agricultural Research Service. 1999. USDA Nutrient Database for Standard Reference, Release 13. Nutrient Data Laboratory Home Page, http://www.nal.usda.gov/fnic/foodcomp.

mineralization The addition of minerals, such as calcium and phosphate, to bones and teeth.

Manganese Toxicity

Manganese toxicity is a greater threat than manganese deficiency. Foundry workers exposed to airborne manganese dust have experienced severe manganese toxicity. Their symptoms included irritability, hallucinations, and severe lack of coordination. Lower doses of airborne manganese can impair memory and cause impaired motor coordination similar to that experienced in Parkinson's disease The UL for manganese is 11 milligrams per day.

Key Concepts: *Manganese is important to the functioning of several enzymes in the human body. Our usual intake of manganese falls within the currently recommended intake range. Food sources for manganese are tea, coffee, cereals, and some fruits. Toxicity is more a threat than deficiency is, primarily to people who are exposed industrially to high levels of manganese dust.*

Fluoride

Fluoride (F), the ionized form of fluorine, has the unique ability to prevent dental caries. Although people first observed this beneficial effect in the early 1800s, scientific proof did not emerge until the time of World War II. In 1945 many U.S. water suppliers began voluntarily fluoridating water to improve the dental health of children. Now that use of fluoridated toothpaste and mouthwash is widespread, some experts are raising concerns about potential harm from excessive fluoride intake.

Functions of Fluoride

Bones and teeth contain nearly 99 percent of the body's fluoride. Fluoride supports the **mineralization** of bone and teeth by promoting the deposition of calcium and phosphate.

Fluoride's cavity-prevention activity is an effect localized in the mouth. Bacteria in the mouth cause dental caries, an infectious disease. When a person eats food, especially carbohydrate foods, these oral bacteria multiply and produce organic acids that eat away tooth enamel, especially beneath plaque. When food leaves the mouth, remineralization begins. If remineralization does not keep pace with demineralization, your teeth become pitted with dental caries. Fluoride decreases the demineralization of tooth enamel and accelerates the subsequent remineralization process. Fluoride also inhibits bacterial activity in dental plaques. These cavity-fighting actions can help make your next trip to the dentist a pleasant one.

Regular ingestion of fluoride is especially important during the eruption of new teeth in children. When administered topically, fluoride's support of tooth enamel remineralization can benefit people of all ages.

Fluoride Absorption and Excretion

Your body absorbs almost all fluoride in water and other liquid beverages. The bioavailability of fluoride in food ranges between 50 and 80 percent. After absorption, the body distributes fluoride in "hard" tissues, mainly the bones and teeth. Excess fluoride is excreted mainly in the urine.

Dietary Recommendations for Fluoride

The Adequate Intake (AI) level for fluoride is 4 milligrams per day for adult men, and 3 milligrams per day for women. As of 1995, the American Dental Association and American Academy of Pediatrics no longer recommend fluoride supplementation from birth, and suggest it only for children

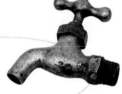

Quick Bites

Accidental Discovery

In the early 1900s people noticed that inhabitants of towns with naturally high levels of fluoride in their water had healthier teeth. To test the correlation between fluoride and tooth decay, in 1945 four cities in the United States and one in Canada took part in a controlled study of water fluoridation. The results were impressive, establishing that fluoride helps to prevent tooth decay.

whose drinking water supplies less than 0.6 milligrams per liter. The AI for fluoride for infants is 0.01 milligram per day for ages 0 to 5 months and 0.5 milligram per day for ages 6 to 11 months.

fluorosis Mottled discoloration and pitting of tooth enamel caused by prolonged ingestion of excessive fluoride.

Sources of Fluoride

Water is the main source of fluoride, whether the fluoride is naturally present or added. Artificially fluoridated water contains 0.7 to 1.2 milligrams per liter. Fluoride naturally present in drinking water may vary from less than 0.1 milligram to more than 10 milligrams per liter. The Environmental Protection Agency's regulations require public drinking water systems to remove excess fluoride so that it does not exceed 4.0 milligrams per liter. Roughly 62 percent of the U.S. population has fluoridated water;[63] most other developed countries do not fluoridate their water.

The balance between the positive effects of just enough fluoride and the negative effects of too much fluoride has become the subject of debate. Some scientists argue that artificial fluoridation is an outdated practice. Fluoridation was instituted 50 years ago when it served as the exclusive source of fluoride for children. Now, however, there are other fluoride sources including ready-to-feed infant formulas, fluoride supplements, mouthwash, toothpaste, and some beverages. The combination of all of these sources may put children at increased risk for excessive fluoride intake and **fluorosis**.

Because there are so many sources of fluoride, it is difficult to determine the current effectiveness of artificial fluoridation of the water supply. Some opponents argue that artificial fluoridation is inappropriate and "equal to mass medication of the population."[64] However, the dramatic decline in dental caries since fluoridation was initiated is undeniable. To retain the benefits yet avoid overconsumption, the American Dental Association recommends the fluoridation of all water supplies and regulation of other fluoride sources.

Quick Bites

Conspiracy Theory

*A*lthough the U.S. Public Health Service and the World Health Organization officially endorsed the fluoridation of water in the 1950s, some groups continue to oppose the practice. Objectors claim that water fluoridation violates civil rights, that fluoride is a "nerve poison," and that fluoride is unwanted compulsory medication that can have dangerous side effects. Some groups even claim that fluoridation is a component of a conspiracy for national destruction. So far, objectors have been unable to substantiate their claims and the courts have upheld the constitutionality of fluoridation.

Fluoride Deficiency, Toxicity, and Pharmacological Applications

Low fluoride intake increases the risk for dental caries, and may hamper the integrity of bone. Adequate fluoride intake in childhood can decrease the incidence of tooth decay by 30 to 60 percent. During tooth development, prolonged excessive fluoride intake can cause fluorosis (**Figure 12.22**). In mild fluorosis, white specks form on the teeth. Severe fluorosis can cause permanent brownish stains and weakened teeth. Consumption of water naturally high in fluoride is the main cause of fluorosis, but children who chronically swallow large amounts of fluoridated toothpaste are also at risk.

Hemodialysis patients who have been given too much fluoride can suffer acute fluoride toxicity with symptoms that include headaches, nausea, and abnormal heart rhythms. Other observed effects of fluorosis include hip fractures, chronic gastritis, and weak, stiff joints.

Researchers have studied fluoride for the treatment of osteoporosis in postmenopausal women. A daily dose of 75 milligrams of sodium fluoride increased spinal bone density, but it also increased the number of nonspine fractures.[65] Subsequent studies using lower amounts of fluoride (25 mg/d) combined with supplemental calcium reduced the risk of fracture. Fluoride is not an approved treatment for osteoporosis.

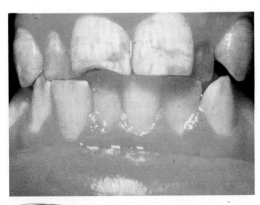

Figure 12.22 **Tooth mottling in fluorosis.**

Key Concepts: *Bones and teeth contain 99 percent of body fluoride. Fluoride supports remineralization and its major function is the prevention of dental caries. Fluoride is unique in that the main dietary source is water, not food. The majority of our nation's municipal water supplies are artificially fluoridated. Excess fluoride can cause fluorosis. Mild fluorosis with mottling of the teeth is primarily a cosmetic problem; severe fluorosis can weaken teeth.*

Chromium

Chromium (Cr) plays an important but poorly understood role in moving glucose into cells, and in lipid metabolism. Although researchers established chromium's essential role in glucose tolerance during the late 1950s and early 1960s, the development of reliable analytical methods took another 20 years. As with many trace minerals, low levels in biological tissues and the potential for sample contamination make chromium assessment particularly challenging.[66]

Functions of Chromium

Chromium enhances the effects of insulin and is important for proper metabolism of carbohydrates and lipids. Chromium may also play a role in metabolism of nucleic acids, and in immune function and growth. Athletes are especially interested in chromium because of its purported effects on body composition.

Chromium Absorption, Transport, and Excretion

Little is known about chromium absorption. Uptake of the inorganic form is thought to be low (about 1 to 2 percent); absorption of organic chromium (a combination of chromium and an organic acid such as chromium picolinate) may be higher (10 to 25 percent). Absorption increases with need and decreases with higher amounts in the diet. Other substances can influence chromium absorption. For example, vitamin C and aspirin increase chromium absorption, and antacids decrease it.[67]

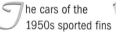

Quick Bites

Chrome-Plated Cars

The cars of the 1950s sported fins and loads of chrome. The chromium in your body is the same metal used for electroplating hard chrome. Using electric current, chromium molecules atoms bond with the original surface, creating a bond between the metals so hard it will remain intact even when subjected to extreme force.

Fyi

Chromium, Exercise, and Body Composition

FOR YOUR INFORMATION

Because chromium supplements are purported to increase lean body mass (LBM) and decrease body fat during resistance training, they have generated a great deal of popular interest. Yet study results are contradictory and chromium's influence on body composition is controversial. The USDA's Human Nutrition Research Center in Beltsville, Maryland, reviewed numerous studies of chromium and body composition.[1] While several of the studies show that chromium supplementation positively affects gains achieved with resistance training, a number of other experiments show no effect.[2]

What are the issues raised by these studies and how are we to understand the contradictory results? After researchers reported the initial positive results, the press and supplement advertisers overstated the benefits of chromium supplementation, thereby creating unrealistic expectations for improvement in muscle mass. Supplement makers marketed chromium picolinate, the form used in most studies, as the healthy alternative to anabolic steroids, and inappropriately extended the research findings to suggest that chromium would be effective as a weight-loss product.[3] Although one study did show a decrease in percentage

of body fat in a group of sedentary subjects, 20 *years* of studies show that chromium has no significant effect as a weight-loss agent.[4] In 1996 the Federal Trade Commission (FTC) ordered the maker of chromium picolinate to stop making unsubstantiated claims of weight loss and health benefits.

Differences in experimental design explain many of these inconsistent results. In some studies the dosage may have been too low and the time period may have been too short to show any effect. One of the limitations of any chromium study is the inability to assess initial status of the subjects.

Transferrin and **albumin** transport chromium in the bloodstream. The body contains approximately 4 to 6 milligrams of chromium, mostly in the liver, spleen, and bone; the remainder is widely dispersed at very low concentrations. The body excretes excess chromium in the urine.

Chromium levels in hair, sweat, and serum decrease with age, but study results raise the question as to whether the decline is normal or an effect of the Western diet on chromium levels.[68] Some researchers speculate that the age-related decline in chromium may contribute to the high incidence of insulin resistance and type II diabetes in Western countries.

Dietary Recommendations and Food Sources for Chromium

In 2001, scientists set an Adequate Intake (AI) level for chromium. For adults 19-50 years of age, the AI is 35 micrograms per day for men and 25 micrograms per day for women. The AI for older adults is 5 micrograms less. More data on actual requirements for chromium and chromium content of foods are needed for more specific dietary recommendations.

Rich sources of chromium are mushrooms, dark chocolate, prunes, nuts, asparagus, whole grains, wine, brewer's yeast, and some brands of beer. Animal products are poor sources; fruits, vegetables, and grains are variable. Cooking acidic foods in stainless steel containers leaches some chromium into the food.

Chromium Deficiency

The difficulty of assessing chromium status makes it hard to determine the effects of deficiency. Nevertheless, studies in animals and humans point to the following signs of chromium deficiency: decreased insulin-mediated glucose uptake by cells, decreased insulin sensitivity, elevated blood glucose and insulin, and blood lipid abnormalities. Doctors have observed more severe signs, such as brain and nerve disorders, in patients who subsist on total parenteral nutrition that has inadequate chromium.[69]

albumin A protein that circulates in the blood and functions in the transport of many minerals and some drugs.

There is no evidence that chromium supplements provide a "quick fix" for athletes, and long-term chromium intake probably has a minimal effect on body composition and body weight. Although the risk of toxicity from supplemental chromium alone is low, chromium can interact with iron and zinc, which raises concern about adverse effects. As is the case with many trace minerals, only further investigation will clarify the role of chromium in human health.

Recent studies have raised safety issues about chromium picolinate supplements. This organic form of chromium is very stable, and cells may acquire it intact. Within cells it can interact with peroxide to form the potentially DNA-damaging hydroxyl radical.[5] Researchers have found that chromium picolinate can cause chromosomal abnormalities in Chinese hamster ovary cells.[6] In addition, absorption rates of chromium picolinate in humans may be high enough to allow tissue levels similar to those shown to produce DNA damage.[7] Numerous health groups advise consumers to avoid chromium picolinate supplements.

The best advice for achieving a healthy, fit body? A varied diet, and regular exercise—not reliance on supplements.

1 Anderson RA. Effects of chromium on body composition and weight loss. *Nutr Rev.* 1998;56:266–270.

2 Evans GW. The effect of chromium picolinate on insulin controlled parameters in humans. *Int J Biosoc Med Res.* 1989;11:163–180.

3 Haymes EM, Clarkson PM. Minerals and trace minerals. In: Berning JR, Steen SN, eds. *Nutrition for Sport and Exercise.* 2nd ed. Gaithersburg, MD: Aspen; 1998:95–98.

4 Anderson RA. Op. cit.

5 Speetjens JK, Collins RA, Vincent JB, Woski SA. The nutritional supplement chromium (III) tris(picolinate) cleaves DNA. *Chem Res Toxicol.* 1999;12:483–487.

6 Stearns DM, Wise JP, Patierno SR, Wetterhahn KE. Chromium (III) picolinate produces chromosome damage in Chinese hamster ovary cells. *FASEB J.* 1995;9:1643–1848.

7 Stearns DM, Belbruno JJ, Wetterhahn KE. A prediction of chromium (III) accumulation in humans from chromium dietary supplements. *FASEB J.* 1995;9:1650–1657.

Chromium Toxicity

The only known cases of chromium toxicity occurred in people exposed to airborne chromium compounds in industrial settings. Since inorganic chromium is so poorly absorbed, extremely high oral intakes would be necessary to attain toxic levels. Numerous experiments show 200 micrograms of inorganic chromium to be a safe dose for supplementation. Recent studies of chromium picolinate supplements show DNA damage in animal cells and have raised safety concerns about this supplemental form (see the FYI feature "Chromium, Exercise, and Body Composition"). To date, no UL has been set for chromium.

Key Concepts: *The primary function of chromium in the body is to potentiate the effects of insulin. Sources of chromium include mushrooms, dark chocolate, prunes, nuts, asparagus, whole grains, wine, brewer's yeast, and some beers. Reliable assessment of chromium status is difficult.*

Molybdenum

Molybdenum (Mo) is essential to both plants and animals. In humans, molybdenum functions as a cofactor for several enzymes that induce oxidation.

Molybdenum Absorption, Use, and Metabolism

The intestine absorbs molybdenum efficiently—some studies suggest up to 80 to 90 percent of the amount consumed. However, the body excretes it rapidly in urine and in bile. Fiber and phytate have no effect on its absorption. Dietary copper is the only significant inhibitor of molybdenum absorption. The body contains about 2 milligrams of molybdenum, 90 percent of which is located in the liver.

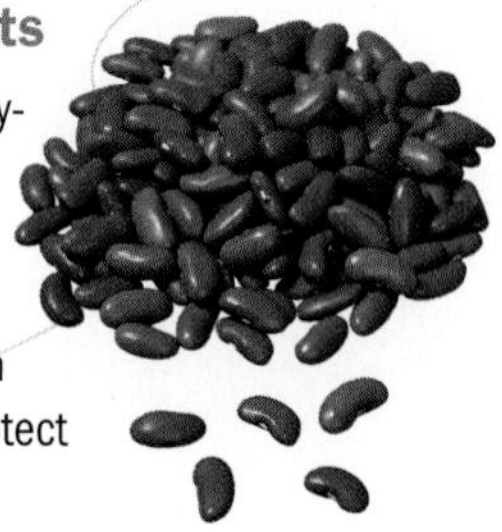

Dietary Recommendations and Food Sources for Molybdenum

For adults, the molybdenum RDA is 45 micrograms per day. Although data is limited, typical intakes in the United States exceed the RDA. Peas, beans, and some breakfast cereals are the richest food sources for molybdenum. Organ meats like liver and kidney also are fairly rich sources, but other meats tend to be poor sources.

Molybdenum Deficiency and Toxicity

Molybdenum deficiency does not occur in people who eat a normal diet. People on total parenteral nutrition who have molybdenum deficiency can suffer weakness, mental confusion, and night blindness. People with a rare congenital disorder have deficient amounts of sulfite oxidase, a molybdenum-dependent enzyme. These people suffer from neurological problems similar to those of severe molybdenum deficiency.

Scientists first recognized the interaction between dietary copper and molybdenum in sheep and cattle that grazed on grass grown on soil either very poor or very rich in molybdenum. If the soil content was low in molybdenum, the animals suffered copper toxicity; if the soil was rich, they were deficient in copper. Doctors exploit this interaction when they use a form of molybdenum to treat patients with Wilson's disease. Despite the possible interaction with copper, molybdenum salts are considered relatively nontoxic. The UL for molybdenum is 2,000 micrograms per day.

Quick Bites

Molybdenum Takes a Stand Against the Elements

Molybdenum is a silvery-gray metal that is not found free in nature. It has properties similar to tungsten and is used as an alloy to strengthen and protect metal from corrosion.

Key Concepts: *Several important enzymes require molybdenum. Good food sources include peas, beans, and some breakfast cereals. Otherwise healthy people with normal diets do not suffer molybdenum deficiency. High intakes of molybdenum may inhibit absorption of copper.*

Other Trace Elements and Ultratrace Elements

The body contains minuscule amounts of "ultratrace" minerals and may require less than 1 milligram per day of each one. At least 18 minerals could be considered "ultratrace": aluminum, arsenic, boron, bromide, cadmium, chromium, fluoride, germanium, iodide, lead, lithium, molybdenum, nickel, rubidium, selenium, silicon, tin, and vanadium.[70] There is substantial research on iodine, fluoride, manganese, molybdenum, and selenium (all discussed previously). The functions of the remaining minerals are less clear. While new evidence and media coverage have focused on arsenic, boron, nickel, silicon, and vanadium, data do not exist for the establishment of AI or RDA for these minerals. ULs are set for boron, nickel, and vanadium.

Arsenic

Although arsenic (As) has been an infamous poison for centuries, inorganic arsenic may actually be an essential ultratrace element. As a colorless, tasteless toxin, arsenic trioxide can be fatal in a dose as low as 2 milligrams.[71] On the other hand, arsenic-deprived laboratory animals have poor growth and abnormal reproduction. Arsenic may also participate in methionine metabolism. Estimates of dietary intake of arsenic range from 15 micrograms per day for children, to 60 micrograms per day for adult males.[72] The most concentrated food sources are oysters, mussels, and fish. In a typical diet, meat and fish supply about 30 percent of dietary arsenic, cereals and breads supply 20 percent, and starchy vegetables provide 15 percent. Given arsenic's highly poisonous nature, much more careful research is required to establish recommended intake levels.

Boron

Boron (B) appears to play an important role in bone metabolism, probably in conjunction with other nutrients such as calcium, magnesium, and vitamin D. Boron deficiency depresses growth and is worsened by a vitamin D deficiency. Conversely, boron supplementation lessens the bone abnormalities observed in vitamin D deficiency.

Fruits, nuts, vegetables, and legumes are the main sources of boron. The body absorbs close to 90 percent of the amount consumed and then promptly excretes most of it in the urine. The usual dietary intake of boron is between 1 and 2 milligrams per day.[73] Based on average consumption as well as supplementation studies, scientists estimate that the daily boron requirement is 1 milligram per day.[74] Chronic boron toxicity symptoms include poor appetite, nausea, weight loss, and decreased sexual activity, seminal volume, and sperm count. More research is needed to set safe lower and upper limits for dietary intake.

Nickel

Nickel (Ni) is widely distributed throughout the body in very low concentrations that add up to a total body content of approximately 10 milligrams. Most of the research on nickel has been conducted in animals, and by extrapolation scientists assume nickel is essential in humans.

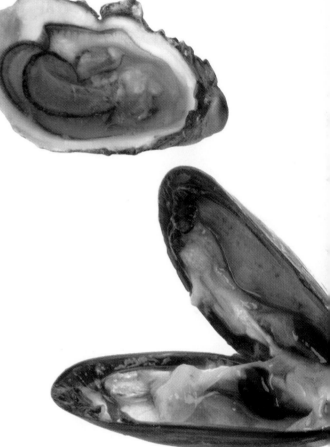

silicosis A disease that results from excess silicon exposure.

Table 12.6 **Tolerable Upper Intake Levels (UL) for Ultratrace Elements**

Arsenic	No UL set
Boron	20 mg/day
Nickel	1 mg/day
Silicon	No UL set
Vanadium	1.8 mg/day

A few nickel-containing enzymes have been identified, and nickel can activate or inhibit a number of enzymes that usually contain other elements. Nickel alters the properties of cell membranes and affects oxidation-reduction systems in cells. Nickel also may function in B_{12} and folate metabolism.[75]

Nuts, legumes, grains, and vegetables are the best sources of nickel. Depending on the amount of plant foods consumed, dietary intake of nickel varies widely. An acceptable dietary intake of 100 to 300 micrograms per day has been proposed.[76] There is no known nickel deficiency in humans. Toxicity has occurred only in workers exposed to nickel dust or nickel carbonyl in industrial settings.

Silicon

Silicon (Si) is the most common element in the earth's crust. The human body contains roughly 1.5 grams of silicon—less than magnesium, but about the same amount as iron and zinc. Connective tissues including the aorta, trachea, tendon, bone, and skin contain much of the body's silicon. From animal studies, scientists hypothesize that silicon helps strengthen collagen and elastin. Experimental diets lacking silicon caused poor growth and skeletal abnormalities in baby chickens. However, there are no known symptoms of silicon deficiency in humans. Recent studies suggest silicon may help prevent atherosclerosis in the elderly. Silicon is relatively nontoxic when ingested orally; however, breathing airborne silicon particles may cause **silicosis**, a type of silicon toxicity.

Unrefined grains, cereals, vegetables, and fruits supply most of our dietary silicon. Animal foods are poor sources. Determining a dietary recommendation is difficult because of the lack of human studies showing signs of deficiency. A balance study conducted in the late 1970s suggests adequate intake is between 21 and 46 milligrams per day.[77] The Total Diet Study conducted in the United States reported silicon intake between 19 and 40 milligrams per day.

Vanadium

In the body, vanadium (V) can exist in a form that is structurally similar to phosphate. Interestingly, in the late 1970s it was noted that in vitro vanadium inhibits ATP synthase, an enzyme required for ATP production. Presumably, vanadium replaces phosphate and blocks the reaction. In rats with experimentally induced diabetes, vanadium has also been shown to mimic insulin. However, a precise function for vanadium in humans has not been found, and given the tiny amounts that we consume, deficiencies have not been observed.

Key Concepts: *Ultratrace minerals are elements with very low estimated requirements. Although specific biochemical functions have not been defined for the minerals arsenic, boron, nickel, silicon, and vanadium, they are thought to be essential for humans.*

Label [to] **Table**

If you looked at a list of minerals, could you pick out the trace minerals? Let's see how well you do! Look at the following Nutrition Facts label from a breakfast cereal and guess how many trace minerals are listed.

You should be able to spot three trace minerals on the label: iron, zinc, and copper. Looking at the "ingredients" and "vitamins and minerals" lists, you can see that the iron and zinc were added but the copper appears to come naturally from the cereal. Why do you think these trace minerals are added to this cereal? Many people (especially children) eat marginal amounts of iron and zinc. The best sources of these minerals are meats, liver, shellfish, and eggs. Most children don't eat much shellfish or liver, so adding the minerals to cereals, which they do eat, is an easy way to make sure they get 45 percent and 25 percent of their iron and zinc Daily Values, respectively.

The last mineral you see listed is copper. There is 2% of the Daily Value for copper in one serving of this cereal. That's 0.04 milligrams (2% of 2 mg).

Nutrition Facts

Serving Size: 1 cup (30g)
Servings Per Container about 9

Amount Per Serving	Cheerios	with ½ cup skim milk
Calories	110	150
Calories from Fat	15	20

		% Daily Value**
Total Fat 2g*	**3%**	**3%**
Saturated Fat 0g	**0%**	**3%**
Polyunsaturated Fat 0.5g		
Monounsaturated Fat 0.5g		
Cholesterol 0mg	**0%**	**1%**
Sodium 280mg	**12%**	**15%**
Total Carbohydrate 22g	**7%**	**9%**
Dietary Fiber 3g	**11%**	**11%**
Soluble Fiber 1g	**11%**	**11%**
Sugars 1g		
Other carbohydrates 1g		
Protein 3g		

Vitamin A	10%	15%
Vitamin C	10%	10%
Calcium	4%	20%
Iron	45%	45%
Vitamin D	10%	25%
Thiamin	25%	30%
Riboflavin	25%	35%
Niacin	25%	25%
Vitamin B₆	25%	25%
Folic Acid	50%	50%
Vitamin B₁₂	25%	35%
Phosphorus	10%	25%
Magnesium	8%	10%
Zinc	25%	30%
Copper	2%	2%

*Amount in Cereal. A serving of cereal plus skim milk provides 2g total fat (0.5g saturated fat, 1g monosaturated fat). less than 5mg cholesterol, 350mg sodium, 300mg potassium, 28g total carbohydrate (7g sugars) and 7g protein.

**Percent Daily Values are based on a 2,000 calorie diet. Your daily values may be higher or lower depending on your calorie needs:

	Calories:	2000	2,500
Total Fat	Less Than	65g	80g
Sat Fat	Less Than	20g	25g
Cholesterol	Less Than	300mg	300mg
Sodium	Less Than	2,400mg	2,400mg
Potassium		3,500mg	3,500mg
Total Carbohydrate		300g	375g
Dietary Fiber	25g	30g	

INGREDIENTS: WHOLE GRAIN OATS (INCLUDES THE OAT BRAN), MODIFIED FOOD STARCH, SUGAR, SALT, OAT FIBER, TRISODIUM PHOSPHATE, CALCIUM CARBONATE, VITAMIN E (MIXED TOCOPHEROLS) ADDED TO PRESERVE FRESHNESS.

VITAMINS AND MINERALS: IRON AND ZINC (MINERAL NUTRIENTS), VITAMIN C (SODIUM ASCORBATE), A B VITAMIN (NIACINAMIDE), VITAMIN B₆ (PYRIDOXINE HYDROCHLORIDE), VITAMIN B₂ (RIBOFLAVIN), VITAMIN B₁ (THIAMIN MONONITRATE), VITAMIN A (PALMITATE), A B VITAMIN (FOLIC ACID), VITAMIN B₁₂, VITAMIN D.

LEARNING *Portfolio* chapter 12

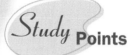

Key Terms

	page
acrodermatitis enteropathica	458
albumin	471
amyotrophic lateral sclerosis (ALS)	467
ceruloplasmin	464
chelation therapy	466
cretinism	459
Crohn's disease	457
cytochromes	445
ferric iron (3+)	444
ferritin	446
ferrous iron (2+)	444
fluorosis	469
galvanize	453
geophagia	453
goiter	462
goitrogens	463
hematocrit	452
heme	444
heme iron	447
hemochromatosis	444
hemodialysis	457
hemosiderin	449
hypogonadism	453
hypothyroidism	459

	page
iron overload	452
Keshan disease	458

	page
Menkes' syndrome	464
metalloprotein	453
metallothionein	454
microcytic anemia	452
mineralization	468
multiple sclerosis	467
myelinization	445
myoglobin	444
non-heme iron	447
polyphenols	448
protoporphyrin	451
selenocysteine	459
selenomethionine	458
silicosis	474
thyroid-stimulating hormone (TSH)	462
thyroglobulin	462
thyroxine (T4)	462
total parenteral nutrition (TPN)	461
transferrin	446
transferrin receptor	449
transferrin saturation	451
triiodothyronine (T3)	462
Wilson's disease	458

Study Points

➤ Trace elements are minerals that the body needs in small amounts. They are involved in a variety of structural and regulatory functions and are found in both animal and plant foods.

➤ Iron functions in oxygen transport as part of hemoglobin and myoglobin. It is also an enzyme cofactor, important for immune function, and involved in normal brain function.

➤ Iron balance is regulated through absorption; absorption increases when body status is low, and decreases when stores are normal. Meat, vitamin C, and stomach acid tend to increase non-heme iron absorption; phytate, phenolic compounds, and high doses of other minerals tend to decrease iron absorption.

➤ Recommendations for iron intake consider the amount needed to replace daily losses, and the bioavailability of iron from a typical mixed diet. Due to regular iron losses via menstrual bleeding, women of childbearing age need more iron than adult men do.

➤ The best sources of iron are meats. Enriched and whole grains are significant sources in the American diet.

➤ Iron deficiency is the most common nutritional deficiency worldwide. The most severe stage of deficiency, following reduction of iron stores and transport iron, results in anemia.

➤ Iron toxicity can result from acute ingestion of high doses, or from chronic excessive iron absorption. Accidental iron overdose is a leading cause of poisoning deaths of children under 6 in the United States.

➤ Zinc is a cofactor for numerous enzymes and is crucial for normal growth, development, and immune function. It is found in protein-rich foods, particularly red meats.

➤ Zinc deficiency results in poor growth, impaired taste, delayed wound healing, and impaired immune response.

➤ Selenium functions as part of the glutathione peroxidases, important antioxidant enzymes. Good sources of selenium are organ meats and seafood. Deficiency of selenium appears to be rare, but has been described in an area of China called the Keshan region.

➤ Iodine is necessary for the formation of thyroid hormones, which regulate metabolic rate and body temperature. Much of the iodide in the American diet comes from iodized salt. Iodine deficiency results in goiter. If severe deficiency occurs during pregnancy, the child may be born with cretinism.

➤ Copper functions in many enzyme systems including those involved with antioxidant mechanisms, iron utilization, and immune function. The richest food sources of copper include organ meats, shellfish, nuts and seeds, peanut butter, and chocolate.

➤ Copper deficiency results in anemia, decreased numbers of white blood cells, and bone abnormalities.

➤ Manganese functions in conjunction with several enzyme systems. The best food sources include tea, coffee, nuts, cereals, and some fruits. Manganese deficiency and toxicity are uncommon; toxicity is usually associated with exposure through manganese mines.

➤ Fluoride promotes mineralization of bones and teeth and protects the teeth from caries. Water is a major source of fluoride, due to either naturally high content or added fluoride. Fluorosis is the result of excessive fluoride intake and results in mottling of the teeth.

➤ Chromium functions in the normal use of insulin to promote glucose use. Rich sources of chromium are mushrooms, dark chocolate, prunes, nuts, asparagus, whole grains, wine, brewer's yeast, and some beers. Chromium deficiency in humans is difficult to assess, and toxicity of inorganic chromium is unlikely.

➤ Although the body contains only about 2 milligrams of molybdenum, it is an important enzyme cofactor. Good food sources are peas, beans, and some breakfast cereals. Molybdenum deficiency and toxicity are both rare.

➤ Ultratrace minerals are those required in extremely small amounts; the specific function of many of these nutrients is unknown. Some ultratrace minerals are arsenic, boron, nickel, silicon, and vanadium.

Study Questions

1. In what two ways do trace minerals differ from major minerals?

2. Name two ways that minerals differ from most vitamins.

3. List five factors that can affect a mineral's bioavailability.

4. Explain the differences between "heme" and "non-heme" iron. Which is absorbed better?

5. List the three stages of iron deficiency and the effects of each.

6. What are some of the main functions of zinc?

7. Describe the common causes of zinc deficiency.

8. What are the main functions of selenium?

9. Iodine is a component of which hormones? What are the functions of these hormones? How is selenium linked to these hormones?

10. What are goitrogens and how are they related to goiter?

11. Define Wilson's disease and Menkes' syndrome.

12. What are the functions of manganese in the body?

13. How does fluoride prevents dental caries?

14. Which foods contain chromium, and why is chromium important?

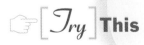 This

A Simple Check on Your Zinc

Reported in the Lancet in the early 1980s, this simple test can provide a rough signal of your zinc status. Buy some zinc sulfate at a health food store. Dissolve it in distilled water to make a 0.1 percent zinc sulfate solution. Refrain from eating, drinking, and smoking for at least an hour before the test. Then swish a teaspoon of the solution around your mouth for 10 seconds. If it tastes unpleasant or metallic, your level of zinc is probably adequate. However, if the solution tastes like water, you may be consuming less zinc than you need.

What About Bobbie?

Let's take a look at Bobbie's intake of the trace minerals iron, zinc, and selenium. Refer to page 28 to review Bobbie's complete food record. Bobbie's intakes of iron, zinc, and selenium exceeded the Recommended Dietary Allowances for her age. This reflects the fact that Bobbie's calorie intake is high enough to satisfy her needs and she selected a wide variety of foods. Below you'll see the foods she ate that contributed the most to her trace mineral intake.

Iron

Bobbie's intake	*8 mg*
Bobbie's RDA	*18 mg*

Most of Bobbie's iron came from enriched grains and red meat. Here are her top four iron sources and the amount each provided:

Spaghetti pasta	*2.9 mg iron*
Bagel	*2.7 mg*
Meatballs	*2.3 mg*
Pizza	*1.5 mg*

Zinc

Bobbie's intake	*14 mg*
Bobbie's RDA	*8 mg*

Bobbie's best source of zinc is red meat—the meatballs she had on her spaghetti. Here are her top four zinc sources and the amount each provided:

Meatballs	*4.9 mg zinc*
Pizza (cheese)	*2.2 mg*
Spaghetti pasta	*1.1 mg*
Bagel	*0.8 mg*

Selenium

Bobbie's intake	*126 µg*
Bobbie's RDA	*55 µg*

Bobbie's best sources of selenium are grain products and meats. Here are her top four selenium sources and the amount each provided:

Spaghetti	*44 µg selenium*
Bagel	*22 µg*
Meatballs	*18 µg*
Turkey	*18 µg*

References

1 Bothwell, TH. Overview and mechanisms of iron regulation. *Nutr Rev.* 1995;53(9):237–245.

2 Walter T, Olivares M, Pizarro F, Munoz C. Iron, anemia and infection. *Nutr Rev.* 1997;55(4):111–124.

3 Kretchmer N, Beard JL, Carlson S. The role of nutrition in the development of normal cognition. *Am J Clin Nutr.* 1996;63:997S-1001S.

4 De Andraca I, Castillo M, Walter T. Psychomotor development and behavior in iron-deficient anemic infants. *Nutr Rev.* 1997;55(4):125-132.

5 Recommendations to Report and Control Iron Deficiency in the United States. *MMWR.* 1998;7(RR-3).

6 Bothwell TH. Op. cit.

7 Beard JL, Dawson BS, Pinero DJ. Iron metabolism: a comprehensive review. *Nutr Rev.* 1996;54(10):295–317.

8 Bothwell TH. Op. cit.

9 Food and Nutrition Board. *Recommended Dietary Allowances.* 10th ed. Washington, DC: National Academy Press; 1989: 195–205.

10 Groff JL, Gropper SS. *Advanced Nutrition and Human Metabolism,* 3rd ed. Belmont, CA: Wadsworth, 2000.

11 Hunt JR, Roughead ZK. Nonheme-iron absorption, fecal ferritin excretion, and blood indexes of iron status in women consuming controlled lactoovovegetarian diets for 8 wk. *Am J Clin Nutr.* 1999;69:944–952.

12 Hunt JR, Roughead ZK. Op. cit.

13 Minihane AM, Fairweather-Tait SJ. Effect of calcium supplementation on daily nonheme-iron absorption and long-term iron status. *Am J Clin Nutr.* 1998;68:96–102.

14 Hallberg L. Does calcium interfere with iron absorption? *Am J Clin Nutr.* 1998;68:3-4.

15 Baynes, RD. Refining the assessment of body iron status. *Am J Clin Nutr.* 1996;64:793–794.

16 Bothwell TH. Op. cit.

17 Recommendations to Report and Control Iron Deficiency in the United States. Op. cit.

18 Stoltzfus RJ, Chwaya HM, Tielsch JM, et al. Epidemiology of iron deficiency anemia in Zanzibari schoolchildren: the importance of hookworms. *Am J Clin Nutr.* 1997;65:153–159.

19 McDowell MA, Briefel RR, Alaimo K, et al. Energy and macronutrient intakes of persons ages 2 months and older in the United States. Third National Health and Nutrition Examination Survey, Phase I, 1988–1991. Huntsville, MD: National Center for Health Statistics publication 255; 1994.

20 Pollitt E. Iron deficiency and educational deficiency. *Nutr Rev.* 1997;55(4):133-140.

21 Zhu YI, Haas JD. Iron depletion without anemia and physical performance in young women. *Am J Clin Nutr.* 1997;66:334–341.

22 Food and Nutrition Board. Op. cit.

23 Preventing Iron Poisoning in Children. *FDA Backgrounder.* Jan 15, 1997.

24 Gordeuk V, Mukiibi J, Hasstedt SJ, et al. Iron overload in Africa: interaction between a gene and dietary iron content. *N Engl J Med.* 1992;326(12):95–100.

25 Prasad AS, Helstead JA, Nadami M. Syndrome of iron deficiency anaemia, hepatosplenomegaly hypogonadism dwarfism and geophagia. *Am J Med.* 1961;31:532–546.

26 Sandstead HH, Prasad AS, Schubert AR, et al. Human zinc deficiency endocrine manifestations and response to treatment. *Am J Clin Nutr.* 1967;20;422–442.

27 Stein, JH. *Internal Medicine.* 4th ed. St. Louis: Mosby Year-Book; 1994.

28 Cousins RJ. Zinc. In: Ziegler EE, Filer LJ, eds. *Present Knowledge in Nutrition.* 7th ed. Washington, DC: ILSI Press; 1996.

29 King JC, Keen CL. Zinc. In: Shils ME, Olson JA, Shike M, Ross AC, eds. *Modern Nutrition in Health and Disease.* 9th ed. Baltimore: Lippincott Williams & Wilkins; 1999.

30 Sandstrom B. Absorption of zinc from soy protein meals in humans. *J Nutr.* 1987;117:321–327.

31 Yan L, Prentice A, Dibba B, et al. Effect of long-term calcium supplementation on indices of iron, zinc, and magnesium status in lactating Gambian women. *Brit J Nutr.* 1996;76(6):821–831.

32 Gibson RS. Content and bioavailability of trace elements in vegetarian diets. *Am J Clin Nutr.* 1994;59(suppl):1223–1232

33 Krebs NF. Overview of zinc absorption and excretion in the human gastrointestinal tract. *J Nutr.* 2000;130:1374S–1377S.

34 Lonnerdal B. Dietary factors influencing zinc absorption. *J Nutr.* 2000;130:1378S–1383S.

35 Cousins RJ. Op. cit.

36 Briefel RR, Bialostosky K, Kennedy-Stephenson J, et al. Zinc intake of the U.S. population: findings from the Third National Health and Nutrition Examination Survey, 1988–1994. *J Nutr.* 2000;130:1367S–1373S.

37 Navert B, Sandstrom B, Cederblad A. Reduction of the phytate content of bran by leavening in bread and its effect on absorption of zinc in man. *Br J Nutr.* 1985;53:47–53.

38 Gerrior SA, Zizza C. Nutrient Content of the U.S. Food Supply, 1909–1990. US Department of Agriculture. Home Economics Research report 52; Sept 1994.

39 Prasad AS. Zinc: an overview. *Nutrition.* 1995;11:93.

40 Tamura T, Goldenberg RL. Zinc nutriture and pregnancy outcome. *Nutr Res.* 1996.

41 Heyneman CA. Zinc deficiency and taste disorders. *Ann Pharmacotherapy.* 1996;30:186–187.

42 Bogden JD, Oleske JM, Lavenhar MA, et al. Effects of one year of supplementation with zinc and other micronutrients on cellular immunity in the elderly. *J Am Coll Nutr.* 1990;9:214–225.

43 King JC, Keen CL. Op. cit.

44 Klevay L. Hypercholesterolemia in rats produced by an increase in the ratio of zinc to copper ingested. *Nutrition.* 1993;9(2):190–198.

45 Hoogenraad T, Van den Hamer C, van Hattum J. Effective treatment of Wilson's disease with oral zinc sulphate: two case reports. *Br Med J.* 1984;289:273–276.

46 Institute of Medicine. Food and Nutrition Board. *Dietary Reference Intakes for Vitamin C, Vitamin E, Selenium, and Beta-Carotene, and other Carotenoids.* Washington, DC: National Academy Press; 2000.

47 Ibid.

48 Ibid.

49 Ibid.

50 Hetzel BS. *The Story of Iodine Deficiency: An International Challenge in Nutrition.* Oxford: Oxford University Press; 1989.

51 World Health Organization Sets Out to Eliminate Iodine Deficiency Disorder. WHO press release; May 25, 1999.

52 Guyton, AC, Hall, JE. *Medical Textbook of Physiology.* 9th ed. Philadelphia: WB Saunders; 1996.

53 Bautista A. Effects of oral iodized salt on intelligence, thyroid status, and somatic growth in school-aged children from an area with endemic goiter. *Am J Clin Nutr.* 1982;35:127–134.

54 Institute of Medicine. Food and Nutrition Board. *Dietary Reference Intakes for Vitamin A, Vitamin K, Arsenic, Boron, Chromium, Copper, Iron, Manganese, Molybdenum, Nickel, Silicon, Vanadium, and Zinc.* Washington, DC: National Academy Press; 2001.

55 Klevay LM, Buchet JP, Bunker VW, et al. Copper in the Western diet. In: Anke M, Meissner D, Mills CF, eds. *Trace Elements in Man and Animals. TEMA-8.* Gersdorf, Germany: Verlag Media Touristik; 1993:207–210.

56 Williams DM. Copper deficiency in humans. *Semin Hematol.* 1983;20:118–128.

57 Keen CL, Uriu-Hare JY, Hawk SN, et al. Effect of copper deficiency on prenatal development and pregnancy outcome. *Am J Clin Nutr.* 1998;67(suppl):1003S–1011S.

58 Turnland JR, Copper. In Shils ME, Olson JA, Shike M, Ross AC, eds. *Modern Nutrition in Health and Disease.* 9th ed. Baltimore: Lippincott Williams & Wilkins; 1999.

59 Kaler SG. Diagnosis and therapy of Menkes' syndrome, a genetic form of copper deficiency. *Am J Clin Nutr.* 1998;67(suppl):1029S–1034S.

60 Greger JL. Dietary standards for manganese: overlap between nutritional and toxicological studies. *J Nutr.* 1998;128:368S–371S.

61 Keen CL, Zidenberg-Cherr S. Manganese. In: Ziegler E, Filer L, eds. *Present Knowledge in Nutrition.* 7th ed. Washington, DC: International Life Sciences Institute; 1996:334–343.

62 Kapaki E, Zournas C, Kanias G, et al. Essential trace element alterations in amyotrophic lateral sclerosis. *J Neurol Sci.* 1997;147(2):171–175.

63 Fluoridation of drinking water to prevent dental caries. *MMWR.* Oct 22, 1999.

64 Simko LC. Water fluoridation: time to reexamine the issue. *Pediatr Nurs.* 1997;23(2):155–159.

65 Riggs BL, Hodgson SF, O'Fallon WM, et al. Effect of fluoride treatment on the fracture rate in women with osteoporosis. *N Engl J Med.* 1990;322:802–809.

66 Mertz, W. Confirmation: Chromium levels in serum, hair, and sweat decline with age. *Nutr Rev.* 1997;55(10):373–375.

67 Nielson, FH. Should you take a chromium supplement? *Healthline.* Dec 1995.

68 Davis S, McLaren HJ, Hunnisett A, Howard M. Age-related decreases in chromium levels in 51,665 hair, sweat, and serum samples from 40,872 patients: implications for the prevention of cardiovascular disease and type II diabetes mellitus. *Metabolism.* 1997;46:469–473.

69 Anderson RA. Effects of chromium on body composition and weight loss. *Nutr Rev.* 1998;56(9):266–270.

70 Nielsen FH. How should dietary guidance be given for mineral elements with beneficial actions or suspected of being essential? *J Nutr.* 1996;126:2377–2385S.

71 Nielsen FH. Ultratrace Minerals. In Shils ME, Olson JA, Shike M, Ross AC, eds. *Modern Nutrition in Health and Disease.* 9th ed. Baltimore: Lippincott Williams & Wilkins; 1999.

72 Dabeka RW, McKenzie AD, Lacroix GM, et al. Survey of arsenic in total diet food composites and estimation of the dietary intake of arsenic by Canadian adults and children. *J AOAC Internat.* 1993;76(1):14–25.

73 Anderson D, Cunningham W, Lindstrom T. Concentrations and intakes of H, B, S, K, Na, Cl, and NaCl in foods. *J Food Comp Anal.* 1994;7:59–82.

74 Nielsen FH. Other trace elements. In: Ziegler E, Filer L, eds. *Present Knowledge in Nutrition.* 7th ed. Washington DC. International Life Sciences Institute; 1996;353–377.

75 Uthus EO, Poellot RA. Dietary folate affects the response of rats to nickel deprivation. *Biol Trac Elem Res.* 1996;52:23–35.

76 Uthus EO, Seaborn CD. Deliberations and evaluations of the approaches, endpoints, and paradigms for dietary recommendations of the other trace elements. *J Nutr.* 1996;126:2452S–2459S.

77 Kelsay JL, Behall KM, Prather E. Effect of fiber from fruits and vegetables on metabolic responses in human subjects. II: Calcium, magnesium, iron, and silicon balances. *Am J Clin Nutr.* 1979;32:1876–1880.

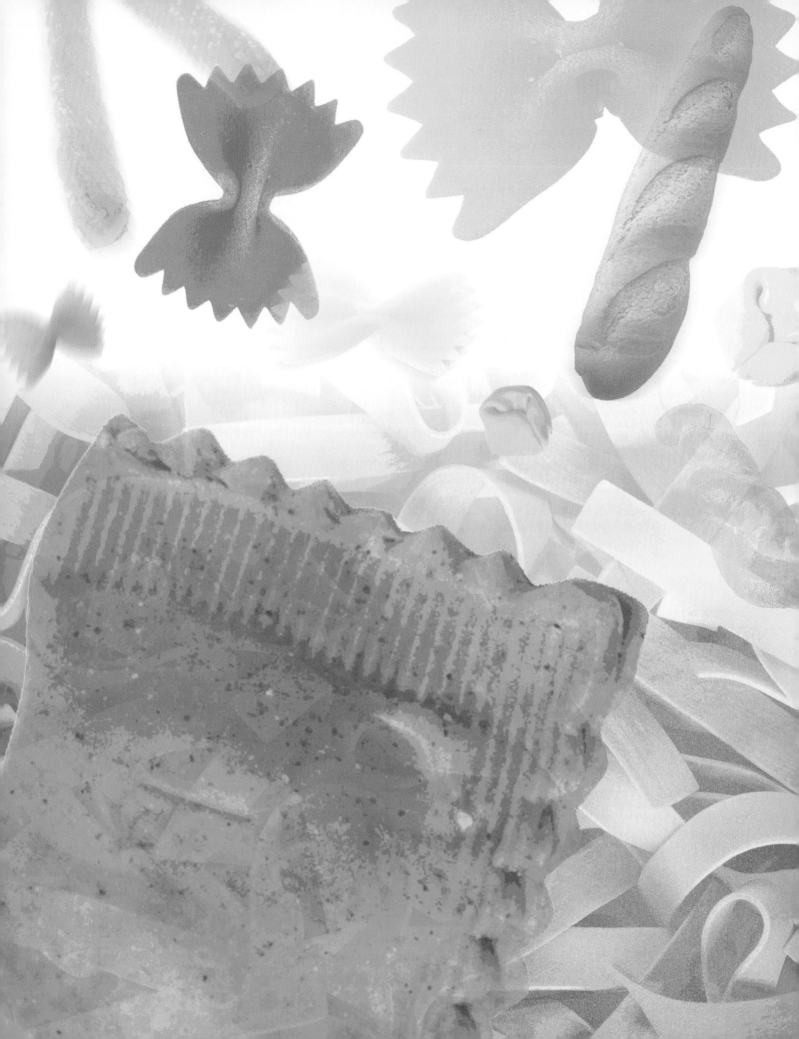

Chapter 13

Sports Nutrition

Think About It

1 How much importance do you place on being physically active?

2 How often do you suffer from muscle fatigue? To what do you attribute it?

3 How often do you think about food choices when you're planning a physical activity?

4 What kind of protein do you emphasize in your diet?

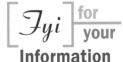
Fyi for your Information

This chapter's FYI boxes include practical information on the following topics:

• Lactate is Not a Metabolic Dead End

• To Zone or Not to Zone? That Is the Question

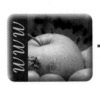

The web site for this book offers many useful tools and is a great source for additional nutrition information for both students and instructors. Visit the site at **nutrition.jbpub.com** for information on sports nutrition. You'll find exercises that explore the following topics:

• Effective Training

• Sports Nutrition from a Sports Drink Company

• The EatRight Web Page of the ADA and CDA

• Scan SCAN

Key to Illustrations

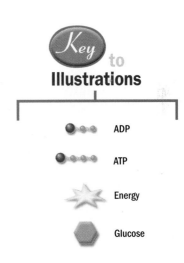

● ● ● ● ADP

● ● ● ● ● ATP

✦ Energy

⬡ Glucose

What About Bobbie?

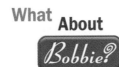

Track the choices Bobbie is making with the EatRight Analysis software.

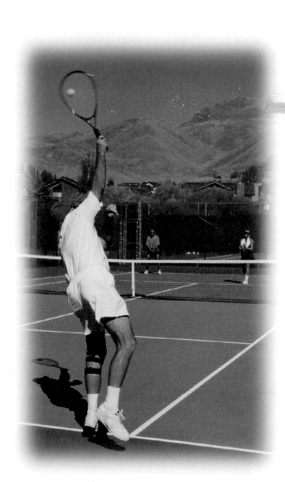

atching a "World's Greatest Athlete" competition on television might cause you to wonder which sports produce the best athletes. How would you answer that question? Who is the most athletic? The most physically fit? Do you value the strength of football players, wrestlers, or weight lifters? The speed of sprinters? The agility of a soccer forward? The balance and coordination of figure skaters or gymnasts? The endurance of marathon runners or distance swimmers?

First, we must define *physical fitness*, and come to realize that fitness is all of these characteristics: strength, speed, agility, balance, coordination, endurance, and more. Fitness is relative—to the sport, to the individual, to the situation. We would certainly consider all Olympic athletes physically fit; but just a slight improvement at that level of fitness may mean the difference between gold and silver medals. Improved fitness in an elderly person can make a difference in how easily that person can move through daily tasks.

In this chapter you will discover how nutrition supports the development of physical fitness. Good nutrition provides the fuel for exercise, and exercise builds fitness. You will also explore specific facets of nutrition that may help give athletes a competitive edge. So are you ready? Get set. Let's GO!

Benefits of Exercise

People of all ages benefit from regular physical activity. In 1996 the U.S. Surgeon General's Report on Physical Activity and Health provided a comprehensive review of the scientific research on physical activity, fitness, and health.[1] This document supports earlier recommendations from the National Institutes of Health (NIH), the Centers for Disease Control and Prevention (CDC), and the American College of Sports Medicine (ACSM) that moderate amounts of physical activity produce health benefits. The report found that physically active people have an increased sense of well-being and a lower risk for developing life-threatening chronic diseases. **Table 13.1** is an excerpt from the Surgeon General's report.

Just how physically active do you need to be? (See **Figure 13.1.**) The ACSM notes an important distinction between physical activity as it relates to health, and exercise for physical fitness.[2] According to the ACSM, the level of physical activity that may reduce the risk of various chronic diseases (e.g., coronary heart disease, diabetes, hypertension, osteoporosis, and obesity) may not be enough—in quantity or quality—to improve physical fitness.

There is not just one measure of physical fitness. Measures may evaluate, among other factors, strength, endurance, flexibility, and breathing capacity. The ACSM defines *physical fitness* as "the ability to perform moderate to vigorous levels of physical activity without undue fatigue and the capability of maintaining this level of activity throughout life."[3] **Table 13.2** gives guidelines for levels of physical activity to promote health and to achieve and maintain fitness.

Nutrition for Physical Performance

Nutrition has taken its rightful place as a vital component of any program that seeks to enhance health, fitness, and athletic performance. In a joint

Think About It 1

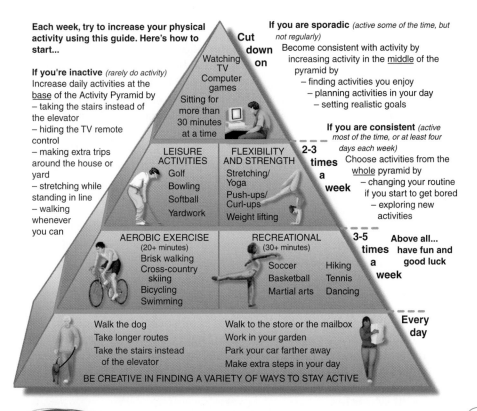

Each week, try to increase your physical activity using this guide. Here's how to start...

If you're inactive *(rarely do activity)*
Increase daily activities at the <u>base</u> of the Activity Pyramid by
– taking the stairs instead of the elevator
– hiding the TV remote control
– making extra trips around the house or yard
– stretching while standing in line
– walking whenever you can

Cut down on
Watching TV
Computer games
Sitting for more than 30 minutes at a time

LEISURE ACTIVITIES
Golf
Bowling
Softball
Yardwork

FLEXIBILITY AND STRENGTH
Stretching/Yoga
Push-ups/Curl-ups
Weight lifting

AEROBIC EXERCISE
(20+ minutes)
Brisk walking
Cross-country skiing
Bicycling
Swimming

RECREATIONAL
(30+ minutes)
Soccer   Hiking
Basketball   Tennis
Martial arts   Dancing

Walk the dog
Take longer routes
Take the stairs instead of the elevator

Walk to the store or the mailbox
Work in your garden
Park your car farther away
Make extra steps in your day

BE CREATIVE IN FINDING A VARIETY OF WAYS TO STAY ACTIVE

If you are sporadic *(active some of the time, but not regularly)*
Become consistent with activity by increasing activity in the <u>middle</u> of the pyramid by
– finding activities you enjoy
– planning activities in your day
– setting realistic goals

If you are consistent *(active most of the time, or at least four days each week)*
Choose activities from the <u>whole</u> pyramid by
– changing your routine if you start to get bored
– exploring new activities

2-3 times a week

3-5 times a week

Every day

Above all...
have fun and good luck

Figure 13.1 **The Physical Activity Pyramid.** Perhaps the most important aspect of increasing physical activity is to have fun.
Source: Adapted from The Activity Pyramid © 1996 Park Nicollet HealthSource® Institute for Research and Education, Park Nicollet HealthSource, Minneapolis. Reprinted by permission.

Table 13.1 **Physical Activity and Health: A Report of the Surgeon General**

Major Conclusions

1. People of all ages, both male and female, benefit from regular physical activity.
2. A person can obtain significant health benefits by including a moderate amount of physical activity (e.g., 30 minutes of brisk walking or raking leaves, 15 minutes of running, or 45 minutes of playing volleyball) on most, if not all, days of the week.
3. Physical activity reduces the risk of premature mortality in general, and of coronary heart disease, hypertension, colon cancer, and diabetes in particular. Physical activity also improves mental health, and health of muscles, bones, and joints.
4. More than 60 percent of American adults are not regularly physically active. In fact, 25 percent of all adults are not active at all.
5. Physical activity declines dramatically during adolescence. Nearly half of American youths 12 to 21 years old are not vigorously active on a regular basis. Moreover, daily enrollment in physical education classes has declined among high school students from 42 percent in 1991 to 25 percent in 1995.
6. Research on understanding and promoting physical activity is at an early stage, but some interventions to promote physical activity through schools, worksites, and health-care settings have been evaluated and found to be successful.

Source: US Department of Health and Human Services. *Physical Activity and Health: A Report of the Surgeon General.* Atlanta, GA: US Department of Health and Human Services, Centers for Disease Control and Prevention, National Center for Chronic Disease Prevention and Health Promotion; 1996:4.

Table 13.2 **Guidelines for Physical Activity: Health and Fitness**

Guidelines for Promoting Health

Frequency: daily activity
Intensity: any level of intensity
Duration: accumulation of a minimum of 30 minutes of total daily activity
Mode: any activity

Guidelines for Achieving and Maintaining Physical Fitness

Frequency: 3 to 5 days a week
Intensity: 50 to 90 percent of maximum heart rate
Duration: 20 to 60 minutes of continuous or intermittent aerobic activity (minimum of 10-minute bouts accumulated during the day)
Mode: activity using large muscle groups maintained continuously in a rhythmic and aerobic manner
Resistance training: minimum of 2 days a week to enhance strength and muscular endurance, and maintain fat-free mass
Flexibility training: minimum of 2 days week, incorporated into overall fitness program to develop and maintain range of motion

Source: American College of Sports Medicine, position stand. The recommended quantity and quality of exercise for developing and maintaining cardiorespiratory and muscular fitness and flexibility in healthy adults. *Med Sci Sports Exerc.* 1998;30:975–991.

Smooth muscle

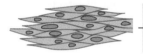

- Bronchi
- Blood vessels
- Small intestine

Cardiac muscle

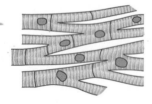

Heart

Skeletal muscle

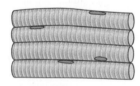

Consciously controlled physical movement

Figure 13.2 **Muscle types.** Smooth muscles, composed of elongated fibers, line blood vessels, bronchial tubes, and most organs. Peristaltic contractions of smooth muscles move food in the GI tract. Cardiac muscle, composed of striated fibers, is your heart muscle. Skeletal muscles, bundles of parallel striated fibers attached to your skeleton, are responsible for physical movement.

position paper, the American Dietetic Association and the Canadian Dietetic Association state that "a proper, well-balanced diet is an essential component of any fitness or sports program."[4] But just what is "a proper, well-balanced diet"? Is it the same for a child who plays recreational softball and for a senior citizen who takes daily walks to prevent type 2 diabetes? What about the competitive athlete who strives to maximize athletic performance and uses nutrition as a competitive edge? To understand the relationship between physical activity and nutrition, you first need to appreciate how we use energy.

Key Concepts: *Exercise provides numerous health benefits including reduced risk of chronic disease. Physical fitness has many elements including strength, endurance, and flexibility. Nutrition is important for optimal physical performance and should be an essential part of all athletes' training programs.*

Energy for Physical Performance

Physical activity and sports performance rely on energy production. Just as a race car depends on a high-performance engine and energy-dense fuel to win in record time, our muscles process fuel in the form of chemical energy to produce power for physical performance.

Types of Muscles

Your body contains hundreds of muscles that help control a myriad of functions from regulating blood pressure to climbing stairs. Yet, as **Figure 13.2** shows, your muscular system contains only three types of muscle:

- smooth muscle
- cardiac muscle
- skeletal muscle

Smooth muscle is composed of elongated, spindle-shaped fibers. They are found in the walls of blood vessels, along the bronchial tubes in your lungs, and in the walls of most organs. The contraction and relaxation of smooth muscle, for example, moves food through the GI tract. Because smooth muscle is not under your conscious control, it also is called **involuntary muscle**.

Cardiac muscle, as the name implies, is your heart muscle. It provides most of the heart's structure and, like smooth muscle, is not under conscious control. Unlike other involuntary muscles, cardiac muscles fibers are striated rather than smooth, and smaller in diameter than skeletal muscle fibers.

Skeletal muscles are bundles of parallel, striated fibers attached to your skeleton (see **Figure 13.3**). These muscles are responsible for your physical movement and are under your conscious control. If you decide to bend your arm, for example, you consciously contract your biceps. Your body contains more than 600 skeletal muscles and uses nine of them just to control your thumb!

Types of Muscle Fiber

Muscles are made up of bundles of muscle fibers, which are the individual muscle cells. There are two primary types of **muscle fiber**:

- **slow-twitch (ST) fibers**
- **fast-twitch (FT) fibers**

They derive their names from the difference in their speed of action. One type of fast-twitch fiber can contract 10 times faster than slow-twitch fibers.[5]

Slow-Twitch Fibers

To power their activity, slow-twitch fibers efficiently produce energy by oxidizing carbohydrate and fat via aerobic pathways-metabolic reactions that require oxygen. As long as the aerobic pathways are active, ST fibers can produce energy to sustain their movement. With a sufficient supply of oxygen, ST fibers can maintain muscular activity for a prolonged time. This ability is known as **aerobic endurance**.

Because ST fibers have high aerobic endurance, your body predominantly relies on them during low-intensity endurance events, such as a marathon, and during everyday activities, such as walking.

Fast-Twitch Fibers

Compared to ST fibers, fast-twitch fibers have poor aerobic endurance. They are optimized to perform anaerobically (when the oxygen supply is limited). FT fibers can efficiently produce energy for their use via metabolic pathways that do not require oxygen. Bundles of FT fibers exert considerably more force than bundles of ST fibers, but due to their limited endurance FT fibers tire quickly.

The body recruits both ST and FT fibers during shorter, higher-intensity endurance events, such as the mile run or the 400-meter swim. During highly explosive events such as the 100-meter dash and the 50-meter sprint swim, the body relies mainly on FT fibers.

Fibers and Fatigue

No matter how much effort you exert, your body does not recruit 100 percent of your muscle fibers. This helps prevent damage to your muscles and tendons. During events that last several hours, your muscles must work at a **submaximal rate** so that you can reach the finish line. You can't sprint the length of a 26-mile marathon course! During such an event, your body recruits a mix of fibers best suited to endurance activities: mostly ST fibers and a few FT fibers. As the event continues, these fibers use up their energy stores (glycogen) so the body recruits more FT fibers to fill the gap. Finally, after the ST fibers and these FT fibers are exhausted, the body recruits another type of FT fiber in order to continue.

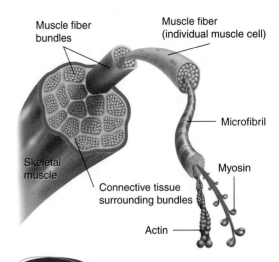

Figure 13.3 Basic structure of skeletal muscle.
A muscle fiber is an individual muscle cell that usually extends the entire length of the muscle. Each muscle fiber contains hundreds to thousands of microfibrils. Each microfibril contains thousands of actin and myosin filaments, large protein molecules responsible for muscle contractions.

Quick Bites

Why is fish meat white?

A large percentage (40 to 60 percent) of a fish's body weight is muscle tissue. Although it spends much of its life slowly cruising, a fish must be able to execute occasional quick bursts of high speed to escape predators or catch a meal. Thus, fish muscle is composed of approximately 75 to 90 percent fast-twitch fibers and fish flesh often is white. The slow-twitch fibers generally are concentrated just under the skin or near fins that are used during slow or high speeds. This arrangement is possible only because fish are buoyant. Land animals could not survive dragging around a large mass of muscle that they used only occasionally in extreme situations.

---

smooth muscle Muscles not under voluntary control that are composed of elongated, spindle-shaped muscle fibers.

involuntary muscle See smooth muscle.

cardiac muscle The heart muscle. Unlike other involuntary muscles, cardiac muscle fibers are striated rather than smooth. These fibers resemble skeletal muscle fibers, but are much smaller in diameter.

skeletal muscle Muscles composed of bundles of parallel, striated muscle fibers under voluntary control. Also called voluntary muscle or striated muscle.

muscle fibers Individual muscle cells.

slow-twitch (ST) fibers Muscle fibers that develop tension more slowly and to a lesser extent than fast-twitch muscle fibers. ST fibers have high oxidative capacities and are slower to fatigue than fast-twitch fibers

fast-twitch (FT) fibers Muscle fibers that can develop high tension rapidly. These fibers can fatigue quickly, but are well suited to explosive movements in sprinting, jumping, and weight lifting.

aerobic endurance The ability of skeletal muscle to obtain a sufficient supply of oxygen from the heart and lungs to maintain muscular activity for a prolonged time.

submaximal rate Less than the greatest possible rate.

ATP-CP energy system A simple and immediate anaerobic energy system that maintains ATP levels. Creatine phosphate is broken down, releasing energy and P_i, which is used to form ATP from ADP.

lactic acid energy system Using glycolysis, this anaerobic energy system rapidly produces energy (ATP) and lactate. Also called glycolytic system or anaerobic glycolysis.

oxygen energy system A complex energy system that requires oxygen. To release ATP, it completes the breakdown of carbohydrate and fatty acids via the citric acid cycle and electron transport chain.

Quick Bites

The Weaker Sex?

Prior to the 1960s, women were banned from running any race longer that 800 meters and could not officially participate in marathon competitions until 1970. The race authorities mistakenly believed that women could harm themselves and were unsuitable for distance running. Imagine their amazement during the 1984 Olympic Games when Joan Benoit won the gold medal for the women's marathon with a time of 02:24:52—a time that would have won 11 of the previous 20 men's Olympic marathons!

Quick Bites

Lactic Acid or Lactate?

Although the terms *lactic acid* and *lactate* often are used interchangeably, they are not identical chemical compounds. Lactic acid ($C_3H_6O_3$), as its name implies, is an acid. Lactate is any salt of lactic acid. When anaerobic glycolysis forms lactic acid, this acid quickly dissociates, releasing hydrogen (H^+). The remaining compound immediately bonds with sodium (Na^+) or potassium (K^+) to form a salt—lactate.

This sequence may explain why fatigue seems to come in stages during an endurance event such as a marathon. It also may explain why a long-distance runner must exert such an extreme effort to maintain her pace near the end of a race.

Fiber Type and the Athlete

Genetics determine the relative proportion of muscle fiber types in athletes. Although distance runners who have a high percentage of ST fibers are well suited for endurance events, they will not succeed as elite sprinters. Conversely, sprinters who have predominantly FT fibers are better equipped for explosive events, but they will not become competitive marathon runners. (See **Figure 13.4**.)

Key Concepts: The body's muscles are of three types: smooth muscle, cardiac muscle, and skeletal muscle. The two main types of muscle fibers are slow-twitch and fast-twitch fibers. Slow-twitch fibers generate fuel through aerobic pathways while fast-twitch fibers produce energy using anaerobic pathways. Fast-twitch fibers can exert more force, but have limited endurance.

Energy Systems and Fuel Sources

ATP, the universal energy currency (see Chapter 7, "Metabolism"), supplies the energy for muscle fiber contraction and relaxation. To produce ATP, your muscles use three energy systems:

- **ATP-CP energy system** (anaerobic)
- **lactic acid energy system** (anaerobic glycolysis)
- **oxygen energy system** (aerobic metabolism)

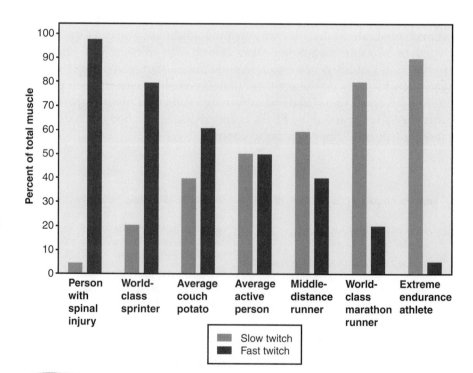

Figure 13.4 What's your mix of muscle fibers?
Source: Adapted from Andersen JL, Scherling P, Saltin B. Muscle, Genes and Athletic Performance, *Scientific American*, September 2000;283(3):49.

ATP-CP Energy System

At rest, your body stores a limited amount of ATP as an immediately available energy source to power activity. Yet, the amount is quite small—only about 3.5 ounces in your entire body. This amount can sustain muscle movements for less than a second, so the body also stores readily available energy in another high-energy phosphate molecule—**creatine phosphate** (also called **phosphocreatine**). The body does not directly use the energy in creatine phosphate. Instead, creatine phosphate helps maintain ATP levels by regenerating ATP from ADP.

Although this reaction can take place in the presence of oxygen, it does not require oxygen. Thus, the ATP-CP system is considered anaerobic. (See **Figure 13.5**.)

Muscle fibers contain four to six times as much creatine phosphate as ATP.[6] During the first few seconds of a high-intensity activity, such as sprinting, levels of creatine phosphate steadily decline as it is used to maintain relatively constant ATP levels. At exhaustion, your body has depleted both CP and ATP to such low levels that they can no longer power further muscle contractions. Your CP and ATP stores can power an all-out effort for only 3 to 15 seconds.[7] To continue the race, your body must call on other energy systems for a continuing supply of ATP.

Lactic Acid Energy System

Another method of fast ATP production is the lactic acid energy system (**Figure 13.6**). Because it involves glycolysis, it is also called the glycolytic system or the anaerobic glycolysis system. Like the ATP-CP system, this energy system does not require oxygen and these two energy systems are the predominant source of ATP during the early minutes of high-intensity exercise. Recall from the Chapter 7 that glycolysis produces small amounts of ATP (a net 2 ATP for each glucose molecule) as it breaks down glucose to pyruvate. If there is a lack of oxygen, the pyruvate is shunted to form lactate. The conversion of pyruvate to lactate also forms NAD^+, which is necessary to continue glycolysis of additional glucose molecules.

Compared to aerobic processing of a glucose molecule via the citric acid cycle and electron transport chain, glycolysis produces small amounts of ATP but at a much faster rate. Stored muscle glycogen is the primary source of glucose for the lactic acid system. Using anaerobic glycolysis, muscle cells can break down thousands of glucose molecules per second to form ATP. Even so, it is not nearly as rapid as the breakdown of CP to form ATP.

Anaerobic glycolysis is an important metabolic pathway, particularly for fast-twitch muscle fibers. It provides energy from ATP for 40 seconds to 2

Creatine phosphate + ADP + H⁺ ↔ ATP + creatine.

> **creatine phosphate** An energy-rich phosphate compound that supplies energy and P_i for the formation of ATP. Also called phosphocreatine.
>
> **phosphocreatine** See creatine phosphate.

LACTIC ACID ENERGY SYSTEM

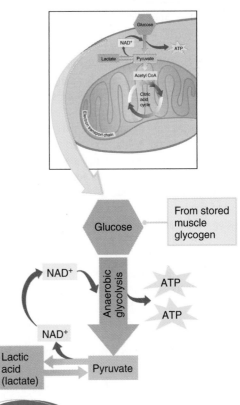

Figure 13.6 **Lactic acid energy system.** Glycolysis rapidly produces small amounts of ATP. Converting pyruvate to lactate supplies the NAD^+ required for glycolysis of additional glucose molecules. This lactic acid energy system does not require oxygen.

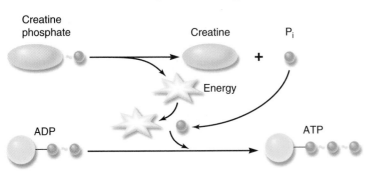

Figure 13.5 **ATP-CP energy system.** To maintain relatively constant ATP levels during the first few seconds of a high intensity activity, creatine phosphate releases energy and Pi to regenerate ATP from ADP. Although this ATP-CP energy system operates in the presence of oxygen, it does not require oxygen.

The Burn to the Finish

The pain a runner feels when approaching the finish line and immediately after the event is called acute muscle soreness. The culprits include a buildup of metabolic byproducts, such as H^+, and tissue edema caused by fluid seeping from the bloodstream into surrounding tissues. This pain and soreness usually disappears within minutes or hours.

minutes of physical activity. However, this rapid formation of ATP causes the accumulation of lactic acid and increases the acidity of the muscle cell. Although lactic acid accumulation is directly related to increased acidity, all the intermediates of glycolysis contribute protons (H^+), which increase acidity. The degradation of ATP to ADP forms additional protons. This acidification of muscle fibers impairs glycolytic enzyme function and inhibits further breakdown of glucose. In addition, this change in pH decreases the fibers' calcium-binding capacity, an important mechanism in muscle contraction, and thus may impede muscle fiber activity. For years, a buildup of lactic acid only has been blamed for muscle fatigue. Rather, the accumulation of H^+ and change in pH are the primary villains that cause muscle fatigue and decreased exercise performance.[8] (See the FYI feature "Lactate Is Not a Metabolic Dead End" for more information about lactate's role in production of energy.)

During exercise, muscle fibers can use energy 200 times faster than at rest.[9] At this rate, our exercise capacity would be limited to only a few minutes if it relied solely on the ATP-CP and lactic acid energy systems. For

Think About It

2

FYI Lactate Is Not A Metabolic Dead End

FOR YOUR INFORMATION

Today's race is 200 meters and you are in the lead. The crowd roars with excitement and your coach screams hoarsely as your feet slam over and over on the hard gray cinder track. Other runners are close behind and you can feel them breathing and pounding at your heels. Air whistles in and out of your wheezing lungs as you doggedly push to stay ahead. Your muscles are screaming, but they carry you across the finish line. A winner!

As you slump in exhaustion, you wonder how your limp muscles carried you through to the end. Each leg seemed to weigh a thousand pounds. As your muscles tire, the pH in your muscle cells drops and lactate levels rise. Scientists, coaches, and athletes have long believed that lactate was a useless, even toxic, dead-end substance. Recent research proves otherwise. It is the overall acidification of the muscle tissue, rather than a buildup of lactate, that primarily causes muscle fatigue. Also, lactate is now recognized as a fuel in its own right. In addition to acting as a metabolic shunt, lactate is a useful fuel, produced and consumed under all conditions of oxygen availability, while exercising or at rest.

Without the energy supplied by the lactic acid energy system, you would never have crossed the finish line. While your body anaerobically burned muscle glycogen, it pro-

duced copious amounts of lactate. Where does this lactate come from and how does your body handle it?

Cori Cycle

Inside your contracting muscle cells during vigorous exercise, glycolysis produces pyruvate and NADH faster than the oxidative metabolic pathways (citric acid cycle and electron transport chain) can accommodate.

The diversion of pyruvate to lactate by a reaction that oxidizes NADH to NAD^+ alleviates the backup. The supply of NAD^+ generated by this reaction is essential for glycolysis to continue.

Lactate easily diffuses through the muscle cell's membrane into the bloodstream. The liver picks up the circulating lactate and converts it back to pyruvate. Using gluconeogenic pathways, the liver transforms the pyruvate

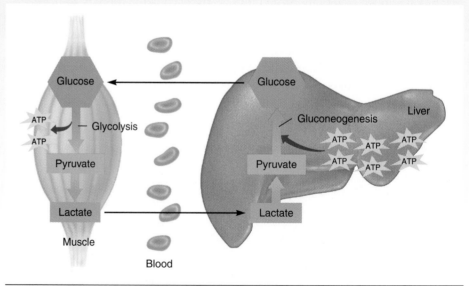

The Cori Cycle. The Cori cycle shifts some of the metabolic burden of contracting muscle to the liver. Lactate formed in contracting muscle travels to the liver which uses it to form glucose. This glucose returns to the muscle to fuel further contractions.

longer activities, the body employs another strategy to generate ATP—the oxygen energy system.

Oxygen Energy System

The oxygen energy system (**Figure 13.7**), as the name implies, involves the aerobic pathways of the citric acid cycle and electron transport chain to supply ATP. (See Chapter 7 for a detailed discussion.) These pathways can operate only when there is a sufficient supply of oxygen. In contrast to the two anaerobic systems (ATP-CP system and lactic acid system), the oxygen energy system can produce a tremendous amount of ATP, but at a much slower rate. Slow-twitch muscle fibers primarily use ATP produced by the oxygen energy system, and endurance events place large demands on the body's ability to supply oxygen to active muscle fibers. As 2 minutes elapse during a distance race, the oxygen energy system is supplying 50 percent of the muscles' energy needs. By the time a runner passes the 30-minute mark, this aerobic system is supplying 95 percent; at 2 hours or more, the oxygen energy system is supplying 98 percent of the muscles' energy needs.[10]

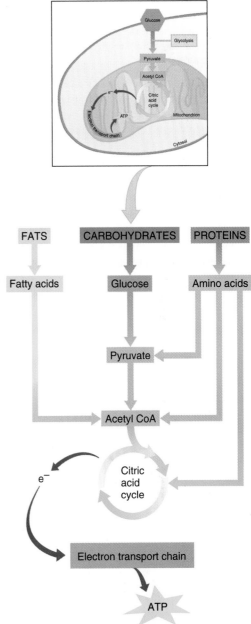

OXYGEN ENERGY SYSTEM

Figure 13.7 **Oxygen energy system.** Complete oxidation of nutrients forms ATP via the citric acid cycle and electron transport chain. This oxygen energy system requires oxygen and primarily relies on fat and carbohydrate as fuels.

into glucose, which the liver exports into the bloodstream. The glucose travels back to the skeletal muscle cells where it reenters the energy-producing glycolytic pathways.

This recurring circular pathway is called the Cori cycle. This cycle essentially buys time with a detour through the liver when pyruvate is backed up in muscle cells. When oxygen becomes readily available, the predominant flow of metabolites returns to the citric acid cycle and electron transport chain.

Lactate Shuttle

The pathways of the Cori cycle are an important, but incomplete, part of the lactate picture. The use of the Cori cycle as a holding pattern led to the mistaken belief that lactate was just a metabolic detour. It was thought that lactate had no direct role as a fuel source and that it was simply waiting for oxygen to become available so it could convert back to pyruvate and reenter the oxidative pathways. Recent studies describe a more extensive role for this long-maligned substrate.

Lactate now is recognized as an important means of distributing carbohydrate energy sources after a meal and during sustained physical exercise. Lactate's advantage is its ability to move rapidly between cells. It is a small mole-

cule and, unlike glucose, does not need insulin to cross a cell membrane.

Under resting conditions of plentiful carbohydrate and oxygen, diverse tissues such as skeletal muscle, liver, and skin produce lactate.[1] In these conditions, the supply of raw materials, rather than limited oxygen, drives the formation of lactate.

According to the lactate shuttle hypothesis, lactate formed in some muscle cells becomes an energy source at other sites, either adjacent or remote. Skeletal muscle, once thought simply to produce lactate, also directly uses lactate as a fuel. At times, skeletal muscle actually removes more lactate than it produces. The heart muscle is fully aerobic, but it both produces and consumes lactate. Studies suggest that during exercise lactate is the major fuel for the heart and the preferred fuel for certain muscle fibers.[2]

The next time you complain about sore, tired muscles, don't vilify lactate. Instead, think about the daily usefulness of lactate and how this little respected substance helped power you to the finish.

1 Brooks GA. Mammalian fuel utilization during sustained exercise. *Comp Biochem Physiol B Biochem Mol Biol.* 1998;(May)120:89–107.
2 Myers J, Ashley E. Dangerous curves: a perspective on exercise, lactate, and the anaerobic threshold. *Chest.* 1997;111:787–795.

VO₂max The greatest amount of oxygen that can be transported from the lungs to muscle tissue during maximal exertion. Also called aerobic power, cardiovascular endurance capacity, maximal oxygen uptake, and maximal oxygen capacity.

Quick Bites

What's your aerobic capacity?

For men, the highest recorded value for VO₂max is 94 for a champion Norwegian cross-country skier. For women, a Russian cross-country skier achieved a VO₂max of 77. In contrast, sedentary adults may have values as low as 20. (Units are milliliters of oxygen per kilogram of body weight per minute.)

The oxygen energy system relies primarily on carbohydrates and fats. When using carbohydrate, this system is an extension of the lactic acid system. Available oxygen allows pyruvate to enter the citric acid cycle and ultimately form ATP via the electron transport chain rather than be shunted to form lactate. The main source of carbohydrate for muscular contraction is glucose from muscle glycogen. When needed, the oxygen system can also form ATP by breaking down muscle triglycerides and circulating free fatty acids. For a given amount of oxygen, carbohydrate releases more energy than fat. However, carbohydrate stores are limited. A 68 kilogram (150-lb) man with 10 to 20 percent body fat, for example, has carbohydrate stores of 1,800 to 2,000 kilocalories in muscle glycogen, liver glycogen, and blood glucose. By comparison, his fat stores hold roughly 63,000 to 120,000 kilocalories depending on his percent body fat.[11]

Key Concepts: *Energy for muscle work comes from production of ATP in the muscle cell. Muscles use three energy systems to produce ATP: the ATP-CP energy system, which does not require oxygen; the lactic acid energy system, which involves glycolysis and is anaerobic; and the oxygen energy system, which relies on carbohydrates and fats. The first two systems are the predominant sources of ATP during the early minutes of high-intensity exercise. The third system produces ATP at a much slower rate and supplies energy for endurance events.*

Contributions of Energy Systems and Fuel Sources

Anaerobic and aerobic metabolism work together to fuel all types of exercise. (See **Figure 13.8**.) During the first few minutes of any activity, anaerobic metabolism (ATP-CP and lactic acid systems) provides most of the energy. As the duration of activity increases but intensity remains low to moderate, aerobic metabolism (oxygen energy system) increases. To meet the demands of aerobic metabolism, your body must deliver oxygen to your muscle fibers. As the demand increases, such as when running increasingly steep hills, you take in ever greater amounts of oxygen until, despite increasing demand, you cannot increase your oxygen uptake further. This capacity is called maximum oxygen uptake, or simply **VO₂max**.

High-intensity exercises performed at greater than 70 percent VO₂max but short in duration (e.g., sprinting and weight lifting) are fueled primarily by muscle glycogen. Exercises performed at 60 percent or less of VO₂max for a longer duration (e.g., long-distance running, cycling, walking, and swimming) are fueled by a higher percentage of fat than carbohydrate. **Table 13.3** lists types of physical activity and the amounts of energy they require from various sources.

Even very lean people have ample fatty acid stores to fuel aerobic activity. The limiting fuel in aerobic metabolism is carbohydrate (and potential carbohydrate sources, e.g., glycogen). The first metabolic reaction in the citric acid cycle requires oxaloacetic acid, which is derived primarily from glucose. After 90 minutes or more of

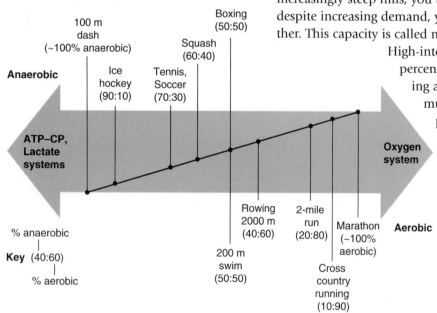

Figure 13.8 **The anaerobic-aerobic continuum.** Most activities use ATP from both anaerobic and aerobic energy systems. The 100 meter dash is considered completely anaerobic and the marathon is considered completely aerobic.

continuous activity at a higher intensity (>70 percent VO₂max), the pool of oxaloacetic acid diminishes. Without sufficient oxaloacetic acid, the citric acid cycle, and ultimately, the electron transport chain cannot produce ATP. When available carbohydrate is exhausted, activity must stop.

Training Influences Fuel Use

Training causes physiological adaptations that can influence the body's use of fuel. Endurance training increases **cardiac output**, which increases oxygen delivery to exercising muscles. (See **Figure 13.9**.) Skeletal muscle also adapts to endurance training with an increase in mitochondria and mitochondrial enzymes. For a given level of work, these adaptations enable an aerobically trained athlete to metabolize fat for energy at a greater rate than an untrained person.

Sprint and power-type workouts also produce training effects that influence fuel use. One study reported that after resistance training, the trained muscles had significant increases in ATP, CP, free creatine, and glycogen, as well as a 28 percent improvement in muscular strength.[12]

In endurance-trained people the **lactate threshold** (the point where lactate production exceeds lactate removal) is approximately 70 to 85 percent VO₂max, compared with 50 to 60 percent VO₂max in untrained people. Why does this training effect occur? Theories are contradictory. Some

> **cardiac output** The amount of blood expelled by the heart. The cardiac output for 1 minute equals the amount of blood ejected by each heart beat multiplied by the number of beats per minute. In resting adults, a normal heart ejects 4 to 8 liters per minute.
>
> **lactate threshold** During exercise of increasing intensity, the point at which muscle lactate levels begin to rise above resting levels.

Table 13.3 Sports Events and Fuel

Event	Typical Duration	ATP-CP System (anaerobic) Creatine Phosphate	Lactic Acid System (anaerobic) Muscle Glycogen (anaerobic)	Oxygen Energy System (aerobic) Muscle Glycogen (aerobic)	Liver Glycogen (blood glucose)	Triglyceride (fatty acids)
Explosive Strength and Power Rapid burst of energy as seen in starting a sprint or lifting a barbell	0–3 sec	nearly 100%				
High Power and Speed	5–30 sec					
100-meter dash	10–12 sec	50%	50%			
200-meter dash	20–25 sec	25%	65%	10%		
Power Endurance	1–2 min					
400-meter race	50–60 sec	12%	63%	25%		
800-meter race	2.0–2.5 min	6%	50%	44%		
Aerobic Power	13–30 min					
5-kilometer race	15–18 min	**	12%	88%		
10-kilometer race	32–35 min	**	3%	97%		
Aerobic Endurance	2+ hr					
marathon (42 km)	2.5–3 hr			75%	5%	20%
ultramarathon (80 km)	5.5–7 hr			35%	5%	60%

** Creatine phosphate is used during the first few seconds and, if resynthesized during the race, in the sprint to the finish.

Note: Recent research indicates that amino acids contribute 3–6% of the fuel for energy metabolism during exercise.

Source: Adapted from McArdle WD, Katch FI, Katch VL. *Exercise Physiology.* Philadelphia: Lippincott Williams & Wilkins; 1999. And Tarnopolski M. Protein metabolism in strength and endurance athletes. In Lamb DR, Murray R, eds. *Perspectives in Exercise Science and Sports Medicine.* Carmel, IN: Cooper Publishing Group. 1999;12.

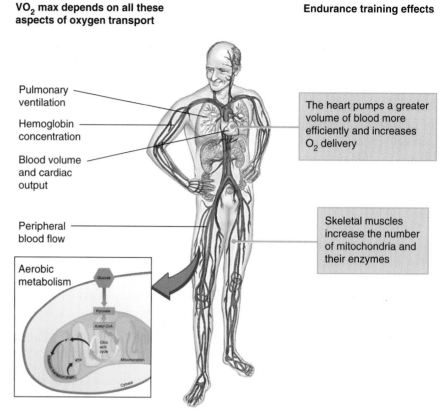

VO$_2$ max depends on all these aspects of oxygen transport

Endurance training effects

Pulmonary ventilation

Hemoglobin concentration

Blood volume and cardiac output

Peripheral blood flow

Aerobic metabolism

The heart pumps a greater volume of blood more efficiently and increases O$_2$ delivery

Skeletal muscles increase the number of mitochondria and their enzymes

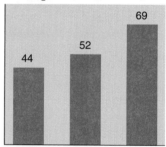

Maximal O$_2$ uptake VO$_2$ max (ml·kg^{-1} min^{-1})

Untrained	Jogger	Marathoner
44	52	69

Figure 13.9 **Oxygen uptake and aerobic training.** Your maximum oxygen uptake, or VO$_2$max, is the maximum rate at which you can take up oxygen no matter how much you further increase the intensity of your exercise.

researchers believe a decrease in lactate production occurs with training. Other investigators propose that the liver and other metabolically active tissues increase their rate of lactate removal.[13]

Glycogen Depletion

After the first few seconds of an event, your muscles rely primarily on muscle glycogen to generate ATP. The intensity of the activity determines the rate of muscle glycogen's depletion. An increase in intensity accelerates the depletion rate dramatically. Sprinting, for example, uses muscle glycogen 35 to 40 times faster than walking.[14] Since the muscle depends on a constant supply of energy fueled by muscle glycogen, the amount of stored glycogen can limit the duration of an activity, even when the effort is mild.

During the first few minutes of an event, the body uses muscle glycogen rapidly. As the event grinds on, the rate of glycogen use markedly slows. **Figure 13.10** illustrates how the sensation of fatigue relates to the depletion of muscle glycogen. Early in the run, when glycogen stores are high, the runner reports that a moderate effort maintains a steady pace. For the first 1.5 hours of the run, the perceived effort does not exceed the moderate level even though glycogen stores are dropping steadily to only one-third of their starting levels. It is not until nearly 3 hours into the run, when glycogen stores are almost entirely depleted, that the runner experiences exhaustive fatigue. Marathon runners commonly experience a sudden onset of fatigue around the 18- to 20-mile mark. Popularly known as "hitting the wall," this sensation is due, at least in part, to glycogen depletion and muscle fatigue.

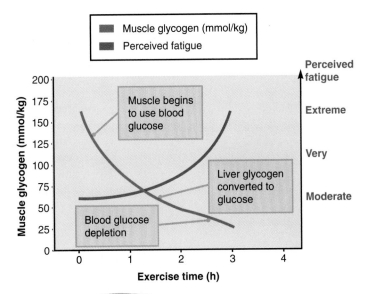

Figure 13.10 Glycogen depletion and the sensation of fatigue.

Glycogen, Blood Glucose, and Fatigue

Since muscle glycogen alone provides insufficient carbohydrate to sustain exercise for several hours, the muscle fibers also rely on blood glucose during endurance events. To maintain a constant level of blood glucose, the liver breaks down its own glycogen stores. Early in an endurance event, blood glucose contributes little to energy production. As the exercise duration increases, the liver must increasingly break down glycogen to keep pace with blood glucose uptake by muscle fibers. During the later stages of an endurance event, the amount of energy obtained from blood glucose can become significant.

The body has limited liver glycogen stores and the liver cannot rapidly produce glucose from other sources. Once the muscles' glucose uptake exceeds the liver's glucose production, blood glucose levels drop. The muscles must then rely on their own nearly empty glycogen reserves, draining them further. The result is total exhaustion.

In activities lasting longer than 30 minutes, glycogen depletion and low blood glucose can limit performance. Larger glycogen reserves at the start of an event extend the time to depletion and improve endurance performance. (See the section "Carbohydrate Loading" later in this chapter). In shorter events, metabolic byproducts in the muscles, such as lactate and H$^+$, are the more likely cause of fatigue.

Key Concepts: *Different types of exercise draw on different energy systems. High-intensity, short-duration activities use anaerobic pathways. As intensity decreases and duration increases, the use of aerobic pathways increases. Training affects fuel use by increasing the efficiency of oxygen delivery to muscles, and increasing the number of muscle mitochondria available for aerobic metabolism. The availability of glucose from muscle and liver glycogen stores is a major factor in endurance.*

Optimal Nutrition for Exercise

The optimal diet for most physically active people—from the college student who plays intramural basketball to the 50-year-old woman who enjoys walking during her lunch break—includes a variety of nutrient-dense foods from the Food Guide Pyramid (See Chapter 2). Food choices should be high in carbohydrate (≥ 60 percent of calories), low in fat (≤ 30 percent of calories), and moderate in protein. Consuming a variety of foods from each of the food groups to meet energy needs will meet micronutrient (vitamins and minerals) needs as well.

Quick Bites

Ouch! But I felt fine yesterday ...

After a bout of heavy exercise, a person may not feel muscle soreness for a day or two. We do not fully understand this painful phenomenon, which is called delayed-onset muscle soreness. Activities that lengthen muscles seem to be the primary cause. The muscles suffer damage with micro-tears in their structure. This leads to an inflammatory response, causing localized muscle pain, swelling, and tenderness.

NCAA National Collegiate Athletic Association.

Nutrition and the Competitive Athlete

Patrice is a 19-year-old soccer player who competes with other top collegiate athletes at an **NCAA** Division I institution. Gary is an NBA basketball player, and Steve is training for the Ironman triathlon competition in Hawaii. Sarah, a 34-year-old accountant, is aiming to break her personal record in a marathon that she has been training for over the past 4 months.

What do these people have in common? They are all competitive athletes who have heavy training schedules. Optimal nutrition is an essential part of every athlete's training program and can make a difference when winning is measured in fractions of seconds or inches. General recommendations for competitive athletes include:[15]

- Consume adequate energy (calories) and nutrients to support health and performance.
- Maintain appropriate sports-specific ranges for percentage of body fat and fat-free body mass.
- Promote optimal recovery from training.
- Maintain hydration status (normal fluid intake).

Studies indicate that athletes are confused about nutrition and do not follow the dietary recommendations for peak sports performance.[16] Let's take a closer look at the nutritional needs of the competitive athlete.

Energy

Adequate energy intake is critical for athletic performance and to maintain- or increase lean body mass. World-class athletes can almost double their energy requirements with 3 to 4 hours of heavy training each day. For some athletes, it is quite challenging to consume enough calories to meet this energy demand.[17]

In contrast, athletes who compete in endurance sports, sports judged by build, and sports with weight classifications often are concerned with avoiding weight gain and, therefore, restrict caloric intake. Studies show that well-trained female athletes tend to have lower energy intake than would be anticipated given the intensity of their workouts.[18] This decrease in energy intake is associated with a lower rate of resting energy expenditure. Sports nutritionists recommend an eating pattern of small, frequent meals to maintain energy metabolism, improve nutrient intake, achieve desired body composition, support training schedule, and reduce injuries.[19]

Carbohydrate

The availability of carbohydrate significantly influences athletic performance. Carbohydrate in the form of muscle and liver glycogen, and blood glucose is the main fuel source for muscle contraction during high-intensity exercise. Carbohydrate is the exclusive fuel for anaerobic glycolysis and the limiting nutrient supporting aerobic ATP production.

Training depletes glycogen stores, with the rate dependent upon the intensity of exercise. Carbohydrate-rich diets can help maximize muscle and liver glycogen stores before exercise and promote faster recovery of stores after exercise.

Carbohydrate Intake Goals for Athletes. Research studies continue to support the need for dietary carbohydrate as the main fuel source for the competitive athlete, with a suggested minimum of 60 percent of total calories from carbohydrate.[20]

Researchers usually recommend carbohydrate-rich diets for endurance athletes who need maximal glycogen stores to prolong endurance. These recommendations may also apply to strength and power athletes, although in this

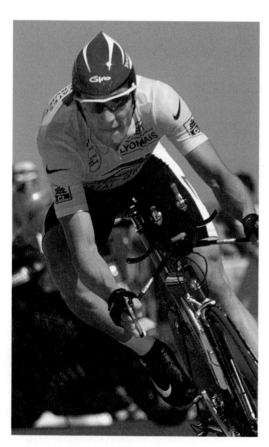

Optimal nutrition is an important part of Lance Armstrong's training.

area the research is less clear. Since strength and power athletes who participate in repetitive bouts of intense activity deplete glycogen stores, a diet high in carbohydrates may improve the performances of these athletes as well.[21]

Type and Form of Carbohydrate. For all athletes, dietary carbohydrates should come from complex carbohydrates, which provide fiber, iron (if enriched), and many of the B vitamins necessary for energy metabolism. Added sugars should supply no more than 10 percent of the day's calories, but some athletes may need to include more simple sugars to meet energy requirements.

Carbohydrate Intake before Training or Competition. Just like "topping off" the gas tank in a car before a long trip, athletes need to fill their glycogen stores prior to training or competition to ensure adequate stores of muscle glycogen and blood glucose concentrations. However, the type of exercise, level of intensity, and time of day can influence an athlete's food choices. Additionally, the amount a person eats before exercising may vary with personal preferences.

In the 1 to 4 hours prior to exercise, a rule of thumb is to consume 1 to 4.5 grams of carbohydrate for each kilogram of body weight.[22] Since many athletes have problems with GI distress, the carbohydrate and caloric content of the meal should be smaller when eaten closer to a workout. For example, if you plan to eat 3 hours before a workout or competition, your meal should contain 3 grams of carbohydrate for every kilogram of body weight. In the 1 to 4 hours before exercising, some athletes can tolerate solid foods; others prefer liquids to avoid GI distress. Since protein and fat take longer to digest and absorb, pre-exercise meals should contain no more than 10 to 15 percent of the calories as protein and less than 20 percent of calories from fat. **Table 13.4** offers guidelines for timing of meals before an event.

> **Before intense exercise**
> 1–4 hours before exercise:
>
> **1–4.5g carbohydrate**
> **per kg body weight**

Table 13.4 **Timing Meals before Events**

Time: 8 A.M. event, such as a road race or swim meet
Meals: The night before, eat a high-carbohydrate dinner and drink extra water. The morning of the event, about 6:00 or 6:30, have a light 200- to 400-calorie meal (depending on your tolerance), such as yogurt and a banana, or one or two sports bars, and extra water. Eat familiar foods. If you want a bigger meal, you might want to get up and eat by 5:00 or 6:00.

Time: 10 A.M. event, such as a bike race or soccer game
Meals: The night before, eat a high-carbohydrate meal and drink extra water. The morning of the event, eat a familiar breakfast by 7:00, to allow 3 hours for the food to digest. This meal will prevent the fatigue that results from low blood sugar. If your body cannot handle any breakfast, eat a late snack before going to bed the night before. This will boost liver glycogen stores and prevent low blood sugar the next morning.

Time: 2 P.M. event, such as a football or lacrosse game
Meals: An afternoon game allows time for you to have either a big, high-carbohydrate breakfast and a light lunch, or a substantial brunch by 10:00, allowing 4 hours for digestion. As always, eat a high-carbohydrate dinner the night before, and drink extra fluids the day before and up to noontime.

Time: 8 P.M. event, such as a basketball game
Meals: A hefty, high-carbohydrate breakfast and lunch will be thoroughly digested by evening. Plan for dinner, as tolerated, by 5:00 or have a lighter meal between 6:00 and 7:00. Drink extra fluids all day.

Time: All-day event, such as a 100-mile bike ride, triathlon training, or long, hard hike
Meals: Two days before, cut back on your exercise; the day before take a rest day to allow your muscles the chance to replace depleted glycogen stores. Eat carbohydrate-rich meals at breakfast, lunch, and dinner. Drink extra fluids. The day of the event, eat breakfast depending on your tolerance—whatever you usually have before exercising. Throughout the day, plan to snack at least every 1.5 to 2 hours on wholesome carbohydrates to maintain a normal blood sugar. At lunchtime, eat a carbohydrate meal. Drink fluids before you get thirsty; you should need to urinate at least three times throughout the day.

Source: Reprinted, by permission, from Nancy Clark, 1997, *Nancy's Clark's Sports Nutrition Guidebook*, 2nd ed. Champaign, IL: Human Kinetics, 169–170.

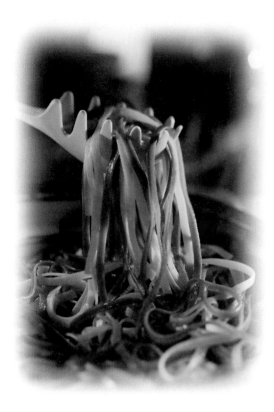

Many athletes are confused about whether to eat less than 1 hour before exercise. Some athletes are unable to fully refuel several hours before a workout and actually rely on carbohydrate intake 1 hour before exercise to decrease hunger and delay fatigue. In fact, some athletes experience an improvement in performance. On the other hand, some athletes experience a sharp drop in blood sugar, which limits performance. To reduce the risk of lowered blood sugar, avoid high-sugar food and drink during this pre-exercise period. Good choices for pre-exercise consumption include spaghetti, milk, some fruits and juices, and most legumes. During exercise, consuming beverages with low to moderate levels of simple carbohydrate can help to maintain the carbohydrate supply to exercising muscle.[23]

Pre-exercise Meals and the Glycemic Index. As you may recall from Chapter 4, individual foods have different effects on blood glucose levels independent of carbohydrate content. The glycemic index of foods is a measure of this effect, and has attracted recent interest in relation to the diets of athletes. High-glycemic-index foods trigger a faster and higher rise in blood glucose. Although research relating glycemic index to athletic performance is limited, researchers have proposed the following guidelines:[24]

- There is no universal recommendation for eating only low-glycemic-index, high-carbohydrate foods prior to a long workout.

- During prolonged exercise, consume moderate- to high-glycemic-index carbohydrates to maintain blood glucose levels and delay fatigue.

- Immediately after exercise, consume moderate- to high-glycemic-index carbohydrates instead of low-glycemic-index carbohydrates to enhance glycogen storage.

- Some athletes experience a detrimental response to carbohydrate-rich foods before exercise and may benefit from a low-glycemic-index pre-exercise meal.

- Overall, athletes should experiment to find the type of carbohydrate foods they can tolerate. Confidence in food choices helps athletes maintain that mental edge critical to peak performance.

Recovery Nutrition. It can take 24 to 48 hours after an event to replenish glycogen stores and the timing and type of carbohydrates are important factors in the refueling process. Athletes who delay the consumption of carbohydrates for more than 4 hours after exercising cut the rate of glycogen synthesis almost in half compared to athletes who consume carbohydrates during the first 2 hours after exercising.[25] Some research shows that the first 15 minutes are critical.[26]

The best way to replenish glycogen stores after intense exercise is to consume 1 to 1.5 grams of carbohydrate per kilogram of body weight within 30 minutes after a workout, followed by an additional 1 to 1.5 grams per kilograms every 2 hours.[27] Carbohydrate intake after exercise also benefits protein metabolism. Several researchers have shown that these levels of carbohydrates taken immediately or 1 hour after resistance exercise decrease protein breakdown and enhance protein retention.[28] (See **Figure 13.11**.)

Consuming high-glycemic-index foods during the first few hours after exercise can improve glycogen synthesis.[29] High-glycemic-index foods include:

- white bread

- processed breakfast cereal

After intense exercise
First 30 minutes, then every 2 hours:

1–1.5g carbohydrate
per kg body weight

- bananas
- potatoes
- jelly beans and hard candy
- sport gels and drinks
- crackers and rice cakes

Carbohydrate Loading. **Carbohydrate loading**, or **glycogen loading**, is a process of manipulating carbohydrate intake and an exercise regimen to maximize muscle glycogen stores. Carbohydrate loading is recommended for athletes who compete in events that last 90 minutes or longer, such as those listed in **Table 13.5**.

The concept of carbohydrate loading has evolved since the original research in the 1960s. Current recommendations for carbohydrate loading include an intake of 60 to 70 percent of calories from carbohydrate along with a decrease in exercise intensity and duration prior to competition.[30] **Table 13.6** is a training plan for endurance athletes that includes carbohydrate loading and exercise for the week before an event. The glycogen content of exercised muscles more than doubles in athletes who adhere to this protocol, and thus extends the duration of higher intensity activity. For example, distance runners who carbohydrate load may be able to keep a faster pace for a longer time and finish a race sooner.[31]

Even though "extra" glycogen prior to competition sounds like a perfect plan, there is a downside to carbohydrate loading. For each gram of glycogen stored in muscle tissue, the body also stores 2.7 grams of water. Many athletes who carbohydrate load complain about this weight gain and subsequent sluggishness. Some opt to train and compete without carbohydrate loading since, for them, the physical discomfort outweighs the benefits of a greater carbohydrate store.

If you participate in an aerobic activity for fewer than 60 to 90 consecutive minutes, carbohydrate loading probably will provide no benefit.

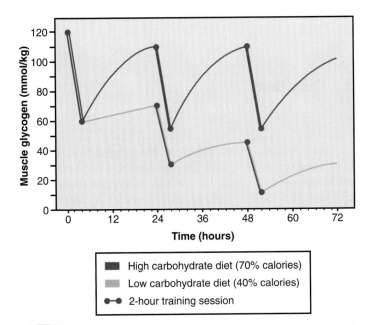

Figure 13.11 A high carbohydrate diet replenishes glycogen stores better than a low carbohydrate diet.
Source: Adapted from Costill DL, Miller JM. Nutrition for endurance sport: Carbohydrate and fluid balance. *Int J Sport Nutr.* 1980;1:2–14.

carbohydrate loading Manipulation of dietary carbohydrate and exercise regimen to maximize glycogen stores in the muscles. It is appropriate for endurance events lasting 60 to 90 consecutive minutes or longer. Also known as glycogen loading.
glycogen loading See carbohydrate loading.

 Table 13.5 **Recommended Events for Carbohydrate Loading**

Marathons
Ultramarathons
Long-distance swimming
Cross-country skiing
30-kilometer runs
Triathlons
Cycling time trails
Long-distance canoe racing

 Table 13.6 **Carbohydrate Loading for Endurance Athletes**

Number of Days before Event	Exercise Duration (min)	Training Diet (g carbohydrate/ kg body weight)
6	90	5
5	40	5
4	40	5
3	20	10
2	20	10
1	Rest day	10
Race	Competition	Precompetition food and fluid

Source: Coleman MA. Carbohydrate and exercise. In: Rosenbloom CA. *Sports Nutrition.* 3rd ed. Chicago, IL: The American Dietetic Association; 2000.

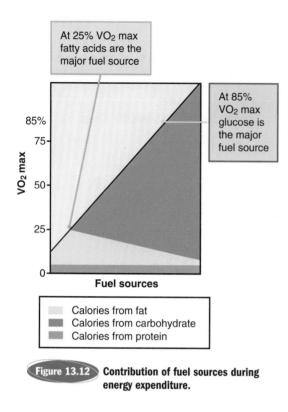

At 25% VO₂ max fatty acids are the major fuel source

At 85% VO₂ max glucose is the major fuel source

85%
75%

50

25

0

VO₂ max

Fuel sources

☐ Calories from fat
☐ Calories from carbohydrate
☐ Calories from protein

Figure 13.12 **Contribution of fuel sources during energy expenditure.**

Instead, experts recommend that you taper your training program a few days before competition and eat a diet that provides 70 percent of its calories from carbohydrate for 1 or 2 days before the event.[32]

Key Concepts: *The most important element of the athlete's diet is energy, and the major source of energy should be carbohydrates. Food rich in complex carbohydrates, which also can provide fiber, iron, and B vitamins, are the best sources. A high-carbohydrate diet before competition helps to maximize glycogen stores and endurance. Consuming carbohydrates soon after exercise enhances the rebuilding of glycogen stores. Carbohydrate loading is a process of adjusting carbohydrate intake and training intensity to maximize glycogen stores just before an event.*

Fat

During exercise, carbohydrates and fats are the two main sources of fuel. Endurance (aerobic) training increases your body's capacity to use fat as a fuel by improving the efficiency of oxygen delivery to the muscle cells, and increasing the number of mitochondria in each cell. In trained athletes, the relative contribution of fatty acids as a fuel source declines as the intensity of exercise increases. At 25 percent VO₂max, fatty acids are the major fuel source; at 85 percent VO₂max, glucose use dominates (**Figure 13.12**).

Although fat is the main source of energy during low- to moderate-intensity exercise, this does not mean that endurance athletes should consume more dietary fat. (See **Figure 13.13**.) High-fat diets usually are lower in carbohydrate, thus limiting muscles' ability to replenish glycogen stores. Carbohydrate also is needed for normal fat mobilization and oxidation during exercise. Additionally, high-fat diets are digested more slowly than high-carbohydrate diets. They also can quickly contribute excess calories, saturated fat, and cholesterol.

Recommendations Regarding Fat Intake. For the general population, dietary recommendations promote a diet with less than 30 percent of calories from fat. At the same time, the popular press defends the benefits of low-carbohy-

---

[*Fyi*] To Zone or Not To Zone? That Is the Question.

FOR YOUR INFORMATION

Barry Sears, creator of Eicotec bars and author of *Enter the Zone* and *Mastering the Zone*, puts forth the theory that insulin response to high-carbohydrate diets reduces performance by interfering with free fatty acid mobilization and lowering blood glucose. He further asserts that the insulin response facilitates the conversion of carbohydrate to fat and increases adipose tissue stores. The Zone diet books recommend a carbohydrate-restricted diet of exactly 40 percent carbohydrate, 30 percent protein, and 30 percent fat.

The Zone diet proponents assert that high insulin levels increase the production of "bad" eicosanoids. Eicosanoids are hormonelike compounds that act in opposition to regulate inflammation, the tendency for blood to clot, and the immune system. The protein content of the Zone diet supposedly increases glucagon levels, which in turn support the production of "good" eicosanoids by counteracting the effects of insulin.

The scientific basis of the theory underlying the Zone diet has many faults. There is no evidence that insulin increases the amount of "bad" eicosanoids or that glucagon makes "good" eicosanoids.[1] A high-carbohydrate diet does elicit an insulin response because insulin is needed for the transport of glucose (energy) into the cells. With insulin-mediated glucose uptake, the synthesis of liver and muscle glycogen leads to a decrease in blood glucose. The body preferentially uses carbohydrates for energy and does not readily convert excess carbohydrate to fat (see the FYI "Do Carbohydrates Turn into Fat?" in Chapter 7). During exercise, the release of catecholamines such as epinephrine and norepinephrine drives an increase in blood glucose and a decrease in insulin. Catecholamines also prompt the adipose tissue to release fatty acids into the bloodstream.

Consuming carbohydrate 30 to 60 minutes before exercise is associated with increased insulin and lowered blood glucose. However,

drate diets that are higher in fat and protein. While the debate continues (see the FYI feature "To Zone or Not To Zone? That Is the Question"), sports nutritionists generally advise athletes to consume 15 to 25 percent of calories as dietary fat.[33] Extreme fat restriction limits food choices, especially sources of protein, iron, zinc, and essential fatty acids. In addition, athletes with high caloric needs (> 5,000 kilocalories per day) may find it difficult to eat enough food without exceeding the general recommendation to get no more than 30 percent of calories from fat. Sports nutritionists recommend that any extra fat calories come from monounsaturated and polyunsaturated sources.

Protein

Historically, many athletes believed that eating muscle from animals would make them strong so they consumed high-protein diets. Early research in the 1800s supported the idea that protein was the major exercise fuel, but subsequent studies showed that exercise had little effect on protein requirements. Beginning in the late 1970s, research data suggested that athletes might require slightly higher protein intakes than sedentary people.[34]

When the book *The Zone* hit bookstores in 1995 with its suggested calorie distribution of 40 percent carbohydrate, 30 percent fat, and 30 percent protein, interest in optimal protein intakes for athletes surged. Athletes—from endurance runners to football players to weekend warriors—are again asking the question, "Do I need to eat more protein and less carbohydrate for optimal performance?"[35]

Protein Requirements of Athletes. The adult Recommended Dietary Allowance (RDA) for protein is 0.8 gram per kilogram of body weight per day,[36] which is based on protein needs of sedentary individuals. The current RDAs do not account for varying levels of activity and the increased protein breakdown that occurs during exercise. People who regularly engage in low-intensity exercise do not need additional protein.[37] However, recent research supports the long-standing idea that athletes who engage in vigorous activities have slightly higher protein needs. The reasons for the increased needs vary from sport to sport.

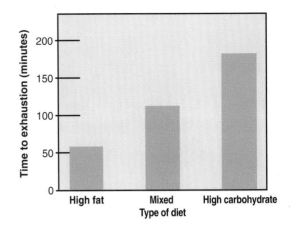

Figure 13.13 **Diet composition and endurance.** Athletes can exercise longer when eating a high carbohydrate diet.

those responses are temporary and do not adversely affect performance. In fact, a high-carbohydrate meal 1 hour before exercise can improve endurance by supplying the exercising muscles with glucose and sparing the loss of glycogen.

Carbohydrates—not fatty acids—are used preferentially for energy during exercise. Muscle glycogen is the body's predominant energy source for most sports at an exercise intensity greater than 65 percent VO_2max. It takes longer for fat to become available to muscles as fuel in the form of free fatty acids. Most athletes do not work out long enough to burn significant amounts of fat during exer-

cise. Rather, the calorie deficit resulting from the exercise session and the negative energy balance during the day promote fat loss. When athletes restrict carbohydrate intake, they compromise the amount of carbohydrate stored in their muscles, which is needed to facilitate exercise performance. The Zone diet is a low-energy diet and does not increase the body's ability to burn fat.

It is not realistic to think that a diet composed of 30 percent protein would contain only 30 percent fat. If you use animal foods to meet these protein recommendations, it is not difficult to exceed the fat recommendations. And, with a restriction of carbohydrate

foods, a vegetarian-based protein intake is largely ruled out.[2] A high-carbohydrate diet is not recommended for some individuals. But athletic individuals are not among them.

1 Coleman E. Carbohydrate and Exercise. *Sports Nutrition.* 3rd ed. In: Rosenbloom CA. Chicago, IL: The American Dietetic Association; 2000.

2 Coleman E. Debunking the "Eicotec" myth. *Sports Med Dig.* 1993;15:6-7.

Aerobic Endurance Training and Performance. Endurance athletes involved in heavy training require from 1.2 to 1.4 grams of protein per kilogram of body weight per day.[38] Endurance athletes who are training for extreme events, such as the Tour de France, need up to 2 grams per kilogram.[39]

This higher protein need reflects increased amino acid oxidation from decreased protein synthesis, increased protein degradation, or a combination of the two.[40] Recent research indicates that amino acids contribute 3 to 6 percent of the fuel for energy metabolism during exercise.[41] The branched-chain amino acids leucine, isoleucine, and valine are the preferred amino acids for oxidative metabolism in skeletal muscle and are used for energy production as muscle glycogen stores decline during prolonged exercise.

Resistance Training and Muscular Strength. It appears that strength athletes need to be in positive nitrogen balance (see Chapter 6) in order to gain muscle mass and strength. This increase in protein synthesis (an indicator of muscle growth) occurs when athletes have sufficient intake of amino acids in combination with a resistance-training program.[42]

Strength athletes consuming 1.4 grams of protein per kilogram of body weight per day showed an increase in body protein synthesis compared to athletes consuming 0.9 grams of protein per kilogram per day. However, when protein intake was increased to 2.4 grams per kilogram, protein synthesis did not increase above what was achieved on the moderate protein intake (1.4 g/kg per day).[43] A final recommendation of 1.6 to 1.7 grams of protein per kilogram per day is based on adding a standard safety margin.[44]

Protein Intake of Athletes. Meeting the protein demands of athletic performance doesn't require protein powders or amino acid supplements. Athletes who are consuming a variety of foods and are meeting their energy needs are probably consuming adequate amounts of protein.

The best way to obtain protein is from high-quality protein foods including low-fat dairy products, egg whites, lean beef and pork, chicken, turkey, and fish. Legumes are also an excellent source of protein. However, many athletes have poor eating habits, lack time to prepare meals, and/or have limited meal-preparation skills, so protein supplements become a convenient way to obtain adequate energy and protein. One downside of regular use of protein supplements is their high cost.

Despite the hype, not all athletes consume too much protein. Certain groups of active people may actually be at risk for inadequate protein intake. Young athletes under 20 years of age have elevated protein requirements to support growth in addition to physical activity. Additionally, athletes who restrict their caloric intake or eliminate certain food groups, such as athletes who are strict vegetarians, may not consume enough protein to support physical activity. **Table 13.7** gives the protein requirements of various levels of physical activity.

Vegetarian athletes can maintain an adequate protein intake by meeting their energy needs and eating a variety of protein-rich foods from plant sources such as grains, nuts, beans, and seeds—on a daily basis. The amount of protein consumed is particularly important because plant proteins are somewhat less digestible than animal foods (85 and 95 percent, respectively).

Protein Intake for Recovery. Along with carbohydrates, protein is important for post-exercise recovery. Protein combined with carbohydrate in a post-exercise meal increases glycogen synthesis.[45] Researchers suggest that the amount of protein should equal about 40 percent of carbohydrate.[46] For example, with post-exercise recommendations of 1.5 grams of carbo-

Quick Bites

Lost in Space

Vigorous weight training can double or triple a muscle's size, whereas the lack of use during space travel can shrink it by 20 percent in 2 weeks.

Table 13.7 **Protein Requirements of Sedentary and Active People**

Activity Level	Protein Requirements (g protein/kg body weight)
Sedentary	0.8
Strength athlete	1.6–1.7
Endurance athlete	1.2–1.4
Maximum usable amount for adults	2.0

Source: Adapted from Snyder AC, Naik J. Protein requirements of athletes. In: Berning JR, Steen SN. *Nutrition for Sport & Exercise.* 2nd ed. Gaithersburg, MD: Aspen; 1998.

Think About It

4

hydrate per kilogram of body weight, a 55-kilogram female athlete would need 82.5 grams of carbohydrate. Forty percent of the carbohydrate intake would then equal 33 grams of protein (82.5 X 0.40 = 33 g). How does this translate to food? A bagel, 2 ounces of string cheese, and 8 ounces of low-fat yogurt would provide a portable snack to enjoy after a hard workout.

Dangers of High Protein Intake. Some athletes believe that protein intake in excess of the recommended amounts will enhance lean muscle mass. Thus, they may be tempted to increase their protein intake with high-protein foods and/or supplements. However, there are several possible side effects of a high protein intake.

First, a diet high in protein is often high in fat, particularly saturated fat. Also, excessive protein intake from food or supplements enhances **diuresis** (loss of body water), thus increasing the risk for dehydration as the body attempts to excrete excess nitrogen through the urine. The extra strain on the kidneys may contribute to kidney disease. However, experts do not believe this is a concern for athletes with normal kidney function.[47] High protein intake may contribute to mineral losses, obesity, osteoporosis, heart disease, and certain types of cancer. (See Chapter 6, "Proteins.")

High intakes of single amino acid supplements also may impair the absorption of other amino acids. Further, the amount of amino acids contained in supplements is very small compared to the amount in food, and the cost of supplements is higher. For example, one pill may contain 500 milligrams of an amino acid, but 1 ounce of meat, poultry, or fish provides more than 7,000 milligrams of essential and nonessential amino acids!

Key Concepts: *Although fat is an important fuel for exercise, a high-fat diet is not necessary. General recommendations that fat not exceed 30 percent of energy intake are appropriate for athletes. Dietary protein is a source of energy, and also a source of amino acids for synthesis of body protein. Protein requirements of athletes are slightly higher than those of sedentary adults, but still within the normal range of protein consumption. High-protein diets are neither recommended nor necessary. Low-fat dairy products, egg whites, lean beef and pork, chicken, turkey, fish, and legumes are good sources of protein.*

Vitamins, Minerals, and Athletic Performance

B Vitamins. B vitamins are essential for energy metabolism (see Chapter 10, "Water-Soluble Vitamins"). It stands to reason then that athletes who need high energy would need a high level of B vitamins as well. This is not, however, a reason to run for the supplement counter. There is little evidence to suggest that athletes are at risk for B vitamin deficiencies if they consume adequate calories and plenty of complex carbohydrates, fruits, and vegetables in the diet. However, athletes can compromise their intake of B vitamins if they consume too few calories or too many refined carbohydrates such as sugar and soft drinks in place of whole-grain breads, cereals, and crackers.

Vitamin B_{12} may be a problem for athletes who follow a vegan diet and do not include foods, such as some soy products and ready-to-eat cereals that are fortified with this vitamin. Athletes who avoid all animal foods should consult a medical advisor or registered dietitian to determine if they need B_{12} supplements.

Calcium. Calcium is essential for normal muscle function and strong bones. Adequate calcium intake coupled with regular exercise slows the

diuresis The formation and secretion of urine.

Table 13.8 A Sample Training Diet

3,300 kcal; body weight = 70-kg; athlete performs prolonged daily training

530 g carbohydrate	63% kcal	7.5 g/kg body weight*
128 g protein	15% kcal	1.8 g/kg body weight**
83 g fat	22% kcal	

Breakfast

8 oz orange juice
2 C Cheerios cereal
8 oz 1% milk
1 large bran muffin

Lunch

2 slices whole-wheat bread
2 oz turkey
2 slices tomato
lettuce leaf
2 tsp mayonnaise
1 med apple
12 oz cranberry juice

Pre-exercise

8 oz Gatorade
1 cereal bar

Post-exercise

1 bagel
2 oz string cheese
16 oz apple juice

Dinner

3 oz chicken breast
1 lg baked potato with
  2 Tbsp low-fat
  sour cream
2 whole-wheat dinner rolls
1 tsp margarine
1 C cooked broccoli
1 C salad greens with
  2 Tbsp Italian salad
  dressing
8 oz 1% milk
1 C low-fat frozen yogurt

* Recommended carbohydrate intake goals for prolonged daily training

** Recommended protein intake goals up to 2 g/kg body weight for extreme training loads

deterioration of the skeleton with age. To promote bone health and slow the development of osteoporosis, exercise planning principles include:

1. Exercise should be weight bearing and stress bones. Examples include walking and running.

2. For continued improvement, exercise intensity should increase progressively.

3. People with small total bone mass have the greatest potential for improvement.

4. There is a maximum achievable bone density. As this is approached, greater efforts are needed to achieve smaller gains.

5. Discontinuing an exercise program reverses the benefits.[48]

Inadequate calcium may increase risk of stress fractures in athletes. This is of particular concern for the amenorrheic athlete (discussed in "The Female Athlete Triad" section later in this chapter). Teen athletes should strive to meet the AI for calcium of 1,300 milligrams per day from a variety of low-fat dairy products and other calcium-rich foods.

Iron. Iron is vital to oxygen delivery and energy production. As an essential part of hemoglobin and myoglobin, iron helps deliver oxygen to active muscle cells. It is also a key component of several enzymes vital to the production of ATP by the oxygen energy system. (For more details about iron's roles, see Chapter 12, "Trace Minerals".)

Female athletes are at higher risk for iron deficiency as a result of menstrual losses and often inadequate intakes of dietary iron. In endurance athletes, the impact of running can cause mechanical trauma to the capillaries in the feet. The increased breakdown of red blood cells in these capillaries coupled with kidney excretion of hemoglobin may contribute to low iron status.[49] Training increases the volume of plasma in the blood without initially changing the amount of hemoglobin. This dilutes the hemoglobin, even though training typically maintains or increases the amount of total hemoglobin. This condition, called **sports anemia**, is a false anemia for most athletes and can be remedied with a few days of rest.

Although many elite athletes, especially endurance athletes, have mild iron deficiency, few are anemic.[50] Although anemia can seriously impair a person's capacity to perform activities, mild iron deficiency has little effect on performance.[51]

Other Trace Minerals. Strenuous exercise also taxes the body's reserves of copper (essential for red blood cell synthesis) and zinc (vital to the proper functioning of many enzymes related to energy production). Endurance runs can increase urinary losses of zinc and cause relatively high losses of copper and zinc in sweat.

Such mineral losses may cause marginal deficiencies, but this does not necessarily call for supplementation. If an athlete takes supplements, he or she must be careful. High-dose supplements of iron, copper, or zinc can interfere with the normal absorption of these and other minerals, so an excess of one can cause a deficiency of the others. **Table 13.8** is an example of a training diet that would meet an athlete's needs for vitamins and minerals through food, which is preferable to taking supplements.

Key Concepts: *Vitamins and minerals are important components of athletes' diets. B vitamins are necessary for normal energy metabolism. Adequate calcium intake can help protect against stress fractures and, coupled with exercise, delays the* *onset of osteoporosis. Iron is needed to carry oxygen. Strenuous exercise can tax the body's reserves of both copper and zinc.*

Fluid Needs during Exercise

Exercise generates heat; heat production can increase 15- to 20-fold during heavy exercise. Most body heat is lost through evaporation of fluid (sweat) from the skin. Sweating rates of elite athletes can range from 1 to 2 liters per hour.[52] That can be as much as 5 to 10 cups of fluid lost every hour! (See **Figure 13.14**.) In fact, sweat production in well-trained athletes begins even before their core body temperature rises, so the body begins to cool itself soon after exercise begins. Sweat rate is affected by environmental temperature (extreme heat or extreme cold), humidity (higher humidity reduces efficiency of evaporation, but increases the rate of sweat production), type of clothing, fitness level, and initial fluid balance.

To keep the body from overheating, blood must flow to the skin where evaporating sweat can dissipate heat. During exercise, the demands for blood flow to the skin for cooling may compete with cardiovascular demands for blood to deliver "fuel" to working muscles. Thus, when body fluids are lost, both systems are stressed, making each less efficient.

sports anemia A lowered concentration of hemoglobin in the blood due to dilution. The increased plasma volume that dilutes the hemoglobin is a normal consequence of aerobic training.

Quick Bites

Sweating a World Record

When Alberto Salazar ran the Olympic Marathon in 1984, he went down in the record books for sweat production. He lost 12 pounds during the 26.2-mile race, despite drinking about 2 liters. His sweat rate was approximately 3.7 liters per hour.

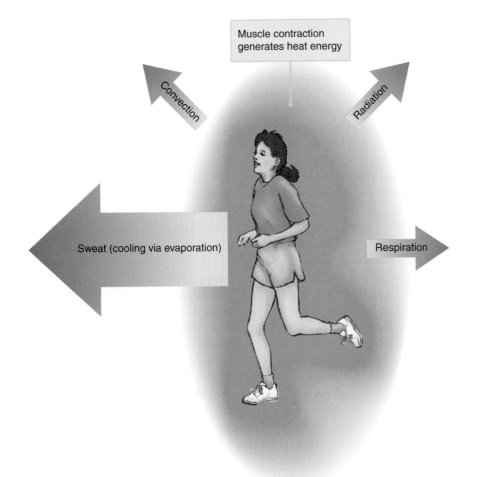

Muscle contraction generates heat energy

Convection

Radiation

Sweat (cooling via evaporation)

Respiration

Figure 13.14 **Dissipation of heat during exercise.** During exercise, radiation, convection and respiration are responsible for some heat loss, but evaporation of sweat dissipates over 80 percent of the heat generated by increased physical activity.

perceived exertion The subjective experience of how difficult an effort is.

palatable Pleasant or acceptable to the palate or taste.

Table 13.9 Typical Fluid Needs

Activity Level	Environment	Fluid Requirements (liters per day)
Sedentary	Cool	2–3
Active	Cool	3–6
Sedentary	Warm	3–5
Active	Warm	5-10+

Note that fluid requirements include fluid from all sources—liquids, food, and metabolic water. See Chapter 11, "Water and Major Minerals," for more information.

Source: Murray, R. Drink more! Advice from a world class expert. *ACSM's Health and Fitness Journal.* 1997;1:19–23, 50.

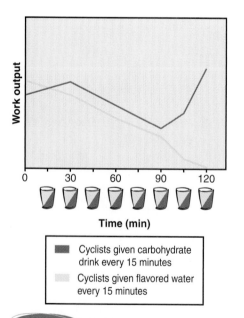

Cyclists given carbohydrate drink every 15 minutes

Cyclists given flavored water every 15 minutes

Figure 13.15 **Sports drinks and performance.** Consuming carbohydrate drinks dramatically increases power output after 90 minutes.

Without fluid replacement, dehydration can occur quickly during heavy exercise. Signs of dehydration include:

- elevated heart rate at a given exercise intensity
- increased rate of **perceived exertion** during activity
- decreased performance
- lethargy
- concentrated urine
- infrequent urination
- loss of appetite

During exercise, adequate fluid consumption helps offset fluid loss, minimize cardiovascular changes, reduce perception of effort, and maintain a supply of fuel to working muscles. Because exercise inhibits the body's thirst signal, drinking only when thirsty rarely offsets fluid loss. Active people must train themselves to consume adequate amounts of fluid before, during, and after exercise. **Table 13.9** shows how much fluid a person should drink at various levels of physical activity.

Hydration: Drink More! Athletes may choose water, sports drinks, or other beverages to meet fluid needs. Water can replace fluid lost in sweat and offset the rise in core temperature resulting from activities that last fewer than 60 continuous minutes. However, water alone may be not be adequate for rehydration because it does not contain energy (calories) or electrolytes, which enhance total voluntary fluid consumption and absorption of fluid.[53]

During exercise that lasts longer than 60 continuous minutes, carbohydrate oxidation normally declines as muscle and liver glycogen stores become depleted. Consuming fluids that contain carbohydrate and sodium can delay fatigue, enhance palatability of fluids, and promote fluid retention. (See **Figure 13.15**.)

Optimal sports drinks provide energy (from glucose, glucose polymers, sucrose) and electrolytes in a **palatable** solution that promotes rapid absorption (<10 percent carbohydrate concentration). Beverages such as fruit juices and soft drinks are concentrated sources of carbohydrates (more than 10 percent) and may slow gastric emptying. The main source of carbohydrate in juice and many soft drinks is fructose, which is associated with slower emptying from the stomach and abdominal cramping. Carbonated soft drinks may decrease the volume of fluid consumed, although this effect varies among individuals. Because beverages that contain alcohol or caffeine are strong diuretics, they do not allow complete rehydration and should be avoided. Some athletes use alcohol for psychological benefits—calming nerves, improving self-confidence, and reducing anxiety, pain, and muscle tremor. This misguided effort fails to recognize alcohol's negative influence on physical performance. Alcohol slows reactions, impairs coordination, and upsets balance. Its diuretic action contributes to dehydration and may impair regulation of body temperature. **Table 13.10** gives the desirable characteristics of a sports drink.

For exercises lasting less than 4 to 5 hours, one reason to drink fluids with electrolytes is to enhance the beverage's palatability. Sodium is the most common electrolyte added to sports drinks, in addition to chloride and potassium. Consuming a beverage that contains sodium and chloride can help ensure an adequate intake of fluid and stimulate greater rehydration following exercise.

Athletes who participate in endurance events that last longer than 4 to 5 hours and do not replace electrolytes put themselves at risk for hyponatremia (abnormally low levels of blood sodium). This life-threatening condition is associated with an excessive loss of electrolytes in sweat, and with the excessive consumption of fluid, such as plain water, that does not replace electrolytes. See **Table 13.11** for a summary of the American College of Sports Medicine's position on the amount and type of fluid to consume before, during, and after activity.

Table 13.10 — Desirable Composition of Sports Beverages

Characteristic	Comment
Fuel/Calories	Contains a source of carbohydrate: glucose, maltodextrin, sucrose, high-fructose corn syrup. Goal intake is 30–60 g/hr (2–4 cups of a 6 percent carbohydrate drink per hour).
Electrolytes	Enhances fluid uptake and palatability. Contains sodium, potassium, chloride, and phosphorus to replace sweat electrolyte loss in activity longer than 4 hours. Not an issue in exercise of shorter duration.
Rapid Absorption	Carbohydrate concentration less than 10 percent. Carbohydrate concentration over 10 percent can slow gastric emptying. Fructose should not be main or sole form of carbohydrate.
Palatability	Flavor may be biggest key to amount consumed. Taste changes can occur during exercise. Carbonation may decrease amount of fluid consumed.

Source: Shi X, Gisolfi CV. Fluid and carbohydrate replacement during intermittent exercise. *Sports Med.* 1998;25:157–172.

Quick Bites

Training: Young at heart or skeletal old age?

With endurance training, younger athletes largely achieve improvements as a result of increased cardiac output. Older athletes show greater improvement in the activities of the oxidative enzymes in their skeletal muscles.

Table 13.11 — American College of Sports Medicine Position on Fluid Replacement

Before Activity or Competition

- Drink adequate fluids during the 24 hours before an event, especially during the meal before exercise, to promote proper hydration before exercise or competition.
- Drink about 500 milliliters (~17 ounces) of fluid about 2 hours before exercise to promote adequate hydration and allow time for excretion of excess ingested water.

During Activity or Competition

- Start drinking early and at regular intervals to consume fluids at a rate sufficient to replace all the water lost through sweating or consume the maximal amount that can be tolerated.
- Fluids should be cooler than ambient temperature and flavored to enhance palatability and promote fluid replacement.

During Competition That Lasts More Than 1 Hour

- To maintain blood glucose concentration and delay the onset of fatigue, the fluid replacement should contain 4 to 8 percent carbohydrate. Electrolytes (primarily salt) are added to make the solution taste better and reduce the risk of hyponatremia. About 0.5 to 0.7 grams of sodium per liter of water replaces sodium lost by sweating.

Following Activity or Competition

- Complete restoration of the extracellular fluid compartment cannot be sustained without replacement of lost sodium.
- For each pound of body weight lost, consume at least 2 cups of fluid.
- Thirst sensation is *not* an adequate gauge of dehydration, and post-exercise consumption stimulates obligatory urine losses. Research shows that drinking an amount of liquid that is 125 to 150 percent of fluid loss is usually enough to promote complete rehydration.

Source: Adapted from American College of Sports Medicine position stand. Exercise and fluid replacement. *Med Sci Sports Exerc.* 1996;28(1):i–vii.

ergogenic aids Substances that can enhance athletic performance.

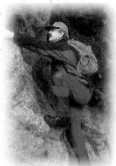

Nutrition Needs of Youth in Sport

Young athletes (younger than 19 years of age) involved in competitive sports need to fuel both physical activity and continued growth. Studies indicate that diets in young athletes are often marginal or inadequate in energy intake.[54] The consequences of chronic low energy intake include:

- short stature and delayed puberty
- nutrient deficiencies and dehydration
- menstrual irregularities
- poor bone health
- increased incidence of injuries
- increased risk of developing eating disorders[55]

Parents and youth need to understand the energy and nutrient demands of growth and training, and many need help in planning meals and snacks to meet those needs. Many youths' sport activities are after school, and some schools serve lunch as early as 10:45 A.M. It is necessary that these young people have meals and snacks before and after exercise in order to provide energy for the activity and nutrients needed for recovery. Easily portable snacks include fruit, pretzels, dry cereal, cereal bars, yogurt, sports drinks, sandwiches, and milk. Young athletes must drink adequate fluids during the day as well as at practice and competition. This is especially important because youths have a high tolerance for exercising in heat, which puts them at increased risk for heat exhaustion and heat stroke.

Key Concepts: *Exercise of any type increases fluid losses through sweat. Evaporation of sweat from the skin allows the body to cool itself. Fluid losses must be replaced in order to avoid dehydration. Athletes need to drink plenty of fluid before, during, and after exercise. Fluid choices depend on the duration of activity and the preferences of the athlete. Optimal sports drinks provide energy and electrolytes in a solution that promotes rapid absorption. Nutrition for athletes of all ages is a key element of the training regimen and should be planned carefully.*

Nutrition Supplements and Ergogenic Aids

The pressure to win contributes to athletes' search for a competitive edge. Many recreational and elite athletes use nutrition supplements and ergogenic aids with the expectation of improved performance. Nutrition supplements and **ergogenic aids** include products that

- provide calories (e.g., liquid supplements and energy bars).
- provide vitamins and minerals (including multivitamin supplements).
- contribute to performance during exercise and enhance recovery after exercise (e.g., sports drinks and carbohydrate supplements).
- are believed to stimulate and maintain muscle growth (e.g., purified amino acids).[56]
- contain micronutrients, herbal, and/or cellular components that are promoted as ergogenic aids to enhance performance (e.g., caffeine, chromium picolinate, creatine, and pyruvate).[57]

Most nutrient supplements are unnecessary for athletes who select a variety of foods and meet their energy needs. For many female athletes, iron and calcium supplements are recommended when diets are low in these nutrients. Liquid supplements and sports bars that contain carbohydrates, proteins, and fats can provide an easy way to increase energy intake.

Sports drinks, gels, and recovery drinks also can contribute to needed fluids and carbohydrates before, during, and after exercise. **Table 13.12** shows the nutrient content of some popular sports bars.

Dietary supplements marketed as performance enhancers are another matter. Herbals, glandulars, enzymes, hormone analogs, and other compounds carry many attractive claims for athletes. Although some products have been well researched, most lack vigorous clinical trials to evaluate efficacy, apply to only one sex (usually males), or are relevant to only one sport (e.g., weight lifting).

Androstenedione and Dehydroepiandrosterone

The adrenal gland synthesizes the testosterone precursors **androstenedione** and **dehydroepiandrosterone (DHEA)**. Manufacturers claim that supplements of "andro" and DHEA increase testosterone levels and enhance muscle building—a kind of "natural" steroid. Studies of DHEA have found increases in androgen levels (including testosterone) in women, but not in men.[58] Two recent studies of androstenedione supplementation in men had mixed results. Low doses of andro (100 milligrams per day) did not raise serum testosterone levels, while 300 milligrams per day did.[59] In the one of these studies that looked at response to strength training, andro was not effective in improving strength or muscle gains.[60] In both studies, andro caused estrogen levels to rise, a potentially serious side effect. No long-term studies have tested the safety of androstenedione or DHEA.[61] Despite the success anecdotally reported by a few high-profile athletes, hormone precursors are not recommended because they have many possible negative effects. In fact, the International Olympic Committee, National Football League, NCAA, and U.S. Tennis Association ban the use of androstenedione.

We know very little about the side effects of these steroidal supplements, but if large quantities of these compounds substantially increase testosterone levels in the body, they also are likely to produce the same side effects as **anabolic steroids**. Anabolic steroid abuse is associated with a wide range of adverse side effects ranging from some that are physically unattractive (e.g., acne and breast development in men), to others that are life threatening (e.g., heart attacks and liver cancer). Most are reversible if the abuser stops taking the drugs, but some are permanent.

Caffeine

Caffeine is a natural stimulant. Research suggests that caffeine may affect athletic performance by facilitating signals between the nervous system and the muscles, and decreasing an athlete's perceived effort during exercise. Caffeine may also increase the body's ability to break down fat (lipolysis)

androstenedione (andro) A steroid precursor secreted by the testes, ovaries, and adrenal cortex.

dehydroepiandrosterone (DHEA) A steroid that is the precursor to androstenedione. DHEA is secreted primarily by the adrenal gland, but also by the testes.

anabolic steroids Several compounds derived from testosterone or prepared synthetically. They promote body growth and masculinization, and oppose the effects of estrogen.

Quick Bites

Placebo Power!

Athletes involved in a heavy weight-lifting program volunteered to participate in a study where they would take what they thought were anabolic steroids. The results were dramatic—during 4 weeks of treatment these experienced weight lifters had a nearly 7.5-fold increase in the rate of their strength gain. However, they were taking a placebo—an inactive substance identical in appearance to the genuine drug. Because there was no pharmacological effect, gains were solely due to their belief in the treatment.

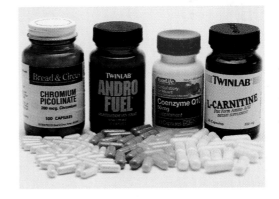

Table 13.12 **Nutrient Content of Sports Bars**

Bar	Calories	Percentage of calories		
		Carbohydrate	Protein	Fat
Power Bar	225	75	17	8
X-Trainer	220	73	18	9
Tiger Sport	230	70	19	11
Ultra Fuel	490	82	12	6
GatorBar	220	87	5	8
PR Bar	190	40	30	30
Gatorade Energy Bar	260	72	11	17

coenzyme Q₁₀ (ubiquinone) An electron and proton carrier abundant in cells and vital to the production of ATP in the electron transport chain.

creatine An important nitrogenous compound found in meats and fish, and synthesized in the body from amino acids (glycine, arginine, and methionine).

for energy. In one well-controlled study, subjects who ingested a high caffeine load 1 hour before exercise used less muscle glycogen and increased endurance when exercising at 80 percent VO_2max.[62]

How practical is this regimen? The dose used in the above study was 9 milligrams of caffeine per kilogram of body weight, which would be 630 milligrams of caffeine for a 70-kilogram person. Considering that one soda has about 30 milligrams of caffeine, and one cup of regular coffee about 150 milligrams, that's quite a lot of caffeine! Enough to be concerned about stomach discomfort, and about increasing the concentration of caffeine in the urine above amounts allowed by the International Olympic Committee. In addition, caffeine is a diuretic, and enhancing urine production is probably not the best course of action right before a competition!

Carnitine

Carnitine, a natural compound in foods, is synthesized in the liver and kidneys from the amino acids lysine and methionine. Carnitine helps transport long-chain fatty acids into the mitochondria for subsequent oxidation. The appeal to athletes is the idea that supplemental carnitine could help move long-chain fatty acids into the mitochondria faster, so they will be oxidized quicker, thus increasing the use of fat as an energy source. Short-term and long-term carnitine supplementation, however, has not been shown to augment muscle use of fatty acids.[63] Even though exercise increases carnitine excretion in the urine, its availability in foods and ready synthesis in the body make it unlikely that supplemental carnitine will benefit athletes.[64]

Chromium

The trace mineral chromium is vital to the movement of glucose into cells. Because of the link between chromium, glucose use, and insulin, chromium has become a popular supplement (typically in the form of chromium picolinate) for both weight loss and athletic performance. The theory is that by enhancing insulin action, chromium increases amino acid uptake, which then increases protein synthesis and promotes a gain in muscle mass. Although the developers of the chromium picolinate supplements had promising results in several studies, subsequent controlled trials have not found chromium picolinate beneficial for body composition changes, strength gains, or performance.[65] Given these results, and the concerns raised in Chapter 12 relative to chromium picolinate supplementation, this supplement cannot be recommended.

Coenzyme Q₁₀ (Ubiquinone)

In the mitochondria of muscle cells, **coenzyme Q₁₀ (CoQ₁₀)** actively helps transfer electrons in the electron transport chain. CoQ_{10} also may function as an antioxidant and spare vitamin E. In both athletes and sedentary people, supplementation with approximately 100 milligrams a day of CoQ_{10} has shown variable effects on aerobic performance. Early studies that showed a positive effect of supplementation had poor study design (no control group). Studies using control groups show no improvement in exercise performance or reduction in oxidative stress induced by exercise.[66]

Creatine

Creatine, a nitrogenous compound in meats and fish, is synthesized by the liver, pancreas, and kidney. Muscles store creatine mainly as creatine phosphate (CP), which functions as part of the ATP-CP energy system.

Creatine has become a popular supplement based on the theory that if a person could increase muscle creatine, this would prolong short-term energy availability, and thus improve performance in short-term, high-intensity activities (such as weight lifting).[67] Several well-controlled studies have shown improvements in muscle strength when creatine supplementation was added to a strength-training regimen.[68] For aerobic training, creatine supplements appear to have no benefit. The main side effect seems to be immediate weight gain attributable to water retention.

Although creatine appears to be effective in some sports situations, questions remain about its long-term use. Increases in muscle mass are probably a response to the increased stress that an athlete can put on muscle tissue by maximal exercise bursts—the supplement without weight training will have no effect. Also, the ability to store more CP may vary widely among people, so supplements may not be effective for everyone. Anecdotal reports of muscle cramps, muscle strains, kidney dysfunction, and GI distress have raised concerns. The American College of Sports Medicine has issued a cautionary statement regarding creatine supplementation and is awaiting the results of more studies that address risks of long-term use before giving the "green light" for use of creatine supplements.[69]

Ginseng

> **ginseng** A collective term that describes several species of plants of the genus Panax.

The root of the ginseng plant has been a popular Chinese health supplement used to treat and prevent numerous disorders for thousands of years. Use of **ginseng** continues because people believe its physiologic activity increases resistance to a wide range of stressors.[70] Ginseng has also become popular among athletes because of reports suggesting improved athletic performance through increased stamina and aerobic capacity.[71]

There is no known mechanism to explain how ginseng might work as an ergogenic aid, and controlled studies do not support ginseng use to improve exercise performance or reduce fatigue. The studies that purportedly show an ergogenic benefit are criticized for their lack of sufficient controls and blinding.[72] In a European study, for example, elite athletes experienced improved physical work capacity and physiological response after 9 weeks of supplementation with 200 milligrams per day of *Panax ginseng*.[73] When this study was repeated by an American laboratory using 200 milligrams or 400 milligrams per day of the same *Panax ginseng*, no effect was noted on heart rate recovery, oxygen use, or aerobic ability.[74] While testimonials continue to drive ginseng supplementation, further research on this popular herb is needed to evaluate the efficacy of ginseng as an ergogenic aid.

Medium-Chain Triglyceride Oil

Medium-chain triglycerides (MCT) are produced from plant oils, primarily coconut oil, and contain saturated fatty acids of medium length (6 to 10 carbons). The body quickly absorbs MCT oil into the blood, where it can become an immediate energy source. One study shows that consumption of carbohydrate combined with MCT may improve cycling performance during endurance events that last more than 2 hours.[75] The majority of research does not support MCT supplementation as an ergogenic aid.[76] The downside of MCT supplementation is that its taste may be unacceptable and it may contribute to gastrointestinal distress.

Pyruvate

Pyruvate and dihydroxyacetone are three-carbon products of carbohydrate metabolism. In animal studies, pyruvate as a dietary supplement or as a

soda loading Consumption of bicarbonate to raise blood pH. The intent is to increase the capacity to buffer acids, thus delaying fatigue. Also known as bicarbonate loading.

partial replacement for dietary carbohydrate enhanced aerobic endurance capacity.[77] The mechanism of action is unclear, but an increased blood glucose concentration, which would spare muscle glycogen, appears to be responsible for the improvements seen after pyruvate-dihydroxyacetone supplementation. These studies only looked at the aerobic endurance of untrained subjects. A study of trained athletes found that pyruvate administered for 5 weeks had no beneficial effect on anaerobic exercise performance.[78] Pyruvate supplementation has been associated with GI distress. Much more research is needed before the claim that pyruvate enhances endurance can be supported.[79]

Sodium Bicarbonate

Some athletes consume sodium bicarbonate (baking soda) in the belief that it will help neutralize the buildup of lactic acid in muscles. Whether **soda loading** actually produces an ergogenic effect is controversial. No improvement in performance has been seen in short-term exercise of 30 to 100 seconds.[80] However, comparative studies that evaluate events lasting from 2 to 10 minutes, where lactic acid buildup is most likely, have shown some positive results related to interval training performance.[81]

Bicarbonate loading can also produce negative effects. Athletes who follow this regimen report side effects such as intestinal discomfort, stomach distress, nausea, cramping, diarrhea, and water retention. Although bicarbonate loading is not banned, it does have serious health-related consequences. Bicarbonate loading increases blood alkalinity and influences blood pressure. Anyone with high blood pressure (hypertension) should not bicarbonate load.

Key Concepts: *Numerous dietary supplements, such as caffeine, chromium, CoQ$_{10}$, and ginseng, are marketed for performance-enhancing effects. However, few have been subjected to rigorous clinical trials or long-term safety evaluation. Athletes should consult a physician before adding dietary supplements to their training regimen.*

Weight and Body Composition

Pete, a bodybuilder, wants to bulk up by gaining 15 pounds of muscle and not fat. Sarah, on the other hand, wants to compete as a lightweight rower and needs to lose 7 pounds. How compatible is gaining or losing weight with a heavy training regimen?

Weight Gain: Build Muscle, Lose Fat

While some athletes struggle to lose weight, others find it nearly impossible to gain weight and muscle mass. Nutritional strategies that support gaining muscle mass include (1) set realistic weight-gain goals, (2) provide adequate energy intake for muscle building, and (3) determine carbohydrate and protein needs.

Setting Weight-Gain Goals

The variety of factors that influence weight gain includes genetics, stage of adolescent development, sex, body mass, diet, training program, prior resistance training, motivation, and use of supplements and anabolic steroids. Complex interactions among these factors make it difficult to predict an athlete's ability to meet a weight goal. However, experience tells us the following:

- Untrained male athletes can gain approximately 3 pounds per month of lean body mass in the early stages of a rigorous resistance-training program. Because of their smaller muscle mass and lean tissue, young women can achieve only 50 to 75 percent of the gains of male counterparts.

- Approximately 20 percent of the increase in lean body mass occurs in the first year of resistance training, tapering to 1 to 3 percent in subsequent years. Scientists believe that the rate declines as muscle mass approaches the maximum possible amount determined by genetics.

- Some high-school-age male athletes have difficulty gaining muscle mass. These athletes may be in the early stages of the adolescent growth spurt and may lack sufficient levels of the male hormones to stimulate muscle development.

- Nutrition plays an important role in increasing lean body mass. Athletes must consume enough calories, along with adequate carbohydrate and protein, to gain the desired muscle mass.[82]

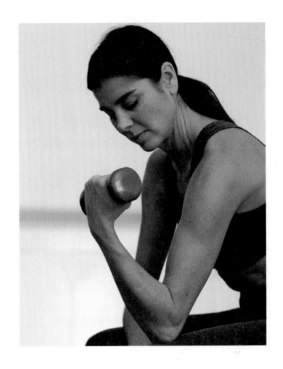

Calories: The Foundation for Building Muscle

Athletes who strive to increase muscle mass are generally seeking to increase their strength and power. Research demonstrates that a well-nourished athlete engaging in a well-designed weight-training program can gain muscle mass and strength. However, for each pound gained as muscle, an athlete must consume about 500 to 1,000 kilocalories per day more than usual energy needs.[83] The athlete needs the extra calories to meet the energy cost of a weight-training program as well as to supply the components for muscle synthesis. The composition of the diet should remain high in carbohydrates, adequate in protein, and sufficient in other nutrients such as zinc and iron that are essential for the growth of new tissue.

Protein: How Much Is Enough?

As mentioned previously, strength-training athletes should consume 1.6 to 1.7 grams of protein per kilogram of body weight per day. For most athletes, eating regular food, rather than relying on protein supplements, meets this level of protein need.

Carbohydrates: Fuel for Growth

Intense weight training depletes glycogen stores, so adequate dietary carbohydrate is essential to replenish and maintain glycogen stores. When carbohydrate intake is insufficient, the body uses protein as a source of energy and glucose. Adequate carbohydrate spares protein, so the body can use it to build muscle. Recommended carbohydrate intake for weight-training programs is 8 to 10 grams carbohydrate per kilogram of body weight per day.

However, many athletes are skeptical that a diet high in carbohydrate combined with a weight-training program will be sufficient to achieve the desired muscular physique. They often incorporate supplements and ergogenic aids into a weight-training program, but with little or no added benefit.

Key Concepts: *Athletes often seek to improve their power and strength by increasing muscle mass. Weight gain as muscle requires increased dietary calories, primarily as carbohydrate, combined with strength training.*

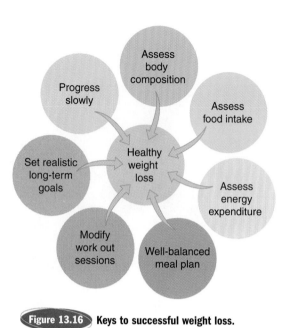

Figure 13.16 Keys to successful weight loss.

Weight Loss: The Panacea for Optimal Performance?

As the pressure to win increases, many coaches and athletes come to believe that weight loss and lower body fat composition will provide that competitive edge. Athletes strive for lower body weight and lower body fat for three reasons: (1) to improve appearance, especially in aesthetic sports (e.g., diving, figure skating, gymnastics); (2) to enhance performance where lower body weight may increase speed (e.g., race walking, running, pole vaulting, jumping, cross-country skiing); or (3) to qualify in a lower weight category (e.g., wrestling, boxing, and rowing).[84] Let's focus on five strategies to maximize chances for healthy weight loss. (See **Figure 13.16**.)

Progress Slowly

Set a realistic target time to achieve your goal weight. Ask yourself if this is the right time to make dietary and lifestyle changes. Is weight loss a personal priority or are outside influences from family, friends, teammates, or coaches pressuring you to lose weight? Consider weight loss during the off season to avoid detrimental effects on athletic performance.

Assess Body Composition, Food Intake, and Energy Expenditure

Many athletes mistakenly interpret "minimal weight" as the "optimal weight" for peak performance and good health. When determining optimal body weight, the first step is an assessment of body composition. Athletes often have additional muscle mass that causes them to exceed weight standards for their height and sex. Standard height-weight tables do not provide reliable information on fat-free body mass and body fat. The body mass index (BMI) better relates body weight and health risks, but it does not consider body composition.[85] It is important that a trained professional evaluate body composition data to provide the most accurate feedback.

Healthy young adults average 15 percent body fat for men 25 percent for women.[86] While these averages provide guidelines for body fat content in athletes, individualized recommendations must also take into account an athlete's genetic background, age, sex, sport, health, and weight history. Male athletes should not go below 5 to 7 percent body fat. Current research data on female athletes suggest that 13 to 17 percent body fat is the minimal level associated with normal menstrual function.[87]

Food and training records provide information on energy intake and expenditure. The best way for athletes to sustain a safe and sensible loss of body fat is to reduce calorie intake moderately and modify the training program. A modest decrease of about 500 kilocalories per day in total energy intake with an increase in aerobic activity is recommended to support a weight loss of 1 to 2 pounds per week.

Establish a Well-Balanced Meal Plan

Athletes, especially athletes who practice daily, should choose foods that replenish glycogen stores and provide adequate protein to maximize protein synthesis. A nutritionally sound weight-reduction meal plan provides the recommended balance of calories: 60 to 65 percent carbohydrate, 15 percent protein, and 20 to 25 percent fat.[88] Daily intake should also provide key micronutrients including calcium, iron, zinc, vitamin A, vitamin C, and B vitamins.

Beware of "fad" weight-loss methods such as ketogenic diets, high-protein diets, and semistarvation diets. These practices can compromise energy reserves, body composition, and psychological well-being, thus leading to decreased performance and increased health risks.

Quick Bites

What's the best "fat-burning" exercise?

It's a common misconception that low-intensity exercise is superior for "fat burning." It is true that aerobic activities use a greater percentage of fat as fuel, but it is the total amount of calories expended during exercise that supports increased mobilization of fat in response to a caloric deficit. In terms of actual energy expenditure, higher intensity exercise requires more calories for a given time period than exercise at a lower intensity. Thus, to lose body fat weight, the fuel (source of calories) is not as important as the amount of energy expended.

Athletes often are alert to the latest supplements to hit the market. Many claim to accelerate the burning of body fat and augment weight loss. In reality, studies show that most "fat burners" are ineffective or cause only very modest weight loss in obese subjects.[89]

Modify Workout Sessions

For many athletes, simply modifying workout sessions achieves their weight-loss goals. Athletes in sports that target skill development such as gymnastics, wrestling, and track, may benefit from training sessions that include aerobic activities such as running, cycling, stair-stepping, and rowing. Adding resistance training to a weight-loss program promotes higher resting metabolism by increasing fat-free mass, which is more metabolically active than body fat.

Set Realistic Long-term Goals

Realistic goals promote permanent behavioral change and maximize the chances for successful weight control. Possible long-term goals include (1) obtain meal-planning and food-preparation skills to support healthy eating habits; (2) complete daily logs of food intake and physical activity; (3) identify family, friends, and professionals who can provide support and guidance in weight-loss efforts; and (4) develop coping strategies and problem-solving skills to work through challenging situations such as social events.

Key Concepts: *Before embarking on a weight-loss program, athletes should evaluate their goals carefully and set a realistic plan for weight loss and maintenance. Safe weight-loss practices include modest changes in food intake accompanied by gradual increases in aerobic activity.*

Weight Loss: Negative Consequences for the Competitive Athlete?

Changing body size and shape can have detrimental effects. An unrealistic perception of optimal body weight, and a belief that weight loss is necessary for improved performance, can contribute to unhealthy weight-loss practices.[90] Athletes risk medical problems when dieting goes awry.

Making Weight

Wrestlers, weight lifters, boxers, jockeys, oarsmen, and coxswains face competitive pressures to "make weight" in order to compete or to be certified in a lower weight classification. Such athletes often resort to **pathogenic** weight-control behaviors such as those summarized in **Table 13.13**. Repeated cycles of rapid weight loss and subsequent regain increase risks of disordered eating, fatigue, psychological distress (anger, anxiety, depression), dehydration, and sudden death.

Studies show that wrestlers, in attempts to gain a competitive advantage, will try to reduce weight a few days before or on the day of competition.[91] Athletes can achieve weight loss up to 22 pounds (10 kg) of body water in one day by fasting, restricting fluids, using diuretics, sitting in a sauna, and exercising in a hot environment using rubber suits. A fluid loss of only 2 percent of initial body weight (3 lb for a 150-lb person) can decrease athletic performance by elevating heart rate, decreasing stroke volume, and lowering cardiac output. Moderate to severe dehydration (> 3 to 5 percent of body weight) can be dangerous because of increased core body temperature, electrolyte imbalances, and cardiac and kidney

pathogenic Capable of causing disease.

Table 13.13 Pathogenic Weight-Loss Practices

Behavior	Consequence
Fasting	Loss of lean body mass and decreased metabolic rate
Diet pills	Medical side effects and weight regained when discontinued
Fat-free diets	Deficient in macronutrients and micronutrients; difficult to maintain
Diuretics	Dehydration and electrolyte imbalance; no fat loss
Laxatives	Dehydration; no fat loss; may be addicting
Sweating	Dehydration; heat injury; no fat loss
Excessive exercise	Risk of injury and overtraining
Enemas	Dehydration and GI problems
Fluid restriction	Dehydration; heat injury
Self-induced vomiting	Dehydration; acid-base and electrolytes imbalance; esophageal tears and GI bleeding; erosion of dental enamel and swollen parotid glands

Source: Adapted from Otis CL. Too slim, amenorrheic, fracture-prone: The female athlete triad. *ACSM's Health and Fitness.* 1998;2:2–25.

hyperthermia A much higher than normal body temperature.

female athlete triad A syndrome in young female athletes that involves restrictive eating, amenorrhea, and lowered bone density.

amenorrhea [A-men-or-Ee-a] Absence or abnormal stoppage of menses in a female; commonly indicated by the absence of three to six consecutive menstrual cycles.

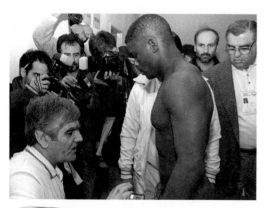

Figure 13.17 **Wrestler weighing in.** The NCAA provides guidelines for weigh-in procedures.

changes. These conditions may result in heat illness including heat cramps, heat exhaustion, or heat stroke.

The deaths of three previously healthy collegiate wrestlers in 1 month highlight the seriousness of rapid weight loss.[92] These athletes had not only dropped significant weight preseason (> 9 kilograms) but lost between 1.6 and 4 kilograms in a period of 1 to 9 hours prior to their deaths. The wrestlers restricted food and fluid intake and attempted to maximize sweat losses by wearing vapor-impermeable suits under cotton warm-up suits and exercising vigorously in hot environments. Their deaths were associated with **hyperthermia** (elevated body temperature) and dehydration.

Since 1998 the NCAA has revised the guidelines for monitoring weight-loss practices and weigh-in procedures. (See **Figure 13.17**.) This includes educating coaches and athletic trainers about healthy weight-control strategies and limiting the amount of preseason and precompetition weight loss.[93]

Female Athlete Triad

While the majority of female athletes benefit from increased physical activity, there are those who go too far and risk developing a trio of medical problems. In 1991 the American College of Sports Medicine coined the term **female athlete triad** to describe the interaction of disordered eating, amenorrhea, and premature osteoporosis.[94] Female athletes who compete in endurance sports, sports judged by build, and sports with weight classifications are at the greatest risk.

Disordered Eating and Eating Disorders: Studies of female athletes indicate that the prevalence of anorexia nervosa appears to be in the same range as that reported for nonathletes. On the other hand, the prevalence of bulimia nervosa or subclinical eating disorders is higher in athletes.[95]

Amenorrhea: In the general population, 2 to 5 percent of women have **amenorrhea**. However, the prevalence is much higher in athletes.[96] Research indicates that amenorrhea in athletic women is related to the synergistic effects of increased physical activity, weight loss, low body fat levels, and insufficient energy intake.

Premature Osteoporosis: Health consequences of amenorrhea include premature osteoporosis. Research shows that amenorrheic athletes experience rapid loss of bone mineral density in the spine, which can spread to other parts of the skeleton if amenorrhea continues for a long time.

Table 13.14 **Combating Eating Disorders in Athletes**

De-emphasize body weight. Do not view the athlete's weight as the primary contributor to, or detractor from, athletic performance. Research indicates that athletes can achieve appropriate weight and fitness when the focus is on physical conditioning and strength development, as well as the cognitive and emotional aspects of performance.

Eliminate group weigh-ins. Often viewed as a way to motivate the team, the practice of group weigh-ins can be destructive to people who are struggling with their body image and disordered eating. If there is a legitimate reason for weighing an athlete, explain the reason and weigh the athlete privately.

Treat each athlete individually. Many athletes have an unrealistic perception of what is an ideal body weight, especially in sports for which leanness is considered important. Additionally, athletes may strive for weight and body composition that may be realistic in only a few genetically endowed people. It is important to understand that genetic and biological processes, rather than one's will power to control food intake, affect a person's weight.

Facilitate healthy weight management. Be sensitive to issues related to weight control and dieting. Because many athletes have limited knowledge of sports nutrition, they resort to pathogenic weight-loss practices. Athletes can benefit from nutrition counseling by a sports nutritionist or a registered dietitian who has experience in working with athletes and disordered eating.

Source: Thompson RA, Sherman RT. Reducing the risk of eating disorders in athletics. *Eating Disorders: Journal of Treatment and Prevention.* 1993;1:65–78.

Treatment involves replacing estrogen, which is low in amenorrheic athletes. Oral contraceptives are the most common method of estrogen replacement and can also serve as a reliable form of birth control. Calcium supplementation is also recommended. Although bone mineralization may never return to normal in amenorrheic athletes, studies indicate that reducing the intensity of training, improving dietary intake, and increasing body weight can help restore menstruation and increase bone density.[97]

Breaking the Triad

Female athletes at risk are perfectionists, driven to excel in a given sport, and believe that a specific athletic body image is required to excel as an athlete. Some reports estimate as many as 60 percent of female athletes in aesthetic sports (e.g., dance, skating, diving, gymnastics) and weight-dependent sports (e.g., rowing, martial arts, horse racing) may be at risk.[98]

Screening, referral, and education are keys to prevention of the female athlete triad. Prevention and treatment strategies are best delivered by a multidisciplinary team of medical, athletic, nutrition, and mental health experts. Proactive sports education includes de-emphasizing body weight, eliminating group weigh-ins, treating each athlete individually, and facilitating healthy weight management. (See **Table 13.14**.)

Key Concepts: *Pathogenic weight-control practices increase risk for dehydration and compromise performance, and may have long-term serious consequences for athletes. The female athlete triad—disordered eating, amenorrhea, and premature osteoporosis—results from excessive weight loss. Often weight loss is driven by unrealistic ideas of appropriate body weight and shape for competition. Education of coaches and athletes is essential to prevent the female athlete triad.*

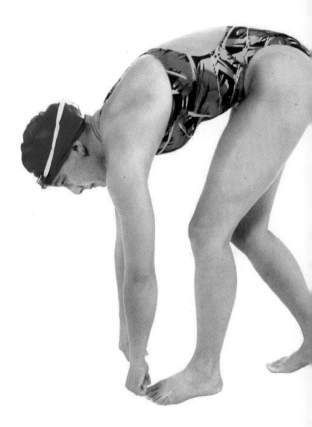

Label [to] **Table**

Sports drinks are often recommended instead of plain water for those who engage in vigorous physical activity. Their proponents claim that they quickly replenish the body's supply of nutrients, particularly electrolytes. Let's take a look at the Nutrition Facts panel from a popular sports drink, Gatorade.

First, look closely at the serving size—it's not the whole container. This is worth noting because many people might drink the whole container and assume they were getting 50 calories. Not true! The whole container has 200 calories (50 × 4 servings). It's always a good idea to look at the serving size when you are studying a nutrition label.

So what makes this sports drink different from plain (and inexpensive) water? This one has added carbohydrate, sodium, and potassium. Replacing carbohydrate during long workouts prevents complete depletion of glycogen stores. Most sports drinks have between 5 and 8 percent simple sugar. Higher amounts would limit water absorption, and replacement of water is more critical than replacement of glucose.

Sodium and potassium are added to sports drinks to improve taste, and help replace electrolytes that are lost during exercise. Gatorade contains 110 milligrams of sodium and 30 milligrams of potassium. For many athletes, and certainly recreational exercisers, water really is the best fluid replacer. Although both sodium and potassium are lost in sweat, water is lost in greater quantities. Sports drinks have been shown to benefit only athletes that are strenuously exercising for longer than an hour. With prolonged exercise and sweat losses, large losses of electrolytes can make a person dizzy and weak, and may even lead to heat exhaustion or heatstroke.

The next time you head out for a bike ride, consider how long you'll be gone and how strenuous your ride will be, and then consider whether you'll need a sports drink. Also consider your personal taste—if a flavored sports drink will encourage you to replace more fluids than plain water, that may be an important advantage. Just don't forget to read the label!

Nutrition Facts
Serving Size 8 fl oz (240mL)
Servings Per Container 4

Amount Per Serving	
Calories 50	

	% Daily Value*
Total Fat 0g	0%
Sodium 110mg	5%
Potassium 30mg	1%
Total Carbohydrate 14g	5%
Sugars 14g	
Protein 0g	

Not a significant source of Calories from Fat, Saturated Fat, Cholesterol, Dietary Fiber, Vitamin A, Vitamin C, Calcium, Iron.

* Percent Daily Values are based on a 2,000 calorie diet.

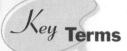

LEARNING *Portfolio* c h a p t e r   1 3

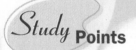

Key **Terms**

	page		page
aerobic endurance	485	hyperthermia	514
amenorrhea	514	involuntary muscle	485
anabolic steroids	507	lactate threshold	492
androstenedione (andro)	507	lactic acid energy system	486
ATP-CP energy system	486	muscle fibers	485
carbohydrate loading	497	NCAA	494
cardiac muscle	485	oxygen energy system	486
cardiac output	491	palatable	504
coenzyme Q_{10} (ubiquinone)	508	pathogenic	513
creatine	508	perceived exertion	504
creatine phosphate	487	phosphocreatine	487
dehydroepiandrosterone (DHEA)	507	skeletal muscle	485
diuresis	501	slow-twitch (ST) fibers	485
ergogenic aids	506	smooth muscle	485
fast-twitch (FT) fibers	485	soda loading	510
female athlete triad	514	sports anemia	503
ginseng	509	submaximal rate	485
glycogen loading	497	VO_2max	490

Study **Points**

➤ Exercise promotes health and reduces risk of chronic diseases.

➤ The ACSM defines *physical fitness* as "the ability to perform moderate to vigorous levels of physical activity without undue fatigue and the capability of maintaining this level of activity throughout life."

➤ The muscular system contains three types of muscles: smooth, cardiac, and skeletal. There are two types of muscle fibers: slow-twitch (ST) and fast-twitch (FT). ST fibers have high aerobic endurance; FT fibers are optimized to perform anaerobically. Your body depends predominantly on ST fibers for low-intensity events and FT fibers for highly explosive events.

➤ The body uses three systems to produce energy for physical activity: (1) the ATP-CP energy system (anaerobic), (2) the lactic acid energy system (anaerobic), and (3) the oxygen energy system (aerobic).

➤ Anaerobic and aerobic metabolism work together to fuel all types of exercise. During the early minutes of high-intensity exercise, the ATP-CP energy system and the lactic acid energy system provide most of the energy. Endurance activities are fueled primarily by the metabolism of glucose and fatty acids in the oxygen energy system.

➤ Training improves use of fat as a fuel by enhancing oxygen delivery and increasing the number of mitochondria in the muscle.

➤ During an activity, muscles depend on muscle glycogen.

➤ Carbohydrates should be the major source of energy in the athlete's diet and should come from complex carbohydrates, which can provide fiber, iron, and B vitamins. Athletes need carbohydrates for adequate stores of muscle glycogen and concentrations of blood glucose before training and competitive events. Likewise, carbohydrates are necessary to replenish glycogen stores after intense exercise.

➤ Carbohydrate loading is a process of reducing activity while increasing carbohydrate intake to maximize glycogen stores, and is most appropriate for endurance athletes.

➤ Fat is a major fuel source for exercise, but high fat intake is not required or recommended.

➤ Protein needs of athletes are higher than those of sedentary individuals, but generally, athletes who consume adequate amounts of energy get enough protein. High protein foods include low-fat dairy products, egg whites, lean beef and pork, chicken, turkey, fish, and legumes.

➤ Other nutrients important to the athlete's diet include B vitamins, iron, zinc, and calcium.

➤ Water is the most essential nutrient and is easily lost from the body with heavy sweating. Replacing fluid with water or sports drinks is important to prevent dehydration. Optimal sports drinks provide energy and electrolytes in a palatable solution that is rapidly absorbed.

➤ Athletes who are still growing have even higher energy and nutrient needs to support both physical activity and normal growth.

➤ Many dietary supplements are promoted as ergogenic aids—substances that enhance performance. Few well-controlled studies on their efficacy and safety have been done, however.

➤ Many athletes strive to either gain or lose weight in order to improve performance. In both cases, realistic goals and gradual changes are necessary for long-term success. Gains in muscle mass requires increased caloric intake and weight training. Successful weight loss requires modest reductions in energy intake and increases in aerobic activity.

➤ Weight-control efforts that involve fasting, excessive sweating, purging, diuretics, or laxatives are detrimental to health.

➤ Disordered eating accompanied by amenorrhea and premature osteoporosis is known as the female athlete triad.

Study Questions

1. Name the three types of muscles in your body.

2. What are muscle fibers and what are the two major types?

3. List the two anaerobic and one aerobic energy systems that your body uses to generate energy during exercise. When is each active during exercise?

4. What are the general recommendations for an athlete (compared to a nonathlete) in terms of the percentage of calories from carbohydrates, proteins, and fats?

5. What is carbohydrate loading? How does it benefit athletes?

6. How do protein recommendations for athletes vary from those for nonathletes?

7. Name three minerals that are of concern for athletes because they may not consume enough.

8. What is sports anemia and why does it happen? How does it compare to other anemias?

9. Define the term *ergogenic aid*. Is there a clear, research-based answer to whether ergogenic supplements work?

10. What is the nutritional strategy for athletes who want to gain muscle mass?

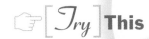 *[Try]* **This**

The Popularity of Ergogenic Aids

Take a trip to a health food store to see just how popular (and expensive!) ergogenic aids are. Try to locate each of the supplements listed in this chapter. Are they all available? What are their prices? Ask a salesperson what he or she knows about each of them. Do their answers match what you read in the text?

Commit to Get Fit

Do you meet the American College of Sports Medicine's (ACSM) definition of fitness? Answer the questions below with a yes or no.
1. Do you exercise consistently three to five days per week?
2. When you exercise, does it include 20 to 60 minutes (20 minutes for intense activity and 60 minutes for less intense activity) of continuous aerobic activity?
3. Does your type of exercise use large muscle groups? Can you maintain it? Is it rhythmical and aerobic?
4. Does part of your activity include strength training of a moderate intensity (a minimum of one set of 8 to 12 repetitions of 8 to 10 exercises) at least two days per week?

If you answered no to any of these questions, you are not following the ACSM's suggestions to develop and maintain cardiorespiratory and muscular fitness. Choose one of the questions to which you answered no and set a specific goal to include that factor in your exercise routine.

What About Bobbie?

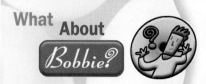

Imagine that Bobbie is training to do a marathon at the end of the semester. She has been exercising consistently and increasing her endurance and mileage times. She hasn't spent much time focusing on her diet though, and wants to know what changes she could make to improve her nutrition and, therefore, performance. Assume that her current diet meets her calorie needs. How would you compare Bobbie's diet to the guidelines you read about in this chapter?

Macronutrient Contributions

Start with her overall contribution of carbohydrates, proteins, and fats. Compare Bobbie's percentage of calories of the macronutrients to the general sports nutrition recommendations.

	Bobbie's	Recommendations
Carbohydrates	48%	60 to 70%
Proteins	16%	~ 15%
Fats	36%	~ 20%

As you can see, Bobbie's diet is higher in fat and lower in carbohydrates than is recommended for an athlete. If she were to reduce her intake of cream cheese, mayonnaise, cookies, and salad dressing and increase her fruits, vegetables, and whole grains, her diet would come closer to the recommendations for sports nutrition.

Protein

Now let's calculate her protein need based on the athlete's guideline and see if she's consuming enough to maintain lean muscle mass and recover well from exercise.

The protein RDA for an athlete is approximately 1.2 to 1.4 grams per kilogram of body weight. Bobbie weighs 155 pounds, so her RDA is as follows:

155 lb ÷ 2.2 kg per lb = 70.45 kg

70.45 kg X 1.3 g/kg = 91.6 g protein

Bobbie's protein intake was 97 grams, which makes her protein intake a near perfect match of her needs.

Minerals

Look at the two primary minerals that might be inadequate in diets of athletes, especially female athletes. Below is a comparison of Bobbie's calcium and iron intake and her daily recommendations.

	Bobbie's	Recommendations
Calcium	745 mg	1,000 mg
Iron	20 mg	8 mg

As you can see, Bobbie did a very good job of consuming iron, but she is short of her calcium need. If she were to replace the diet soda she had with lunch with 1 cup of nonfat or 1% milk, her intake of calcium would rise to just above 1,000 milligrams. Or she could change her afternoon snack of chips and salsa to a cup of yogurt to accomplish the same thing.

Hydration

Check out Bobbie's intake of fluids in Chapter 1. How many ounces of plain water did she consume? That's right, she only had 16 ounces! Bobbie is making the same mistake that many athletes do—not drinking enough water; poor hydration status will probably affect her performance adversely. Bobbie's biggest change should be to increase her fluid intake. She'd be smart to drink at least 12 to 16 ounces of caffeine-free fluids at all of her meals and snacks. This way she'll stay hydrated and be able to perform at an optimal level!

References

1 US Department of Health and Human Services. *Surgeon General's Report on Physical Activity and Health.* Atlanta, GA: US Department of Health and Human Services, Centers for Disease Control and Prevention, National Center for Chronic Disease Prevention and Health Promotion: 1996.

2 American College of Sports Medicine. Position stand: the recommended quantity and quality of exercise for developing and maintaining cardiorespiratory and muscular fitness and flexibility in healthy adults. *Med Sci Sports Exerc.* 1998;30:975–991.

3 Ibid.

4 Position of the American Dietetic Association and The Canadian Dietetic Association: nutrition for physical fitness and athletic performance for adults. *J Am Diet Assoc.* 1993;93:691.

5 Andersen JL, Scherling P, Saltin B. Muscle, genes and athletic performance. *Sci Am.* 2000;283(3):48–55.

6 Connolly-Schoonen J. Physiology of anaerobic and aerobic exercise. In: Rosenbloom CA, ed. *Sports Nutrition.* 3rd ed. Chicago, IL: The American Dietetic Association; 2000.

7 Wilmore JH, Costill DL. *Physiology of Sport and Exercise.* 2nd ed. Champaign, IL: Human Kinetics; 1999.

8 Brooks GA, Fahey TD, White T. *Exercise Physiology.* Mountain View, CA: Mayfield; 1996.

9 Wilmore JH, Costill DL. Op. cit.

10 McArdle WD, Katch FI, Katch VL. *Essentials of Exercise Physiology.* Baltimore, MD: Lippincott Williams & Wilkins; 1999.

11 Ibid.

12 Ibid.

13 Bassett DR, Nagle FJ. Energy metabolism in exercise and training. In: Wolinsky I, Hickson JF, eds. *Nutrition in Exercise and Sport.* 2nd ed. Boca Raton, FL: CRC Press, 1994.

14 Wilmore JH, Costill DL. Op. cit.

15 Berning JR., Steen SN. *Nutrition for Sport & Exercise.* 2nd ed. Gaithersburg, MD: Aspen Publishers; 1998.

16 Hawley J, Dennis SC, Lindsay FH, Noakes TD. Nutritional practices of athletes: re they sub-optimal? *J Sports Sci.* 1995;13:S75–S87.

17 Vinci DM. Effective nutrition support programs for college athletes. *Int J Sports Nutr.* 1998;8:308–320.

18 Hawley J, Dennis SC, Lindsay FH, Noakes TD. Op. cit.

19 Benardot D, Thompson WR. Energy from food for physical activity: enough and on time. *ACSM's Health & Fitness.* 1999;3:14–18.

20 Coleman, EJ. Carbohydrate and exercise. In Rosenblum CA. Op. cit.

21 Walberg-Rankin J. Dietary carbohydrate as an ergogenic aid for prolonged and brief competitions in sport. *Int J Sport Nutr.* 1995;5:S13–S28.

22 Coleman EJ. Op. cit.

23 Walton P, Rhodes EC. Glycemic index and optimal performance. *Sports Med.* 1997;23:164–172.

24 Burke LM, Collier GR, Harbreaves M. Glycemic index—A new tool in sports nutrition? *Int J Sport Nutr.* 1998;8:401–415.

25 Ivy JL, Lee MC, Broznick JT, Reed MJ. Muscle glycogen storage after different amounts of carbohydrate ingestion. *J Appl Physiol.* 1988;65:2018–2023.

26 Storlie, J. The art of refueling. *Training and Conditioning.* 1998;8:29–35.

27 Coleman EJ. Op. cit.

28 Roy B, Tarnopolosky M, MacDougall J, et al. Effect of glucose supplement timing on protein metabolism after resistance training. *J Appl Physiol.* 1997;82:1882–1888.

29 Hawley J, Burke L. *Peak Performance: Training and Nutritional Strategies for Sport.* Leonards, Australia: Allen & Unwin; 1998.

30 Coleman EJ. Op. cit.

31 Ibid.

32 Walberg-Rankin J. Op. cit.

33 Kleiner SM, Greenwood-Robinson M. *Power Eating: Build Muscle, Gain Energy, Lose Fat.* Champaign, IL: Human Kinetics; 1998.

34 Lemon PWR. Effects of exercise on dietary protein requirements. *Int J Sport Nutr.* 1998;8:426–447.

35 Clark N, Rosenbloom C. To zone or not to zone: people respond to The Zone diet plan. *SCAN'S PULSE.* 1997;16:5–7.

36 Food and Nutrition Board. *Recommended Dietary Allowances.* 10th ed. Washington, DC: National Academy Press; 1989.

37 Carroll C. Protein and exercise. In: Rosenbloom CA. Op. cit.

38 Lemon PW. Dietary protein requirements in athletes. *J Nutr Biochem.* 1997;8:52.

39 Hawley J, Burke L. Op. cit.

40 Lemon PW. Op. cit.

41 Tarnopolsky M. Protein metabolism in strength and endurance athletes. In: Lamb DL, Murray R, eds. *Perspectives in Exercise Science and Sports Medicine. 12: The Metabolic Basis of Performance in Exercise and Sport.* Carmel, IN: Cooper Publishing Group; 1999.

42 Snyder AC, Naik J. Protein requirements of athletes. In: Berning JR, Steen SN. Op. cit.

43 Tarnopolsky MA, Atkinson SA, MacDougall JD, et al. Evaluation of protein requirements for trained strength athletes. *J Appl Physiol.* 1992;73:1986.

44 Lemon, PW. Op. cit.

45 Storlie J. The art of refueling. *Training & Conditioning.* 1998;8:29–30, 32, 34–35.

46 Storlie J. From fork to muscle. *Training & Conditioning.* 1998;8:26, 28–29, 32–33.

47 Snyder AC, Naik J. Op. cit.

48 McArdle WD, Katch FI, Katch VL. Op. cit.

49 Clarkson PM, Haymes EM. Exercise and mineral status of athletes: calcium, magnesium, phosphorus, and iron. *Med Sci Sports Exerc.* 1995;27:831–843.

50 Fogelholm M. Indicators of vitamin and mineral status in athletes' blood: a review. *Int J Sport Nutr.* 1995;5:267–284.

51 Zhu YI, Haas JD. Iron depletion without anemia and physical performance in young women. *Am J Clin Nutr.* 1997;66:334–341.

52 Guyton AC, Hall JE. *Textbook of Medical Physiology.* 9th ed. Philadelphia: WB Saunders; 1996.

53 Convertino VA, Armstrong LE, Coyle EF, et al. American College of Sports Medicine position stand. Exercise and fluid replacement. *Medic Sci Sports Exerc.* 1996;28:i–vii.

54 Thompson JL. Energy balance in young athletes. *Int J Sport Nutr.* 1998;8:160–174.

55 Ibid.

56 Skinner R, Coleman E, Rosenbloom O. Ergogenic aids. In Rosenbloom CA. Op. cit.

57 Ibid.

58 Clarkson PM, Rawson ES. Nutritional supplements to increase muscle mass. *Crit Rev Food Sci Nutr.* 1999;39:317-328; and Kreider RB. Dietary supplements and the promotion of muscle growth with resistance exercise. *Sports Med.* 1999;27:97–110.

59 King DS, Sharp RL, Vukovich MD, et al. Effect of oral androstenedione on serum testosterone and adaptations to resistance training in young men. *JAMA.* 1999;281:2020–2028; and Leder BZ, Longcope C, Catlin DH, et al. Oral androstenedione administration and serum testosterone concentrations in young men. *JAMA.* 2000;283:779–782.

60 King DS, Sharp RL, Vukovich MD, et al. Op. cit.

61 Sarubin A. *The Health Professional's Guide to Popular Dietary Supplements.* Chicago, IL: The American Dietetic Association; 2000.

62 Spriet L. Caffeine and performance. *Int J Sport Nutr.* 1995;5(suppl):S84–S99.

63 Kanter M, Williams M. Antioxidants, carnitine, and choline as putative ergogenic aids. *Int J Sport Nutr.* 1995;5(suppl): S120–S131.

64 Ibid.

65 Campbell WW, Joseph LJ, Davey SL, et al. Effects of resistance training and chromium picolinate on body composition and skeletal muscle in older men. *J Appl Physiol.* 1999;86:29–39.

66 Sarubin A. Op. cit.

67 Toler SM. Creatine is an ergogen for anaerobic exercise. *Nutr Rev.* 1997;55:21–25.

68 Engelhardt M, Neumann G, Berbalk A, Reuter I. Creatine supplementation in endurance sports. *Med Sci Sports Exerc.* 1998;30:1123–1129.

69 American College of Sports Medicine. Current Comment: creatine supplementation. Indianapolis, IN; 1998.

70 Williams MH. *The Ergogenics Edge: Pushing the Limits of Sports Performance.* Champaign, IL: Human Kinetics; 1998.

71 Engles HJ, Wirth JC. No ergogenic effects of ginseng (Panax ginseng C.A. Meyer) during graded maximal aerobic exercise. *J Am Diet Assoc.* 1997;97:1110–1115.

72 Sarubin A. Op. cit.

73 Engles HJ, Wirth JC. Op. cit.

74 Ibid.

75 Van Zyl CG, Lambert EV, Hawley JA, et al. Effects of medium-chain triglyceride ingestion on fuel metabolism and cycling performance. *J Appl Physiol.* 1996;80:2217–2225.

76 Skinner R, Coleman M, Rosenbloom C, Op. cit.

77 Ivy JL. Effect of pyruvate and dihydroxyacetone on metabolism and aerobic endurance capacity. *Med Sci Sports Exercise.* 1998;6:837–843.

78 Stone MH, Sanborn K, Smith LL, et al. Effects of in-season (5 weeks) creatine and pyruvate supplementation on anaerobic performance and body composition in American football players. *Int J Sport Nutr.* 1999;9:146–165.

79 Sarubin A. Op. cit.

80 Horswill CA. Effects of bicarbonate, citrate, and phosphate loading on performance. *Int J Sport Nutr.* 1995;5(suppl): S111–S119.

81 Ibid.

82 Storlie J. From fork to muscle. Op. cit.

83 Kleiner SM, Greenwood-Robinson M. Op. cit.

84 McArdle WD, Katch FI, Katch VL. Op. cit.

85 Ibid.

86 Ibid.

87 Ibid.

88 Mole PA. Exercise and the fat balancing act. *ACSM's Health & Fitness.* 1997;1:18–26.

89 Clarkson PM. The skinny on weight loss supplements and drugs. *ACSM's Health & Fitness,* 1998;2:18–26, 55.

90 Thompson JL. Op. cit.

91 Metz G. The NCAA weighs in. *Training & Conditioning.* 1998;8:16–17, 19, 21–23.

92 Rapid weight loss in wrestlers results in death. *MMWR.* 1998;47(6):105–108.

93 Metz G. Op. cit.

94 Otis CL, Drinkwater B, Johnson M, et al. American College of Sports Medicine position stand: the female athlete triad. *Med Sci Sports Exerc.* 1997;29:i–ix.

95 Sundgot-Borgen J. Risk and trigger factors for the developing of eating disorders in female elite athletes. *Med Sci Sports Exerc.* 1994;4:414–419.

96 Smith AD. The female athlete triad: causes, diagnosis, and treatment. *Physician Sportsmed.* 1996;24:67–70, 75–76, 86.

97 Dueck CA, MM Manore, Matt KS. Role of energy balance in athletic menstrual dysfunction. *Int J Sport Nutr.* 1996;6:165–190

98 Otis CL, Drinkwater B, Johnson M, et al. Op. cit.

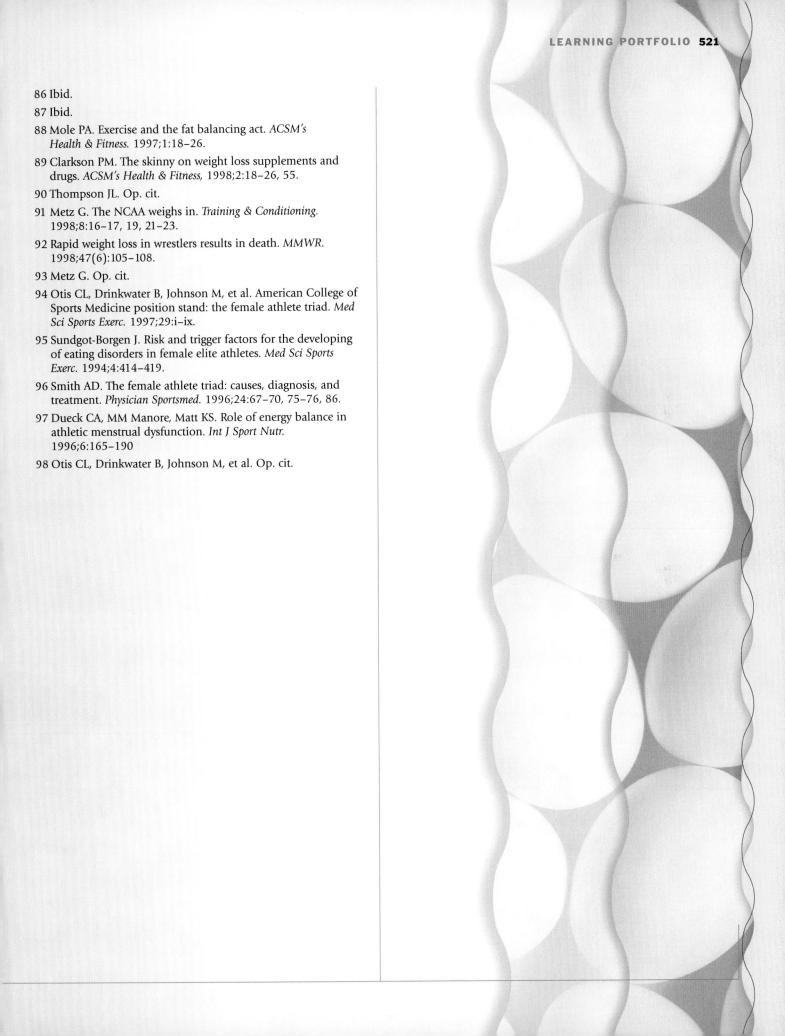

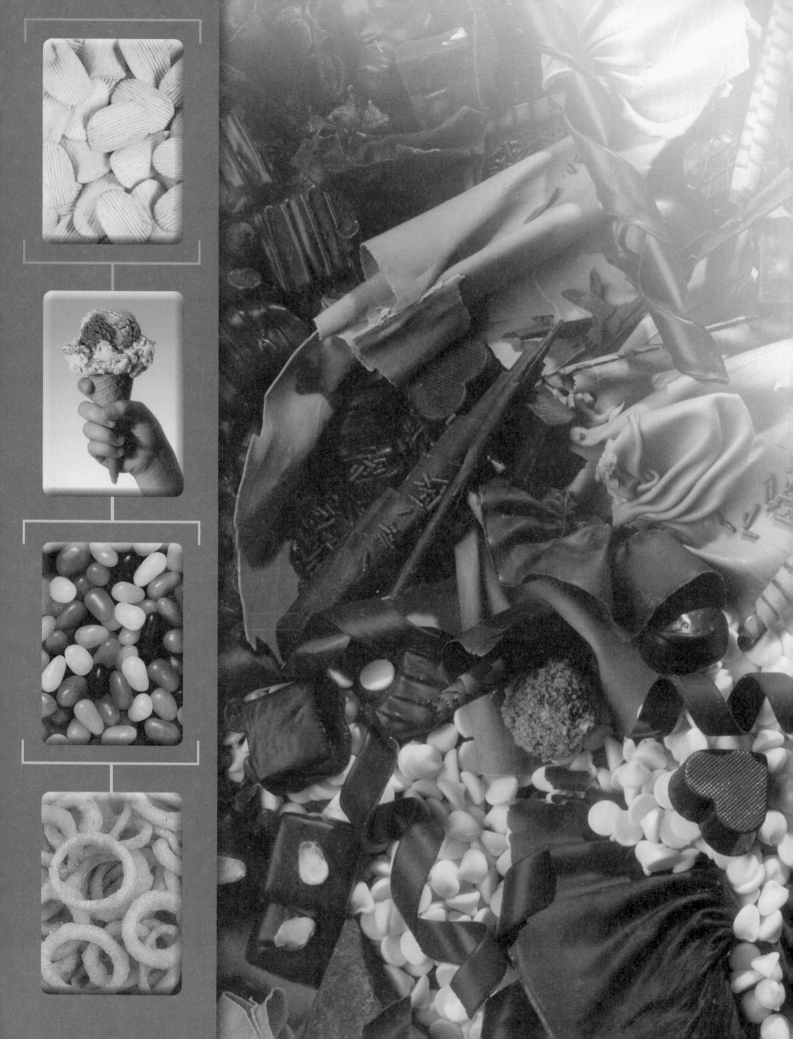

Spotlight on

Eating Disorders

Think About It

1. What's your view of the ideal female body?
2. When should you be concerned about obsessive dieting?
3. Given the right situation, what foods are you likely to binge on?
4. How many magazines do you read that promote dieting or encourage thinness?

Fyi for your Information

This chapter's FYI box includes practical information on the following topic:
- Diary of an Eating Disorder

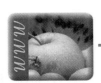

The web site for this book offers many useful tools and is a great source for additional nutrition information for both students and instructors. Visit the site at nutrition.jbpub.com for information on eating disorders. You'll find exercises that explore the following topics:
- Age and Eating Disorders

- Body Image

- The Genetics of Eating Disorders

- Cultural Roles

What About Bobbie?

Track the choices Bobbie is making with the EatRight Analysis software.

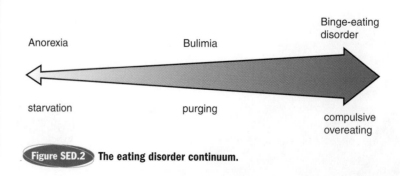

A gaunt, hollow-cheeked, college freshman confides to her roommate that she feels chubby. After an enormous lunch, a secretary works her way through a bag of cookies, followed by a box of chocolates. A swimming champion who obsesses over every calorie becomes concerned that she hasn't had a period in two months. Disordered eating? Very likely! Eating disorder? Possibly!

Eating disorders and **disordered eating** are not the same. An eating disorder such as anorexia nervosa or bulimia nervosa is an illness that can seriously interfere with daily activities. Disordered eating is usually a temporary or mild change in eating patterns. Although it can occur after an illness or stressful event, it often is related to a dietary change intended to improve one's health or appearance. Unless disordered eating persists, it rarely requires professional intervention. Disordered eating, however, can lead to an eating disorder.

For most of us, eating is a pleasure. For people with an eating disorder, however, food is a source of continual stress and anxiety. Eating disorders require professional intervention. They include a spectrum of emotional illnesses ranging from self-imposed starvation to chronic binge eating. These illnesses involve severe distortions of the eating process, with physical consequences that are often life-threatening.[1] (See **Figure SED.1**.)

Most of us have eaten to the point of discomfort on particular occasions. (Thanksgiving dinner comes to mind.) And many of us have cut out desserts at one time or another, hoping to fit into a special outfit or to make weight for an athletic event or job interview. But stuffing yourself at a holiday meal or going on an *occasional diet* does not constitute an eating disorder. According to the *Manual of Clinical Dietetics,* a defining characteristic of an eating disorder is a persistent inability to eat in moderation.[2]

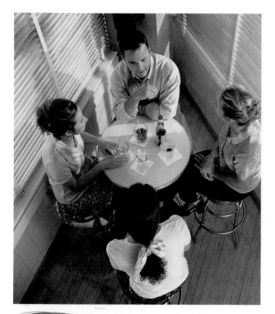

Figure SED.1 Can you spot the person with the eating disorder?

The Eating Disorder Continuum

The 1994 edition of the American Psychiatric Association's *Diagnostic and Statistical Manual of Mental Disorders (DSM-IV)* divides eating disorders into three categories, with small but significant areas of overlap. These categories form a continuum, with self-starvation at one end and compulsive gorging at the other (**Figure SED.2**). **Anorexia nervosa** is at the self-starvation end of the continuum. Anorexia is a self-imposed starvation syndrome that is triggered by a severely distorted **body image**. People with anorexia are at war with their bodies. Even when they are dangerously underweight,

eating disorder A spectrum of abnormal eating patterns that eventually may endanger a person's health or increase the risk for other diseases. Generally, psychological factors play a key role.

disordered eating An abnormal change in eating pattern related to an illness, a stressful event, or a desire to improve one's health or appearance. If it persists it may lead to an eating disorder.

anorexia nervosa [an-OREX-ee-uh ner-VOH-sah] An eating disorder marked by prolonged decrease of appetite and refusal to eat, leading to self-starvation. It results in part from a distorted body image and intense fear of becoming fat, often linked to social pressures.

body image A person's mental concept of his or her physical appearance, constructed from many different influences.

Anorexia   Bulimia   Binge-eating disorder

starvation   purging   compulsive overeating

Figure SED.2 **The eating disorder continuum.**

people with anorexia typically see themselves as fat. Severely restricted food intake is another symptom of anorexia nervosa. It may also involve purging (self-induced vomiting) and excessive exercise. Anorexia is most prevalent among adolescent females.

At the opposite end of the continuum is **binge-eating disorder**, formerly known as **compulsive overeating**. People with this disorder chronically consume massive quantities of food. Sufferers are typically obese; however, all obese people are not binge eaters. Diagnosis of binge-eating disorder is based on a person's having an average of two binge-eating episodes per week for six months. Such episodes often are triggered by emotions such as frustration, anger, depression, and anxiety.

In the middle of the continuum is **bulimia nervosa**. Like those with binge-eating disorder, people with bulimia nervosa compulsively gorge themselves. Like those with anorexia, bulimics desperately want to be thin and resort to purging to attain this goal. After gorging, bulimic people often become disgusted with themselves and terrified of getting fat. To compensate, bulimic people make themselves vomit, use laxatives, exercise excessively, and take other action to avoid gaining weight. It is important to realize that few people who suffer from eating disorders are purely anorexic, bulimic, or binge eaters. Many swing from one disordered eating pattern to another, alternately starving and gorging themselves. People may suffer from binge-eating disorder at one point in their lives, and anorexia or bulimia at another.[3]

History of a Modern Malady

Contrary to public perception, eating disorders are not New-Age diseases. In fact, the first formal report of anorexia nervosa appeared in the medical literature in the 1870s.[4] Informal reports of a "voluntary starvation syndrome" were published as early as 1694.[5] And some nutritional anthropologists argue that eating disorders can be traced to even more ancient times. During the Middle Ages, for instance, early Christian ascetics, who led lives of contemplation and rigorous self-denial, shunned worldly pleasures, including food, to show obedience and become closer to God. These people alternated periods of semi-starvation with frequent fasts. Was this anorexia disguised as religious devotion? Some scholars think so.[6]

Early Greeks and Romans, in contrast, exhibited exaggerated bingeing and purging behavior at banquets that lasted for days. Guests gorged to the point of physical pain, then tickled the back of their throats with feathers to induce vomiting. Once their stomachs were empty, they returned to the table. Rather than finding this behavior repulsive or shameful, the ancient Romans glorified it. They even built areas known as vomitoriums into their banquet halls.[7] Interestingly, in ancient Rome only upper-class males attended banquets.[8]

Some scholars contend these ancient Romans had bulimia. Others disagree, arguing that the Roman men ate for pleasure in the company of others and purged only so they could rejoin the feast. In contrast, modern bulimia sufferers are usually females who gorge and purge in isolation—and in hopes of attaining an unrealistic cultural standard of beauty. Furthermore, today's bulimia sufferers invariably feel shame, low self-esteem, and even self-hate connected with their eating habits.

Although eating disorders are not an exclusively modern malady, it's clear that eating disorders have become increasingly common in the past three decades. A British model named Twiggy, nicknamed for her sticklike

binge-eating disorder An eating disorder marked by repeated episodes of binge eating and a feeling of loss of control. The diagnosis is based on a person's having an average of at least two binge-eating episodes per week for 6 months.

compulsive overeating See binge-eating disorder.

bulimia nervosa [bull-EEM-ee-uh] An eating disorder marked by consumption of large amounts of food at one time (binge eating) followed by compensatory behavior such as self-induced vomiting, use of laxatives, excessive exercise, fasting, or other practices to avoid weight gain.

Quick Bites

Scary Statistics

About 5 million Americans have anorexia nervosa, bulimia, or binge-eating disorders. Researchers estimate that 15 percent of young women have disordered eating attitudes and behaviors. Every year an estimated 1,000 people die from anorexia nervosa.

Quick Bites

Were underweight Romans dangerous?

Let me have men about me that are fat; ...
Yon Cassius has a lean and hungry look:
   such men are dangerous...
I do not know the man I should avoid
So soon as that spare Cassius.

—Shakespeare, *Julius Caesar*, Act 1, Scene II

Perhaps Caesar should have listened to his instincts. He was stabbed to death by Cassius and other conspirators.

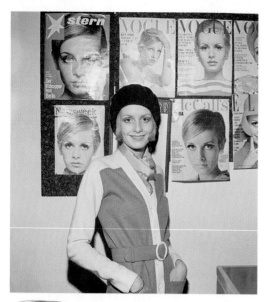

Figure SED.3 In the 1960s, Twiggy became the new role model for young women who wanted to be thin and glamorous.

appearance, ushered in the epidemic in the early 1960s. Admiring fashion magazine stories reported that she subsisted on water, lettuce, and a single daily serving of steak, and that she had learned to suppress her hunger pangs. Rather than condemn these clearly dangerous eating habits, the magazines held Twiggy up as a model of self-control for girls and young women. (See **Figure SED.3**.)

Our national denial regarding the dangers of semistarvation ended abruptly and dramatically in 1983 with the highly publicized death of 32-year-old pop singer Karen Carpenter from complications of anorexia. Widespread media coverage of Ms. Carpenter's death highlighted the lethal potential of eating disorders, and made the terms *anorexia* and *bulimia* household words. Soon, other stars of film, TV, sports, and the fashion world revealed that they, too, suffered from eating disorders, and described the physical, emotional, and social damage these diseases caused in their own lives. But ironically, increased visibility and knowledge has not stemmed the tide of eating disorders. To the contrary, the prevalence of eating disorders and disordered eating continues to increase.[9]

Key Concepts: *Eating disorders are ancient conditions that have become alarmingly common in industrialized countries, particularly the United States. A primary explanation is that our society combines an abundance of food, and food-oriented advertising, with an obsession for thinness.*

No Simple Causes

Certain people appear to have a predisposition to eating disorders. This vulnerability may be psychological. A person who suffers from depression or obsessive-compulsive disorder, for example, may have an increased risk of developing an eating disorder. The vulnerability also may be biological. Indeed, there is evidence that genetic factors may create an increased risk for eating disorders. Another important factor in the development of eating disorders is society's emphasis on extreme thinness. It is clear that eating disorders are complex problems, with multiple causes. Social, psychological, and biological factors all play roles.

Social pressure to attain an unrealistic standard of thinness is a well-recognized factor in the development of eating disorders, particularly for women. Modern Western culture would have women weigh less than is considered healthy. This means that for most women, the current "ideal" female form simply cannot be attained without significant food deprivation. These pressures affect even very young girls, starting with their first Barbie doll (see **Figure SED.4**) and her unnatural shape, if not before.[10]

Psychological factors are important as well. These encompass everything from peer relationships to relationships with parents. In one recent study of peer relationships, Dr. L. Kris Gowen of the Stanford Center on Adolescence found that pre-adolescent girls who were teased or bullied by peers had a more negative image of their bodies and a greater concern about their weight than other girls.[11] This was true regardless of the girls' actual weight. Studies also have linked more severe forms of emotional trauma to disordered eating. For example, researchers at Texas A&M University detected symptoms of **post-traumatic stress disorder (PTSD)** in more than half of the anorexia and bulimia patients they studied.[12] PTSD occurs in people who have endured a significant trauma, such as child abuse or rape. Dysfunctional family relationships are associated with eating disorders as well. Some psychologists believe that people with anorexia and bulimia are

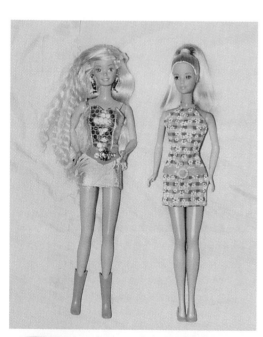

Figure SED.4 In 1998, Mattel overhauled Barbie's look for the millennium, giving her slimmer hips, a wider waist, and smaller breasts. Barbie's periodic overhauls are meant to fit the fashion of the times. Does the new Barbie (right) represent a realistic role model for today's young girls?

Think About It

1

trying to fulfill unrealistic parental expectations of perfection, in part by succumbing to societal pressure to be very thin.

In recent years, scientists have made major advances in understanding the biological underpinnings of eating disorders. Particularly important are studies linking the neurotransmitters serotonin and norepinephrine to eating behavior. (See **Figure SED.5**.) Researchers, for example, have shown that bulimia patients experience spontaneous improvement in eating habits when they take an antidepressant medication that increases brain levels of serotonin.[13] Interestingly, anti-obesity drugs like Redux, PhenFen, and Meridia also affect serotonin levels.[14]

Neurotransmitters are just one focus of research into the biology of eating disorders. Another line of investigation focuses on genes. Recently, researchers have confirmed what they had long suspected: eating disorders run in families. In addition, eating disorders occur most frequently in families with a history of obsessive-compulsive disorders, anxiety disorders, and depression.[15] Significantly, both depression and obsessive-compulsive behavior have been linked to atypical levels of serotonin and norepinephrine in the brain.[16]

Most likely, many genes are involved in the development of eating disorders. Two recently discovered genes are involved in the synthesis and release of the hormones leptin and **orexin**.[17] The leptin gene regulates the body's production of leptin, a hormone that causes rapid weight loss in genetically obese mice. (Unfortunately, leptin has not stimulated the same reaction in humans.) The orexin gene regulates production of two appetite-stimulating hormones, orexin A and orexin B (after the Greek word *orexis*, for "appetite"). In experiments, rodents injected with either hormone increased their food consumption 8- to 10-fold.[18] The discoveries of leptin and orexin are significant advances in our understanding of brain chemistry and eating disorders, and may eventually lead to new classes of more effective drugs. Drugs that mimic orexin, for example, might help patients with anorexia or other wasting syndromes by increasing their appetites. Conversely, drugs that block orexins might help patients struggling with obesity and binge eating. Or, a leptin-like drug may eventually be used to stimulate weight loss. At the very least, discovery of these genes underscores the idea that biological factors probably contribute to the development of eating disorders in vulnerable people.

Key Concepts: *The precise causes of eating disorders remain obscure. Some researchers believe that eating disorders are primarily psychological in origin. Others have championed the theory that eating disorders have an important genetic basis. The current view is that eating disorders are a result of the complex interaction of biological and psychological factors. In other words, eating disorders occur in biologically susceptible individuals exposed to particular types of environmental stimuli.*

Anorexia

Until the 1960s, anorexia nervosa was a relatively obscure disease. Physicians learned about the condition in medical school, but few doctors ever saw a case in their own practices. By the mid-1970s, however, anorexia was widely reported, particularly among young women. Today an estimated 1 in 100 females between the ages of 13 and 19 suffers from anorexia.

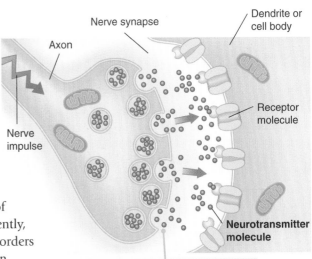

The end of a stimulated nerve cell releases neurotransmitter molecules, like serotonin and norepinephrine, which transfer the signal to the beginning of the next nerve cell

Figure SED.5 **Neurotransmitters in action.** Neurotransmitters, such as serotonin and norepinephrine, may not function correctly in some people with eating disorders.

post-traumatic stress disorder (PTSD) An anxiety disorder characterized by an emotional response to a traumatic event or situation involving severe external stress.

orexin A class of hormones in the brain with receptors in the lateral hypothalamus that may affect food consumption.

Quick Bites

A Skinny Trend

In 1970 the average Playboy Playmate weighed 11 percent below the national average. Only 8 years later, in 1978, the average weight of Playboy Playmates was 17 percent below average. Today, the average model is 22 to 23 percent leaner than the average American woman.

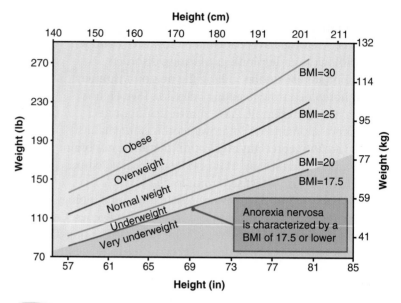

Figure SED.6 **BMI and underweight.**

In comparison, fewer than 1 in 1,000 males younger than 20 have the problem.[19] Up to 10 percent of sufferers die from this disease.

The term anorexia nervosa, which translates to "nervous loss of appetite," is misleading. People diagnosed with anorexia do not lose their appetite except in the final stages of the disorder. Instead, they are obsessed with food. But their obsession with thinness is even greater. The German term for the disorder, *pubertätsmagersucht*, or "mania for leanness," is much more accurate.[20] Anorexia is more prevalent in industrialized societies that share an abundance of food and an attitude that equates beauty, particularly feminine beauty, with thinness. (See **Figure SED.6.**)

Nine of 10 anorexia sufferers are female. We do not understand fully the cause of this disparity between the sexes, but a chief suspect is Western society's greater emphasis on thinness for women than for men.[21] Until recently, the typical anorexia sufferer was an upper-class Caucasian female adolescent. Unfortunately, during the past decade anorexia has become a more equal-opportunity disorder. Physicians are reporting cases of the disorder in young women from all social and ethnic backgrounds, especially women who participate in activities that emphasize leanness, including modeling, ballet, and gymnastics. Also, anorexia has increased significantly among African American women.[22]

Causes of Anorexia

On the surface, anorexia usually seems to result from a weight-loss program gone awry. A high school freshman may go on a diet after her boyfriend or gymnastics coach tells her she is too heavy An eighth grader may want to lose weight in hopes of being more popular at a new school. The diet may start out just fine, but it never stops.

Beneath the surface, psychological issues are typically at work. Because most cases of anorexia begin around the age of puberty, some psychologists theorize that anorexic behavior is an attempt to prevent or delay sexual maturation. By retaining a child's body, a young girl may hope to avoid the pressures of the teen years and the responsibilities of adulthood. In addition, psychologists report that anorexia sufferers tend to be rigid, perfectionistic, all-or-nothing thinkers. Sufferers tend to lack a sense of independence and control over their own destiny. They may attempt to compensate for this through acts of intense self-discipline. Parents may facilitate this syndrome by being overly protective or rigid or by holding a child to excessively high standards of achievement.[23]

Several lines of evidence suggest a predisposition to anorexia. For example, obsessive-compulsive behaviors, depression, and anxiety frequently precede anorexia. In fact, a major depressive disorder or **obsessive-compulsive disorder** has been reported in up to half of anorexia sufferers.[24] All these disorders involve abnormalities in neurotransmitters, suggesting that brain chemistry contributes to anorexia. Although it is likely that biological factors predispose an individual to anorexia, psychological and social factors are critical in precipitating the disease. The current view is that complex biological, social, and psychological factors contribute to anorexia.

Warning Signs

Parents and friends of people with anorexia often miss the early signs of the disease. It can be easy to mistake a loved one's obsession with dieting, avoidance of particular foods, or rigorous exercise schedule for a reasonable desire to lose weight.[25]

When asked about a child who has been diagnosed with anorexia, most parents will describe a "wonderful" daughter—one who has always been cooperative, obedient, an exceptional student, and unusually neat and organized. When she started to diet, she did so with the same zeal and dedication she exhibited in other areas of her life.[26]

Initially, anorexia provides a sense of power. Sufferers enjoy a feeling of control as they learn to deny their hunger and limit their food intake. Early warning signs include obsessively counting calories, developing lists of "safe" foods and foods to avoid, cutting foods, including things like peas, into small pieces, and spending a great deal of time rearranging food on a plate. To suppress hunger, a person with anorexia may drink up to 30 cups of water or diet soda a day. Anorexia sufferers also may channel their obsessions with food into the preparation of elaborate meals for others without partaking of the food themselves.[27] **Table SED.1** shows the warning signs of anorexia.

As the disease progresses, anorexia sufferers become increasingly disillusioned, withdrawn, and hostile. Success always seems beyond their grasp. No matter how thin they are, they perceive themselves as overweight. (See **Figure SED.7**.) When they eat more than they think they should, they may induce vomiting or use **emetics**, **enemas**, **diuretics**, or **laxatives**. Or they may exercise relentlessly. Eventually, their efforts to avoid obesity take over their lives. They start to avoid social situations that may expose their behaviors, withdrawing more and more from friends and family. Groggy and irritable from food deprivation and sleep disturbances, people with advanced anorexia spend so little time on their schoolwork or jobs that their performance deteriorates. Yet when confronted with their obsessive dieting or deteriorating behavior, they will deny that anything is unusual.[28]

Treatment

Just as there is no one cause for anorexia nervosa, there is no single way to cure it. In fact, most experts doubt that patients with anorexia can ever be cured. Research suggests that with intensive therapy, most patients can

Think About It 2

obsessive-compulsive disorder A neurological disorder characterized by a tendency to repeat certain acts continuously and without practical need and by ritualistic behavior to relieve anxiety.

emetic An agent that induces vomiting.

enema An infusion of fluid into the rectum usually for cleansing or other therapeutic purposes.

diuretic [dye-u-RET-ik] A drug or other substance that promotes the formation and release of urine. Diuretics are given to reduce body fluid volume in treating such disorders as high blood pressure, congestive heart disease, and edema. Both alcohol and caffeine act as diuretics.

laxative A substance that promotes evacuation of the bowel by increasing the bulk of the feces, lubricating the intestinal wall, or softening the stool.

Table SED.1 **Warning Signs of Anorexia**

Anorexia nervosa is a disorder in which preoccupation with dieting and thinness leads to excessive weight loss. The anorexic person may not acknowledge that weight loss or restricted eating are problems. Family and friends can help by recognizing that the following are warning signs:

- Loss of a significant amount of weight
- Continuing to diet (although thin)
- Feeling fat, even after losing weight
- Fear of weight gain
- Cessation of monthly menstrual periods
- Preoccupation with food, calories, nutrition, and/or cooking
- Preferring to eat in isolation
- Exercising compulsively
- Bingeing and purging

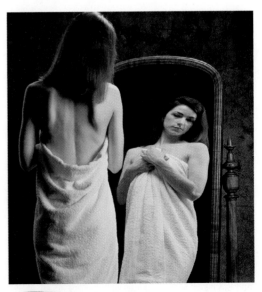

Figure SED.7 **Distorted body image.**

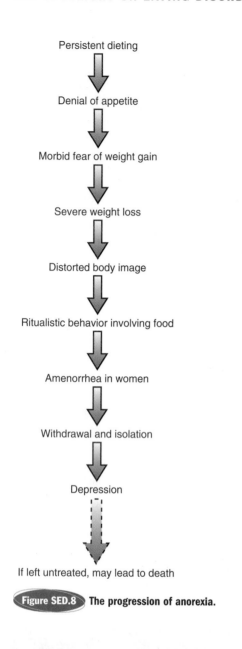

Persistent dieting

Denial of appetite

Morbid fear of weight gain

Severe weight loss

Distorted body image

Ritualistic behavior involving food

Amenorrhea in women

Withdrawal and isolation

Depression

If left untreated, may lead to death

Figure SED.8 **The progression of anorexia.**

Table SED.2 **When Hospitalization Is Needed**

Suggested criteria for hospitalization for individuals with anorexia nervosa include:

- Weight loss of greater than 30 percent over 3 months
- Severe metabolic disturbance
- Severe depression or suicide risk
- Severe bingeing and purging
- Failure to maintain outpatient weight contract
- Psychosis
- Family crisis

Source: American Psychiatric Association. Diagnostic and Statistical Manual of Mental Disorders. 4th ed. Washington, DC: Author; 1994.

achieve normal weight. However, they may struggle all their lives with a moderate to severe preoccupation with food and body weight, poor social relationships, and depression. The earlier a patient begins treatment, the better the prognosis.

The course of anorexia varies greatly among patients. In rare instances, a sufferer recovers spontaneously without treatment. More typically, a patient recovers only after a variety of treatments, or enters a cyclical pattern of weight gain and relapse. From 30 to 50 percent of anorexia patients also have symptoms of bulimia, which can complicate diagnosis and treatment.[29] Tragically, in 6 to 18 percent of cases, the disease proves fatal. (See **Figure SED.8.**) Patients who have other emotional disorders, such as major depression or substance abuse, are the most likely to die from complications of the disease. Potentially fatal complications of anorexia include starvation and suicide.[30]

As with many other behavioral disorders, people with anorexia usually deny the danger of their situation. Hence, it falls to family and friends to ensure that sufferers get treatment. They may get together and supportively confront the person with evidence that something is seriously wrong. This common technique sometimes helps people accept the need for at least an initial medical screening. The complex and multifaceted nature of anorexia requires a team of experienced health-care professionals, including physicians, clinical dietitians, and psychotherapists, so that both the physical and psychological aspects of the disorder can be addressed. One of the best places to find an experienced team of therapists is at an eating disorder clinic associated with a major medical facility.[31]

The first goal of treatment is to stabilize the patient's physical condition. The second is to convert the patient, who is typically reluctant, into a willing participant in the treatment plan. A combination of hospitalization, psychotherapy, and pharmacotherapy is often necessary.

The foremost consideration in the treatment of anorexia is restoring the patient's nutritional status. Otherwise, dehydration, starvation, and electrolyte imbalances can lead to serious health problems and even death. (See **Figure SED.9.**) If a patient has lost more than 30 percent of body weight over a three-month period, or weighs 70 percent or less of the standard weight considered healthy for height, hospitalization is essential. (See **Table SED.2.**) Once the patient's physical condition has stabilized and some of the physical symptoms of starvation have disappeared, psychotherapy can begin in earnest. Many clinicians use a cognitive behavioral therapy approach to help the patient challenge irrational beliefs, and establish healthy attitudes and behaviors for gaining and maintaining weight.

The early phases of weight gain are fraught with challenges for both patient and clinician. Patients must gain a certain amount of weight to prevent death or permanent damage, while the psychotherapeutic portion of their treatment is still in the very early phases. At first, the patient is encouraged to simply eat enough food to minimize or stop weight loss. Next, the patient is started on a very slow process of weight gain, all the while receiving intensive psychotherapy. The first sign of weight gain can precipitate a crisis. Phobia of obesity may return with renewed vengeance. Many patients refuse to eat. Others resist treatment in covert ways. If not restricted to bed and closely supervised, they may try to burn off calories through relentless exercise or by purging. To avoid detection, they adopt a series of behaviors to conceal their lack of weight gain. These include wearing concealing clothes, or "bulking up" prior to weigh-ins by filling their pockets with coins or drinking large amounts of water or diet soda.[32]

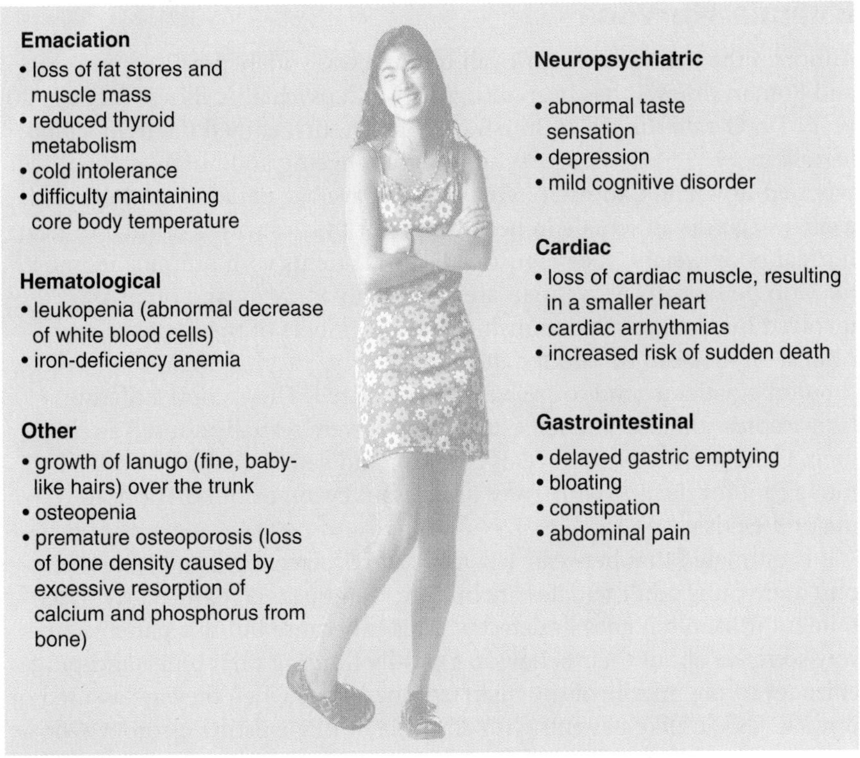

Emaciation
- loss of fat stores and muscle mass
- reduced thyroid metabolism
- cold intolerance
- difficulty maintaining core body temperature

Hematological
- leukopenia (abnormal decrease of white blood cells)
- iron-deficiency anemia

Other
- growth of lanugo (fine, baby-like hairs) over the trunk
- osteopenia
- premature osteoporosis (loss of bone density caused by excessive resorption of calcium and phosphorus from bone)

Neuropsychiatric
- abnormal taste sensation
- depression
- mild cognitive disorder

Cardiac
- loss of cardiac muscle, resulting in a smaller heart
- cardiac arrhythmias
- increased risk of sudden death

Gastrointestinal
- delayed gastric emptying
- bloating
- constipation
- abdominal pain

Figure SED.9 **Anorexia and the side effects of excessive weight loss.**

Psychologists use a variety of psychotherapeutic techniques to help the patient deal with underlying emotional issues, such as depression. Treatment programs generally use a combination of behavioral therapy, individual psychotherapy, patient education, family education, and family therapy. Frequently, therapists find family conflicts at the heart of the eating disorder. Ongoing therapy for the patient and family are key to successful recovery. As the patient's symptoms resolve, she or he must find new ways of relating to and communicating with family members. Family members must remain open and willing to change their behavior toward the person with the eating disorder.

Dietitians work closely with the psychotherapist to help patients develop a realistic view of food and to reshape their food selection and eating behaviors. Although no pharmaceutical agent has been developed specifically to treat anorexia, certain antidepressants have proved useful in its treatment.

The vast majority of patients with anorexia nervosa require continued intervention after discharge from the hospital or treatment program. Support groups for people with eating disorders and their families can be an important link in the recovery process. Support groups also can be a useful technique for easing a resistant patient into treatment. With expert help and ongoing therapy, patients with anorexia can develop new mechanisms for coping with life's stresses, eventually replacing their disordered relationship with food with new, healthier interpersonal relationships.

Key Concepts: *The hallmark symptoms of anorexia nervosa are a mania for thinness and self-imposed starvation. Sufferers have a body weight as much as 15 percent below normal, a severely distorted body image, withdrawal from family and friends, and various physical and psychological changes related to starvation.*

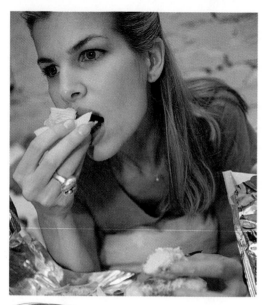

Figure SED.10
The typical person suffering from bulimia is a single, Caucasian woman in her 20s or 30s.

$\mathcal{Q}$*uick* $\mathcal{B}$*ites*

I'm so hungry I could eat an ox!

$\mathcal{T}$he term bulimia is derived from the Greek word *bous* meaning "ox" and *limos* meaning "hunger."

Bulimia Nervosa

Although the behavior we now call bulimia was widely practiced in Greek and Roman times, it has been recognized as a psychiatric illness for only 20 years. Dr. Gerald Russell, a British psychiatrist, first coined the term *bulimia nervosa* in 1979 to describe a syndrome of bingeing and purging being reported in young Caucasian females.[33] The average patient with bulimia is a single, Caucasian female in her twenties or thirties with a normal or near-normal body weight. (See **Figure SED.10**.) Patients with bulimia are more likely to be sexually active than are those with anorexia and often are involved in destructive relationships with members of the opposite sex. Almost anyone can be affected, however.

Bulimic patients tend to feel very disorganized. They report suffering from depression and low-self esteem. Many were sexually abused as children. Food was often a source of comfort, and eating gradually evolved into a tool for dealing with every unpleasant event, from boredom to major life crises.

It is estimated that between 1 percent and 3 percent of American adolescent and young adult females are bulimic. But bulimia, particularly in its milder forms, often goes undetected. This is because bulimic patients are very secretive about their behavior, typically limiting their binge-and-purge episodes to the middle of the night or other times when they are assured of privacy. Also, unlike patients with anorexia or binge-eating disorder, whose body weights may hint at their underlying psychiatric disorder, the body weight of a patient with bulimia is usually average or only slightly above average. Several studies have found that as many as 40 percent of college-age women occasionally binge and purge (too infrequently for an official diagnosis of bulimia but often enough to raise concern).[34] **Table SED.3** lists the warning signs of bulimia.

Causes of Bulimia Nervosa

Bulimia seems to occur most often in people who have an intense desire to nurture themselves with food but are also strongly influenced by our

$\mathcal{E}$very time I leave one of my sessions I feel better. We talk about stuff; I feel, express, and even cry. Today was the third time since I left her office to come home and throw up. I think things are getting better despite the fact that my mind focuses 80 percent of the time on food during the 55 minutes. But it's like the kitchen is a refuge for my mind. I always know it will be there, waiting to embrace me when I get home.

Alone is how I hope to find it. I have been thinking of what I will sink my teeth into first. Usually I go for the fat-free chocolate cake, then to the frozen yogurt (which makes it all come up much smoother). I don't think this is normal, though I am not really concerned. I feel like a million-pound weight has been swept away by the effortless flush of the toilet. The hardest thing is to look in the mirror after I have thrown up. Sometimes I wipe my face before I look. Other times I leave the spit, bile, and food on my mouth and hands. I just stand there holding my hands up, with my shoulders slumped over. I produce this expression of absolute helplessness—then I laugh.

I guess I am amazed by the act I've just committed. I can't explain why, I can't believe that it is really me doing this. Why would I do something like throw up? I really have no reason to torture myself. Bulimia was always *them*—I can't possibly be like that. I throw up, but I am not a bulimic. I sure as hell don't have an eating disorder.

I am totally for this whole counseling thing because I feel sad a lot and I want to feel better. But I can't leave there and not feel that I have to get this crap out. All this stuff that we talk about.

Table SED.3 **Warning Signs of Bulimia**

Bulimia nervosa involves frequent episodes of binge eating, almost always followed by purging and intense feelings of guilt or shame. The sufferer feels out of control, and recognizes that the behavior is not normal. The signs that a person may be bulimic include:

- Bingeing, or eating uncontrollably
- Purging by strict dieting, fasting, vigorous exercise, vomiting, or abusing laxatives or diuretics in an attempt to lose weight
- Using the bathroom frequently after meals
- Preoccupation with body weight
- Depression or mood swings
- Irregular menstrual periods
- Dental problems, swollen cheeks or glands, heartburn, or bloating
- Personal or family problems with drugs or alcohol

binge Consumption of a very large amount of food in a brief time (e.g., 2 hr) accompanied by a loss of control over how much and what is eaten.

purge Emptying of the GI tract by self-induced vomiting and/or misuse of laxatives, diuretics, or enemas.

societal obsession with thinness. People with bulimia have been described as being obsessed with food but repulsed by fat. In contrast to people with anorexia, people with bulimia focus more on food than on thinness.

Psychologists who have worked with bulimic patients have found that sufferers typically did not receive sufficient nurturing during their formative years. Whereas families of anorexic patients tend to have a lot of rigidly defined roles and rules, families of bulimic patients tend to lack structure. Roles may be loosely defined. Parents are often described as distant and judgmental. Significant family conflict usually exists. Patients often feel that their families failed to provide an adequate sense of security and protection.

Diagnostic and Clinical Features

A person with bulimia chronically **binges** and **purges**. To meet the official DSM-IV definition of the disorder, bingeing and purging must occur at least twice a month for at least three months. Purging may be accompanied or replaced by other compensatory behaviors such as fasting and excessive

Today, Dr. Tant asked me when this all began. My first thought was, "Oh this throwing up thing? I can't remember." But I do recall one time when my ex-boyfriend Matt and I had gone to a really nice dinner. My recollection of the evening was that it was perfect. I remember thinking about how this food was really fattening, though, and how it would make me fat if I kept it down. I didn't know or have the willpower to just not eat it. Over and over I tortured and berated myself about the effects this dinner would have on my body. I couldn't bear it. This dinner was

no longer one meal; it was going to ruin my body and make me fat. I couldn't stand that food being inside me another moment. Looking back I can't imagine how I could have thrown up right there on the side of the road. It was like I had no couth. I told Matt to pull over, and I just stuck my hand down my throat. Rationalizing the act while engaging in it, I then jumped back in the truck to carry on with the night. We never discussed my vile act other than Matt saying, "I can't believe you just did that."

"I know," I responded, "but it just was making me feel so sick. I mean, my stomach was really nauseous [sic]." Basically I don't know when I began this war with myself, but I know it caused me to fear myself. The rest is a blur—its beginning, its incentive. I heard Dr. Tant's question. I just didn't have the answer.
Chelsea Browning Smith

Source: Smith, C. *Diary of an Eating Disorder.* Dallas, TX: Taylor Publishing Company, 1998.

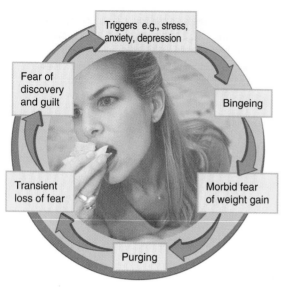

Figure SED.11 The binge-purge cycle of bulimia.

exercise. Between binges, bulimics *typically* restrict their dietary intake to a limited number of low-calorie foods they consider "safe." This dietary control is an illusion, however. The average bulimic sufferer is obsessed by thoughts of food and spends a great deal of time both planning the next binge and trying to resist the urge to binge. **Figure SED.11** illustrates the binge-and-purge pattern of bulimia.

Just what triggers a binge is not clear. People with bulimia tend to be all-or-nothing thinkers. If they eat a single piece of food from their forbidden list, say a cookie, they feel driven to consume the entire box. Some researchers believe that hunger caused by very restrictive dieting, combined with a buildup of everyday stresses, overwhelms the person's resolve and precipitates a binge.

During a binge, individuals with bulimia typically consume massive quantities of highly palatable "forbidden" foods like pastry, ice cream, and candy. This gorging takes place over a relatively short time span, say an hour or two. Binges have been reported that contain up to 10,000 kilocalories. Afterward, feeling physically ill from overindulgence, sufferers use a variety of purging techniques, such as self-induced vomiting or excessive quantities of laxatives, to rid themselves of the food. Or, they may follow a binge with a period of very strict fasting and heightened exercise.

Bulimic patients who purge frequently develop a variety of physical symptoms. Over time, gastric acid in vomit burns the lining of the pharynx, esophagus, and mouth, erodes tooth enamel, and may even result in loss of teeth. Repeated vomiting also can enlarge the salivary glands and erode the lining of the stomach and esophagus.

Excessive self-induced vomiting and diarrhea can upset the body's delicate biochemical balance through loss of electrolytes and body water. Among other dangers, changes in electrolyte balance can trigger an irregular heartbeat and precipitate a life-threatening medical crisis. Excessive use of emetics (drugs to induce vomiting) and laxatives carries its own risks. Repeated use of emetics is toxic to the liver and kidneys, and abuse of laxatives can damage the lining of the large intestine. **Figure SED.12** shows the side effects of bulimic purging.

Treatment

Little research has been done on the long-term course of bulimia. It appears, however, that bulimia is easier to treat than anorexia, perhaps because bulimic patients tend to recognize that their behavior is abnormal. Following treatment, more than half of patients report an improvement in their binge-eating and coping behaviors. About 30 percent of patients eventually become symptom-free. The rest, however, struggle with the disorder to some degree throughout their lives. To reduce the risk of relapse, therapists encourage patients to stay involved in support groups after completing formal therapy.

Cognitive behavior therapy is key to helping patients reshape their attitudes about food and identify situations that trigger bingeing. The therapist's goal is to help patients let go of their need to categorize foods as safe or dangerous, good or bad. Patients must learn techniques for dealing with stress and uncomfortable or painful memories and feelings. Depression, which typically accompanies this disorder, must be treated as well. Many bulimic patients also require treatment for substance abuse. A patient is hospitalized only when severely depressed or when purging is so frequent that physical damage has occurred or is imminent.

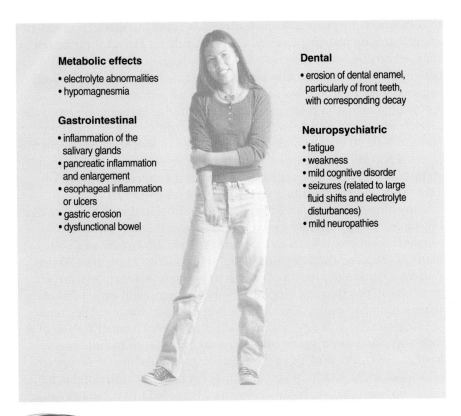

Metabolic effects

- electrolyte abnormalities
- hypomagnesmia

Gastrointestinal

- inflammation of the salivary glands
- pancreatic inflammation and enlargement
- esophageal inflammation or ulcers
- gastric erosion
- dysfunctional bowel

Dental

- erosion of dental enamel, particularly of front teeth, with corresponding decay

Neuropsychiatric

- fatigue
- weakness
- mild cognitive disorder
- seizures (related to large fluid shifts and electrolyte disturbances)
- mild neuropathies

Figure SED.12 Bulimia and side effects of purging.

Medication can be an effective adjunct to psychotherapy. Serotonin-enhancing antidepressants have been used successfully to treat bulimia. In 1997 the FDA approved the antidepressant Prozac for this purpose.

Key Concepts: *Key symptoms of bulimia nervosa are binge-eating episodes at least twice a week for a month, followed by compensatory behavior like severe dieting, purging, or a combination of dieting and purging. The body weight of people with bulimia is typically close to or slightly above that considered healthy for their heights.*

Binge-Eating Disorder

Overeating has been reported in the medical literature since scribes first put stylus to tablet. And over the generations, societies, including our own, have considered obesity a sign of good health, wealth, and even fertility.[35] Our present society is not among these. In 1994 the American Psychiatric Association recognized binge-eating disorder as an emotional illness. Binge eating is the most common eating disorder in industrialized nations. It occurs only in societies where people have access to an abundant supply of food. Precise causes of this disorder are unclear. However, the condition seems to be related to an intense desire to nurture oneself with food or to reduce stress by eating.[36]

Diagnostic and Clinical Features

A person with binge-eating disorder consumes excessive quantities of food in a relatively short time at least twice a week. Unlike the bulimia sufferer, however, the person with binge-eating disorder does not attempt

Table SED.4 **Warning Signs of Binge-Eating Disorder**

Binge eaters, like bulimia sufferers, experience periods of uncontrolled eating that they usually keep secret. Binge eaters often are depressed and sometimes have other psychological problems. Signs that a person may have a binge-eating disorder include:

- Episodes of binge eating
- Eating when not physically hungry
- Frequent dieting
- Feeling unable to stop eating voluntarily
- Awareness that eating patterns are abnormal
- Weight fluctuations
- Depressed mood
- Attribution of social and professional success and failures to weight

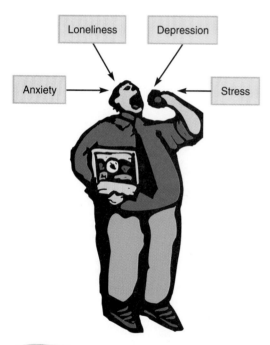

Figure SED.13 Feelings of loneliness, depression, anxiety, or stress can trigger a binge-eating episode.

Quick Bites

When Plumpness Was Valued

In centuries past, extra pounds displayed one's wealth and prosperity. The wealthy could afford abundant food and didn't perform physical labor.

to compensate by purging or other means. In some instances, binge eaters adopt a grazing pattern. "Grazers" eat constantly for extended periods of time, eventually consuming an exceptionally large quantity of food. This pattern of overindulgence may be seen in people who restrict their food intake at work or school but seek solace in food at home.

Not all people who binge are obese. But bingeing is common among the severely obese and people with a history of weight cycling. In the United States at least 30 percent of the people enrolled in weight-management programs report behaviors consistent with a diagnosis of binge-eating disorder, compared with only 3 percent to 5 percent of the general population.[37] **Table SED.4** lists the warning signs of binge-eating disorder.

Many binge eaters begin dieting in grade school and start bingeing during adolescence or in their early twenties. Typically, they try numerous weight-loss programs without long-term success. Binge eaters exhibit many of the same characteristics as bulimic patients. More than 50 percent have clinical depression. Feelings of depression, loneliness, anxiety, or stress can precipitate a binge. Like other patients with eating disorders, those with binge-eating disorder are all-or-nothing thinkers. They tend to categorize foods as safe or dangerous. Eating even a small serving of a forbidden food can trigger a binge. Typical binge foods include sweets, pastries, ice cream, and high-fat snacks like nuts and chips. However, if junk foods aren't handy, binge eaters may eat large quantities of starchy foods, such as potatoes, bread, and pasta. **Figure SED.13** illustrates some things that trigger binge eating.

Most binge eaters are people who have not learned to express or even acknowledge their feelings. During therapy sessions, many binge eaters report feeling helpless to change the course of events or behaviors of others around them. Rather than acknowledge their feelings, they swallow them—aided by large quantities of food. They become addicted to the behavior itself because it is the only way they can get relief from stress. (See **Figure SED.14**.)

Binge eating often is a learned response to stress or conflict, passed down from one generation to the next. In such families, the parents use food rather than affection and discussion to direct their children's behavior. Food is used for celebration and consolation, for reward and punishment. Children growing up in such environments learn to eat in response to emotions rather than hunger. As adults, they turn to food to satisfy all their emotional needs.

Treatment

Little is known about the course and prognosis of binge-eating disorder. However, people who become obese as a result of this disorder are at risk of developing weight-related health problems, including type 2 diabetes, hypertension, degenerative joint disease, heart disease, and even certain cancers.

People who have binge-eating disorder are rarely able to control the condition themselves. Typically, they require therapy to help them identify their long-buried emotions and learn techniques for giving voice to their feelings. Therapists experienced in treating this disorder discourage patients from trying to lose weight initially. Any attempts to restrict food intake can backfire by creating anxiety and provoking a binge. The major focus of therapy is to help patients identify their emotions and separate true biological hunger from emotional hunger. Once significant progress is made in these areas, the patient is better equipped psychologically to address weight issues.

Long-term support is key to keeping binge eaters from relapsing. Self-help groups like Overeaters Anonymous are one source of support. These groups are organized according to the 12-step philosophy of Alcoholics Anonymous. In addition, many hospitals in large urban areas have support groups led by trained therapists. Hospitals and clinics that provide medically supervised fasting programs such as Optifast often supply this type of service as well. (See Chapter 8, "Energy Balance, Body Composition, and Weight Management," for further information on this type of weight-control program.)

Many patients with binge-eating disorder benefit from antidepressant medications. These drugs, presumably by altering the brain's serotonin levels, reduce the urge to binge. Various weight-management medications are now in development. These also may curb the urge to binge.

Key Concepts: *Diagnostic criteria have recently been established for binge-eating disorder, the most common eating disorder. People of all ages and backgrounds suffer from this disorder. Like people with bulimia, those with binge-eating disorder consume significantly more food than is typically eaten in a given period. In contrast to individuals with bulimia, those with binge-eating disorder do not engage in compensatory behaviors to limit weight gain. Not all binge eaters are obese, although many obese people binge eat. Some people with binge-eating disorder tend to graze; that is, they eat a large amount of food over a prolonged period, rather than all at once.*

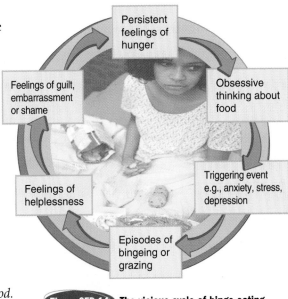

Persistent feelings of hunger

Feelings of guilt, embarrassment or shame

Obsessive thinking about food

Feelings of helplessness

Triggering event e.g., anxiety, stress, depression

Episodes of bingeing or grazing

Figure SED.14 The vicious cycle of binge eating.

Males: An Overlooked Population

As many as a million men struggle with eating disorders.[38] Yet males with eating disorders have been "ignored, neglected or dismissed because of statistical infrequency of the disease, combined with the pervasive myth that eating disorders are a female disease," according to Arnold E. Andersen, MD, former director of the Eating and Weight Disorders Clinic at Johns Hopkins and scientific editor of the book, *Males with Eating Disorders.*[39]

Women who develop eating disorders feel fat, but they typically are near average weight. In contrast, most men who develop these diseases are medically overweight. Many were seriously teased about their weight as children. While women are concerned predominately with weight, men are concerned with shape and muscle definition. Indeed, men often develop disordered eating habits while trying to improve their athletic performance. Finally, more men than women diet to prevent medical consequences associated with being overweight.

Why do fewer males than females develop full-blown eating disorders? Anderson contends there is a "dose-response" relationship between the amount of sociocultural pressure to be thin and the probability of developing an eating disorder. Consider that articles and advertisements that promote dieting usually are targeted at young women rather than young men. When men are exposed to activities that require leanness, such as wrestling, swimming, running, and horse racing, they exhibit a substantial increase in anorexic behavior. It seems clear that cultural conditioning, not sex, contributes to the incidence of eating disorders.

Furthermore, the degree of thinness held up as desirable for women is 15 percent below a healthy body weight; whereas the degree of thinness held up as desirable for men is well within the healthy limits of normal weight. Thus, women are more likely than men are to alter their eating habits to achieve the desired appearance.

Diagnostic and Clinical Features

Like women, most men develop eating disorders during adolescence. But males can develop eating disorders during preadolescence and young adulthood as well. The diagnostic criteria for anorexia and bulimia in men and women are similar. (See **Tables SED.5** and **SED.6**.) But doctors are so conditioned to viewing eating disorders as a female phenomenon that they often miss eating disorders in males. Likewise, the patient, his family, and friends may not recognize disordered eating patterns. Binge eating in particular may go unrecognized in men, because our culture accepts overeating among men more readily than in females. Another reason anorexia may elude diagnosis in men more often than in women is that malnourished men don't experience definitive symptoms like a woman's loss of menstrual periods, which can alert professionals and others to the problem. Additionally, men tend to view eating disorder behaviors as a "woman's disease," so they often are hesitant to seek medical attention.[40]

Key Concepts: *Men also suffer from eating disorders, although at rates much lower than that of females. Like women, men typically develop eating disorders during adolescence and young adulthood but are more often overweight, and striving for a particular body shape and muscularity. Although the diagnostic criteria are the same, with the exception of amenorrhea, men's eating disorders are often undiagnosed due to societal conditioning that eating disorders are "female" diseases.*

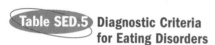

Table SED.5 Diagnostic Criteria for Eating Disorders

Anorexia nervosa

- Body weight <85% of expected weight (or BMI<17.5)
- Intense fear of weight gain
- Inaccurate perception of own body size, weight, or shape
- Amenorrhea (in females after menarche)

Bulimia nervosa

- Recurrent binge eating (at least two times per week for 3 months)
- Recurrent purging, excessive exercise, or fasting (at least two times per week for 3 months)
- Excessive concern about body weight or shape
- Absence of anorexia nervosa

Binge-eating disorder

- Recurrent binge eating (at least two times per week for 6 months)
- Marked distress with at least three of the following:
  - Eating very rapidly
  - Eating until uncomfortably full
  - Eating when not hungry
  - Eating alone
  - Feeling disgusted or guilty after a binge
  - No recurrent purging, no excessive exercising, and no fasting
  - Absence of anorexia nervosa

Table SED.6 Signs of an Undisclosed Eating Disorder

People with eating disorders usually exhibit several of the following signs:

Physical

- Arrested growth
- Marked change or frequent fluctuations in weight
- Inability to gain weight
- Fatigue
- Constipation or diarrhea
- Susceptibility to fractures
- Delayed menarche
- Calcium or phosphorus imbalances, abnormal blood pH, or high serum amylase levels

Behavioral

- Change in eating habits
- Difficulty in social settings
- Reluctance to be weighed
- Depression
- Social withdrawal
- Repeated absence from school or work
- Deceptive or secretive behavior
- Stealing (e.g., to obtain food)
- Substance abuse
- Excessive exercise

Anorexia Athletica

Participation in competitive athletics seems to be a common link in the development of eating disorders among male and female athletes, regardless of their social or ethnic backgrounds. Sports-related eating disorders are known as **anorexia athletica**. Some studies suggest that as many as 30 percent of competitive athletes exhibit some degree of disordered eating.[41] A study focusing on the incidence of eating disorders in female athletes found a higher incidence among gymnasts. Some 62 percent of college-age female gymnasts reported disordered eating patterns. Anorexia is also seen frequently in swimmers, dancers, wrestlers, and bodybuilders. Athletes who have anorexia athletica are seeking to attain an unrealistic body size that they consider desirable for purposes of competition. In many cases, athletes with mild eating disorders are able to disguise their disease as attention to fitness. People who seem to be addicted to their exercise routine are at greater risk of developing eating disorders.[42]

According to the American College of Sports Medicine, coaches and trainers play a significant role in the development of eating disorders among athletes. The attitude that leanness equals performance, exemplified by sayings such as "get down to your fighting weight," still prevails.[43]

The Female Athlete Triad

Women athletes who fall prey to the "thin-at-any-cost" philosophy are at risk of developing a condition known as the female athlete triad. (See **Figure SED.15**.) This syndrome is characterized by restrictive eating disorder, amenorrhea (absence of menstruation), and abnormally low bone density. This triad occurs especially in young women who participate in sports that involve appearance (e.g., gymnastics) and endurance (e.g., long distance running). Once body fat falls below 20 percent, many women's estrogen levels drop significantly. As a result, their bodies enter a quasi-menopausal state years ahead of time. Their periods become irregular or cease altogether. Bone loss accelerates, just as it would after natural menopause. Many female athletes who suffer from this triad have the bone density of women in their fifties and sixties. Weakened bones are more likely to fracture during exercise or daily activities. And because much of this bone loss is irreversible, women who suffer from the female athlete triad are at increased risk of developing osteoporosis.[44]

To help combat this alarming trend, The American College of Sports Medicine and the National Collegiate Athletic Association (NCAA) has an eating disorders awareness campaign aimed at coaches and trainers. The NCAA also has a three-part video series, *Nutrition and Eating Disorders*, to acquaint coaches and trainers with the causes and effects of eating disorders, as well as the steps to take when they suspect an athlete has an eating disorder.[45]

Key Concepts: *Athletics can be a gateway to eating disorders. Women athletes who develop restrictive eating habits are at risk for developing a more severe syndrome known as the female athlete triad. Restrictive eating disorder, amenorrhea, and abnormally low bone density characterize this syndrome. If not corrected, the female athlete triad can hinder athletic performance and set the stage for lifelong health problems.*

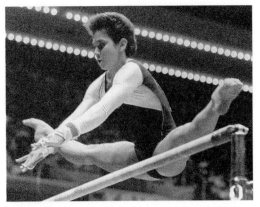

Christie Henrich, a top Olympic gymnast, weighed only 60 lbs at her death in 1994.

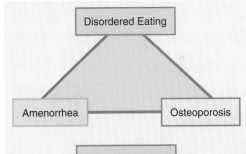

Disordered Eating

The athlete develops one or more harmful eating behaviors in an attempt to lose weight. The result is an energy deficit.

Amenorrhea

An energy deficit leads to a reduction in body fat. Once body fat falls below about 20 percent, the athlete's body stops producing the hormones needed to make estrogen, resulting in menstrual cycle irregularities.

Osteoporosis

The lack of estrogen decreases calcium absorption and retention. Dietary deficiency of calcium also is common. Left untreated, this lack of calcium leads to bone loss, stress fractures and osteoporosis.

 Figure SED.15 **Female athlete triad.** Stress fractures are a red flag for female athlete triad.

anorexia athletica Eating disorder associated with competitive participation in athletic activity.

baryophobia [barry-oh-FO-bee-ah] An uncommon eating disorder that stunts growth in children and young adults as a result of underfeeding.

infantile anorexia Severe feeding difficulties that begin with the introduction of solid foods to infants. Symptoms include persistent food refusal for more than 1 month, malnutrition, parental concern about the child's poor food intake, and significant caregiver-infant conflict during feeding.

Vegetarianism and Eating Disorders

Some researchers have found a strong correlation between vegetarianism and eating disorders in teenagers. A recent study conducted in Minnesota schools found 81 percent of the students who classified themselves as vegetarians were female. Compared with nonvegetarian peers, these self-described vegetarians were twice as likely to participate in frequent diets, four times as likely to report intentional vomiting, and eight times as likely to report laxative use.[46] Some people with eating disorders try to disguise a change in eating habits by adopting a strict vegetarian diet.

Smoking and Eating Disorders

A British medical researcher, Sir Arthur Crisp, Ph.D, recently described a new variation on eating disorders. His previous studies showed that smoking is more common among teens with eating disorders than in the general teenage population. His new research indicates that despite ample knowledge of the health risks of smoking, girls of average or slightly above-average weight are taking up smoking in record numbers to cut their appetites. Though not frankly anorexic or bulimic, many of the young subjects report they periodically combine smoking with self-induced vomiting to enhance weight-control efforts.[47] This combined behavior is of particular interest and concern to researchers.

Baryophobia

Baryophobia, a disorder characterized by fear of fat, was virtually unheard of until the late 1970s, when pediatricians began reporting a surprising number of young patients from affluent backgrounds whose growth appeared to be stunted due to poor nutrition. In some instances, the stunting occurs when a child secretly starts to diet in order to fit in better with his or her trimmer classmates. More often, however, the child's parents are at the root of the problem. Many well-intentioned parents underfeed their children in an attempt to "protect" them from inheriting their family's tendency toward obesity, heart disease, or diabetes. But the low-fat, high-carbohydrate diet beneficial to many adults may supply too few calories to meet the energy demands of active, growing children. In such instances, the entire family needs nutritional counseling to help them understand what constitutes a healthful diet and realistic body weight for a growing child.[48]

Infantile Anorexia

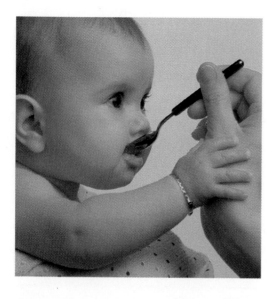

Unwitting parents can even create disordered eating in infants, perhaps setting the stage for eating disorders later in life.[49] Childhood nutrition specialist Ellyn Satter, RD, MSW, has analyzed videotapes of infant feedings. Satter examined whether parents responded to—or ignored—their babies' nonverbal eating readiness cues. She concluded that many parents fail to recognize their babies' body language: They feed their babies too rapidly or too slowly; they offer foods the baby doesn't care for; or they persist in trying to feed a clearly full baby who is turning away from food. These well-meaning parents may inadvertently teach their babies to ignore hunger and satiety (fullness) cues and, instead, to eat in response to outside influences.

Reports of a new disorder called **infantile anorexia** lend support to Satter's observations.[50] A team of child psychiatrists at the National Medical Center in Washington, D.C., described this disorder in which severe feeding difficulties begin as an infant is introduced to solid foods. Symptoms include persistent food refusal for more than one month, malnutrition, parental concern about the child's poor food intake, and significant conflict between caregiver and infant during feeding. The disorder typically starts or worsens during the transition from nursing to spoon-feeding and self-feeding, between six months and three years of age.

Babies with infantile anorexia should not be confused with "picky" eaters. Picky eaters may initially refuse all foods but allow themselves to be coaxed into eating. Picky eaters have strong food likes and dislikes but are not malnourished. And the relationship between the picky eaters and their parents or caregivers lacks the element of frustration and conflict seen in infantile anorexia.

Infantile anorexia has many serious consequences. Malnutrition can impair the developing brain and adds special stress to the parent-infant relationship. Furthermore, early conflict around meals may herald a life-long unhealthy relationship with food.

Key Concepts: *Researchers are continuously recognizing associated markers of behavioral traits, such as vegetarianism and smoking, that may signal the development of an eating disorder. Even babies and young children may suffer from disordered eating patterns.*

Combating Eating Disorders

Eating disorders are extremely difficult to treat, although advances in neurochemistry and scientific understanding of the mind-body connection may provide new avenues of treatment. Most experts agree that emphasis should be placed on preventing eating disorders.

The NIH believes that health-care professionals should lead efforts to prevent eating disorders by learning to promote self-esteem in their patients and teaching patients that people can be healthy at every size. (See **Table SED.7**.) Ideally, this approach would have a ripple effect: patients would transmit these beliefs to others. A variety of public information campaigns aimed at parents and people who work with children and adolescents have evolved over the past decade to promote awareness of eating disorders. One of the most prominent examples is the Body Size Acceptance campaign coordinated through the University of California, Berkeley, under the direction of Joanne Ikeda, MA, RD.[51]

Table SED.7   **Preventing Eating Disorders**

To join the effort to prevent eating disorders, follow some of these tips from the Body Size Acceptance campaign:

- Celebrate the diversity of human body shapes and sizes.
- Present accurate information about nutrition, weight management, and health.
- Discourage restrictive eating practices, including skipping meals.
- Encourage people to eat in response to hunger, not emotions.
- Reinforce messages about good eating and activity patterns at school and at home.
- Carefully phrase comments about a person's weight, body, or fitness level.
- Teach children and young people how to constructively express negative emotions.
- Encourage parents, teachers, coaches, and other professionals who work with children to do likewise.
- Encourage people of all ages to focus on personal qualities rather than physical appearance, of themselves and others.
- Find and promote images of fit people of all sizes and shapes.

Source: Excerpted from The Body Size Acceptance Campaign coordinated through the University of California, Berkeley under the direction of Joanne Ikeda, MA, RD.

LEARNING *Portfolio*

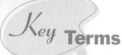

Key Terms

Study Points

> An eating disorder is a complex emotional illness, the primary symptom of which is significantly altered eating habits. Eating disorders occur in biologically susceptible people exposed to particular types of environmental stimuli.

> The typical person with a restrictive eating disorder is a young Caucasian female from an upper-class, achievement-oriented family.

> Although eating disorders existed even in ancient times, they have become alarmingly common in industrialized countries.

> Eating disorders may involve highly restrictive eating patterns as seen in anorexia nervosa, a combination of compulsive overeating and purging as seen in bulimia, or unrestricted binge eating.

> Eating disorders are common in people who participate in body-conscious activities such as dance, wrestling, gymnastics, and bodybuilding.

> One to five percent of people with eating disorders are male.

> Anorexia nervosa is an obsession for thinness manifested in self-imposed starvation.

> Victims of anorexia nervosa have a body weight 15 percent below normal, a distorted body image, and physical and psychological symptoms related to starvation.

> The body weight of people with bulimia is close to or even slightly above that considered healthy for their height.

> Key symptoms of bulimia nervosa are binge eating episodes at least twice a week for a month, followed by severe dieting, purging, or a combination of dieting and purging.

> Binge-eating disorder is the most common eating disorder.

> Like those with bulimia, people with binge-eating disorder consume more food than is typically eaten in a given period.

> Athletics can be a gateway to eating disorders for both men and women.

> Restrictive eating disorder, amenorrhea, and abnormally low bone density characterize the "female athlete triad."

> The best treatment for eating disorders is prevention. Once an eating disorder has become entrenched, intensive and prolonged treatment is typically required. Many people require life-long support to maintain healthful eating and lifestyle habits.

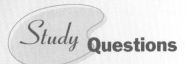

Study Questions

1. **What three factors play a role in most, if not all, eating disorders?**
2. **What are the warning signs of anorexia nervosa?**
3. **What is the usual treatment for people with anorexia nervosa and what do most experts say about their recovery?**
4. **What is the typical profile of a person with bulimia nervosa?**
5. **Describe an eating binge and all the behaviors that constitute purging.**
6. **List some common traits of people with binge-eating disorder.**
7. **What are the three components of the female athlete triad?**

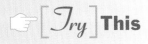 **This**

Is there any help out there?

How much help is available in your community for people with eating disorders? Scan the telephone directory (Yellow Pages) for eating disorders clinics, programs, and centers. Call them to inquire about their services. Do they have a psychologist, medical doctor, dietitian, nurse, and/or social worker on staff? Is it an inpatient or outpatient program? What is their philosophy of therapy? What is their success rate? What are their payment plans?

What About Bobbie?

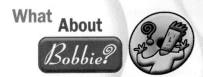

Bobbie's friend Janet has been struggling with anorexia nervosa for some time. Bobbie recently expressed concern again and asked Janet about her eating habits. Janet told Bobbie she eats the following foods in a typical day:

"Breakfast"
1 head of iceberg lettuce, with salt and pepper but no dressing
(If she wakes up really hungry, she'll have another with vinegar on it.)

"Snack"
6 to 8 white mushrooms

"Lunch"
3 or 4 dill pickles

"Dinner"
1 12-ounce can artichoke hearts (rinsed)

Fluids include mineral water, diet cola, and/or caffeinated tea.

Let's compare this intake to Bobbie's (see page 28 to review Bobbie's one-day diet). First, Janet's daily intake is just under 300 kilocalories compared to Bobbie's 2,440. Not only is Janet at risk due to her lack of calories but her intake of protein is approximately 0 grams. Her body has already used any glycogen it had as reserve fuel. In addition, at 5'3" and 89 pounds, she has very little reserve fat tissue for future energy needs. Without intake of dietary protein, her organ and muscle tissues have become prime targets for degradation. Even though Janet takes a multivitamin and a mineral supplement, if she doesn't seek help soon she may suffer the typical symptoms and effects of starvation and malnutrition.

References

1 ADA Reports: Position of the American Dietetic Association: Nutrition intervention in the treatment of anorexia nervosa, bulimia nervosa, and binge eating. *J Am Diet Assoc.* 1994;94:902–911.

2 American Dietetic Association. *Manual of Clinical Dietetics.* 5th ed. Chicago: Author; 1996.

3 Westenhoefer J, Stunkard AJ, Pudel V. Validation of the flexible and rigid control dimensions of dietary restraint. *Int J Eat Disord.* 1999;26:53–64.

4 Leutwyler, K. Treating Eating Disorders. The History of Anorexia Nervosa. http://www.sciam.com/explorations/1998/030298eating/anorexia.html. Accessed 8/1/00.

5 Ibid.

6 Suraf, M. Holy anorexia and anorexia nervosa: society and the concept of disease. *Pharo.* 1998;61(4):2–4.

7 Reid TR. The world according to Rome. *National Geographic.* 1997;8:54–83.

8 Casson L. *Everyday Life in Ancient Rome.* Baltimore: Johns Hopkins University Press; 1998.

9 National Institutes of Health. National Center for Health Statistics. www.nih.gov. Accessed 8/1/00.

10 Strauss R. Adolescents' perception of their body weight is dependent on social, cultural, and family pressures. *Arch Pediatr Adolesc Med.* 1998;153:741–747.

11 Gowan C. Teasing and body image: a predictor of eating disorders? Paper presented at the American Psychiatric Association annual meeting in San Francisco, CA; Aug 1998.

12 Gleaves DH. Scope and significance of posttraumatic symptomatology among women hospitalized for an eating disorder. *Int J Eat Disord.* 1998;2:147–156.

13 Mayer LE, Walsh BT. The use of selective serotonin reuptake inhibitors in eating disorders. *J Clin Psychiatry.* 1998;59(suppl 15):28–34.

14 Kaye W, Gendall K, Strober M. Serotonin neuronal function and selective serotonin reuptake inhibitor treatment in anorexia and bulimia nervosa. *Biol Psychiatry.* 1998;44:825–838. Review.

15 Lilenfeld LR, Kaye WH, Greeno CG, et al. A controlled family study of anorexia nervosa and bulimia nervosa: psychiatric disorders in first-degree relatives and effects of proband comorbidity. *Arch Gen Psychiatry.* 1998;55:603–610.

16 Aragona M, Vella G. Psychopathological considerations on the relationship between bulimia and obsessive-compulsive disorder. *Psychopathology.* 1998;31:197–205.

17 Leutwyler K. Treating Eating Disorders. http://www.sciam.com/explorations/1998/030298eating/index.html. Accessed 8/1/00.

18 Sakurai T, Amemiya A, Ishii M, et al. Orexins and orexin receptors: a family of hypothalamic neuropeptides and G protein-coupled receptors that regulate feeding behavior. *Cell.* 1998;92:573–585.

19 National Institutes of Health, National Center for Health Statistics. Op. cit.

20 American Anorexia and Bulimia Association. General Information on Eating Disorders http://www.aabainc.org/home.html. Accessed 8/1/00.

21 American Psychiatric Association. *Diagnostic and Statistical Manual of Mental Disorders.* 4th ed. Washington, DC: American Psychiatric Association; 1994, Reaffirmed until 2000.

22 le Grange D, Telch CF, Tibbs J. Eating attitudes and behaviors in South African Caucasian and non-Caucasian college students. *Am J Psychiatry.* 1998;155:250–254.

23 Anderson AE. Recognizing eating disorders. *Nutrition & the MD.* 1998;24(7):5–7.

24 Logsdail S, Marks I, OSullivan G. Eating disorders and obsessive-compulsive disorder. *Am J Psychiatry.* 1988;145:899.

25 Anderson AE. Op. cit.

26 Strauss R. Op. cit.

27 Anderson AE . Op. cit.

28 ADA Reports. Op. cit.

29 American Anorexia and Bulimia Association. Op. cit.

30 American Psychiatric Association. Op. cit.

31 Brownell K, Fairburn M. *Eating Disorders and Obesity: A Comprehensive Handbook.* New York: Guilford; 1995.

32 Anderson AE. Op. cit.

33 Leutwyler K. Op. cit.

34 Anderson AE. Op. cit.

35 Leutwyler K. Op. cit.

36 American Psychiatric Association. Op. cit.

37 Ibid.

38 Olivardia R, Pope HG Jr, Mangweth B, Hudson JI. Eating disorders in college man. *Am J Psychiatry.* 1995;152:1279–1284.

39 Andersen EA. *Males with Eating Disorders.* New York: Brunner Mazel; 1990.

40 Olivardia R, et al. Op. cit.

41 Eating disorders and exercise: the connection. *Nutrition & the MD.* 1998;24(7):5–6

42 Benyo R. *The Exercise Fix.* Berkeley, CA: Leisure Press; 1991.

43 Otis CL, Drinkwater B, Johnson M, et al. American College of Sports Medicine position stand. The female athlete triad. *Med Sci Sports Exerc.* 1997;29:i–ix.

44 Rosenbloom, CA, ed. *Sports Nutrition,* 3rd ed. Chicago, IL: The American Dietetic Association, 2000.

45 Mermel V. A review of contemporary sports nutrition. *Athletic Training.* 1995;1:228–244.

46 Martins Y. Restrained eating among vegetarians: does a vegetarian eating style mask concerns about weight? *Appetite.* 1999;32:145–154.

47 Crisp AH, Halek C, Sedgewick P, et al. Smoking and pursuit of thinness in schoolgirls in London and Ottawa. *Postgrad Med J.* 1998;74:473–479.

48 Leifshiz F. Children on adult diets: is it harmful? Is it hurtful? *J Am Coll Nutr.* 1992;11:845–850.

49 Ibid.

50 Satter E. The Feeding Relationship: Implications for Dietitians. Paper presented at the American Dietetic Association Annual meeting, Washington, DC; Oct 1992.

51 Parham ES. Promoting body size acceptance in weight management counseling. *J Am Diet Assoc.* 1999;99:920–925.

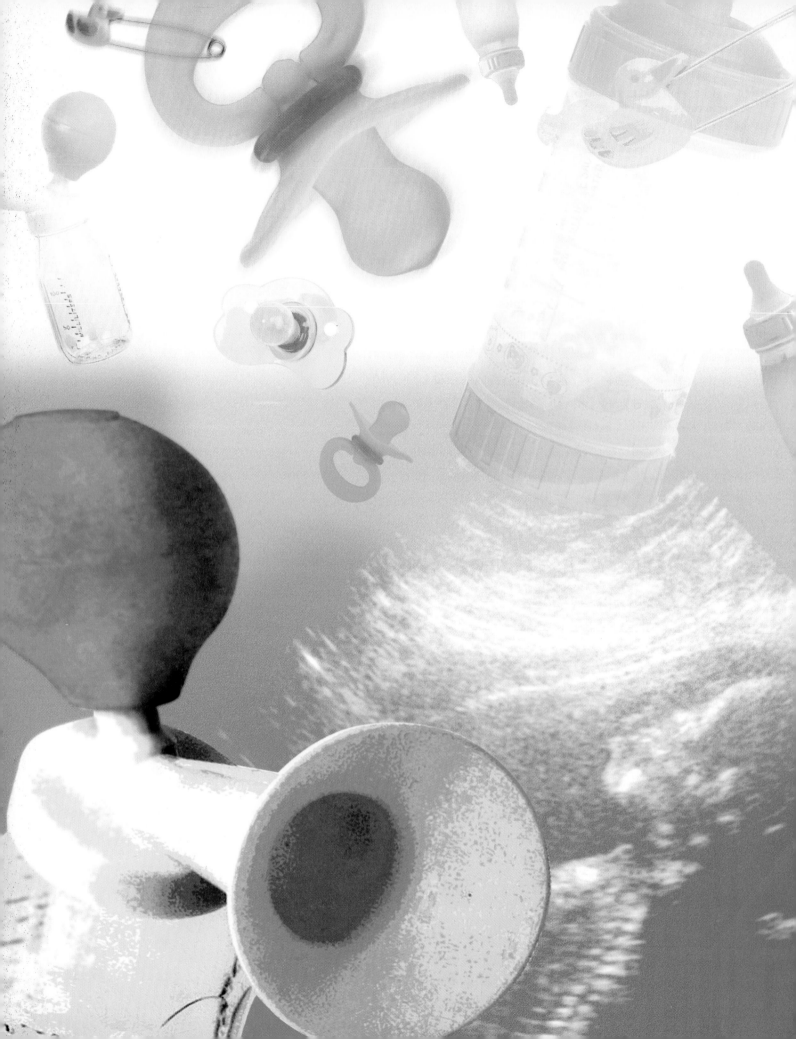

Chapter 14

Life Cycle: Pregnancy and Lactation

Think About It

1 Saying she is eating for two, your pregnant friend can't stop eating. What do you think about this?

2 Think about the eating habits of any pregnant woman you have known. What are your thoughts about what a pregnant woman should eat?

3 Your best friend tells you she is pregnant. You know that she enjoys wine with dinner. What do you say to her?

4 Were you breast-fed? Do you know of any benefits?

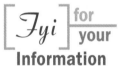

[Fyi] for your Information

This chapter's FYI boxes include practical information on the following topics:

• Vegetarianism and Pregnancy

• Pregnancy and Postpartum Exercise

The web site for this book offers many useful tools and is a great source for additional nutrition information for both students and instructors. Visit the site at **nutrition.jbpub.com** for information on nutrition for pregnancy and lactation. You'll find exercises that explore the following topics:

• Iron Supplementation in Canada

• Don't Even Mention Food: Eating During Morning Sickness

• Spicy Breast Milk?

• The Lactational Amenorrhea Method

What About Bobbie?

Track the choices Bobbie is making with the EatRight Analysis software.

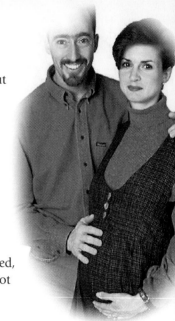

*I*magine waking up tomorrow and finding out you are pregnant! Although for many of you this is a physical impossibility, play along for a moment. Consider what being pregnant would mean to you. What changes would you need to make in your life? Think about your diet for a moment—would you change your eating habits if you found out you were pregnant? What changes would you make and why? What about other aspects of your lifestyle? Smoking, alcohol, exercise? What about after the baby is born? How would you feed your baby? If you chose to breastfeed, your dietary choices would continue to influence not only your health, but your baby's health as well.

Pregnancy

Pregnancy is a time of tremendous physiological changes, and these changes demand healthful dietary and lifestyle choices. The need for almost every nutrient increases, and in the case of iron, the recommended intake levels for the pregnant woman are *double* those of the nonpregnant woman. Although energy needs increase as well, the need for calories increases by a smaller percentage than the need for vitamins and minerals, meaning that food choices during pregnancy must be nutrient-dense.

What about tobacco and alcohol? Research clearly shows that both have damaging effects on a developing fetus; avoiding both during pregnancy is recommended. Although research about the effects of caffeine is less conclusive, most health-care professionals also recommend limiting caffeine intake during pregnancy.

As you read this chapter, think about the effects of pregnancy on nutrition and diet, and the changes a pregnant woman would need to make.

Preconceptional Nutrition

Everyone knows a woman needs to eat well once she becomes pregnant. But her nutrition status at the moment of conception is also critical. Vitamin status at conception, for example, can mean the difference between a healthy baby and one with a devastating birth defect. In addition, a woman's weight at conception can influence her pregnancy and delivery, and the baby's health.

For these reasons, many experts recommend extending prenatal care—the routine health care that a woman receives during her pregnancy—to include the preconception period as well (**Figure 14.1**). Two prestigious public health bodies, the Institute of Medicine and the U.S. Public Health Service Expert Panel on the Content of Prenatal Care, advocate routine preconception care for all prospective mothers.[1] While this position is certainly the ideal, it is important to realize that about half of pregnancies in the United States are unplanned. Hence, good nutrition for all women of childbearing age is an important public health objective.

Preconception care has three main components: risk assessment, health promotion, and intervention. Nutrition is an important aspect of all three components (**Table 14.1**). For example, risk assessment includes an evaluation of a prospective mother's vitamin status and weight, as well as her health habits—including use of alcohol, tobacco, and other substances—and her overall medical condition. Health promotion means providing the

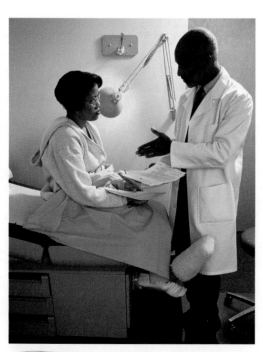

Figure 14.1 Preconception care is recommended for all prospective mothers.

would-be mother with information about the steps she can take to maximize her chances of a trouble-free pregnancy, an uneventful delivery, and a healthy, full-term baby. The third component of preconception care, intervention, can be as simple as prescribing a folic acid supplement, or as complex as treating an eating disorder or substance abuse. The goal is to resolve before conception the nutrition and health issues that could harm a mother or her baby.

Weight

For a woman contemplating pregnancy, weight is more than a cosmetic issue. Maternal obesity can complicate pregnancy and delivery, and may compromise a baby's health. Being too thin, meanwhile, carries its own risks.

Body Mass Index (BMI) is an index of a prospective mother's weight status. (See Chapter 8 to review how to calculate BMI.) Lean women with a BMI less than 20 have an increased risk of delivering a **low-birth-weight infant** and of **preterm delivery**.[2] At the other end of the spectrum, overweight and obese women have an increased risk of several adverse pregnancy outcomes, including preterm delivery and stillborn fetus.[3] For obese women, the risks include:

- high blood pressure
- impaired blood sugar metabolism (resulting in occasional low or high blood sugar
- **gestational diabetes** (a form of diabetes that is associated with pregnancy; it often is controlled through diet alone)
- **preeclampsia** (a condition marked by high blood pressure, fluid retention, and protein in the urine)
- prolonged labor
- unplanned cesarean section
- difficulty initiating and continuing breastfeeding[4]

Of course, the time to lose or gain weight is well before a pregnancy gets under way. It is not a good idea for pregnant women, even obese pregnant women, to diet. And a thin woman who finds it hard to put on weight

> **low-birth-weight infant** A newborn who weighs less than 2,500 grams (5.5 lb) as a result of either premature birth or inadequate growth in utero.
>
> **preterm delivery** A delivery that occurs before the 37th week of gestation.
>
> **gestational diabetes** A condition that results in high blood glucose during pregnancy.
>
> **preeclampsia** A condition of late pregnancy characterized by hypertension, edema, and proteinuria.

Quick Bites

Would it be healthier to menstruate *less* often?

Women in industrialized countries, who start menstruating at an average age of 12.5 years, will go through 350 to 400 menstrual cycles in their lifetimes. In populations where birth control is not used, however, women spend the majority of their fertile years either pregnant or lactating. Menarche in these populations occurs at an average age of 16. In addition, since menstrual cycles do not occur during pregnancy and may not occur during lactation, women in natural-fertility populations, like the Dogon of West Africa, experience only about 110 menstrual cycles in a lifetime. Women who go through fewer menstrual cycles are exposed to less estrogen and other steroid hormones. Researchers hypothesize that this may partly explain why nonindustrialized societies have lower cancer rates than industrialized societies.

Table 14.1 **Nutrition-Related Components of Preconception Care**

Risk Assessment

Age, diet, substance use (tobacco, alcohol, illicit drugs)
Existing medical condition(s)
Barriers to prenatal care and primary health care

Health Promotion

Healthful diet and refraining from substance use
Compliance with prenatal care

Interventions

Referral to high-risk pregnancy programs if necessary
Referral to treatment of adverse health behaviors
Nutrition counseling, supplementation, or referral to improve diet as needed

Source: Adapted in part from Jack B, et al. *Perspectives on Prenatal Care.* New York: Elsevier Science; 1990.

trimester One of the three periods of pregnancy, each lasting approximately 3 months.

cleavage The rapid cell divisions that occur in the ovum immediately after fertilization. This process transforms a single-celled zygote to a multicellular embryo.

blastogenic stage The first stage of gestation, during which tissue proliferation by cleavage begins.

placenta The organ formed during pregnancy that produces hormones for the maintenance of pregnancy and across which oxygen and nutrients are transferred from mother to infant, and waste materials are transferred from infant to mother.

SPINE AFFECTED BY SPINA BIFIDA

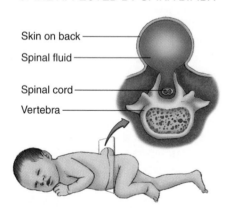

Skin on back
Spinal fluid
Spinal cord
Vertebra

Figure 14.2 **Spina bifida: a neural tube defect.**

Table 14.2 **Folate in Grain Products**

Foods	Folate (µg DFE)
Ready-to-eat cereals (25% DV), 1 C	170
Pasta, enriched, cooked, 1 C	140–160
Rice, enriched rice, cooked, 1 C	170
Tortilla, flour, enriched, 1 (10" diameter)	140
Bagel, enriched, 2 oz (3" diameter)	70
Bread, white, enriched, 1 slice	25–40

Source: Data compiled from Suitor CW, Bailey LB. Dietary folate equivalents: Interpretation and application. *J Am Diet Assoc.* 2000;100:88–94.

under normal circumstances is unlikely to find it easy when she's pregnant, especially if she experiences morning sickness.

Women with eating disorders have their own pregnancy-related risks. Ideally, anorexia nervosa or bulimia nervosa is diagnosed and treated well before conception, to give the prospective mother's body plenty of time to recover and prepare for the rigors of pregnancy, birth, and breastfeeding. A woman who enters pregnancy with an active eating disorder may not gain enough weight—or may vomit too much—to sustain a growing fetus. Results can include premature delivery, a low-birth-weight infant, and even fetal death.

Vitamins

Pregnancy, labor, delivery, and breastfeeding place increased demands on a mother's body. A good diet goes a long way toward meeting those demands, but even a carefully balanced diet may not be adequate nutritionally. This is especially true for folic acid, a nutrient needed to prevent neural tube defects, which are birth defects that involve the spinal column.[5] One of the most common neural tube defects is spina bifida, a birth defect in which part of the spinal cord protrudes through the spinal column, causing varying degrees of paralysis and lack of bowel and bladder control. Spina bifida and other neural tube defects affect approximately 4,000 pregnancies each year in the United States. (See **Figure 14.2**.)

In 1992, to reduce the incidence of these preventable birth defects, the U.S. Public Health Service made the following recommendation:

All women of childbearing age in the United States who are capable of becoming pregnant should consume 0.4 milligrams of folic acid per day for the purpose of reducing their risk of having a pregnancy affected with spina bifida and other neural tube defects.[6]

This recommendation covers *all* women of childbearing age—not just pregnant women—because neural tube development occurs before the sixth week of fetal life, when a woman may not know she is pregnant or may not have made appropriate dietary changes.

The revised RDA values for folate, published in 1998, state that all women capable of becoming pregnant should consume 0.4 milligrams of synthetic folic acid from fortified foods (such as enriched grain products) or supplements in addition to their consumption of folate in other foods. **Table 14.2** presents the folate content of selected grain products.

While it is important to get enough folic acid, it is also crucial to avoid getting too much vitamin A (retinol) during pregnancy. Some vitamin A is good for you; too much may be teratogenic. A teratogen is a substance that causes birth defects—literally, the term means "monster-producing." In one study of more than 22,000 pregnant women, one of every 57 who consumed more than 10,000 IU (3,000 RAE, or 3.75 times the RDA) of retinol daily during pregnancy gave birth to a child with birth defects of the head, heart, brain, or spinal cord.[7]

To avoid these tragedies, some scientists recommend that "women who are, or might become pregnant should avoid consuming supplements containing more than 8,000 IU (2,400 RAE) of retinol."[8] The FDA recommends that women limit their intake of retinol to 100 percent of the Daily Value (5,000 IU or 1500 RAE) and further, that they choose fortified foods that contain vitamin A in the form of beta-carotene rather than retinol.[9] Finally, any woman who might become pregnant must avoid using drugs that contain vitamin A or vitamin A analogs such as the cystic acne medications isotretinoin (Accutane) and tretinoin (Retin-A). These medications are potent teratogens.[10] Because of this, doctors typically prescribe such drugs to women of childbearing age only if they provide evidence of a negative pregnancy test, and practice birth control.

Pregnant women can—and should—eat as much as they like of fruits and vegetables rich in beta-carotene and other carotenoids. These foods pose no risk of birth defects, and offer many health benefits.

Substance Use

Many women plan to give up cigarettes, alcohol, or other drugs when they get pregnant. (See **Figure 14.3**.) A better plan is to give up the substances well before becoming pregnant. A woman who uses or abuses tobacco, alcohol, or illicit drugs prior to conception is likely to enter pregnancy with a low BMI and deficient nutritional stores.[11]

Key Concepts: *Ideally, the time to prepare nutritionally for pregnancy is well before conception. Adequate maternal nutrient stores, particularly of folic acid, along with healthy weight can reduce the risk for maternal and fetal complications during pregnancy. In addition to healthful diet selections, avoidance of cigarettes, alcohol, and other drugs is important when contemplating pregnancy.*

Physiology of Pregnancy

Pregnancy is an awe-inspiring process of growth and development that affects both mother and fetus. An understanding of the physiological changes that occur in the mother during pregnancy, along with the growth and development of the fetus, will help to explain the nutrient needs of a pregnant woman.

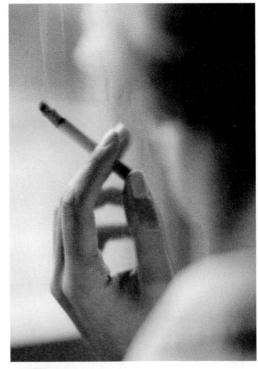

Figure 14.3 Avoid substance use before becoming pregnant.

Stages of Human Fetal Growth

How long does pregnancy last? Nine months, right? Well, it depends on when you start counting. When a health-care provider gives an expectant mother a due date, it is typically calculated as 40 weeks from the date of the start of her last menstrual period, roughly 10 to 14 days before the date of conception. This 40-week period is often divided into three **trimesters** of 13 or 14 weeks each; however, this division is somewhat arbitrary, and does not reflect specific stages of fetal development. **Figure 14.4** illustrates how conception occurs.

Following fertilization of the egg, or ovum, is the **blastogenic stage**—a period of rapid cell division known as **cleavage**. As these cells divide, they begin to differentiate. The inner cells in this growing mass will form the fetus; the outer layer of cells will become the **placenta**. During this stage, about 2 weeks long, the fertilized ovum implants itself in the wall of its mother's womb. The implanted ovum begins to secrete the hormone human chorionic gonadotropin (HCG), which can be detected in the mother's urine within a few days of implantation, but in most cases the mother does not yet suspect she is pregnant.

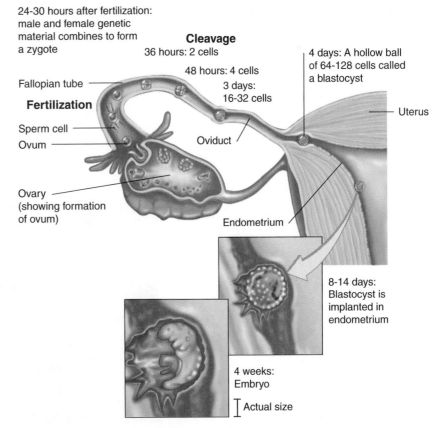

Figure 14.4 **How conception occurs.** The fertilized egg divides rapidly and begins to differentiate. The inner cells become the fetus and the outer cells become the placenta.

embryonic stage The developmental stage between the time of implantation (about 2 weeks after fertilization) through the 7th or 8th week; the stage of major organ system differentiation, and development of main external features.

critical period of development Time during which the environment has the greatest impact on the embryo.

fetal stage The time of rapid growth from the end of the embryonic stage until birth.

The next period of pregnancy, the **embryonic stage**, extends from the end of the second week through the eighth week after conception. The placenta, a vital organ that serves as a conduit between mother and child, forms on the uterine wall during this stage. Attached to the placenta by the umbilical cord, the embryo now receives its nourishment from its mother, and nearly everything the mother eats, drinks, or smokes reaches the embryo. This is the period of organogenesis. By the time the embryo is 8 weeks old, all of the main internal organs have formed, along with the major external body structures (**Figure 14.5**). Because nutrient deficiencies or toxicities and intake of harmful substances can result in congenital abnormalities (birth defects) or spontaneous abortion (miscarriage), this stage is a **critical period of development**. At the end of this stage, the embryo is still minute, only about 1 inch long. The mother has missed one menstrual period, and may have just confirmed her pregnancy using a home pregnancy test, or at a trip to the doctor. Because of all of the development that occurs in this early stage, the importance of preconception care cannot be overemphasized.

The longest period of pregnancy is the **fetal stage**. During this period, the fetus is growing rapidly, with dramatic changes in body proportions. From

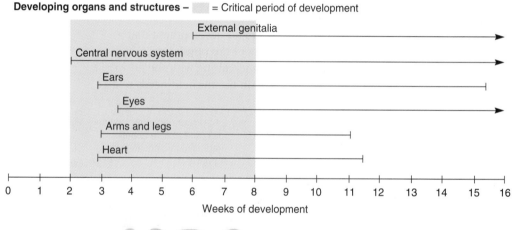

Developing organs and structures – ▨ = Critical period of development

External genitalia

Central nervous system

Ears

Eyes

Arms and legs

Heart

Weeks of development
0 1 2 3 4 5 6 7 8 9 10 11 12 13 14 15 16

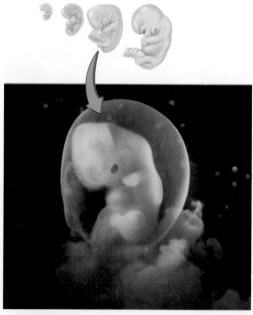

Figure 14.5 **Embryonic development.** During the embryonic stage—week two through week eight—the embryo is highly vulnerable to nutrient deficiencies and toxicities as well as harmful substances such as tobacco smoke.

the end of the third month of pregnancy until delivery at full-term, fetal weight increases nearly 500-fold. The typical newborn is about 20 inches long, and weighs approximately 7 pounds 7 ounces.

Key Concepts: *From conception to full-term baby, the process of fetal development is typically divided into three stages. The blastogenic stage involves rapid cell division of the fertilized ovum and implantation of the fertilized ovum in the uterine wall. Cells differentiate and organ systems and body structures are formed during the embryonic stage. The fetal stage is marked by growth and by change in body proportions, and is the longest stage of pregnancy.*

Maternal Physiological Changes and Nutrition

While the fertilized ovum develops from blastocyst to embryo to fetus, changes are occurring in the mother's body as well. (See **Figure 14.6**.) These changes occur as the result of various hormones, such as estrogen, progesterone, and human placental lactogen, secreted in response to pregnancy. The placenta is the major source of these hormones.

Growth of Maternal Tissue Maternal tissues, including the breasts, uterus, and adipose stores, increase in size during pregnancy. The hormone progesterone relaxes the smooth muscles of the uterus so that it can grow and expand as the fetus grows. Progesterone also affects the smooth muscles of the GI tract. Other hormones promote both growth and changes in the breast tissue that prepare for lactation. Fat stores increase to provide energy for late pregnancy and for lactation, and are a major component of maternal weight gain.

Maternal Blood Volume During the course of pregnancy, blood volume expands by nearly 50 percent. Production of red blood cells also increases.

Quick Bites

Who am I?

Our entire collection of genes, the human genome, contains about 30,000 genes. These genes are made of building blocks called base pairs. The human genome contains about three billion base pairs. Your mother supplied half of your genes and your father supplied the other half to create your unique combination. Unless you are an identical twin, no other person has your combination of genes.

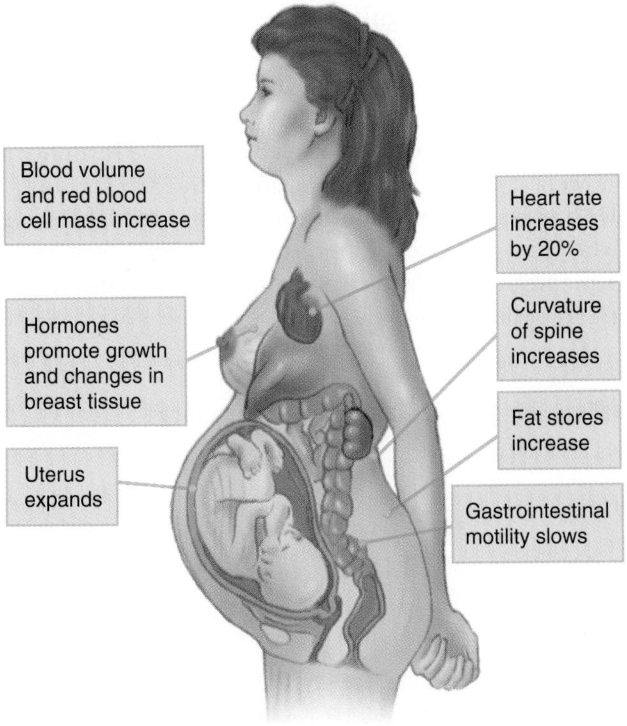

Blood volume and red blood cell mass increase

Hormones promote growth and changes in breast tissue

Uterus expands

Heart rate increases by 20%

Curvature of spine increases

Fat stores increase

Gastrointestinal motility slows

Figure 14.6 **Maternal changes during pregnancy.** Hormones released throughout pregnancy influence the growth of the baby and alter the way the mother's organs function. In addition, the growing baby displaces abdominal organs.

The new mother has about 20 percent more red blood cells than she had prior to pregnancy. Iron, folate, and vitamin B_{12} are all key nutrients in red blood cell production. Hemoglobin and hematocrit values during pregnancy are lower than when not pregnant, but this is more often due to the dilution of the blood cells (also known as hemodilution) than to nutrient deficiency. Still, regular monitoring of such markers of hematological status is an important component of prenatal care so that true deficiencies can be identified and treated early.

Gastrointestinal Changes During pregnancy, gastrointestinal motility slows, and food moves more slowly through the intestinal tract. On the plus side, because nutrients spend more time in the small intestine, nutrient absorption is increased. On the other hand, slower motility can contribute to nausea, heartburn, constipation, and hemorrhoids.

Key Concepts: *The mother's body undergoes various changes during pregnancy, guided by changing levels of hormones. Uterine, breast, and adipose tissues grow, blood volume expands, and gastrointestinal motility slows. All of these changes have nutritional and dietary implications for pregnant women.*

Maternal Weight Gain

How much weight should a woman gain during pregnancy? Doctors' recommendations have varied over time from minimal weight gain to unlimited weight gain, to more recent recommendations based on prepregnancy BMI, as shown in **Table 14.3**. For women of normal weight (BMI 19.8–26), the recommended weight gain is 25 to 35 pounds (12.5–18 kg).[12] For the heaviest women—those with BMIs greater than 29 at the start of pregnancy—the Institute of Medicine recommends a weight gain of at least 15 pounds (6 kg), but not much more. When maternal weight gain is within these limits, the infant is more likely to be born healthy and at term. These more flexible recommendations recognize that weight gain varies widely among women who give birth to healthy, full-term infants.[13]

Twin births account for one of every 90 live births in the United States. Of course, women who carry two or more fetuses need to gain more weight than women who carry just one. Based on available data, the Institute of Medicine suggests a weight gain of 35 to 45 pounds (16–20.5 kg) for women pregnant with twins. The institute also recommends higher weight gains for women who were underweight prior to pregnancy. When an expectant mother's prepregnancy BMI is less than 19.8, the recommended weight gain is 28 to 40 pounds (13–18 kg).

Table 14.3 Guidelines for Weight Gain during Pregnancy

Prepregnancy BMI (kg/m²)	Weight Gain* (kg)	(lb)
Low (< 19.8)	12.5–18	28–40
Normal (19.8–26)	11.5–16	25–35
High (>26–29)	7.0–11.5	15–25
Obese (> 29)	≥ 6	≥ 15

*Young adolescents should strive for gains at the upper end of the recommended range. Short women (<157 cm or 62 in.) should strive for gains at the lower end of the range.

Source: Adapted with permission from *Nutrition During Pregnancy.* Copyright 1990 by the National Academy of Sciences. Courtesy of the National Academy Press, Washington, DC.

The pattern of weight gain is also important to a healthy pregnancy outcome. During the first trimester, average weight gain is low, less than 5 pounds for most women. Over the second and third trimester, the suggested weight gain is a little less than 1 pound a week (0.4 kg per week); with more gain suggested for underweight women and those carrying twins, and a lower gain for women who are overweight.[14] Monitoring the amount and rate of weight gain is an important component of prenatal care.

The weight gained during pregnancy can be divided into two major parts: the fetus and associated tissues and fluids, and maternal tissue growth. In a typical final weight gain of 27.5 pounds (12.5 kg), the fetus, placenta, and **amniotic fluid** account for nearly 40 percent of that weight. Maternal tissues (i.e., adipose stores, breast and uterine growth, and expanded blood and extracellular fluid volumes) account for the remaining 60 percent (see **Figure 14.7**).

Key Concepts: *Weight gained during pregnancy is a combination of fetal and maternal tissues and fluids. Weight gain recommendations are based on BMI prior to pregnancy. Women of normal weight (BMI = 19.8–26) should gain 25 to 35 pounds over the course of pregnancy. Most of this weight gain occurs during the second and third trimesters.*

Energy and Nutrients during Pregnancy

Growing a baby takes energy. A pregnant woman requires added calories to grow and maintain not just her developing fetus, but also the placenta, increased breast tissue, and fat stores, and to fuel other metabolic changes. Growth and development of the fetus also requires nutrients—carbohydrates and fat as a source of energy, and protein, vitamins, and minerals to support growth and cell differentiation.

Energy

The current RDA for energy suggests that during the second and third trimesters, when fetal growth is the greatest, pregnant women need 300 kilocalories per day more than they did prior to pregnancy. This figure is based on estimations that a full-term pregnancy demands roughly 80,000 kilocalories above a woman's usual calorie intake.[15]

Recent evidence suggests that this recommendation is too simplistic, and does not reflect the wide variation in energy expended by pregnant women.[16] A prospective study of 16 women measured the components of energy expenditure, energy intake, and fat mass before pregnancy, in each trimester, and 4 to 6 weeks postpartum. Although the average estimated total energy cost of pregnancy was similar to other estimates, the actual variation in energy balance among these subjects was substantial. When compared to nonpregnant values, total energy expenditure throughout pregnancy ranged from a decrease of 25 kilocalories per day to an increase of more than 800 kilocalories per day. On average, the increase in total energy expenditure was about 24 percent. Energy intake, however, increased by an average of only 9 percent. The researchers speculated that women's bodies may compensate for increases in metabolism during pregnancy by minimizing fat deposition, or reducing the energy required for activity and the thermic effect of food.[17] Weight gain during pregnancy is probably the best indicator of adequate calorie intake.

As mentioned in the discussion of preconception care, dieting to lose weight or sharply restrict weight gain during pregnancy is never advisable. Severe energy restriction may result in ketosis, which may harm the fetus.[18]

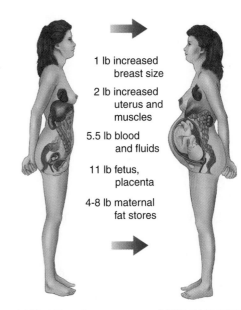

1 lb increased breast size

2 lb increased uterus and muscles

5.5 lb blood and fluids

11 lb fetus, placenta

4-8 lb maternal fat stores

(a) First trimester   (b) Third trimester

Figure 14.7 **Components of maternal weight gain.** During the first trimester, most women gain less than five pounds. Over the second and third trimester, the suggested weight gain is a little less than 1 pound a week.

amniotic fluid The fluid that surrounds the fetus contained in the amniotic sac inside the uterus.

In the first trimester, severe energy restriction is associated with higher rates of premature delivery, fetal death, and malformations of the infant's central nervous system. During the second and third trimesters, the primary consequence of maternal energy restriction is slowed fetal growth so that the fetus is underdeveloped for his or her age.

Key Concepts: *The RDA for energy is increased by 300 kilocalories per day for pregnancy, although current evidence suggests that the actual increase in need varies substantially among women. Determination of weight gain is an important tool for assessment of the adequacy of energy intake. Weight loss is not advised during pregnancy, even for obese women.*

Nutrients to Support Pregnancy

Most healthy women who eat a well-balanced diet have no trouble meeting the majority of their nutrient requirements in pregnancy without vitamin and mineral supplements. It is still routine, however, for health-care providers to prescribe specially formulated prenatal multivitamin/mineral supplements. The Institute of Medicine's (IOM) Nutrient Supplement Subcommittee concluded that there is no need for routine multivitamin/mineral supplements among healthy pregnant women. However, because some pregnant women are unlikely to get enough iron and folate through diet alone, the IOM recommends routine iron and possibly folate supplementation.[19] At the time of the IOM report, the RDA for folate during pregnancy was 400 micrograms. It is now 600 micrograms. At this newer recommended intake level, the subcommittee would probably have concluded that routine supplementation was warranted.

Essential nutrients can be divided into two broad categories: macronutrients (proteins, fats, and carbohydrates) and micronutrients (vitamins and minerals). **Figure 14.8** shows the nutrient recommendations for pregnant women compared to nonpregnant women.

Macronutrients Macronutrients supply energy and provide the building blocks for protein synthesis. The recommended balance of energy sources does not change during pregnancy. A low-fat, moderate-protein, high-carbohydrate diet is still appropriate.

Protein. A pregnant woman's RDA for protein is 60 grams—about 10–15 grams a day higher than that recommended for women in the general population. This amount of protein is needed for the synthesis of new maternal, placental, and fetal tissues, and is easily supplied in typical American diets consumed by nonpregnant women. Thus many women need not increase their protein intake to reach the levels recommended. Pregnant women who are vegetarians, including vegans, also should be able to meet their protein needs from food sources alone—as long as they select a variety of protein sources and consume enough total calories

Only one group of women is at risk of inadequate protein intake during pregnancy: women whose total calorie intake is low.[20] The solution is to increase calorie intake from a variety of foods, not just those high in protein. Because taking high-protein supplements may increase the risk of premature delivery and low birth weight, they are not recommended.[21]

Fats. In the course of a normal pregnancy, bloodstream levels of fatty compounds are elevated significantly by the end of the third trimester. These fats provide vital fuel for the mother and for the development of placental tissues. The pregnant woman's body also stores fats that can support breastfeeding after childbirth. *Very* low-fat diets (in which fewer than 10

NUTRITIONAL RECOMMENDATIONS FOR PREGNANCY

	Nonpregnant	Pregnant	% increase
Energy (kcal)	2,200	2,500	14
Protein (g)	46	60	30
Vitamin A (μgRAE)	700	770	10
Vitamin D (μg)	5	5	0
Vitamin E (mg)	15	15	0
Vitamin K (μg)	90	90	0
Thiamin (mg)	1.1	1.4	27
Riboflavin (mg)	1.1	1.4	27
Niacin (mg)	14	18	29
Vitamin B_6 (mg)	1.3	1.9	46
Folate (μg)	400	600	50
Vitamin B_{12} (μg)	2.4	2.6	8
Choline (mg)	425	450	6
Vitamin C (mg)	75	85	13
Calcium (mg)	1,000	1,000	0
Phosphorus (mg)	700	700	0
Magnesium (mg)	310	350	13
Iron (mg)	18	27	50
Zinc (mg)	8	11	38
Selenium (μg)	55	60	9
Iodine (μg)	150	220	47
Fluoride (mg)	3	3	0
Copper (μg)	900	1000	11
Chromium (μg)	25	30	20
Manganese (mg)	1.8	2	11
Molybdenum (μg)	45	50	11

Figure 14.8 **Nutritional recommendations for pregnancy.** Needs for most nutrients increase during pregnancy. Generally, vitamin and mineral needs increase more than energy needs, which means that food choices should be nutrient dense. Values shown are RDA or AI values for ages 19–30.

percent of daily calories come from dietary fats) are not recommended for pregnancy. Such diets are unlikely to supply sufficient amounts of essential fatty acids or fat-soluble vitamins. Moreover, because fats are the most calorie-dense of the macronutrients, a woman who eats a very low-fat diet may find it difficult to consume as many calories as she needs to support a healthy pregnancy.

Carbohydrates. Carbohydrates provide the main source of extra calories during pregnancy. Food choices should emphasize complex carbohydrates such as breads, fortified cereals, rice, and pasta. In addition to supplying vitamins and minerals, these foods increase fiber intake substantially. A fiber-rich diet is recommended during pregnancy to help prevent constipation and hemorrhoids.

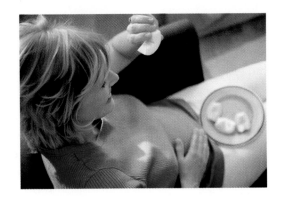

Key Concepts: *Most healthy women with well-balanced diets meet the majority of their nutrient requirements in pregnancy without supplements. Although protein needs increase during pregnancy, the basic balance of energy sources should still emphasize complex carbohydrates. As long as energy intake is adequate, and a variety of foods are eaten, protein intake should be more than adequate to support prenatal growth and development.*

Fyi Vegetarianism and Pregnancy

FOR YOUR INFORMATION

Can pregnant women meet all of their nutritional needs on a vegetarian diet? A fair question. Common vegetarian practices include the avoidance of meat, poultry, and fish (lacto-ovo-vegetarian and lactovegetarian) and the avoidance of all animal foods (vegan). These foods are important sources of iron, zinc, calcium, and other nutrients. Although vegetarian diets can provide reasonable quantities of trace elements, animal-derived foods frequently contribute larger amounts that the body absorbs more easily. To meet the demands of pregnancy, supplementation may be in order.

Supplemental iron is generally recommended for all pregnant women. Supplemental vitamin B$_{12}$ (2.0 micrograms per day) is also recommended for vegan mothers. If their sun exposure is limited, they also may need daily supplementation of 10 micrograms of vitamin D.[1] Vegetarians with low calcium intake (<600 milligrams per day) should consume a supplement that provides at least 500 milligrams per day. Some vegan foods, such as fortified soy milks, may contain these important nutrients.

The overall nutrient content of a vegetarian diet depends on both the energy content and the variety of the foods consumed. The suggested dietary patterns in Table A will meet the average energy levels recommended for pregnant women.

1 Institute of Medicine. *Dietary Reference Intakes for Calcium, Phosphorus, Magnesium, Vitamin D, and Fluoride.* Washington, DC: National Academy Press; 1997.

Table A: **Suggested Servings for Pregnant Vegans**

Food Group	2,200 kcal	2,800 kcal
Bread, grains, cereals (50% whole-grain products)	10	12
Legumes, plant proteins	2	3
Vegetables	3	4
Dark-green leafy vegetables	2	2
Fruits	4	6
Nuts, seeds	1	1
Fortified soy drinks* and tofu	3	3
Added fats and oils	4	6
Approximate Composition		
Protein (g)	76	95
% Kcal as fat	24	25
% Kcal as carbohydrate	62	61

* Milk alternatives fortified with calcium, vitamin D, and vitamin B$_{12}$

Source: Adapted from Haddad, EH. Development of a vegetarian food guide. *Am J Clin Nutr.* 1994;59(suppl.):1248S–1254S.

Micronutrients A pregnant woman has an increased need for many vitamins and minerals that support growth and development. In addition, her increased energy needs require higher amounts of nutrients, such as the B vitamins thiamin, riboflavin, niacin, and pantothenic acid, which are essential for energy metabolism.

Needs for the other B vitamins (except biotin) also increase. Folate and vitamin B_{12} are used in synthesis of DNA and red blood cells, and vitamin B_6 is crucial for metabolism of amino acids. Of these vitamins, folate needs increase the most. For nonpregnant women, the RDA for folate is 400 micrograms per day of dietary folate equivalents (DFE). For pregnant women, the RDA is 600 micrograms per day as DFE. Vitamin C needs increase slightly during pregnancy, from 75 to 85 milligrams per day for women ages 19 to 50 years. For the fat-soluble vitamins, the RDA for vitamin A increases during pregnancy, while the recommended intake levels for vitamins D, E, and K are unchanged.

When the DRI committee completed its review of calcium and related nutrients (phosphorus, magnesium, fluoride, and vitamin D), they increased only the magnesium recommendations for pregnancy. Pregnancy enhances calcium absorption and the committee determined that pregnant women maintain their calcium balance with calcium intake levels similar to those of nonpregnant women. To support growth of lean tissue, the RDA for magnesium increases by 40 milligrams per day during pregnancy.[22]

For the other minerals, recommended intakes are higher during pregnancy, most dramatically for iron. The RDA for iron increases from 18 milligrams per day to 27 milligrams per day. Iron is necessary to make red blood cells and is important for normal growth and energy metabolism. Iron deficiency, and its associated anemia, is the most common nutrient deficiency in pregnancy. Because hemoglobin and hematocrit levels normally decline in pregnancy as the blood volume increases, doctors use different standards to evaluate these parameters in pregnant women.[23] **Table 14.4** lists the characteristics of women who are at particularly high risk for iron deficiency during pregnancy.

Getting 27 milligrams of iron in the daily diet is not easy, so experts recommend iron supplementation for the general population of pregnant women.[24] A single-salt iron supplement such as ferrous sulfate is best. A woman can maximize absorption of an iron supplement by eating it on an empty stomach (between meals or at bedtime), and washing it down with liquids other than milk, tea, or coffee, which inhibit absorption.

Higher iron doses are not recommended. Too much iron can cause diarrhea, constipation, nausea, and heartburn. In addition, excess iron consumption may result, paradoxically, in decreased iron absorption by the body. Finally, consuming iron supplements may reduce the body's absorption of zinc, another essential mineral, and is dangerous for those with hemochromatosis (see Chapter 12, "Trace Minerals").

Key Concepts: *Needs for vitamins and minerals increase during pregnancy, some more than others. Extra micronutrients are needed to support growth and development, and increased energy use. Recommended intake levels increase most dramatically for folate and iron.*

Table 14.4 **Factors Associated with Increased Risk for Iron Deficiency during Pregnancy**

Young age (e.g., 15 to 19 years)
Multiple gestation
Diets low in meat and ascorbic acid
Diets high in coffee and tea
Low socioeconomic status
Low level of education
Black or Hispanic ethnicity

Source: Adapted from Puolakka J, Janne O, Pakarinen A, Vihko R. Serum ferritin in the diagnosis of anemia during pregnancy. *Acta Obstet Gynecol Scand.* 1980;95(suppl.):57–63.

Food Choices for Pregnant Women

Think
About It
2

You may be surprised to learn that the recommended diet for a pregnant woman is not much different from that for adults in the general population. The familiar Food Guide Pyramid recommendations apply to pregnant women.

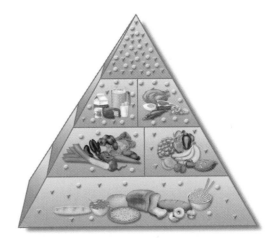

Food Group	Food Pyramid Servings	2,200 kcal Servings	2,800 kcal Servings
Bread, cereal, rice, and pasta	6–11	9	11
Vegetables	3–5	4	5
Fruits	2–3	3	4
Milk, yogurt, and cheese	2–3	3	3
Meat, poultry, fish, dried beans, eggs, and nuts	2–3	6 oz	7 oz
Fats, oils, and sweets	——Use sparingly——		

The only specific advice for pregnant women is to consume at least three servings of milk or other dairy products each day. Sample menus using the Food Guide Pyramid for 2,200 and 2,800 kilocalories can be planned that meet all the nutrient needs for pregnant women, with the exception of folate and iron.[25] Variety is the key to a well-balanced diet. The extra calories needed for pregnancy are easy to obtain from an additional serving of grains, vegetables, fruits, and low-fat milk. Because the increased need for energy is proportionately less than the increased need for most nutrients, nutrient-dense foods are important. There is little room in the diet plan for high-calorie, high-fat, low-nutrient "extras."

Supplementation

Other than iron and probably folate, a pregnant woman can get all of the nutrients she needs by making healthful choices using the Food Guide Pyramid. Ideally, health-care providers should evaluate the dietary intake of all prenatal patients and recommend dietary changes to improve nutrient intake where needed. In reality, this seldom happens, and pregnant women in the United States routinely receive prescriptions for prenatal vitamin/mineral supplements. The amount and balance of nutrients in prenatal formulations is appropriate for pregnancy. Because toxic levels can be reached quickly, especially for vitamins A and D, pregnant women should avoid high-dose and multiple supplements. In addition, because most herbal preparations have not been evaluated for safety during pregnancy, they are not recommended.

Foods to Avoid

Generally, no foods are completely off-limits to pregnant women, with the exception of alcohol. If a mother-to-be is experiencing problems with nausea and vomiting, she may want to abstain for a while from foods that aggravate these symptoms. Cultural traditions may dictate changes in diet, but these tend to reflect traditional beliefs and practices rather than physiological relationships.

The need to restrict or eliminate caffeine during pregnancy remains controversial. High caffeine intake has been shown to be teratogenic in animal studies, and has been linked to low birth weight in humans. Recent studies suggest that low birth weight with high caffeine consumption occurs only in combination with smoking. Nonetheless, since caffeine sources tend to be low in nutrients, it is prudent to limit caffeine intake during pregnancy.

Key Concepts: A well-balanced, varied diet can easily meet all of a pregnant woman's nutrient needs, with the exception of iron and folate. Pregnant women should choose nutrient-dense and high-carbohydrate foods, in the balance found in the Food Guide Pyramid. Although vitamin/mineral supplementation is common during pregnancy, other than for iron and folate, it is probably not needed. When supplements are used, they should be designed for pregnant women. Pregnant women should avoid alcohol and moderate their intake of caffeine.

Substance Use and Pregnancy Outcome

When a pregnant woman eats, she eats for two. When she smokes, drinks, or uses drugs, she does so for two as well. The consequences of these behaviors may be felt for generations.

Tobacco and Alcohol

Smoking during pregnancy increases the risks of miscarrying, delivering a stillborn infant, giving birth prematurely, and delivering a low-birth-weight baby.[26] Women in lower socioeconomic groups have the highest rates of cigarette use before, during, and after pregnancy. Women in the highest socioeconomic groups, meanwhile, are the most likely to quit smoking during pregnancy, but are as likely as other women to take up the habit again after giving birth.

Alcohol is a powerful drug that crosses the placenta and enters the baby's bloodstream in the same concentration as its mother's. Moreover, because the fetus's immature liver does not produce the necessary enzymes, the fetus cannot metabolize the alcohol effectively.[27]

Fetal alcohol syndrome (FAS) describes a consistent pattern of physical, cognitive, and behavioral problems in infants born to women who use alcohol heavily during pregnancy. The incidence of fetal alcohol syndrome has been estimated at 10 percent for women consuming 1.5 to 8 drinks per

[*Fyi*] Pregnancy and Postpartum Exercise

FOR YOUR INFORMATION

Maintenance, rather than improvement, of fitness should be the goal during pregnancy.[1] Generally, women can continue to participate at their current level of activity as long as there are no contraindications. Necessary modifications to an exercise plan depend on the maternal and fetal response to the type of exercise, and any exercise plan should be discussed with the health-care provider. For example, pregnant women should avoid exercise in the supine position (lying down) after the fourth month of gestation. As pregnancy progresses, intensity of running should be decreased. The following maternal and fetal responses to exercise are adapted from animal and human studies:[2]

Maternal Physiology at Rest and during Exercise

- Resting heart rate increases by approximately 15 beats per minute during pregnancy.
- Distribution of blood to the mother's muscles is decreased due to increased uterine blood flow.
- Ventilation rate increases.

Fetal Responses to Exercise

- Animal studies have reported decreases in arterial oxygen and carbon dioxide during maternal exercise.
- Circulation remains stable; heart rate may increase or decrease initially, but then stabilizes.

Concerns Related to Exercise during Pregnancy

- Any decrease in uterine blood flow can compromise fetal blood flow.
- Utero-placental oxygen insufficiency could retard fetal oxygen supply.
- Maternal or fetal hypoglycemia could compromise maternal and fetal glucose supply.

The American College of Obstetrics and Gynecology offers the following guidelines for exercise during pregnancy and postpartum. A controversy exists regarding maternal target heart rate during exercise. The individual's prepregnancy fitness level is considered a better predictor of the maximum allowable

week and 30 to 40 percent for women who consume more than 8 drinks per week.[28] Children severely afflicted by the syndrome show marked growth deficiencies before and after birth, physical anomalies such as a small head, certain characteristic facial irregularities, heart defects, and joint and limb irregularities; mental retardation; and central nervous system disorders. The greater a mother's alcohol use during pregnancy, the more severe the symptoms of FAS tend to be in the child. (See **Figure 14.9**.) A woman suffering from alcoholism may have a poor diet as well, resulting in energy and nutrient deficiencies that can further harm a developing fetus.

There is no known safe threshold for alcohol use in pregnancy. Low to moderate levels of alcohol consumption may result in offspring with possible fetal alcohol effects including cognitive and behavior problems.[29] The only way to avoid alcohol-related risks to a fetus is to avoid all alcohol during pregnancy. In 1981 the U.S. Surgeon General advised pregnant women to abstain completely from alcohol. This recommendation still stands.

Drugs

The main active ingredient of marijuana, 9-tetrahydrocannabinol, crosses the placenta and enters the fetal bloodstream. A pregnant woman who smokes marijuana increases the risk for miscarriage, premature delivery, and low birth weight. In addition, maternal marijuana use may result in some of the same physical abnormalities seen in infants with FAS. Effects on the fetus vary depending on the mother's diet, frequency of her marijuana use, and whether she uses other drugs.

Cocaine use has reached epidemic proportions among women of childbearing age in the United States, with the greatest use among African American and Hispanic women.[30] In addition to addicting the newborn, cocaine use increases risks of stroke, prematurity, fetal growth retardation, miscarriage, and certain congenital anomalies.[31] Some of these problems may stem from the mother's nutritional deficiencies both before and

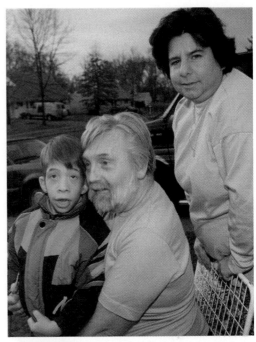

Figure 14.9 **Fetal alcohol syndrome.** The facial characteristics of a child with fetal alcohol syndrome include a short nose with a flattened bridge, eyelids with extra folds, and a thin upper lip with no groove below the nose.

---

exercise heart rate than is an absolute rate of 140 to 150 beats per minute[3].

Guidelines for Exercise
- Precede exercise with a 5- to 10-minute warm-up.
- Follow exercise with a cool-down period of gentle stretching that does not reach maximum extension.
- Regular exercise at least three times per week is preferred to less regular activity.
- Do not exercise vigorously in hot, humid weather or with a fever.
- Avoid reaching maximum exertion and deep flexion or extension of joints.

- Establish target heart rates in consultation with a physician.
- Stand up gradually to avoid lightheadedness. Do not exercise in the supine position after the fourth month of gestation.
- If unusual symptoms appear, stop activity and consult a physician.
- To prevent dehydration, drink fluids liberally before, during, and after exercise.
- Ascertain that caloric intake is adequate to meet the extra needs of pregnancy *and* exercise.
- Avoid hot tubs and saunas.

1 Kullick K, Dugan L. Exercise and pregnancy. In: Rossenbloom CA, ed. *Sports Nutrition.* 3rd ed. Chicago, IL: The American Dietetic Association; 2000.

2 Ibid.

3 Ibid.

morning sickness A persistent or recurring nausea that often occurs in the morning during early pregnancy.

during pregnancy, as well as from concurrent tobacco and alcohol use, which is common among cocaine users. **Figure 14.10** illustrates the possible effects of a woman's using drugs while she is pregnant.

Key Concepts: *Smoking, alcohol, and illicit drug use during pregnancy can all have devastating effects on fetal development. Low birth weight, preterm delivery, and congenital malformations are some of the consequences. Fetal alcohol syndrome is a set of physical, mental, and behavioral consequences of alcohol consumption during pregnancy. A pregnant woman should avoid all these substances.*

Special Situations during Pregnancy

Most women progress through pregnancy with no more than a mild period of morning sickness or problems with constipation or heartburn. However, complications such as abnormal glucose tolerance or elevated blood pressure may affect dietary choices or nutrition status. Also, some women have unique nutritional needs during pregnancy. These include women with certain chronic illnesses such as diabetes, and adolescents, who are themselves still developing.

Gastrointestinal Distress

Morning sickness, or nausea associated with pregnancy, is most common early in pregnancy as the mother's body adjusts to changes in hormone levels. Many pregnant women find they experience less "morning sickness" if they eat dry cereal, toast, or crackers about half an hour before getting out of bed. Keeping some food in the stomach throughout the day helps, too. This means eating smaller, more frequent meals, and drinking liquids between meals instead of with food. Avoiding food aromas that trigger nausea is another useful tactic.

Heartburn and constipation are the result of slowed GI movement. Remaining upright for at least an hour after eating, and having smaller, more frequent meals may prevent heartburn. Getting plenty of fiber and fluids in the diet, and getting regular mild to moderate exercise can limit constipation. Of course, a pregnant woman should always consult her

Figure 14.10 **Substance use can lead to birth defects.** When a pregnant woman smokes, drinks, or uses drugs, so does her growing baby. The consequences of these behaviors may be felt for generations.

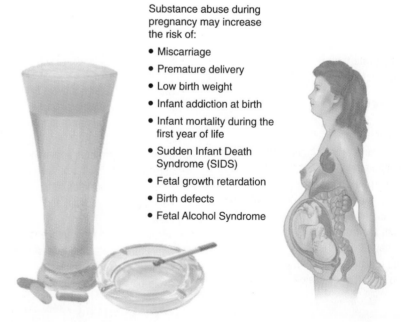

Substance abuse during pregnancy may increase the risk of:

- Miscarriage
- Premature delivery
- Low birth weight
- Infant addiction at birth
- Infant mortality during the first year of life
- Sudden Infant Death Syndrome (SIDS)
- Fetal growth retardation
- Birth defects
- Fetal Alcohol Syndrome

health-care provider before using a prescription drug, over-the-counter medicine, or home remedy for nausea, vomiting, heartburn, or constipation.

Food Cravings and Aversions

Many pregnant women experience specific food cravings and/or aversions, and we often laugh at stories about unusual combinations such as pickles and ice cream. These changes in food preference may be linked to taste and metabolic changes, but they rarely have a physiological basis such as a nutrient deficiency. Most cravings and aversions do not affect the quality of the diet unless food choices become very narrow.

Some pregnant women crave nonfood items such as starch or clay. Pica is the routine consumption of nonfood items such as dirt, clay, laundry starch, ice, or burnt matches. Although to some this behavior seems outlandish, it is in many cases a culturally-accepted practice that affects significant numbers of pregnant women, especially in rural areas of the Southeastern United States. Pica could be harmful if nonfood items crowd nutritious foods out of the diet. In addition, nonfood items may contain toxins, bacteria, and parasites, and in the case of laundry starch, a significant number of calories may be consumed without providing any micronutrients.

Hypertension

Measurement of blood pressure is a routine part of prenatal care. When uncomplicated by other symptoms, increased blood pressure during pregnancy is usually a transient condition with little risk. However, the combination of hypertension, edema, and proteinuria (protein in the urine) indicates the condition known as preeclampsia. If preeclampsia progresses to eclampsia, it can be life-threatening for both mother and baby.

Preeclampsia is more common in women who are pregnant for the first time, adolescents, and women older than 35, and those with pre-existing diabetes or hypertension. In mild cases, bed rest and close monitoring are the treatments of choice. Sodium restriction and drug therapy are not recommended. Severe cases may require more aggressive treatment. Studies show that preventive measures such as aspirin or calcium supplementation offer no benefit. Early identification of preeclampsia through routine prenatal care is important for good maternal and fetal outcomes.

Diabetes

A woman with diabetes faces special challenges in pregnancy. She has an increased risk of developing preeclampsia and a greater-than-average chance of problems that affect the fetus, including fetal death. However, with early prenatal intervention and careful control of blood sugar levels, these risks can be reduced to the same level as that in nondiabetic pregnancies.[32]

Pregnancy may require frequent adjustments of both diet and insulin to keep blood sugar in check. Insulin requirements often decrease during the first half of pregnancy, but increase during the second half. Some diabetic women who did not need insulin before they became pregnant and were able to control their blood sugar through diet alone, may begin to need insulin during their pregnancy.

Gestational Diabetes

Gestational diabetes is a condition in which abnormal glucose tolerance exists only during pregnancy and resolves after delivery. The hormones of pregnancy tend to be antagonistic to the action of insulin, and in about four percent of pregnancies, this results in a rise in blood glucose.

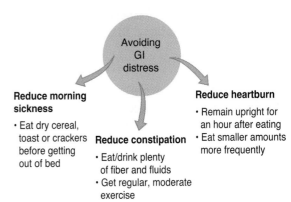

Avoiding GI distress

Reduce morning sickness
- Eat dry cereal, toast or crackers before getting out of bed

Reduce constipation
- Eat/drink plenty of fiber and fluids
- Get regular, moderate exercise

Reduce heartburn
- Remain upright for an hour after eating
- Eat smaller amounts more frequently

Table 14.5 **Factors Associated with Gestational Diabetes**

Age > 25 years
Obesity, at any age
Family history of diabetes mellitus
Previous poor pregnancy outcome
History of abnormal glucose tolerance
Ethnicity associated with high incidence
of diabetes

Gestational diabetes often can be controlled through diet. Although screening of all women has been routine, current policy of the American Diabetes Association is to screen only those at high risk through an oral glucose tolerance test between the 24th and 28th weeks of pregnancy.[33] **Table 14.5** lists factors associated with an increased risk of gestational diabetes.

Phenylketonuria

Phenylketonuria (PKU) is an inherited defect in which the body is unable to metabolize phenylalanine, an essential amino acid found in egg whites, milk, some other protein-containing foods, and the artificial sweetener aspartame. People born with PKU require a carefully planned diet with enough phenylalanine to satisfy essential amino acids requirements while preventing excess phenylalanine from building up to toxic levels in the bloodstream. High blood levels of phenylalanine can cause mental retardation.

Women with PKU who become pregnant must minimize dietary sources of phenylalanine, while ensuring adequate protein intake—no easy task. They also need to look for the required warning label on foods and beverages that are sweetened with aspartame, and avoid those products. (The American Medical Association states that consumption of aspartame in "customary" amounts in normal pregnancy is not likely to be toxic to the fetus.)

AIDS

Women with AIDS are likely to have multiple nutrition problems, including protein-energy malnutrition, vitamin and mineral deficiencies, and inadequate weight gain. All of these can pose risks for the fetus. A pregnant woman with AIDS requires intensive nutrition management. Approximately 25 to 30 percent of pregnant women with HIV transmit the AIDS virus to their newborns, but medical intervention can reduce this number substantially.

Adolescence

Despite prevention efforts, adolescent pregnancy rates in the United States are among the highest in the developed world.[34] Pregnant adolescents are nutritionally at risk. Their own needs for growth and development are compromised by the extra demands posed by the growth and development of the fetus. Risks for preeclampsia, anemia, premature birth, low-birth-weight babies, infant mortality, and sexually transmitted diseases are all increased for pregnant adolescents under the age of 16.[35]

Prior to becoming pregnant, many teenagers do not demonstrate healthful eating patterns. Their diets are likely to be inadequate in total energy intake, calcium, iron, zinc, riboflavin, folic acid and vitamins A, D, and B_6. Poverty, smoking, and abuse of alcohol and other substances compound the negative effects of adolescent nutritional inadequacies.

Nutrition care for pregnant teens starts with determining daily energy needs. The Institute of Medicine recommends that pregnant adolescents be encouraged to strive for weight gains toward the upper end of the range recommended for adult mothers (see **Table 14.3**).[36] Need for supplemental vitamins and minerals is also greater in this age group.

Key Concepts: *Numerous factors affect the dietary needs and choices of pregnant women. Routine prenatal care is important to identify unhealthful eating behaviors and potential complications such as preeclampsia and gestational diabetes. Pregnant women with diabetes, PKU, or AIDS need special dietary intervention. Pregnant teens have especially high nutrient needs to fuel not only fetal growth, but also their own adolescent growth.*

Lactation

During pregnancy, physiological changes in breast tissue and fat stores prepare the woman's body for the demands of lactation. Preparation for lactation also involves education. Although breastfeeding is one of the most natural functions of a woman's body, there is much to learn about lactation so that breastfeeding is a success for both mother and infant.

Breastfeeding Trends

Public health goals since the late 1970s have been to increase the percentage of infants who are breast-fed. The goal of *Healthy People 2010* is to increase the proportion of newborns who are initially breast-fed to at least 75 percent. Efforts have been moderately successful; approximately 60 percent of infants are now breast-fed initially, up from a low of 20 percent in the early 1970s.[37] **Figure 14.11** illustrates trends in breastfeeding since 1900.

However, only about 30 percent of infants are still being breast-fed at 6 months of age, much lower than the *Healthy People 2010* goal of 50 percent. What are the reasons for this trend? Lack of knowledge about the benefits of breastfeeding for both mother and baby surely plays a role. Societal attitudes regarding the acceptability of breastfeeding are certainly influential, and vary across cultural and demographic groups. Some states have actually had to pass laws stating that breastfeeding in public is not indecent exposure! In addition, the decline in breastfeeding through the 1950s and 1960s affected the attitudes and knowledge base of today's grandmothers.

Decisions about infant feeding must take place from an informed perspective. Information about the mechanics of breastfeeding along with the benefits for both mother and baby should be an integral part of prenatal care.

Key Concepts: *Increasing the proportion of infants who are breast-fed is an important public health goal. Although more than half of infants born in the United States are breast-fed initially, only 20 percent are still being breast-fed at 6 months of age.*

Quick Bites

Breastfeeding and Birth Control

Does breastfeeding prevent pregnancy? No. But under certain conditions, breastfeeding can dramatically reduce the chances of becoming pregnant. During the first 6 months after giving birth, a woman who has not yet had a period and fully breastfeeds her baby (no other liquids or solids), has less than a 2 percent chance of pregnancy.

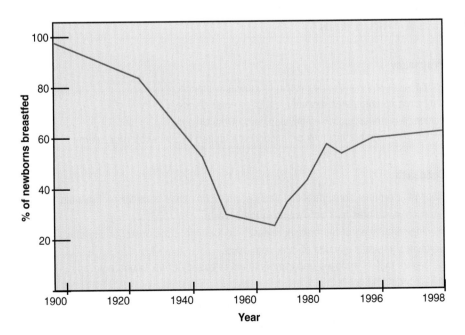

Figure 14.11 **Trends in breastfeeding.**
Source: Data compiled from the American Dietetic Association. Promotion of breastfeeding—Position statement. *J Am Diet Assoc.* 1997;97: 662–666; Ryan AS. The resurgence of breastfeeding in the United States. *Pediatrics.* 1997;99(4); and U.S. Department of Health and Human Services. Healthy People 2010. http://www.health.gov/healthypeople.

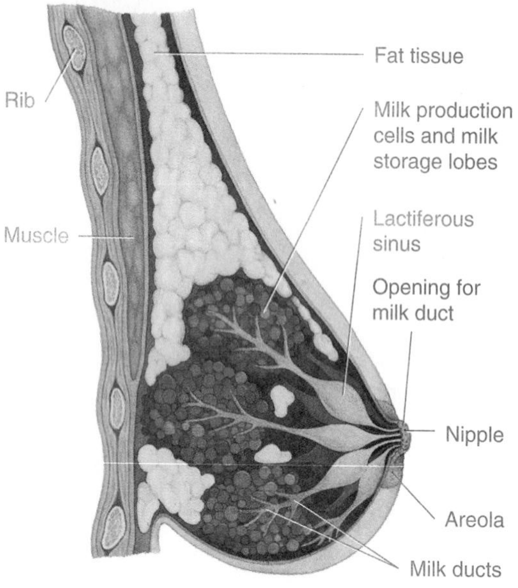

Fat tissue

Rib

Milk production cells and milk storage lobes

Muscle

Lactiferous sinus

Opening for milk duct

Nipple

Areola

Milk ducts

Figure 14.12 Anatomy of the breast. During pregnancy, the breast increases in size and undergoes internal development. By the start of the third trimester, the breast is capable of producing milk.

Physiology of Lactation

Virtually every woman who wants to breastfeed her newborn can do so. All that is needed for successful initiation of breastfeeding is an intact mammary gland and the physiological processes that produce and release milk in the breast tissue. The size or shape of the breast has no impact on the lactation process. **Figure 14.12** shows the anatomy of a normal breast.

Adolescent Breast Development

Although newborns have mammary tissue, it does not grow and develop until the onset of puberty. Throughout adolescence, the breast tissue grows as the mammary glands and ducts develop. An adolescent who becomes pregnant shortly after her first period or who has had only irregular periods prior to becoming pregnant may have underdeveloped mammary glands and insufficient breast tissue to support lactation. **Table 14.6** outlines the hormonal influences on the development of mammary glands from puberty to childbirth and on secretion of milk for breastfeeding.

Changes during Pregnancy

The final changes in the breast tissue that make milk production possible occur during pregnancy. Not only does the breast change in size, but the structure of the glands and ducts becomes more intricate and secretory cells are formed. The mammary tissue is mature and capable of producing milk by the start of the third trimester.

After Delivery: Stages of Lactation

Although birth triggers a rapid increase in milk production and secretion, full lactation does not begin as soon as the baby is born. One of the best ways to establish lactation is to put the newborn to the breast as soon after delivery as possible. During the first 2 or 3 days after birth, a nursing infant receives **colostrum**, an immature milk that is quite high in protein and

Table 14.6 **Hormonal Control of Mammary Gland Development and Milk Secretion**

Puberty

Estrogen and *progesterone* stimulate development of alveolar glands and ducts of mammary glands.

Pregnancy

Estrogen causes the ductile system to grow and branch.
Progesterone stimulates development of alveolar glands.
Placental lactogen promotes development of the breasts.
Prolactin is secreted but milk production is inhibited by *placental progesterone*.

Childbirth

Placental hormone concentrations decline; *prolactin* action is no longer inhibited.
Prolactin stimulates milk production in the breasts.
Nursing stimulation of the breasts releases *oxytocin* from the posterior pituitary.
Oxytocin stimulates ejection of milk from ducts.
As long as milk is removed, more *prolactin* is released; if milk is not removed, milk production ceases.

Source: Shier D. Reproductive systems. In: Hole's *Anatomy and Physiology* 8th ed. Boston:WCB/McGraw-Hill; 1999. Reproduced with the permission of the McGraw-Hill Companies.

immunoglobulins (immunoprotective factors). By about the end of the first week, colostrum has changed in composition. This **transitional milk** still has more protein than mature milk, but less than the early colostrum. Within 2 or 3 weeks postpartum, if the newborn has been fed regularly at the breast, lactation is firmly established and mature milk is being produced. **Figure 14.13** illustrates the stages of lactation.

Hormonal Controls

Maturation of breast tissue and the production and release of breast milk are controlled by various hormones. During lactation, two important hormones, **prolactin** and **oxytocin**, are produced by the pituitary gland. (See **Figure 14.14**.) Prolactin stimulates the production of milk in the breast tissue. Its release from the pituitary gland is stimulated by the infant suckling at the breast. Milk production operates on an efficient supply-and-demand process. The more frequently the infant nurses, the more milk is produced. Giving water or infant formula to the baby reduces the time spent nursing at the breast, and milk production declines. Establishment of lactation depends on frequent opportunities for the infant to nurse.

The second hormone, oxytocin, allows milk to be released from the mammary glands to the nipple, and therefore to the hungry infant. It would be inconvenient and messy if milk were released from the breast as soon as it was produced! So, the infant suckling at the breast signals the pituitary gland to release oxytocin, which in turn stimulates the release of milk. This process is often called the **let-down reflex**, and may be accompanied by a tingling sensation in the breast letting the mother know that the infant is receiving milk. Let-down can be inhibited by anxiety, stress, and fatigue. It can also sometimes be stimulated by thoughts of the baby, or hearing the baby cry.

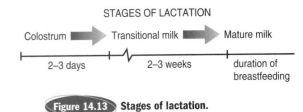

STAGES OF LACTATION

Colostrum ➡ Transitional milk ➡ Mature milk

2–3 days | 2–3 weeks | duration of breastfeeding

Figure 14.13 **Stages of lactation.**

colostrum A thick yellow fluid secreted by the breast during pregnancy and the first days after delivery.

transitional milk A milk that is whiter and thinner than colostrum and is produced beginning about 5 to 7 days after delivery. This transitional milk signals the gradual development of mature milk.

prolactin A pituitary hormone that stimulates the production of milk in the breast tissue.

oxytocin A pituitary hormone that stimulates the release of milk from the breast.

let-down reflex The release of milk from the breast tissue in response to the stimulus of the hormone oxytocin. The major stimulus for oxytocin release is the infant suckling at the breast.

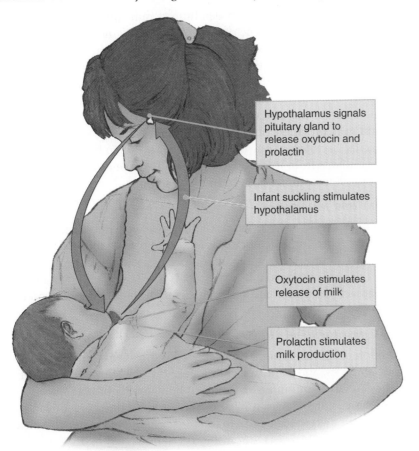

Hypothalamus signals pituitary gland to release oxytocin and prolactin

Infant suckling stimulates hypothalamus

Oxytocin stimulates release of milk

Prolactin stimulates milk production

Figure 14.14 **Hormonal control of lactation.** During the let-down reflex, the infant's suckling stimulates the nipple which sends nerve signals to the hypothalamus. In turn, the hypothalamus signals the pituitary gland to release hormones that stimulate milk production and release.

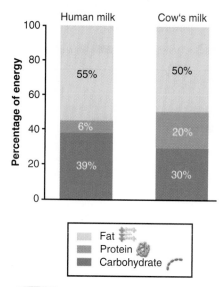

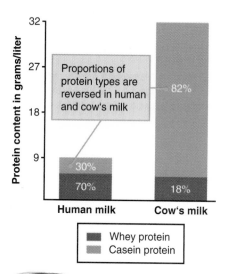

Figure 14.15 Energy nutrients in human and cow's milk.

Figure 14.16 Proteins in human and cow's milk. The amount of protein in one liter of human milk is less than in cow's milk. In addition, the protein in human milk is mainly whey protein, while most of the protein in cow's milk is casein.

But the Breast Milk Looks Weak...

*M*ature breast milk looks similar to nonfat milk—thin, pale, and bluish. Not to worry! This appearance is normal and breast milk always contains the right amount of nutrients for the baby. It is never too weak.

Key Concepts: *Changes in breast tissue that allow lactation begin during adolescence, and culminate at delivery. Breast milk changes in the 2 or 3 weeks following the infant's birth. The first milk, colostrum, is high in protein and immune factors. Prolactin and oxytocin are the hormones that regulate milk production and release.*

Composition of Human Milk

Breast milk is considered the ideal food for infants; after all, it is the food specifically designed to meet their needs! The components of human milk represent both substances that are synthesized in the breast tissue and substances that are taken directly from the maternal circulation. **Figure 14.15** compares the energy nutrients in human and cow's milk.

Carbohydrates and Lipids

The main carbohydrate in human milk is lactose. The breast tissue takes up glucose from the maternal circulation. Some of that glucose is converted to galactose, and then glucose and galactose are joined to make lactose.

Triglycerides are the major energy source in human milk, providing about 50 to 55 percent of the calories. Breast milk is rich in essential fatty acids and two long-chain omega-3 fatty acids: eicosapentaenoic acid and docosahexaenoic acid. These fatty acids have roles in neurological development, so some researchers have suggested that they should be considered provisionally essential for human infants.[38] Infants also need cholesterol for brain development. Human milk is rich in cholesterol, with about 20 to 30 milligrams per 100 milliliters.

Proteins

One of the major differences between human milk and milk of other mammals (such as cows) is the type of protein each contains Milk proteins can generally be divided into two types: casein and whey. The balance of milk proteins in human milk is the reverse of that found in cow's milk: whey proteins predominate in human milk. One advantage of this balance is that humans can digest whey more easily than casein. **Figure 14.16** compares the proteins in human and cow's milk.

Human milk provides complete protein; it contains all of the essential amino acids. Lactoferrin, one of the unique proteins in human milk, helps to protect infants from infection. Other helpful proteins are immunoglobulins that provide immune protection to the infant.

Vitamins and Minerals

Human milk provides the amounts of vitamins and minerals that human babies need. Therefore, the micronutrient composition of human milk is the reference point for designing infant formula. Although the absolute content of some nutrients in human milk is low (e.g., vitamin D and iron), infants absorb these nutrients more efficiently from breast milk than from formula.

Other Constituents of Human Milk

In addition to nutrients, human milk contains digestive enzymes such as lipases, amylases, and proteases, which assist the newborn's digestion of breast milk. Other anti-infective factors in human milk protect against infectious disease. Human breast milk also contains hormones and growth factors, although their specific roles in infant development are not completely understood. **Table 14.7** lists the advantages of human milk over cow's milk.

Key Concepts: *The components of human milk are synthesized in breast tissue or extracted from the mother's bloodstream. Breast milk is designed to nourish infants and, as such, contains optimal nutrition for them. Fat is the main source of energy, and proteins in human milk are complete and easily digested. Enzymes, immune factors, and hormones in human milk contribute to its unique composition.*

Nutrition for Breastfeeding Women

To provide adequate nutrition for her baby while protecting her own nutrition status, a breastfeeding mother must choose a varied, healthful, nutrient-dense diet. Her needs for energy and most nutrients are higher or the same as for pregnancy. For a few nutrients—iron, folate, magnesium, and niacin—recommended intake levels are lower during lactation than for pregnancy.

Energy

The energy RDA for breastfeeding women is 500 kilocalories per day higher than the RDA for nonpregnant, nonlactating women, but this may be an overestimation of actual needs, especially for sedentary women. Nursing mothers typically lose weight gradually, about 0.5 to 1 kilogram per month; however, some gain and others maintain weight.[39] Many new mothers are in a hurry to lose their "baby fat." But to ensure adequate milk production and avoid nutrient deficiencies, a nursing mother should consume at least 1,800 kilocalories a day. Consuming fewer than 1,500 kilocalories a day may decrease milk volume to a level that cannot support infant growth and development. In addition, losing more than 0.5 kilogram per week, even for a woman with good fat stores, can reduce milk production.

Protein

Adequate protein intake is also important while nursing. For the first 6 months of exclusive breastfeeding, milk production uses up to 15 grams of protein a day; during the next 6 months, it uses 12 grams a day. Thus, the RDA for protein rises to 65 grams per day for the first 6 months of lactation, and then is 62 grams per day for the second 6 months. Lack of dietary protein is uncommon among American women, unless calorie intake is very low.

Vitamins and Minerals

Demand for most vitamins during lactation is even greater than during pregnancy. Exceptions include vitamins D and K, for which the recommended intake is the same during lactation and pregnancy; and niacin and folate, for which the RDA is lower during lactation than during pregnancy (although still higher than for women in the general population). When vitamin intake is inadequate, the vitamin content of breast milk can diminish, which puts the infant at risk for deficiency.

For minerals, current RDA and AI values suggest increased needs during lactation (as compared to pregnancy) for all minerals except calcium, phosphorus, magnesium, fluoride, and molybdenum. Iron needs decrease below nonpregnant values because iron losses from menstruation are not present during the early months of exclusive breastfeeding. Maternal intake of minerals has less influence on levels in breast milk than is true for vitamins.

Water

Breastfeeding women require plenty of fluids. A nursing mother should drink about 2 liters (~8 cups) of water per day, and at least one cup of

Table 14.7 Advantages of Human over Cow's Milk

Protein

More whey protein
Less casein
Less phenylalanine
More peptidase

Lipids

More lipase enzyme
More linoleic acid
Higher polyunsaturated-to-saturated fatty acids ratio
More cholesterol

Minerals

Less calcium
Less sodium
Higher calcium-to-phosphorus ratio
Iron and zinc in more available forms

Source: Riordan J, Auerbach KG. *Breastfeeding and Human Lactation.* 2nd ed. Sudbury, MA: Jones and Bartlett Publishers, 1999.

colic Periodic inconsolable crying in otherwise healthy infants that appears to result from abdominal cramping and discomfort.

bifidus factor A compound in human milk that stimulates the growth of *lactobacillus bifidus* bacteria in the infant's intestinal tract.

Quick Bites

Flavored Breast Milk

When lactating mothers exercise vigorously, the amount of lactic acid in breast milk can increase. Some babies dislike the taste, and tend to nurse less. Alcohol can also cause a taste that babies dislike. What flavors do babies like? When mothers consume vanilla, mint, or garlic, some babies nurse more.

water each time she breast-feeds her baby. Coffee and other caffeinated beverages are acceptable if limited to one or two cups a day—and if they do not replace other fluids. Because caffeine passes into the breast milk, caffeine can make some breast-fed infants wakeful and jittery.

Key Concepts: *Need for energy and many nutrients is higher during lactation than during pregnancy. RDA values suggest an additional 500 kilocalories and 12 to 15 grams of protein each day. Recommended intake levels for minerals are generally higher during lactation than during pregnancy. Fluids are also important for adequate milk production.*

Food Choices

Choosing a variety of foods from the USDA Food Guide Pyramid is the best way to meet the nutritional demands of lactation. Following the pyramid guidelines, diets of 2,200 to 2,800 kilocalories per day can easily meet most nutrient needs.

Nursing mothers should eat plenty of vegetables, the source of many essential micronutrients. But vegetables in the cabbage family, including broccoli, cauliflower, kale, and Brussels sprouts, have long been considered causes of **colic** symptoms in breast-fed infants. However, these cruciferous vegetables may have an unwarranted bad reputation. Scientific evidence that these vegetables cause distress for infants remains weak. Other foods with a bad reputation among nursing mothers are peanut butter, chocolate, egg whites, and nuts. If colic is a problem in a breast-fed newborn, a new mother might eliminate any suspected offending food from her diet for a while to see if there is any effect on colic symptoms.[40] Removal of numerous foods from the diet should be done only under the supervision of a registered dietitian.

Supplementation

Breastfeeding women do not generally need routine vitamin/mineral supplementation. The exceptions are those women who do not follow dietary guidelines, and vegan women, who avoid all animal products. Vitamin B_{12} is likely to be too low in the milk of nursing vegans, and they should take a B_{12} supplement.[41] For breastfeeding women who do not get regular sun exposure and do not drink milk or other fortified products, a vitamin D supplement may be warranted. For most nursing mothers, though, dietary counseling is the preferred way to address nutrient imbalances.

Practices to Avoid during Lactation

When a nursing mother smokes or uses alcohol or other drugs, these substances wind up in her breast milk. Nicotine-laced milk may be harmful to the infant. In addition, cigarette smoking can decrease production of breast milk.[42] It is best to avoid alcohol while nursing. It is a myth that drinking alcohol enhances the let-down reflex, making it easier to nurse. Rather, alcohol inhibits the milk-ejection reflex so that the baby gets less milk with a higher concentration of alcohol.

Illicit drugs also show up in breast milk and can be transferred to the infant. If a new mother cannot abstain from using these drugs, she should not breastfeed. Legal drugs can be harmful to babies, too. A woman should discuss over-the-counter and prescription medicines, and herbal products with her health-care providers before taking them. In the rare case where the drug is essential for the mother but harmful to the baby, the mother may pump and discard her milk. After the drug has cleared her system, she can resume breastfeeding safely. Women who are undergoing radiation therapy or chemotherapy treatment for cancer should not breastfeed.

Key Concepts: *Food choices during lactation should follow the USDA Food Guide Pyramid and emphasize nutrient-dense foods. With good choices and adequate calories, a lactating woman may not need vitamin and mineral supplements. During pregnancy and lactation, a woman should avoid tobacco, alcohol, and illicit drugs. She should consult a health-care professional before taking medications or dietary supplements.*

Benefits of Breastfeeding

Breast milk is the optimal food for the health, growth, and development of infants.[43] Both mother and infant benefit from breastfeeding; in fact, the larger society benefits through reduced infant illness and health-care costs.

Benefits for Infants

Human milk provides optimal nutrition for babies. The specific nutritional needs for infants are discussed in Chapter 15. Breast milk provides more than nutrients, however, and the health-promoting factors in breast milk are difficult, if not impossible, to replicate in infant formula.

Immune Factors Breast milk has been shown to reduce the incidence of respiratory, gastrointestinal, and ear infections, allergies, diarrhea, and bacterial meningitis. Recent evidence suggests that these effects occur in a dose-response relationship, with the best outcomes for infants who are exclusively breast-fed for at least 6 months.[44] Colostrum contains substantial amounts of antibodies, including immunoglobulin A (IgA), the first line of defense against most infectious agents.[45] Another beneficial biochemical in human milk is **bifidus factor**. This factor fosters the growth of the bacteria *Lactobacillus bifidus*, which in turn interfere with the growth of harmful bacteria in the baby's digestive system. **Table 14.8** lists other factors in breast milk that contribute to infant health.

Psychological and Emotional Benefits Breastfeeding promotes a close bond between mother and infant that may be important to normal psychologic development.[46] It is virtually impossible to breastfeed without holding an infant close and gazing into his or her eyes. It is important for mothers (and fathers) who bottle-feed to promote the same type of closeness while feeding. Recently, it has been suggested that breastfeeding enhances psychological and intellectual development, although in many studies it is difficult to control for factors such as maternal IQ and level of education.[47]

Other Benefits As long as mother and baby are in reasonably close proximity, breast milk is always ready when the baby is ready to eat. Nothing to prepare, mix, or heat; and for a hungry infant, that's an important advantage! Breast milk is always the perfect temperature, and is sterile. In addition, links between breastfeeding and reduced risk of disorders such as type 1 diabetes, certain cancers, and Crohn's disease, have been suggested, and need further study. **Table 14.9** lists some of the protective benefits of human milk.

Benefits for Mother

Breastfeeding speeds maternal physiologic recovery by stimulating uterine contractions, which help to return the uterus to its normal size. These same contractions (an effect of oxytocin) can also help control blood loss if the baby is put to the breast immediately after delivery. Exclusive breastfeeding suppresses ovulation in many women, although this cannot be counted on as an effective method of birth control.

Table 14.8 **Protective Factors in Human Milk**

Factor	Description and Function
Bifidus factor	Present in both colostrum and mature milk; favors the growth in the GI tract of *Lactobacillus bifidus*, the bacteria that prevent the growth of harmful *E. coli* bacteria
Immunoglobulins	Proteins found in colostrum and mature milk that act as antibodies; secretory IgA is the most common
Lysozyme	An enzyme in human milk that attacks the cell wall of bacteria, thereby inhibiting growth of harmful bacteria
Lactoferrin	An iron-binding protein in human milk; enhances the bioavailability of iron from human milk; reduces available iron needed for growth of harmful bacteria
Intestinal growth factor	Growth factor in human milk that stimulates the replacement of damaged cells in the intestinal tract

Source: Adapted from Worthington-Roberts BS, Williams SR. *Nutrition Through the Life Cycle.* 4th ed. New York: McGraw-Hill, 1999.

Table 14.9 **Suggested Protective Benefits of Human Milk**

Breastfeeding may reduce a baby's risk of these disorders during infancy or later in life:

- Sudden infant death syndrome (SIDS)
- Type 1 diabetes mellitus
- Crohn's disease
- Ulcerative colitis
- Chronic digestive diseases

Source: Adapted from Lawrence A. *A Review of the Medical Benefits and Contraindications to Breastfeeding in the United States.* (Maternal and Child Health Technical Information Bulletin). Arlington, VA: National Center for Education in Maternal and Child Health; 1997.

galactosemia [gah-LAK-toh-see-mee-ah]
An inherited disorder of galactose metabolism marked by high levels of galactose in the blood and the buildup of toxic substances.

Quick Bites

Breastfeeding to Control Blood Pressure?

Oxytocin, the hormone produced while breastfeeding, can lower the blood pressure of nursing mothers. A recent study showed that breastfeeding mothers had lower blood pressures after nursing than did bottle-feeding mothers. When asked to discuss stressful events, nursing mothers also showed smaller increases in blood pressure than the bottle-feeders showed. Mothers often claim that they feel relaxed during breastfeeding, which may account for the difference in blood pressure.

Breastfeeding is as convenient for mother as it is for baby, and is certainly less expensive than formula feeding. Although more comprehensive studies are needed, there is some evidence that breastfeeding reduces a woman's risk of ovarian cancer, breast cancer, and osteoporosis.[48] If, as expected, a breast-fed baby has fewer episodes of infectious illness, this saves health-care costs, and reduces employee absence and lost income for working mothers.

Contraindications to Breastfeeding

Nearly all women who want to breastfeed can do so successfully. There are times, however, when breastfeeding is inappropriate because of infant or maternal disease, or drug use. Breast surgery may or may not preclude breastfeeding depending on the specifics of the operation.[49]

If an infant has **galactosemia**, an inborn error in carbohydrate metabolism, the infant cannot metabolize galactose. Unless given a galactose-free diet, the afflicted infant will fail to develop mentally and physically in a normal way. Since the digestion of human milk produces galactose, infants with galactosemia must consume a special lactose-free formula. Infants with PKU, however, can be breast-fed and receive supplemental low-phenylalanine formula. Breastfeeding is also contraindicated if the mother has certain illnesses. For example, a woman with untreated tuberculosis should not breastfeed because she may transmit the illness to her child. Individual situations should be discussed with the health-care provider. In the United States, women infected with the human immunodeficiency virus (HIV) are advised not to breastfeed because HIV can be transmitted to baby through breast milk. In developing countries, where the risks of infectious diseases and infant mortality are high, the benefits to the baby of breastfeeding may outweigh the low risk of contracting HIV from the mother's milk.[50]

Finally, some medications pass directly into human milk. Some prescribed medications may preclude breastfeeding. Illegal drugs pass into human milk as well. If the mother is using illegal drugs such as cocaine, she should not breastfeed. Women taking prescription or over-the-counter medicines or herbal supplements should discuss the effects of these products on breast milk with their health-care providers.

Key Concepts: *Health benefits and convenience are the advantages of breastfeeding. For the infant, breastfeeding has been linked to reduced incidence of many types of infectious diseases, as well as other conditions. For a mother, breastfeeding speeds recovery of normal uterine size, and may reduce her disease risk. Although breastfeeding is the preferred method of infant feeding, there are times that breastfeeding is contraindicated. These situations should be identified and discussed as part of prenatal care.*

Resources for Pregnant and Lactating Women

The Special Supplemental Nutrition Program for Women, Infants, and Children (WIC) is a much-acclaimed program of the Food and Nutrition Service of the U.S. Department of Agriculture (USDA). WIC provides food assistance, nutrition education, and referrals to health-care services to low-income pregnant, postpartum, and breastfeeding women, as well as infants and children up to the age of 5. Compared with at-risk women and children who are eligible for WIC but do not participate in the program, WIC participants have significantly fewer problems such as low-birth-weight infants.[51] The number of pregnant women who participate in WIC has tripled during the past 15 years, up to 6 million participants.

Since its inception in 1972, the WIC program has provided infant formula as part of its food assistance for infants. However, stronger promotion of breastfeeding began in the late 1980s. WIC services now include intensive breastfeeding education and support. Peer counselors not only encourage pregnant women to choose breastfeeding, but also work to convince new mothers to continue breastfeeding throughout the baby's first year of life.[52] Over the first six months of life, breast-fed infants enrolled in WIC use about $500 less in WIC and Medicaid services than do formula-fed infants enrolled in WIC, according to a study conducted in Colorado.[53] Continued promotion of breastfeeding by WIC and other public health programs can have both health and economic benefits.

The La Leche League is a voluntary health and education organization that offers programs and educational materials to help breastfeeding mothers learn about the benefits and practice of breastfeeding.

The March of Dimes provides educational materials regarding perinatal nutrition and healthy pregnancy. The organization has produced programs and materials to promote optimal nutrition during pregnancy.

The American College of Obstetrics and Gynecology provides patient education materials, including pamphlets that address breastfeeding.

The American Dietetic Association (ADA), through its National Center for Nutrition and Dietetics, provides services, programs, and materials for the public. A nutrition hotline, staffed by registered dietitians, provides consumers with up-to-date information about nutrition. The center also publishes fact sheets on topics related to women's health, including tips for pregnant teens.

Label [to] **Table**

A pregnant woman requires more nutrients than usual. The RDA for both iron and folate increases by 50 percent during pregnancy. Iron, especially, is difficult to get in this quantity from the diet. Enriched grains and fortified foods, like cereals, make it easier to obtain these essential nutrients. Let's take a look at the Nutrition Facts label from a popular breakfast cereal.

Take a look at how much folic acid a one-cup serving of this breakfast cereal contains—50% DV (DV = 400 micrograms). The DV for folate is the same as the RDA for nonpregnant women; for pregnancy, the RDA increases to 600 micrograms. Because the folate in ready-to-eat cereal is almost all added folic acid, one serving actually provides 340µg DFE (400µg [DV] X 0.50 X 1.7 = 340). If orange juice accompanies the cereal, another 15% DV (60µg) is added for a one-cup serving. So, these two foods provide a total of 500µg DFE, or more than two-thirds of what a pregnant woman would need.

Iron is also extremely important for pregnancy because of its role in growth and its importance as blood volume increases during pregnancy. One serving of this breakfast cereal provides almost half of the DV (45 percent of the 18 milligrams, or about 8 milligrams). However, during pregnancy, the RDA for iron is 27 milligrams. So, one serving of this cereal provides nearly one-third of the iron needed each day—a good start. Having orange juice with the cereal will enhance iron absorption.

Nutrition Facts
Serving Size: 1 cup (30g)
Servings Per Container about 9

Amount Per Serving	Cheerios	with ½ cup skim milk
Calories	110	150
Calories from Fat	15	20

		% Daily Value**
Total Fat 2g*	3%	3%
Saturated Fat 0g	0%	3%
Polyunsaturated Fat 0.5g		
Monounsaturated Fat 0.5g		
Cholesterol 0g	0%	1%
Sodium 280mg	12%	15%
Total Carbohydrate 22g	7%	9%
Dietary Fiber 0g	11%	11%
Sugars 1g		
Protein 3g		

Vitamin A	10%	15%
Vitamin C	10%	10%
Calcium	4%	20%
Iron	45%	45%
Vitamin D	10%	25%
Thiamin	25%	30%
Riboflavin	25%	35%
Niacin	25%	25%
Vitamin B₆	25%	25%
Folic Acid	50%	50%
Vitamin B₁₂	25%	35%
Phosphorus	10%	25%

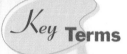

Key Terms

	page		page
amniotic fluid	555	gestational diabetes	549
bifidus factor	570	let-down reflex	567
blastogenic stage	550	low-birth-weight infant	549
cleavage	550	morning sickness	562
colic	570	oxytocin	567
colostrum	567	placenta	550
critical period of development	552	preeclampsia	549
embryonic stage	552	preterm delivery	549
fetal stage	552	prolactin	567
galactosemia		transitional milk	567
[gah-LAK-toh-see-mee-ah]	572	trimester	550

Study Points

➤ Nutrition status before pregnancy is an important part of having a healthy baby. Moreover, it is an integral part of all aspects of preconception care: risk assessment, health promotion, and intervention. Being either overweight or underweight prior to pregnancy increases risk of complications.

➤ Folic acid supplementation before pregnancy has been shown to reduce the risk of neural tube defects such as spina bifida.

➤ Excessive intake of some vitamins (vitamin A, in particular), and use of tobacco, alcohol, and drugs all increase the risk of poor pregnancy outcomes. These practices should be discontinued before pregnancy.

➤ Pregnancy can be divided into three stages: blastogenic, embryonic, and fetal. In the blastogenic stage, the fertilized ovum begins rapid cell division and implants itself in the uterine wall. During the embryonic stage, organ systems and other body structures form. During the fetal stage, the longest period of pregnancy, the fetus grows in size and changes in proportions.

➤ While the baby develops, changes are occurring in the mother's body such as growth of uterine, breast, and fatty tissue and expansion of blood volume. During pregnancy, gastrointestinal motility slows to allow enhanced absorption of nutrients.

➤ Women who enter pregnancy at a normal BMI should gain 25 to 35 pounds during pregnancy. Underweight women should gain more weight and overweight women less.

➤ The energy RDA during pregnancy increases by 300 kilocalories per day for the second and third trimesters.

➤ Protein needs of pregnant women increase by about 10 grams per day, for a total recommended intake that is well within normal protein consumption in the United States. The diet should contain carbohydrates and fats in the same proportions as recommended for nonpregnant women.

➤ Using the Food Guide Pyramid, pregnant women who consume enough energy should be able to meet all their nutrient needs with the exception of iron and folate. They should get extra calories mainly from grains, fruits, and vegetables.

➤ Limiting caffeine intake during pregnancy is recommended. Smoking during pregnancy increases the risk of preterm delivery and low birth weight. Alcohol and drug use can interfere with normal fetal development and should be avoided during pregnancy.

➤ Gastrointestinal distress such as morning sickness, heartburn, and constipation are common during pregnancy and results from the action of various hormones on the GI tract. Although most food cravings or aversions present no problems, excessive consumption of nonfood items, known as pica, interferes with adequate nutrition.

➤ The combination of high blood pressure, protein in the urine, and edema is called preeclampsia, a life-threatening condition for both mother and infant.

➤ Regulation of blood sugar levels is very important for women with diabetes who become pregnant. Gestational diabetes is an elevation of blood glucose levels during pregnancy that can usually be controlled by diet.

➤ Pregnant women with PKU must monitor phenylalanine intake. Pregnant women with AIDS face substantial nutritional challenges. Teen pregnancy poses significant nutritional challenges to meet the demands of both pregnancy and normal adolescent growth.

➤ During pregnancy hormones control the development of breast tissue in preparation for milk production. Colostrum, the first milk, which is rich in protein and antibodies, is produced soon after delivery. By two to three weeks after delivery, lactation is well established, and mature milk is being produced.

➤ The pituitary hormone, prolactin, stimulates milk production. Oxytocin, another pituitary hormone, stimulates milk release, which is known as the let-down reflex.

➤ The main carbohydrate in breast milk is lactose, synthesized in the breast tissue. Triglycerides are the main source of energy in breast milk.

➤ The vitamin and mineral content of breast milk is considered optimal for infant growth and development. Other factors in human milk reduce disease risk, enhance development, and improve digestion.

➤ Unless they reduce their physical activity, breastfeeding women need about 500 more kilocalories per day than they did when they were not pregnant. Obtaining adequate energy and using the Food Guide Pyramid to balance choices, most lactating women can obtain all the nutrients they need from their diet. Cigarettes, alcohol, and illicit drugs should not be used while breastfeeding.

➤ Mothers benefit from breastfeeding through enhanced physiologic recovery, convenience, and emotional bonding. Contraindications to breastfeeding include infants with galactosemia, mothers infected with HIV or active tuberculosis, and chronic use of certain medications.

➤ Numerous resources for support and education of pregnant and breastfeeding women exist including La Leche League, the March of Dimes, and the WIC program.

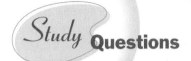

Study Questions

1. What are the main components of preconception care?
2. What are the stages of human fetal growth?
3. What are some the physiological changes that occur to a woman during pregnancy?
4. How do the RDA values for protein, iron, folate, and calories change for pregnancy?
5. How do the recommendations of the Food Guide Pyramid change during pregnancy? Why?
6. What contributes to "morning sickness" and how can a woman minimize its effects?
7. List five common nutrition-related conditions associated with pregnancy.
8. What is gestational diabetes?
9. What are the calorie guidelines for lactation? How few calories can be consumed if a woman wants to lose her pregnancy weight?
10. What are the nutrient needs of breastfeeding mothers?
11. What are some of the benefits of breastfeeding?

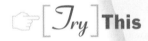

Try This

Can You Eat Like You're Expecting for Just One Week?

The purpose of this exercise is to see if you can follow the nutrition guidelines for pregnancy for just one week. Keep in mind that pregnant women attempt to do this for 38 to 40 weeks! Your goal is to reduce or eliminate caffeine, alcohol, and over-the-counter medications. If necessary, increase your Dairy Food Group servings to at least three per day. You should also take a basic multivitamin/mineral tablet (in place of a woman's prenatal) daily. Make your choices from each food group wisely so that you select some of the most nutrient-dense foods. This will ensure that you consume the amounts of protein, vitamins, and minerals recommended for pregnancy.

Can You Drink Like You're Nursing for Just One Week?

The purpose of this exercise is to see if you can follow the fluid guidelines recommended for breastfeeding mothers. Remember that adequate hydration is key for proper milk formation and to prevent a new mother from becoming dehydrated. Experts recommend that most nursing mothers consume about 2 liters of water per day, not including caffeinated drinks like coffee, tea, or soda. Can you drink that much? Two liters is approximately 8 1/2 cups of water (or 68 fluid ounces). Here's a suggestion for keeping track. Start your day with 8 pennies in a pocket. Each time you drink 8 to 10 ounces of noncaffeinated fluid, move one penny from that pocket to another. When you get undressed at the end of the day, you'll be able to estimate your water consumption by how many pennies you've moved!

What About

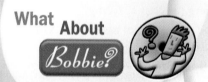

Let's pretend that Bobbie is pregnant and in her second trimester. She wants to know whether she's meeting her basic nutrient needs by following her usual diet. Refer to Chapter 1 to review her one-day intake. How do you think she's doing? Let's compare Bobbie's intake of nutrients to the recommendations for pregnant women.

Calories

The recommended calorie intake for women in their second and third trimesters is an extra 300 kilocalories per day over the nonpregnant RDA. Using the RDA value for an average female, this is 2,500 kilocalories. Bobbie's intake for this one day was 2,440 kilocalories, which may be enough for her growing baby. Bobbie's energy needs may be higher or lower than the RDA of 2,200 for her age group.

Protein

If you remember reviewing Bobbie's diet after reading Chapter 6, "Protein," you may recall that it is quite high in protein. Her intake was 97 grams and her nonpregnancy RDA (based on her weight) was 51 grams. During pregnancy, however, Bobbie should have an extra 10 grams of protein to ensure her body can handle the demands of tissue growth. Even with the added protein need of pregnancy (61 grams total protein per day), Bobbie's current intake is more than adequate, and could be reduced.

Folate

Bobbie's intake of folate was 470 micrograms, which is short of her pregnancy RDA of 600 micrograms. Although she meets the nonpregnancy recommendations (400 micrograms per day), she would be advised to add folate-rich foods such as spinach, legumes, and orange juice. If Bobbie is adhering to proper prenatal/pregnancy care, then she is consuming a prenatal supplement with folic acid as well. Bobbie's folate intake is not reported as DFE. Because her diet included several enriched grain products, her actual consumption of

folate in terms of µg of DFE would be higher due to the higher bioavailability of folic acid added to enriched grains.

Iron

Bobbie's intake of iron for 1 day was 20 milligrams. This is substantially lower than her pregnancy RDA of 27 milligrams. This places Bobbie at greater risk for iron deficiency, a common condition in pregnancy. In addition to taking a prenatal supplement that contains iron, Bobbie is advised to continue choosing iron-rich lean red meats like the beef meatballs for dinner. She would also benefit from adding more dark green, leafy vegetables to her diet, along with a squeeze of lemon (or other source of vitamin C) to increase the absorption of the non-heme iron. With these additions to her diet, Bobbie will lower her chances of having iron deficiency during her pregnancy.

References

1 Keen CL, Zidenberg-Cherr S. Should vitamin mineral supplementation be recommended for all women with childbearing potential? *Am J Clin Nutr.* 1994;59:532S.

2 Cnattingius S, Bergstrom R, Lipworth L, Kramer MS. Prepregnancy weight and the risk of adverse pregnancy outcomes. *N Engl J Med.* 1998;338:147–152.

3 Ibid.

4 Cnattingius S, et al. Op. cit.; and Goldenberg RL, Tamura T. Prepregnancy weight and pregnancy outcome. *JAMA.* 1996;275:1127–1128.

5 Institute of Medicine. Food and Nutrition Board. *Dietary Reference Intakes for Thiamin, Riboflavin, Niacin, Vitamin B6, Folate, Vitamin B12, Pantothenic Acid, Biotin, and Choline.* Washington, DC: National Academy Press; 1998.

6 US Department of Health and Human Services, Public Health Service, Centers for Disease Control. Recommendations for the use of folic acid to reduce the number of cases of spina bifida and other neural tube defects. *MMWR.* 1992;41:1.

7 Rothman KJ, Moore LL, Singer MR, et al. Tetratogenicity of high vitamin A intake. *N Engl J Med.* 1995;333:1369.

8 Oakley GP, Erickson JD. Vitamin A and birth defects-continuing caution is needed. *N Engl J Med.* 1995;333:1414.

9 Food and Drug Administration. Vitamin A and Birth Defects. October 6, 1995. Press release.

10 Worthington-Roberts B. The role of maternal nutrition in the prevention of birth defects. *J Am Diet Assoc.* 1997;97:S184.

11 Piyathilake CJ, Macaluso M, Hine RJ, et al. Local and systemic effects of cigarette smoking on folate and vitamin B12. *Am J Clin Nutr.* 1994;60:559–566.

12 Institute of Medicine. *Nutrition during Pregnancy.* Washington, DC: National Academy Press; 1990.

13 Ibid.

14 Ibid.

15 Picciano MF. Pregnancy and lactation. In: Ziegler EE, Filer LJ, eds. *Present Knowledge in Nutrition.* 7th ed. Washington, DC: ILSI Press; 1996.

16 Pitkin RM. Energy in pregnancy. *Am J Clin Nutr.* 1999;69:583.

17 Kopp-Hoolihan LE, van Loan MD, Wong WW, King JC. Longitudinal assessment of energy balance in well-nourished, pregnant women. *Am J Clin Nutr.* 1999;69(4):697–704.

18 Dewey KG, McCroy MA. Effects of dieting and physical activity on pregnancy and lactation. *Am J Clin Nutr.* 1994;59(2 suppl):446S–452S.

19 Institute of Medicine. Op. cit.

20 Dewey KG, McCroy MA. Op. cit.

21 Institute of Medicine. Op. cit.

22 Institute of Medicine. *Dietary Reference Intakes for Calcium, Phosphorus, Magnesium, Vitamin D, and Fluoride.* Washington, DC: National Academy Press; 1997.

23 Picciano MF. Op. cit.

24 Institute of Medicine. *Nutrition during Pregnancy.* Op. cit.

25 Shaw A, Fulton L, Davis C, Hogbin M. *Using the Food Guide Pyramid: A Resource for Nutrition Educators.* USDA: www.usda.gov/cnpp/using.htm. Accessed 10/30/00.

26 Lowe JB, Balanda KP, Clare G. Evaluation of antenatal smoking cessation programs for pregnant women. *Austral New Zeal J Pub Health.* 1998;22:55–59.

27 Gabriel K, Hofmann C, Glavas M, Weinberg J. The hormonal effects of alcohol use on the mother and fetus. *Alcohol Health Res World.* 1998;22:3.

28 Picciano MF. Op. cit.

29 Worthington-Roberts BS, Williams SR. *Nutrition in Pregnancy and Lactation.* 6th ed. Madison, WI: Brown & Benchmark; 1997.

30 Pamuk E, Makuc D, Heck K, et al. *Socioeconomic Status and Health Chartbook. Health, United States, 1998.* Hyattsville, MD: National Center for Health Statistics; 1998. Updated Oct 1999.

31 Institute of Medicine. *Nutrition during Pregnancy.* Op. cit.

32 Story M, Alton I. Nutritional guidelines during pregnancy and lactation. In: Wolinsky I, Klimis-Tavantzis D, eds. *Nutritional Concerns of Women.* New York: CRC Press; 1996.

33 American Diabetes Association. Gestational diabetes. *Diabetes Care.* 1998;21:S60–S61.

34 Assessing adolescent pregnancy. *MMWR.* 1998;47:433.

35 Story M, Alton I. Nutrition issues and adolescent pregnancy. *Nutr Today.* 1995;30:142.

36 Institute of Medicine. *Nutrition during Pregnancy.* Op. cit.

37 American Dietetic Association. Position of The American Dietetic Association: Promotion of breast-feeding. *J Am Diet Assoc.* 1997;97:662–666.

38 Uauy R, Peirano P, Hoffman D, et al. Role of essential fatty acids in the function of the developing nervous system. *Lipids.* 1996;31:S167–S176.

39 Picciano MF. Op. cit.

40 Lust KD, Brown JE, Thomas W. Maternal intake of cruciferous vegetables and other foods and colic symptoms in exclusively breastfed infants. *J Am Diet Assoc.* 1996;96:47–48.

41 Institute of Medicine. *Nutrition during Pregnancy.* Op. cit.

42 Story M, Alton I. Op. cit.

43 American Dietetic Association. Op. cit.

44 Raisler J, Alexander C, O'Campo P. Breast-feeding and infant illness: a dose-response relationship? *Am J Public Health.* 1999;89:25–30.

45 American Dietetic Association. Op. cit.

46 Worthington-Roberts BS, Willams SR. *Nutrition Throughout the Life Cycle.* 4th ed. New York: McGraw-Hill; 1999.

47 Lawrence A. *A Review of the Medical Benefits and Contraindications to Breastfeeding in the United States.* (Maternal and Child Health Technical Information Bulletin). Arlington, VA: National Center for Education in Maternal and Child Health; 1997.

48 Ibid.

49 Riordan J, Auerbach KG. *Breastfeeding and Human Lactation.* 2nd ed. Sudbury, MA: Jones and Bartlett; 1999.

50 Worthington-Roberts BS, Willams SR. Op. cit.

51 Owen GM. Maternal nutrition. In: Owen AL, Splett PL, Owen GM, eds. *Nutrition in the Community: The Art and Science of Delivering Services.* 4th ed. Boston, MA: WCB-McGraw-Hill; 1999:208.

52 Kistin N, Abramson R, and Dublin P. Effect of peer counselors on breast-feeding initiation, exclusivity, and duration among low-income urban women. *J Human Lactation.* 1994;10:11–15.

53 Montgomery DL, Splett PL. Economic benefits of breast-feeding infants enrolled in WIC. *J Am Diet Assoc.* 1997;97:379–386.

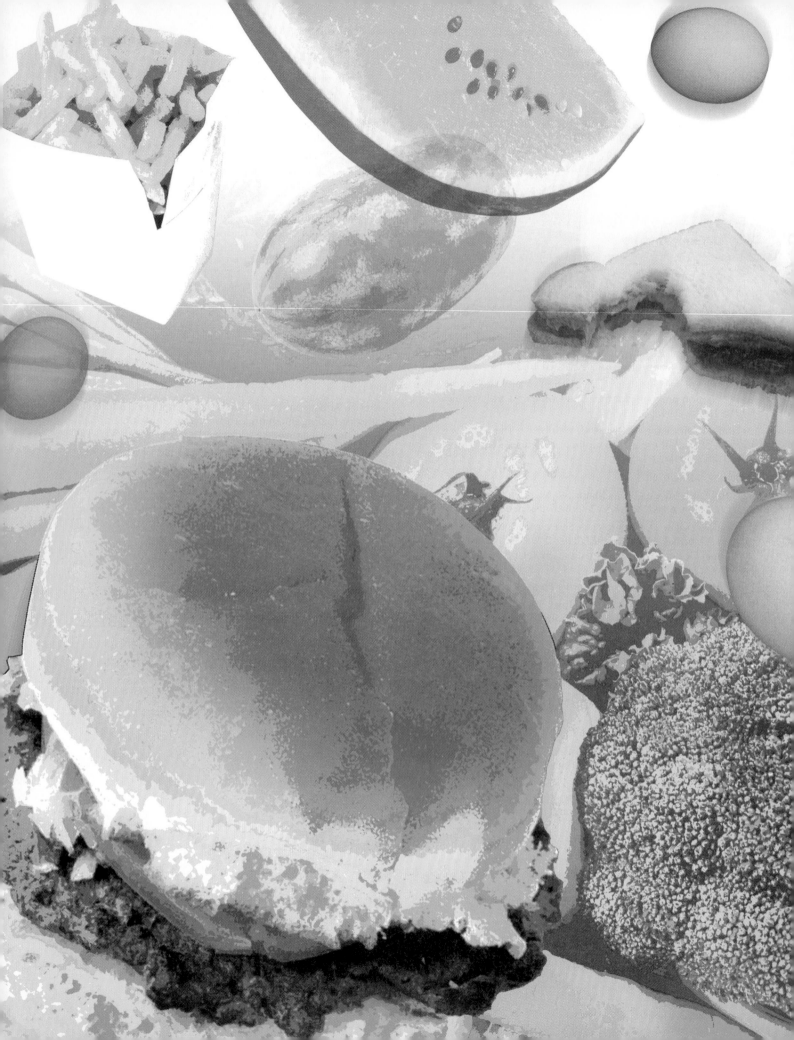

Chapter 15

Life Cycle: Infancy, Childhood, and Adolescence

Think About It

1 What can your parents tell you about your birth weight and your first year of life?

2 Can you predict your height from your parents' height?

3 What's your experience with acne and eating particular foods?

4 What were your eating habits like during adolescence?

Fyi for your Information

This chapter's FYI boxes include practical information on the following topics:

- Preterm Infant Needs

- Fruit Juices and Drinks

- Food Hypersensitivities and Allergies

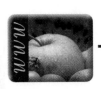

The web site for this book offers many useful tools and is a great source for additional nutrition information for both students and instructors. Visit the site at **nutrition.jbpub.com** for information on nutrition during infancy, childhood, and adolescence. You'll find exercises that explore the following topics:

- Female Athletes and Meatless Diets

- Got Milk—Allergy?

- Lead

- Childhood Malnutrition

Key to Illustrations

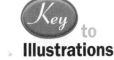

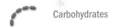 Carbohydrates

Energy

Fat-Soluble Vitamins

Proteins

Triglyceride

Water-Soluble Vitamins

Water

What About Bobbie?

Track the choices Bobbie is making with the EatRight Analysis software.

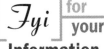

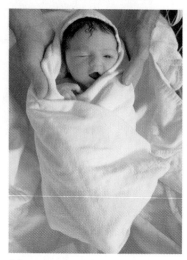

(a)

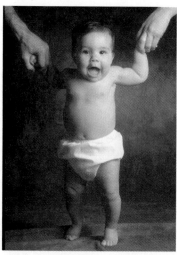

(b)

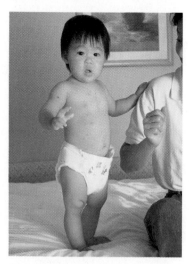

(c)

Figure 15.1 **Different stages of infancy.** (a) Newborn. (b) 4–6 months. (c) 12 months.

id you know that your most rapid period of growth occurs in **infancy**, with adolescence in second place? If so, did you realize just how *rapid* that infant growth is? During the first year of life, a typical newborn's birth weight triples and length increases by 50 percent. Just imagine, if we kept growing at that rate, our children would be ready for the NBA or WNBA before their fourth birthdays!

Fortunately, growth is never as rapid, nor are nutrient needs as high as in the first year of life. But this rapid growth rate makes nutrition a critical element of caring for infants. What to feed and how much to feed are questions every parent faces.

By the time babies become teenagers, parents are less worried about what to feed their children than *how* they are going to pay for it! Adolescent growth is not nearly so rapid as during infancy, but the adolescent growth spurt sparks a tremendous surge in hunger, which is particularly noticeable among teenage boys. The average teen grows 6 to 8 inches and gains 35 to 45 pounds during puberty. Whether that growth is fueled with burgers and fries, black beans and rice, or chips and soft drinks determines a lot about the future health of that teen.

This chapter explores the physiologic and developmental growth that occurs during infancy, childhood, and adolescence, and it discusses nutritional needs during each of these stages. In addition, this chapter addresses feeding practices, meal planning, and obstacles to healthful eating for each age group.

Infancy

Infancy is the period of a child's life between birth and 1 year. Feeding an infant requires little more than logic and love. Human milk provides all of the nutrients an infant needs, and is the model for all alternative milk feedings for infants. By 4 to 6 months, the infant's physical development and physiological maturation signals readiness for the addition of "solid" foods to the diet. For example, because the gastrointestinal tract usually is mature enough to digest complex carbohydrates by this age, infant rice cereal often is introduced. At about this time, the infant's iron stores, developed during fetal growth, are becoming depleted, so dietary iron sources become more important.

Human infants need love as much as they need food. Without love and nurturing, a baby can fail to thrive even if she is offered all of the right nutrients. If an infant is not nourished emotionally, nutrition recommendations and requirements become meaningless.[1]

Infant Growth and Development

Immediately after birth, a newborn is evaluated by **Apgar scores**, weighed, and measured for length. The Apgar score is a quick method of assessing an infant's status 1 minute and 5 minutes after delivery. The score is made up of five parts: heart rate, respiratory effort, muscle tone, reflex irritability, and color; each part is given a score of 0, 1, or 2. Birth weight is the best predictor of the child's health in the first year of life; however, it is important to correlate weight with **gestational age**. The risk profile of an infant who has a low birth weight because of **prematurity** is different from that of a **full-term** baby with a low birth weight.

Immediately after birth, an infant loses about 6 percent of his body weight. This is normal and expected. By 10 to 14 days, the infant should return to his birth weight. Over the next 12 months, his growth will be phenomenal. In early infancy, for example, a baby may gain as much as an ounce a day. Proportional to body weight, his calorie intake at this stage is more than twice that of an adult. By the age of 4 to 6 months, a healthy infant has doubled his birth weight. By his first birthday, the infant has tripled his birth weight, and increased his length by about 50 percent. (See **Figure 15.1**.) During the first year of life, body water content decreases while lean body mass and head circumference increase. The infant's body proportions change, too, so that by age 1 he is looking less like a baby and more like a toddler.

Growth Charts

Length (used instead of height because infants can't stand) and **head circumference** are more sensitive measures than weight for assessing a baby's growth and nutritional status. Weight alone reflects just recent nutritional intake. Head circumference measures brain growth and development. Chronic malnutrition can limit this growth, and is reflected in inadequate gains in head size. Regular measurements of head circumference, therefore, can verify proper growth. Head circumference measurements are useful in infants and children up to age 2.

During routine checkups throughout childhood and adolescence, health-care practitioners measure weight, height (or length), and head circumference and plot these values on **growth charts**. Each growth chart consists of a set of curves called percentiles that show the distribution of values for American children based on a certain measurement (**Figure 15.2**). New growth charts released in 2000 have separate charts for weight, length (height), head circumference, and body mass index (BMI) for ages 2 to 20. Separate charts for each of these measures are available for boys and girls, and for two age ranges: birth to 36 months, and 2 to 20 years. (See Appendix I.) Health-care practitioners use these charts to plot the growth of an individual child, and to compare one child's growth to that of children in the general population. Where the child's measurement falls on the percentile curves shows how that individual child ranks among 100 of her peers. For example, if an infant is at the 75th percentile for length, it means that this child, compared to 100 other infants of the same age, is longer than 75 and shorter than 25. Parents can become preoccupied with percentile rankings, comparing these numbers to grades in school, for instance. It is important to remember that the percentiles are only a means of tracking a child's growth. If a child begins life at the 10th percentile for weight and length, and continues to progress at this same percentile throughout infancy and childhood, there is no cause for alarm. While this particular child may be "small" or petite, he or she is growing well. Genetic predisposition—parental height, for example— plays a large role in determining a child's growth pattern. Concern should be raised only when an infant or older child crosses two or more percentile curves in a short time.

infancy The period between birth to 12 months of age.

Apgar scores Quantitative rating system to measure vital signs of a newborn immediately after birth based on heart rate, respiration rate, color, muscle tone, and response to stimuli.

gestational age Age of the fetus measured from the first day of the mother's last menstrual period until birth.

prematurity Birth before 37 weeks of gestation.

full-term The normal period of human gestation, between 38 and 41 weeks.

length Appropriate measure of an infant not yet capable of standing; differentiated from height.

head circumference Measurement of the largest part of the infant's head (just above the eyebrow and ears); used to determine brain growth.

growth chart Charts that plot the weight, length, and head circumference of infants and children as they grow.

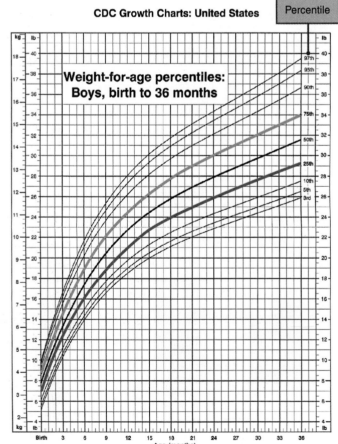

Figure 15.2 **Growth chart from the CDC.**
Source: Developed by the National Center for Health Statistics in collaboration with the National Center for Chronic Disease Prevention and Health Promotion (2000).

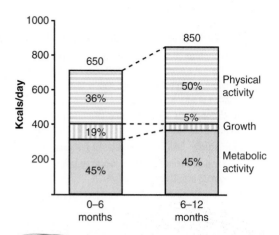

Table 15.1 **Energy RDA for Infants**

Age (mo)	Median Weight		kcal/kg	kcal/d*
	lb	kg		
0–6	13	6	108	650
6–12	20	9	98	850

* The values for kilocalories per day are based on median weights of infants. Needs of individual infants vary.

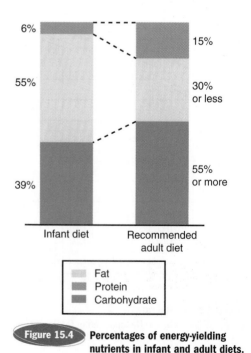

Figure 15.4 **Percentages of energy-yielding nutrients in infant and adult diets.**

Catch-up Growth

Infants are capable of catch-up growth following illness or periods of inadequate nutrition. Rapid weight gain is first, followed by a jump in length. Resolution of the illness or resumption of adequate nutrition must occur in order for catch-up growth to take place.

Key Concepts: *A full-term infant is expected to lose about 6 percent of her weight immediately after birth. The infant will regain this lost weight within 10 to 14 days, and will continue to gain weight rapidly thereafter. A typical infant doubles her birth weight by age 4 to 6 months, and triples it by 12 months. Infant length increases about 50 percent during the first year. Health-care practitioners use growth charts to follow and assess an infant's growth in weight, length, and head circumference.*

Energy and Nutrient Needs of Infancy

How do you suppose scientists determine the nutrient needs of newborns and young infants? Studies with babies as subjects are rare—the logistical and ethical questions are daunting! So how else can we know what babies need? It's simple; we just look at the food that was designed especially for babies—breast milk. The composition of human milk is the gold standard by which infant nutrient needs are determined. Babies who are not breast-fed are given infant formula. To ensure that formula meets all of an infant's nutrient needs, federal regulations require that the formula's composition comply with nutritional standards. In the United States, most infant formulas have a base of modified cow's milk or soy protein.

Energy

An infant's energy need is the amount of energy she requires for basal functions such as respiration and metabolism, in addition to growth and activity. An infant's basal energy needs, relative to her size, are about twice that of an adult. This is partly because infants, for their size, have a greater surface (skin) area than adults do, and therefore lose proportionately more body heat. The amount of energy an infant needs for activity varies throughout the first year of life, increasing as the child becomes more mobile. (See **Figure 15.3**.) Activity typically increases sharply during the second 6 months of life. In general, an infant requires about 100 kilocalories per kilogram of body weight.[2] **Table 15.1** lists the specific RDA values.

The appropriate balance of energy sources (carbohydrate, fat, and protein) is different for infants and adults (**Figure 15.4**). The best diet for infants (as modeled by human milk) is high in fat, and moderate in carbohydrate. Feeding infants poses the situation of high-calorie needs but low volume of consumption. An infant's stomach is quite small; a newborn can consume only about 1 to 2 ounces of liquid at a feeding. Because fat is the most concentrated source of calories, a high-fat diet supplies adequate calories in a smaller volume. A high-fat diet also is necessary for normal brain growth, which continues until about 18 to 24 months of age. **Figure 15.5** shows the primary functions of energy-yielding nutrients in infants, which we discuss in the next sections.

Protein

Protein needs during infancy are higher than at any other time in the life cycle. In fact, protein needs (measured in grams per kilogram of body weight) throughout the first year of life are at least twice as high as an adult's needs. Nine essential amino acids are required in infancy. Deficiency in any of them can retard growth. During times of stress, such as illness, three conditionally essential amino acids—cysteine, tyrosine, and taurine—may become essential to an infant. In addition, these nutrients may be essential for premature infants and for babies who suffer from certain **inborn errors of metabolism**. The carnitine and glycine content of human milk suggests that these amino acids are required in higher amounts during infancy as well. **Table 15.2** lists the protein RDA for infants.

The protein content of human milk is lower than that of unmodified cow's milk. This is appropriate for the **neonate**, whose kidneys and GI tract are still immature. Indeed, excessive protein may disturb an infant's fragile hydration status, which is one reason that regular cow's milk is inappropriate for infants. The types of protein in human and cow's milk also differ. The main types of proteins in any milk are casein (phosphorus-containing proteins) and whey proteins. Human milk has larger amounts of the whey protein **alpha-lactalbumin**, for example. This protein contains all of the essential amino acids infants need, and human babies easily digest and absorb it. Cow's milk, in contrast, contains larger amounts of casein, a large protein that forms hard curds in the infant's stomach. Infants cannot digest or absorb casein easily, and it may cause intestinal blood loss. The whey-to-casein ratio of human milk is 80:20, and the whey-to-casein ratio of cow's milk is 20:80.

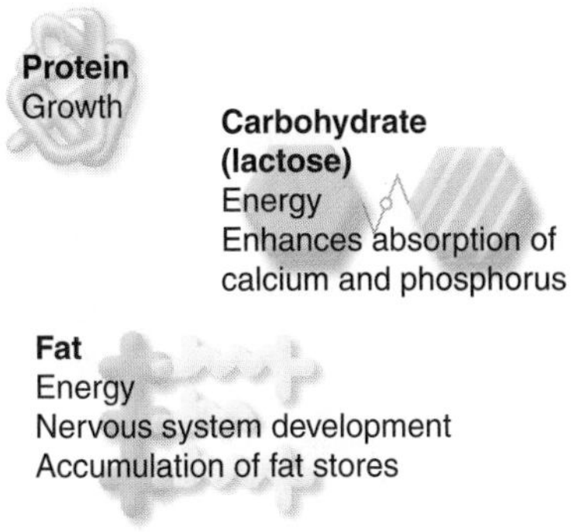

Carbohydrate and Fat

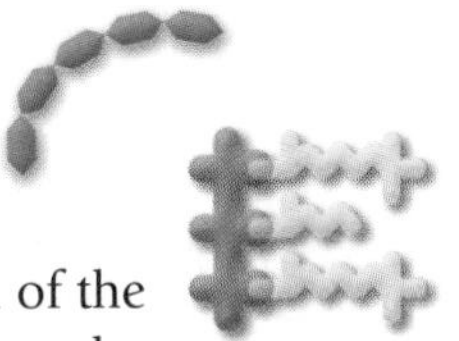

Carbohydrates and triglycerides are the major energy sources for infants. This allows protein to be used primarily for growth and not as an energy source. Nearly all of the carbohydrate in human milk, and in the infant formulas made from cow's milk, is lactose. Infants digest lactose easily and tolerate it well.

Fat is the major energy source in the infant's diet, and is important for development of the central nervous system, and accumulation of body fat stores. Fats in milk also enhance a baby's sense of fullness between feedings. Although formula manufacturers try to mimic the composition of human milk, formula remains an imperfect copy. For example, alpha-linolenic acid, an essential omega-3 fatty acid, is missing from many formulas. In addition, formulas lack two related fats found in human milk, eicosapentaenoic acid (EPA) and docosahexaenoic acid (DHA).

Water

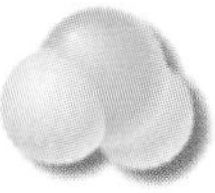

Because water as a percentage of body weight is higher in babies than in adults, infants have higher fluid needs. Infants need 1.5 milliliters per kilocalorie consumed; the value for adults is 1.0 milliliters per kilocalorie. Human milk fulfills not only the nutrient needs of the neonate, but also the fluid requirements. Properly prepared formula accomplishes the same task. During the first 4 to 6 months, supplemental water is not necessary for healthy infants who are exclusively breast-fed or who receive properly mixed formula. This is true even in hot, humid weather.[3] Hospitals frequently provide glucose water to newborns, but this practice is unnecessary and may interfere with breastfeeding.[4] Once solid foods are introduced, a baby's water needs change and additional water may be required.

Vitamins and Minerals

As long as an infant is receiving adequate calories from breast milk or infant formula, nearly all vitamin and mineral needs also are being met.

PRIMARY FUNCTIONS OF ENERGY-YIELDING NUTRIENTS IN INFANTS

Protein
Growth

Carbohydrate (lactose)
Energy
Enhances absorption of calcium and phosphorus

Fat
Energy
Nervous system development
Accumulation of fat stores

Figure 15.5 Primary functions of energy-yielding nutrients in infants.

Table 15.2 Protein RDA for Infants

Age (mo)	g/kg	g/d*
0–6	2.2	13
6–12	1.6	14

* The values for grams per day are based on median weights of infants.

Source: Food and Nutrition Board. *Recommended Dietary Allowances.* 10th ed. Washington, DC: National Academy Press; 1989.

inborn error of metabolism Biological defect (e.g., PKU) that prevents proper metabolism of a specific nutrient.

neonate An infant from birth to 28 days.

alpha-lactalbumin Primary protein in human milk.

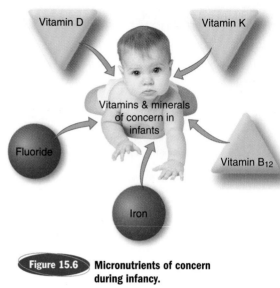

Figure 15.6 **Micronutrients of concern during infancy.**

Infant formula is fortified with all essential vitamins and minerals according to guidelines established by the American Academy of Pediatrics (AAP) and enforced by the Food and Drug Administration. Human milk provides all of the necessary vitamins and minerals for infant growth and development, with a few important exceptions. This section focuses on these exceptions, and other nutrients of concern for infants (see **Figure 15.6**).

Vitamin D Vitamin D is a key nutrient for calcium absorption and mineralization of bone. Human milk is low in vitamin D; however, most infants make enough vitamin D from exposure to sunlight, so inadequate vitamin D is rarely a problem. It may be a concern, though, for infants who are not exposed to sunlight, as well as those with darkly pigmented skin. These babies make less vitamin D from the same amount of sunlight exposure than do lighter-skinned infants. If a breast-fed baby does not get adequate sunlight exposure, and if the baby's mother is deficient in vitamin D, the infant's risk is especially high. At-risk babies should receive supplements of 10 micrograms (400 IU) of vitamin D per day.[5]

Vitamin K Vitamin K is necessary for the production of prothrombin, a substance needed in order for blood to clot. An important source of vitamin K for the body is intestinal bacterial synthesis of this vitamin. Babies, however, are born with minimal stores of vitamin K and since the gut is sterile at birth, limited vitamin K is available. It is therefore recommended that a single dose of vitamin K be given at birth. Both human milk and infant formula provide adequate vitamin K, and as feeding begins, helpful bacteria begin to flourish in the infant's intestinal tract.

Vitamin B$_{12}$ Vitamin B$_{12}$ is essential for cell division and normal folate metabolism. Mothers who include meat, fish, and dairy products in their diets produce milk that is adequate in vitamin B$_{12}$. This may not be true of strict vegetarians, whose diet—and milk—may be deficient in vitamin B$_{12}$. Breast-fed infants of vegan mothers may need a vitamin B$_{12}$ supplement.

Iron Iron is essential for growth and development, and iron-deficiency anemia is the most common nutritional deficiency in the United States. Human milk is not a rich source of iron, but it does not need to be. Approximately 50 percent of the iron in breast milk is absorbed, compared to only 4 percent of the iron in infant formula. If the mother has consumed an iron-rich diet during pregnancy, the fetus builds large enough iron stores during gestation to meet most of its iron needs for the first few months of life. These stores begin to diminish during the fourth month of life. By the age of 6 months, a breast-fed infant needs an additional iron source. Iron-fortified infant cereals can meet this need. For formula-fed babies, iron supplementation is needed from birth. The AAP therefore recommends iron-fortified formula for all formula-fed babies.[6]

Fluoride Human milk also is low in fluoride, a mineral important for dental health. Current research has led the American Dental Association and the AAP to recommend fluoride supplements for breast-fed infants after the age of 6 months.[7] If the local water supply has adequate fluoride, and the formula is mixed with tap water, formula-fed infants do not need fluoride supplements. If the water used to mix formula has inadequate fluoride, fluoride supplements are indicated. Fluoridation policies and the fluoride content of tap water vary among municipalities.

Key Concepts: *Energy and nutrient needs for infancy are estimated based on the composition of human milk. Compared to adults, the energy and nutrient needs of infants, per kilogram of body weight, are quite high, in order to support rapid growth and development. Vitamin D, iron, and fluoride need a bit of special attention to ensure the infant obtains enough. If breast milk or formula (properly mixed) is meeting energy needs, fluid needs of the infant also are being met.*

Newborn Breastfeeding

The AAP has identified breastfeeding as the ideal method of feeding to achieve optimal growth and development of the infant,[8] and recommends that breastfeeding begin as soon after birth as possible. Whenever newborns show signs of hunger, they need to be fed. These signs include **rooting** (turning its head when stroked on the cheek) and alertness. Preferably, feeding should begin before the infant cries. It can be difficult for a crying, frantic newborn to **latch on** to its mother's breast (nipple and areola), and the anxiety created in the mother may inhibit letdown. Feedings should occur every 2 to 3 hours, for a total of 8 to 12 feedings a day. Duration of feedings is guided by the infant's behavior, and may last from 10 to 15 minutes per breast. Hospitals should provide every opportunity for breastfeeding to begin before the baby goes home. "Rooming-in," in which the baby stays in its mother's hospital room instead of in a nursery, makes breastfeeding easier. Nurses or **lactation consultants** should be available to offer professional breastfeeding support to new mothers. The AAP recommends that no supplements be given to breast-fed neonates unless medically indicated. Also, the AAP discourages such common hospital practices as presenting the neonate to the mother with supplemental bottles of glucose water or formula, and giving breastfeeding mothers emergency supplies of infant formula when they are discharged from the hospital.

Alternative Feeding: Infant Formula

Chapter 14 presents the benefits of breastfeeding, so let's look at alternative feeding. Women may decide not to breastfeed, or to breastfeed only briefly. Their infants need infant formulas designed to provide adequate nutrition.

Standard Infant Formulas

Infant formula is manufactured under strict government standards to reflect the nutritional needs of the infant. Standard infant formulas have cow's milk as a base. In making infant formula, manufacturers first remove the fat and replace it with vegetable oils. They add vitamins and minerals to approximate the nutritional content of human milk. Energy content mirrors human milk, providing 20 kilocalories per ounce. Popular infant formula brands include Enfamil, Good Start, and Similac. Infant formulas are available with or without added iron, but because of the decreased bioavailability of iron in infant formulas and the infant's high needs, the AAP recommends only iron-fortified formulas.

Soy-Based Formulas

Formula-fed infants who develop vomiting, diarrhea, constipation, abdominal pain, or colic are frequently switched to soy formulas. In these formulas, soy is the source of protein. To compensate for the inferior digestibility of soy protein, soy formulas contain more protein than formulas based on cow's milk. Soy formulas are lactose-free and iron-fortified. Corn syrup and sucrose are the carbohydrate sources. Examples of soy formulas are Alsoy, Isomil, and Prosobee.

rooting The infant's response to stimuli around the mouth—turning the head expecting to suckle.

latching on Successful attachment of the infant to the breast, taking in the nipple and as much areola as possible.

lactation consultant Health professional trained to specialize in education about and promotion of breast-feeding; may be certified as an International Board Certified Lactation Consultant (IBCLC).

Quick Bites

What's a biberon?

Many people consider Dr. Nils Rosen von Rosenstein the father of pediatrics. In his 1764 textbook, he describes a "biberon," a leather nipple used for artificial infant feeding. He also describes 14 types of infant diarrhea.

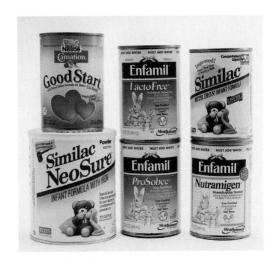

Popular infant formulas.

Hypoallergenic Protein Hydrolysate Formulas

Infants who are allergic to both cow's milk and soy protein may receive special formulas that use hydrolyzed protein. Enzymes hydrolyze protein to amino acids and small peptides. Examples of protein hydrolysate formulas include Alimentum, Enfamil Nutramigen, and Pregestimil. Fat sources vary among these formulas. Infants who have difficulty absorbing fat should have formulas with medium-chain triglycerides. Although these formulas are expensive and taste bad, they are essential for many infants.

Preterm Infant Formulas

Special formulas are made for preterm infants—those born before 37 weeks gestation. Human milk is still best for these infants but is not always available. Most preterm formulas are used only until the infant achieves the desired weight for hospital discharge. Compared to standard formulas, these formulas are more concentrated in calories (22 to 24 kilocalories per ounce) and higher in protein, vitamin E, calcium, and phosphorus. Because preterm infants have less lactase in their digestive systems than full-term babies, preterm formulas have low lactose content and use glucose polymers as a source of carbohydrates. These products contain 60 percent whey proteins, and provide the conditional amino acid cysteine. Medium-chain triglycerides supply 40 to 50 percent of the fats. Examples of preterm formulas are Enfamil Premature, Similac NeoSure, and Similac Special Care.

Formula Preparation

Formulas come in three forms: ready-to-feed, concentrate, and powdered. Although the ready-to-feed is the most convenient, it is also the most expensive. As the name implies, the formula can be poured directly from the can into a bottle and fed to the baby. For at least the first few months, the AAP recommends sterilizing all equipment used for feeding. Liquid concentrate formula is mixed with an equal amount of water before feeding. Powdered formula also is mixed with water and is the least expensive. Again, before making formula for infants, all equipment should be steril-

Fyi | Preterm Infant Needs

FOR YOUR INFORMATION

Preterm describes infants born before 37 weeks gestation. Preterm infants are not fully mature or developed. Depending on their gestational age at birth, the infant may require intensive care. During the last trimester, the fetus is gaining weight rapidly and building stores of such nutrients as calcium, phosphorus, and iron. Calcium and phosphorus are required for bone mineralization during the third trimester. If the fetus is delivered preterm, much of this bone development and nutrient storage must be accomplished through feeding after birth.

For the infant who weighs more than 1,500 grams at birth, human milk or standard formula that delivers 20 calories per fluid ounce is adequate to support growth.[1] Very low-birth-weight infants require fortified human milk or preterm formula that contains 24 calories per fluid ounce. Because of the immaturity of a preterm infant's GI tract, preterm formulas contain increased medium-chain triglycerides, protein, glucose polymers, calcium, and phosphorus.

Mothers of preterm infants are strongly encouraged to breastfeed. Human milk is easily digested and absorbed. In addition, both colostrum and human milk contain factors useful in preventing infection. These factors are particularly important for preterm

infants, whose immunological systems are especially immature. Because a preterm infant may not be able to suck vigorously enough, the mother may need to use a breast pump to express her milk. The milk can then be delivered through a tube to the baby's stomach. Liquid human milk fortifiers are added to provide the supplemental calcium and phosphorus required by preterm babies. As the baby gains weight and becomes stronger, efforts are made to get the baby to the breast for feedings.

1 American Academy of Pediatrics. Committee on Fetus and Newborn. *Guidelines for Perinatal Care.* 4th ed. Elk Grove, IL; 1997.

ized and water for mixing with the formula should be boiled for 5 minutes and allowed to cool for at least 20 minutes. Individual bottles or a day's supply can be mixed at one time.

People who use infant formulas must observe principles of food safety. Infants have an immature immune system, and may develop infections from improperly prepared or stored formula. Bacteria grow best in warm, wet, sugar-rich environments, making improperly stored formula an ideal breeding ground for germs. If not fed to the infant immediately, prepared formula should be refrigerated immediately and kept in the refrigerator until needed. After formula is made, it may stay in the refrigerator for 48 hours. After that time it should be discarded. In countries and areas where the purity of the water supply is questionable, or aseptic technique is impossible, preparation may contaminate the formula. Bacteria or other microorganisms in contaminated water can cause serious illness and can be fatal. Improperly mixed formula is another danger, whether a result of ignorance in following instructions or of economics. Some caregivers on limited budgets might purposefully overdilute formula to make it last longer. This deprives the infant of necessary calories and protein, and provides too much water. Other caregivers overconcentrate the formula in the misguided belief that this might encourage faster growth. Overconcentrated formula provides too much protein and too little water, and may impair an infant's kidney function and hydration status.

Breast Milk or Formula: How Much Is Enough?

It is fairly simple to use RDA values and breast milk or formula composition to estimate an infant's needs based on body weight. For example, a newborn who weighs 7 pounds, 11 ounces (3.5 kg) requires approximately 378 kilocalories (108 kcal/kg × 3.5 kg) and 7.7 grams of protein each day. This amount is provided by approximately 550 milliliters (~ 19 oz) of breast milk or infant formula. It's easy to keep track of how much formula an infant has consumed, but what about the breast-fed baby?

Although you can't see how much breast milk a nursing infant is consuming, there are other markers that baby is getting enough to eat. An adequately fed newborn will breastfeed 8 to 12 times, wet at least 6 diapers, and have at least 3 loose stools each day in the first week of life. The newborn will also regain its birth weight within the first 2 weeks. Normal growth, regular elimination patterns, and a satisfied demeanor are the best indicators that a baby is getting enough to eat.

Feeding Technique

A breastfeeding mother holds her baby close, at a distance that encourages mother-baby eye contact (see **Figure 15.7**). Nature also encourages a nursing mother to breastfeed in a quiet setting, when she is calm. Milk simply doesn't "let down" if a mother is tense or distracted. While nursing, a baby is doing much more than merely filling his stomach. He is gazing into his mother's eyes, nuzzling her breast with his cheek, and snuggling close to her body, enveloped in Mom's smell and warmth. When motor coordination allows it, the baby reaches up to explore his mother's face as he nurses, tracing the outline of her lips, putting a tiny finger into her mouth, patting and stroking her cheek, playing with her hair. These are intensely rewarding times for both mother and baby, and are usually accompanied by much maternal smiling, cooing, and talking. Bottle-feeding can, and should, be just as emotionally nurturing. Feeding should

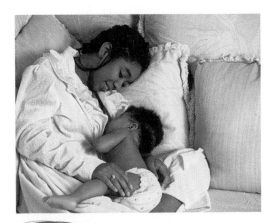

Figure 15.7 Breastfeeding nutures an infant emotionally as well as physically.

take place in a loving and warm environment. During bottle-feeding, the caregiver needs to hold the baby close and make eye contact. Propping the bottle against a pillow or other object, so that the baby can feed alone, should be avoided.

Babies swallow air while feeding, whether at the breast or with a bottle, and they need to be burped. Some caregivers place the baby over a shoulder, so that the shoulder places gentle pressure on the baby's belly. Another method is to sit the baby up and gently lean her forward. Babies generally need to be burped after 15 minutes or 2 to 3 ounces of formula. Just as the infant sends signals of readiness for feeding, she also signals fullness. Fullness cues include fussiness, playfulness, sleep, or just turning away. Parents need to learn these cues, and follow them.

WIC: Support for Infants

As described in the previous chapter, the Special Supplemental Nutrition Program for Women, Infants, and Children (WIC) is a much-acclaimed program of the Food and Nutrition Service of the U.S. Department of Agriculture (USDA). WIC provides food vouchers to support the nutritional needs of breastfeeding women, while educational programs and peer support answer questions and encourage new moms. WIC also provides vouchers to low-income families whose infants require formula. Clients present these vouchers to their local stores for the purchase of infant formula. The vouchers cover all formula needs for the first few months of life; clients must bear some of the cost as the child grows. Periodically, WIC participants are required to bring their infants into the local WIC office. These visits give WIC staff an opportunity to evaluate the infant's growth and provide the caregiver with additional nutrition education.

Key Concepts: *Human milk provides all necessary nutrients for growth and development and enhances the immune system of the maturing infant. Infants who are not breast-fed receive infant formula, which should be fortified with iron. There are four general categories of infant formula: standard, soy, hypoallergenic hydrolyzed protein, and preterm. Careful preparation and storage of the formula ensures proper nutrient composition and food safety. Formula feedings should nourish the baby emotionally as well as nutritionally.*

Introduction of Solid Foods into the Infant's Diet

Solid foods are introduced based on an infant's physiological needs, such as depletion of iron stores, and on physical development, such as the ability to sit up. To say that we are introducing solid foods is a bit of a misnomer; we are really referring to pureed and liquefied cereals, fruits, vegetables, and meats that are added to the infant's diet of breast milk or infant formula. Currently, the American Academy of Pediatrics recommends that solid foods be introduced between the age of 4 and 6 months.[9] This age range is purposefully broad to allow for differences in growth and development among babies.

Physiological Indicators of Infant Readiness for Solid Foods

Before a baby reaches 4 to 6 months of age, solid food is not necessary for nutrition; in fact, early introduction of supplemental foods can be detrimental. At the age of 4 to 6 months, however, an infant is physiologically ready to expand his diet. For example, a baby has increased levels of digestive enzymes by this age, so that foods other than human milk or formula can be digested with ease. In addition, the infant is able to maintain adequate hydration better by the age of 6 months. Before this, adding cereals or other solid foods to the diet can negatively affect an infant's hydration. It is probably no coincidence that the iron stores acquired in the mother's womb become depleted at the same time the baby is physiologically ready to expand his diet. However, solid food is a supplement to, not a replacement for, human milk or formula at this stage.

It is wise to proceed slowly with the introduction of solid foods. It has been shown that delaying the introduction of common food allergens, particularly cow's milk, egg whites, and wheat, can prevent food allergies for many infants. Because the infant's immune and digestive systems are still immature, these foods should be avoided for the first 12 months of life. If these foods are introduced prematurely, the infant may mount an immunological response, or allergic reaction. In addition to its allergic potential, whole cow's milk provides too much protein and too little iron, is low in essential fatty acids, may impair kidney function and lead to dehydration, and has been linked to development of insulin-dependent diabetes mellitus.[10] Although the existence of a link between early introduction of unmodified cow's milk and diabetes has not been clarified, the AAP recommended in 1994 that families with a strong history of type 1 diabetes mellitus breast-feed their infants, and avoid introducing intact cow's milk protein during the first year of life.[11]

Developmental Readiness for Solid Foods

If you attempt to spoon-feed a very young infant, for example, at 3 weeks of age, the infant's tongue will push the spoon and food right back out. This **extrusion reflex** is a sign that the infant is not ready for solid foods. By 4 to 6 months of age, the infant will no longer push the food out, and is capable of transferring food from the front of the mouth to the back, an ability necessary to swallow solid foods. Also, the infant can purposefully bring its hand to its mouth, an ability necessary for self-feeding. In addition, if the baby is able to control its head and neck while sitting with minimal support, she is ready to be fed solids.

Feeding Schedule for Infants

The first food introduced is usually an iron-fortified, hypoallergenic infant cereal: baby rice cereal. The cereal should be mixed with human milk, formula, or water. Feeding a baby solids is easier using a spoon appropriately sized for the infant. Still, feeding solids takes practice, for both baby and adult! Once the infant is taking rice cereal two or three times each day, other foods such as vegetables and fruits can be introduced. New foods are introduced one at a time, at intervals of about 1 week to see how well the infant tolerates each food, and to be on the lookout for allergic reactions. If the infant appears disinterested in a food, or seems to dislike it, try it again another time. If a rash or other sign of reaction develops, the pediatrician should be consulted before trying that food again.

Although convenient, commercially prepared baby foods are not necessary. Baby foods can be prepared at home using a grinder, food mill, blender, or food processor. Seasonings should be avoided. Caregivers should allow the baby to develop personal food preferences, rather than feed the baby only the foods the caregivers enjoy. Even throughout the first year, breast milk or infant formula still forms the major portion of the infant's diet. Ideally, however, the child has been introduced to a variety of foods by its first birthday. **Table 15.3** is a guide to feeding infants up to 12 months old.

extrusion reflex Response by an infant to thrust the tongue forward when a spoon is put in its mouth; indicates that an infant is not ready for spoon feeding.

Quick Bites

Pumping Iron

The use of cow's milk for children younger than 1 year is a common cause of iron deficiency. Cow's milk is low in iron, and drinking cow's milk can cause intestinal bleeding in infants. The amount of iron in breast milk is low, but this iron is very bioavailable. Breast milk also contains proteins that bind iron, thereby inhibiting the growth of diarrhea-causing bacteria that feed on iron. If formula is used, the AAP recommends that it be iron-fortified.

palmar grasp Infant's use of entire palm to pick up items; an early gross motor skill.

pincer grasp Infant's use of fingers to manipulate items; indicates readiness to handle finger foods.

By 6 to 7 months of age, the child demonstrates advances toward self-feeding. Allowing the baby to hold an infant spoon and cup (preferably one with a cap and spout) during feeding encourages eventual self-feeding. At this age, the baby is not capable of manipulating either item successfully, but wants to mimic the caregiver's behavior. Babies of this age use a **palmar grasp** to pick up items, allowing them to hold large items like infant teething biscuits. Picking up small pieces of food is still difficult. It is important to allow the child to experience feeding time with as many senses as possible. Tactile senses are heightened at this time, and most exploration is accomplished through the mouth. As you might imagine, feeding time for infants and toddlers can get a bit messy!

At 8 months, the infant has more manual dexterity. The child may demonstrate the **pincer grasp**, using fingers to pick up objects. He is able to participate in the feeding process, and may be able to pick up small particles of food. It is important that caregivers monitor the child's eating to make sure the youngster does not choke on food, or on nonfood items.

By 9 to 12 months of age, a greater proportion of the child's nutrient needs are being met through solid foods. Consequently, intake of either human milk or formula decreases. Now the child is demonstrating a limited proficiency with both cup and spoon, and self-feeding is under way. If the texture is soft and the pieces are small, most table foods are appropriate for the child at this stage. The exceptions are cow's milk, egg whites, and wheat, which should be avoided. **Table 15.4** lists the developmental patterns for infants during the first year.

Table 15.3 Infant Feeding Guide (0 to 12 months)

Age (mo)	Human Milk or Iron-fortified formula	Cereals & Breads	Vegetables	Fruits	Other Protein Foods
0–4	8–12 feedings per day 16–32 oz	None	None	None	None
4–6	4–7 feedings per day 24–32 oz	Iron-fortified baby cereal, rice, barley, oatmeal; feed by spoon; Mix 2–3 tsp with human milk or formula	None	None	None
6–8	3–4 feedings per day 24–32 oz Begin to offer cup	Add mixed cereal after previous plain ones; 2 servings per day; dry toast or teething biscuit	Plain strained or mashed vegetables 2 times per day	Fresh or cooked fruits: mashed bananas, applesauce; strained plain fruits; 2 times per day	
8–10	3–4 feedings per day 16–32 oz Offer formula in cup	Infant iron-fortified cereals; Cream of Rice; dry toast, teething biscuit	Plain cooked mashed vegetables;	Peeled soft fruit wedges: bananas, pears, oranges, apples, peaches	Lean meat and chicken: strained, chopped, or small tender pieces
10–12	3–4 feedings per day 16–32 oz Formula in a cup	Infant cereals, unsweetened cereals, bread, rice, noodles and pasta	Cooked vegetable pieces	All fresh fruits peeled and seeded; canned fruit in water	Small tender pieces of meat, chicken, or fish; eggs, mild cheeses, yogurt, cooked dried beans

Feeding time should be a set time to communicate with and enjoy the child at a slow pace. Equipment such as a highchair or a booster seat attached to the table allow the child sufficient space to enjoy the meal, and help to define the mealtime environment. Without proper equipment, many infants merely graze all day, moving from one activity to another without the opportunity to develop good feeding skills. Interacting with the child during a meal can be as important to the child's development as the foods provided.[12] Slower-than-expected growth, or failure to thrive, during the second 6 months of life frequently is related to feeding practices and progression of food introduction. Questions to ask in these cases include the following: Is the mealtime defined? Has the child become "stuck" on a limited selection of foods? Does the child drink too many of his or her calories as milk or juice? **Table 15.5** gives pratical tips on feeding babies; **Table 15.6** lists foods and practices to avoid when feeding babies.

This chapter does not attempt to define the caregiver for the infant. In today's society, it is inappropriate to assume that the caregiver is the mother, father, grandparent, or even a relative of the child. Infant nutrition is influenced by all adults or caregivers in the child's life. Many children spend the majority of their feeding time in a child-care setting. Nutrition education and training for child-care workers enhances the likelihood of proper feeding practices in these settings.[13]

Table 15.4 Developmental Patterns and Feeding Recommendations for Infancy

	Birth	1mo	2mo	3mo	4mo	5mo	6mo	7mo	8mo	9mo	10mo	11mo
Mouth Pattern	Suck and swallow reflex Extrusion reflex				Transfer food from front to back Drooling				Begin chewing Side to side movement of tongue Mashing food with jaws			Biting Chewing
Hand Coordination	Random motion of hands Hand to mouth to signal hunger				Hand to mouth purposefully		Palmar grasp	Pincer grasp	Grabs spoon		Spoon to mouth turned over	
Body Control	Minimal head control				Sits supported, loses balance when reaching		Sits unsupported and while reaching Hand manipulation		Continued improvement of balance while sitting Begins to stand and possibly walks			
Digestive Ability	Can digest appropriate milk				Intestinal amylase increases			Gastric acid volume increases			Can handle balanced amount of unseasoned family food	
Homeostatic Ability	Low, needs breast milk or carefully adapted formula							Increased ability to maintain hydration and chemical balance				
Nutritional Requirements	High nutrient needs for rapid growth	Iron stores depleted for preemies					Iron stores depleted for term infants		Needs gradually being met with solid diet over breast milk/formula			Move to table food and cup
Feeding Style	Nipple feeding				Begin spoon feeding	Spoon feeding	Introduce cup with meals		Begin self-feed with cup; begin proficiency with spoon			Cup and spoon self-feed
Food Selection	Breast or formula				Begin solids, iron source		Semi-solid foods	Increase texture			Pieces of soft cooked foods	

Source: Adapted from Satter E. *Child of Mine: Feeding With Love and Good Sense.* 3rd. ed. Palo Alto, CA: Bull Publishing Co.; 2000.

Table 15.5 Practical Feeding Tips

4–6 months old

Avoid seasonings. Babies enjoy plain foods. Added sugar and salt are unnecessary.

Commercially prepared foods are acceptable, but so are home-prepared foods. Mash plain, cooked vegetables or fruit.

Add one new food each week.

Work up to a total of one-half cup of cereal per day.

Feed the baby from a dish, not the jar.

Throw out leftovers from the baby's dish.

Once introduced, aim for 2 tablespoons per day of vegetables and fruit.

Use baby-sized spoons, cups, and bowls.

7–9 months old

Cook fruits with a little water to soften them.

Add more finger foods to the diet. Examples include dry unsweetened oat or rice cereal, rice cakes, and cooked rice.

Grate fresh fruits and vegetables, and allow the child to pick them up and self-feed.

Offer a variety of cooked vegetables that can be either mashed or picked up in tiny pieces.

Offer a variety of protein sources: cooked fish; chicken; turkey; beef; mashed, cooked beans.

10–12 months

Allow the child to self-feed with a spoon and cup.

Have the child join the rest of the family at meals.

Feed the child both meals and healthful snacks, sometimes just smaller versions of the meal, to fulfill his or her energy needs.

Remember to offer the child water from a cup.

Table 15.6 Feeding Practices and Foods to Avoid

Practice to Avoid	Rationale
Leaving baby alone during feeding	Infants and toddlers need to be supervised at all times. Children can accidentally choke during mealtime.
Adding salt, seasonings, and spices	Children prefer plain foods and do not need additional seasoning. Excessively salty foods can place a burden on the developing kidney system.
Egg whites and wheat	A common source of food allergies. Neither is necessary in the diet before age 1.
Cow's milk	Neither necessary nor well tolerated until age 1. Associated with increased allergic potential and iron-deficiency anemia.
Honey and corn syrup	Both products contain spores of *Clostridium botulinum*. In infants, these spores can cause botulism, a deadly food-borne illness.
High-risk choking foods	Foods that are choking hazards for infants and toddlers include hot dogs, nuts, peanuts, raw carrots, sausage pieces, raisins, apple chunks, popcorn, hard candy, potato chips, gum, hard pretzels or pretzel nuggets, chicken bones and wings, grapes, and plain peanut butter from a spoon. Because peanuts are a common food allergen, peanut butter should not be introduced in the first year.
Heating foods on the stove/microwave	Accidental injury or burns can occur with uneven and excessive overheating of infant foods. The baby cannot tell the caregiver that the food is too hot.
Excessive amounts of breast milk or formula	During the second half of the first year, the child gradually decreases consumption of breast milk and formula in order to increase the amount of solid foods needed for energy and iron.
Excessive intake of fruit juices/drinks	Both failure to thrive and overweight have been seen from excessive consumption of juice or other drinks. See the FYI feature "Fruit Juices and Drinks."
Goat's milk	Goat's milk is too low in folate, iron, vitamins C and D, and is not a suitable substitute for either human milk or formula.

Key Concepts: *Usually between the ages of 4 and 6 months an infant's physiological needs and developmental readiness indicate the appropriate time to introduce solid foods. Semisolid and solid foods are introduced slowly to assess for food intolerances. The caregiver should choose foods that meet the child's nutritional needs and suit his or her developmental capabilities. Iron-fortified rice cereal is the ideal first food. As the infant's oral dexterity increases, foods with texture and shape can be introduced. Self-feeding techniques develop from the palmar grasp to pick up large items to the pincer grasp to pick up small items.*

Feeding Problems during Infancy

Colic

Colic is a term that describes continuous crying and distress in a healthy infant, and appears to be due to abdominal cramping and discomfort. Infants with colic usually cry for hours, despite efforts to comfort them. In addition, these infants tend to sleep poorly, appear to pass gas frequently, and often want to be held and cuddled. Sometimes holding the baby and gentle, regular motion can give temporary relief. Parents need support and reassurance that it is not their parenting skills affecting the baby. In some cases, a change in formula or a change in the breastfeeding mother's diet provides some relief; however, diet is not considered a cause of colic. Most often, colic goes away on its own, usually by the age of 3 to 4 months.

Nursing Bottle Tooth Decay

Extensive tooth decay (**Figure 15.8**) can result if baby teeth are bathed too long in formula or juice, which nourish decay-producing bacteria. The problem usually occurs when a baby is routinely put to bed with a bottle, so that the baby's teeth are awash in formula or juice for much or all of the night. Another dental concern is that prolonged sucking through the night can affect the development and position of the teeth and jaw.

Iron-Deficiency Anemia: Milk Anemia

Human milk and cow's milk both are low in iron. As discussed earlier, this is usually not a problem—the iron in breast milk is well absorbed, and regular cow's milk is not recommended for babies under the age of 1 year. However, an infant who switches to solid foods but does not eat enough foods that are rich in iron, may develop iron-deficiency anemia. This also may occur when milk feedings supply too much of an infant's daily energy intake.

Gastroesophageal Reflux

Gastroesophageal reflux is the regurgitation of the stomach contents into the esophagus after a feeding. The relaxation or the incompetence of the lower esophageal sphincter can cause this problem. This type of spitting up occurs in 3 percent of newborns, predominantly males. Reflux typically disappears within 12 to 18 months. Spitting up small amounts of a feeding is normal, and not worthy of treatment or concern. Concern is warranted if reflux makes a child difficult to feed or results in coughing, choking, or frequent vomiting. Although some babies with severe reflux problems need surgery to repair their lower esophageal sphincter, adjustments in feeding practices can eliminate most reflux problems. For example, it can be helpful to feed the baby in an upright position; hold the baby upright after a feeding; offer smaller, more frequent feedings; burp more frequently; elevate the head of the crib; switch formulas; or thicken the formula with rice cereal.[14] (See **Table 15.7**.) Adding cereal to bottle feedings is not recommended for a baby who has reflux.

gastroesophageal reflux A backflow of stomach contents into the esophagus, accompanied by a burning pain because of the acidity of the gastric juices.

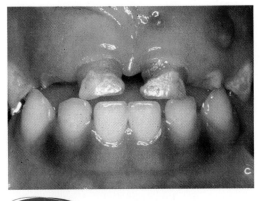

Figure 15.8 **Nursing bottle tooth decay.**

Table 15.7 **Mealtime Tips for an Infant with Reflux**

- Feed the infant in a place that is easy to clean.
- Try not to wear your favorite clothes while feeding the baby.
- Plan bath and play times for at least 1 hour after feeding.
- When changing the diaper, never raise the infant's legs above the head.
- Elevate the head of the infant's crib (place a wedge under the mattress; do not put pillows in a baby's crib).
- Enjoy your baby, but be prepared for messy feeding times.
- Be reassured that as long as the baby continues to grow, reflux is primarily a nuisance.

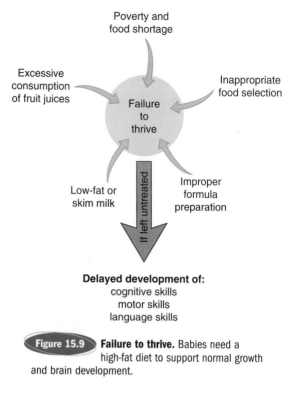

Figure 15.9 **Failure to thrive.** Babies need a high-fat diet to support normal growth and brain development.

Diarrhea

Stool patterns vary from infant to infant, as well as in the same infant over time. Healthy, thriving breast-fed infants may have up to 12 stools a day—or only 1 a week. Formula-fed infants usually have 1 to 7 bowel movements per day. Diarrhea, the frequent passage of loose, watery stools, can rapidly dehydrate an infant. Infants with diarrhea require increased fluids and caregivers should consult the child's pediatrician for specific advice about how meet this need. For example, the doctor may recommend oral rehydration therapy, using a special electrolyte-rich solution such as Enfalyte or Pedialyte.

Failure to Thrive

Full-term infants who experience poor growth in the absence of disease or physical defect suffer from **failure to thrive (FTT)**. (See **Figure 15.9**.) Although FTT can occur at any age, in infancy it usually occurs in the second half of the first year. Common causes include poverty and a resulting shortage of food, feeding inappropriate foods to an infant, and improper formula preparation. Excessive consumption of fruit juice or fruit drinks also can be the problem. The juice or drinks can cause chronic diarrhea, resulting in poor growth, or may replace meals, resulting in inadequate nutritional intake. In addition, well-meaning parents may introduce low-fat or skim milk in an attempt to prevent obesity. Babies need a high-fat diet to support normal growth and brain development. As stated, regular cow's milk should not be introduced before age 1. Low-fat milks are inappropriate for children younger than 2 years old.

Fyi **Fruit Juices and Drinks**

FOR YOUR INFORMATION

Fruit juices are popular beverages for children aged 6 months to 5 years. Juices do have benefits to the diet. They are refreshing and sweet, accessible and affordable, more healthful than soft drinks, and provide energy, water, and selected minerals and vitamins.[1] A glass of 100 percent fruit juice counts as one fruit serving. If juice is being used as a source of vitamin C, only 3 to 6 fluid ounces per day are needed for this purpose.

Fruit juices vary greatly in fiber, pectin, sorbitol, and carbohydrate composition. White grape juice is probably the easiest to digest (it contains similar amounts of glucose and fructose, and no sorbitol). Apple and pear juice, while more popular, are less well absorbed due to higher amounts of sorbitol and fructose.[2]

Fruit juice consumption can be a factor in obesity, if excess juice is consumed on top of a well-rounded diet. Paradoxically, fruit juice consumption can also be a factor in failure to thrive. Failure to thrive may result if fruit juices replace other food sources (particularly milk), or if high amounts of sorbitol and fructose cause diarrhea and malabsorption.[3] Excessive fruit juice consumption has been linked not only to failure to thrive but also to short stature and obesity.[4]

The vast array of juice drinks and fruit beverages available in the marketplace make it difficult for parents to find nutritious choices. At best, these beverages contain added vitamin C and in some cases, vitamin A and calcium. However, beverages that are less than 100 percent fruit juice are more like soft drinks than fruits, and as such should be severely limited in the diets of young children.

Recommendations for keeping intake of fruit juices to a healthy level include

- Delay the provision of juice through the WIC program (typically beginning at 4 months) to a later age.
- Limit consumption of fruit juice to 12 fluid ounces per day, and ideally no more than 3 to 6 fluid ounces per day.
- Encourage caregivers to offer fruit rather than juice to children.
- Dilute fruit juice with water.
- Delay introduction of juices in the diet until the child can drink from a cup, thus avoiding using juice in bottles.
- Research further the effects of fruit juice in the diets of children, specifically focusing on obesity and malabsorption.

1 Lifshitz F. Weaning foods...the role of fruit juice in the diets of infants and children. *J Am Coll Nutr.* 1996;15(suppl):15–35.

2 Ibid.

3 Nobugrot T, Chasalow F, Lifshftz F. Carbohydrate absorption from one serving of fruit juice in young children: age and carbohydrate composition effects. *J Am Coll Nutr.* 1997;16:152–158.

4 Dennison BA, Rockwell HL, Baker SL. Excess fruit juice consumption by preschool-aged children is associated with short stature and obesity. *Pediatrics.* 1997;99:15–22.

Untreated, FTT can delay cognitive, motor, and language development. Studies indicate, however, that intensive intervention can correct FTT and catch-up growth is possible. Such intervention includes nutrition education for caregivers, maintenance of food records by the caregiver, frequent weight checks of the infant, and perhaps social service intervention for the family.

Phenylketonuria

Phenylketonuria (PKU) is an inborn error of amino acid metabolism, in which the essential amino acid phenylalanine cannot be degraded to the amino acid tyrosine (see also Chapter 6). This disease occurs in 1 out of every 10,000 to 15,000 births, predominately among Caucasians and Asians. By law, newborns must be screened for PKU in the first two weeks of life. Children with untreated PKU suffer from profound mental retardation, brain damage, seizures, skin lesions, and neurological impairment. Treatment centers upon diet. The dietary goal is to provide enough phenylalanine for normal protein synthesis, but not so much that blood phenylalanine levels increase and affect intellectual development. Too little phenylalanine will limit growth, but too much may cause intellectual deterioration.[15] A special infant formula is available for young infants with PKU. Breastfeeding may be combined with the low-phenylalanine formula. As the child grows, caregivers must carefully calculate and balance dietary phenylalanine, protein, and calories. Professional assistance is required to maintain the diet and monitor blood phenylalanine levels.

Toddler Feeding

A **toddler** is an older infant or young child who is mobile and in the early stages of self-feeding. This is more of a developmental term than a **chronological age**. Toddlers are busy, active, messy, clumsy—and require constant supervision. A toddler's job is to explore the world and learn by mimicking. This is a wonderful yet exhausting time for caregivers. There can be a struggle between the child's need to explore and the caregiver's hope for order.

Toddlers start to exhibit unique feeding practices and styles. For some, this means that one food cannot touch another, or that foods cannot be green, or that all foods must be green. All of these preferences are merely the toddler's way of exhibiting control over his or her environment while experimenting and exploring. Although it may seem like an eternity to even the most patient caregiver, these food habits usually are temporary. The wise caregiver allows this process to occur naturally, rather than wage food-battles that the child always wins. Toddlers are ready for most table foods and can eat the same foods as the family, but with constant mealtime supervision so they avoid choking. **Table 15.8** lists patterns of eating behaviors that are normal for toddlers; **Table 15.9** offers suggestions for making toddlers' mealtimes less frustrating and more pleasant, especially for the caregiver.

While there is nothing complex about the nutrient needs and food choices appropriate for babies, it is important for caregivers to receive some education about proper feeding. Some of the practices we learn from friends, parents, and other family members, or remember from our own childhood, are inappropriate for babies. Studies show that even people who receive nutrition education in the WIC program introduce solid foods much too early, and feed infants sweet tea, colas, and other inappropriate foods. It would be nice if newborns came with instructions, but in the absence of that, a pediatrician or registered dietitian can answer feeding questions.

failure to thrive (FTT) Abnormally low gains in length (height) and weight during infancy and childhood; may result from physical problems or poor feeding, but many affected children have no apparent disease or defect.

toddler A child between 12 and 36 months of age.

chronological age Age calculated by calendar years from birth.

Table 15.8 **Common Food Habits of Toddlers**

- *Playing with food:* Toddlers frequently appear disinterested in food, merely playing with it, and refusing to let the caregiver feed them. They actually need to play with food to discover its texture, smell, and taste.

- *Food jags:* A toddler may want nothing but macaroni and cheese for dinner for a while, or refuse foods that aren't white. Nothing lasts forever, however. The caregiver should continue to offer new foods, but allow the toddler to refuse them. One day both the caregiver and the toddler may be surprised when a new food is eaten and enjoyed!

- *Food protests:* A toddler's communication skills are not as developed as his opinions or strength, which means unwanted food may end up on the floor or walls. Although this behavior is normal, it does not have to be tolerated. The toddler needs to know that the caregiver is disappointed in her. The caregiver should model positive, corrective behavior.

- *Irregular eating patterns:* Toddlers are active and need energy. However, their growth has slowed considerably by this stage, and energy requirements per unit of body weight have decreased. Toddlers will slow down their food intake, and may skip meals. It is important to continue to offer both regular meals and snacks, but the caregiver should not be disappointed when the child refuses to eat. Toddlers and children do regulate their caloric intake over time: they eat when they need to, and don't when they are not hungry, yet their average caloric intake remains fairly constant. Forcing children to eat only diminishes the importance of internal signals of hunger, satiation, and satiety.

Table 15.9 **Survival Guidelines for Toddler Mealtimes**

- Prepare for a mess. Feed the toddler in the kitchen or a part of the home that is easy to clean.

- High chairs or booster seats help define the place and time of meals and keep the toddler focused on exploring only the meal, not the entire environment.

- Keep food for meals, not for punishment or reward. This sets a foundation for healthful food habits and associations.

- Continue to present new foods to picky eaters. Then stand back and observe. Try again if necessary.

- Try not to show frustration. Keep mealtime as positive as possible.

- Learn to trust the toddler's hunger cues. If he or she doesn't seem hungry, wait until the next meal or snack.

- Allow the toddler to choose as many foods as possible, carefully framing and limiting the choices: "Would you like a banana or applesauce?"

- Encourage self-feeding with cup and child-sized utensils.

- Remember, it is the parent's job to present a healthful nutritious diet and a safe eating environment, and it's the child's job to eat it or not!

Source: Satter E. *Child of Mine: Feeding with Love and Good Sense.* 3ʳᵈ ed. Palo Alto, CA: Bull Publishing Co.; 2000; used with permission.

Key Concepts: *Feeding-related problems of infancy include colic, nursing bottle tooth decay, iron-deficiency anemia, gastroesophageal reflux, diarrhea, failure to thrive. Usually minor adjustments in food choices or feeding techniques solve these problems; however, caregivers may need the guidance of a pediatrician or registered dietitian. Feeding Infants and toddlers can be messy, and it's important to remember that exploration of food is part of the learning process. Toddlers can eat most table foods, but with supervision to avoid choking.*

Childhood

Childhood is the term that covers the years from age 1 through the beginning of **adolescence**. Growth in childhood, while continuous, occurs at a significantly slower rate than in infancy. During the childhood years, a typical child will gain about 5 pounds and grow 2 to 3 inches annually. Children can be divided into three groups based on their age and development: toddlers (ages 1–3); preschoolers (ages 4–5); and school-aged children (ages 6–10).

Energy and Nutrient Needs during Childhood

Energy and Protein

An average 1-year-old requires about 1,000 to 1,300 kilocalories per day. This daily energy requirement gradually increases until it almost doubles by around age 10. (See **Table 15.10.**) While total energy requirements increase, the kilocalories needed per kilogram of body weight slowly decrease as children move through childhood. The same is true for protein requirements.

Vitamins and Minerals

With the cooperation of a healthy child, a well-planned diet during childhood should provide most nutrients. One exception is iron. (See **Figure 15.10.**) The RDA for iron during childhood is 7 milligrams for ages 1-3 and 10 milligrams for ages 4-8. Children may not get that amount without careful meal planning. As mentioned earlier, high consumption of milk can contribute to inadequate iron intake. During childhood, milk, a low source of iron, should be limited to 3 to 4 cups per day. This allows room in the diet for high-iron food sources such as lean meats, legumes, fish, poultry, and iron-enriched breads and cereals. (See **Table 15.11.**) Iron deficiency not only affects growth, but also can impair the child's mood, attention span, focus, and ability to learn.

A child's diet also may be low in other micronutrients. A study of the diets of middle- and upper-income Caucasian toddlers found low intakes of zinc, vitamin D, and vitamin E. The authors attribute these deficiencies in part to the fact that the toddlers followed their parents' low-fat diets, including low-fat dairy products, which are poor sources of zinc and vitamin E. In addition, the toddlers demonstrated a dislike of vegetables.[16]

Vitamin and Mineral Supplements

Many caregivers would rather give a child a vitamin/mineral pill than engage in the planning and food preparation necessary to ensure an adequate diet. However, the balanced diet a child needs is not much different from the diet an adult needs. In fact, the USDA Food Guide Pyramid for

childhood The period of life from the age of 1 to the onset of puberty.

adolescence The period between onset of puberty and adulthood.

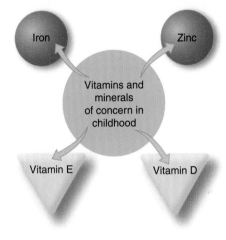

Figure 15.10 **Micronutrients to emphasize in childhood.**

Table 15.11 Iron-Rich Foods and Snacks

Iron-Rich Foods

Ground beef
Poultry
Fish
Legumes
Dark green vegetables
Enriched breads, cereals, rice, and pasta

Iron-Rich Snacks

Cream of Wheat
Cooked macaroni or pasta
Enriched cereals, either dry or with milk
Tortillas filled with refried beans
Dried apricots
Raisins (for older children)
Bean dip
Chili, mildly seasoned
Peanut butter on enriched bread
    or graham crackers
Sloppy Joe
Casseroles with meat (many children
    do not like plain meats)

Table 15.10 Energy and Protein RDAs for Children

Age (yr)	Kcal/kg	Kcal/d*	Protein g/kg	Protein g/d*
1–3	102	1,300	1.2	16
4–6	90	1,800	1.1	24
7–10	70	2,000	1.0	28

*The values per day are based on median weights of children.

Source: Food and Nutrition Board. *Recommended Dietary Allowances.* 10ᵗʰ ed. Washington, DC: National Academy Press; 1989.

children ages 2 to 6 years (**Figure 15.11**) shows approximately the same balance of food groups as is recommended for adults. With this in mind, there may be less temptation to rely on supplements for the benefits of a balanced diet.

Some children's diets require supplementation. These include children whose diets are restricted for medical reasons, those with food allergies that require avoidance of multiple foods or food groups, those with chronic dis-

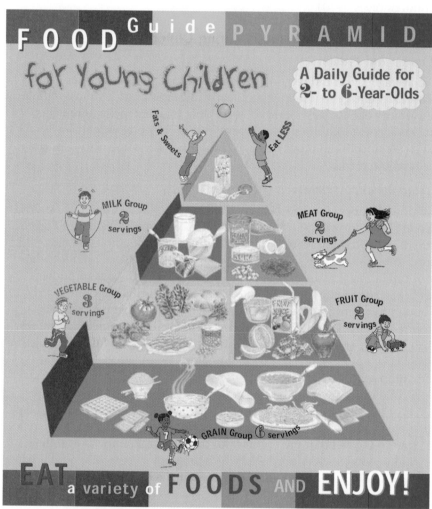

U.S. DEPARTMENT OF AGRICULTURE
CENTER FOR NUTRITION POLICY AND PROMOTION

WHAT COUNTS AS ONE SERVING?

GRAIN GROUP
1 slice of bread
½ cup of cooked rice or pasta
½ cup of cooked cereal
1 ounce of ready-to-eat cereal

VEGETABLE GROUP
½ cup of chopped raw or cooked vegetables
1 cup of raw leafy vegetables

FRUIT GROUP
1 piece of fruit or melon wedge
¾ cup of juice
½ cup of canned fruit
¼ cup of dried fruit

MILK GROUP
1 cup of milk or yogurt
2 ounces of cheese

MEAT GROUP
2 to 3 ounces of cooked lean meat, poultry, or fish.
½ cup of cooked dry beans, or 1 egg counts as 1 ounce of lean meat.
2 tablespoons of peanut butter count as 1 ounce of meat.

FATS AND SWEETS
Limit calories from these.

Four- to 6-year-olds can eat these serving sizes. Offer 2- to 3-year-olds less, except for milk.
Two- to 6-year-old children need a total of 2 servings from the milk group each day.

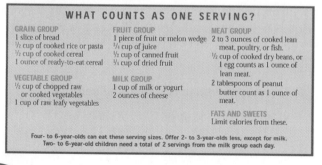 **Figure 15.11** **Food Guide Pyramid for Young Children.** Young children have unique food patterns and needs in comparison to older children and adults. Also, many young children are not eating healthful diets, and early food experiences are crucial to food preferences and patterns throughout life. To help improve the diets of young children two to six years old, the USDA has developed the Food Guide Pyramid for Young Children.

eases, and those who are malnourished.[17] Caregivers need to be reminded that vitamin and mineral supplements for children are dangerous in large doses. Vitamin and mineral preparations must be treated like all medicines, and kept safely out of children's reach. Iron-containing supplements, especially, present grave threats to children if consumed in doses over 30 milligrams. Accidental consumption of vitamin and mineral or iron supplements should be treated as a poisoning emergency.

Influences on Childhood Food Habits and Intake

Children develop food preferences at an early age. As their environment expands, so do the number of external factors influencing their diet. It is estimated that children spend more time watching television than doing most other activities. Recognizing the influence that children have on household purchases, advertisers target commercials specifically at children during prime children's viewing hours. Saturday morning cartoons, for example, feature countless ads for sweetened cereals, fast foods, candy, and other foods high in sugar or fat, none of which is necessary or desirable.[18]

Social events and parties often promote unhealthful eating habits. No matter what the occasion, the menu for children's parties rarely varies. The staples are pizza, ice cream, soft drinks, and candy. None of these foods alone is a problem, but the fact that these foods are offered at the majority of social gatherings is. Popular snacks and beverages also tend to be too high in sugar and fat. Serving healthful, but child-friendly snacks, such as those in **Table 15.12**, breaks this tradition.

Key Concepts: *Children ages 1 through 10 grow at a slower rate than they did as infants, but still gain 2 to 3 inches and about 5 pounds per year. They should be able to obtain adequate energy and nutrients from their meals and snacks. Iron-deficiency anemia is the most common nutritional deficiency among American children. Cow's milk is not an adequate source of iron, and should be limited to 3 or 4 cups per day to allow for other, high-iron foods. Outside influences, such as television viewing, affect children's preferences for low-nutrient-density foods.*

Nutritional Concerns of Childhood

Malnutrition and Hunger in Childhood

Of all of the issues facing children with respect to growth and nutrition, there is none so devastating as hunger and subsequent malnutrition. Throughout the world, hunger and malnutrition are responsible for nearly half of the deaths of preschool children. Deficiencies in vitamin A, zinc, iron, and protein also result in illness, stunted growth, and limited development, and in the case of vitamin A, possibly permanent blindness.

In the United States, an estimated 2.5 to 3 million people are homeless. Of this group, 43 percent are families with children.[19] About 25 percent of children younger than 3 years old live in poverty—a higher percentage than in any other age bracket of the population.[20] Nearly 12 million children grow up in so-called **food-insecure households** (where calories are adequate, but diet quality has suffered), and more than 2.7 million children experience hunger.[21] Data to measure household food security are collected annually by the Census Bureau[22] and households are characterized as one of the following:

- *Food Secure:* No evidence of food insecurity; food is available or can be obtained readily.
- *Food Insecure without Hunger:* Concern about inadequate resources to buy food, quality of the diet is reduced, but actual intake is not reduced.

Table 15.12 **Healthy Snacks**

Cereal and milk
Yogurt shake: plain yogurt, fresh fruit
Peanut butter on celery
Popcorn sprinkled with Parmesan cheese
Fresh vegetables and a yogurt dip
Pretzels
Bananas with peanut butter
Graham crackers and peanut butter
Sliced apples with cheese
Bagel and melted cheese
Bran muffins
Pumpkin, banana, or zucchini bread
Mini pizza on English muffin
Homemade pita pocket sandwiches
Yogurt and mini bagel
Vegetable soup
Fresh fruit
Hot chocolate (made with milk)

Quick Bites

Television Tubbies

The number of obese children in America doubled in the past 20 years, and one in five American children is now overweight. Today's kids spend more time watching TV and playing video games than engaging in physical activity. Advertisers know it. When programs for children are broadcast, 80 percent of commercials advertise food, most of it high-sugar or high-fat foods.

food-insecure household A household in which the diet is characterized by adequate energy intake but reduced quality so that not all daily nutritional requirements are met.

- *Food Insecurity with Moderate Hunger:* Food insecurity has led to reduced intake by the adult members of the household, but not the children.

- *Food Insecurity with Severe Hunger:* All members of the household including the children are experiencing the uneasy or painful sensations caused by a lack in food.[23]

Because their bodies need to grow, children are more vulnerable than adults to the effects of malnutrition. In addition to limited *quantities* of food, many households with food insecurity suffer from poor *quality* of foods. Children in poverty may not have food at home or refrigeration. This limits their food choices to easy-to-prepare foods or fast foods, high in both fat and sugar.[24] Children are more likely to be underweight in the winter when families may decide that heating fuel is more necessary than eating.[25]

Federal programs such as the WIC program, National School Lunch Program, School Breakfast Program, and Summer Feeding Program help to create a safety net for these children (**Figure 15.12**). The WIC program, designed to follow children through the fifth birthday, provides vouchers for milk, eggs, cereal, juice, cheese, and either peanut butter or dried beans. However, participation rates in WIC are less than they could be. Many caregivers do not understand that WIC is still available after a child is off formula, or do not have transportation to the WIC site or grocery store. The National School Lunch and School Breakfast programs offer free or reduced-cost breakfast and lunch at school. Lunches must provide at least one-third of a child's RDA for energy, protein, vitamins A and C, and the minerals iron and calcium; breakfasts must supply one-fourth of the RDA for these nutrients. In addition, school meals must now conform to the *Dietary Guidelines for Americans* and limit total fat calories to 30 percent and saturated fat calories to 10 percent. The Summer Feeding Program was created after the realization that many children who depend on the breakfast and lunch programs during the school year were experiencing hunger during the summer months. For many children, these meals are the major, and in some cases the only, sources of calories and other nutrients. Those who plan and serve meals have the challenge of balancing popular foods that children will eat, and good nutrition.

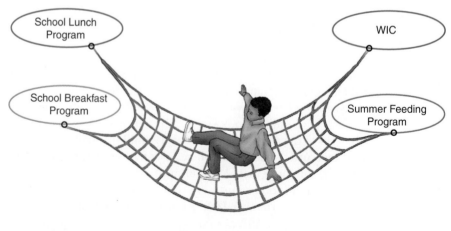

Safety Net for Children

Figure 15.12 **Federal safety net for children.** Children are more vulnerable than adults to the effects of malnutrition. For many children, these federal programs provide the major, and in some cases the only, sources of calories and other nutrients.

Food and Behavior

Many parents and caregivers mistakenly believe that consuming sugar-laden foods causes **hyperactivity** in children. The myth persists despite a number of carefully controlled studies that found no cause-and-effect relationship.[26] The term *hyperactivity* usually is defined as an abnormal increase in activity that is maladaptive and inconsistent with developmental level, but common usage has blurred its meaning. Parents often use this term to describe what they view as unruly behavior of children, particularly in social settings like parties. Many people also believe that certain food additives, including preservatives and colorings, can cause or exacerbate behavioral disorders. However, no studies conclusively link food to behavior. Children typically react to situations surrounding foods or parties (where high-sugar foods are often served) in excitable ways. This is not proof of a cause-and-effect relationship between those foods and those behaviors.

Caffeine products can make children jittery and interfere with their sleep. Children's smaller body sizes enhance the effects of a caffeinated beverage. Many soft drinks are high in caffeine; examples include Mountain Dew (55 mg per 12-oz. can), Surge (51 mg per 12-oz. can), and Coca-Cola (47 mg per 12-oz. can).

Nutrition and Chronic Disease in Childhood

When is it appropriate to adopt adult dietary guidelines for children? It is well documented that early signs of chronic disease appear in children. Evidence of early plaque development has been seen in the coronary arteries of adolescents, and is associated with adult cardiovascular diseases. However, the low-fat, high-fiber diet advocated for adults may jeopardize a very young child's growth. Infants and young toddlers younger than 2 years old need fat in their diets for growth, organ protection, and central nervous system development. Dietary restrictions at this age are not appropriate.

For children older than 3, efforts to lower fat, saturated fat, and cholesterol intake may reduce risks of chronic disease. The American Heart Association, National Heart, Lung and Blood Institute, and the AAP all support such efforts.[27] However, it is important that parents and caregivers do not misinterpret the recommendations and restrict children's energy intake. During the preschool and school years, gradual changes can bring food choices in line with the *Dietary Guidelines for Americans*.

Many experts feel that before puberty, a low-fat diet has no demonstrated benefits to children. Health Canada, the Canadian government's health promotion department, recommends making energy intake a priority, as well as the intake of nutrients required for proper growth. It recommends against restricting food choices during preschool and childhood. Health Canada recommends gradually adjusting fat intake so it approaches adult recommendations at adolescence or puberty.[28] Caregivers should present healthful choices for children and, as they grow, educate them about proper adult nutrition.

Using a variety of food sources, children can increase their fiber intake without negatively affecting growth.[29] Increasing fiber does not appear to adversely affect vitamin and mineral intake or absorption. Adding fiber from a variety of foods is consistent with the goals to increase intake of whole grains and cereals and to consume five servings of fruits and vegetables per day.

hyperactivity A maladaptive and abnormal increase in activity that is inconsistent with developmental levels. Includes frequent fidgeting, inappropriate running, excessive talking, and difficulty in engaging in quiet activities.

Quick Bites

Are minority children at high risk for cardiovascular disease?

Early risk factors for cardiovascular disease are increasing in America. Among children, African American and Mexican American children are more likely to exhibit high blood pressure and high Body Mass Index and to consume a higher percentage of calories from fat than Caucasians. The three ethnic groups have similar blood cholesterol levels, however, and Caucasian children are more likely to smoke.

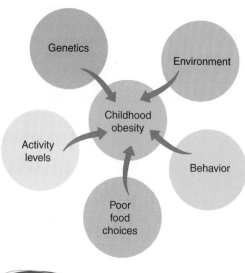

Figure 15.13 Factors that contribute to childhood obesity.

Childhood Obesity

In the United States, obesity in childhood is increasing at an alarming rate Obese children run a high risk of becoming obese adults, and suffering the ensuing health problems. An obese child is likely to reach maturity earlier than a child of normal weight, but perhaps at the expense of height. Some obese children already deal with cardiovascular consequences of obesity, such as lipid abnormalities and hypertension. Finally, obese children are not immune to the psychological trauma associated with obesity in our culture. Factors involved in the development of obesity in childhood include genetics, environment, behavior, and activity levels. (See **Figure 15.13**).

Programs designed to treat childhood obesity generally provide behavior modification, exercise counseling, psychological support or therapy, family counseling, and family meal-planning advice. The goal is not weight loss, but to allow the child's height to catch up with his or her weight. Rather than restrict caloric intake or food choices, the strategy is usually to increase activity and improve food choices.

Lead Toxicity

Lead toxicity can result in slow growth and iron-deficiency anemia, and can damage the brain and central nervous system, leading to a host of learning disabilities and behavior problems. Lead is present in the plumbing of old homes, old paint, house dust in homes with cracked or peeling lead-based paint, and in some areas, the soil. Children can ingest lead by drinking contaminated water, eating paint chips, or sucking their fingers

⌈*Fyi*⌋ Food Hypersensitivities and Allergies

FOR YOUR INFORMATION

Food allergies, or food hypersensitivities, are allergic reactions to food proteins. Allergies are different from food intolerances (such as lactose intolerance) that may involve digestive problems rather than an immune response. Allergies are less likely than intolerances to be transient, and tend to have more serious consequences. Proteins that trigger allergies are known as allergens. The most common food allergens are found in milk, eggs, tree nuts, peanuts, soy, wheat, fish, and seafood.

Food allergies occur when the immune system mounts a specific reaction to a food protein. Surveys suggest that about 25 percent of people in the general population think they suffer from food allergies. But studies show that only 1 to 2 percent of adults, and 6 to 8 percent of children under the age of 3, truly do.[1]

In a true allergic reaction, the immune system responds to an allergen with a cascade of chemical reactions that can cause wheezing, difficulty breathing, and hives as well as a host of other symptoms (see Table A: Symptoms of Food Allergies). Food allergy symptoms often affect more than one body system, and may change in severity from one reaction to the next.

Anaphylaxis, the most severe allergic reaction, usually takes place within the first hour after eating the offending food. Shock and respiratory failure can rapidly ensue. Anaphylaxis can be fatal, so immediate emergency care is essential.

Allergy symptoms that occur immediately after a food is eaten makes for easier detective work. If symptoms are slow to evolve, a child may suffer chronic diarrhea and even experience failure to thrive before the problem is identified.

An elimination diet can help determine allergic responses to foods when identification of the food culprit is difficult. All suspected foods are eliminated from the diet and slowly re-introduced, one by one, on a specific schedule. Both intake and reactions are carefully recorded. Prolonged or improper use of such a diet can have severe nutritional consequences. A registered dietitian can help with diet planning to ensure nutritional adequacy.

The double-blind, placebo-controlled food challenge is the gold standard of food allergy testing. Although definitive, it can be dangerous for people prone to anaphylactic reactions. In this test, increasing amounts of a suspected food are given to the child under the supervision of a physician, who looks for allergy symptoms and signs. This test must be done by trained personnel with emergency equipment handy.

The treatment for food allergy is avoidance of the offending allergen. Each child with a food allergy needs a nutrition assessment, with specific attention paid to the specific nutrients missing as a result of the avoided

after playing in or around lead-contaminated house dust or soil. Lead toxicity occurs more frequently in areas of poverty, where lead sources are higher, and where iron-deficiency anemia is present.

Low intakes of iron, calcium, and zinc tend to result in increased lead absorption. Children with an adequate intake of these micronutrients show less incidence of lead toxicity. Therefore, many of the programs established to reduce the incidence of lead toxicity in children include promotion of proper nutrition, with an emphasis on adequate iron, calcium, and zinc consumption.

Vegetarianism in Childhood

A lacto-vegetarian or a lacto-ovo-vegetarian diet can supply adequate levels of protein, iron, calcium, vitamin B_{12}, and vitamin D. Without careful planning, however, a vegan diet, which contains no animal products, may not supply all of the nutrients needed to support a child's growth. For a vegan child, legumes and nuts should be substituted for meats, and calcium- and vitamin B_{12}-fortified soy milk should be substituted for cow's milk. At least 20 to 30 minutes of sunlight exposure three times a week should provide enough vitamin D.[30]

Key Concepts: *Hunger and malnutrition affect a significant number of our nation's children; nearly 14 million children grow up in "food-insecure" households. To combat the growing number of hungry children, programs such as WIC, the National School Lunch Program, and the National School Breakfast Program are vital. Other concerns common to childhood include obesity, lead toxicity, and*

Quick Bites

Tragedy in Lead

About 5 percent of American children demonstrate signs of lead toxicity, defined as a blood level of 10 micrograms of lead per deciliter. When children are exposed to lead on a continuous or regular basis, brain function is affected.

foods. For example, if a baby is avoiding milk and milk products due to a cow's milk allergy, the nutrients most at risk would be protein, vitamin D, and calcium. As a baby's diet includes more and more foods, the key becomes careful label reading to identify allergen-containing foods. As late as 1992, anaphylactic reactions were documented from ingestion of foods containing sodium caseinate, a milk protein derivative; the food labels had not listed sodium caseinate separately, but included it only under the heading "natural flavorings." Organizations such as the Food Allergy Network provide materials for deciphering food labels.[2] The Food Allergy Network also offers tips for successful traveling and dining with a child who has food allergies.

Many children naturally outgrow food allergies by the time they are 3 years old. Once outgrown, the food allergy will not return.

Table A **Symptoms of Food Allergies**

Gastrointestinal Tract	*Respiratory Tract*
Itching of the lips, mouth, and throat	Runny or stuffed-up nose, sneezing, post-nasal discharge
Swelling of the throat	Recurrent croup
Abdominal cramping and distention	Chronic pneumonia
Diarrhea	Middle-ear infections
Colic	
Gastrointestinal bleeding	
Protein-losing enteropathy	*Systemic*
	Anaphylaxis
Skin	Heart rhythm irregularities
	Low blood pressure
Hives	
Swelling	
Eczema, contact dermatitis	

1 Sampson HA. Food allergy. *JAMA.* 1997;278:1888–1894.

2 The Food Allergy Network. http://www.foodallergy.org. Accessed 11/2/00.

puberty The period of life during which the secondary sex characteristics develop and the ability to reproduce is attained.

menarche First menstrual period

epiphyses The heads of the long bones that are separated from the shaft of the bone until the bone stops growing.

chronic disease prevention. Infants and toddlers should not be given low-fat, high-fiber diets; when children reach the age of 3, appropriate dietary guidelines should begin to be introduced. For children, strict vegetarian diets may be limited in calcium, vitamin D, and vitamin B₁₂.

Adolescence

An adolescent appears to grow overnight. Many caregivers complain that they cannot keep enough food in the house to feed an adolescent's appetite. Indeed, the rate of growth during adolescence—and the energy intake to support it—are impressive. Adolescence commonly is defined as the time between the onset of **puberty** and adulthood. This maturation process involves both physical growth and emotional maturation.

Physical Growth and Development

Growth through adolescence is hormone driven, and varies from child to child. In general, growth spurts begin between ages 10.5 and 11 for girls, with a peak in the rate of growth at around age 12. For boys, growth spurts usually begin between ages 12.5 and 13, and peak at around age 14. This spurt, or period of maximal growth, lasts about 2 years.

Height

The first phase of adolescent growth is linear. On average, boys grow 8 inches and girls grow 6 inches during puberty. This growth is uneven. The hands and feet enlarge first. The calves and forearms lengthen next, followed by expansion of the hips, chest, shoulders, and trunk. As a result, adolescents often appear awkward or clumsy. After the main growth spurt, growth continues for 2 to 3 years, but at a much slower rate.

For girls, peak growth occurs about 1 year prior to **menarche**, the onset of menstruation. A typical girl has achieved about 98 percent of her adult height by menarche, and grows only 2 to 4 inches during the remainder of adolescence. With some exceptions, girls who reach menarche at an earlier age tend to grow more after menarche than do girls with late menarche. Growth rates are closely related to sexual maturation, reflected in breast development (girls), change of voice (boys), development of sexual organs, and growth of pubic hair. A trained clinician can estimate an adolescent's future growth based on the stage of sexual maturation. For example, a very tall boy at the early stages of sexual maturation may be expected to grow much taller. Conversely, a short boy who is sexually mature may not grow much more. Skeletal growth is completed when the growth plates, or **epiphyses**, at the ends of the long bones, close. This is a critical point in development. An adolescent who is malnourished and of small stature at the point of epiphysis closure may not achieve his or her full potential height.

Weight

The second growth phase of adolescence involves lateral growth. Here, the adolescent "fills out," or gains weight. External factors such as diet and exercise affect weight gain more than linear growth, so weight gain can vary widely among adolescents. However, a typical healthy girl will gain 35 pounds during adolescence; a typical boy will gain 45 pounds. In our weight-sensitive society, adolescents should be prepared for this normal, expected weight gain. Although the bulk of an adolescent's lateral growth occurs after the linear growth spurt, a significant portion of the two growth stages overlap. For girls, for example, peak weight gain usually occurs around the time of menarche.

Body Composition

Before puberty, the body composition of boys and girls does not differ greatly. This changes dramatically during adolescence. Boys experience greater increases in lean body mass, resulting in more obvious muscle definition. Girls accumulate greater stores of body fat, specifically around the hips and buttocks, upper arms, breasts, and upper back. By adulthood, a typical woman's body composition is 23 percent fat; a typical man, in contrast, has 12 percent body fat.

As adolescents grow in height and weight, so do their internal organs—heart, lungs, liver, spleen, kidneys, thyroid, and sexual organs. Blood pressure increases, while heart rate decreases, eventually reaching adult levels.

Emotional Maturity: Developmental Tasks

To complicate matters, adolescence is a time of tremendous emotional growth. This psychological development affects food choices, eating habits, and body image. Many teens become more interested in the healthful aspects of nutrition. Others experiment with unhealthful food choices, as an exercise in independence or in an attempt to achieve an idealized body.

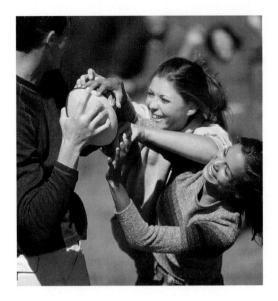

Nutrient Needs of Adolescents

Although growth, not age, should be the ultimate indicator of nutrient needs, RDAs are established based on age. One of the changes in the DRI revisions was a change in age groupings for children and adolescents. The separate recommendations for males and females reflect their differences in growth rates and body composition seen during adolescence.

Energy and Protein

Energy needs, as total kilocalories per day, are greater during adolescence than at any other time of life, with the exception of pregnancy and lactation. Recommended energy intakes are guidelines only; adjustments often are needed to meet individual requirements. For example, the recommendations do not take into account activity levels. An active teen involved in regular exercise or sports will exceed the recommendations for energy. Conversely, a physically mature teen, with no regular exercise or fitness plan, will not need this much energy for weight maintenance.

To support growth, an adolescent's protein needs per unit body weight are higher than an adult's but less than a rapidly growing infant's. For females aged 15 to 18, the protein RDA declines to adult levels (as g/kg body weight), reflecting the cessation of linear growth in most teen girls. American teens rarely have a problem with adequate protein intake (**Table 15.13**), but teen girls may risk a lack of protein if they cut calories too drastically in attempts to control weight.

	Age Categories (years)	
1989 RDA		DRI
1–3 years		*1–3 years*
4–6 years		*4–8 years*
7–10 years		
11–14 years, male		*9–13 years, male*
11–14 years, female		*9–13 years, female*
15–18 years, male		*14–18 years, male*
15–18 years, female		*14–18 years, female*

Table 15.13 **Energy and Protein RDAs for Adolescence**

	Age (yr)	Kcal/kg	Kcal/d*	Protein g/kg	Protein g/d*
Males	11–14	55	2,500	1.0	45
	15–18	45	3,000	0.9	59
Females	11–14	47	2,200	1.0	46
	15–18	40	2,200	0.8	44

* The values for grams per day are based on median weights of adolescents.

Source: Food and Nutrition Board. *Recommended Dietary Allowances.* 10th ed. Washington, DC: National Academy Press; 1989.

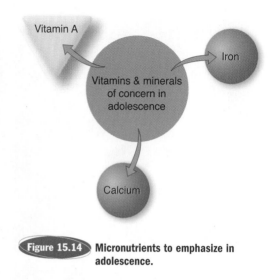

Figure 15.14 Micronutrients to emphasize in adolescence.

Table 15.14 Information Resources for Calcium

- NIH Consensus Statement: Optimal Calcium Intake. Bethesda, MD: US Department of Health and Human Services, National Institutes of Health, 1994. Free copies of this statement are available via Internet at http://www.nih.gov/niams/news/calsum.htm.

- 1-800-WHY-MILK: A Crash Course on Calcium. Toll-free hotline provides educational materials, including videos. Developed by the National Dairy Council.

- Power Up From the Inside Out! Brochure designed for teens: National Dairy Council, Power Up From the Inside Out! Department Teens, 10255 West Higgins Road, Suite 900, Rosemont, IL 60018-5616.

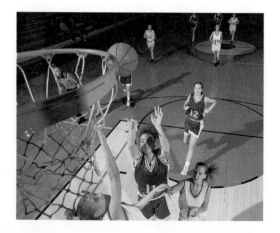

Vitamins and Minerals

Along with increased needs for energy and protein, adolescents have higher vitamin and mineral needs as compared to most other life cycle stages. Three nutrients of particular concern for adolescents are vitamin A, calcium, and iron, each of which plays an important role in growth. (See **Figure 15.14**.)

Improving fruit and vegetable intake among teens will help them obtain adequate vitamin A. Adequate calcium, essential for bone formation and maximal bone density, can be harder to obtain.[31] During puberty, adolescents gain 15 percent of their full adult height, and accumulate half of their ultimate adult bone mass. Adults gradually begin to lose bone mass in midlife. Adolescents that do not achieve sufficient bone density have a greater risk of developing osteoporosis later in life. The AI for calcium in adolescence is 1,300 milligrams of calcium every day. Dairy products are rich in calcium and convenient to eat; without these or calcium-fortified products, meeting the AI is difficult indeed. **Table 15.14** lists resources for more information about adolescents and calcium.

Adolescent boys need added iron to support growth of muscle and lean body mass. Teenage girls need added iron to replace blood lost during menstruation. The recommended intake for boys ages 14-18 is 11 milligrams per day throughout adolescence; for teen girls, it is 15 milligrams per day. Provided their energy intake is adequate, both groups should be able to obtain this iron from nutrient-dense foods. During adolescence, however, food selection often is less than optimal. Careful meal planning is required to maximize teenagers' iron consumption.

Key Concepts: *Humans need more calories and nutrients during adolescence than at any other stage of life, with the exception of pregnancy and lactation. Boys grow about 8 inches, gain about 45 pounds, and increase their lean body mass. Girls grow about 6 inches, gain about 35 pounds, and increase their body fat. These changes do not come at scheduled intervals or at a given chronological age, but at individual rates. As at earlier ages, calcium, iron, and vitamin A are nutrients that are often lacking in adolescent diets.*

Nutritional Concerns for Adolescents

Fitness and Sports

For many adolescents, an interest in fitness becomes the catalyst for learning about nutrition and improving dietary habits. Others, unfortunately, become obsessed with their athletic performance, food intake, and body appearance and go to extremes that can jeopardize not only their current athletic performance but also their long-term health.

Energy needs grow as activity increases. Active adolescents need additional carbohydrates, iron, calcium, B vitamins, and especially fluids. Careful counseling is required to motivate the young athlete to follow proper diet recommendations and to plan meals accordingly. Sports that require attention to body size, such as gymnastics, wrestling, skating, and dancing, also need adequate calories for both growth and for training. Although not all athletes fall in the trap, disordered eating is evident among many adolescent athletes who are preoccupied with body image and who exercise as a means toward thinness.[32] As always, water is the most important nutrient for athletic performance. Attention to fluid intake before, during, and after exercise maintains hydration and enhances performance. It is vital for young athletes to understand that thirst is not an adequate indicator of fluid needs during exercise. For most athletic events, water is the ideal fluid replacement.[33]

Athletes concerned with both performance and body sculpting may feel pressured to use anabolic steroids, derivatives of the male sex hormone testosterone that can increase lean body mass. Side effects of anabolic steroid use include alteration in mood, including psychotic behavior; increased body hair; severe acne; changes in the size and function of internal organs; blood disorders; and reproductive abnormalities. Other serious consequences of steroid use include heart attacks and liver cancer. Even "natural" steroids like DHEA and androstenedione can cause serious side effects (see Chapter 13). Both the AAP and the American College of Sports Medicine condemn the use of anabolic steroids by athletes.

Acne

acne An inflammatory skin eruption that usually occurs in or near the sebaceous glands of the face, neck, shoulders, and upper back.

Acne is so common during puberty that it often is labeled as normal. Myths surrounding acne and diet abound, but research has not found any correlation between acne and chocolate, greasy foods, soft drinks, nuts, or milk. Unfortunately, acne cannot be cured or prevented through diet. People who suffer from acne, therefore, should not be made to feel guilty about their food choices. Effective treatments for acne include topical benzoyl peroxide; low-dose oral antibiotics; and two medications derived from vitamin A—Retin-A and Accutane. Although both of these medications are derivatives of vitamin A, there is no correlation between dietary vitamin A and acne.

Behaviors Incompatible with Good Health

Tobacco, Alcohol, and Recreational Drugs

Developmentally, adolescence is a period of experimentation. Many adolescents experiment with illegal substances or drugs. Despite national efforts, tobacco use continues to grow, especially among young females who smoke to control appetite and weight. An adolescent who smokes tobacco has a lower energy intake and subsequently decreased nutrient intake.

Marijuana has the opposite effect on hunger. Many teens who smoke marijuana will experience "the munchies," a desire to snack and munch—usually on high-calorie, low nutrient-density snack foods. Dangers in smoking marijuana include those of tobacco. In addition, marijuana frequently is laced with other drugs, including LSD and amphetamines.

Adolescents who drink alcohol are at greater risk of harming themselves or others through violence and accidental injury.[34] In addition, teens who drink are replacing needed nutrients with empty alcohol calories. Finally, alcohol can interfere with the absorption and metabolism of necessary nutrients. (For more information about nutrition and alcohol, see the "Spotlight on Alcohol," especially the section "Alcohol and Malnutrition.") Growing adolescents cannot afford to have nutrients replaced or poorly absorbed during growth.

Other drugs, such as cocaine, pose further risks. In using illegal drugs, the adolescent becomes preoccupied with both the acquisition and use of the drug; these activities take priority over food intake or selection. Teens who use drugs are usually underweight and report poor appetites.

Eating Disorders

Eating disorders, discussed more thoroughly in the "Spotlight on Eating Disorders," frequently begin during adolescence. It is not uncommon for adolescents to become preoccupied with their weight, appearance, and eating habits. Although eating disorders still affect more girls than boys, the prevalence in males is increasing so it shouldn't be ignored or dismissed as only a "girl's problem." Eating disorders are seen in people as young as 7

Quick Bites

The Dangers of Teenage Smoking

The Centers for Disease Control and Prevention estimates that one-third of high-school students smoke regularly. They predict that one-third of the three million American teenage smokers will die of smoking-related diseases. New research shows that the earlier a person begins to smoke, the greater the damage.

Quick Bites

Early Abusers

These days, youngsters seem to start abusing substances earlier and earlier. Use of alcohol, cigarettes, and inhalants is increasing among fourth, fifth, and sixth graders. By sixth grade, 15 percent of children have tried alcohol and cigarettes. Many children say that peer pressure is their reason for experimentation.

Table 15.15 Risk Factors for Obesity in Adolescents

Risk Factors	Explanations
Social Variables	
Socioeconomic status	Direct relationship for males; inverse relationship for females
Parental obesity	Strong correlation between obese parents, siblings, and the adolescent
Race	Higher in white children; and African American female adolescents
Family size	Less obesity with larger family size
Television watching	Increased viewing correlates with increasing obesity
Physical Environment	
Region	Greater incidence of obesity in Northeast; urban areas
Seasonal	Higher in winter
Genetic and Metabolic Factors	
Reduced energy expenditure	

Source: Bandini, L. Obesity in the Adolescent, *Adolescent Medicine: State of the Art Reviews.* 3(3):459–472, Hanley & Belfus, Inc. Philadelphia, 215-546-4995, www.hanleyandbelfus.com.

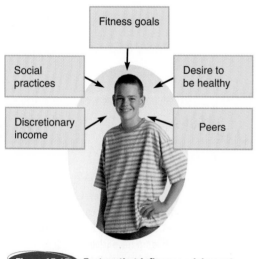

Figure 15.15 Factors that influence adolescent food choices.

years old. Registered dietitians need to be involved in both the prevention and treatment of eating disorders.[35]

Obesity

As in childhood, obesity rates in adolescence are climbing. Obese adolescents have an increased risk of developing high blood pressure and abnormal glucose tolerance. They also suffer psychologically from teasing, being ostracized by peers, and from longing to be slimmer. In addition, adolescent obesity sets the stage for adult obesity, with all of its attendant health consequences (see Chapter 8). Finally, adolescents who engage in unhealthful weight loss methods are more likely to engage in other risky behaviors, such as tobacco, alcohol, or other drug use, unprotected sex, suicide attempts, and delinquency.[36] **Table 15.15** lists the factors that can put an adolescent at risk for obesity.

Programs that address body image, stress obesity prevention, and promote early intervention seem to have the best chances of success. Successful programs need to include family members and be culturally sensitive.[37] Intervention strategies that focus on nutrition, exercise, eating patterns, snack choices, attitudes, and family support will be more effective than strict diets or programs solely based on caloric deficits. When behavior modification and psychological counseling are also offered, programs appear especially promising.[38] Interdisciplinary teams composed of a physician or nurse, a psychologist or therapist, and a nutritionist are most capable of providing a program that promotes lifelong fitness goals, appropriate food habits, self-acceptance and psychosocial adjustments.

Meal Planning for Adolescents

Teenagers want and need to make their own food choices and purchases, and may want to take over preparation of their own food. While the parent can set a good example, parental influence is much weaker now. Factors that influence an adolescent's food selection and consumption include the desire to be healthy, fitness goals, amount of discretionary income, social practices, and peers (see **Figure 15.15**).

Meal Schedules

Teens generally do not follow standard meal times and schedules. They frequently skip breakfast in lieu of sleep or grooming. Snacks make up a large portion of the diet, but do not provide sufficient nutrients. Food of low nutrient density, such as soft drinks, chips, and candy, are frequent snack choices. Teens often obtain meals from vending machines or fast-food restaurants. As a result, adolescent diets frequently are low in fruits and vegetables. Up to 40 percent of the adolescents from low socioeconomic backgrounds have diets that contain inadequate servings of fruits and vegetables. Additional groups at risk for inadequate fruit-and-vegetable intake include adolescents with low family connectedness, teens who are dissatisfied with their weight, and teens who do poorly in school.[39]

Vitamin/mineral supplements are increasingly popular among adolescents, who use the preparations to ensure healthy growth, to treat illness, or to enhance athletic performance. Although equal numbers of boys and girls take vitamins, boys are more likely to associate supplement use with performance enhancement in sports.[40]

Teens have more access to foods than children do. Teens usually have their own money and even access to independent transportation. Along with this increased freedom comes spending power. Teens enjoy spending money on food, and making their own selections. Food manufacturers and the food industry respond accordingly by marketing directly to teens. Advertised products may not be nutritionally adequate, but the message is for enjoyment and pleasure. Snack foods and convenience store products such as subs and cheese steaks, chips, soft drinks, and fruit drinks are popular. Teens attending school are faced with more food choices than ever before. In addition to the standard school lunch or breakfast program outlined earlier, middle schools and high schools may have vending machines, snack carts, school stores, or even private vendors supplying foods such as pizza for cafeteria meals. Policies are needed in the school system to address issues of nutritional messages and food availability on the school grounds.[41]

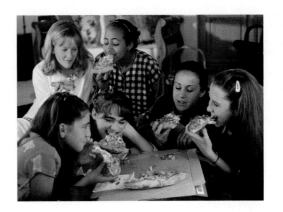

Key Concepts: *Adolescence is an uncomfortable time for the teen who is concerned with body image or body changes or athletic activities. Increased independence allows the teen to wield more control or power over his own meal planning and food consumption. This power is not always exercised wisely; low nutrient snacks are a large part of the diet, and adequate amounts of fruits and vegetables are missing. Factors that determine food selection and consumption include the desire to be healthy, fitness goals, amount of discretionary income, social practices, and peers.*

Label [to] **Table**

What is it about fruit snacks that attracts kids? The sweet flavors, bright colors, shapes, and logos of favorite movie or TV characters? Probably all of them. Parents may be attracted by claims for vitamins. So are these nutritious snacks or little more than candy? Let's have a look at the label.

On the positive side, this is a fat-free snack and contains little sodium. However, most of the calories, 56 out of 80, come from sugar (14 g X 4 kcalories per gram), and the remainder from starch and protein. The ingredient list shows that the first three ingredients are sugars: corn syrup, sucrose, and fruit juice from concentrate.

The vitamins added to fruit snacks are the only redeeming feature of the product, providing 25% of the DV for vitamins A, C, and E. But is there a better way to get these nutrients? One-half cup of orange juice provides two-thirds of the DV for vitamin C, and significant amounts of thiamin, folate, and potassium as well. Just a handful of baby carrots provides more than 100% DV for vitamin A, along with some fiber. Vitamin E is widespread in the food supply—a small amount of salad dressing as a dip for the carrots would add vitamin E.

So, the fruit snacks are not as devoid of nutrients as candy, but are not as nutrient dense as fruits and vegetables. The fruit snacks may have some nutrient value, but they are high in sugar and, like all sugary snacks, should be used sparingly.

Nutrition Facts

Serving Size: 1 pouch (26g/0.9 oz)
Servings Per Container 10

Amount Per Serving

Calories 80

	% Daily Value*
Total Fat 0g	
Sodium 15mg	0%
Total Carbohydrate 19g	1%
Sugars 14g	6%
Protein 1g	

Vitamin A 25%
(100% as beta carotene)

Vitamin C 25% • Vitamin E 25%

Not a significant source of calories from fat, saturated fat, cholesterol, dietary fiber, calcium, or iron.

*Percent Daily Values are based on a 2,000 calorie diet. Your daily values may be higher or lower depending on your calorie needs:

		Calories:	2000	2,500
Total Fat	Less Than		65g	80g
Sat Fat	Less Than		20g	25g
Cholesterol	Less Than		300mg	300mg
Sodium	Less Than		2,400mg	2,400mg
Total Carbohydrate			300g	375g
Dietary Fiber			25g	30g

Calories per gram:
Fat 9 • Carbohydrate 4 • Protein 4

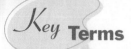

LEARNING *Portfolio* c h a p t e r 1 5

Key Terms

	page		page
acne	607	hyperactivity	601
adolescence	597	inborn error of metabolism	583
alpha-lactalbumin	583	infancy	580
Apgar scores	580	lactation consultant	585
childhood	597	latching on	585
chronological age	595	length	581
epiphyses	604	menarche	604
extrusion reflex	589	neonate	583
failure to thrive (FTT)	595	palmar grasp	590
food-insecure household	599	pincer grasp	590
full-term	581	prematurity	581
gastroesophageal reflux	593	puberty	604
gestational age	581	rooting	585
growth chart	581	toddler	595
head circumference	581		

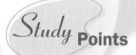

Study Points

➤ Growth is the key determinant of nutrient needs for infants, children, and adolescents.

➤ Infancy is the fastest growth stage in the life cycle; infants double their birth weight in 4-6 months and triple it by one year of age. The nutritional status of infants is primarily assessed through measurements of growth.

➤ Infants' energy needs must be met through a high-fat diet, which includes the maximum calories in minimal volume. Infants' protein and fluid needs are likewise high.

➤ Human milk is low in vitamin D; breast-fed babies need regular sun exposure or supplemental vitamin D. Likewise, for breast-fed infants, iron-fortified foods need to be introduced by 6 months of age. Formula-fed infants should be given iron-fortified formula.

➤ Infant formulas are either cow's milk based, soy-protein based, or made from hydrolyzed proteins. Unmodified cow's milk is inappropriate for infants throughout the first year of life.

➤ The FDA regulates the vitamin and mineral composition of infant formulas to ensure adequate infant nutrition. Formula is available in ready-to-feed, liquid concentrate, and powdered forms.

➤ A nurturing environment is important to the feeding of infants, no matter what the milk source.

➤ Solid foods are introduced to the infant one at a time, usually beginning with iron-fortified infant cereal. Potential allergens, such as cow's milk, egg whites, and wheat should be delayed until the baby is 12 months old. Developmental markers such as head and body control and the absence of the extrusion reflex show readiness for solid foods.

➤ Colic, although troublesome to infant and caregiver, is not caused by diet. Iron-deficiency anemia is common in infants who lack-iron rich foods. Infants are susceptible to dehydration, especially when diarrhea is prolonged. Failure to thrive describes an infant who is not growing well; it may require intervention to correct feeding practices of caregivers. Infants with PKU and other inborn errors of metabolism usually need special formulas.

➤ Growth rates slow in toddlers and children, and this may be reflected in reduced appetites and irregular feeding patterns. If diets are planned carefully, children do not need vitamin/mineral supplementation.

➤ Federally funded nutrition and feeding programs reduce malnutrition and hunger among American children.

➤ Adoption of adult-style diets to reduce risk of chronic disease should begin gradually after the age of 3.

➤ Obesity rates and eating disorders are rising among American children; treatment programs should address food choices and activity levels rather than impose strict calorie limits. Vegetarian diets for children need to be planned carefully to avoid nutrient deficiencies.

➤ Growth spurts in adolescence begin earlier for girls than for boys. As adolescents grow, boys add both lean and fat tissue while girls gain primarily fat mass, resulting in a significant difference in body composition.

➤ Total energy and nutrient needs of adolescents are high in order to support growth and maturation. Girls need more iron than boys do to compensate for losses after the onset of menstruation.

➤ Active teens need more calories and nutrients than sedentary teens; fluid intake is also a priority.

Study Questions

1. Is it okay for an infant to experience weight loss immediately after birth? If an infant does lose weight, does it mean he or she is at nutritional risk?

2. What is a better indicator of chronic malnutrition in children: a small head circumference or being underweight?

3. How much water does a breast-fed or formula-fed infant need each day?

4. Is it necessary to give breast-fed infants supplements of vitamins and/or minerals? If so, which ones?

5. Describe the process for introducing solid foods into an infant's diet.

6. List the feeding problems that may occur during infancy.

7. Which vitamins and minerals are most likely to be deficient in a child's diet?

8. Describe the hunger and malnutrition that occur in U.S. households. What federal programs help to address these problems?

9. Identify several chronic nutrition problems that can affect children. How can these problems be avoided?

10. Besides pregnant and lactating women, what age group has the highest total energy needs?

11. What are typical nutritional concerns for adolescents?

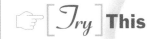 [Try] This

Eat Like a Kid

Children, especially toddlers, tend to be exploratory, and take in the sensory nature of food—the textures, smells, and tastes. In fact, you were probably once this way. The purpose of this exercise is to eat a meal like a kid and gain an appreciation of food's textures and taste. Make some mashed potatoes, macaroni and cheese, buttered peas, or spaghetti (favorite "kid food") and eat it with your fingers. Explore your food and play with it. Try mixing foods. How does this experience make you feel?

Infant Formulas

The purpose of this exercise is to learn about the variety of infant formulas on the market today. Spend some time at the grocery store and see how many brands of infant formula are on the shelf. Can you find at least one of the following: a standard infant formula, a soy-based formula, and a hypoallergenic protein hydrosylate formula? Compare not only the nutrient content of these formulas, but the prices too!

What About Bobbie?

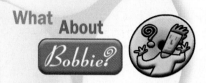

To gain perspective of the nutrient demands of teenagers, let's pretend that Bobbie is a 14-year-old girl. Consider her 1-day intake (see Chapter 1) as typical of her eating habits. How do you think she faired in her intake of the bone minerals needed in the greatest amounts during the teen years? Below you'll see her intake of phosphorus, magnesium, and calcium compared to the Dietary Reference Intakes (DRIs) for females between the ages of 14 and 18 years.

Bobbie's intake of the bone minerals phosphorus and magnesium were consumed in adequate amounts at approximately 92 percent of the RDA, each. However, Bobbie's calcium intake was quite low at 745 milligrams, which is a little more than half of her Adequate Intake (1,300 mg). Remember if Bobbie were 14 years old, she would be at a critical time for bone growth. To optimize her bone mass so that she achieves peak levels later, she would benefit by increasing her intake of low-fat dairy products and/or calcium-fortified foods.

Phosphorus

Recommended Dietary Allowance (RDA)	1,250 mg
Bobbie's intake	1,145 mg

Magnesium

Recommended Dietary Allowance (RDA)	360 mg
Bobbie's intake	330 mg

Calcium

Adequate Intake (AI)	1,300 mg
Bobbie's intake	745 mg

References

1 American Dietetics Association Commentary. Why children must play while they eat: an interview with T. Berry Brazelton. *J Am Diet Assoc.* 1993;93:1385–1387.

2 Institute of Medicine. Food and Nutrition Board. Committee on Nutritional Status during Pregnancy and Lactation. *Nutrition during Lactation.* Washington, DC: National Academy Press; 1990.

3 Sachdev HP., Krishna J, Puri RK, et. al. Water supplementation in exclusively breast-fed infants during summer in the tropics. *Lancet.* 1991;337(8747)929–933.

4 American Academy of Pediatrics. Breastfeeding and the use of human milk. *Pediatrics.* 1997;100:1035–1039.

5 American Academy of Pediatrics. Committee on Fetus and Newborn. *Guidelines for Perinatal Care.* 4th ed. Elk Grove, IL: Author; 1997.

6 Ibid.

7 Ibid.

8 American Academy of Pediatrics. Breastfeeding and the use of human milk. Op. cit.

9 Kleinman RE, ed. *Pediatric Nutrition Handbook.* 4th ed. Elk Grove, IL: American Academy of Pediatrics; 1998.

10 American Academy of Pediatrics. Infant feeding practices and their possible relationship to the etiology of diabetes mellitus. *Pediatrics.* 1994;94:752–754.

11 Ibid.

12 Rickert CP, DeBrie K. Parent-child relationships and feeding in infants and young children: a developmental perspective. *Clin Appl Nutr.* 1992;2(2):1–10.

13 Nahikian-Nelms M. Influential factors of caregiver behavior at mealtime: a study of 24 child care programs. *J Am Diet Assoc.* 1997;97:505–509.

14 Berube M, Parrish R. Home care of the infant with gastroesophageal reflux and respiratory disease. *J Pediatric Health Care.* 1994;8:173–180.

15 Fisch RO, Matalon R, Weisberg S, Michals K. Phenylketonuria: current dietary treatment practices in the US and Canada. *J Am Coll Nutr.* 1997;16:147–151.

16 Skinner JD, Carruth BR, Houck KS, et. al. Longitudinal study of nutrient and food intakes of infants aged 2 to 24 months. *J Am Diet Assoc.* 1997;97:496–504.

17 Kleinman RE, ed. Op. cit.

18 Kotz K, Story M. Food advertisements during children's Saturday morning television programming: are they consistent with dietary recommendations? *J Am Diet Assoc.* 1994;94:1296–1300.

19 American Academy of Pediatrics. Committee on Community Health Services. Health needs of homeless children and families. *Pediatrics.* 1996;98:789–791.

20 Zuckerman B, Parker S. Preventive pediatrics: new models of providing needed health services. *Pediatrics.* 1995;95:758–762. Editorials.

21 Andrews M, Nord M, Bickel G, Carlson S. Household Food Security in the United States, 1999. *Food Assistance and Nutrition Research Report No. 8 (FANRR-8).* USDA. Fall 2000.

22 USDA, Economic Research Service. "Domestic Food Security and Hunger Briefing Room." http://www.ers.usda.gov/briefing/foodsecurity/measurement.htm. Accessed 9/6/00.

23 Ibid.

24 American Academy of Pediatrics, Committee on Community Health Services. Health needs of homeless children and families. *Pediatrics.* 1996;98:789–791.

25 Zuckerman B, Parker S. Op. cit.

26 Wolraich ML, Lindgren SD, Stumbo PJ, et al. Effects of diets high in sucrose or aspartame on the behavior and cognitive performance of children. *N Engl J Med.* 1994;330:301–307.

27 Gaull G, Giombetti T, Yeaton Woo R. Pediatric dietary lipid guidelines: A policy analysis. *J Am Coll Nutr.* 1995;14:411–418.

28 Zlotkin S, reviewer. Review of the Canadian nutritional recommendations update: dietary fat and children. *J Nutr.* 1996;126 (suppl):1022S–1027S.

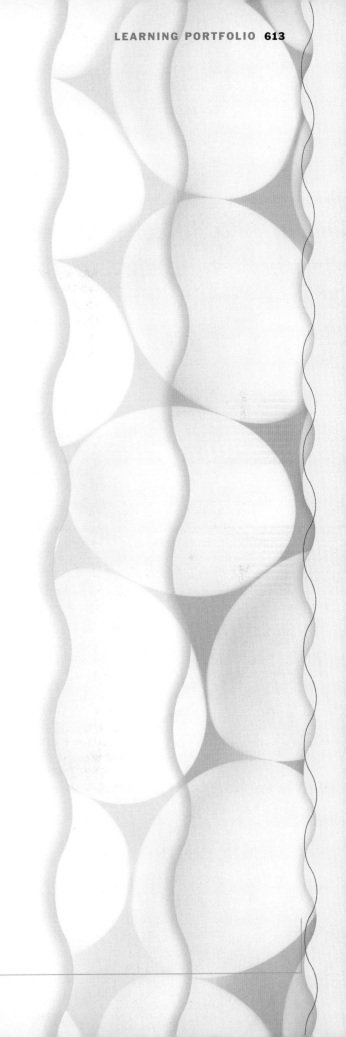

29 Williams C. Is a high-fiber diet safe for children? *Pediatrics.* 1995;96:1014–1019.

30 Novak P. Nutrition counseling for the vegetarian child. *Pediatric Nutrition—A Building Block for Life.* 1991;14(4):5–9.

31 Ragalie J. Improving the calcium intake of adolescents. *Pediatric Nutrition-A Building Block for Life.* 1998;22(3):1–9.

32 Yeager KK, Agostini R, Nattiv A, et. al. The female athlete triad: disordered eating, amenorrhea, osteoporosis. *Med Sci Sports Exerc.* 1993;25:775–777.

33 Convertino VA, Armstrong LE, Coyle EF, et al. American College of Sports Medicine Position Stand. Exercise and fluid replacement. *Med Sci Sports Exerc.* 1996;28:i–iv.

34 Wechsler H., Lee, JE, Kuo M, Lee H. College binge drinking in the late 1990s: A Continuing Problem. *J Am Coll Health.* March 2000;48:199–210.

35 American Dietetics Association Reports. Position statement of the American Dietetic Association: Nutrition intervention in the treatment of anorexia nervosa, bulimia nervosa, and binge eating. *J Am Diet Assoc.* 1994;94:902–907.

36 Neumark-Sztainer D, Story M, French SA. Covariations of unhealthy weight loss behaviors and other high-risk behaviors among adolescents. *Arch Pediatr Adolesc Med.* 1996;150:304–308.

37 Mlenyk MG, Weinstien E. Preventing obesity in black women by targeting adolescents: a literature review. *J Am Diet Assoc.* 1994;94:536–540.

38 Foreyt JP, Poston WS. The role of the behavioral counselor in obesity treatment. *J Am Diet Assoc.* 1998;98(Suppl):S27–S30.

39 Neumark-Sztainer D, Story M, Resnick, MD, Blum RW. Correlates of inadequate fruit and vegetable consumption among adolescents. *Prevent Med.* 1996;25:497–505.

40 Sobal J, Marquart LF. Vitamin/Mineral supplement use among high school athletes. *Adolescence.* 1994;29:835–843.

41 Story M, Hayes M, Kalina B. Availability of foods in high schools: is there cause for concern? *J Am Diet Assoc.* 1996;96:123–126.

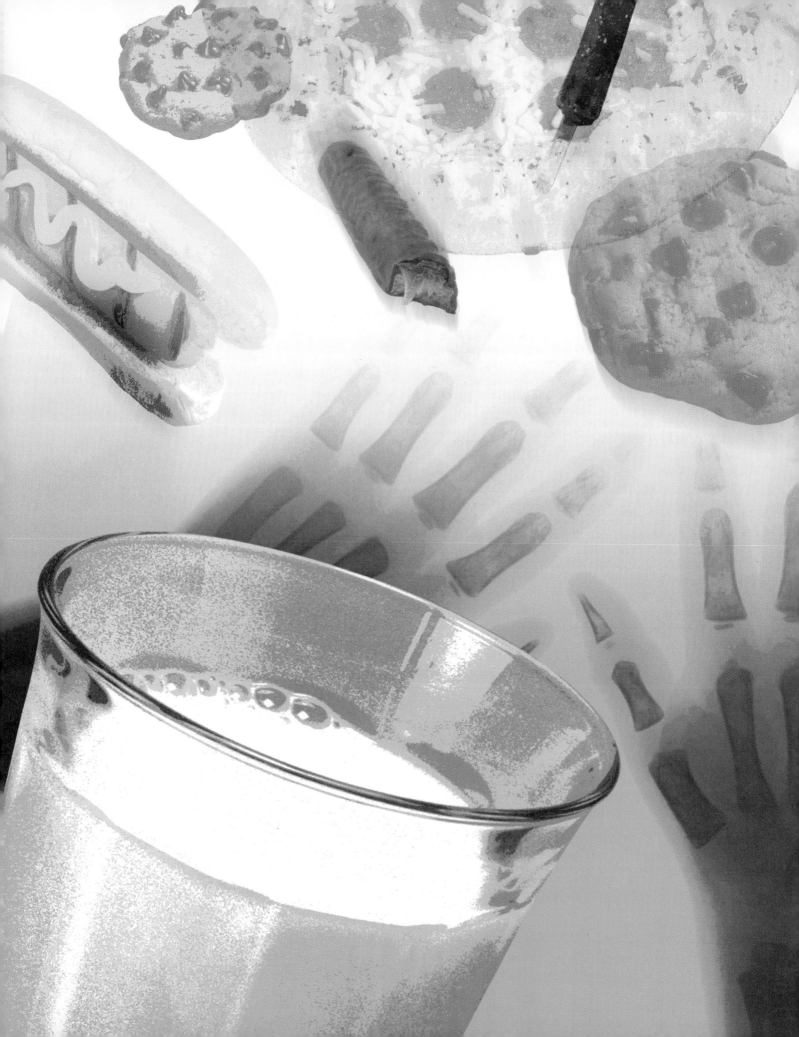

Chapter 16

Life Cycle: The Adult Years

Think About It

1 What behavior changes would you consider making now that would help you live longer?
2 You notice your slender grandparents have stopped drinking milk. What do you think?
3 Your grandmother takes numerous vitamin supplements. Do you have any concerns about this?
4 Your grandfather lives by himself and relies on frozen foods for his nutritional needs. How do you feel about this strategy?

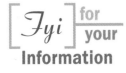

Fyi for your Information

This chapter's FYI boxes include practical information on the following topics:
- Are Dietary Recommendations to Lower Cholesterol Really Necessary for Elders?
- Vulnerability to Nutrition Quackery

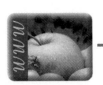

The web site for this book offers many useful tools and is a great source for additional nutrition information for both students and instructors. Visit the site at **nutrition.jbpub.com** for information on nutrition through the adult years. You'll find exercises that explore the following topics:
- The Elderly Nutrition Program
- Older Women and B$_{12}$
- Arthritis and Nutrition
- Crohn's Disease

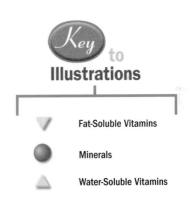

Key to Illustrations

▽ Fat-Soluble Vitamins

● Minerals

△ Water-Soluble Vitamins

What About Bobbie?

Track the choices Bobbie is making with the EatRight Analysis software.

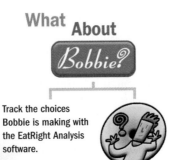

*I*t's the year 2050. Who are you? Where do you live? What is your life like? How healthy are you? If projected trends played out, you are part of the largest segment of the population: in 2050 between one-third and one-fourth of Americans are older than 65. Perhaps you have retired recently, or maybe you continue to work in your profession. Think about how technology has changed in your lifetime; new methods of communication have been developed that make e-mail and the Internet seem so old-fashioned, so late 20th century!

Consider your health status in 2050. If you continued your eating habits as they were in college, would you have controlled your weight, blood cholesterol, and blood pressure? Or perhaps in the year 2050 these conditions will no longer be of concern. Advances in genetics may have allowed gene therapy to replace diet therapy and medications for chronic diseases.

So what will be the health and nutritional concerns in the future? Will we still prepare a variety of foods, or subsist on dietary supplements and not bother with shopping and cooking? Although it's fun to speculate about the future, at the present we must consider nutritional needs of aging adults in terms of the impact of nutrition on the aging process, and the impact of the aging process on nutrition.

Staying Young while Growing Older

Just when does old age begin? The answer is increasingly elusive, as more people remain healthy and active well into their 70s, 80s, and even 90s. Today, older people represent the fastest-growing segment of the U.S. population. (See **Figure 16.1**.) The size of the older population (age 65 or older) is projected to double between 2000 and 2030. It is estimated that by the year 2030, nearly one in four Americans will be older than 65. The population aged 85 and older is growing fastest. In fact, the number of persons aged 100 or older is expected to increase nearly sixfold from 2000 to 2030.[1]

These aging people, and the people who love and care for them, need to understand the nutritional and physical needs of late adulthood. Fortunately, this task is becoming easier. Until the 1990s, health and nutrition surveys barely addressed the needs of people older than 50. And, before the development of the Dietary Reference Intakes (DRIs), nutrient recommendations grouped together all adults older than 50. Now, DRI values have categories for adults aged 51 to 70, and for those older than 70. This allows more accurate analysis of survey data pertaining to the health and nutrition of elders.

Many of our choices—food, exercise, smoking, and alcohol—affect not only our risk for chronic disease, but also the rate at which we age. Although it is not possible to stop the aging process, we can control aspects of our lifestyle that contribute to a healthier old age. (See **Figure 16.2**.)

Nutrition and Weight

As we age, body weight has many effects on our health. People who are overweight when they enter their later years, or who gain weight after age 50, have

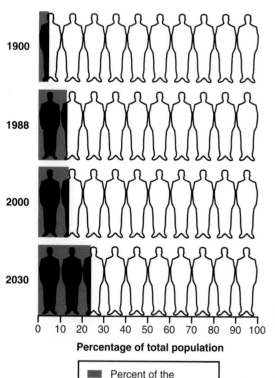

1900

1988

2000

2030

0 10 20 30 40 50 60 70 80 90 100
Percentage of total population

■ Percent of the population 65 or older

Figure 16.1 **The aging U.S. population.**
Source: U.S. Department of Health and Human Services. *Healthy People 2010: Tracking Healthy People 2010.* http://web.health.gov/healthypeople/

a significantly increased risk of developing cardiovascular disease.[2] In addition, heavier weights are often associated with diabetes, high blood pressure, and possibly some types of cancer. However, although excess body weight is a health risk up through age 74, the relative risk associated with excess weight is higher among younger people.[3] Ironically, heavier weight may offer protection against osteoporosis, especially in women after menopause.

On the other hand, people who enter their mature years lean—and who remain lean due to a healthy, active lifestyle—increase their chances of enjoying a healthy old age. Numerous studies have consistently shown that reducing calorie intake while maintaining adequate protein and micronutrient intake increases the life span of laboratory animals. Although scientists suspect that humans respond similarly, more studies are needed.[4] But thinness alone is not always a health advantage. Obviously, older adults who drop weight due to illness enjoy no health benefits from losing these pounds. To the contrary, losing weight compromises their nutritional status and immunity. This puts them at increased risk for further illness, including cardiovascular disease and osteoporosis—especially if the original illness also limits activity. Of course, leanness is no virtue if it is due to tobacco use or alcoholism. Safe, deliberate, and modest weight loss, however, can reduce cardiovascular risks for older people who are overweight but otherwise healthy.

Think About It 1

Immunity

Nutrition influences our immunity from the time we are born until we die. Immune function declines with age, and inadequate nutrition can be responsible for part of that decline.

Quick Bites

Animal Lifetimes

In general, larger animals live longer than smaller animals, but there are many interesting exceptions. For instance, a mouse, a parakeet, and a bat are approximately the same size, but the mouse has a life span of 2 years, the parakeet 13 years, and the bat up to 50 years!

Quick Bites

Longevity Champions

In the United States, women live an average of 7 years longer than men do.

Chronic diseases	Dietary risk factors						Non-dietary risk factors					
	High fat diet	Excessive alcohol	Low complex carbohydrate/fiber	Low vitamin and/or mineral	High sugar	High intake of salty or pickled foods	Genetics	Age	Sedentary lifestyle	Smoking and tobacco use	Stress	Environmental contaminants
Cancers	?*	X	X	X		X	X	X	X	X		X
Hypertension	X	X		X		in salt sensitive people	X	X	X	X	X	
Diabetes (NIDDM)	X		X				X	X	X			
Osteoporosis		X		X			X	X	X	X		
Atherosclerosis	X		X	X			X	X	X	X	X	
Obesity	X	X	X		X		X					
Stroke	X			X			X	X	X	X	X	
Diverticulosis	X		X	X					X	X		
Dental and oral diseases				X	X		X			X		

* The Nurses' Health Study, a large prospective study, found no evidence linking higher total fat intake with increased risk of breast cancer. These results call into question theories that link dietary fat to other cancers.

Figure 16.2 **Risk factors for chronic disease.**

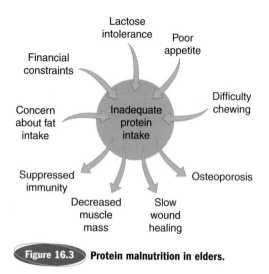

Figure 16.3 Protein malnutrition in elders.

Inadequate consumption of protein is one of the nutritional factors that compromises immunity and health in elders. Older people may eat less meat and dairy products because of poor appetite, difficulty chewing, financial constraints, concerns about fat intake, or lactose intolerance. Reduced consumption of meat and dairy products can make it difficult for older adults to get all the calories and essential nutrients they need. Lack of protein, and many of the vitamins and minerals commonly associated with animal foods (i.e., vitamins B_6, B_{12}, and D, calcium, iron, and zinc) can lead to suppressed immunity, decreased muscle mass, slowed wound healing, and osteoporosis.[5] (See **Figure 16.3**.)

Mobility

Today's mature adults are more mobile than the senior citizens of past generations. However, much of their increased mobility is due to modern conveniences like cars, escalators, and elevators. By reducing the need for everyday physical activity, these conveyances may impair later mobility by exacerbating obesity, insulin resistance, heart disease, and risk of stroke. In addition, the less people move around on their own, the more quickly they lose flexibility, balance, muscle mass, and bone density. These changes, in turn, can cause falls and fractures, mishaps that can turn an active older adult into an invalid.

Obesity also decreases mobility. Excess fat, especially excess abdominal fat, causes shortness of breath, and moving a large body requires extra energy. This becomes a vicious cycle because as people age, they burn fewer calories, which often causes weight gain, which leads to less activity.

Muscle mass and strength decline naturally with age. Indeed, physiological functions that affect our mobility begin to decline (see **Figure 16.4**) at the rate of about 1 percent or more per year beginning about age 30.[6] Due to a decrease in muscle tone, bone loss, and bad habits, our posture begins to deteriorate in our 50s. This can affect pulmonary and cardiovascular function, mobility, and balance. Diseases such as stroke, arthritis, and diabetes become more common, and may cause severe physical disability. Medications and nutritional deficiencies may lead to impaired motor function.

Fortunately, exercise can offset much of this decline. In fact, the benefits of physical activity and strength training may be most profound during aging. Increased self-confidence, better balance and mobility, enhanced mental acuity, and improved appetite and nutrient intake are but a few of the physical and psychological benefits of exercise during our older years.

Key Concepts: *Lifestyle choices, such as diet and exercise, affect how we age. Control of body weight can reduce our risk for many chronic diseases associated with aging. Adequate protein, vitamins, and minerals can protect our immune status. Regular exercise not only enhances our mobility, but also reduces disease risk and improves mental health.*

How People Age

As the body ages, cells and tissues degenerate. Much like a cellular phone dropping a call, communication between cells is interrupted. The ability to adapt to physiological and psychological stress decreases. Because these age-related changes occur gradually, most of us are able to compensate for them. With advancing age, however, adapting becomes more challenging. If we live long enough, age-related changes inevitably become obvious.

Decrease in exercise leads to loss of

Mobility

Muscle mass

Flexibility

Balance

Bone density

Obesity

Increased muscle mass

Better nutrient intake

Better appetite

Improved confidence and mental acuity

Greater mobility

Better balance

Increase in exercise leads to

Figure 16.4 Effects of exercise in elders.

Physiologic Changes Accompanying Aging

Normal aging causes multiple physiologic changes that affect our nutrient needs and nutritional status (see **Table 16.1**). Environmental, pharmacological, and psychological stresses often compound age-related changes in body composition, sensory abilities, organ systems, and immune function. (See **Figure 16.5**.) Individuals age at different rates, and many of the declines in physiological functions have little impact on the day-to-day lives of many elders. Also, with aging, physical responsibilities may decline so that gradual changes in strength do not pose problems until the loss is severe and the person is quite old. Obviously, the circumstances of the person matter. The grandmother who is raising two of her grandchildren may be more highly affected than a retired individual with no regular responsibilities.

Changes in Body Composition

Human growth hormone stimulates skeletal and muscle growth. Production of this hormone declines with age, contributing to a gradual loss of bone, muscle mass, and strength. Beginning at about age 30, we annually lose about 1 to 2 percent of our lean body mass—muscles, organs, and skeletal tissue. This subtle decline continues until about age 45, then the rate of loss slows. From then on, our lean body mass decreases by 5 to 8 percent each decade. Bone loss in women accelerates after menopause. With this loss of body mass comes decreased strength, reduced resting energy expenditure, and increased proportion of body fat, even when weight is unchanged (see **Figure 16.6**). These changes can contribute to declines in mobility and balance as well as to osteoporosis, all of which can diminish an older person's ability to cook, bathe, dress, and get around. In addition, increases in body fat and decreases in physical activity can lead to glucose intolerance and insulin resistance, problems that adversely affect the cardiovascular system and kidneys. Adequate intake of dietary calcium and vitamin D, together with regular

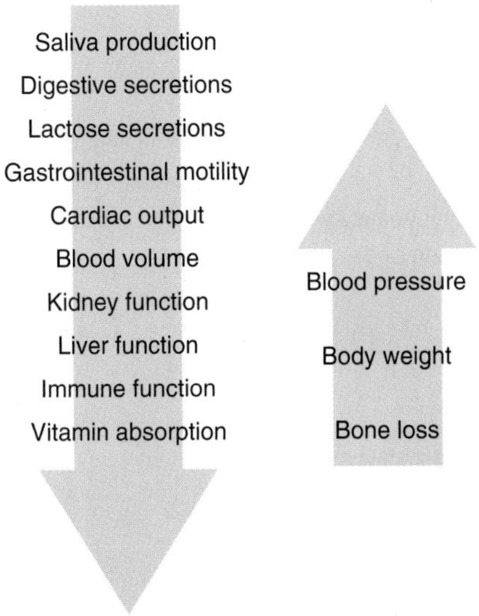

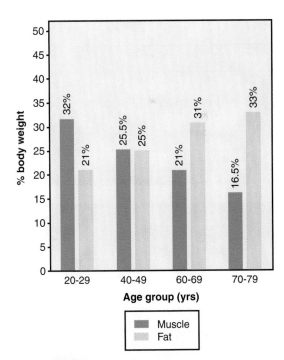

Figure 16.5 Age-related physiological changes.

Figure 16.6 Age-related changes in body composition.

Source: Adapted from Cohen SH, et. al. Compartmental body composition based on the body nitrogen, potassium, and calcium. *Am J Physiol.* 1980;239:192–200.

Table 16.1 Age-Related Changes and Nutrient Needs

Change in Body Composition or Physiologic Function	Impact on Nutrient Requirement
Decreased muscle mass	Decreased need for calories
Decreased bone density	Increased need for calcium, vitamin D
Decreased immune function	Increased need for vitamin B_6, vitamin E, zinc
Increased gastric pH	Increased need for vitamin B_{12}, folic acid, calcium, iron, zinc
Decreased skin capacity for cholecalciferol synthesis	Increased need for vitamin D
Increased wintertime parathyroid hormone production	Increased need for vitamin D
Decreased calcium bioavailability	Increased need for calcium, vitamin D
Decreased hepatic uptake of retinol	Decreased need for vitamin A
Decreased efficiency in metabolic use of pyridoxal	Increased need for vitamin B_6
Increased oxidative stress status	Increased need for beta-carotene, vitamin C, vitamin E
Increased levels of homocysteine	Increased need for folate, vitamin B_6, vitamin B_{12}

Source. Blumberg J. Nutritional needs of seniors. *J Am Coll Nutr.* 1997;16(6):517–523.

Quick Bites

Losing Water

At birth, 75 percent of the body is composed of water. By the time a person reaches old age, that number has dwindled to 50 percent due to changes in body composition.

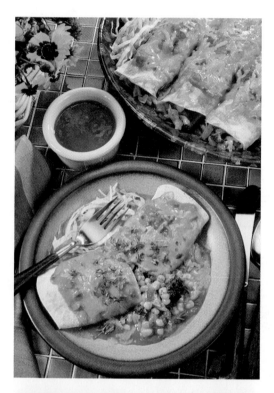

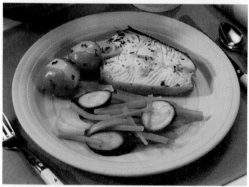

Figure 16.7 **Elders need stronger flavors.** A more highly spiced meal as opposed to a bland one may encourage an elder to eat more.

taste threshold The minimum amount of flavor that must be present for a taste to be detected.

weight-bearing exercise, can help prevent some age-related bone loss. An exercise program that increases fat-free mass can also help to reverse or lessen risks of osteoporosis and glucose intolerance.

Sensory Changes

Our taste buds decrease in both size and number as we get older. Sensitivity to sweet and salty tastes goes first, so older adults often increase their intake of foods high in sugar and sodium—exacerbating health problems that stem from overconsumption of these nutrients. In older adults, the **taste threshold**—the minimum amount of a flavor that must be present in order to detect the taste—is more than double that of college-age adults. Along with taste, our sense of smell also diminishes with age, especially in the seventh decade of life and beyond. Ideas that older people should be served bland foods are rather misguided; in fact, foods need more flavor to be palatable. Enhancement of flavors and odors has increased food consumption (and therefore nutrient intake) by both healthy and ill elders.[7] (See **Figure 16.7**.)

Key Concepts: *Body composition changes as we age. In general, we lose lean body mass and gain fat mass. Loss of lean tissue compromises strength, reduces resting energy expenditure, and increases risk of osteoporosis. Also declining with age is the perception of taste. It takes a higher concentration of a flavor for an older person to detect it. This loss of taste may contribute to loss of appetite and poor food intake.*

Gastrointestinal Changes

Numerous changes occur all along the GI tract as we age. Changes in GI function can interfere not only with food intake, but also with absorption, and elimination of wastes.

Saliva production tends to decrease as we age, especially in people who take medications for conditions such as congestive heart failure. Too little saliva affects chewing, swallowing, taste, and speech. Lack of saliva also affects the preparation of food for digestion and contributes to gum disease—a breach in one of the immune system's first lines of defense against infection. These age-related changes increase the risk of periodontal disease and tooth loss, especially in those who are unable to tend adequately to oral hygiene. With tooth loss comes the inability to chew food well, which increases the risk of choking and aspiration. Dentures that fit comfortably can solve this problem. Reduced salivary production and tooth loss may have a significant effect on the types of foods included and excluded from the diet.

Subtle, age-related changes occur in swallowing, but these changes usually go unnoticed in healthy individuals. Significant swallowing problems may accompany such illnesses as stroke, Parkinson's disease, and dementia.

With age, digestive secretions decline. Most significant are reductions in the stomach secretions of hydrochloric acid and pepsin. These reductions accompany atrophic gastritis—a chronic inflammation of the stomach lining that is common among elders. Atrophic gastritis can affect protein digestion as well as interfere with normal absorption of iron, calcium, vitamin B_{12}, vitamin B_6, and folate.[8] Although reduced lactase also is associated with aging, a complete intolerance to milk and dairy products is less common than older people often suspect. Most people with reduced lactase production can include some milk, cheese, and yogurt in their diets.

Constipation, gas, and bloating are common complaints in old age. These problems are due to a slowing of gastrointestinal motility with aging, along with decreased physical activity, a diet low in or lacking high-fiber fruits and vegetables, and low fluid intake. Feelings of fullness may cause older people to eat less and reduced digestive secretions lower the amount of nutrients they absorb from the foods they do eat.

Myths and misinformation about GI effects of various foods, even among the medical community, may steer a person away from nutrient-dense foods such as dairy products, legumes, broccoli, cauliflower, tomatoes, and citrus products. While many elders mistakenly blame these foods for causing problems with gas, others may be sensitive to lactose in dairy products, or have had an adverse reaction to members of the cabbage family or "acid" containing foods. GI distress also may be caused by factors totally unrelated to the food itself—inappropriate food preparation, lack of adequate fluid, and physical inactivity. Regardless of the cause, once people have an adverse reaction, they may associate it with a recently consumed food and become reluctant to try it again, thus eliminating it from their diets.

Changes in Other Organ Systems

As we advance in years, the workload on the heart increases as the heart loses some of its pumping efficiency. Plaque deposits and loss of elasticity increase the resistance to blood flow in peripheral blood vessels. Resting cardiac output declines with age, and blood pressure tends to rise.

With age, the kidneys less effectively excrete such metabolic products as acid, sodium, and potassium. This alters water balance, putting older people at risk for overhydration or underhydration. In addition, a declining

Quick Bites

Hardy Hearts

By the end of a normal life span, the human heart has pumped more than three billion times. Despite this heavy use, heart failures are usually caused by problems with blood vessels and valves; heart muscle itself rarely wears out.

Fyi

FOR YOUR INFORMATION

Are Dietary Recommendations to Lower Cholesterol Really Necessary for Elders?

Coronary heart disease remains the number one cause of morbidity and mortality in the United States. While concern surrounding cholesterol and fat intake in elders continues, there is some speculation that overemphasizing restriction of these two dietary components may be unwarranted, and for some, unhealthful. People between the ages of 50 and 70 may benefit from blood lipid screening and intervention; however, those older than 70 may not.

Research has shown that there is little relationship between serum cholesterol values and coronary heart disease in those older than 70. Seniors who are overweight or who have coexisting chronic diseases such as diabetes may benefit more from controlling these conditions than from reducing cholesterol. Maintaining weight at a healthy level and controlling blood sugar may do more to

bring cholesterol into line than a low-fat, low-cholesterol diet. Many older individuals are fat- and cholesterol-phobic, thanks to the media and popular press, and set themselves up for problems associated with osteoporosis and possibly protein-energy malnutrition.

Low blood cholesterol levels are associated with malnutrition, morbidity, and mortality, especially among frail elders. Adequate protein and calorie intake is necessary to prevent unintended weight loss. When older people restrict their intake of foods that are good sources of protein (e.g., meat, poultry, and dairy products) because they believe these foods are too high in fat, they risk depressing their immune system and causing irreversible, unintended weight loss.

For some, unintentional weight gain and associated health problems (e.g., increased triglycerides, blood glucose, and obesity)

may arise from restricting fat in the diet. It is widely known that those who focus on fat-free and reduced-fat foods often increase their intake of carbohydrates, particularly sugar. These empty calories are of little use for those whose caloric needs are lower and nutrient needs higher.

Rather than focus on dietary restriction for those over the age of 70, it is more appropriate to focus on nutrients that are important for maintaining health and vitality, which in turn, reduces the risk of debilitation and disease. The proposed trend is away from diets that focus on reducing fat and cholesterol and toward those that include foods from all of the food groups in moderate amounts.

Sources: Heart Disease in Older Adults: Are Dietary Restrictions Effective? Presented at: The American Dietetic Association 81st Annual Meeting and Exhibition; October 19, 1998; Kansas City, Missouri; and Position statement: liberalized diets for older adults in long-term care. *J Am Diet Assoc.* 1998;98:201.

T-cell A type of immune cell involved in mediating the cellular immune response.

warfarin A prescription anticoagulant medicine.

ability to concentrate urine means that an older person requires more water to excrete the same amount of solute. Reduced thirst sensation compounds the potential for dehydration.

As we age, the liver less efficiently clears prescription and over-the-counter drugs and their metabolites. This change leaves older people susceptible to overmedication and dangerous drug interactions.

Key Concepts: *The aging process affects all of the organ systems. In the GI tract, reduction in hormonal, acid, and enzyme secretions affects nutrient absorption. Reduced motility contributes to constipation. The functional capacity of the heart, liver, and kidneys decline, which can result in a number of problems.*

Changes in Immune Function

In the fifth decade of life, the body's defense mechanisms begin to weaken. Changes are most notable in **T-cell** function. These cells assist in the body's response to viruses, bacteria, and other foreign bodies. Such changes leave elders more vulnerable to upper-respiratory infections, including influenza and pneumonia; urinary tract infections; pressure sores; and food-borne illnesses. Physical barriers to infectious agents, foreign bodies, and chemicals weaken as well. These barriers include the skin, the acid environment in the stomach, and swallowing and coughing reflexes. Declines in immune function can also be related to chronic diseases such as diabetes.

Changes in Vitamin Status

In late adulthood, peripheral tissues in the body become less efficient at taking up circulating fat-soluble vitamins (A, D, E, and K) that are essential to tissue health. Other physiologic and behavioral changes of old age often compound this problem. For example, many older adults are concerned about cardiovascular health so they restrict their dietary fat intake, thereby reducing their intake of fat-soluble vitamins, especially vitamin E. Elders are at particular risk for vitamin D deficiency, which contributes to osteoporosis. Not only are aging tissues less able to take up vitamin D from the blood, but aging skin is less able to synthesize vitamin D when exposed to sunlight. In addition, many elders spend more time indoors and have reduced exposure to sunlight. When they go outside, many avoid the sun and use sunscreens—a good strategy for skin cancer prevention but it also reduces vitamin D synthesis. Lactose intolerance often leads to avoidance of dairy products and a reduction in vitamin D intake, further compromising vitamin D status. Vitamin K deficiency is a hazard for older people who take **warfarin**, a medication that decreases blood-clotting time. People who take warfarin must keep their vitamin K intake consistent, which often means limiting foods that are very high in vitamin K. Limiting these foods, which include green leafy vegetables, may further jeopardize vitamin status and put such people at risk for inadequate intake of vitamin A, vitamin C, fiber, and other needed nutrients.

Key Concepts: *Immune function declines with age. As a result, elders are more susceptible than younger people to infections and illness. Absorption, transport, storage, and use of fat-soluble vitamins are also affected by aging. These effects, in turn, have an impact on many body systems.*

Psychological Impact of Aging

As we get older, many of us fear loss of mental function even more than loss of physical function. Yet, as the years advance most people maintain cognitive function with only subtle changes.

When there is a cognitive decline, people often have difficulty remembering names or retrieving the right words. It becomes harder to focus attention, especially in the face of distracting stimuli. This inability to concentrate puts elders at risk for falls and accidents, for example, while cooking in the kitchen or driving a car. In most cases, slight changes involving sensory acuity, secondary memory, and information-processing speed do not affect quality of life or lead to progressive or rapid declines in mental function. On the other hand, when depression or dementia is suspected, professional evaluation becomes necessary. Changes in behavior of elders may not be the result of disease, but of overmedication or drug interactions.

Changes in Appetite

Many older people experience decreased appetite and an inability to recognize hunger sensations. For most people, these are not inevitable consequences of aging. Depression, dementia, and social isolation, rather than the aging process itself, often are responsible.

Stress

Continued stress, as observed in people who experience lifelong economic hardship, can cause earlier physical, cognitive, and mental health declines.[9] Chronic stress may impair memory and even lead to brain damage over time. Chronic stress increases the secretion of stress hormones and leads to changes in the autonomic nervous system. Over time, these changes can affect cardiovascular function, food intake, and metabolism, as well as the immune system. Chronic stress is also a risk factor for depression.

Depression

Many studies of elders report high levels of well-being among elders, especially those who remain independent. Although depression is one of the most common psychological effects of aging, it is most common among institutionalized and low-income elders. Researchers believe that depression is related to the loss of receptors for the neurotransmitter serotonin. Loss of these receptors also may cause cognitive difficulties. Critical age-related stress can become concentrated and frequent in later life, increasing the likelihood and severity of depression. Among these stressors are the loss of loved ones, including spouse and friends; physical disability; perceived loss of physical attractiveness; inability to psychologically defend oneself from unpleasant events; inability to care for oneself, which forces dependence upon caregivers and long-term care; social isolation; and, inevitably, the approach of death. In elders, depression often leads to malnutrition, and may manifest itself as either anorexia (loss of appetite) or obesity. Anorectic elders lose weight and muscle mass, putting them at risk for chronic conditions such as osteoporosis.

Alcoholism

Alcoholism may be prevalent, especially among socially isolated or depressed elders. A diet low in essential nutrients often accompanies excessive alcohol consumption. Over time, excessive alcohol use can cause chronic liver disease, pancreatitis, secondary vitamin and mineral deficiencies, and protein-energy malnutrition.

Dementing Illnesses

Dementing illness, which becomes more common after age 80, can interfere with food preparation and prevent eating. A person with dementia, for example, may suffer **apraxia**—the inability to perform purposeful movements—

apraxia The impairment or inability to use objects correctly.

agnosia The inability to recognize sensory stimuli, which may include smells, taste, visual stimuli, and tactile stimuli.

Alzheimer's disease A presenile dementia characterized by accumulation of plaques in certain regions of the brain and degeneration of a certain class of neurons.

and lack the ability to prepare food safely and adequately. Another common disorder in dementia is **agnosia**—an inability to appreciate sensory impressions. People with agnosia may lose their desire for food.

Alzheimer's Disease

Among its other ravages, **Alzheimer's disease** (AD) eventually destroys the ability to obtain, prepare, and consume an optimal diet. While genetic factors can affect the risk for Alzheimer's disease, other risk factors include age, head trauma, and possibly exposure to environmental toxins. Although much more research is needed, estrogen, and a combination of nonsteroidal anti-inflammatory drugs and antioxidants may provide protection from the disease.[10]

Most cases of Alzheimer's disease begin after age 70, but it can strike genetically predisposed people at a younger age. During the first stage of the disease, the afflicted person can have difficulty recalling names, frequently lose possessions, and easily become lost. Sensory sensitivity, such as loss of the sense of smell, begins to change gradually, and so may not be readily noticed. As the disease progresses, the person becomes unable to complete simple tasks that require learned motor movement, such as using a can opener. There is an increase in behavior problems, including wandering, aggression, and sleep disorders. These behaviors, if they occur frequently, can affect the person's ability to maintain weight and nutritional status. The late stages of the disease are marked by inability to communicate, and about one-third of those with AD develop overactivity that drains the nutritional reserve and increases calorie needs. Eventually, people with AD become unable to walk and become chair- or bed-bound. At this time, the caregiver must carefully plan the person's diet to meet psychological and physical needs, with particular attention to optimum nutrition without excess weight gain.

Key Concepts: *Psychological changes associated with aging also affect food intake and nutritional status. Depression, stress, and dementing illness can interfere with appetite and normal food intake. Alzheimer's disease can lead to a loss of independent feeding and changes in nutritional needs.*

Nutrient Needs of the Mature Adult

To live life to its fullest, you need good nutrition. A lifestyle that incorporates the Dietary Guidelines for Americans, together with regular physical activity, is essential to a long and productive life. **Figure 16.8** shows the Food Guide Pyramid modified for older adults.

Nutritional Status of Our Aging Nation

Data are currently being evaluated regarding the eating habits and nutritional status of older Americans. The third National Health and Nutrition Examination Survey (NHANES III) obtained information for three groups of older Americans: those aged 60 to 69; those aged 70 to 79; and those aged 80 and above. NHANES III further divided these groups by ethnicity, with separate analyses for non-Hispanic whites, African Americans, and Mexican Americans. Some of the studies reveal the following:

- For older Americans overall, mean energy intake is below the RDA. Energy intake of whites is higher than that of African Americans and Mexican Americans.

- Fat intake as a percentage of total daily calories ranges from 31 to 34 percent—slightly higher than the recommended 30 percent.

- Both men and women in all groups take in less cholesterol than the recommended limit of 300 milligrams per day.

- On average, older women consume about two-thirds of the RDA for folate, while older men consume approximately 80 percent of the RDA. On the other hand, both women and men consume more than the RDA for vitamin B_{12}.

- Average calcium intake is below the current AI of 1,200 milligrams per day (670 mg/d for women and 830 mg/d for men), as are intakes of vitamin E, magnesium, and zinc. Intake of vitamin D (a nutrient of concern for elders) was not reported. Other nutrients met or exceeded the current recommended values.

- Intake of total calories, cholesterol, and vitamin B_{12}, as well as percentage of calories from fat all decrease with advancing age.

- Energy and mineral intakes among African Americans and Mexican Americans are lower than among non-Hispanic whites, while cholesterol intakes are higher.[11]

A similar study evaluated the dietary intake of nearly 2,000 elders participating in the **Elderly Nutrition Program (ENP)** and compared them to nonparticipants living in the same areas.[12] This program provides nutrition services to more than three million low-income and minority elders at increased health and nutritional risk. Subjects in this study were primarily female (70 percent) with an average age of 77 years. Although their calorie intake was less than the RDA of 1,900 kilocalories per day for

Elderly Nutrition Program (ENP) A federally funded program that provides older persons with nutritionally sound meals through meals-on-wheels programs or in senior citizen centers and similar congregate settings.

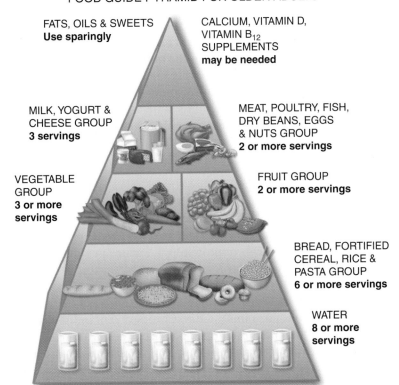

FOOD GUIDE PYRAMID FOR OLDER ADULTS

FATS, OILS & SWEETS
Use sparingly

CALCIUM, VITAMIN D, VITAMIN B_{12} SUPPLEMENTS **may be needed**

MILK, YOGURT & CHEESE GROUP
3 servings

MEAT, POULTRY, FISH, DRY BEANS, EGGS & NUTS GROUP
2 or more servings

VEGETABLE GROUP
3 or more servings

FRUIT GROUP
2 or more servings

BREAD, FORTIFIED CEREAL, RICE & PASTA GROUP
6 or more servings

WATER
8 or more servings

Figure 16.8 **Food Guide Pyramid for older adults.**
While not an official USDA pyramid, the Food Guide Pyramid for Older Adults reflects the nutrition needs of seniors. Its narrower profile reflects reduced energy needs and the base recommends water to combat the chronic dehydration that is common in seniors.
Source: Adapted from Russell R, Rasmussen H, Lichtenstein A. Modified Food Guide Pyramid for people over 70 years of age, *J Nutr.* 1999;129:752.

women and 2,300 kilocalories per day for men, the program participants nevertheless had nutrient-dense diets that met or exceeded recommended intakes for most nutrients. Average intakes of vitamin D, vitamin E, folate, calcium, magnesium, and zinc were less than current recommended intake levels. Of these, intake of vitamin D raised the most concern, with an average of 5 micrograms per day for women and 6 micrograms per day for men (the AI for vitamin D is 10 micrograms per day for those aged 51 through 70 years and 15 micrograms per day for those over 70 years of age). Congregate (group) or home-delivered meals (at least one meal must be provided each day, 5 days per week) contributed 40 to 50 percent of the daily intake for most nutrients. Compared to older people not served by the ENP, the participants' diets generally contained more vitamins and minerals, but with total fat and sodium levels closer to the *Dietary Guidelines for Americans.*

Key Concepts: *While nutrition studies do not show widespread malnutrition among elders, they do indicate dietary practices of concern. High fat intakes are common, while low calcium intakes occur frequently. Caloric intake, as assessed in national surveys, is below the RDAs.*

Dietary Requirements of Older Adults

Energy

Primarily because of decreases in metabolically active lean body mass and reductions in physical activity, our energy requirements decline as we age. Physical activity can delay some of this loss, thus allowing us to eat more without gaining weight, and increasing the likelihood that our diets will be adequate in essential nutrients.

The RDA for energy reflects the average requirement for individuals aged 51 and older. For men this value is 2,300 kilocalories per day, and for women the RDA is 1,900 kilocalories. Older men expend about 20 percent less energy than younger men. On the other hand, older women experience minimal changes in energy expenditure. One proposed explanation is that men tend to reduce their physical activity significantly when they retire, but women continue doing the bulk of the housework throughout their lives. In addition, resting metabolic rate decreases by 20 percent in men, but only 13 percent in women. Individual energy needs change based on activity, lean body mass, and concurrent disease; a person who is bed- or chair-ridden, for example, usually requires fewer calories than a mobile person.

Protein

Protein needs (as grams per day) do not change as we age, but may be somewhat harder for us to meet as our overall energy needs decrease and our tastes change. As our caloric needs decrease and our protein needs remain constant, an adequate diet must contain relatively more protein. For healthy older people, the RDA for protein is 0.8 grams per kilogram of body weight, or 50 grams per day for women, and 63 grams per day for men using median body weights. Data from the studies cited earlier show that, on average, men consume approximately 75 grams per day and women consume about 60 grams per day. Chronically ill individuals may need more protein to maintain nitrogen balance. Trauma, stress, and infection also may increase protein needs. However, there are risks associated with high levels of protein intake, including dehydration, nitrogen overload, and adverse effects on the kidney.

Carbohydrate

After infancy, carbohydrates should make up more than half of the calories in the diet. Because foods with primarily simple carbohydrates provide little nutrient value, the best choices are foods with complex carbohydrates.

Fiber, a complex carbohydrate, has many potential benefits, including preventing constipation and diverticulitis, and possibly reducing the risk of colon cancer. (See Chapter 4 for more information about fiber.) There are no specific fiber recommendations for elders; the typical recommendation for the general population is 20 to 35 grams per day. Fiber also can help to reduce blood cholesterol, making these recommendations especially important for those who are at risk for heart disease. Five or more servings of fruits and vegetables daily, accompanied by whole-grain breads or a serving of a cereal high in bran, will supply this amount easily. To avoid abdominal discomfort, increase dietary fiber intake gradually. When increasing dietary fiber intake, it is essential to consume adequate fluids—ideally water—to avoid dehydration and constipation.

Fat

Excess dietary fat can lead to obesity, which in turn increases the risk for diabetes, heart disease, and some types of cancer. Younger people should limit their dietary cholesterol and fat, but severe restrictions in elders may be counterproductive. Some older people make extreme attempts to avoid dietary fat and consume a very low-fat diet, which is high in simple carbohydrates. This strategy may exacerbate insulin resistance, elevate triglycerides, decrease HDL cholesterol levels, or create more weight problems. Extreme fat phobia may contribute to nutritional deficiencies among older people who are afraid to drink milk, eat red meat, or even eat poultry or fish. Too few animal products in the diet may contribute to a lack of dietary protein, deficiency of minerals such as calcium, iron, and zinc, and poor vitamin B_{12} intake and absorption.

Think About It 2

Healthy people who are at low risk for heart disease should obtain a maximum of 30 percent of their daily calories from fat, with no more than 10 percent of the calories from saturated fat. They should limit their cholesterol intake to 300 milligrams per day. People at increased risk for heart disease should limit saturated fat and cholesterol even more, according to their physicians' advice.

Water

Nutritionists often call water the forgotten nutrient. Water is essential to all body functions and if intake is inadequate, cellular metabolism becomes difficult, if not impossible. In elders, a decreased thirst response and the kidney's reduced concentrating capacity can lead to dehydration. Diuretic medications, alcohol, and caffeine all increase fluid excretion and are contributors to dehydration. Scientists estimate water needs at 1 milliliter per kilocalorie of food consumed, or about 30 milliliters per kilogram of body weight per day.

Key Concepts: *Although caloric needs decline with loss of lean tissue and reduced physical activity, protein needs do not change as we grow older. A high-carbohydrate, moderate-fat diet is still recommended for elders. Water is important, and because of their diminished thirst response, older people may not drink enough of it.*

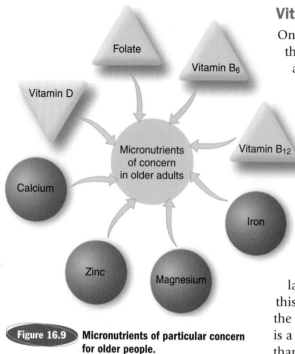

Figure 16.9 **Micronutrients of particular concern for older people.**

Vitamins and Minerals

One of the significant changes in the Dietary Reference Intakes (DRI) is the expansion of age categories to include one for ages 51 through 70 and a second category for those older than 70. With this revision, nutritionists can make more precise recommendations for older citizens and better evaluate their diets. The setting of Tolerable Upper Intake Levels (UL) is important for older people who take high-dose dietary supplements.

As we age, our micronutrient status changes, especially our needs for vitamin D, vitamin B_{12}, and calcium. (See **Figure 16.9**.) In many cases, our vitamin needs remain stable while our energy needs decline. In other cases, age-related declines in absorption, use, or activation of nutrients increase dietary vitamin and mineral needs. Therefore, it is especially important for elders to eat nutrient-dense foods. Adequate dietary calcium can reduce bone loss and risk of fractures. Although other minerals such as zinc may be needed in larger amounts during late adulthood, conclusive evidence to support this view is lacking. The potential role of increased dietary magnesium in the reduction of high blood pressure, cardiovascular disease, and diabetes is a top research priority. The new adult RDA values are slightly higher than those set in 1989, but do not change with aging.[13]

Vitamin D

Vitamin D promotes bone health; too little dietary vitamin D can lead to brittle and porous bones that are susceptible to fracture. Because of decreased exposure to sunlight, age-related decreases in synthesis and activation, and low dietary intake, elders often have low vitamin D.

DRI values released in 1997 reflect the increased intake elders need to maintain optimal bone health. These recommendations assume that elders have limited exposure to sunlight. The AI for vitamin D for adults aged 51 though 70 is 10 micrograms per day. For adults 70 and older, the AI is 15 micrograms

[*Fyi*] Vulnerability to Nutrition Quackery

FOR YOUR INFORMATION

Snake oil salesmen pedaled their tonics from town to town in the nineteenth century. Today's snake oil salesmen are a little more sophisticated and cunning, with numerous marketing tools at their fingertips. They prey on those who are suffering from chronic illness, are terminally ill, or have other debilitating conditions. Even well-educated people may turn to worthless products with the belief that anything is better than their current treatment regimen. Besides, there is the eternal hope that these products will provide a cure. Some believe that these "magic bullets" will enhance performance, improve memory, impart beauty, or prevent aging.

While people of all ages fall victim to questionable methods and products, at least 60 percent of victims of health fraud are elders. More people in this group tend to be chronically ill and are looking, if not for a cure, at least for something to make them feel better.[1]

Quacks promise youth. In a society that prizes youth and physical attractiveness, it is no wonder that many elders are in search of the fountain of youth. Many older persons are vulnerable to claims made in print and broadcast media. Testimonials for products from seemingly reliable salespeople or admired celebrities make the quick cure even more believable. Little do people real-

ize that magic pills and potions costing hundreds of dollars are unnecessary; a healthful diet, physical activity, and not smoking are the best strategies for preventing or delaying many of the diseases of aging.

People vulnerable to quackery should avoid promotions for remedies and cures. This is easier said than done, however, since well-meaning friends and relatives may offer questionable products and advice in hopes of helping the infirm to get better. Unfortunately, most magazine and newspaper editors and producers of infomercials do not screen their advertisements for truth or accuracy. These media reach large audiences vulnerable to questionable products. The

per day. For adults aged 31 through 50, the AI is 5 micrograms per day, the same value that was recommended for all adults in the 1989 RDA.

B Vitamins

The B vitamins deserve special consideration in adults and the aged. Extensive research links inadequate folate, vitamin B_{12}, and vitamin B_6 to elevated levels of plasma homocysteine, a factor associated with an increased risk for cardiovascular disease in elders.[14]

The current RDA for folate is 400 micrograms per day for all adults over 51 years of age. This is an increase from the 200 micrograms per day for men and 180 micrograms per day for women called for in the previous (1989) RDA. Meeting folate intake recommendations became easier after January 1, 1998, when the government began requiring all enriched cereal grains to be fortified with 1.4 milligrams of folic acid per kilogram of grain.[15]

At least 15 percent of elders may have vitamin B_{12} deficiency.[16] Although most adults consume adequate amounts of dietary vitamin B_{12}, from 10 to 30 percent of elders lose their ability to absorb protein-bound vitamin B_{12} from foods. This inability to absorb vitamin B_{12} may be due to a decrease in gastric acidity, which affects the breakdown of protein, or to competition with increased numbers of bacteria, particularly *Helicobacter pylori*.[17] A reduction in the production of intrinsic factor, also impairs B_{12} absorption. An intake of 2.4 micrograms per day of vitamin B_{12} is now recommended for all adults older than 51 years, an increase over the 1989 RDA of 2.0 micrograms per day.[18] Because B_{12} is absorbed more easily from B_{12}-fortified foods or B_{12}-containing supplements, scientists suggest that adults older than 50 use these sources to meet their requirements for vitamin B_{12}.

In the over 50 category, the RDA for vitamin B_6 is 1.7 milligrams per day for men and 1.5 milligrams per day for women, values that are slightly higher than the 1.3 milligrams per day recommended for younger adults. While very high protein diets might increase vitamin B_6 requirements, not

best adage to remember is, "if it seems too good to be true, it probably is." In addition, any of the following claims, statements, and behaviors signal that the product is unlikely to deliver what it promises:

- It is an undiscovered cure for a disease, or a cure that is not understood or supported by the medical community.
- The manufacturer or salesperson belittles the medical community for their lack of support of the product or procedure.
- Advertisements or salespeople state that the product is effective against a wide range of diseases; it is a cure-all.
- Claims are made for widespread deficiency of a particular nutrient; the only way to treat the deficiency is by using the product.
- The product is said to prevent illness.
- Advertisements include testimonials and/or case histories from satisfied medical providers or patients.
- The product is made from a "secret" formula, usually available from only one company, and usually only by mail or from door-to-door solicitations.
- Information about ingredients is unclear or absent.
- The research that supports use of the product is done with animals rather than humans. (Before principles can be established for the treatment of diseases in humans, studies on humans are necessary.)
- Supporting research is based on one or two small clinical trials, and the results have not been replicated, or even published in peer-reviewed journals.[2]

1 National Institute on Aging. Age Page, Health Quackery. http://www.nih.gov/nia/health/agepages/healthqy.htm Accessed 9/9/00.

2 Jarvis WT, Barrett, S. How Quackery Sells. http://www.quackwatch.com/01QuackeryRelatedTopics/quacksell.html. Accessed 9/9/00.

all studies support this relationship.[19] Excessive consumption of vitamin B_6 may result in peripheral neuropathies (reduced sensation or pain in the extremities), so caution is warranted when using supplements. The UL for vitamin B_6 is 100 milligrams per day.

Key Concepts: *Vitamin D, folate, vitamin B_{12}, and vitamin B_6 are key nutrients for elders. Vitamin D status can decline due to reduced intake, synthesis, and activation. Poor folate, B_{12}, and B_6 status may result in high homocysteine levels, a risk factor for heart disease. Vitamin B_{12} absorption declines with age; B_{12} is more easily absorbed from fortified foods and supplements, so these become important sources for elders.*

Calcium

Maintaining adequate calcium intake reduces the rate of age-related bone loss and the incidence of fractures, especially of the hip.[20] For all adults aged 51 and older, the AI for calcium is 1,200 milligrams per day, an increase of 400 milligrams per day over previous recommendations, and 200 milligrams per day higher than the AI for adults 31 to 50 years old.[21]

A loss of vitamin D receptors in the gut appears to be partly responsible for the age-related decline in calcium-absorbing ability. Atrophic gastritis also reduces calcium absorption, as does an increase in the consumption of fiber—a practice that doctors recommend for its laxative effects. Because of lactose intolerance, many older people have a low intake of dairy foods, and therefore of calcium.

Zinc

Although clinical zinc deficiencies are uncommon, older adults frequently have marginal zinc intakes.[22] Stress, especially in hospitalized elders, appears to increase the risk of zinc deficiency and suppress immune function. Studies show that zinc supplementation hastens wound healing, but only in those who are zinc deficient. Because zinc may interfere with immune function and the absorption of other minerals, and possibly lower HDL cholesterol, people of all ages should avoid excessive and continuous zinc supplementation.

Magnesium

Magnesium plays an essential role in many cellular reactions. Evidence is beginning to accumulate regarding the relationship between low serum magnesium and atherosclerosis.[23] Magnesium-deficiency has been observed in people with malabsorption syndromes, those with malnutrition or alcoholism, and in elders. However, pure magnesium deficiency due to inadequate intake is rare. The body absorbs magnesium from food more efficiently than from supplements. Although magnesium supplements seem to have few side effects, large doses can cause adverse effects, particularly in people with renal insufficiency. The UL for supplemental magnesium is 350 milligrams per day.

Iron

Iron remains an important nutrient throughout the life cycle. Following menopause, the RDA for women drops to the same level as for men, 8 milligrams per day. Iron deficiency is a concern for elders who have limited intake of iron from the best sources—red meats, fish, and poultry. Reduced meat consumption may result from taste changes, economics, poor dentition, or a combination of factors.

To Supplement or Not to Supplement

Use of dietary supplements, including vitamins, minerals, and herbal and botanical products, is growing fast. Although food is "the best medicine," some elders may think they need a supplement in order to meet their nutrient needs. Food is more than the sum of its known nutrients, however, and replacing food with supplements may be a poor trade-off. In addition, some nutrients in large amounts can be toxic, affect the absorption of other nutrients, or interfere with the absorption and metabolism of prescription medications.

Excessive use of vitamin supplements by elders may result in **hypervitaminosis**. The need for vitamin A decreases with age, increasing the chances that supplementation may lead to liver dysfunction, bone and joint pain, headaches, and other problems. Also, taking large amounts of vitamin C can increase the likelihood of renal stones and gastric bleeding. Because we know that many older people use vitamin supplements, and that megadoses may have negative effects on health, it is important to inform elders of the ULs for micronutrients. For most nutrients, the UL represents a level of intake from a combination of food and dietary supplements that should not be exceeded on a routine basis.

Key Concepts: *Important minerals for elders are calcium, zinc, magnesium, and iron. Calcium is important to reduce the risk for osteoporosis. Marginal zinc deficiency has been suspected in many elders, and may be the result of reduced intake of red meats. Magnesium may have a role in cardiovascular disease. Iron needs decline for women as they go through menopause. Excessive supplementation with certain vitamins or minerals can lead to health problems.*

Nutrition-Related Concerns of Mature Adults

Many factors can interfere with intake or use of nutrients by older adults. Therefore, it is extremely important to monitor the nutritional health of seniors. Simple screening tools can identify risks for poor nutritional status. (See **Figure 16.10**.) To manage acute or chronic nutrition-related conditions, seniors may need to make specific dietary changes.

Nutrition Screening

To identify malnutrition risk factors among the aging population, the American Academy of Family Physicians, the American Dietetic Association, and the National Council on Aging collaborated on the Nutrition Screening Initiative (NSI). This five-year project focused on nutrition screening and interventions that help prevent and manage nutrition-related problems before a person becomes ill or a condition worsens. They designed the first step, a "Determine Your Nutritional Health" checklist, to be self-administered. A dietitian, physician, nurse, or other health-care provider can review the resulting score to determine the person's nutritional risk and, if indicated, recommend a more in-depth Level I screen.

The Level I screen assesses four areas in which elders may be able to improve their diet and health:

- physical measurements (e.g., current weight and recent weight loss or gain),
- dietary intake,
- living environment (e.g., whether cooking facilities are available,), and
- functional status, including activities of daily living (ADLs) and instrumental activities of daily living (IADLs).

hypervitaminosis High levels of vitamins in the blood, usually a result of excess supplement intake.

UL Values for Vitamins and Minerals

Vitamin A	3000 mg RAE/d
Vitamin D	50 µg/d
Niacin	35 mg/d
Vitamin B₆	100 mg/d
Folic acid	1,000 µg/d (from fortified foods and supplements only)
Choline	3.5 g/d
Vitamin C	2,000 mg/d
Vitamin E	1,000 mg/d
Calcium	2,500 mg/d
Phosphorus	4,000 mg/d (for > 70 yr, 3,000 mg/d)
Magnesium	350 mg/d (from nonfood sources only)
Copper	10,000 µg/d
Fluoride	10 mg/d
Iodine	1,100 µg/d
Iron	45 mg/d
Manganese	11 mg/d
Molybdenum	2000 µg/d
Selenium	400 µg/d
Zinc	40 mg/d

Determine Your Nutritional Health

Read the statements below. Circle the number in the yes column for those that apply to you or someone you know. For each yes answer, score the number in the box. Total your nutritional score.

	YES
I have an illness or condition that made me change the kind and/or amount of food I eat.	2
I eat fewer than 2 meals per day.	3
I eat few fruits or vegetables, or milk products.	2
I have 3 or more drinks of beer, liquor, or wine almost every day.	2
I have tooth or mouth problems that make it hard for me to eat.	2
I don't always have enough money to buy the food I need.	4
I eat alone most of the time.	1
I take 3 or more different prescribed or over-the-counter drugs a day.	1
Without wanting to, I have lost or gained 10 pounds in the last 6 months.	2
I am not always physically able to shop, cook, and/or feed myself.	2
TOTAL	

Total Your Nutrition Score. If it's—

0–2 *Good! Recheck your nutritional score in 6 months.*

3–5 *You are at moderate nutritional risk. See what can be done to improve your eating habits and lifestyle. Your office on aging, senior nutrition program, senior citizens center, or health department can help. Recheck your nutritional score in 3 months.*

6 or more *You are at high nutritional risk. Bring this checklist the next time you see your doctor, dietitian, or other qualified health or social service professional. Talk with them about any problems you may have. Ask for help to improve your nutritional health.*

Figure 16.10 Nutrition screening checklist.

Source: Adapted from the Nutrition Screening Initiative, *Nutrition Applications in the Life Cycle.* The American Academy of Family Physicians, the American Dietetic Association, and the National Council on Aging, Inc., and funded in part by a grant from Ross Products Division, Abbott Laboratories; with permission.

A more comprehensive Level II screen identifies people with potentially serious nutrition or medical problems, such as protein-energy malnutrition. This tool employs more detailed anthropometric measurements, including triceps skinfold, mid-arm muscle circumference, and body mass index. Laboratory tests identify clinical or subclinical nutrient deficiencies and the health professional evaluates cognitive and emotional status. The drug-use questionnaire is an important component of this screening, since **polypharmacy**, the use of multiple medications, is common among people and can interfere with food intake and nutrient absorption.

The NSI assessment can indicate minor and major signs of poor nutritional status and the need for intervention. Because both deficiencies and excesses contribute to health risks, the health-care provider who is devising an older person's nutrition plan must consider not only the possibility of nutrient deficiencies, but also the likelihood of excessive nutrient intake.

Key Concepts: The tools developed by the Nutrition Screening Initiative can identify nutritional risks that can be corrected before they become debilitating. Many older people use multiple medications, which can interfere with food intake and nutrient absorption. People who plan menus for seniors must consider nutrient excesses along with nutrient deficiencies.

Drug-Drug and Drug-Nutrient Interactions

Drugs affect the way the body uses nutrients and can alter the activities of other drugs. In turn, foods and nutrients can enhance or interfere with the effects of drugs. (See **Table 16.2**.) Some drugs interfere with appetite; others cause a dry mouth. Because many elders take several medications or are on long-term drug therapy, these factors often put elders at increased nutritional risk.

For example, aspirin, vitamin E, wide variations in vitamin K intake, and several herbal supplements interfere with the effectiveness of warfarin (Coumadin), a common blood thinner. Foods that contain large amounts of the amino acid tyramine (e.g., aged cheeses, beer, and Chianti wine) can interfere with a group of antidepressant drugs called MAOIs (monoamine oxidase inhibitors). Potassium supplements and salt substitutes that contain potassium chloride can be a problem for people who take certain types of diuretics for treatment of hypertension.

People should view herbal supplements and vitamins or minerals in high doses as drugs, particularly when they take them in conjunction with prescription or over-the-counter medications. Although herbals almost certainly interact with other medicines, such interactions are not

polypharmacy The use or prescription of two or more different drugs to treat one or more health problems.

Table 16.2 **Examples of Food-Drug Interactions**

Drug	Food That Interacts	Effect of the Food	What to Do
Analgesic			
acetaminophen (Tylenol)	Alcohol	Increases risk for liver toxicity	Avoid alcohol.
Antibiotic			
tetracyclines	Dairy products; iron supplements	Decreases drug absorption	Do not take with milk. Take 1 hr before or 2 hr after food or milk.
amoxicillin, penicillin,	Food	Decreases drug absorption	Take 1 hr before or 2 hr after meals.
zithromax, erythromycin	Food	Decreases drug absorption	Take 1 hr before or 2 hr after meals.
nitrofurantoin (Macrobid)	Food	Decreases GI distress, slows drug absorption	Take with food or milk.
Anticoagulant			
warfarin (Coumadin)	Foods rich in vitamin K	Decreases drug effectiveness	Limit foods high in vitamin K: liver, broccoli, spinach, kale, cauliflower, and Brussels sprouts.
Antifungal			
griseofulvin (Fulvicin)	High-fat meal	Increases drug absorption	Take with high-fat meal.
Antihistamine			
diphenhydramine (Benadryl), chlorphenira-mine (Chlor-Trimeton)	Alcohol	Increases drowsiness	Avoid alcohol.
Antihypertensive			
felodipine (Plendil), nifedipine	Grapefruit juice	Increases drug absorption	Consult physician or pharmacist before changing diet.
Anti-inflammatory			
naproxen (Naprosyn)	Food or milk	Decreases GI irritation	Take with food or milk.
ibuprofen (Motrin)	Alcohol	Increases risk for liver damage or stomach bleeding	Avoid alcohol.
Diuretic			
spironolactone (Aldactone)	Food	Decreases GI irritation	Take with food.
Psychotherapeutic (MAO inhibitors)			
tranylcypromine (Parnate)	Foods high in tyramine: aged cheeses, Chianti wine, pickled herring, Brewer's yeast, fava beans	Risk for hypertensive crisis	Avoid foods high in tyramine.

Note: Grapefruit juice contains a compound not found in other citrus juices. This compound increases the absorption of some drugs and can enhance their effects. It's best to not take medications with grapefruit juice. Drink it at least 2 hours before or after you take your medication. If you often drink grapefruit juice, talk with your pharmacist or doctor before changing your routine.

Source: Bobroff LB, Lentz A, Turner RE. *Food/Drug and Drug/Nutrient Interactions: What You Should Know about Your Medications.* Gainesville, FL: University of Florida; March 1999. Publication FCS 8092 in a series of the Department of Family, Youth and Community Sciences, Florida Cooperative Extension Service, Institute of Food and Agricultural Sciences.

well documented. In addition to the health and safety issues, many supplement therapies can be costly.

Timing of medication and meals can enhance or impair the absorption of drugs and change the way they are metabolized by the body. It is imperative to follow directions regarding how to take medications. If fluid restriction is not an issue, medications generally should be taken with a full glass of water in order to enhance absorption and prevent dehydration.

Anorexia of Aging

Poor food intake can lead to **anorexia of aging**. When older people become ill, anorexia puts them at high risk for developing protein-energy malnutrition. Protein-energy malnutrition, in turn, can contribute to immune deficiencies, anemia, falls, cognitive deficits, osteopenia (decreased bone mass), altered drug metabolism, **sarcopenia** (excessive loss of muscle mass), and prolonged hospital stays.[24] Researchers also link weight loss among elders with increased mortality.[25]

Sarcopenia frequently is accompanied by a decline in immune function, which puts elders at risk for secondary infections during periods of acute and chronic illness. In addition, failure to thrive syndrome (FTT) often is thought to accompany sarcopenia, either as a cause or result of lean tissue loss.[26] With these problems comes an increase in frailty, loss of independence, reduced food intake, and poor prognosis in the presence of chronic or acute illness.

It can be difficult to pinpoint treatment strategies for anorexia in older people. However, treating even one aspect of the problem can provide at least temporary improvement. Ideally, wasting syndromes should be prevented and a regular regimen of exercise, both aerobic and strength training, can slow the progression of muscle wasting in elders. Exercise has the additional benefit of increasing appetite and, therefore, the amount of food eaten. Nutritional supplementation can decrease the incidence of protein-energy malnutrition and decrease morbidity and mortality of hospitalized patients.[27] Unfortunately, lifelong inappropriate food habits, social factors, living conditions, and fear of injury may interfere with a person's ability and desire to stay or become healthy.

Key Concepts: *Use of medications and lack of appetite are more common among older people. Medicines have the potential to interact with food and nutrients in the diet, and a lack of knowledge of these possibilities increases the risk for harmful effects. Lack of appetite and associated reduction in food intake can contribute to wasting syndromes.*

Arthritis

Arthritis is a general term that describes more than 100 diseases that cause pain and swelling of joints and connective tissue. (See **Figure 16.11**.) Nearly 43 million Americans have arthritis, making it one of the most prevalent chronic health problems in the United States. The three most common forms of arthritis are osteoarthritis, fibromyalgia, and rheumatoid arthritis. Of the three, osteoarthritis is the most common, affecting some 20.7 million people, most of them older than 45 years.[28] Gout is another form of arthritis that may affect older people; this complaint usually involves the big toe and other small joints.

Arthritis is a chronic, lifelong affliction that, at its worst, can make movement difficult or even impossible. Unfortunately, there is no proven cure for arthritis. At best, appropriate treatment programs reduce symptoms.

anorexia of aging The loss of appetite and wasting associated with old age.

sarcopenia A syndrome of aging that includes a loss of lean body tissue, and often accompanied by decreased immune function.

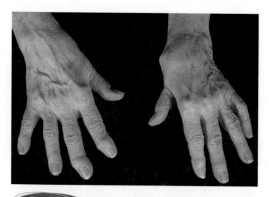

Figure 16.11 Degeneration of the finger joints causes mild to extreme lack of function.

Arthritis pain may impair appetite or make it hard to prepare meals, and some arthritis medications may interfere with nutrient absorption. These factors underscore the importance of a nutrient-dense diet for arthritis sufferers.

Weight management is important in treating arthritis. Excess weight puts undue pressure on the hips and knees. Weight loss in overweight and obese individuals may reduce the risk of developing osteoarthritis, particularly of the knee.[29]

People who have rheumatoid arthritis may benefit from adding foods that are high in unsaturated fatty acids, particularly the omega-3 fatty acids in flaxseed and cold-water fish. There is some evidence that these fatty acids may have beneficial effects on the immune system of people with rheumatoid arthritis, thus lessening the discomfort of the disease.[30]

Among the many kinds of arthritis, gout stands out because of the intensity of its pain. The classic attack occurs in someone who goes to bed feeling well and then awakens in the middle of the night with excruciating pain that has been likened to having someone walk on your eyeballs. This often leads to a visit to the emergency room.

Gout is directly linked to hyperuricemia, an excess of uric acid in the blood. Uric acid, a natural breakdown product of the purines (organic compounds) found in all foods and body tissues, is normally dissolved in blood. But excess uric acid can precipitate as microscopic crystals in hand or foot joints, where it leads to painful inflammation, or gouty arthritis. Age-related degenerative osteoarthritis, particularly in the big toe, also enhances the risk of gout.

Certain medications, drinking alcohol, overeating, and an unusual increase in exercise can trigger an attack of gout, but it often strikes without warning. After the attack passes, medications can help control uric acid levels. To reduce the risk of future attacks, overweight people should gradually lose weight, cut down on alcohol, and reduce their consumption of foods high in purines, such as organ meats, red meat, shellfish, and beans.

Bowel and Bladder Regulation

As a result of physiological changes and lifestyle, older people are susceptible to problems with their bowels and bladder. Hospitalized or institutionalized elderly patients who require catheters for urine excretion run an increased risk of **urinary tract infection (UTI)**, both during and after the procedure. Poor hygiene by free-living elders, particularly women, also may increase the frequency of UTIs.

Cranberry juice has been a popular home remedy for UTIs since at least 1914. Contrary to popular belief, its effect cannot be attributed to an increase in the acidity of the urinary tract. Rather, cranberry juice contains a protein that may prevent bacteria from attaching to the inner lining of the bladder.[31]

Urinary incontinence becomes more common as the muscle walls of the bladder weaken; in attempts to control urinary incontinence, some people severely restrict fluids, resulting in inadequate fluid intake. People with disorders of fluid metabolism and congestive heart failure also may refuse fluids in an attempt to prevent or reduce edema (swelling).

Inadequate hydration not only affects the bladder, but also increases the likelihood of constipation. Age-related decreases in intestinal motility and transit time, accompanied by poor food intake, may exacerbate the problem. In addition, lack of physical activity contributes to loss of muscle tone

urinary tract infection (UTI) An infection of one or more of the structures in the urinary tract, usually caused by bacteria.

needed for elimination. Diseases such as diabetes and Parkinson's disease, and the use of medications for heart disease, anemia, and depression may cause changes in bowel habits as well.

Chronic constipation is one of the most common health complaints among elders. If they do not have at least one bowel movement per day, many elders wrongly consider themselves constipated and quickly self-prescribe laxatives. Laxative use and abuse is common, with approximately $725 million spent on laxatives in the United States each year.[32] Excessive use of laxatives may cause nutritional deficiencies by decreasing transit time and preventing adequate absorption of nutrients. Decreased transit time also reduces water reabsorption by the GI tract and contributes to dehydration.

For some elders, the problem is diarrhea rather than constipation. Although laxative abuse and prescription medications that stimulate the intestinal tract can cause diarrhea, foodborne bacteria are the most common culprits. Food-related illness can exacerbate urinary tract and yeast infections, hypotension (low blood pressure), and dehydration, leading to more serious illness and hospitalization.

Increasing dietary fiber and fluid is one of the most effective treatments for bowel and bladder problems. Elders should gradually switch to—and then maintain—a high-fiber diet. They also should be careful to maintain adequate fluid intake.

Key Concepts: *Arthritis and changes in bowel and bladder habits are common problems in elders. Weight management is an important component of arthritis treatment. With the increased risk of dehydration and constipation among elders, they should be encouraged to follow a high-fiber diet and consume plenty of fluids.*

Dental Health

The mouth is the gateway to the rest of the gastrointestinal system. Poor oral health impairs the ability to eat and obtain adequate nutrition. Missing teeth or poorly fitting dentures make some elders self-conscious about eating, which leaves them unable to eat comfortably in public. Mouth pain and difficulty swallowing interfere with the process of eating, and tooth loss can alter choices and quality of food. Oral infections affect the whole body, and may increase the risk of other chronic diseases, including heart disease. Information regarding changes in oral health and their impact on some body processes was discussed earlier in this chapter.

To identify problems in oral health, dentists and other health-care practitioners use a checklist adapted from the Nutrition Screening Initiative checklist. The questions target the most common factors that place people at risk for nutrition problems.[33] (See **Figure 16.12.**)

Vision Problems

An estimated 1.6 million people in the United States are disabled by blindness and vision problems.[34] Poor vision and blindness interfere with the ability to procure and prepare food; visually impaired people cannot read food labels, cookbooks, or the settings on stoves or microwave ovens.

Macular degeneration is a common disease of the eye that gradually leads to loss of vision. It affects about 6 percent of people between the ages of 65 and 74, and about 20 percent of those aged 75 to 85. Research has found that people with a higher intake of green, leafy vegetables are less likely to develop this sight-robbing disorder. Foods that contain antioxidants, including carotenoids but not vitamin E, are most strongly associated with a

macular degeneration Progressive deterioration of the macula, an area in the center of the retina, that eventually leads to a loss of central vision.

reduced risk. Greens, such as collards and spinach, show the most promise when consumed five or more times a week. By preventing free-radical damage, antioxidants in these foods may protect the eye and the blood vessels that supply it. Retinol supplements do not appear to decrease risk of age-related macular degeneration, and vitamin C from foods had only a marginally beneficial effect on development of the disease.[35]

Determine Your Oral Health

Oral health can affect your nutritional health. A healthy mouth, teeth and gums are needed to eat.

If you answered "yes" to "I have tooth or mouth problems that make it hard for me to eat," on the Determine Your Nutritional Health Checklist, answer the questions below.

Check all that apply

___ Do you have tooth or mouth problems that make it hard for you to eat, such as loose teeth, ill-fitting dentures, etc.

___ Is your mouth dry

___ Do you have problems with:

- ___ lips (soreness or cracks in corners of your mouth)?
- ___ tongue (pain/soreness?
- ___ sores that do not heal?
- ___ bleeding or swollen gums?
- ___ toothaches or sensitivity to hot or cold?
- ___ pain or clicking in your jaw?

Have you visited a dentist:

- ___ within the past 12 months
- ___ in the last 2 years
- ___ never been to a dentist

If you have visited a dentist, was the main reason for your visit:

- ___ regular checkup
- ___ to have a denture made
- ___ to have teeth cleaned
- ___ bleeding or sore gums
- ___ to have a tooth filled
- ___ loose teeth/loose tooth
- ___ to have a tooth pulled or other surgery
- ___ oral or facial pain
- ___ to have a root canal
- ___ adjustments or repair of denture
- ___ other

Discuss with your care provider what can be done to correct the problems you have indicated. Also bring this checklist to your dentist the next time you visit. Remember that warning signs suggest risk, but do not represent diagnosis of any condition.

Figure 16.12 **"Determine Your Oral Health" checklist.** **Source:** Adapted from Nutrition Screening Initiative; *Incorporating Nutrition Screening and Interventions into Medical Practice: A Monograph for Physicians.* The American Academy of Family Physicians, the American Dietetic Association and the National Council on the Aging, Inc. Funded in part by a grant from Ross Products Division, Abbott Laboratories, 1994; with permission.

Quick Bites

Why Elephants Don't Need Dentures

Elephants are the only mammals with a built-in tooth replacement system. As they age, elephants go through six sets of teeth, changing about every 10 years. When elephants are around 70 years old, about the maximum life span, the last set of molars wears out.

estrogen replacement therapy (ERT) Use of hormonal preparations containing estrogen (and sometimes progestins) before, during, and after menopause to reduce menopausal symptoms, slow bone loss, and lower the risk for heart disease.

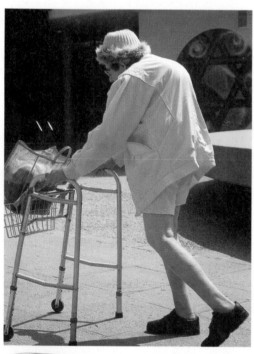

Figure 16.13 A hunched back due to collapsed vertebrae is a visible symptom of osteoporosis.

Osteoporosis

Although osteoporosis affects older adults of both sexes, it is most common in postmenopausal women. Osteoporosis is the deterioration of bone structure (**Figure 16.13**), until often without warning, the fragile bone breaks upon the slightest impact. Such fractures often precipitate a need for long-term care and in 12 to 20 percent of cases, death occurs within 1 year of the fracture.[36]

Genetic as well as environmental conditions affect bone mass. Nutritional factors, particularly early in life, are thought to play an important role in the development of osteoporosis. The two nutrients that most affect bone, vitamin D and calcium, are discussed elsewhere in this chapter. (See Chapter 11, "Water and Major Minerals," for more on osteoporosis including risk factors.)

Estrogen replacement therapy (ERT) can help prevent and treat bone loss in postmenopausal women. It can also reduce menopausal symptoms and the risk of cardiovascular disease in older women. Although epidemiological studies suggest that low-dose estrogen decreases frequency of fractures, estrogen therapy is not without risks. It may increase the risk of certain types of cancer, particularly breast cancer.

Estrogen, bisphosphonates (medications such as etidronate or alendronate), and newer drugs like raloxifene are the most common drug therapies for osteoporosis. These drugs, alone or in combination, help maintain bone mass and can be effective in women up to 20 years past menopause.

While regular weight-bearing exercise helps prevent osteoporosis, inactivity increases osteoporosis risk. Lack of physical activity for long periods of time, such as may be imposed by complete bed rest or illnesses that limit mobility, can promote the disease.

Although prevention is the best treatment for osteoporosis, many people enter later life with poor dietary and physical activity patterns that put them at risk. Adopting a diet that is rich in calcium and vitamin D, along with engaging in regular physical activity, particularly weight-bearing exercises, minimizes osteoporosis risks.

Key Concepts: *Oral health, vision, and bone health all decline with aging. Tooth loss and oral pain can reduce food intake and nutrient quality. Loss of vision can make food shopping and preparation difficult. Osteoporosis, most common in postmenopausal women, can cause debilitating fractures. Management of these conditions depends first on their identification by health-care professionals.*

Meal Management for Mature Adults

Many elders are at nutritional risk because of economics, social isolation, physical restrictions, inability to shop for or prepare food, and medical conditions. Fortunately, there are a number of ways that older people can remain independent and have access to an adequate diet.

Managing Independently

Independent and assisted-living programs allow people to live relatively carefree yet independent lives. Senior-citizen apartment buildings and retirement villages offer a variety of services, including balanced meals. Programs like **Meals on Wheels** and the Elderly Nutrition Program (ENP) provide meals to homebound people, as well as those in congregate (group) settings. Most programs provide meals at least five times per week.

The ENP is supported primarily with federal funds; volunteer time, in-kind donations, and participant contributions make up the remainder.

People without the means to purchase food may be eligible for hot meals at community "food kitchens." These are similar to congregate meal sites, but serve a broader population. Although these programs are free, most require determination of eligibility. Some food kitchens and emergency food banks also offer groceries or vouchers to purchase food. The Food Stamp program is another option that provides low-income elderly households with the means to purchase food. Unfortunately, because Food Stamps carry a "welfare" stigma, some elders are reluctant to use them. In addition, many people who need some help buying food cannot meet the eligibility requirements.

Although they can live independently, 77 percent of the participants in the ENP are unable to perform or have much difficulty in one or more **Activities of Daily Living (ADLs)** or **Instrumental Activities of Daily Living (IADLs)** without the assistance of another person or the use of physical devices.[37] Home health services can help these people avoid institutionalization due to illness or recurrence of a previous illness. Homemaker services provide assistance with meal preparation, transportation, bathing, and shopping. As the number of elders in our society increases, the number and variety of services are likely to increase.

Wise Eating for One or Two

Preparing meals that are healthful and tasty is a challenge for those living alone, or in small households. As discussed earlier in this chapter, our nutrition needs—with the exception of calories—do not decrease as we age, but our ability to meet these needs does. Reliance on convenience foods, fast foods, and eating out can adversely affect the nutritional status of older persons. Males who live alone are especially likely to eat out or skip meals rather than prepare foods for themselves. For both men and women, physical disability or illness can quash the desire to prepare meals and eat.

Some simple changes in appliances and food-preparation techniques can help elders overcome common obstacles to food preparation. Those who can't or won't cook can use microwave or toaster ovens and small appliances to prepare simple meals. A meal based on a lower-sodium, low-fat convenience entree can meet nutritional needs if accompanied by vegetables, whole-grain bread, milk, and fruit.

Adaptive equipment helps people with physical disabilities. Older people can use reaching devices, for example, to get items that otherwise would be out of reach. Special can and jar openers make it easier to open containers and special accessories make it easier to grasp eating and cooking utensils. Another useful product is a dinner plate with a wide, curved lip to keep food on the plate while eating.

Food Safety

Maintaining food safety in the homes of independently living elders can be a challenge. Because of their compromised immune status, and diminished vision and sense of smell, many elders are at risk for foodborne illness. Most foodborne illness is caused by

- improper personal hygiene, particularly after using the toilet,
- improper cooking,
- inappropriate delay in refrigerating hot foods for storage,

Meals on Wheels A voluntary, not-for-profit organization established to provide nutritious meals to homebound people (regardless of age) so they can maintain their independence and quality of life.

Activities of Daily Living (ADLs) Activities one needs to perform daily, including personal grooming, eating, getting in and out of bed, walking, taking a bath or shower, using the toilet, and dressing.

Instrumental Activities of Daily Living (IADLs) Activities necessary to facilitate daily living, including using the telephone, taking medication, managing money, preparing meals, doing housework, and grocery shopping.

holding A common food-service term, usually referring to time between preparation of food and eating.

- cross-contamination of cooked and uncooked foods, and
- improper **holding** of hot and cold foods.

Elders can take precautions to lower their risk of foodborne illness. Precautions include thoroughly washing hands after going to the toilet, and regularly cleaning food-preparation areas with dilute chlorine bleach. To decrease the risk of contamination from pesticides, dirt, and fertilizers, elders should carefully wash all produce. Thorough washing also reduces the potential for contamination by *Salmonella* and other pathogens that have been found on the surface of such produce as watermelon. Finally, cooked foods must be handled properly and cold foods must be stored correctly. All dishes and utensils used to prepare food, including knives and cutting boards, should be washed thoroughly after use to prevent cross-contamination.

Finding Community Resources

An older person's need for community support typically changes from decade to decade. Often, a hospitalization marks a significant change. Hospitals usually help identify an older patient's physiological, psychological, and social needs at the time of discharge, and work with the patient and caregivers to identify community resources. The goal of this discharge planning process is to enhance the patient's quality of life.

For homebound elders who have not been hospitalized recently—as well as for the family members who care for them—identifying community resources can be challenging. Financial considerations may further limit access to resources that can assist older people in their own homes.

The Resource Directory for Older People is a cooperative effort of the National Institute on Aging and the Administration on Aging. This directory provides resources for elders, their caregivers and family members, and those in the legal and health-care professions. It is available via the Internet at http://www.aoa.dhhs.gov/aoa/dir/intro.html. This Web site provides telephone numbers (some toll-free), names, addresses, and fax numbers for organizations that work with older adults.

Another resource is The Eldercare Locator, a public service of the Administration on Aging, U.S. Department of Health and Human Services, administered by the National Association of Area Agencies on Aging and the National Association of State Units on Aging. The Eldercare Locator is a nationwide directory-assistance service that helps older persons and their families identify resources for aging Americans. The Eldercare Locator can be reached toll-free at (800) 677-1116 or on the Internet at http://www.aoa.dhhs.gov/elderpage/locator.html.

Within local communities, Area Agencies on Aging, Social and Rehabilitation Services, Cooperative Extension Services, churches, and extended-care facilities also may have lists of resources and educational programs for elders.

Key Concepts: *Older adults who obtain adequate food and nutrient intake while living independently may require assistance from time to time. This assistance may take the form of help with food shopping or preparation, or identification of community resources that can stretch the food dollar. Because elders are at higher risk for foodborne illness due to weakened immune systems, food safety information is important. Numerous resources exist to assist elders in maintaining a productive, high-quality life.*

Label [to] **Table**

You may have seen advertisements for nutritional supplements like Ensure. At one time, these products were not advertised to the general public, but were used in hospitals and long-term care centers as a meal supplement or the sole source of nutrition for individuals with very poor appetites or with disease conditions that made eating solid food difficult. Now, however, these products are being promoted as a convenient, nutritious addition to the diets of healthy elders. Let's look at the Nutrition Facts from a can of Ensure to see what's in it.

This supplement provides about one-quarter of the DV for vitamins and minerals in 250 kilocalories, and that certainly would qualify Ensure as a "nutrient-dense" product. Look at the ingredient list. Although the list is long, most of the names should be familiar to you now. This list shows you that Ensure is more of a formulation than a food.

So, why not just buy Ensure, and drink our diet, instead of bothering with shopping and preparing a variety of foods? First, Ensure may contain all the vitamins and minerals we currently consider essential, but it is far from a complete diet. What's missing? Fiber and phytochemicals aren't present in these types of formulated supplements. Although we don't currently have recommended intake levels for phytochemicals (nor do we know what all of them are!), we do know that diets that include a wide variety of fruits, vegetables, and whole grains are associated with reduced disease risk, not diets that contain the DV of all the vitamins and minerals.

Another reason to choose foods over formulas is the pleasure that we get from eating. Ensure always has the same taste, aroma, texture, and mouthfeel. Our enjoyment of a variety of sensory properties makes eating interesting, and our pleasure in eating continues while we age. While products like Ensure have their place in medically indicated situations, they are no replacement for the pleasure we get from our favorite foods.

Nutrition Facts

Serv. Size 1 can (8 fl oz)
Calories 250
Calories from Fat 50

	% Daily Value*		% Daily Value*
Total Fat 6g	9%	**Total Carb.** 40g	13%
Saturated Fat 0.5 g	3%	Dietary Fiber <1g	4%
Cholest. <5mg	<2%	Sugars 18g	
Sodium 200 mg	8%	**Protein** 9g	18%
Potassium 410 mg	12%		

Vitamin A 25% • Vitamin C 50% • Calcium 30% • Iron 25% • Vitamin D 25%
Vitamin E 25% • Vitamin K 25% • Thiamin 25% • Riboflavin 25%
Niacin 25% • Vitamin B$_6$ 25% • Folate 25% • Vitamin B$_{12}$ 25% • Biotin 25%
Pantothenic Acid 25% • Phosphorus 30% • Iodine 25% • Magnesium 25%
Zinc 25% • Selenium 25% • Copper 25% • Manganese 60% • Chromium 25%
Molybdenum 50% • Chloride 10%

*Percent Daily Values based on a 2000 calorie diet

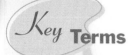

LEARNING *Portfolio* c h a p t e r 1 6

Key Terms

Study Points

➤ Nutrition and physical activity are two important, controllable components of a healthy life and healthful aging. Moreover, numerous physiological and psychological aspects of the aging process affect food intake and nutritional status.

➤ Lean body mass normally declines with age while body fat increases. Our senses of taste and smell also decline, making enhancements to flavors and odors important.

➤ Reduction in GI secretions affects swallowing, digestion, and absorption, and reduction in intestinal motility leads to constipation. In addition, functional changes occur in all organs of the body, including the heart, liver, and kidneys.

➤ Loss of appetite due to stress, depression, and/or medications is common. Debilitating illnesses such as Alzheimer's disease can interfere with normal food intake and affect nutrient needs.

➤ National surveys show that elders tend to consume fewer calories, more fat, and less calcium than is recommended. While widespread nutrient deficiencies are not apparent, marginal vitamin and mineral status may be common.

➤ Energy needs decline with age, reflecting loss of lean body mass and reduced physical activity. The protein RDA, and the recommended balance of carbohydrate and fat calories in the diet are similar for young and older adults. Fluid intake needs special attention due to the reduced thirst response that occurs with age.

➤ Because of reduced intake, synthesis, and activation, vitamin D status declines with age; recommended intake levels are therefore raised. Vitamin B_{12} status may be compromised due to inadequate absorption.

➤ Calcium and zinc intakes are likely to be marginal in the diets of elders. Magnesium and iron remain important.

➤ Dietary supplements, both vitamin/mineral and herbal/botanical, should be used with caution, preferably with professional advice.

➤ The Nutrition Screening Initiative developed tools for the identification of factors that can lead to nutritional risk.

➤ Because many elders take multiple medications, they are at risk for drug-nutrient, food-drug, and drug-drug interactions. Anorexia of aging is also a major public health problem.

➤ Arthritis is a prevalent chronic health problem in this age group. Weight management is a key element of arthritis treatment.

➤ Chronic constipation is a common complaint among older adults. Fluids, fiber, and regular exercise can reduce the likelihood of constipation.

➤ Both poor oral and visual health can compromise the ability of elders to consume a nutritionally adequate diet.

➤ Osteoporosis is a major health problem that can be addressed through adequate calcium, vitamin D, regular weight-bearing exercise, and medication if needed.

➤ Food safety is an important issue for older adults. Most foodborne illnesses are caused by factors such as improper personal hygiene and cooking habits.

➤ Maintaining independence while aging may require special assistance with food procurement and preparation. Community resources exist to respond to these needs of elders and those of their caretakers and family.

Study Questions

1. List 10 common physiological changes associated with aging.

2. What are some of the consequences of decreased immunity among elders?

3. Based on recent studies, which nutrients are most likely to be low in the diets of older Americans?

4. How does the fact that most older people have less lean mass affect their need for protein? Compared to a younger adult, does a person older than 65 need more, less, or about the same amount of protein?

5. Why are elders at risk for vitamin D deficiency?

6. Discuss minerals that may need special attention in assessment of an elder's nutritional status.

7. What problems might elders encounter with dietary supplements?

8. What do the letters *NSI* stand for and what are its goals? How does NSI approach these goals?

9. What are some of the foods that may help prevent macular degeneration?

10. What is the role of estrogen in osteoporosis prevention? What other factors are important?

11. List some of the meal/food programs that are available to assist older persons.

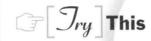 **This**

Aging Simulation

The purpose of this exercise is to simulate what it can be like to age and experience age-related declines in health. Have you ever thought of how difficult it is to be an older person with health problems and do routine activities? Invite a few friends over and do the following:
  * Put gloves on to simulate the difficulty of losing sensitivity in your hands.
  * Use cotton balls in your ears to decrease your hearing ability.
  * Apply some petroleum jelly to a pair of glasses or sunglasses to give yourself poor vision.

Now try a simple activity. Make a salad or put a CD in your CD player and listen to it. After completing the activity, switch disabilities with your friends so that everyone has experienced each of the limitations. What is it like to do these everyday activities with your impairment?

Volunteering at a Community Agency for Elders

The purpose of this exercise is to learn about the local programs to help elders. Look in a phone book to see how many agencies offer services in your community for older adults. Inquire about volunteering some time with any of these agencies to gain experience working with elders. Perhaps you can assist with delivering food or can help with a congregate meal program.

What About Bobbie?

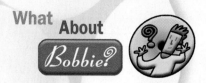

Let's pretend that Bobbie is in her 60s and just read a newspaper article about how older people may have low intakes of vitamins E and B$_6$, magnesium, calcium, and iron. How do you think her diet compares to the needs of a 65-year-old woman? You may want to review her one-day intake in Chapter 1. Although her calorie intake is probably much higher than that of most women in their 60s, let's look at her intake of these vitamins and minerals.

Bobbie met or exceeded her RDA or AI for each nutrient except vitamin E and calcium. This low value for vitamin E probably reflects a lack of complete data for the vitamin E content of foods since Bobbie's fat intake was ample. True of many women in their 60s who don't have an adequate intake of calcium, this increases Bobbie's risk of osteoporosis.

Vitamin E
RDA	15 mg
Bobbie's intake	9 mg

Vitamin B$_6$
RDA	1.5 mg
Bobbie's intake	1.9 mg

Magnesium
RDA	320 mg
Bobbie's intake	330 mg

Calcium
AI	1,200 mg
Bobbie's intake	745 mg

Zinc
RDA	8 mg
Bobbie's intake	14 mg

References

1 Older Americans 2000: Key indicators of well-being. Federal Interagency Forum on Aging-Related Statistics. http://www.agingstats.gov/chartbook2000/population.html. Accessed 9/8/00.

2 Harris TB, Savage PJ, Grethe ST, et al. Carrying the burden of cardiovascular risk in old age: association of weight and weight change with prevalent cardiovascular disease, risk factors, and health statistics in the Cardiovascular Health Study. *Am J Clin Nutr.* 1997;66:837–844.

3 Stevens J, Cai J, Pamuk ER, et al. The effect of age on the association between body-mass index and mortality. *N Engl J Med.* 1998;338:1–7.

4 Weindruch R, Sohal RS. Caloric intake and aging. *N Engl J Med.* 1997;337:986–994.

5 Lesourd BM. Nutrition and immunity in the elderly: modification of immune responses with nutritional treatments. *Am J Clin Nutr.* 1997;66(suppl):478S–484S.

6 Worthington-Roberts BS, Williams SR. *Nutrition Throughout the Life Cycle.* 3rd ed. St. Louis, MO: Mosby-Year Book; 1996.

7 Schiffman SS, Warwick ZS. Effect of flavor enhancement on nutritional status: food intake, biochemical indices, and anthropometric measures. *Phys Behav.* 1993;53:395–402; and Schiffman SS. Intensification of sensory properties of foods for the elderly. *J Nutr.* April 2000;130(suppl):927S–930S.

8 Worthington-Roberts BS, Williams SR. Op. cit.

9 McEwen BS. Stress and the aging hippocampus. *Front Neuroendocrinol.* 1999;20:49–70.

10 Cyr M, Calon F, Morissette M, et al. Drugs with estrogen-like potency and brain activity: potential therapeutic application for the CNS. *Curr Pharm Des.* 2000;6:1287–1312; and Prasad KN, Hovland AR, Cole WC, et al. Multiple antioxidants in the prevention and treatment of Alzheimer disease: analysis of biologic rationale. *Clin Neuropharmacol.* 2000: 23:2–13.

11 Marwick C. NHANES III: Health data relevant for aging nation. *JAMA.* 1997;277:100–102; and Alaimo K, McDowell MA, Briefel RR, et al. *Dietary Intake of Vitamins, Minerals, and Fiber of Persons Age 2 Months and Over in the United States: Third National Health and Nutrition Examination Survey, Phase 1, 1988–91.* Advance Data from Vital and Health Statistics, No. 258. Hyattsville, MD: National Center for Health Statistics; 1994.

12 Serving Elders at Risk: The Older Americans Act Nutrition Programs—National Evaluation of the Elderly Nutrition Program, 1993–1995. Volume I: Evaluation Findings. http://www.aoa.dhhs.gov/aoa/nutreval/fulltext/textpage.html. Accessed 9/9/00.

13 Institute of Medicine. Food and Nutrition Board. *Dietary Reference Intakes for Calcium, Phosphorus, Magnesium, Vitamin D, and Fluoride.* Washington, DC: National Academy Press; 1999.

14 Blumberg J. Nutritional needs of seniors. *J Am Coll Nutr.* 1997;16:517–523.

15 US Department of Health and Human Services: FDA Announces Name Changes for Lower-Fat Milks and Folic Acid Fortification for Bakery Products. *HHS News;* December 31, 1997.

16 Stabler SP, Lindenbaum J, Allen RH. Vitamin B$_{12}$ deficiency in the elderly: current dilemmas. *Am J Clin Nutr.* 1997;66:741–749.

17 Carmel R. Cobalamin, the stomach, and aging. *Am J Clin Nutr.* 1997;66:750–759.

18 Institute of Medicine. Food and Nutrition Board. *Dietary Reference Intakes for Thiamin, Riboflavin, Niacin, Vitamin B$_6$, Folate, Vitamin B$_{12}$, Pantothenic Acid, Biotin, and Choline.* Washington, DC: National Academy Press; 2000.

19 Ibid.

20 Blumberg J. Op. cit.

21 Institute of Medicine. *Dietary Reference Intakes for Calcium, Phosphorus, Magnesium.* Op. cit.

22 Blumberg J. Op. cit.

23 Liao F, Folsom AR, Brancati FL. Is low magnesium concentration a risk factor for coronary heart disease? The Atheroclerosis Risk in Communities (ARIC) study. *Am Heart J.* 1998;136:480–490.

24 Morley JE. Anorexia of aging: physiologic and pathologic. *Am J Clin Nutr.* Oct 1997; 66:760–773.

25 Diehr P, Bild DE, Harris TB, et al. Body mass index and mortality in nonsmoking older adults: the Cardiovascular Health Study. *Am J Public Health.* Apr 1998; 88:623–629.

26 Roubenoff MD, Harris TB. Failure to thrive, sarcopenia, and functional decline in the elderly. *Clin Geriatric Med.* 1997;13:613–622.

27 Morley JE. Op. cit.

28 Osteoarthritis (OA). Arthritis Foundation. http://www.arthritis.org/answers/diseasecenter/oa.asp. Accessed 9/9/00.

29 Ibid.

30 James MJ, Cleland LG. Dietary n-3 fatty acids and therapy for rheumatoid arthritis. *Semin Arthritis Rheum.* 1997;27:84–97.

31 Monane M, Avorn J. Cranberry juice and urinary tract infections. *Healthline;* August 1994.

32 National Digestive Diseases Information Clearinghouse, National Institute of Diabetes and Digestive and Kidney Diseases. Constipation. NIH publication 95-2754; July 1995. http://www.niddk.nih.gov/health/digest/pubs/const/const.htm. Accessed 9/9/00.

33 Erickson L. Oral health promotion and prevention for older adults. *Dental Clin N Am.* 1997;41:727–750.

34 Macular Degeneration Foundation. All about MD. http://www.eyesight.org/All_About_MD/all_about_md.html. Accessed 9/9/00.

35 Diets high in carotenoids may lower risk of macular degeneration. Reprinted from *Med Sci Bull.* Feb 1995. Pharmaceutical Associates Limited. http://www.eyesight.org/All_About_MD/Reports_Index/Report-Carotenoids/report-carotenoids.html. Accessed 9/9/00.

36 Lyles, KW Osteoporosis: Pathophysiology, clinical presentation and management. In: Kelly WN, ed. *Textbook of Internal Medicine.* 3rd ed. Philadelphia: Lippincott-Raven; 1997.

37 Serving Elders at Risk. Op. cit.

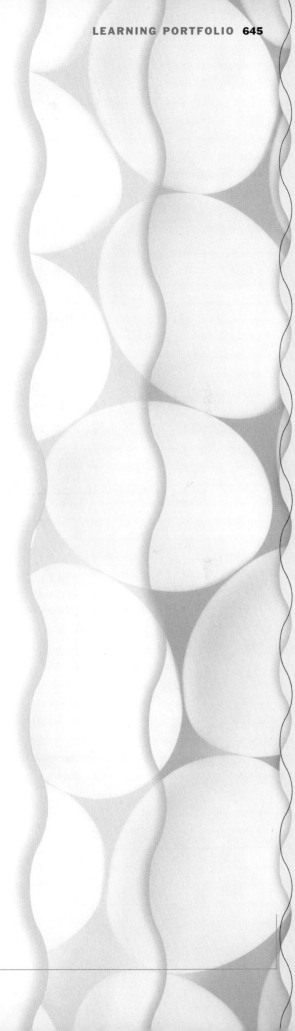

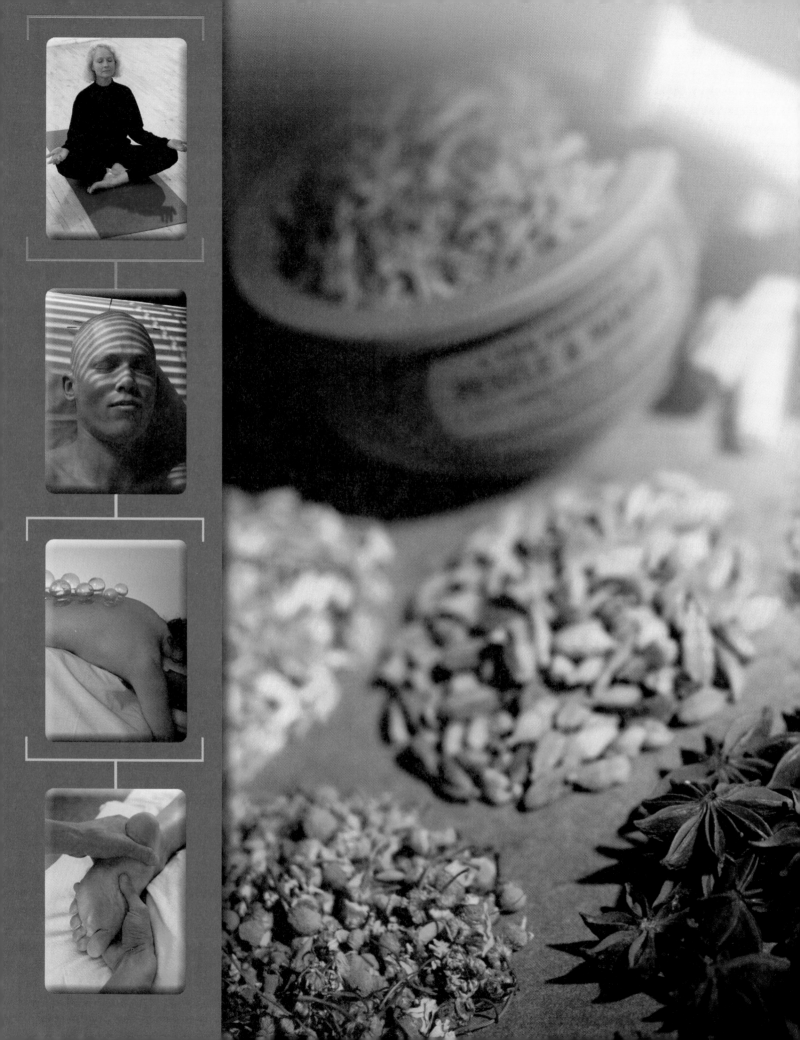

Spotlight on

Complementary and Alternative Nutrition

Think About It

1 Have you ever been the victim of quackery?

2 What are your feelings about the safety of megadose nutrient supplements?

3 Would you tell your physician if you were taking an herbal supplement?

4 If a friend told you about a new licorice extract that is guaranteed to tone muscles, would you try it?

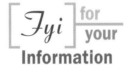

Fyi for your Information

This chapter's FYI boxes include practical information on the following topics:
• Do You Need a Vitamin E Supplement?

• Talking with Your Doctor

The web site for this book offers many useful tools and is a great source for additional nutrition information for both students and instructors. Visit the site at **nutrition.jbpub.com** for information on complementary and alternative nutrition. You'll find exercises that explore the following topics:

• The ADA's Dietetics Practice Groups

• The ADA and Diets versus Supplements

• Complementary and Alternative Therapies

• The Office of Dietary Supplements

*M*arcie visits a chiropractor twice a month for relief of chronic back pain. Seema takes the herbal St. John's wort, hoping it will pull her out of the doldrums. Emil swears by the use of creatine in his muscle-building regime. Jason is into orthomolecular medicine, taking megadoses of many vitamins and minerals to ward off cancer and heart disease. Others in search of better health turn to massage therapy, magnets, macrobiotic diets, homeopathy, acupuncture, and many other practices.

The use of therapies such as these is growing rapidly. More frequently than ever, people are seeking treatments and preventive measures outside the medical mainstream, and spending millions of dollars each year for services and supplements. Why? What factors are driving the interest in alternative therapies? Some say it's dissatisfaction with prevailing health-care practices and costs. Others point to philosophical and spiritual reasons. Still others note that scientific investigation is beginning to support many therapies that were once dismissed as quackery.

This chapter examines **complementary and alternative medicine (CAM)**, and the role of nutrition, including the growing use of dietary supplements. We discuss CAM from the perspective of current claims and knowledge, along with regulatory and safety issues, and do not attempt to include all known therapies. Making decisions about nutrition and health requires consumers and professionals alike to stay informed and consult reliable sources before embarking on a new health regime.

complementary and alternative medicine (CAM) A broad range of healing philosophies, approaches, and therapies that include treatments and health-care practices not taught widely in medical schools, not generally used in hospitals, and not usually reimbursed by medical insurance companies.

phytotherapy The therapeutic use of herbs and other plants to promote health and treat disease.

orthomolecular medicine The preventive or therapeutic use of high-dose vitamins to treat disease.

Complementary and Alternative Medicine

Complementary and alternative medicines are therapies and treatments outside the medical mainstream. They tend to be based mainly or solely on observation or anecdotal evidence rather than controlled research. One widely used definition is "treatments or health-care practices neither taught widely in U.S. medical schools nor generally available in U.S. hospitals."[1] This definition, however, may need updating; many medical schools and conventional health-care providers have begun to teach or integrate these therapies, sometimes with insurance reimbursement.[2]

The term *alternative* suggests practices that *replace* conventional ones. *Complementary* implies practices that are used *in addition* to conventional ones. For example, using only herbs and megavitamins to treat AIDS would be "alternative," whereas using herbs to combat diarrhea caused by conventional AIDS medications, and taking supplements to replace lost vitamins, would be "complementary." Many people find the terms *complementary* or *integrative* more acceptable than *alternative*, although all these terms often are used interchangeably. CAM includes a broad range of healing therapies and philosophies. Several among them involve nutrition, including special diet therapies, **phytotherapy** (herbalism), **orthomolecular medicine** (nutrient megadoses), and other biologic interventions (see **Table SAN.1**).

Popularity of Complementary and Alternative Medicine

In 1990 about 34 percent of the adult U.S. population used CAM;[3] by 1997 that number had grown to 42 percent.[4] As **Table SAN.2** shows, the increases

Table SAN.1 Kaleidoscope of Complementary Therapies

CAM includes a broad range of disparate healing therapies and philosophies. The Office of Alternative Medicine (OAM) in the U.S. National Institutes of Health (NIH) has attempted to categorize these.

Field of Practice	Description	Examples
Alternative Systems of Medical Practice	Health care ranging from self-care according to folk practices, to care rendered in an organized health-care system based on alternative traditions or practices.	Acupuncture Homeopathic and naturopathic medicine Shamanism
Bioelectromagnetic Applications	The unconventional use of electromagnetic fields, such as pulsed fields, magnetic fields, or alternating current or direct current fields, to treat diseases (e.g., asthma, cancer) or manage pain (e.g., migraine headaches).	Blue light treatment Electromagnetic fields
Diet, Nutrition, Lifestyle	Dietary or nutritional intervention to prevent illness, maintain health, and reverse the effects of chronic disease.	Changes in lifestyle and diet Macrobiotics Megavitamins
Herbal Medicines	Pharmacological use of plant and plant products according to some traditional folk medicines. .	Echinacea Ginkgo biloba St. John's wort
Manual Healing	Use of touch and manipulation with the hands as a diagnostic and therapeutic tool.	Chiropractic medicine Massage therapy
Mind-Body Control	Using the mind's capacity to affect the body; based on traditional medical systems that make use of the interconnectedness of mind and body.	Biofeedback Meditation Yoga
Pharmacological and Biological Treatments	Drugs and vaccines not yet accepted by mainstream medicine.	Chelation therapy Metabolic therapy

Source: Adapted from Barrocas A. Complementary and alternative medicine: Friend, foe, or OWA? *J Am Diet Assoc.* 1997;97:1373-1376.

 Table SAN.2 Use of Alternative Medicine, 1990 and 1997

Use of alternative medical practices is growing. Numbers reflect the percent of those surveyed who had used each method.

Type of Therapy	1990	1997	Type of Therapy	1990	1997
Relaxation techniques[a]	13.1%	16.3%	Commercial diet[d]	3.9%	4.4%
Herbal medicine	2.5	12.1	Folk remedies	0.2	4.2
Massage	6.9	11.1	Lifestyle diet[e]	3.6	4.0
Chiropractic	10.1	11.0	Energy healing[f]	1.3	3.8
Spiritual healing by others[b]	4.2	7.0	Homeopathy	0.7	3.4
Megavitamins[c]	2.4	5.5	Hypnosis	0.9	1.2
Self-help groups	2.3	4.8	Biofeedback	1.0	1.0
Imagery	4.2	4.5	Acupuncture	0.4	1.0

a. Relaxation techniques include meditation and the relaxation response.
b. Prayer or spiritual healing by others is separate from prayer or spiritual practice by the individual surveyed.
c. Megavitamins are distinct from daily vitamins or vitamins prescribed by a doctor.
d. Commercial diet programs are "the kind you have to pay for, but not including trying to lose or gain weight on your own."
e. Lifestyle diet includes practices like vegetarianism and macrobiotics.
f. Energy healing includes use of magnets, energy-emitting machines, and the "laying on of hands."

Source: Adapted from Eisenberg DM, Davis RB, Ettner SL, et al. Trends in alternative medicine use in the United States, 1990–1997: results of a follow-up national survey. *JAMA.* 1998;280:1569–1575.

were significant for relaxation techniques, herbal medicine, massage, spiritual healing, megavitamins, self-help groups, folk remedies, energy healing, homeopathy, and acupuncture. The most popular therapies in 1997 were relaxation techniques, herbal medicine, massage, and chiropractic. People seek out CAM for numerous reasons including fear of aging, personal beliefs, and distrust of institutional medicine.

Demographics

Ours is an aging population, one with a focus on health, well-being, and quality of life. There is great interest in the ways diet can help us feel better, stay well, even live longer. But some expectations are unrealistic. From sexual, intellectual, or athletic prowess to freedom from wrinkles and age spots, promotions portray a dream, then sell products that promise to attain it. Baby boomers would rather focus on health than disease and often are more interested in adding something (e.g., an herbal supplement) than restricting their behavior (e.g., eating less fat).

Many older people have chronic illnesses like arthritis, Alzheimer's disease, Parkinson's disease, and cancer—conditions for which conventional therapies often are unsatisfactory. People who have chronic conditions are more apt to try any alternative that gives them hope for alleviation or cure. Difficult-to-treat conditions have spawned a plethora of alternative treatments and afflicted people are vulnerable to health fraud and quackery. Understandably, people desperate to feel better or regain their health may be willing to try anything.

Mass Media and Ease of Communication

Health sells! Newspaper editors, radio and television broadcasters, and Web site managers understand this. With the need to compete with other media, to fill air time on all-news radio and 24-hour news television, and to win limited attention on-line, there's more health-related news than ever. But when compressed into sound bites or hyped to ensure audience attention, information is easily distorted or misunderstood. Add to the mix infomercials, commercials, and advertisements, and the latest health fact or fad discussed on talk shows. The ubiquitous Internet, with Web sites of variable quality, further complicates the process of obtaining valid information.

Economic Incentives

Consumers expect that alternative medicine will save money by keeping them healthy or, if they do get sick, it will reduce the need for costly conventional treatments. For practitioners, producers, and suppliers, alternative medicine is a burgeoning billion-dollar industry, fueled by loose regulations and expanding sales opportunities. In 1997 consumers spent an estimated $27 billion on alternative therapies, a figure comparable to out-of-pocket expenditures for all U.S. physician services.[5]

Holistic Approaches to Health

Many people choose alternative treatments because these therapies seem more compatible with spiritual and philosophical approaches that view the body in total; they usually subscribe to the belief that the health of body, mind, and spirit are interrelated. Advocates praise CAM for emphasizing wellness and prevention, and for treating the whole person, while they criticize conventional medicine for focusing on one or two diseased body parts. CAM practitioners often spend more time with their patients to uncover and address the emotional, social, and family factors that affect health. However, conventional physicians also take a **holistic**, preventive approach when they counsel patients to eat wisely, exercise routinely, and control stress.

holistic An approach to health care in which the practitioner considers the whole person, including physical, mental, emotional, and spiritual aspects.

Environmental Concerns

Many people perceive alternative medicine as "natural" and "friendly" to the environment. Alternative practitioners, particularly herbalists, have a strong stake in preserving the environment—the source of their therapies—and they often are vocal advocates for conservation. Concerned herbalists worry that the current popularity of herbs such as goldenseal or ginseng will deplete the forests of these plants.[6]

But herbalists are not the only ones worrying about loss of plant habitats. Pharmaceutical companies first isolated many medicines from plants, and they understand the importance of preserving natural environments. Large pharmaceutical firms often support conservation efforts, and help fund studies of indigenous healers, hoping to get ideas for new medicines.

People who follow strict vegetarian diets, and take supplements as well, are sometimes surprised by the number of products that have animal origins. Some examples are chitosan, glucosamine, whey protein, some enzymes, and glandular extracts. Gelcaps that contain supplements are usually gelatin from animal collagen. Some traditional medicines include reptile or insect parts, or other animal tissue.

Use of animal parts in some alternative traditions has been criticized severely for depleting rare species: tigers, rhinoceros, and tortoises. The popularity of shark cartilage supplements raising concerns about the exploitation and depletion of fragile shark populations.[7]

New Government Regulations and Institutions

Historically, idealism and commitment to health characterized alternative medicine, but the field also included shoddy science, quackery, and outright fraud. Recent governmental actions attempt to eliminate these negative elements, and encourage commercial and scientific opportunities. In 1992 the creation of the Office of Alternative Medicine (OAM) within the National Institutes of Health (NIH) legitimized the field and provided a structure for review, evaluation, and research. In 1998 OAM established the National Center for Complementary and Alternative Medicine (NCCAM) to conduct and support research and training. NCCAM maintains an extensive database of published research, available to the public. So far, published results from OAM-funded research have been limited, however.[8]

Where Does Nutrition Fit In?

A number of alternative therapies involve nutrition, and sometimes the line between standard and alternative nutrition is not clear. Nutrition practices can include special diets and vitamin, mineral, and other nutrient supplements. Other types of dietary supplements, including herbals and botanicals, also can be considered part of nutrition. The growing use of supplements requires that all health-care providers, dietitians and nutritionists included, be aware of claims and scientific support for supplements, in addition to their state's professional licensing regulations that deal with advising patients or clients about their use.[9]

Key Concepts: *The term complementary and alternative medicine (CAM) refers to therapies outside the medical mainstream such as herbal medicine, acupuncture, and nutrient megadosing. The growth of CAM is due to many factors including more widespread acceptance, changes in regulations, economics, marketing, demographics, and scientific validation of many therapies.*

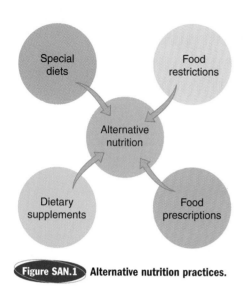

Figure SAN.1 **Alternative nutrition practices.**

macrobiotic diet A highly restrictive dietary approach applied as a therapy for risk factors or chronic disease in general.

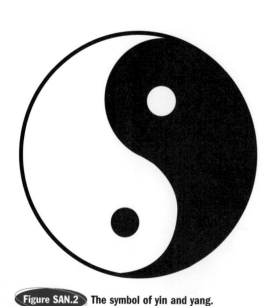

Figure SAN.2 **The symbol of yin and yang.**

Alternative Nutrition

Special dietary regimens are components of conventional treatments for a variety of health conditions such as diabetes, GI disorders, and kidney disease. Alternative nutrition practices include diets to prevent and treat diseases not shown to be diet-related. (See **Figure SAN.1**.) What often makes these practices "alternative" is the limited nature of the diet, the lack of rigorous scientific evidence to support efficacy, and the divergence from established health-promoting eating patterns such as the Food Guide Pyramid. Other practices outside the nutritional mainstream include reliance on only organically grown foods, use of herbal and botanical supplements, and megadoses of vitamin/mineral supplements.

Special Diets, Food Restrictions, and Food Prescriptions

Vegetarian Diets

The specifics of vegetarianism are described in Chapter 6. Most nutritionists consider vegetarianism a routine variation of a normal diet, particularly if the vegetarian's motivation is religious, philosophical, concern for animals, or aversion to animal products. When a meat eater goes vegetarian to prevent or cure disease, that's "alternative."

Macrobiotic Diet

Aside from vegetarianism, the **macrobiotic diet** probably is the best-known alternative diet. As originally proposed, this primarily vegetarian diet progressed in ten increasingly restrictive stages, with the "highest level" consisting of little more than brown rice and water. The diet has since evolved to a simpler one-level regimen based on whole-grain cereals and vegetables, a small amount of fish, no other animal products, and no fruit.[10]

Proponents tout the macrobiotic diet as a cure for a variety of illnesses, most notably cancer. To use it as a cancer treatment, the practitioner individualizes the diet based on Eastern philosophy (yin and yang, whose symbol is shown in **Figure SAN.2**) and location of the cancer. Critics say macrobiotic restrictions interfere with legitimate cancer treatment by causing weight loss in people who are already too thin from their illness. The diet is so limited, it just can't meet the increased nutritional needs of the cancer patient. Advocates of macrobiotics, on the other hand, argue that undernutrition may help fight the cancer by starving it.[11] It looks like neither opinion is correct: macrobiotic diets appear to have no clear effect, good or bad, on cancer progression or survival.

Compared to the general public, macrobiotic adherents tend to have healthier blood lipid levels, and higher blood levels of phytochemicals (plant chemicals), which reflects vegetable intake.[12] However, the diet is low in calcium and vitamin D, which contributes to the risk for osteoporosis. Pediatricians caution against this diet for children.

Gerson Diet

Another diet proposed for cancer treatment is the Gerson Diet. Dr. Gerson developed this dietary strategy in the 1920s to treat tuberculosis, and later modified it for use by advanced cancer patients. The regimen includes potassium and thyroid gland supplements, salt and fat restrictions, periodic protein restrictions, and coffee enemas.[13] After more than 70 years and thousands of patients, there is no clear evidence of its effectiveness, but the Mexican clinic that dispenses Gerson treatments continues to attract desperate cancer victims.

Kelley Regimen

In the 1960s Dr. Kelley, an orthodontist, claimed he successfully treated his own cancer through dietary changes. Pancreatic enzyme supplements play a big role in this regimen. Although basically vegetarian, the Kelley regimen uses coffee enemas and practitioners tailor the diet to a patient's needs, sometimes even including red meat. Although he was convicted of practicing medicine without a license in 1970, Dr. Kelley continued to promote his ideas until the mid-1980s. Dr. Kelley no longer participates in his own program, but the Kelley diet is still used in the United States.[14]

Food Restrictions and Food Prescriptions

Societies throughout the world commonly use dietary changes to treat or prevent illness. The specifics vary from place to place, however, which suggests that they are based on cultural factors rather than science.

In recent years we have seen yeast-free diets, dairy-free diets, sugar-free diets, white-flour-free diets, both low-carbohydrate and high-carbohydrate diets, both low-red-meat and high-red-meat diets, caffeine-free diets, salicylate-free diets, and more. We have been advised to load up on molasses, yogurt, honey, vinegar, oysters, mushrooms, and soy nuts. People with subjective symptoms like headaches, fatigue, or back pain have been instructed to avoid irrational lists of "allergenic foods" based on "blood screening." We've also seen illogical instructions on how to combine foods, such as "don't eat applesauce and asparagus at the same meal." For weight loss, we've had grapefruit diets, hard-boiled-egg diets, cottage-cheese diets, water diets, high-fat diets, low-fat diets, and blue-foods-only diets; the list goes on and on.

Such diets come and go. They are not based on science, and eventually fall out of style when they don't work. Those few that prove effective and have a scientific basis become integrated into conventional nutrition and diet therapy. (See **Figure SAN.3**.)

Key Concepts: *Many types of diet can be described as alternative. Their origins and claims vary, and many have no proof of efficacy. Some alternative diets can actually be harmful by restricting foods and thereby lowering the body's intake of necessary nutrients.*

Dietary Supplements

Dietary supplements come in various forms—vitamins, minerals, amino acids, herbals, glandular extracts, enzymes, and many others. As a result of recent regulatory changes, an avalanche of new products has exploded onto the market, together with claims for everything from enhancing immune function to improving mood. **Table SAN.3** shows many of the popular supplements along with suggested claims and important cautions.

Vitamin and Mineral Supplementation

"Should I take vitamin and mineral supplements?" Apparently a significant number of people already have answered that question for themselves: one-quarter of American adults buy supplements.[15] In our discussion, we consider two levels of supplementation: (1) moderate doses that are in the range of the Daily Values (DV) or levels you might eat in a nutrient-rich diet and (2) megadoses or high levels that are typically multiples of the DVs, and much greater amounts than diet alone could supply.

Quick Bites

The Yin and Yang of Food

The early theory of yin and yang had its genesis during the Yin and Zhou dynasties (16th century-221 B.C.E.). The yin force is passive, downward flowing, and cold. Conversely, the yang force is aggressive, upward raising, and hot. The concept of balance and harmony of these life forces is the basis upon which food and herbs are used as medicine. In traditional Chinese healing methods, disease is viewed as the result of an imbalance of these energies in the body. To balance these energies, your diet should balance yin foods and yang foods, according to this view. Yin (cold) foods include milk, honey, fruit, and vegetables and yang (hot) foods include beef, poultry, seafood, eggs, and cheese. Foods are also classified as sweet (earth), bitter (fire), sour (wood), pungent (metal), and salty (water). Each class supposedly has specific effects on different parts of the body.

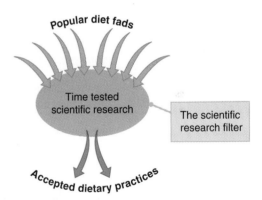

Figure SAN.3 **Many apply but few are chosen.** Dietary practices with a scientific basis and proven efficacy are incorporated into conventional nutrition and diet therapy.

Table SAN.3 **Examples of Dietary Supplements and Their Claims**

Supplement	Claimed Benefits	Current Reaserch Caveats
Beta carotene	Prevents cancer and heart disease and boosts immunity.	Diets rich in beta carotene-containing fruits and vegetables reduce heart disease and cancer risk. Supplements have not been shown to be beneficial. Taking supplements may increase lung cancer risk in smokers.
Chromium picolinate	Builds muscle, prevents and cures diabetes, promotes weight loss.	No solid evidence that chromium picolinate supplements perform as claimed or benefit healthy people. Some evidence that they may harm cells.
Coenzyme Q_{10}	Cure-all; prevents heart disease.	May have value in pre-existing heart disease but benefits for healthy people unproven.
Creatine	Improves athletic performance.	May enhance power and strength for some athletes but meaningless for casual exercisers and distance athletes.
Echinacea	Cures colds, boosts immunity.	Inconsistent evidence of benefit. Products on the market are unstandardized.
Ephedra	Weight control, herbal "high," decongestant.	Ephedrine raises heart rate and blood pressure, and is dangerous for people with diabetes, high blood pressure, heart disease.
Garlic	Lowers blood pressure and blood cholesterol, prevents stomach cancer.	Some evidence that garlic reduces cholesterol.
Ginkgo biloba	Improves blood flow and circulatory disorders, and prevents or cures absent-mindedness, memory loss, dementia	Limited benefits for some Alzheimer's patients. No proven benefit for others. Products on the market are unstandardized.
Ginseng	Improves athletic performance, fights fatigue, cures cancer and heart disease.	No evidence that ginseng has any beneficial effects. Many products on the market contain no ginseng.
Glucosamine & chondroitin sulfate	Halt, reverse, or cure arthritis.	Some evidence of reduced pain, although more studies are needed. Does not reverse arthritis.
Melatonin	Promotes sleep, counters jet lag, improves sex life, etc.	Studies are contradictory relative to sleep/jet lag. No evidence for anti-aging or sex drive claims. No data on long-term safety.
Saw palmetto	May shrink prostate, reduce symptoms of benign prostatic hyperplasia.	May improve urinary tract symptoms. No evidence for prevention of prostate cancer. May affect PSA test and diagnosis of prostate cancer.
St. John's wort	Alleviates depression.	Studies in Europe suggest efficacy for mild depression. Clinical trial underway in U.S. Should not be taken with prescription antidepressants.

Source: Adapted from *The Wellness Guide to Dietary Supplements.* UC Berkeley Wellness Letter. August 1998 and Sarubin A. *The Health Professional's Guide to Popular Dietary Supplements.* Chicago, IL: The American Dietetic Association 2000.

Moderate Supplementation Conventional health-care practitioners often recommend moderate dietary supplementation for people with elevated nutrient needs and for people who may not always eat well enough. Some examples include:

- *Pregnant and breastfeeding women.* Women who take supplemental folic acid prior to and during pregnancy can reduce the incidence of neural tube defects in their babies. The increased needs for iron during pregnancy are difficult to meet from diet alone. "Morning sickness" makes it even harder to fill the increased nutrient requirements of pregnancy. For many nutrients, needs are higher during lactation than pregnancy.

- *Women with heavy menstrual bleeding.* Lab tests can show if blood-building nutrients are inadequate, and if so, which ones. Women should not take high doses of iron unless their doctors recommend that they do so.

- *Children.* A supplement can help balance the diets of picky eaters or children on a food jag, and it can ease parental worries.

- *Infants.* If their access to sunlight is restricted, infants may need supplemental vitamin D. Doctors may prescribe fluoride in nonfluoridated areas.

- *People with severe food restrictions, either self-imposed or prescribed.* Supplements may help people on a strict weight-loss diet, those who have eating disorders, those who have mental illnesses, and those who limit their eating because of social or emotional situations.

- *Vegans.* Because they abstain from animal foods and dairy products, vegans may need supplemental vitamin B_{12}, and maybe calcium, zinc, iron, and other minerals.

- *Elders.* Inadequate stomach acid is common in this group, so they may need extra vitamin B_{12}. Supplements of calcium, vitamin D, and other nutrients help maintain bones if their diets lack dairy products and they have limited exposure to the sun.

Many people take nutrient supplements to "ensure" that they meet their nutritional needs. However, simply shoring up a habitually poor diet is a bad idea. Foods not only provide nutrients, but fiber and other health-promoting phytochemicals. Whenever possible, it is best to meet nutritional needs with food.

Most supplements sold in the United States are multiple vitamin/minerals. These supplements should contain at least 20 vitamins and minerals, each no more than 150 percent of its Daily Value.[16] For balance, the minimum for most supplement nutrients should be 50 to 100 percent of its Daily Value. (See **Figure SAN.4**.) Although most products have nutrient levels in this range, some formulas are irrational and unbalanced, with some nutrients less than 10 percent of its Daily Value, others more than 1,000 percent.

Key Concepts: *Vitamins and minerals are popular dietary supplements; however, it is better to obtain nutrients from food. Some conditions and circumstances make it difficult to get adequate nutrition from food or consume enough to accommodate increases in nutrient needs. Multivitamin/mineral supplements should be well balanced not contain doses greater than about 150% DV of each nutrient.*

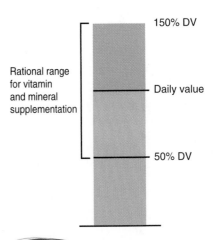

Figure SAN.4 **Moderate supplementation.**

Megadoses in Conventional Medical Management High doses of single vitamins and minerals are used surprisingly often in the conventional care of patients. Some vitamins and minerals have become so integrated into medical management that many physicians regard their use as "standard medical practice" rather than as "practicing nutrition." Usually these nutrients are purchased by prescription rather than over the counter. Here are some situations in which megadosing is used:

- A medication may dramatically deplete or destroy vitamin and mineral stores, or block vitamin and mineral activity. Megadosing overcomes these effects. For example, folic acid and vitamin B_6 are used during long-term treatment with some tuberculosis drugs. Also, B vitamins may also be prescribed along with seizure medications, or medicines that work by blocking metabolism of nucleic acids.[17]

- People with malabsorption syndromes often take large nutrient doses to compensate for losses and to override intestinal barriers to absorption. Colitis and cystic fibrosis are conditions routinely treated with megadoses.

- Megadoses of vitamin B_{12} can treat pernicious anemia typically caused by malabsorption of B_{12}. Ordinarily an intricate series of steps during digestion prepares B_{12} for normal intestinal absorption; if any of these steps malfunctions, the vitamin is lost. Megadoses allow a small amount of the vitamin to diffuse across the intestine, thus overriding the normal mechanism and preventing deficiency.[18]

- A vitamin at megadose levels can have "pharmacological activity," that is, it acts as a drug. Nicotinic acid (niacin) is the best example. At usual levels (around 10 or 20 mg), it functions as a vitamin, but at levels 50 or 100 times that, it acts as a drug to lower LDL cholesterol and triglycerides. Like any drug, though, it can have serious side effects.[19]

Benefits from high doses of other vitamins are not clear-cut. The B vitamins, including niacin, have been tried for emotional disturbances and mental illnesses; they work well when there's an underlying deficiency, but otherwise results have been mixed, and often disappointing. Vitamin E has been tried for some neurological illnesses, to minimize complications of diabetes mellitus, and to prevent coronary artery disease. Megadoses of vitamin C cannot effectively prevent common colds or treat cancer, but the vitamin may help prevent other conditions such as cataracts.[20] Further research into the links between heart disease, homocysteine, and certain B vitamins is needed before specific recommendations for supplements can be made.

Megadosing beyond Conventional Medicine: Orthomolecular Nutrition The term orthomolecular medicine was coined in 1968 by Dr. Linus Pauling, the best-known advocate of megadosing. To him, "orthomolecular" meant achieving the optimal nutrient levels in the body.[21] Few nutritionists argue with the importance of optimum nutrition. In fact, some nutritionists share many of Pauling's concerns, such as that the typical diet is too refined to provide adequate nutrients, and that earlier RDA values may not be high enough to achieve optimal body levels.

Most nutritionists would argue, however, with the high doses Dr. Pauling recommended to attain those optimal body levels, and with the therapeutic value he and his followers attributed to those doses. Most notably, Pauling's

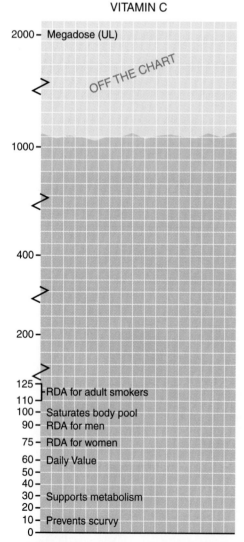

VITAMIN C

2000 – Megadose (UL)

OFF THE CHART

1000 –

400 –

200 –

125 – RDA for adult smokers
110 –
100 – Saturates body pool
90 – RDA for men
75 – RDA for women
60 – Daily Value
50 –
40 –
30 – Supports metabolism
20 –
10 – Prevents scurvy
0 –

Figure SAN.5 Megadoses of vitamin C are much higher intakes than currently recommended.

followers continue to recommend vitamin C in levels more than 100 times the Daily Value. (See **Figure SAN.5**.) Some advocates of vitamin C give even greater doses, relying on intravenous administration to avoid causing diarrhea. Dr. Pauling claimed megadose vitamin C prevented or cured the common cold. Many researchers attempted to confirm this theory. Although a few found marginally reduced severity or frequency of colds in specific groups of people,[22] most studies found no beneficial effect.[23] The most controversial claim for vitamin C was its purported ability to prevent and treat cancer. Well-controlled studies have now disproved this claim.[24]

Drawbacks of Megadoses Megadose vitamins and minerals remain popular. But when taken without recommendation or prescription from a qualified health professional, they can be problematic. Since high-dose nutrients can have pharmacological effects with the inherent risk of adverse side effects, people who choose to take megadoses should always check first with their doctors.

Excesses of some nutrients can create deficits of other nutrients. High doses of supplemental minerals, especially calcium, iron, zinc, and copper, can interfere with absorption of the others. In general, dosing with minerals has a smaller margin of safety than dosing with vitamins.

High-dose supplementation with fat-soluble vitamins A, D, and K can easily reach toxic levels. Vitamin E appears relatively safe, even at doses 10 or 20 times the DV, although its tendency to reduce blood clotting merits caution. Megadosing with water-soluble vitamin B_6 at 50 to 100 times the DV can do nerve damage. You may want to review the DRI tables for tolerable upper intake levels (UL) for vitamins and minerals.

Megadoses often are recommended for sick people, but sick people may be least able to tolerate them. Iron is very hard on a sensitive digestive system, for example. Vitamin C causes diarrhea. Although people who drink a lot of alcohol often are deficient in vitamin A, supplements not much greater than the DV produce undesirable liver changes in alcoholics.[25]

Megadoses can also interfere with medications and treatments. Although some people who take antiseizure medications also may need folic acid supplementation, too much folic acid can allow "breakthrough seizures." Vitamin K interferes with medication to control blood clotting, and should be taken only under a doctor's direction. People undergoing surgery should describe their nutritional supplements to their doctor, because high-dose vitamin E, especially if accompanied by blood thinners like gingko biloba, aspirin, or fish oil, can cause bleeding problems in the operating room. Antioxidant nutrients may be counterproductive during chemotherapies or radiation therapies that rely on oxidative destruction of cancer cells.

Key Concepts: *High doses (megadoses) of vitamins or minerals turn nutrients into drugs—chemicals with pharmacological activity. While there may be medical reasons for prescribing high-dose supplements, they should be taken under a physician's supervision. Many claims for high-dose supplements, such as that vitamin C prevents cancer, are not supported by clinical studies.*

Herbal Supplements

Supplementation with herbal products is growing in popularity. Survey data suggest that the use of herbals grew from 2.5 percent of adults in 1990 to 12.1 percent in 1997 (see **Table SAN.2**). Herbal therapy is nothing new, however. Most cultures have long traditions of using plants (and some animal products) to treat illness or sustain health. For centuries there were no

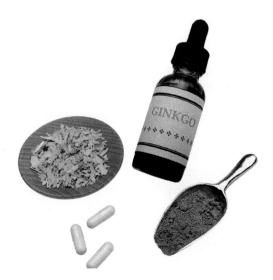

other medicines. Even now, most of the world's people depend primarily on herbs for medications, and in some remote areas, modern medicines are just not obtainable.

Contemporary herbalists in the United States prefer to use natural plant parts rather than (or in addition to) synthesized or highly purified medications. They reason that natural products are likely to contain a complex of healing ingredients, whereas a purified pharmaceutical product contains only one or two. They believe when active ingredients are combined with many other plant components, their side effects may be blunted or neutralized. (Although many herbal products are plant extracts, they generally are not highly purified, and often are blended with whole plant mixtures.)

Using herbal medicine sounds simple and easy. But in fact, herbalism calls for a great deal of skill. Traditional healers typically serve long apprenticeships, and acquire a subjective "feel" for their therapies after much experience. They must learn to judge the safety and potency of individual plants, which vary from season to season, location to location, age of the plant, and plant part. They must know how to prepare the plant, whether to extract it and with what, or how to make it into a salve or into an oral preparation. They must know how to blend it with other herbs and with other therapies. In traditional Chinese medicine, for example, a blend of herbs, sometimes 30 or more, can be used at once; they usually are sim-

 Do You Need a Vitamin E Supplement?

FOR YOUR INFORMATION

For decades vitamin E has been touted as a remedy for everything from graying hair to a sluggish libido. While most claims remain unproved, preliminary research shows that large doses bolster immune function as well as help prevent such chronic conditions as heart disease, cancer, and Alzheimer's disease.

Vitamin E ranks as one of the most popular vitamin supplements in the United States, second only to vitamin C.[1] Still, no major health organization has endorsed widespread use of vitamin E supplements because the science on the matter, though encouraging, is still not definitive.

Vitamin E and Heart Disease

One of the most promising uses for vitamin E may be preventing heart disease, the number one killer of both men and women. Epidemiological studies, animal research, and human clinical trials suggest that the nutrient inhibits oxidation of LDL cholesterol.

Although the findings are promising, many major health organizations want confirmation by clinical trials before recommending vitamin E supplements. In a recent study of individuals with either cardiovascular disease or diabetes, 400 IU of supplemental vitamin E daily had no apparent effect on cardiovascular events such as heart attack or stroke.[2] Only randomized, placebo-controlled clinical trials can determine whether long-term use of vitamin E—say, over the course of decades—causes side effects that haven't occurred in trials lasting only several years.

Vitamin E and Immunity

Some research suggests that daily doses of vitamin E may help reverse age-related declines in immune function. One study conducted at the Jean Mayer USDA Human Nutrition Research Center on Aging at Tufts University, for example, suggests that vitamin E positively affects the immune system. In the study, people who took 200 milligrams of vitamin E exhibited a substantially better response than people who took either 60 or 800 milligrams of vitamin E. It may be that 200 milligrams was effective because it is just at or below a threshold after which vitamin E confers no benefits to the immune system. This is one of many questions that remain unanswered.[3]

mered in water and taken as a tea or "soup." Other herbal traditions use only one or two carefully chosen herbs at a time.

Traditional herbalists know their patients and individualize the herbal approach. In the United States that includes knowing results of diagnostic testing; in other cultures it includes recognizing and understanding symptoms. Such care is rare in the U.S. mass market for herbal supplements.

Helpful Herbs, Harmful Herbs People who decide to use herbs instead of conventional medicines must choose their practitioners carefully. Herbalists must know their herbs, but they also must know when to tell patients to seek conventional care. People who use both an herbalist and a conventional doctor should tell both practitioners about the other, and disclose all treatments.

Most research on herbs has been published in obscure or foreign language journals that are hard to locate or read. In addition, traditional herbal medicine uses plants to make teas or soups, a far cry from the purified extracts and herbal blends sold in a supermarket. Nevertheless there is enough data for some herbs to warrant carefully controlled studies. OAM has funded a large study of St. John's wort, based on preliminary evidence that it fights mild depression and sleeplessness.[26] Milk thistle appears helpful for liver disease.[27] Gingko biloba appears to help blood circulation, and a preliminary study suggests it may help in treating Alzheimer's disease.[28] In short-term studies, saw palmetto extract improves urinary tract function in

Quick Bites

Culinary herbs are not medicinal herbs. Or are they?

Herbs used in cooking are called culinary herbs to distinguish them from medicinal herbs. But culinary herbs are also rich in phytochemicals. Some examples are beta-carotene in paprika, the antioxidants in rosemary, the mild antibiotic allicin in garlic, and the mild antiviral curcumin in turmeric.

Vitamin E and Alzheimer's Disease

Scientists suspect that vitamin E's antioxidant properties may be useful in treating people with Alzheimer's disease. Research at Columbia University indicates that vitamin E may slow the rate of deterioration in people with moderately severe Alzheimer's disease.[4] The findings prompted the American Psychiatric Association to include the therapeutic use of vitamin E in their 1997 guidelines for the treatment of moderately impaired Alzheimer's patients.[5]

Experts caution, however, that the 2,000 IU dose of vitamin E used in this research should not be taken without a physician's supervision. In addition to the risks of hemorrhagic stroke and decreased ability of blood to clot, vitamin E may also interfere with other medications often administered to people with Alzheimer's disease.

Vitamin E and Prostate Cancer

One study has associated vitamin E with a decreased risk of prostate cancer, the most commonly diagnosed cancer in men in the United States.[5] The prostate glands of most older men harbor microscopic areas of cancerous cells that may progress into a cancerous tumor. Because men who took vitamin E experienced a reduction in detectable cancer within 2 years of taking the supplement, scientists believe that vitamin E may block a prostate's cancerous cells from progressing into malignant masses.

While this study is promising, most experts hesitate to raise hopes until its results are replicated, particularly in other groups such as nonsmokers and people of different ethnic backgrounds.

1 Richman A, Witkowski JP. Sixth Annual Dietary Supplement Survey. *Whole Foods.* June 1998:23–28.

2 The Heart Outcomes Prevention Evaluation Study Investigators. Vitamin E supplementation and cardiovascular events in high-risk patients. *N Engl J Med.* 2000;342:154–160.

3 Meydani SN, Meydani M, Blumberg JB, et al. Vitamin E supplementation and in vivo immune response in healthy elderly subjects. *JAMA.* 1997;277:1380–1386; and Chandra RK. Graying of the immune system: can nutrient supplements improve immunity in the elderly? *JAMA.* 1997;277:1398–1399.

4 Sano M, Ernesto C, Thomas RG, et al. A controlled trial of selegiline, alpha-tocopherol, or both as treatment for Alzheimer's disease. *N Engl J Med.*1997;336:1216–1222.

5 Practice guidelines for the treatment of patients with Alzheimer's disease and other dementias of late life. *Supplement Am J Psychiatry.* 1997;154(5 suppl):1–39.

6 Heinonen OP, Albanes D, Virtamo J, et al. Prostate cancer and supplementation with alpha-tocopherol and beta-carotene: incidence and mortality in a controlled trial. *J Nat Cancer Inst.* 1998;90:440–446.

Table SAN.4 **Popular Herbal Supplements**

Gingko biloba to combat cerebral vascular insufficiency

Ginseng (Asian) for energy and mood improvement

Garlic to reduce cholesterol and blood pressure; has anticoagulant properties

Echinacea to stimulate the immune system prior to and during the cold and flu season

St. John's wort to treat mild to moderate depression

Saw palmetto to promote prostate health and to treat benign prostatic hyperplasia

Cranberry to treat urinary tract irritations and infections

Valerian as a mild sedative and to treat insomnia

Kava as a tranquilizer and sedative

Milk thistle to detoxify the liver

Feverfew to relieve migraine headaches

men with benign prostate enlargement.[29] Drinking cranberry juice discourages urinary tract infections by inhibiting harmful bacteria from sticking to the urinary tract's lining.[30]

The suggested benefits of other herbs are based not on scientific study, but on years of informal observation: mint helps indigestion; ginger helps nausea and motion sickness; lemon perks appetite; chamomile helps insomnia. See **Table SAN.4** for popular supplements and claimed benefits.

If you're considering using an herb, remember this important rule of thumb: any herb that is strong enough to help you can be strong enough to hurt you. Like any medicine, herbs can have side effects, and herbs can be contraindicated. The FDA has issued a public health advisory warning of interactions between St. John's wort and some prescription medications.[31] Gingko biloba is a blood thinner, and has caused harmful bleeding in some people.[32] Just like any other new, unusual substance, herbs can cause sudden allergic reactions.

Herbs can interfere with standard medicines, and they can make people with underlying health problems quite sick. For example, licorice extract—even as a flavoring in chewing tobacco—flushes potassium from the body, raises blood pressure, and can interfere with blood pressure medication.[33] (Most licorice candy is now flavored synthetically; naturally flavored licorice has little effect unless routinely eaten in large amounts.) **Table SAN.5** lists some possible interactions of herbs and drugs.

Some herbs and herbalist treatments are downright dangerous. Some hazardous therapies even use lead or arsenic.[34] Yohimbe, ephedra (ma huang), chaparral, and comfrey are herbs that have been shown to be dangerous.[35] Senna, cascara, and rhubarb are powerful laxatives used in products described as "colon cleansers," "colon purifiers," or even "blood purifiers"; their overuse is as damaging as overuse of conventional laxatives. (See **Table SAN.6**)

Herbal blends marketed for specific conditions, such as "healthy bone formula" or "female blend," do not always make sense in light of current scientific knowledge. For example, pennyroyal and St. John's wort—herbs

Think About It

4

Table SAN.5 **Possible Herb-Drug Interactions**

Herb	Drug	Interaction
Feverfew, Garlic, Ginger, Gingko Biloba, Guarana, and Pau d' Arco	warfarin, aspirin	Increases anticoagulant effect by inhibiting platelet aggregation.
Hawthorne and Horse Chestnut	digoxin, diuretics	Affects cardiac function and blood pressure; should not be taken with digoxin and diuretics.
Aloe, Senna (laxative), Cascara, and Licorice	digoxin, diuretics	Causes electrolyte imbalance; true licorice increases blood pressure. Do not take with diuretics and digoxin.
Kava and Valerian	anxiolytics, narcotics, and alcohol	Increases sedative effects.
St. John's Wort	antidepressants, crixivan (indinavir) and other protease inhibitors, cyclosporine	Should not be taken with prescription antidepressants; risk of hypertensive crisis if taken with antidepressants. St. John's Wort makes several prescription medications used in the treatment of AIDS less effective. The herb speeds up activity in a key pathway responsible for breaking these drugs down in the body. When the medications are taken with St. John's Wort, blood levels of the drugs decrease because the body breaks them down faster.

contraindicated during pregnancy—have shown up in some "prenatal formulas." Also, a popular blend used to treat prostate cancer actually had the estrogenic activity contraindicated for this condition.[36]

Quality control is a big issue in herbal medicines. Contaminants have caused acute illness and death.[37] A common problem is poorly standardized strength or potency. The potency of the popular, over-the-counter St. John's wort supplements varies as much as 17-fold.[38] In another analysis, the quantity of active ingredient in ginseng supplements varied from the amount stated on the label by as much as 10-fold.[39]

Manufacturers and practitioners are working with the FDA to establish standards and procedures to ensure potency and to prevent adulteration and contamination. To guarantee quality, each step from field to market must be monitored carefully. However, monitoring the production of herbal supplements poses special challenges. Herbs are grown and harvested in far-flung, sometimes remote areas of the world. Extraction or preparation of the herbs may take place elsewhere. Mixing the herbs and putting them in capsules, tonics, or teas is typically done by yet another party in yet another location.

Other Dietary Supplements

The supplement market used to be vitamins, minerals, and a handful of other products like brewer's yeast and sea salt. Today there are dozens more

Table SAN.6 **Possible Adverse Effects of Selected Herbs**

Herb	Possible Adverse Effects
Chamomile (tea)	Allergic reaction; digestive upset
Chaparral	Liver toxicity
Comfrey	Liver and kidney disease
Echinacea	Allergic reaction; stimulation of immune system: not for use by those with systemic/autoimmune diseases
Ephedra	Insomnia, headaches, nervousness, seizures, increased blood pressure, stroke, death
Gingko biloba	Inhibits blood clotting; do not take with aspirin, anticoagulants, vitamin E
Ginseng	Headaches, insomnia, diarrhea, heart palpitations, vaginal bleeding
Kava	Slowed reaction time; scaly dermatitis
Licorice	Headaches, fluid retention, increased blood pressure, electrolyte imbalance, heart failure
Pau d'Arco	Severe nausea, vomiting; anemia; bleeding tendencies
Pennyroyal	Liver damage, convulsions, abortions, coma, death; oil is very toxic
St. John's wort	Adverse interactions with antidepressant medication; possible photosensitivity
Senna	Laxative dependency, diarrhea, cramps, electrolyte disturbances
Valerian	Headache, excitability, insomnia

Sources: McGuffin M, Hobbs C, Upton R, Goldberg A. *American Herbal Products Association Botanical Safety Handbook.* Boca Raton, FL: CRC Press; 1997; and Sarubin A. *The Health Professional's Guide to Popular Dietary Supplements.* Chicago, IL: The American Dietetic Association; 2000; and Foster S, Tyler VE. *Tyler's Honest Herbal: A Sensible Guide to the Use of Herbs and Related Remedies.* Binghamton, NY: Haworth Herbal Press; 1999.

products, with new ones continuously popping up. Although some are useful, many are of dubious benefit.

Supplement categories now include protein powders, amino acids, carotenoids, bioflavonoids, digestive aids, fatty acid formulas and special fats, lecithin and phospholipids, probiotics, products from sharks and other seafood, algae, human metabolites such as coenzyme Q_{10} and nucleic acids, glandular extracts, garlic products, and fibers such as guar gum. Supplement producers also blend these products with herbs and nutrients, resulting in a countless array of individual and combination supplements sold today. In most cases, labeling and advertising claims go beyond current knowledge about these products.

Key Concepts: *Herbal products are among the many dietary supplements available today. Herbal medicine has a long history in many cultures. Although there is anecdotal support for the use of many herbal products, there is little scientific evidence to back it up. The FDA and manufacturers are working to set standards for production and sale of herbal supplements. It is important to remember that any herb that is strong enough to help you can also be strong enough to hurt you. Before taking any supplements, it's a good idea to consult your health-care practitioner.*

[Fyi] Talking with Your Doctor

FOR YOUR INFORMATION

Unfortunately, people do not generally disclose their use of alternative therapies to their physicians.[1] This lack of candor is a cause for concern because an estimated 15 million Americans in 1997 took prescription medications and herbal remedies concurrently. Because one in five people who take prescription medications is also taking herbs, high-dose vitamin supplements, or both, millions of adults may be at risk for unintended interactions.[2]

In an effort to increase communication between patients and their physicians regarding the use of alternative remedies, David Eisenberg, M.D., Director of the Center for Alternative Medicine Research at Boston's Beth Israel Deaconess Medical Center, has developed an approach that includes the following advice to consumers:

- Always keep your doctor informed of any alternative therapies you're pursuing or thinking of trying.
- Listen to your doctor's reaction, even if it's not what you want to hear. It might be that your physician knows of serious side effects, feels that the treatment will interfere with a traditional treatment which he or she knows works well, or knows of factors in your medical history that make an alternative therapy risky for you.
- If you plan to pursue the alternative against your doctor's advice, say so. The discussion should be noted in your chart. This information may be useful later in preventing unnecessary tests or in identifying treatment interactions.
- Assuming your doctor agrees to work with you, ask whether he or she has any questions for your alternative-care provider. It is best if the two practitioners can communicate directly. Let your doctor know if the alternative provider is advising you to do something that directly conflicts with medical recommendations. Review the alternative provider's professional credentials, training, and experience. Try to find out if any complaints have been filed against the provider.
- Take steps to track your progress, and make an appointment with your conventional doctor to reassess your situation. Start by keeping a daily diary in which you record your symptoms (e.g., back pain on a scale from 1 to 10).
- Whether therapy was effective or not, ask your doctor to note the results in your chart.
- Remember that your doctor may not have enough time to read up on every kind of alternative treatment that's out there, so the responsibility of researching the treatment will most likely rest with you.[3]

1 Eisenberg DM, Davis RB, Ettner SL, et al. Trends in alternative medicine use in the United States, 1990–1997. *JAMA.* 1998;280:1569–1575.

2 Considering alternative medicine? *Tufts University Health and Nutrition Letter.* Nov 1998.

3 Ibid.

Dietary Supplements in the Marketplace

Although some dietary supplements have druglike actions (e.g., reducing cholesterol levels), government agencies regulate supplements differently from drugs. The freedoms of speech and press prevail; in practical terms, almost anything goes. Promotional books, magazine articles, audio- and videotapes, lectures, staged interviews, and messages posted on Internet chat lines—all are protected by the First Amendment, and have the freedom to inform or to deceive. It's up to the listener or reader to distinguish fact from fiction. (See **Figure SAN.6**.)

The FTC and Supplement Advertising

The Federal Trade Commission (FTC) in the U.S. Department of Commerce is responsible for ensuring that advertisements and commercials are truthful and do not mislead. The agency depends on and encourages self-monitoring by the supplement industry. In pursuing companies that skirt the regulations, the FTC gives priority to cases that put people's health and safety at serious risk, or that affect sick and vulnerable consumers.[40]

The FDA and Supplement Regulation

The Food and Drug Administration (FDA) has primary responsibility for regulating labeling and content of dietary supplements, under the Federal Food, Drug, and Cosmetic Act, as amended by the Dietary Supplement Health and Education Act of 1994, or DSHEA.[41]

Defining Dietary Supplements

How do you know a product is a "dietary supplement?" Simple. DSHEA defines any product intended to supplement the diet as a dietary supplement, and requires that the word *supplement* be clearly stated on the label.

Dietary supplements are *not drugs*. A drug is intended to diagnose, cure, mitigate, treat, or prevent disease. Before marketing, drugs must undergo

(Beware the exclamation point)

Prevents Osteoporosis!
Prevents Heart Disease!
Promotes Joint Health!

Maintains a healthy circulatory system
Maintains a healthy immune system

Helps you relax
Enhances libido
For muscle enhancement

For common symptoms of PMS
For hot flashes
For morning sickness

Figure SAN.6 None of these claims has received FDA approval.

extensive studies of effectiveness, safety, interactions with other substances, and dosing. The FDA gives formal premarket approval to a drug, and monitors its safety after the drug is on the market. None of this is required of dietary supplements. A dietary supplement with a label claiming to cure or treat a specific condition is, in reality, an unauthorized drug.

Dietary supplements are *not food additives*. Before using a new food additive, manufacturers must do considerable safety testing, which the FDA reviews before granting premarket approval. For new ingredients in dietary supplements, the manufacturer finds information (usually not scientific proof) to show the supplement is safe if used as directed, and submits this information to the FDA 75 days prior to first marketing the supplement. However, formal approval by the FDA is not required. New dietary supplements that contain ingredients already in use do not require such advance notification. Unlike pharmaceutical manufacturers who must prove the safety of their products before they sell them, supplement manufacturers can market their products without the FDA's approval. To restrict sale and use of a dietary supplement, the FDA must prove that it isn't safe after it is on the market.

Supplement Label Claims

Regulations limit claims on supplement labels to the following:

- *Nutrient-content claims* describe the level of a nutrient, such as "high in calcium." These claims must be consistent with definitions approved for foods.

- *Health claims* show a link between a supplement and a disease or a health-related condition. The FDA authorizes these claims based on a review of the scientific evidence (as they do for food labels, see Chapter 2) or on an authoritative statement from recognized scientific agencies. For example, a supplement with sufficient calcium could carry a statement about the link between calcium and osteoporosis.

- *Nutrition-support claims* describe the link between a nutrient and a deficiency disease. For example, the label of a vitamin C supplement could state that vitamin C prevents scurvy, but these claims must also mention the prevalence of the deficiency disease in the United States.

- *Structure-function claims* describe the supplement's effect on body structure or function, including its overall effect on well-being. An example might be "calcium builds strong bones." Manufacturers can use structure-function claims without FDA authorization, and can base their claims on their own review and interpretation of the scientific literature. Structure-function claims are easy to spot because they are accompanied with the disclaimer "This statement has not been evaluated by the Food and Drug Administration. This product is not intended to diagnose, treat, cure, or prevent any disease." There is often a fine line between structure-function claims and claims that would make the product an unauthorized drug. For example, the claim "promotes urinary tract health" on a bottle of cranberry extract capsules would be allowable, while "prevents urinary tract infections" would not.

Supplement Facts

Since March 1999 all labels on dietary supplements must include ingredient information and a **Supplement Facts panel**.[42] You'll notice in **Figure SAN.7** that the format is similar to the Nutrition Facts on food labels. An

Supplement Facts panel Content label that must appear on all dietary supplements.

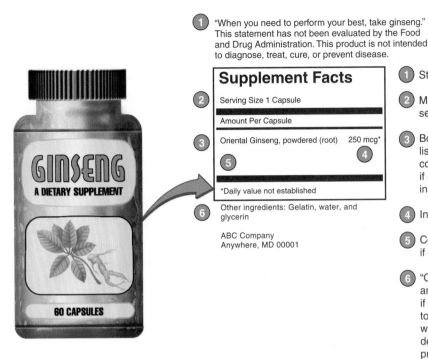

① "When you need to perform your best, take ginseng." This statement has not been evaluated by the Food and Drug Administration. This product is not intended to diagnose, treat, cure, or prevent disease.

Supplement Facts

② Serving Size 1 Capsule

Amount Per Capsule

③ Oriental Ginseng, powdered (root)   250 mcg*

⑤   ④

*Daily value not established

⑥ Other ingredients: Gelatin, water, and glycerin

ABC Company
Anywhere, MD 00001

① Structure/function claim

② Manufacturer's suggested serving size

③ Botanical supplements must list part of plant present and common name (Latin name if common name not listed in "Herbs of Commerce")

④ Information listed per "serving"

⑤ Conventional food nutrients, if present, must be listed

⑥ "Other" dietary ingredients and quantities listed here, if present. For proprietary blends total weight only may be listed, with components listed in descending order of predominance by weight

Figure SAN.7 **Supplement facts panel.**
Source: Food and Drug Administration. http://www.fda.gov.

important difference is that a Supplement Facts panel includes substances for which no Daily Value has been established. In combination products the panel separates these substances from established nutrients and displays them at the bottom. Herbal ingredients must list the plant part, such as root or leaf.

Key Concepts: *Dietary supplements are neither foods nor drugs, and their manufacture and sale are regulated differently from foods, food additives, and drugs. The FTC and FDA monitor advertising and labeling of dietary supplements. A Supplement Facts panel is now required on labels.*

Choosing Dietary Supplements

DSHEA has made many improvements, such as the Supplement Facts panel, to help consumers of dietary supplements. By loosening previous restrictions, DSHEA has made many more products available to consumers. However, with the resulting proliferation of supplements, it is challenging to effectively monitor claims, quality, and safety. In an environment in which manufacturers can market their products without prior approval, it is wise to be wary. Knowledge of nutrition science is your most valuable tool for evaluating a supplement. Read each label and judge each implied claim in light of what you know. Ask the following questions.

Is the quantity enough to have an effect or is it trivial? Consider amino acids, for example. A product contains 25 milligrams of glycine. Compare it to the amount of glycine you'd obtain from a diet with 70 grams of protein. Has glycine been added to the product or is it a component of the gelatin capsule? Is glycine an essential or a nonessential amino acid? What will happen if you take more than you need? Is it a problem if you get less than you need?

Is the product new to you? Learn about it from the many reliable resources listed in Appendix K. Evaluate the product in light of scientific research. Has it been studied in humans, rodents, or other animals, or only in cell cultures or *in vitro*? If in humans, was the study controlled to eliminate a placebo effect? For case report studies, could the placebo effect influence the results? Consider also the type of preparation and the route of administration. An injected herbal extract may have a very different effect than the same herb in a pill.

Consider the dose used in the study. Is it a reasonable amount, an amount found in over-the-counter products? For example, serious researchers studied the testosterone precursor DHEA and found it may help some immune disorders, but at doses 20 to 50 times greater than DHEA sold in health-food stores.[43] A consumer who chooses to take 20 of these pills daily to match that used in studies would risk side effects, and magnify effects of potential contaminants. Another example is shark cartilage. In the best-controlled study to date of shark cartilage and cancer, the dose was equivalent to about 75 capsules of shark cartilage daily; even at that high dose, patients with advanced cancer were not helped.[44]

Can the supplement cross the intestine and travel to its presumed site of action in the body? The body digests enzyme preparations, for example, along with other proteins. Herbal preparations and other types of non-nutrient supplements lack bioavailability data. Does the product promise too much? A product touted to control hypercholesterolemia, hang nails, psoriasis, and insomnia, is unlikely to do much of anything. Neither will a "low-calorie, high-energy" drink. It's possible that the same results can be achieved less expensively and more enjoyably by eating regular foods. Why take lycopene capsules when you can eat tomatoes, even catsup? Why take bilberry extract when blueberries (the American equivalent to European bilberries) are delicious and low in kilocalories?

Who is selling the product? Alternative practitioners, dietitians, and even physicians sometimes sell the supplements they recommend,[45]—which is a possible conflict of interest that could compromise their objectivity. Expect to pay extra for supplements sold via **multilevel marketing**, because each level in the system takes a commission on the product you buy. When you buy supplements over the phone, by catalogue, or over the Web, you lose the chance to examine it before you buy it.

A good indicator of quality is the **USP (U.S. Pharmacopoeia)** notation, which certifies that the product meets the U.S. Pharmacopoeia's standards for quality, strength, purity, packaging, and labeling. Established in 1820, the USP is a voluntary, not-for-profit organization that sets quality standards for a range of health-care products, including prescription and non-prescription medicines, biotechnology drugs, home test kits, medical devices, vitamins and minerals, and dietary supplements. Nationally known food and drug manufacturers have established standards, quality control, and manufacturing practices that they are likely to apply to their dietary supplements as well.

Contact the company with your questions; you'll learn a lot, although maybe not what you expected. The "technical representative" may be unable to give you any more information than a brief readout from a computerized database. Some companies respond to queries by sending a long printout of journal citations, most of them inappropriate, without text or even abstracts; many references are in a foreign language. On the other hand, some dietary-supplement companies have on-site quality control, and on-site nutritionists who are knowledgeable and happy to supply helpful information.

Even the best-intentioned, most carefully considered supplement can prove ineffective or even risky. Take the example of beta-carotene. Despite a good theoretical basis for assuming it reduces cancer risk, several large well-controlled

multilevel marketing A system of selling in which each salesperson recruits assistants who then recruit others to help them. The person at each level collects a commission on sales made by the later recruits.

U.S. Pharmacopoeia (USP) Established in 1820, the USP is a voluntary, not-for-profit health-care organization that sets quality standards for a range of health-care products.

studies found it had no protective effect. For some groups of people, it actually increased risk.[46] The results disappointed advocates of beta-carotene, but these studies demonstrate the value of carefully controlled studies and the risk of unproved assumptions about dietary supplements.

Fraudulent Products

Some health advocates consider the burgeoning market of dietary supplements an unwelcome return to the "snake oil" era of the late nineteenth and early twentieth centuries, when "magic" potions and cures were sold door to door and at county fairs and markets. Most manufacturers work hard to assure the quality of their products, yet some supplements on the market are nothing more than a mixture of ineffective ingredients.

In a recent issue of *FDA Consumer*, the agency had this to say about fraudulent products:

Fraudulent products often can be identified by the types of claims made in their labeling, advertising, and promotional literature. Stephen Barrett, M.D., a board member of the National Council Against Health Fraud, points to the following indicators of possible fraud:

- *Claims that the product is a secret cure and use of such terms as breakthrough, magical, miracle cure, and new discovery. "If the product were a cure for a serious disease, it would be widely reported in the media and used by health-care professionals," he says.*
- *Pseudomedical jargon, such as detoxify, purify, and energize to describe a product's effects. "These claims are vague and hard to measure," Barrett says. "So, they make it easier for success to be claimed, even though nothing has actually been accomplished," he says.*
- *Claims that the product can cure a wide range of unrelated diseases. "No product can do that," he says.*
- *Claims that the supplement has only benefits—and no side effects. "A product potent enough to help people will be potent enough to cause side effects," Barrett says.*
- *Claims that a product is backed by scientific studies, but with no list of references or references that are inadequate. For instance, if a list of references is provided, the citations cannot be traced, or if they are traceable, the studies are out-of-date, irrelevant, or poorly designed.*
- *Accusations that the medical profession, drug companies, and the government are suppressing information about a particular treatment. "It would be illogical," Barrett says, "for large numbers of people to withhold information about potential medical therapies when they or their families and friends might one day benefit from them."[47]*

Supplement users who suffer a serious harmful effect or illness that they think is related to supplement use should call a doctor or other health-care provider. Practitioners can report to FDA MedWatch by calling 1-800-FDA-1088 or by going to www.fda.gov/medwatch/report/hcp.htm on the MedWatch Web site. Consumers can call the toll-free MedWatch number or go to www.fda.gov/medwatch/report/consumer/consumer.htm on the MedWatch Web site to report an adverse reaction.

Key Concepts: *When considering a dietary supplement, it is important to consider the product and its claims carefully. Be aware that some products may promise more than they can deliver. A good indicator of quality is the USP notation, but even this does not guarantee efficacy.*

Quick Bites

Jell-O and Your Nails

You may have heard that taking gelatin can make your nails stronger. Not true. Fingernails get their strength from sulfur in amino acids. Gelatin has no sulfur-containing amino acids.

Label [to] **Table**

If you picked up a multivitamin/mineral container from your drugstore shelf, would you know how to read it? Look at the following Supplement Facts label from a basic multivitamin/mineral and see how well you can answer these questions.

1. If you were a 20-year-old woman who knew she wasn't consuming enough calcium, would this supplement allow you to get your recommended intake?
2. If 25 percent of the vitamin A in this supplement comes from beta-carotene, where does the rest come from?
3. What trend do you see in the amounts of B vitamins?
4. What trend do you see in the amounts of bone minerals?
5. What trend do you see in the amounts of antioxidant vitamins?
6. Does the USP statement make this supplement "legitimate"?

Supplement Facts
Daily Multivitamin/Mineral Dietary Supplement

USP Made to U.S. Pharmacopoeia (USP) quality, purity, and potency standards. Laboratory tested to dissolve within 60 minutes.

Serving Size 1 tablet

Each Tablet Contains	% DV	Each Tablet Contains	% DV
Vitamin A 10,000 I.U. 25% as beta-carotene	200%	Iodine 150 mcg	100%
Vitamin C 120 mg	200%	Magnesium 100 mg	25%
Vitamin D 400 IU	100%	Zinc 22.5 mg	150%
Vitamin E 60 IU	200%	Selenium 45 mcg	64%
Vitamin K 25 mcg	31%	Copper 3 mg	150%
Thiamin (vit. B$_1$) 1.5 mg	100%	Manganese 2.5 mg	125%
Riboflavin (vit. B$_2$) 1.7 mg	100%	Chromium 100 mcg	83%
Niacin 20 mg	100%	Molybdenum 25 mcg	33%
Vitamin B$_6$ 2 mg	100%	Chloride 36.3 mg	1%
Folate (folic acid) 400 mcg	100%	Sodium less than 5 mg	less than 1%
Vitamin B$_{12}$ 6 mcg	100%	Potassium 40 mg	1%
Biotin 30 mcg	10%	Nickel 5 mcg	*
Pantothenic acid 10 mg	100%	Tin 10 mcg	*
Calcium 162 mg	16%	Silicon 2 mg	*
Iron 9 mg	50%	Vanadium 10 mcg	*
Phosphorus 109 mg	11%	Boron 150 mcg	*

* Daily Value (%DV) not established

Answers to Questions

1. No. This supplement only provides 162 milligrams and the Adequate Intake (AI) for a 20-year-old female is 1,000 milligrams. She may need a calcium supplement if she can't eat enough calcium-rich foods.
2. The other 7,500 IU of vitamin A is most likely retinol in the form of retinyl acetate or retinyl palmitate; check the list of ingredients.
3. With the exception of biotin, this supplement provides 100% Daily Value of the B vitamins. And the 30 micrograms of biotin provides 100 percent of the current AI.
4. This supplements contains very low percentages of the Daily Values for calcium, magnesium, and phosphorus (16%, 11%, and 25%, respectively). Adding more of these minerals would make the pill huge and impossible to swallow! A nutritious diet should provide the rest of these minerals.
5. This supplement contains 200 percent of the Daily Value for each of the three vitamin antioxidants (vitamins A, C, and E).
6. By listing the U.S. Pharmacopoeia "stamp of approval," you can be confident that this supplement underwent a test to see how quickly it dissolves. If pills do not dissolve, their contents cannot be absorbed. In this case, the supplement took 60 minutes to dissolve. The USP sets standards for the quality, purity, and potency of supplements.

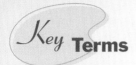 **LEARNING** *Portfolio*

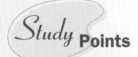 **Key Terms**

	page		page
complementary and alternative medicine (CAM)	648	orthomolecular medicine	648
holistic	650	phytotherapy	648
macrobiotic diet	652	Supplement Facts panel	664
multilevel marketing	666	U.S. Pharmacopoeia (USP)	666

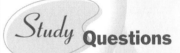 **Study Points**

➤ Complementary and alternative medicine (CAM) comprises practices outside the medical mainstream that are becoming increasingly popular. CAM includes a broad range of therapies, many of which include nutrition. People seek them for a variety of reasons including a fear of aging and environmental concerns.

➤ There is little scientific support for the use of restrictive diets such as the macrobiotic diet, Gerson diet, and Kelley regimen in the treatment of cancer.

➤ Dietary supplements encompass vitamins, minerals, herbals, amino acids, glandular extracts, enzymes, and many other products.

➤ Vitamin and mineral supplements may be warranted in certain circumstances, although the preferred mode of obtaining adequate nutrition is through foods.

➤ Megadose vitamin or mineral therapy has not been proved effective in the treatment of cancer, colds, or heart disease. Moreover, such megadoses act more like drugs than nutrients in the body and should be approached with caution.

➤ Herbal medicine is a traditional form of healing in many cultures. Some herbal medicines have shown enough promise to warrant large-scale clinical studies involving supplements. However, herbal products can have side effects and can interfere with prescription medications.

➤ Dietary supplements are regulated based on the provisions of the Dietary Supplements Health and Education Act of 1994. But dietary supplements do not need premarket approval.

➤ Claims for dietary supplements can include nutrient-content claims, disease claims (like health claims on food), nutritional-deficiency claims, and structure-function claims.

➤ Dietary supplements must have a Supplement Facts panel on the label.

➤ Consumers should carefully evaluate claims and evidence for dietary supplements and consult their physician before taking a supplement.

Study Questions

1. Discuss some of the reasons for the popularity of complementary and alternative medicine therapies.
2. What is a macrobiotic diet?
3. How do you know a product is a dietary supplement?
4. What things should someone consider before purchasing supplements?
5. If a product label contains the words "High in vitamin E," what type of health claim is it making? What other claims can a food product make?
6. How does the government regulate the sale of dietary supplements that have druglike actions?
7. Why is it a bad idea for physicians to sell the products they recommend?
8. What are some of the complications involved in using herbal medicines?

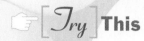

Try **This**

Supplement Savvy

This exercise will familiarize you with the many supplements available to consumers. Take a trip to your local drug store and spend some time in the supplements section. Pick out about 10 different supplements and try to identify how many have nutrient-content claims, disease-related claims, and structure-function claims. Note the prices of these supplements. Do any of them have the USP stamp of approval?

Take a Walk on the "Web Side"

This exercise will familiarize you with various Web sites that promote and sell supplements. Log on to the Internet and start doing searches with the key words affiliated with supplements. Try *vitamins*, *minerals*, *supplements*, *herbs*, and even some specific terms like *chromium picolinate* and *ginseng*. In the Web sites you visit, how is the nutrition information presented? Do the supplement benefits sound too good to be true? See if you can spot a fraud. Use the information in the "Fraudulent Products" section of this chapter to identify the accuracy of the product information you find.

References

1 Eisenberg DM, Kessler RC, Foster C, et al. Unconventional medicine in the United States: prevalence, costs, and patterns of use. *N Engl J Med.* 1993;328:246–252.

2 Pelletier KR, Marie A, Krasner M, Haskell WL. Current trends in the integration and reimbursement of complementary and alternative medicine by managed care, insurance carriers, and hospital providers. *Am J Health Promotion.* 1997;12:112–123.

3 Eisenberg DM, Kessler RC, Foster C, et al. Op. cit.

4 Eisenberg DM, Davis RB, Ettner SL, et al. Trends in alternative medicine use in the United States, 1990–1997. *JAMA.* 1998;280:1569–1575.

5 Ibid.

6 Bannerman JE. Goldenseal in world trade: pressures and potentials. *HerbalGram.* 1997;41:51–52.

7 Fleming EH, Papageorgiou PA. Shark fisheries and trade in Europe. *Traffic Europe Report.* March 1997. (Published in Brussels, Belgium, by TRAFFIC, the joint wildlife trade monitoring program of WWF-World Wide Fund For Nature and IUCN-The World Conservation Union.)

8 Angell M, Kassirer JP. Alternative medicine-the risks of untested and unregulated remedies. *N Engl J Med.* 1998;339:839–40.

9 Ephraim RJ. Dietary supplementation: the newest specialty. *Nutrition in Complementary Care Newsletter.* 1999;1(2):6.

10 Alternative Medicine, Expanding Medical Horizons: A Report to the National Institutes of Health on Alternative Medical Systems and Practices in the United States. Bethesda, MD: NIH publication 94-066. Dec 1994:230–232, 237.

11 Ibid.

12 Ibid.

13 Ibid.

14 Ibid.

15 Slesinski MJ, Subar SF, Kahle LL. Trends in use of vitamin and mineral supplements in the United States: The l987 and l992 National Health Interview Surveys. *J Am Diet Assoc.* 1995;95:921–923.

16 Vitamin Supplements. http://www.intelihealth.com. Accessed 11/5/00.

17 *Physicians' Desk Reference.* 53rd ed. Montvale, NJ: Medical Economics Company; 1999.

18 Lederle FA. Oral cyanocobalamin for pernicious anemia: medicine's best kept secret? *JAMA.* 1991;265:94–95.

19 *Physicians' Desk Reference.* 53rd ed. Op. cit.

20 Jacques PF, Taylor A, Hankinson SE, et al. Long-term vitamin C supplement use and prevalence of early age-related lens opacities. *Am J Clin Nutr.* 1997;66:911–916.

21 Alternative Medicine, Expanding Medical Horizons. Op. cit.

22 Hemila H. Vitamin C intake and susceptibility to the common cold. *Br J Nutr.* 1997;77:59–72.

23 Chalmers TC. Effects of ascorbic acid on the common cold: an evaluation of the evidence. *Am J Med.* 1975;58:532–536.

24 Byers T, Guerrero N. Epidemiologic evidence for vitamin C and vitamin E in cancer prevention. *Am J Clin Nutr.* 1995;62(suppl):1385S–1392S.

25 Leo MA, Lieber CS. Alcohol, vitamin A, and beta-carotene: adverse interactions, including hepatotoxicity and carcinogenicity. *Am J Clin Nutr.* 1999;69:1071–1085.

26 St. John's Wort Study Launched. Bethesda. MD: NIH news release; Oct 1, 1997.

27 Flora K, Hahn M, Rosen H, Benner K. Milk thistle (silybum marianum) for the therapy of liver disease. *Am J Gastroenterol.* 1998;93:139–143.

28 Le Bars PL, Katz MM, Berman N, et al. A placebo-controlled, double-blind, randomized trial of an extract of Ginkgo biloba for dementia. North American EGb Study Group. *JAMA.* 1997;278:1327–1332.

29 Wilt TJ, Areef I, Stark G, et al. Saw palmetto extracts for treatment of benign prostatic hyperplasia. *JAMA.* 1998; 280:1604–1609.

30 Schmidt DR, Sobota AE. An examination of the anti-adherence activity of cranberry juice on urinary and nonurinary bacterial isolates. *Microbios.* 1988;55:173–181.

31 FDA Public Health Advisory. Risk of Drug Interactions with St. John's Wort, Indinavir and Other Drugs. Feb. 10, 2000. http://www.fda.gov/cder/drug/advisory/sjwort.htm.

32 Rosenblatt M, Mindel J. Spontaneous hyphema associated with ingestion of Gingko biloba extract. *N Engl J Med.* 1997;336:15, 1108.

33 Edwards C. Lessons from licorice. *N Engl J Med.* 1991;325:1242–1243.

34 Gallagher RE. Arsenic: new life for an old potion. *N Engl J Med.* 1998;339:1389–1390; Lead poisoning associated with use of traditional ethnic remedies-California, 1991–1992. *MMWR.* 1993;42:521–523.

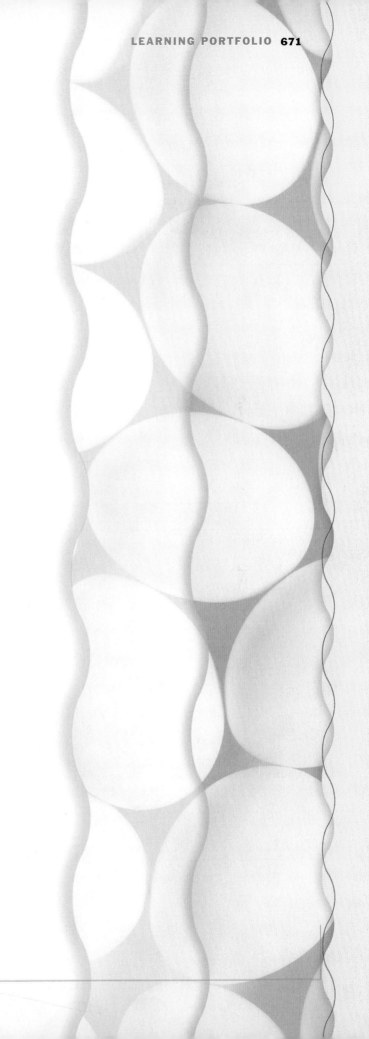

35 Gordon DW, Rosenthal G, Hart J, et al. Chaparral ingestion: the broadening spectrum of liver injury caused by herbal medications. *JAMA.* 1995;273:489–490.

36 DiPaola RS, Zhang H, Lambert GH, et al. Clinical and biologic activity of an estrogenic herbal combination (PC-SPES) in prostate cancer. *N Engl J Med.* 1998;339:785–791.

37 Anticholinergic poisoning associated with herbal tea-New York City, 1994. *MMWR.*1995;44:193–195; and Plantain Adulteration with Foxglove. FDA press release; June 12, 1997.

38 Good Housekeeping Consumer Safety Symposium on Dietary Supplements and Herbal Remedies. New York, NY. March 3, 1998.

39 Herbal roulette. Consumer Reports. Nov 1995:698.

40 Business Guide for Dietary Supplement Industry. Washington DC: Federal Trade Commission press release; Nov 18, 1998.

41 Dietary Supplement Health and Education Act of 1994. US Food and Drug Administration, Center for Food Safety and Applied Nutrition. Dec 1, 1995.

42 Kurtzweil P. An FDA guide to dietary supplements. *FDA Consumer.* Sept-Oct 1998, revised January 1999. http://www.fda.gov/fdac/features/1998/598_guid.html. Accessed 11/5/00.

43 Salvato P, Thompson C, Keister R. Viral load response to augmentation of natural dehydroepiandrosterone (DHEA). Presented at: International Conference on AIDS; July 7–12, 1996; Vancouver, B.C., Canada.

44 Miller DR, et al. Phase I/II trial of the safety and efficacy of shark cartilage in the treatment of advanced cancers. Presented at: The 33rd annual meeting of the American Society of Clinical Oncology; May 17–20, 1997; Denver, CO.

45 Washburn L. Are doctors' side deals prescription for trouble? *Hackensack (NJ) Sunday Record;* Aug 22, 1999: p. A1.

46 The Alpha-Tocopherol, Beta-Carotene and Cancer Prevention Study Group. The effect of vitamin E and beta-carotene on the incidence of lung cancer and other cancers in male smokers. *N Engl J Med.* 1994;330:1029–1035.

47 Kurtzweil P. Op. cit.

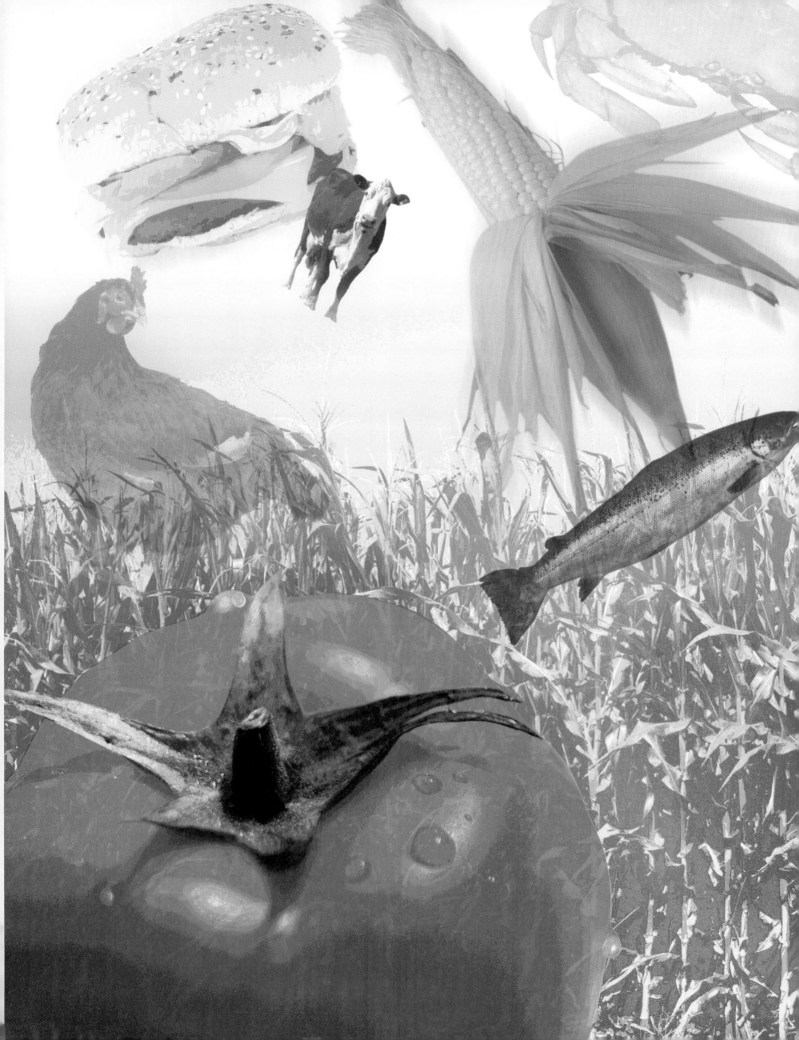

Chapter 17

Food Safety and Technology

Think About It

1 Do you worry about getting sick from the food you eat?

2 To what extent do you rely on organically grown food to avoid pesticides?

3 What food safety measures, such as thawing meat in the refrigerator, do you practice at home?

4 How welcome would genetically modified rice be at your dinner table?

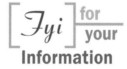

Fyi for your Information

This chapter's FYI boxes include practical information on the following topics:

• Seafood Safety

• Safe Food Practices

• The Saccharin Story

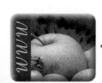

The web site for this book offers many useful tools and is a great source for additional nutrition information for both students and instructors. Visit the site at nutrition.jbpub.com for information on food safety and technology. You'll find exercises that explore the following topics:

• The HACCP Approach to Food Safety

• Genetically Modified Food

• Irradiated Food

• What's Swimming with Your Seafood?

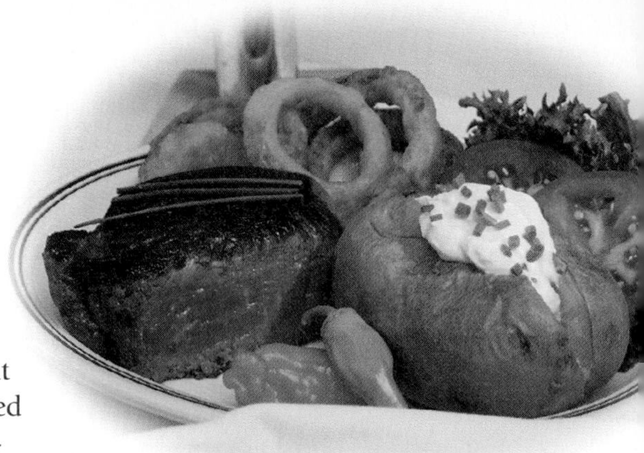

*Y*ou pick up the newspaper and the headline screams, "POORLY COOKED HAMBURGER MEAT PROVES FATAL." You read further and discover that a child's death has been traced to thriving bacteria in under-cooked hamburger meat. Additionally, several adults have become sick from the same source. This worries you. You hate well-done meat. You especially like your hamburgers blood red and your steaks rare. "Well," you ponder, "maybe I'll move my preferences up a notch to pink hamburgers and medium rare steaks." Have you made the right choice? Or should you investigate this issue further?

Once confined mainly to cookbooks and textbooks, food safety advice is showing up in all kinds of places—the popular press, the classroom, even the *Dietary Guidelines for Americans*. What has prompted such enthusiasm? Headlines of recent years tell part of the story. In the 1990s, microbial contamination of such foods as hamburger, apple juice, eggs, raw sprouts, and frozen berries, seriously sickened thousands and killed many, especially those most susceptible: young children, people with compromised immune systems, and seniors.

Consumers are also voicing their concerns about other food safety issues. These concerns include fears about excessive pesticide residues in plant foods, antibiotics and hormones in animals used for food, and hidden food allergens (e.g., nuts, milk, or eggs) in prepared foods. People often fail to recognize that a prepared food contains an ingredient they are allergic to (e.g., caseinates as milk protein) or the allergen may be an unintentional food additive (e.g., peanut residue in a milk chocolate candy from previous processing of peanut butter cups). Other less frequently discussed food hazards include physical contamination with glass fragments and other sharp objects, heavy metals, and naturally occurring toxins in seafood and some agricultural products (**Figure 17.1**).

Food Safety

This chapter reviews major food safety hazards and touches on controversial issues such as the merits of organic foods, the use of food irradiation, and the production of genetically modified foods.

Harmful Substances in Foods

Pathogens

Most food safety experts agree that the chief cause of **foodborne illness** in this country is pathogenic (disease-causing) microorganisms, including bacteria, viruses, and parasites. (See **Table 17.1** for a list of common foodborne microbes and the serious illnesses they cause.) Researchers at the Centers for Disease Control and Prevention (CDC) estimate that foodborne microbes cause 76 million illnesses, 325,000 hospitalizations, and 5,000 deaths in the United States each year.[1] In deriving these figures, researchers corrected for the estimated number of unrecognized and unreported food-caused illnesses. The U.S. Department of Agriculture (USDA) estimates that the seven most common foodborne pathogens

Quick Bites

A Morbid Margin Note

*E*very day 16,000 Americans get sick from something they ate. Twenty-five of them die.

foodborne illness A sickness caused by food contaminated with microorganisms, chemicals, or other substances hazardous to human health.

are responsible for $6.5 billion to $34.9 billion in medical costs and productivity losses each year.[2] Illnesses can range from relatively mild stomach upset to severe symptoms that can be fatal.

Foodborne illnesses can result directly from infection with a pathogen or from toxins produced by a pathogenic microorganism. For example, the bacterium *Staphylococcus aureus* creates havoc with the gastrointestinal tract by producing a toxin. When food containing *S. aureus* stands unrefrigerated, the bacteria begin multiplying. After several hours the expanding bacterial population can produce quantities of a nasty toxin sufficient to cause nausea, vomiting, and abdominal cramps. Staphylococcal food poisoning is extremely common, causing more than a million illnesses each year. Fortunately, the illness usually resolves with no further deleterious effects after a day or so of vomiting and feeling miserable. Another toxin-producing bacterium, *Clostridium botulinum*, causes the rare but deadly illness, botulism. Improperly canned foods, as well as garlic in oil preparations, are sources of **botulism**. Honey can be contaminated with botulinum, but the acid in adult stomachs kills the bacteria. Infants produce insufficient amounts of stomach acid to kill *botulinum*, so even small amounts of contaminated honey can be fatal.

Salmonella bacteria cause many cases of foodborne illness each year. *Salmonella* bacteria are prevalent on poultry and in eggs as well as in a wide

botulism An often fatal type of food poisoning caused by a toxin released from *Clostridium botulinum*, a bacterium that can grow in improperly canned low-acid foods.

Salmonella Rod-shaped bacteria responsible for many foodborne illnesses.

Quick Bites

Saucy *Salmonella*

Hollandaise and Béarnaise sauces may pose health risks because of the infamous *Salmonella* bacteria. Cooks traditionally make these sauces with raw eggs, and even apparently pristine Grade A eggs may harbor the bacteria. Raw cookie dough and certain homemade salad dressings such as Caesar have the same problem.

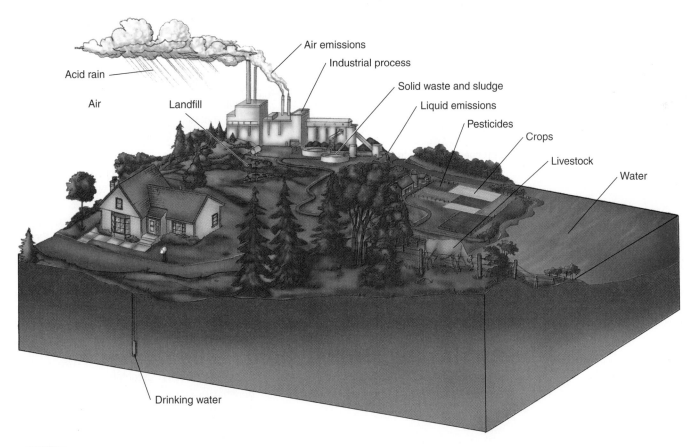

Figure 17.1 **Heavy metals and other contaminants can be found in foods.** Industrial plants and automobiles release heavy metals and other contaminants into the air. Rainfall carries these contaminants to the soil. Plants for food crops and animal feed absorb contaminants from the soil. Runoff can pick up contaminants from pesticides, fertilizer and animal manure. This pollutes surface water (lakes and streams), ground water, and coastal water. Polluted water contaminates seafood and other fish that people eat.

Escherichia coli (E. coli) Bacteria that are the most common cause of urinary tract infections. Because they release toxins, *E. coli* can rapidly cause shock and death.

variety of other foods. Choosing eggs cooked "over easy" could be disastrous because inadequate cooking can leave you vulnerable to the misery of salmonellosis. (See the FYI feature "Safe Food Practices" for more information on how to protect yourself from foodborne illness.)

Scientists long have know that pathogens, such as *Salmonella* and *Clostridium botulinum*, cause foodborne illness, but other microbes, such as *Escherichia coli* (*E. coli*), did not emerge as foodborne pathogens until the past decade. Also, some foods that had not been known to harbor pathogenic microorganisms are now recognized as possible sources.

Table 17.1 **Common Foodborne Pathogens and Illnesses**

Organism	Sources	Diseases and Symptoms
Bacteria		
Campylobacter jejuni	Raw poultry and meat and unpasteurized milk	Campylobacteriosis **Onset:** usually 2 to 5 days after eating **Symptoms:** diarrhea, stomach cramps, fever, bloody stools. Lasts 7 to 10 days
Clostridium botulinum—illness is caused by a toxin produced by this organism	Improperly canned foods such as corn, green beans, soups, beets, asparagus, mushrooms, tuna, and liver pate; also, luncheon meats, ham, sausage, garlic in oil, lobster, and smoked and salted fish	Botulism **Onset:** usually 4 to 36 hours after eating **Symptoms:** nerve dysfunction, such as double vision, inability to swallow, speech difficulty, and progressive paralysis of respiratory system; can lead to death
Escherichia coli O157:H7	Raw or undercooked meat, raw vegetables, unpasteurized milk, minimally processed ciders and juices, water	*E. coli* infection **Onset:** few days after eating **Symptoms:** watery and bloody diarrhea, severe stomach cramps, dehydration, colitis, neurological symptoms, stroke, and hemolytic uremic syndrome (HUS), a particularly serious disease in young children that can cause kidney failure and death
Listeria monocytogenes	Soft cheeses, unpasteurized milk, imported seafood products, frozen cooked crab meat, cooked shrimp, surimi (imitation shellfish) Note: resists salt, heat, nitrite and acidity better than most microorganisms	Listeriosis **Onset:** from 7 to 30 days after eating, but symptoms have been reported 2 to 3 days after eating **Symptoms:** fever, headache, nausea, and vomiting; primarily affects pregnant women and their fetuses, newborns, older adults, people with cancer and compromised immune systems; can cause death in fetuses and babies
Salmonella species	Meats, poultry; eggs, milk, ice cream, and other dairy products; seafood; fresh produce, including raw sprouts; coconut; pasta; chocolate; foods containing raw eggs	Salmonellosis **Onset:** usually 6 to 48 hours after eating **Symptoms:** nausea, abdominal cramps, diarrhea, fever, and headache
Shigella bacteria	Undercooked liquid or moist food that has been handled by an infectious person	Shigellosis (bacillary dysentery) **Onset:** 1 to 7 days after eating **Symptoms:** stomach cramps, diarrhea, fever, sometimes vomiting, and blood, pus, mucus in stools

Unpasteurized fruit and vegetable juices, for example, can contain harmful bacteria that make some people sick. Contaminated water also has gained greater recognition as a source of foodborne pathogens.[3] Today we know that many foods, including eggs, dairy products, meat and poultry, seafood, fresh produce, juices, and cereal grains, can harbor disease-causing bacteria.

Because bacteria and other infectious organisms are pervasive in the environment, the contamination of food can occur anywhere from the farm to your plate. Many organisms capable of causing foodborne illness in humans are naturally present in food-producing animals and their environ-

Table 17.1 **Common Foodborne Pathogens and Illnesses—continued**

Organism	Sources	Diseases and Symptoms
Bacteria		
Staphylococcus aureus—illness is caused by a toxin produced by this organism	Meat and poultry; egg products; tuna, potato, and macaroni salads; cream-filled pastries and other foods left unrefrigerated for long periods *S. aureus* is frequently found in cuts on skin and in nasal passages.	Staphylococcal food poisoning **Onset:** 30 minutes to 8 hours after eating **Symptoms:** diarrhea, vomiting, nausea, stomach pain, and cramps; lasts 1 to 2 days
Vibrio vulnificus	Raw seafood, especially raw oysters	*Vibrio* infection **Onset:** 6 hours to a few days **Symptoms:** chills, fever, nausea and vomiting, and possibly death, especially in people with underlying health problems
Viruses		
Hepatitis A	Raw shellfish from polluted water, food handled by an infected person	Hepatitis A **Onset:** average about 1 month after exposure **Symptoms:** at first, malaise, loss of appetite, nausea, vomiting, and fever; after 3 to 10 days, jaundice and darkened urine; severe cases can result in liver damage and death
Norwalk virus	Raw shellfish from polluted water; salads, sandwiches, and other ready-to-eat foods handled by an infected person	Gastroenteritis **Onset:** 1 to 3 days **Symptoms:** nausea, vomiting, diarrhea, stomach pain, headache, and low-grade fever
Protozoa		
Anisakis	Raw fish	Anisakis infection **Onset:** 12 to 24 hours **Symptoms:** abdominal pain, can be severe
Cryptosporidium	Food that comes in contact with sewage-contaminated water; foods handled by a person who did not wash hands after using the toilet	Cryptosporidiosis **Onset:** 1 to 12 days **Symptoms:** profuse watery stools, stomach pain, loss of appetite, vomiting, and low-grade fever
Giardia lamblia	Consumption of contaminated water, contamination of food by infected food worker	Giardiasis **Onset:** 1 to 3 days **Symptoms:** diarrhea, abdominal cramps, nausea
Toxoplasma gondii	Raw or undercooked meat, and, under certain conditions unwashed fruits and vegetables; also cats shed cysts in their feces during acute infection—organism may be transmitted to humans, if feces are handled.	Toxoplasmosis **Onset:** 10 to 13 days **Symptoms:** fever, headache, rash, sore muscles, diarrhea; can kill a fetus or cause severe defects, such as mental retardation

How many *Salmonella* does it take?

In 1994, 224,000 people in 41 states came down with *Salmonella* food poisoning from eating ice cream. The amazing part? The ice cream contained only about six *Salmonella* bacteria per serving.

ment. For example, *Salmonella enteritidis* enter eggs directly from the egg-laying hen,[4] and *E. coli* are normally present in the intestines of cattle. Microorganisms natural to the marine environment, but toxic to humans, can contaminate seafood. (See the FYI feature "Seafood Safety.")

Exposure to animal manure or sewage runoff can contaminate crops. Sewage runoff into rivers and streams also can contaminate fish that live there. In the food-processing stage, contamination can occur from food contact with dirty equipment, rodent droppings, improper food storage, and infectious employees who fail to wash their hands adequately or take proper precautions when handling food. Poor food safety practices in retail facilities and at home also can contaminate food.

Patterns of foodborne illness have changed dramatically over the last several decades as our food production has become more centralized. When food animals and produce were grown, prepared, and eaten on the family farm, the consequences of errors in food handling were generally limited to a single family. Now, much of the food we eat is mass produced at central locations and distributed widely to restaurant chains and supermarkets. Although most food poisoning cases arise from poor food handling in homes and restaurants, if a processing plant contaminates food, hundreds or even thou-

Fyi Seafood Safety

FOR YOUR INFORMATION

Seafood can be a delicious and heart-healthy part of our diets. However, as with all food, contamination can have serious consequences. Seafood is one of the most rapidly perishable foods, so proper refrigeration and rapid processing and transport to the consumer are essential. Although certain types of microbial contaminants and toxins are unique to seafood, properly handled and cooked seafood is as safe to eat as most other foods.

Eating raw seafood, on the other hand, is risky business. Despite the popularity of such dishes as sashimi, sushi, and raw oysters, uncooked fish, no matter how carefully prepared, poses a risk for infection. People with liver disease, diabetes, cancer, or other diseases that impair immune function should be especially careful to stay away from raw seafood. Pregnant women also should avoid uncooked seafood; some physicians recommend that pregnant women avoid seafood altogether. The rest of us should think twice before enjoying those raw oysters and sashimi, and at the very least, make sure they are fresh and from a reliable source before letting those slippery delicacies pass our lips.

Seafood-related illness falls into several categories. Sources of infections include bacteria, viruses, and parasites. Toxins occur naturally in some fish, and human pollution may contaminate seafood. The following are several examples of seafood-caused illness:

- Raw or undercooked shellfish such as oysters, clams, and mussels may be contaminated with bacteria such as *Salmonella*, *Vibrio* species, and *Staphylococcus aureus*. Hepatitis A (caused by a virus) and gastroenteritis are other illnesses that can be contracted by eating uncooked shellfish from polluted waters.
- Fish such as mahi-mahi, tuna, and bluefish that have begun to spoil can cause scombroid poisoning. A toxin in these decomposing fish causes flushing, itching, and headache. Cooking does not destroy the toxin, so the best prevention is proper refrigeration and rapid use of fresh fish.
- Some tropical fish such as red snapper and barracuda may contain ciguatera toxin, which can cause gastrointestinal and neurological problems in humans.

Larger warm-water fish are most often implicated in this illness. The toxin is actually produced by tiny plants that are eaten by small fish. When larger fish consume many small fish, the toxin can accumulate. The flesh of these large fish may contain enough of the toxin to make humans very ill. Heating or freezing does not destroy this toxin.

- *Anisakis* is a parasite found in raw fish. After a person eats an infected fish, the larvae of this roundworm can invade the human stomach, causing severe abdominal pain. Cooking or freezing the fish for at least 72 hours can kill this parasite.
- Red tide is a well-known phenomenon in which huge numbers of tiny toxic organisms called dinoflagellates infest seawater. Shellfish in the area become poisonous as a result. The effects of eating shellfish from red tide areas can include respiratory paralysis and death.
- Human pollution is a serious problem, especially near population centers where industrial wastes and human sewage flow into the water. Heavy metals such as mercury can accumulate in

sands of people can be made ill. This can have nationwide implications and, therefore, receives intense national media attention.

Key Concepts: *Foodborne pathogens are a major cause of illness in North America. Pathogenic (disease-causing) microorganisms include bacteria, viruses, and parasites. Contamination of food can occur at many points along the chain from farm to table.*

Chemical Contamination

Food safety experts view chemical contamination of food as a less significant public health hazard than contamination with pathogenic microorganisms. Yet surveys and retail trends suggest that consumers think otherwise. To avoid foods exposed to chemicals, more and more people are turning to **organic foods**. (See the section "Organic Alternatives" on p. 681.) Chemical contaminants include pesticides, drugs, pollutants, and natural toxins.

Pesticides **Pesticides** play an important role in food production—controlling plant diseases, weeds, insects, and other pests. Pesticides protect crops and ensure a substantial yield, thus assuring consumers of a wide variety of foods at affordable prices. Without these chemicals, many argue that crop production would fall and prices for food would rise.

organic foods Foods that originate from farms or handling operations that meet the standards set by the USDA National Organic Program.

pesticides Chemicals used to control insects, diseases, weeds, fungi, and other pests on plants, vegetables, fruits, and animals.

larger fish (e.g., sharks and swordfish) that have been exposed to mercury in their environment for long periods. Since commercially caught fish generally contain minimal amounts of mercury, even large fish are safe to eat, although pregnant women are advised to avoid eating shark or swordfish more than once a month.

- Dioxin and polychlorinated biphenols (PCBs) also can accumulate in fish living in polluted water. Commercial seafood companies tend to avoid contaminated areas, but local fishers who frequently catch and eat fish from these waters may be at some risk.[1]

1 US Food and Drug Administration. FDA and Seafood Safety. Washington, DC: Author; 1991.

Table A: **Understanding Seafood Safety**

Condition	Explanation
Scombroid poisoning	Scombroid poisoning is a type of food intoxication caused by the consumption of scombroid and scombroid-like marine fish species that have begun to spoil with the growth of particular types of food bacteria. Fish most commonly involved are members of the *Scombridae* family (tunas and mackerels), and a few nonscombroid relatives (bluefish, dolphin or mahi-mahi, and amberjacks). The suspect toxin is an elevated level of histamine generated by bacterial degradation of substances in the muscle protein.
Anisakis	*Anisakis simplex* (herring worm) and *Pseudoterranova* (*Phocanema, Terranova*) *decipiens* (cod or seal worm) are anisakid nematodes (roundworms) that have been implicated in human infections caused by the consumption of raw or undercooked seafood. Anisakiasis is the term generally used to refer to the acute disease in humans.
Red tide	When temperature, salinity, and nutrients reach certain levels, algae grow very fast or "bloom" and accumulate into dense, visible patches near the surface of the water. "Red tide" is a common name for such a phenomenon where certain species of phytoplankton contain reddish pigments and "bloom" such that the water appears to be colored red. The term red tide is a misnomer because it is not associated with tides. A small number of species produce potent neurotoxins that can cause illness and even death.
Polychlorinated biphenols (PCBs)	A group of toxic, persistent chemicals used as insulation for transformers and capacitors and as lubricants in gas pipeline systems. PCBs are a serious health problem because of their persistence in the environment, accumulation in the body, and potential for a long-term negative effect on health. In the U.S., their manufacture was stopped in 1976.

Every year, the U.S. Food and Drug Administration (FDA) collects about 10,000 samples of domestic and imported food and analyzes them for pesticide residues.[5] Since 1987 the FDA has found no illegal residues in more than 99 percent of domestic and more than 95 percent of imported samples. When a violation occurred, it usually involved the use of a pesticide on crops for which it had not been approved, rather than an excessive level. In 1999 the FDA found no residues in more than 60 percent of the samples.[6]

The FDA also samples and analyzes domestic and imported animal feeds for pesticide residues. This monitoring focuses on feeds for livestock and poultry—animals that become or produce foods for human consumption. In 1999 the FDA analyzed 463 domestic and 61 imported feed samples. Only two of these samples exceeded an established EPA tolerance or a FDA requested maximum level.[7]

Despite these reassuring results, concerns about pesticides in food persist. Processing methods can either reduce or concentrate pesticide residue in foods (see **Figure 17.2**). Infants and young children are particularly susceptible to the hazards of pesticides. Their small size and rapid growth make them especially vulnerable to pesticide residues, which can accumulate in their bodies over their lifetimes. Enacted in 1996, the Food Quality Protection Act includes landmark protections for the young. For the first time, manufacturers must show that pesticide levels are safe for infants and children. In addition, when determining a safe level for a pesticide in a food, the Environmental Protection Agency (EPA) now must account for the cumulative effect of exposures to similar pesticides and toxic chemicals.[8]

Consumers Union (the nonprofit publisher of Consumer Reports) issued a report stating that legally permitted pesticide levels in some foods are much higher than the levels that scientific data show are safe for children.[9] Consumers Union analyzed data collected by the USDA's Pesticide Data Program and concluded that a relatively small number of highly toxic

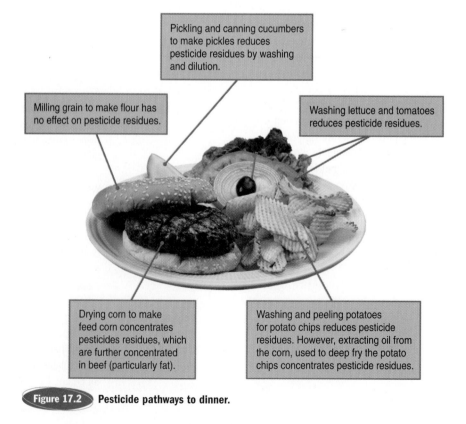

Pickling and canning cucumbers to make pickles reduces pesticide residues by washing and dilution.

Milling grain to make flour has no effect on pesticide residues.

Washing lettuce and tomatoes reduces pesticide residues.

Drying corn to make feed corn concentrates pesticides residues, which are further concentrated in beef (particularly fat).

Washing and peeling potatoes for potato chips reduces pesticide residues. However, extracting oil from the corn, used to deep fry the potato chips concentrates pesticide residues.

Figure 17.2 Pesticide pathways to dinner.

insecticides accounted for most of the toxicity in foods. Consumers Union suggests that focusing on reducing or eliminating these high-risk pesticides may be the best way to reduce toxicity from our foods.

To decrease pesticide intake, Consumers Union recommends washing and peeling (if possible) fruits and vegetables, and eating a variety of produce.[10] Because the benefits of these foods far outweigh the risks from the pesticides they might contain, Consumers Union emphasizes that it does not recommend eating fewer fruits and vegetables.

Excessive use of synthetic pesticides, herbicides, and fertilizers contributes substantially to the pollution of soil and water. Overuse can be particularly hazardous to farm workers whose exposure to these chemicals typically is much higher than that of general consumers. Overuse also threatens wildlife. Today, many farmers use alternatives to reduce pesticide use. (See **Figure 17.3.**) Their methods include crop rotation, use of natural rather than synthetic pesticides, and planting nonfood crops nearby that lure pests away from food crops. Releasing sterile fruit flies into orchards also allows reductions in pesticide use. Because fruit flies produce no offspring when they mate with sterile partners, the overall fruit fly population drops.

Organic Alternatives   Organic foods are grown or produced without synthetic pesticides and without synthetic fertilizer. Sales of organic foods totaled $3.5 billion in 1996, and the market is growing at least 20 percent a year.[11] Growth of the industry reflects, in part, America's distrust of technology, and a desire to return to a simpler, more "natural" way of food production.

The Organic Foods Production Act and the National Organic Program (NOP) are intended to assure consumers that the organic foods they purchase are produced, processed, and certified to consistent national standards. The labeling requirements of the new program apply to raw, fresh produce and to processed foods that contain organic ingredients. Foods that are sold, labeled, or represented as organic must be produced and processed in accordance with the NOP standards.[12] **Table 17.2** outlines the requirements for labeling organic food.

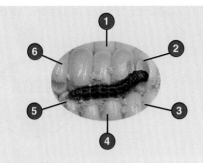

1. **Legal control**
   State and federal guidelines are designed to limit the spread of pests.

2. **Biological control**
   Beneficial organisms, such as predators, parasites, and viruses, are released into the environment to suppress pest organisms.

3. **Cultural control**
   Rotation, sanitation, and other good farming techniques are employed to help reduce pest populations.

4. **Physical control**
   Barriers, traps, and the location and timing of planting are all used to control pest infestations.

5. **Genetic control**
   Resistant plant strains are developed to reduce the impact of pests.

6. **Chemical control**
   Conventional pesticides, biopesticides, pheromones, and other chemicals are used to prevent or suppress pest outbreaks. The chemical controls are specific to a pest species and are ideally short-lived in the environment. In addition, the chemicals are used at their lowest effective rate and may be alternated to help prevent the development of pest resistance.

Figure 17.3   Integrated pest management.

Table 17.2   **Labeling Requirements for Organic Food**

Labeling requirements are based on the percentage of a product's ingredients that are organic.

Foods labeled "100 percent organic" and "organic"

- Products labeled "100 percent organic" must contain only organically produced raw or processed products (excluding water and salt).
- Products labeled "organic" must consist of at least 95 percent organically produced ingredients (excluding water and salt). Any other ingredients must consist of nonagricultural substances or non-organically produced agricultural products approved and on the National List maintained by the USDA National Organic Program.
- Products that meet the requirements may display these terms on their principal display panel.
- The USDA seal and the seal or mark of certifying agents may appear on product packages and in advertisements.

Processed products labeled "made with organic (specified ingredients)"

- Products that contain 50 to 95 percent organic ingredients can use the phrase "made with organic (specified ingredients)" and list up to three of the organic ingredients on the principal display panel. For example, organic beef stew can be labeled stew, "made with organic beef, potatoes, and carrots."
- The certifying agent's seal or mark may be used on the package. However, the USDA seal cannot be used anywhere on the package.

Processed products that contain less than 50 percent organic ingredients

- The packaging of these products can make no organic claim except on the information panel, and must specify the ingredients that are organically produced.

Other labeling provisions

- The package information panel of any product labeled "organic" must state the actual percentage of organic ingredients and use the word *organic* to modify each organically produced ingredient.
- The name and address of the certifying agent of the final product must be displayed on the information panel.
- There are no restrictions on labeling claims such as "pesticide free," "no drugs or growth hormones used," or "sustainably harvested."

Source: USDA. National Organic Program, Agricultural Marketing Service. Washington, DC. June 2000.

Under the NOP, farm and processing operations that grow and process organic foods must be certified by the USDA. The certification process includes an on-site inspection that must verify that the applicant's operation is in compliance with strict national organic standards. Certifying agents may collect and test soil, water, waste, plant and animal tissues, and processed products. A certified operation may label its products or ingredients as organic and may use the "USDA Certified Organic" seal.

Despite a lack of scientific evidence that genetic engineering and irradiation of foods present unacceptable risks, public opposition led the NOP to prohibit use of these technologies with organic foods. While these methods have been approved for use in general agricultural production and may offer certain benefits for the environment and human health, consumers strongly oppose their use in organically grown foods. Since the use of these methods runs counter to consumer expectations, foods produced with these techniques are prohibited from carrying the organic label.[13]

Organic food advocates claim that using natural fertilizer, such as manure, produces a soil that is richer in a range of nutrients, as opposed to chemical fertilizers that typically contain only a few basic nutrients. They reason that organically fertilized soils produce foods that contain more nutrients. Analyses, however, find no evidence of consistent nutritional differences between organic and conventionally grown foods.[14]

Organic farming has its drawbacks. The use of manure raises food safety concerns. The organic producer must manage animal and plant waste materials so they do not contribute to contamination of crops, soil, or water. Manure runoff can pollute nearby lakes and streams. Other critics charge that organic farming is "elitist," that synthetic fertilizers and pesticides are necessary to meet the food needs of an expanding world population. They also point out that complete freedom from pesticides cannot be guaranteed, no matter how carefully a food is produced, since pesticide residues may still exist in soil, water, and air.[15]

Organic foods are not pesticide-free foods. Organic farmers can use natural and approved synthetic pesticides to control weeds and insects.[16] Microbial contaminants that cause foodborne illness can be found in organic as well as conventional foods. Consumers must handle all food appropriately, whether organically or conventionally grown.

Think About It

2

Animal Drugs Current agricultural practice depends heavily on the use of drugs in food animals and food-producing animals raised specifically to provide meat, milk, and eggs. Producers use drugs to maintain animal health and well-being, as well as increase production. Maintenance of good animal health reduces the chance that disease will spread from animals to humans. But drugs used in animals could enter human food and possibly increase the risk of ill health in humans. Many researchers fear that overuse of animal antibiotics could contribute to the emergence of antibiotic-resistant microorganisms that could threaten human health. A less widespread problem is the potential for humans with drug allergies to have reactions to drug residues in food-producing animals. Some people worry that the widespread use of hormones may impair animal health or the quality of the food obtained from treated animals.

There are five major classes of drugs used in animals raised for food:

1. topical antiseptics, bactericides, and fungicides used to treat skin or hoof infections, cuts, and abrasions;

2. ionophores, which alter stomach microorganisms to digest feeds more efficiently and to help protect against some parasites;

3. hormone and hormonelike production enhancers (anabolic hormones for meat production and bovine somatotropin for increased milk production in dairy cows);

4. antiparasite;

5. antibiotics used to prevent infections, treat disease, and promote growth. Healthy animals can use nutrients for growth and production rather than to fight infection.[17]

The FDA is responsible for ensuring that drugs approved for use in animals are safe not only for the animals but also for humans who eat food produced from the animals. In addition, the FDA enforces regulations to ensure that drugs are used properly in cows, chickens, and seafood. However, FDA surveillance is not perfect; government investigations have revealed that a few U.S. veterinarians and farmers illegally use animal drugs that are known to be dangerous to humans.

Pollutants Pollutants from animal manure and other wastes, factories, human sewage, and other runoff can contaminate food-production areas. For example, some scientists theorize that **dioxin** contamination of foods may cause human cancer. Dioxins are chemical compounds created in the manufacturing, combustion, and chlorine bleaching of pulp and paper, and in other industrial processes.[18] Dioxins can accumulate in the food chain, and are potent animal carcinogens. Fish from dioxin-polluted waters can contain significant amounts of dioxin. The commercial fishing industry avoids areas of known dioxin pollution. Dioxins in tiny amounts are found in food packages, paper plates, and coffee filters made of bleached paper. Because the quantity of this toxic chemical is minimal, however, the FDA has concluded that use of these products poses no significant risk to human health.

Natural Toxins Other chemical contamination of food can occur from **natural toxins.**[19] Examples include

- **aflatoxins** in contaminated food or animal feed. Aflatoxins are produced by certain strains of *Aspergillus* fungi under certain conditions of temperature and humidity. The most pronounced contamination has been found in tree nuts, peanuts, and other oilseeds, such as corn and cottonseed. Aflatoxins have been implicated as a factor in the development of liver cancer, particularly in parts of the world where food and water are frequently contaminated with this fungus.

- **ciguatera** and other marine toxins. These toxins can accumulate in seafood (mainly in large tropical fish) and when ingested, cause serious problems including paralysis, amnesia, and nerve toxicity. Commercial fishers avoid waters known to harbor ciguatera toxin. Ciguatera poisoning sometimes occurs when these fish are caught as part of recreational fishing. Cooking does not destroy these toxins.

- **methyl mercury.** Mercury occurs naturally in the environment and is produced by human activities. It is soluble in water, where bacteria can cause chemical changes that transform mercury to methyl mercury, a more toxic form. Fish absorb methyl mercury from water passing over their gills and by eating other contaminated aquatic species. Because larger predatory fish can consume many contaminated smaller fish, they accumulate higher levels of methyl mercury. (See **Figure 17.4.**)

- **poisonous mushrooms.** These plants produce toxic substances that can cause stomach upset, dizziness, hallucinations, and other neurological symptoms.[20] The more lethal mushroom species can cause liver and kidney failure, coma, and death.

dioxin A contaminant of a widely used herbicide. Because of its toxicity, the herbicide is no longer manufactured in the United States.

natural toxins Poisons that are produced by or naturally occur in plants or microorganisms

aflatoxins Carcinogenic and toxic factors produced by food molds.

ciguatera A toxin found in more than 300 species of Caribbean and South Pacific fish. It is a nonbacterial source of food poisoning.

methyl mercury A toxic compound that results from the chemical transformation of mercury by bacteria. Mercury is water soluble in trace amounts and contaminates many water bodies.

poisonous mushrooms Mushrooms that contain toxins that can cause stomach upset, dizziness, hallucinations, and other neurological symptoms.

Quick Bites

Well-Traveled Dioxin

In Nunavut, Canada's newest province, the breast milk of native Inuits has twice the average concentration of dioxin than milk of women in southern Quebec. Native Inuits primarily eat fatty animals high on the food chain. They accumulate dioxin, but where did the dioxin originate? Not Canada. Most comes from industrial combustion in eastern and midwestern United States and some originates as far away as Mexico.

solanine A potentially toxic alkaloid that is present with chlorophyll in the green areas on potato skins.

Food Allergy Network A nonprofit organization devoted to increasing public awareness of food allergy and anaphylaxis (a life-threatening reaction), educating the public about food allergies, and advancing research on food allergies.

- **solanine,** a toxic substance in raw potato skins.[21] Solanine develops in the greenish layer of improperly stored potatoes. It can be removed by thoroughly peeling the potato.

A variety of compounds in herbs and spices also can be toxic. However, foodborne illness caused by these and other natural toxins is relatively rare compared with illness from pathogenic microorganisms.

Other Food Contaminants For people allergic to certain food substances, the inadvertent addition of an allergenic substance to a food whose labeling does not identify the ingredient can constitute a major hazard. The most common food allergens, according to the **Food Allergy Network**, are milk, eggs, wheat, peanuts and other nuts, fish, shellfish, and soy.[22] (See **Figure 17.5.**) In an allergic person, these foods can cause a variety of reactions, including gastrointestinal problems, skin irritation, breathing difficulty, shock, and even death.

Whether intentionally added through tampering or unintentionally during food production, glass, metal, and other objects also are food contaminants that can have serious health consequences. Misuse of cleaning agents in food-contact areas such as refrigerator trucks, food-production lines, and storage units can introduce undesirable chemicals into food. While generally not a health hazard, insects, dirt, and other undesirable items also can contaminate a food.

Figure 17.4 **Toxins become concentrated as you move up the food chain**.

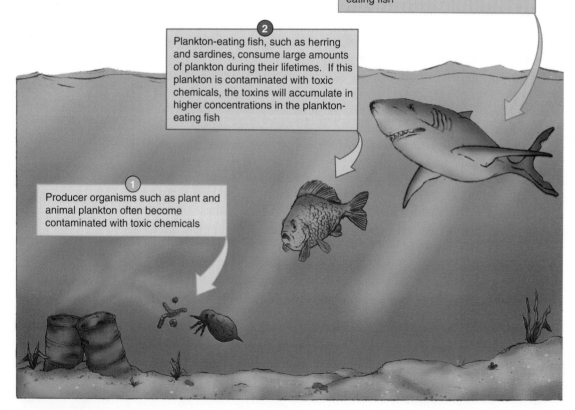

Carnivorous fish, such as swordfish and tuna, consume plankton-eating fish thus accumulating toxins in still higher concentrations. Carnivorous fish are therefore likely to contain higher concentrations of toxins than plankton-eating fish

Plankton-eating fish, such as herring and sardines, consume large amounts of plankton during their lifetimes. If this plankton is contaminated with toxic chemicals, the toxins will accumulate in higher concentrations in the plankton-eating fish

Producer organisms such as plant and animal plankton often become contaminated with toxic chemicals

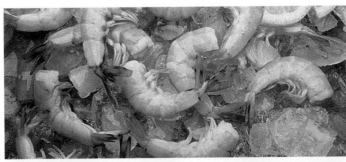

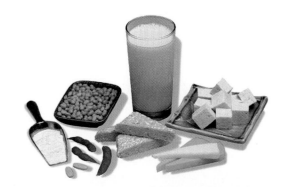

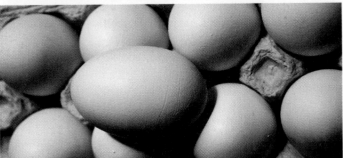

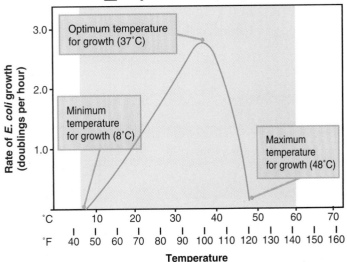

Figure 17.5 Foods that commonly cause allergic reactions.

Key Concepts: *Chemical contaminants in foods include pesticides, natural toxins, and contamination related to pollution. Organic foods, like conventionally grown foods, can still be contaminated.*

Keeping Food Safe

The fifth edition of the *Dietary Guidelines for Americans*, released in 2000, contains a new guideline: "Keep food safe to eat." Having safe foods to eat requires the efforts of a great many people along the way from the farm to your plate. Imagine yourself enjoying a nice piece of broiled chicken. Consider that harmful contamination of that chicken could have occurred at the farm, in the processing plant, or during transportation to the supermarket. Once at the supermarket, the chicken might have been underrefrigerated or kept too long before being sold. After buying the chicken, you might have left it in a warm car, or kept it in a refrigerator that was not cold enough. Your kitchen hygiene might not have been the best, and finally, you could have undercooked the chicken. Considering the many opportunities for contamination, it is truly amazing that most of the time our food does not make us sick. **Figure 17.6** illustrates the growth of microbes that can contaminate food.

Keeping foods free from contamination is a job that falls to many parties. It is not only the responsibility of government officials at the national, state, and local levels, but of everyone who comes in contact with food—the producer, the manufacturer, the retailer, and ultimately the consumer.

Government Agencies

The basis of modern food law is the Federal Food, Drug, and Cosmetic (FD&C) Act of 1938, which gives the FDA authority over food and food ingredients and defines

Quick Bites

Early Food Laws

In 1202 King John of England proclaimed the first English food law, the Assize of Bread, which prohibited adulteration of bread with such ingredients as ground peas or beans. Regulation of food in the United States dates from early colonial times. In 1785 Massachusetts enacted the first general food-adulteration law in the United States.

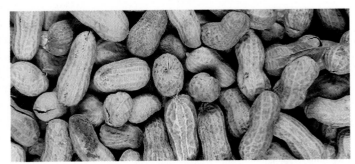

Figure 17.6 **Growth of microorganisms.** *E. coli* bacteria grow best between 8°C and 48°C (46°–118°F). Because most microbial growth occurs between 40°–140°, this is called the "Danger Zone."

requirements for truthful labeling of ingredients. Today at the federal level, six agencies (**Figure 17.7**) share responsibility for food safety:

1. *The Food and Drug Administration (FDA)* enforces laws governing safety of domestic and imported food, except meat and poultry.
2. *The Centers for Disease Control and Prevention (CDC)* monitors outbreaks of foodborne diseases, investigates their causes, and determines proper prevention.
3. *The USDA Food Safety and Inspection Service (FSIS)* enforces laws governing safety of domestic and imported meat and poultry products.
4. *The USDA Cooperative State Research, Education, and Extension Service (CSREES)* develops research and education programs on food safety for farmers and consumers.
5. *The USDA Agricultural Research Service (ARS)* conducts research to extend knowledge of various agricultural practices, including those involving animal and crop safety.
6. *The Environmental Protection Agency (EPA)* regulates public drinking water and approves pesticides and other chemicals used in the environment.

Figure 17.7 Government agencies that help protect our food supply.

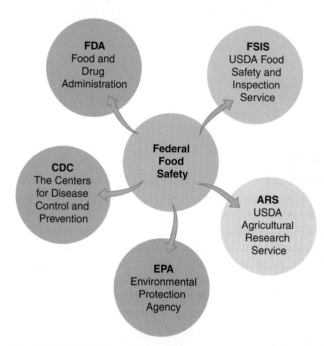

OTHER AGENCIES WITH FOOD SAFETY RESPONSIBILITIES

FTC
- Regulates the advertising and marketing of food products.
- Has the authority to take legal action against unwarranted advertising claims.

Department of Justice
- Seizes products when federal food safety laws are violated.
- Prosecutes suspected violators of food safety laws.

Bureau of Alcohol, Tobacco and Firearms (BATF)
- Enforces laws that involve the production, distribution, and labeling of most alcoholic beverages.
- Sometimes shares responsibilities with FDA when alcoholic beverages are adulterated or contain food or color additives, pesticides, or contaminants.

National Marine Fisheries Service (NMFS)
- Responsible for seafood quality and identification, fisheries management and development, habitat conservation, and aquaculture production.

State and Local Governments
- Inspects restaurants, retail food outlets, dairies, grain mills, and other food establishments within their area of jurisdiction.
- Embargoes illegal food products in many situations.

State and local health and agricultural departments oversee food safety in their jurisdictions, often in conjunction with federal agencies.

The public's heightened concern about food safety is evident in the creation of new consumer advocacy groups such as **S.T.O.P. (Safe Tables Our Priority)**, a national organization that works with government agencies and industry to prevent foodborne illnesses and deaths. In addition, the federal **Food Safety Initiative** calls on the federal government to take the lead in expanding research, training, and education about safety at all levels of food production.[23] The Food Safety Initiative has expanded the use of the food industry safety system called **Hazard Analysis Critical Control Point, or HACCP** (pronounced "hassip"). The Food Safety Initiative has also created a campaign to educate consumers, health professionals (such as doctors), and retail establishments about food safety. Other goals of the Food Safety Initiative include improved detection of foodborne pathogens and prevention of microbial growth during food production and distribution.[24]

Hazard Analysis Critical Control Point

Hazard Analysis Critical Control Point is a food industry program that focuses on preventing contamination by identifying areas in food production and retail where contamination could occur. HACCP is intended to replace the traditional system of spot-checks of food manufacturing conditions and random sampling of final products. The old system could uncover problems only after they had occurred, whereas HACCP works by preventing contamination.

Companies and retailers analyze their food-production processes and determine "**critical control points**" (CCP)—points at which hazards could occur. They then determine measures that they can institute at these points to prevent, control, or eliminate the hazards. (See **Figure 17.8**.) Critical control points can occur anywhere in a food's production—from its raw state through processing and shipping to purchase by the consumer. Preventive measures can include proper cooking, chilling, and sanitizing, as well as preventing cross-contamination and improving employee hygiene.

The USDA requires HACCP for meat and poultry, the food products it regulates.[25] The FDA, which regulates all other foods, requires HACCP in the seafood and low-acid canned-food industries and has proposed it for the juice industry.[26] Also, the FDA has incorporated HACCP principles in its **Food Code**,

Safe Tables Our Priority (S.T.O.P.) A national organization devoted to preventing illness and death from foodborne illness by working with government agencies and industry to encourage practices and policies that promote safe food.

Food Safety Initiative A 1996 presidential directive to three Cabinet members to identify specific steps to improve the safety of the U.S. food supply.

Hazard Analysis Critical Control Point (HACCP) A modern food safety system that focuses on preventing contamination by identifying potential areas in food production and retail in which contamination could occur and taking steps to ensure contaminants are not introduced at these points.

critical control points (CCP) An operational step or procedure in a process, production method, or recipe, at which control can be applied to prevent, reduce, or eliminate a food safety hazard.

Food Code A reference published periodically by the Food and Drug Administration for restaurants, grocery stores, institutional food services vending operations, and other retailers on how to store, prepare, and serve food to prevent foodborne illness.

HACCP: HAZARD ANALYSIS CRITICAL CONTROL POINT

Step 1: Analyze hazards. Identify the potential hazards associated with a food. The hazard could be biological (e.g., a microbe), chemical (e.g., mercury), or physical (e.g., ground glass or metal).

Step 2: Identify critical control points (CCPs). Identify points in a food's production path—from its raw state through processing and shipping to consumption —where a potential hazard can be controlled or eliminated. Examples of CCPs are cooking, chilling, handling, cleaning, and storage.

Step 3: Establish preventative measures with critical limits for each control point. An example is setting the minimum cooking temperature and time to ensure safety for a particular food (the temperature and time are critical limits).

Step 4: Establish procedures to monitor the control points. Such procedures might include determining how and by whom cooking time and temperature should be monitored.

Step 5: Establish corrective actions to be taken when a critical limit has not been met—for example, reprocessing or disposing of food if the minimum cooking temperature is not met.

Step 6: Establish effective record keeping to document the HACCP system.

Step 7: Establish procedures to verify that the system is working consistently—for example, testing time-recording and temperature-recording devised to verify that a cooking unit is working properly.

Figure 17.8 **HACCP anticipates and prevents problems.**

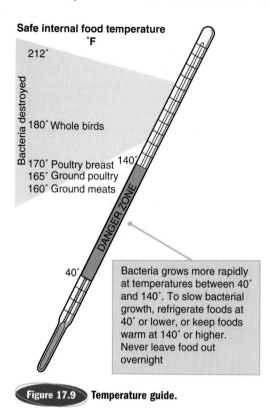

Safe internal food temperature
°F

212°

Bacteria destroyed

180° Whole birds

170° Poultry breast   140°
165° Ground poultry
160° Ground meats

DANGER ZONE

40°

Bacteria grows more rapidly at temperatures between 40° and 140°. To slow bacterial growth, refrigerate foods at 40° or lower, or keep foods warm at 140° or higher. Never leave food out overnight

Figure 17.9 **Temperature guide.**

a reference for restaurants, grocery stores, institutional food services, vending operations, and other retailers on how to store, prepare, and serve food to prevent foodborne illness.[27] The FDA updates and publishes the Food Code periodically as model recommendations for states to adopt and use to regulate retail food establishments in their jurisdictions.

Key Concepts: *Food safety is the responsibility of many agencies at the federal and state levels. The use of the Hazard Analysis Critical Control Point system allows government and industry to identify possible sites of food contamination and correct problems before they occur.*

The Consumer's Role in Food Safety

Food safety advice to consumers used to consist of a simple message: "Keep hot foods hot and cold foods cold (see **Figure 17.9**)." Now food safety experts urge consumers to follow the following four rules:

- *Clean.* Wash hands and surfaces often.
- *Separate.* Don't cross-contaminate.
- *Cook.* Cook to proper temperatures.
- *Chill.* Refrigerate promptly.[28]

𝓕𝔂𝒊 | Safe Food Practices

FOR YOUR INFORMATION

Because bacteria grow rapidly between 40°F and 140°F (4°C–60°C), most food should be kept out of this temperature range, known as the Danger Zone. Cold temperatures keep bacteria from multiplying; the fewer bacteria, the less the risk of illness. Proper cooking (or other heat treatment, such as pasteurization) kills the bacteria. These principles serve as the basis for many of the following recommended food-handling practices.

Buying Food

- Buy from reputable dealers and grocers who keep their selling areas and facilities clean and sanitary, and keep food at the appropriate temperature; for example, holding dairy foods, eggs, meats, and seafood, and certain produce such as cut melons and raw sprouts at refrigerator temperatures.
- Don't buy canned goods with dents or bulges. Don't select torn, crushed, or open food packages. Also, avoid buying packages that are above the frost line in the store's freezer. If the package cover is

transparent, look for frost or ice crystals, signs that the product has been stored for a long time, or thawed and refrozen.

Storing Food

- Refrigerate perishable items as quickly as possible after purchase. The refrigerator temperature should be 40°F or colder. Check it periodically with a thermometer to make sure the correct temperature is being maintained.
- Keep eggs in their original carton and store them in the refrigerator itself, not the door, where the temperature is warmer.
- If raw meat, poultry products, or fresh seafood will be used within two days, store them in the coldest part of the refrigerator, usually under the freezer compartment or in a special "meat keeper." Store the packages loosely to allow air to circulate freely around each package, and be sure to wrap them tightly so that raw juices can't leak out and contaminate other foods.

- If raw meat, poultry, and seafood will not used within two days, store them in the freezer, which should have a temperature of 0°F. Check this temperature periodically, too, and adjust as needed.
- Read label directions for storing other foods; for example, mayonnaise and ketchup need to be refrigerated after they have been opened.
- Store potatoes and onions in a cool dark place, but not under the sink because leakage from pipes can contaminate and damage them. Keep them away from household cleaning products and other chemicals, as well.

Preparing Food

- Wash hands thoroughly with warm, soapy water for at least 20 seconds before beginning food preparation and every time after handling raw foods, including fresh produce.
- Defrost meat, poultry, and seafood products in the refrigerator, microwave oven, or in a water-tight plastic bag

Once a consumer takes possession of a food, food safety becomes his or her responsibility. (See **Figure 17.10**.) Unfortunately, studies show that a large percentage of consumers fail to follow safe food practices in the home. Current public health efforts focus on teaching consumers—from young children to older Americans—safe food practices in the home. (See the FYI feature "Safe Food Practices.")

Some food handling practices are so important that the federal government requires specific instructions or warnings on labels of certain foods. Following outbreaks of illness from E. coli O157:H7 from contaminated hamburger in 1993, the USDA mandated instructions on labels of raw meat and poultry to encourage consumers to follow recommendations for safe handling and cooking of these products.[29]

In 1998 the FDA established a rule requiring labels of unpasteurized or otherwise untreated packaged juice products to carry a statement about the product's possible danger to children, older adults, and people with weakened immune systems.[30] The warning states that the product has not been pasteurized, and therefore may contain harmful bacteria that can cause serious illness in these high-risk groups. This requirement was made after a number of people were made seriously ill after drinking unpasteurized apple juice that was contaminated with E. coli.

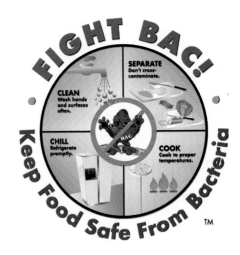

Clean: Wash hands and surfaces often
Separate: Don't cross-contaminate
Cook: Cook to proper temperatures
Chill: Refrigerate properly

Figure 17.10 Keeping harmful bacteria at bay.

submerged in cold water (the water must be changed every 30 minutes). Never defrost at room temperature—an ideal temperature for bacteria to grow and multiply.
- Marinate foods in the refrigerator. Discard the marinade after use because it contains raw juices, which may harbor bacteria; make a separate batch for basting food while cooking.
- Always use a clean cutting board. Wash cutting boards with hot water, soap, and a scrub brush. Then sanitize them in an automatic dishwasher or by rinsing with a solution of 5 milliliters (1 teaspoon) chlorine bleach to about 1 liter (1 quart) of water. If possible, use one cutting board for fresh produce and a separate one for raw meat, poultry, and seafood. Once cutting boards become excessively worn or develop hard-to-clean grooves, you should replace them.
- Before opening canned foods, wash the top of the can to prevent dirt from com-

ing in contact with the food.
- Wash fresh fruits and vegetables thoroughly with water only.
- Avoid eating dough or batter containing raw eggs because of the risk of *Salmonella enteritidis*, a bacterium that can be in shell eggs. Cooking the egg to at least 140°F (60°C) kills the bacteria.

Cooking Food
- Cook foods to the appropriate minimum internal temperature:
  Seafood
    145°F (63°C)
  Beef, lamb, and pork
    160°F (71°C)
  Ground chicken and turkey
    165°F (74°C)
  Poultry breasts
    170°F (77°C)
  Whole poultry and thighs
    180°F (82°C)
- Always use a thermometer to ensure that the product has reached the correct internal temperature. Color is not always a good guide.

- When microwaving foods, rotate the dish and stir its contents several times to ensure even cooking. Follow recommended standing times, then check meat, poultry, and seafood products with a thermometer to make sure they have reached the correct internal temperature.
- Cook eggs until the white is firm and the yolk begins to harden.

Serving Food
- Keep hot foods at 140°F (60°C) or higher, and cold foods at 40°F (4°C) or lower.
- Do not keep leftovers at room temperature for more than two hours. Refrigerate as quickly as possible.
- Date leftovers so that they can be used within a safe time—generally, three to five days in the refrigerator.

Quick Bites

How good are your food safety habits?

Do Americans practice food safety in their own kitchens? Apparently not. A study conducted by the FDA and the Centers for Disease Control and Prevention showed that one-half of people surveyed ate undercooked eggs in the past year. Twenty percent of people ate undercooked hamburger, and 25 percent of men and 14 percent of women failed to wash their hands with soap after handling raw meat.

Quick Bites

Wood vs. Plastic: The Cutting Controversy

Which type of cutting board is safer to use while cutting meat, wood or plastic? They both have drawbacks. A wood cutting board tends to absorb bacteria, sucking them down into the wood fibers. This may be safer than a plastic board, which keeps bacteria on the surface, in an easy position to rub off onto food and other objects. But used wooden cutting boards tend to keep more on the surface than new wooden boards, acting more like plastic boards. What's the solution? Keep cutting boards clean, by heating wooden boards in the microwave or putting plastic boards in the dishwasher.

In 1999 the FDA proposed rules requiring safe handling statements on egg cartons.[31] The proposed statement reads:

SAFE HANDLING INSTRUCTIONS: Eggs may contain harmful bacteria known to cause serious illness, especially in children, the elderly, and persons with weakened immune systems. For your protection: Keep eggs refrigerated; cook eggs until yolks are firm; and cook foods containing eggs thoroughly.

Food manufacturers may voluntarily place other safe handling instructions on the label, such as proper cooking and storage of the item. Consumers should always follow these instructions.

Who's at Increased Risk for Foodborne Illness?

People with certain diseases and conditions need to be especially careful about following safe food practices. Their condition or the drugs they use may compromise their immune systems, making it more difficult for them to fight off infections. People who are at risk include those with these conditions:

- immune disorders, such as HIV infection
- cancer
- diabetes
- long-term steroid use, such as for asthma or arthritis
- liver disease
- hemochromatosis, an iron storage disorder that affects the liver
- stomach problems, including previous stomach surgery and low stomach acid (for example, from chronic antacid use).

Because these conditions are more common in older adults, seniors have an increased risk of foodborne illness. Young children do not have fully developed immune systems, so they are particularly vulnerable to serious illness from foodborne disease. Also, pregnant women and their fetuses are at special risk from the bacterium *Listeria monocytogenes* and the parasite *Toxoplasma gondii*. Both of these microorganisms can harm, even kill, fetuses and young babies.

Final Word on Food Safety

A totally risk-free system of food production is an unreasonable and unattainable goal. The United States and Canada enjoy a reputation as having food supplies that are among the safest in the world. We expect our food to be clean, fresh, and not contaminated with debris, chemicals, or organisms that cause sickness or discomfort. To make sure it stays that way, food safety experts are continually trying to instill in every participant in the food production chain—from the farmer who produces the food, to the manufacturer who processes it, to the retailer who sells it, and to the consumer who buys it—the need for improved measures to help reduce and perhaps even eliminate foodborne disease in this country. That's one reason food safety advice today is turning up in so many places—to ensure that everyone gets the word on food safety.

Key Concepts: *Consumers play a huge role in food safety. They can avoid foodborne illness by following a few simple food-handling and preparation rules: keep hands and food-preparation areas clean; avoid cross-contamination of foods; cook foods adequately; refrigerate foods promptly. People who have weak or less-developed immune systems are at high risk for foodborne illnesses.*

Food Technology

At the start of the twenty-first century, technology is having a larger and larger impact on the food we eat. Our use of additives, preservation techniques, and genetic engineering have implications for our food supply in the years to come and have triggered debates about their risks and benefits.

Food Additives

Food **additives** serve a variety of functions that help give us a safe, plentiful, varied, and relatively inexpensive food supply. The FDA requires rigorous testing of all new food additives and scientific experts believe the benefits of food additives far outweigh the minimal or nonexistent health risks associated with their use.

Food additives can be either direct or indirect. **Direct additives** are added to a food for a specific reason. The artificial sweeteners aspartame, saccharin, and sucralose are direct food additives. Direct additives are identified in the ingredient list on the food label. **Indirect additives** are substances that become part of the food in trace amounts as a result of the food coming in contact with the substance—for example, migration of chemicals from a food's packaging. The FDA evaluates both direct and indirect additives for safety.

Additives are used in foods for five main reasons:

1. *To maintain product consistency.* Emulsifiers give products such as peanut butter a consistent texture and prevent them from separating. Stabilizers and thickeners give ice cream a smooth, uniform texture. Anticaking agents help substances such as salt to flow freely.

2. *To improve or maintain nutritional value.* Vitamins and minerals are added to many common foods such as milk, flour, cereal, and margarine to make up for elements likely to be lacking in a person's diet, replace those lost in processing, or improve shelf life. Such fortification and enrichment has reduced nutrient deficiencies among the U.S. population. (See Chapter 2 for more on fortification and enrichment.) Added nutrients are listed in the ingredient list and Nutrition Facts panel.

3. *To maintain palatability and wholesomeness.* Preservatives retard product spoilage caused by mold, air, bacteria, fungi, or yeast. Bacterial contamination can cause foodborne illness, including life-threatening botulism. Antioxidants are preservatives that prevent fats and oils in baked goods and other foods from becoming rancid or developing an off-flavor. They also prevent cut fresh fruits, such as apples, from turning brown when exposed to air.

4. *To provide leavening or control acidity and alkalinity.* Leavening agents that release acids when heated can react with baking soda to help cakes, biscuits, and other baked goods to rise during baking. Other additives modify the acidity and alkalinity of foods for flavor, taste, and color.

5. *To enhance flavor or impart desired color.* Many spices and added flavors enhance the taste of foods. Colors, likewise, enhance the appearance of certain foods to make them more appealing or meet consumer expectations.

additives Substances added to food to perform various functions, such as adding color or flavor, replacing sugar or fat, improving nutritional content, or improving texture or shelf life.

direct additives A substance added to a food for a specific purpose.

indirect additives Substances that become part of the food in trace amounts due to its packaging, storage, or other handling.

color additive Any dye, pigment, or substance that can impart color when added or applied to a food, drug, or cosmetic, or to the human body.

Generally Recognized As Safe (GRAS) Substances that are "generally recognized as safe" for consumption and can be added to foods by manufacturers without establishing their safety by rigorous experimental studies. Congress established the list of substances in 1958.

prior-sanctioned substance All substances that the FDA or the U.S. Department of Agriculture (USDA) had determined were safe for use in specific foods prior to the 1958 Food Additives Amendment were designated as prior-sanctioned substances. These substances are exempted from the food additive regulation process.

Delaney clause The part of the 1960 Color Additives Amendment to the Federal Food, Drug and Cosmetic Act that bars FDA from approving any products shown in laboratory tests to cause cancer.

Although most people think additives are complex chemicals with unfamiliar names, the three most common additives are sugar, salt, and corn syrup. These three, plus citric acid (found naturally in oranges and lemons), baking soda, vegetable colors, mustard, and pepper account for more than 98 percent by weight of all food additives used in the United States. (See **Figure 17.11.**)

Regulation by the FDA

Food additives serve important functions; however, many consumers are skeptical about their safety. Additives fall into four regulatory categories: food additives, color additives, GRAS (Generally Recognized As Safe) substances, and prior-sanctioned substances. A new additive requires premarket approval by the FDA. The process requires the manufacturer to provide convincing research evidence that the additive not only performs its intended function, but is not harmful at expected consumption levels. Based on this and other scientific information, the FDA decides whether to approve the additive, the types of foods that may contain the additive, the quantities that can be used, and the way the substance will be identified on labels.

A **color additive** is any dye, pigment, or substance that can impart color when added to a food, drug, or cosmetic or to the human body. Colors allowed for use in food are classified as either certified or exempt from certification. Certified colors are synthetic. The manufacturer and the FDA test each batch to ensure their purity. Certified colors added to a food must be listed on the food's ingredient list by common name. Colors exempt from certification include natural substances derived from vegetables, minerals, or animals. These colors also must be produced according to specifications that ensure purity.

A third type of additive falls under the category **Generally Recognized As Safe**, or **GRAS**. Congress first defined GRAS substances in 1958 when it passed the Food Additives Amendment to the FD&C Act. GRAS substances are those

Fyi The Saccharin Story

FOR YOUR INFORMATION

The granddaddy of all sugar substitutes is saccharin. Discovered in 1879, it was used during both world wars to sweeten foods, helping to compensate for sugar shortages and rationing. It is 300 times sweeter than sugar.

In 1907 an early attempt to ban saccharin was thwarted when President Theodore Roosevelt proclaimed the top safety official behind the effort to be "an idiot." Safety questions resurfaced in 1911 when a board of federal scientists called the artificial sweetener "an adulterant" that should not be used in foods. This same board later decided to limit saccharin just to products "intended for invalids," a restriction that was lifted after

sugar shortages developed during World War I.

In 1958, when Congress passed the Food Additives Amendment to the Food, Drug, and Cosmetic Act, saccharin was one of the ingredients "generally recognized as safe," or GRAS. That same year the saccharin-based product Sweet 'N Low took the public by storm. Food and beverage companies scrambled to offer saccharin-sweetened products that came to include the diet soda Tab and a plethora of gelatins, candies, and baked goods.

By the early 1970s, studies of rats that had been fed saccharin raised concerns about the sweetener's role in causing bladder cancer, but scientists later suggested that impurities, not saccharin, may have caused the tumors.

Then in 1977, a Canadian study looked specifically at the role of saccharin in test animals. Researchers fed rats high doses of saccharin equivalent to 5 percent of their diet. The results again showed that saccharin caused bladder cancer in rats.

Because the Delaney Clause prohibits the use of any food additive shown to cause cancer in animals or humans, the FDA proposed an immediate ban on saccharin. The FDA proposal prompted a public outcry, fueled in part by media reports that the test rats were fed the equivalent of as many as 800 diet sodas a day.[1]

Congress responded by passing the Saccharin Study and Labeling Act, which

whose use is generally recognized by experts as safe, based on their extensive history of use in food before 1958 or based on published scientific evidence. Salt, sugar, spices, vitamins, and monosodium glutamate (MSG), along with several hundred other substances, are considered GRAS. Manufacturers may petition FDA for a new food additive to be considered GRAS.

Yet another type of additive is the **prior-sanctioned substance**, which the FDA or USDA had determined was safe for use in a specific food before the 1958 legislation. Examples include sodium nitrite and potassium nitrite to preserve luncheon meats.

Delaney Clause

Regulations governing food additives and color additives include a provision that prohibits the approval of an additive if it is found to cause cancer in humans or animals. This clause is often referred to as the **Delaney Clause**, named for its sponsor, Congressman James Delaney (D., New York).

While the Delaney Clause sounds good in principle, it has become one of the most controversial food laws on the books. Animal cancer tests frequently involve giving rodents massive doses of the chemical to be tested. Many experts question whether an additive should be banned from use at low levels because it may cause cancer at extremely high levels. Critics argue that feeding animals large doses of a substance over their entire lifetimes may have little relevance to human consumption of trace amounts of that same substance.

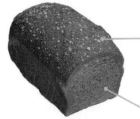

Maturing and bleaching agents such as bromates, peroxides, and ammonium chloride speed up the natural aging and whitening processes of milled flour, allowing it to be used more quickly for baking products.

Leavening agents such as yeast, baking powder and baking soda produce carbon dioxide bubbles, which create a light texture in breads and cakes.

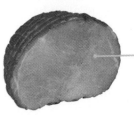

Vitamin D is added to milk to improve its nutritional quality. Many other vitamins and minerals are added to a variety of other foods.

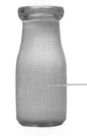

Curing and pickling agents such as nitrates and nitrites are added to bacon, ham, hot dogs, and other cured meats primarily to prevent the growth of *Clostridium botulinum*, the bacterium that causes botulism. Nitrates also give these meats their characteristic pink color. When consumed, nitrates are converted by the body to nitrosamines, which are carcinogenic. Other additives, such as vitamin C, inhibit this conversion.

Figure 17.11 **Common foods that contain additives.**

---

placed a two-year moratorium on any ban of the sweetener while additional safety studies were conducted. Congress has extended the moratorium several times, most recently renewing it until 2002. The law also required that any foods containing saccharin must carry a label that reads *"Use of this product may be hazardous to your health. This product contains saccharin which has been determined to cause cancer in laboratory animals."* In 1996 Congress repealed the saccharin notice requirements.

In May 2000, the National Toxicology Program delisted saccharin as a possible human carcinogen. The NTP concluded that the types of tumors caused by saccharin in rats arose from a mechanism that is not relevant to humans. This ruling is in keeping with the opinion of other scientific bodies. The National Cancer Institute states in its "Cancer Facts" that "epidemiological studies do not provide clear evidence" of a link between saccharin and human cancer. Regina Ziegler, Ph.D., an NCI epidemiologist, says, "Typical intakes of saccharin at normal levels for adults show no evidence of a public health problem."[2] Other health groups, including the American Medical Association, the American Cancer Society, and the American Dietetic Association, agree that saccharin use is acceptable.

Saccharin remains on the market and continues to have a fairly large appeal as a table-top sweetener, particularly in restaurants, where it is available in single-serving packets under trade names such as Sweet 'N Low. The familiar warning label on the "pink stuff" may soon be a thing of the past!

1 Henkel J. Sugar substitutes: Americans opt for sweetness and lite. *FDA Consumer.* Nov/Dec 1999.
2 Ibid.

pasteurization A process for destroying pathogenic bacteria by heating liquid foods to a prescribed temperature for a specified time.

preservatives Chemicals or other agents that slow the decomposition of a food.

Quick Bites

Where do *E. coli* hang out?

Ground beef is the most common source of *E. coli* bacteria, but *E. coli* also have been found in apples and lettuce.

When the Delaney Clause was first enacted in 1960, scientists could detect substances only in parts per thousand. Current technology enables scientists to detect substances in parts per billion or even per trillion. One part per trillion is equivalent to about one grain of sugar in an Olympic size swimming pool! Critics charge that the Delaney Clause combined with modern detection techniques has created a situation in which even very pure substances can be shown to be contaminated with traces of one carcinogen or another.

What margin of safety is appropriate? Generally, an additive is permitted in foods at 1/100 the level that causes no harmful effect in animals.[32] This is an extremely large margin of safety. In comparison, many natural toxins in foods appear at levels that bring their margins of safety closer to 1/10.

Many food safety experts recommend revision of the law to allow approval of a potential cancer-causing food substance, as long as the risk of cancer is extremely low. This would be in line with current laws regulating food pesticides. In 1996 the Food Quality Protection Act stated that the approval of any food pesticide must be based on a standard of "reasonable certainty of no harm," which is usually interpreted to mean less than one cancer per million people exposed over their lifetimes. Special care must be taken to determine that infants and children, who are more vulnerable than adults to the risks of chemical substances, would not be harmed.

But proponents of the Delaney Clause say that any risk for cancer, even minimal, is too high. They point out that even if the cancer risk for an individual chemical is extremely low, we must take into account the fact that people are exposed to a great many cancer-causing substances, whose effects over a long period of time may be additive. In addition, they say, the absolute zero risk in the Delaney Clause is good because it lessens the opportunity for legal or political interference in the decision to approve a food substance.

For now, the Delaney Clause remains part of our food safety laws. Future scientific techniques might decrease reliance on animal testing and improve accuracy in predicting the effects of food additives on human health.

Key Concepts: *Direct food additives serve specific functions. Indirect food additives become part of the food in trace amounts when the food comes in contact with the substance. Food additives serve a variety of purposes including improving product quality, maintaining freshness, and improving nutritional value. Unless determined to be a prior-sanctioned ingredient or GRAS, new additives undergo extensive testing to prove their safety and efficacy to the FDA. The FDA is responsible for approving and regulating food additives. The Delaney Clause prohibits the approval of an additive if it is found to cause cancer in humans or animals.*

Food Preservation

In our modern society, few people grow their own vegetables, fruits, and grains, or keep livestock as a source of meat and milk. Rather, we shop for our food, typically at a large, full-service supermarket. Because we do not consume our food at the point of harvest or slaughter, various means of food preservation help maintain the quality of the foods we purchase. Food preservation methods range from the addition of chemical preservatives, to canning or freezing, to **pasteurization**, to more recent methods such as irradiation.

Preservatives

As mentioned earlier, **preservatives** are added to foods to prevent spoilage and increase shelf life. The most common antimicrobial agents are salt and sugar. Other preservatives such as potassium sorbate and sodium propionate extend the shelf-life of baked goods and many other products. Antioxidants are a class of preservatives that prevent the changes in color and flavor caused by exposure to air. Common antioxidants include vitamin C and vitamin E, sulfites, and BHA and BHT.

Preparation for Preservation

Some preservation techniques, such as salting and fermenting, date to ancient times and are still practiced along with their modern counterparts—freezing, canning, pasteurization, and others. Salting, drying, or fermenting foods creates an environment in which bacteria cannot multiply, and therefore, cannot cause food spoilage. Canned foods are heated quickly to a temperature that kills microbes, and then sealed airtight to prevent both contamination and oxidative damage. Freezing temperatures not only keep bacteria from multiplying, but also prevent normal enzymatic changes in food that would cause spoilage. Pasteurization of milk or other beverages uses a very high temperature for a very short time to kill bacteria, but minimize changes that would result from longer heating. The food industry and the American public readily accept these food-preservation methods. One of the most modern preservation techniques—irradiation—is also the most controversial, in part because of our fear of anything that has to do with radiation.

Irradiation

Food **irradiation** has the longest history, more than 40 years, of scientific research and testing of any food technology before approval.[33] In this process foods are exposed to a measured dose of radiation to reduce or eliminate pathogenic bacteria, including *E. coli* O157:H7, *Salmonella*, and *Campylobacter*, the chief causes of foodborne illness today.[34] Irradiation also can destroy insects and parasites, reduce spoilage, and inhibit sprouting and delay ripening of certain fruits and vegetables. Irradiation can reduce pathogens in raw poultry or meat by 99.9 percent.[35] Some people fear irradiation will make the food radioactive. This concern is unfounded. The energy used to irradiate foods passes through the food and leaves no residue, similar to the way microwaves pass through food. Despite its benefits, use of irradiation remains rare in the United States.

Food manufacturers have been reluctant to use irradiation on their products for fear of consumer rejection.[36] Some consumers and advocacy groups protest its use because they are concerned that irradiation may compromise a food's nutritional value and change its texture, taste, or appearance. According to the American Dietetic Association (ADA), the nutritive loss associated with irradiation is actually less than for most conventional methods of food preservation.[37] The ADA also states that at appropriate doses, irradiation of food does not significantly change its flavor, texture, or appearance. Many organizations including the ADA, the American Medical Association, and the World Health Organization endorse irradiation as a means of providing the public with a safer food supply.

The FDA has approved irradiation for

- spices and dry vegetable seasoning to decontaminate and control insects and microorganisms,
- dry or dehydrated enzyme preparations to control insects and microorganisms,
- fruits and vegetables to inhibit maturation,
- poultry and red meat to control spoilage and pathogenic microorganisms, and
- to control insects, mites and other arthropod pests in all of the foods above.

irradiation A food preservation technique in which foods are exposed to measured doses of radiation to reduce or eliminate pathogens and kill insects, reduce spoilage, and, in certain fruits and vegetables, inhibit sprouting and delay ripening.

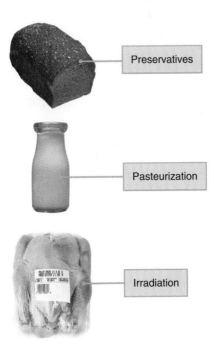

Preparing food for safe consumption.

Figure 17.12 **Irradiation.** Irradiation can retard spoilage and reduce risk of foodborne illness.

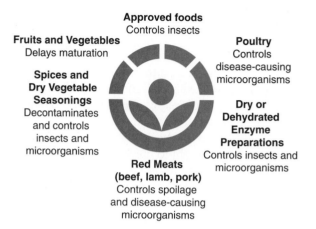

FDA APPROVED USES OF IRRADIATION

Approved foods
Controls insects

Fruits and Vegetables
Delays maturation

Poultry
Controls disease-causing microorganisms

Spices and Dry Vegetable Seasonings
Decontaminates and controls insects and microorganisms

Dry or Dehydrated Enzyme Preparations
Controls insects and microorganisms

Red Meats (beef, lamb, pork)
Controls spoilage and disease-causing microorganisms

Quick Bites

Bacteria at the Supermarket

Bacteria abound on the surface of supermarket meat. A piece of pork, on average, may harbor a few hundred bacteria per cubic centimeter, and a piece of chicken may have 10,000 in the same area.

genetically modified (GM) foods Foods produced using plant or animal ingredients that have been modified using gene technology.

The FDA requires labels of irradiated foods to state that the product was "treated with irradiation" or "treated by irradiation" and to display the international symbol for irradiation, the radura. (See **Figure 17.12**.) In May 2000, the USDA proposed the use of irradiation for fruits and vegetables imported into the United States in order to control fruit flies and mango seed weevil.

Some experts believe the time is right for food irradiation to become more widespread. The recent media attention to deaths related to foodborne illness has made the public more aware of the need to protect against contamination of food. As more consumers become aware of the benefits of irradiation, the demand for irradiated foods is expected to increase. Studies have shown that education about irradiation significantly improves customers' attitudes.[38]

Key Concepts: *Various processing methods help protect us from contamination of food with pathogens. Drying, salting, canning, freezing, and pasteurizing are methods that consumers accept. Irradiation is a process in which foods are exposed to a measured dose of radiation to reduce or eliminate pathogenic bacteria. While government and professional organizations deem irradiation a safe procedure, consumers are still wary.*

Genetically Modified Foods

Genetically modified (GM) foods have arrived, and many of us are already dining on them. When you prepare a dinner of broccoli and tofu, some of the soybeans used to make the tofu probably came from plants genetically modified to resist herbicide sprays, or insect pests, or both. And although your broccoli is currently "natural," you can be sure that in a lab somewhere genetically modified broccoli seeds are sprouting, perhaps with enhanced nutrient or other phytochemical levels. If you are eating tenderloin tonight, the steak probably came from a steer fed on genetically modified corn that had its DNA altered by the addition of foreign genes to allow the plant to resist insect pests and herbicides.

Should you be indignant that these new foods are showing up on your table without any indication on the label, or should you be grateful that these high-tech crops are keeping crop yields high and food costs low?

An informed answer to this question requires some understanding of how genetic engineering works, how new crops and foods are regulated, and how gene modification of crops and animals differs from the classical methods of agricultural breeding that have been practiced for thousands of years.

A Short Course in Plant Genetics

How do GM food plants differ from those developed through traditional cross-pollination and hybridization? The answer, surprisingly, is that most crop modifications achieved by DNA manipulation and associated techniques of **biotechnology** could also be achieved with classical techniques, but the time scale and expense are very different.[39] (See **Figure 17.13**.)

The classical techniques for breeding a plant with new characteristics have been practiced for hundreds of years. They involve crossing two plants with different characteristics, then growing the resulting hybrid seeds and looking for plants with the desired combination of characteristics. Hybrid plants get half of their genes from one parent and half from the other. Though the hybrid may combine favorable qualities from both parents, a lot of undesirable genetic baggage must be sorted out after formation of such a hybrid. It usually takes dozens of additional crosses, and many years, to separate the desirable genes from the undesirable, and the process has a large element of chance.

Genetic engineering, on the other hand, allows scientists to transform a plant one gene at a time, using well-established methods for manipulating DNA sequences and integrating them into the plant **genome** (its set of genes). Since many plant genes have already been identified, and complete DNA sequences of plant genomes soon will be available, we can anticipate that the genetic engineering of plants will become increasingly powerful and precise. Designing a new GM plant should come to resemble a manufacturing process rather than the tedious guessing game of classical genetics. In some cases, a gene can be selected and introduced into plant cells, and new GM seeds can be prepared within a year or two. When we consider that it took centuries of selection and breeding to transform the weedy wild maize plant of pre-Columbian Mexico into our modern varieties of corn, the scale and speed of the gene revolution in agriculture is both astounding and a little frightening.

Genetically Modified Foods: An Unstoppable Experiment?

How extensive is the shift to gene-modified crops and how many different crops are involved? About 50 percent of soybeans and over 33 percent of cotton grown in the United States are genetically modified.[40] In addition to soybeans, the few types of genetically modified food crops in commercial production include corn, potatoes, and rapeseed (the source of canola oil). However, the amount of acreage involved is substantial, roughly equal to the land area of Oregon. Most of these genetically engineered crops are being grown in the United States, Canada, and South America. The increased yields and lower costs associated with GM crops make them attractive to farmers. There is now strong, perhaps unstoppable, momentum to continue and expand GM crop plantings. However, European countries have been slow to accept gene-modified crops. They are concerned about possible ecological damage from such crops and fear potential unintended consequences of genetic "tampering" with the food

biotechnology The set of laboratory techniques and processes used to modify the genome of plants or animals, and thus create desirable new characteristics. Genetic engineering in the broad sense.

genetic engineering Manipulation of the genome of an organism by artificial means for the purpose of modifying existing traits or adding new genetic traits.

genome The total genetic information of an organism, stored in the DNA of its chromosomes.

supply. In 1999 the Gerber Products Company decided to stop using GM corn and soy in its baby foods. While some consumer groups voice similar concerns, agribusiness and the U.S. federal government have been quite supportive of the trend toward GM foods.

The GM crops mentioned above are just the tip of the genetic modification iceberg; hundreds more are under development in university laboratories and in the labs of giant agribusinesses like Monsanto,

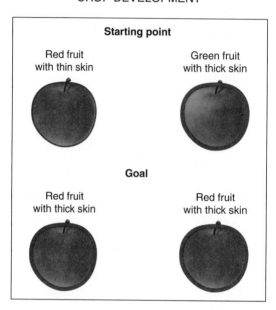

CROP DEVELOPMENT

Starting point

Red fruit
with thin skin

Green fruit
with thick skin

Goal

Red fruit
with thick skin

Red fruit
with thick skin

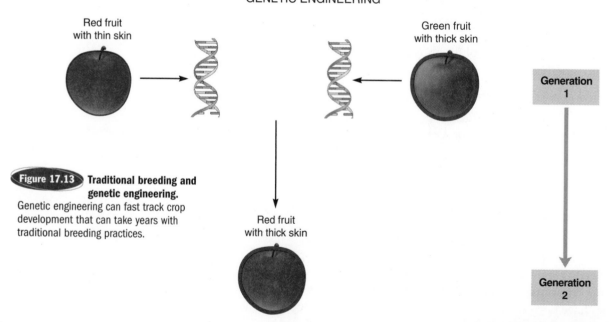

GENETIC ENGINEERING

Red fruit
with thin skin

Green fruit
with thick skin

Generation
1

Red fruit
with thick skin

Generation
2

Scientists can use genetic engineering to
combine certain traits in a single generation

Figure 17.13 **Traditional breeding and genetic engineering.** Genetic engineering can fast track crop development that can take years with traditional breeding practices.

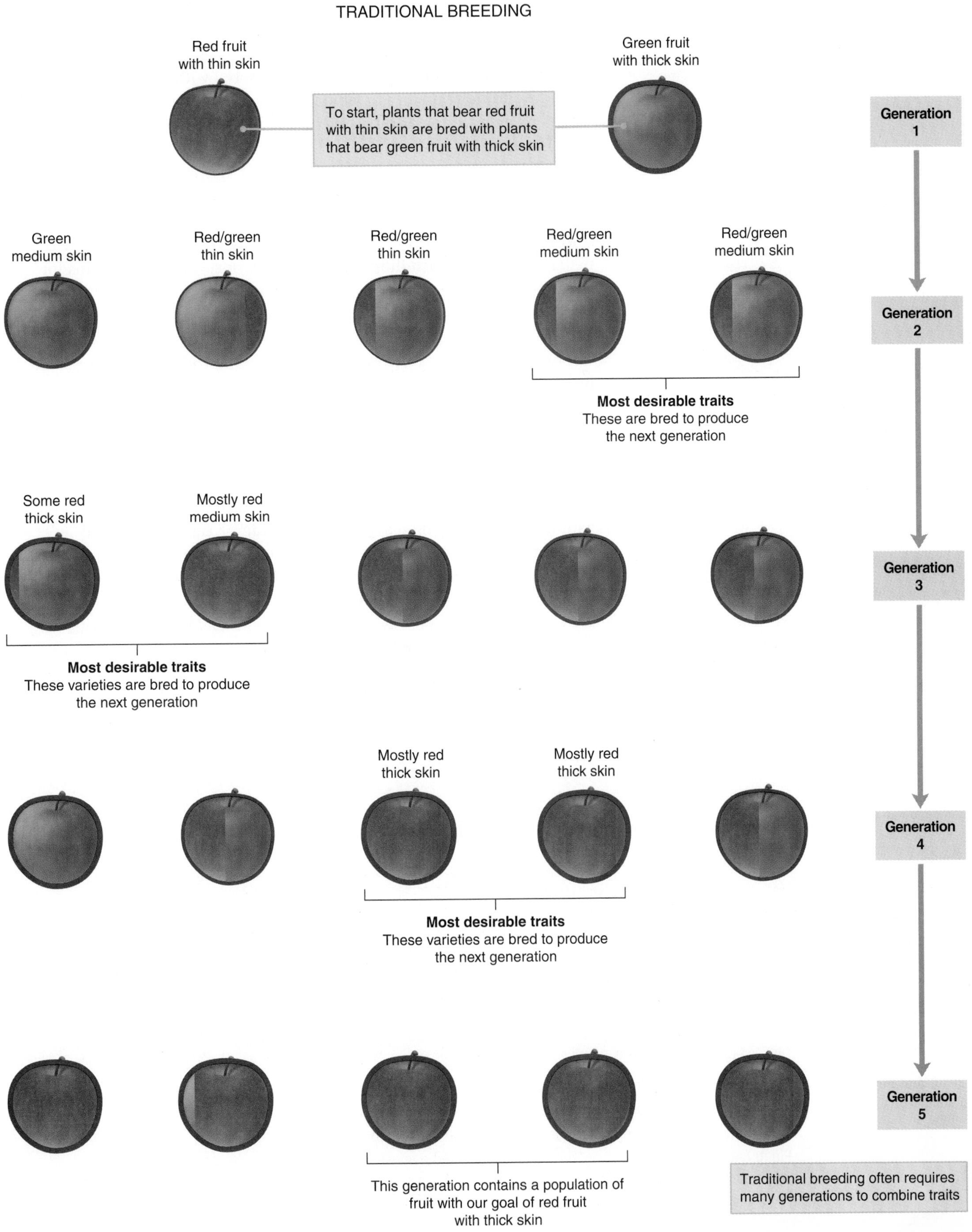

TRADITIONAL BREEDING

Red fruit
with thin skin

Green fruit
with thick skin

To start, plants that bear red fruit
with thin skin are bred with plants
that bear green fruit with thick skin

Generation 1

Green
medium skin

Red/green
thin skin

Red/green
thin skin

Red/green
medium skin

Red/green
medium skin

Most desirable traits
These are bred to produce
the next generation

Generation 2

Some red
thick skin

Mostly red
medium skin

Most desirable traits
These varieties are bred to produce
the next generation

Generation 3

Mostly red
thick skin

Mostly red
thick skin

Most desirable traits
These varieties are bred to produce
the next generation

Generation 4

This generation contains a population of
fruit with our goal of red fruit
with thick skin

Traditional breeding often requires
many generations to combine traits

Generation 5

Novartis, and DuPont. **Table 17.3** shows the emergence of GM foods. The goals of these modifications are higher yields, increased amounts of critical nutrients, and a healthier mix of plant oils. Many of these goals would be achievable with classical selection techniques, but with genetic engineering they move from laboratory to table in decades, rather than centuries.

Genetic engineering also has affected the food-processing industry. The cheese-making industry uses genetically modified bacteria to produce the widely used enzyme chymosin. Chymosin has virtually replaced the natural milk-clotting enzyme, rennet, which is extracted from the stomachs of calves.

In the future we will see GM plants that have been modified to yield better textile fibers including colored cotton, or specialized proteins for use in human pharmaceuticals, or even plants that produce the starting materials for manufacture of plastics. In economic terms, these nonfood GM crops may become even more important than GM foods.

If only plant genes were involved in GM food production, there would be much less controversy. However *any* gene, including genes from bacteria and animals, can be introduced into a plant genome. Some people find this frightening, and an imaginative term, *Frankenfoods*, has been coined to express the "unnatural" nature of some GM products. But how unnatural is the exchange of DNA between species? It may be reassuring to realize that organisms have been swapping DNA for eons, with no help from humans. Foreign DNA can be carried from one species to another by a variety of viruses, for example. Nature has already performed millions of "gene modifications" on its own, and exchange of DNA is an established part of the evolutionary process. Now that we can do our own experiments with DNA manipulation, we hope the benefits will be increased.

Benefits of Genetic Engineering

Whatever the risks, no one can argue with the success of these GM techniques. For instance, a bacterial gene was used to create Monsanto's new insect-resistant varieties of corn, potatoes, and soybeans. This gene, the

Table 17.3	Genetically Modified Crops and Plants, 1994-2000 and Beyond
1994	FlavrSavr Tomato
1996	Herbicide-tolerant soybeans and rapeseed Insect-resistant corn and cotton
1998	Herbicide-tolerant corn Virus and insect-resistant potatoes
1999	Virus-resistant tomatoes
2000	High-lysine soybeans, modified-oil soybeans, and high-sucrose soybeans, beta-carotene containing rice
2001	Disease-protected potatoes and high-methionine soybeans
2002 and beyond	Cotton with improved fiber, and colored fiber Plants producing special proteins for medical use, such as human hormones Plants producing precursor molecules for plastics (normally made from petroleum) Plants producing human and animal vaccines, directed against bacterial diseases Vegetables with higher amounts of calcium

Bt gene, was taken from the soil bacterium *Bacillus thuringiensis*. When inserted into a plant genome, the Bt gene specifies an insecticidal protein throughout the plant, and thus makes the plant toxic to insects. Such crops have been extremely successful, and produce high yields without use of insecticides. Bt-modified crops, which are now grown in the United States over an area larger than Rhode Island, are a boon both to the economy and the environment. Because chemical insecticides are not necessary, many benign insects are spared and insect **biodiversity** is preserved. Similarly, other plants can be genetically modified to resist the effects of common herbicides. Chemical sprays that are lethal to most plant life have no effect on these GM plants. The crop plant grows larger in the absence of weeds, and the farmer gets a better yield with less effort and expense.

The economic benefits of GM foods are clearly substantial. Increased yields of important food plants can help feed increasing populations without the need for putting more land under the plow, or increasing the use of toxic insecticides. In the coming century, this may be the difference between starvation and adequate nutrition in many developing countries. It is also easy to imagine how manipulation of plant amino acids and plant oils could yield superior foods, which would be able not only to satisfy calorie requirements, but also to address protein and vitamin needs. A strain of rice, genetically modified to be rich in beta-carotene, could benefit the million plus children in developing countries who die or are weakened by vitamin A deficiency.[41] In developed countries, where heart disease and cancer loom as greater risks than malnutrition, the ability to adjust the saturation level of plant lipids or to boost beneficial phytochemicals would be of great value to public health. But do these undoubted benefits outweigh the risks?

Think About It
4

Risks

What are the specific risks of GM foods? Many consumers are concerned about whether these new foods are safe to eat. The answer to this concern is a fairly unequivocal yes. When a new protein or other substance is introduced into a food, the FDA requires substantial testing to demonstrate its safety. With GM foods, the principal risk appears to be the possibility of introducing a new allergen into a GM food. To be cautious, the FDA has focused on allergy issues. Under the law and the FDA's biotech food policy, companies must tell consumers on the food label when a product includes a gene from a food that commonly causes an allergic reaction. The only exception is when the company can show that the protein produced by the added gene does not make the genetically modified food cause allergies.[42]

Of greater concern, and more difficult to predict, are environmental effects, though no ecological disasters have occurred thus far. What if the Bt-containing plants lead to the development of insects resistant to Bt and to other insecticides? Would the appearance of Bt-resistant insects spell the doom of a large portion of our crops of soybeans, or maize? In a study of Bt cotton plants, scientists estimated that 1 in 350 pests carried resistance to the Bt gene,[43] but further research shows that genetic engineering can also be used to overcome or at least delay development of Bt resistance.[44] Scientists suggest that planting a certain percentage of normal plants alongside the Bt-modified plants should delay the appearance of such resistant

---

Bt gene *Bacillus thuringiensis* (Bt) is a bacterium that produces a protein called the Bt toxin. One of the bacterium's genes, the Bt gene, carries the information for the Bt toxin. Inserting a copy of the Bt gene into plants enables them to produce Bt toxin protein and resist some insect pests. The Bt protein is not toxic to humans.

biodiversity The countless species of plants, animals and insects that exist on the earth. An undisturbed tropical forest is an example of the biodiversity of a healthy ecosystem.

mutants. If populations of such mutants became significant, farmers could fall back on conventional pest-control techniques. Meanwhile, we could have better crop yields with a reduction in pesticide use.

A related concern is the development of herbicide-resistant weeds, or "superweeds." When herbicide-resistant crops are planted in proximity to related wild plants, pollen may drift from food plant to weed, and the resistance genes might be passed to the weedy cousins of the GM plants. In the presence of herbicide, this might lead to the rapid selection of herbicide-resistant weeds. Although transfer of the herbicide-resistant gene to a related weed can occur, so far the effects have been minor, and the "superweeds" have rapidly lost the resistance gene once the herbicide was removed.

A final concern is that the herbicide-resistant food plants may become so successful that they are planted over a vast acreage in developing countries, and sprayed with excessive amounts of herbicides. In the worst scenario, this could lead to a loss of many species of unmodified plants as well as the insect and animal communities that depend on them. Many scientists believe that the loss of biodiversity is one of the greatest threats to the planet today. Because of the complexity and interdependence of the biosphere, this is perhaps the greatest unknown, and the greatest danger of unmonitored use of GM crops.

Regulation

The FDA regulates foods and food safety, and it oversees genetically modified foods as well as conventional foods. For foods derived from new varieties of plants, the FDA takes the position that whether modified by traditional breeding or genetic engineering, testing for safe human consumption is the legal responsibility of the producer or manufacturer of the foods. Crops like Bt-modified soybeans do not require special testing or labeling, or FDA approval. Although the plant expresses the Bt protein, the beans do not contain it. Except for some foreign DNA sequences, the beans are identical to unmodified soybeans. However, when a new substance is added to a food, FDA review and approval are necessary. Thus, if a new substance is produced or introduced into a food by genetic means, it must be tested as though it were a food additive.

The generally conservative approach of the FDA is based on decades of experience with food plants, which contain thousands of different substances. The plants we eat every day produce a variety of compounds that, if eaten in sufficient quantity, are toxic to humans. Potatoes, for instance, produce variable amounts of solanine, a fairly toxic alkaloid. These naturally occurring toxins may be inadvertently increased by classical breeding and selection, and so monitoring levels of toxins in plants is neither new nor unusual. If there are unexpected consequences of gene modification, the FDA is in an excellent position to evaluate them, and alter food-testing procedures where necessary. Many groups from government agencies like the FDA, to professional organizations like the ADA, to consumer advocacy groups are monitoring developments in biotechnology. Web sites for these organizations can be a source of policy statements and breaking news in this area. Regardless of our views on genetic manipulation of food plants, we are likely to see an explosion of new GM foods in the coming years.

Key Concepts: *Genetic engineering allows scientists to transform a plant one gene at a time, using well-established methods for manipulating DNA sequences. The goals of genetic modification of foods are higher yields, lower costs, increased amounts of critical nutrients, and a healthier mix of plant oils. Because of the complexity and interdependence of the biosphere, loss of genetic biodiversity is perhaps the greatest unknown, and the greatest danger of unmonitored GM crops.*

Label [to] **Table**

Many people are apprehensive about eating foods that have unfamiliar ingredients. You may say to yourself, "What is this chemical-sounding stuff and what is it doing in my food?" Unless you are a food scientist, it may be difficult to know exactly why certain additives are in food. However, it is important to remember that one of the major reasons for using additives is to enhance food safety. Preservatives can retard the growth of pathogenic bacteria by decreasing the moisture in food or by increasing the acidity of food. Other additives are used to improve the color and flavor of foods. While the chemical names on ingredient labels may sound foreign, consider that all foods are chemicals, and many additives are in fact natural substances. Let's take a look at the following ingredient list on a label from canned tomatoes.

The first three ingredients are all familiar. But what about calcium chloride and citric acid? Citric acid is a natural constituent of citrus fruits and a common food additive. It helps control the pH (acidity/alkalinity) as well as maintain palatability and wholesomeness. Remember, most pathogenic bacteria love a neutral or basic pH, and in particular the very dangerous bacteria *Clostridium botulinum* likes an anaerobic environment, like the one provided by a sealed can.

So what about the calcium chloride? Calcium chloride is a humectant (a compound that retains water) and can increase both the firmness and tenderness of a product. Wouldn't you rather open a can of firm, diced tomatoes to add to your spaghetti sauce than a can of mushy tomatoes? The calcium chloride is added to make sure you can!

Once you realize what these compounds are used for, you can see that they are added for our benefit. Many times, the purpose of the additive is listed right after the ingredients. If you are curious about other food additives that you see on ingredient labels, check the International Food Information Council's (IFIC) Web site at http://ificinfo.health.org for further information.

Nutrition Facts

Serving Size: $1/2$ cup (121g)
Servings Per Container about 3.5

Amount Per Serving

Calories 25	Calories from Fat 0

	% Daily Value*
Total Fat 0g	0%
Saturated Fat 0g	0%
Cholesterol 0mg	0%
Sodium 220mg	9%
Total Carbohydrate 4g	1%
Dietary Fiber 1g	4%
Sugars 3g	
Protein 1g	

Vitamin A	10%	Vitamin C	15%
Calcium	2%	Iron	4%

*Percent Daily Values are based on a 2,000 calorie diet.

INGREDIENTS: TOMATOES, TOMATO JUICE, SALT, CALCIUM CHLORIDE (FIRMING AGENT) AND CITRIC ACID.

LEARNING *Portfolio* c h a p t e r 1 7

Key Terms

	page		page
additives	691	Genetically modified (GM) foods	697
aflatoxins	683	genome	697
biodiversity	700	Hazard Analysis Critical Control Point (HACCP)	687
biotechnology	697	indirect additives	691
botulism	675	irradiation	695
Bt gene	700	methyl mercury	683
ciguatera	683	natural toxins	683
color additive	692	organic foods	679
critical control points (CCP)	687	pasteurization	695
Delaney clause	694	pesticides	679
dioxin	683	poisonous mushrooms	683
direct additives	691	preservatives	695
Escherichia coli (E. coli)	676	prior-sanctioned substance	694
Food Allergy Network	684	Safe Tables Our Priority (S.T.O.P.)	687
Food Code	687	*Salmonella*	675
Food Safety Initiative	687	solanine	684
foodborne illness	674		
Generally Recognized As Safe (GRAS)	692		
genetic engineering	697		

Study Points

➤ Foodborne illness is extremely common; it affects millions of Americans each year. Estimates of the frequency of foodborne illness are difficult because the vast majority of foodborne illnesses go unreported.

➤ The incidence of foodborne illness may be on the rise in the United States. Numerous factors are responsible including the increased centralization of food preparation, importation of many foods, increasing population of especially susceptible individuals (such as the elderly and immunocompromised), and failure of consumers and retail establishments to follow appropriate food safety measures.

➤ Microorganisms cause most foodborne diseases in the United States. Most of these illnesses are preventable.

➤ *Staphylococcus aureus* is one of the most common causes of foodborne illness. Onset of illness is rapid, typically occurring between 30 minutes and a few hours of consuming the contaminated food.

➤ Common symptoms of foodborne illness are diarrhea, nausea, abdominal cramps, and sometimes fever. The severity of the illness depends on the type of organism and the amount of contaminant eaten.

➤ Ensuring a safe food supply is a farm-to-table continuum involving producers, manufacturers, retailers, and consumers.

➤ Pesticides, animal drugs, natural toxins, and pollutants are the major forms of chemical food contamination.

➤ The government monitors imported and domestic foods for pesticide residues by testing food samples for both amounts and types of pesticides. Efforts are under way to lower the allowable amounts of certain pesticides to avoid harm to infants and children.

➤ The FDA evaluates drugs used in food-producing animals for safety in both animals and humans. Overuse of animal antibiotics could contribute to the emergence of antibiotic-resistant microorganisms that could threaten human health.

➤ The government and the food industry use the Hazard Analysis Critical Control Point system to prevent food contamination.

➤ Consumers must take responsibility for food safety in their homes. Cleaning hands and surfaces, avoiding cross-contamination, cooking adequately, and refrigerating foods promptly are important steps to prevent foodborne illness.

➤ The federal government reviews the safety of new food additives before they can be used in foods sold on the market.

➤ The Delaney Clause is a controversial food law that prohibits the approval of a food additive if it has been found to cause cancer in humans or laboratory animals, even if massive doses are required to produce the disease.

➤ Food-preservation techniques inhibit growth of microorganisms. Canning, drying, freezing, fermentation, and pasteurization are common.

➤ Although the FDA has approved food irradiation for numerous uses, it is rarely used primarily due to consumer fears. Food irradiation does not make foods radioactive. It can kill insects and most microorganisms. Appropriate doses of radiation extend the shelf-life of many foods.

➤ Genetically modified (GM) foods are most likely already on your table. Soybeans, corn, and potatoes are some of the GM foods being commercially produced. Concerns about GM foods include worries about decreasing biodiversity and the development of herbicide-resistant weeds.

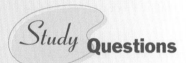

Study Questions

1. **What are the two main ways that pathogenic bacteria can cause foodborne illness?**

2. **Why shouldn't your 97-year-old great-grandmother drink homemade eggnog made from raw eggs?**

3. **How can you limit your intake of pesticides, according to the Consumers Union?**

4. **List four naturally occurring toxins.**

5. **List the most common food allergens. What are some symptoms of a food allergy?**

6. **What does "HACCP" stand for and what is its purpose?**

7. **The home kitchen can be a breeding ground for pathogenic bacteria; what are some ways to keep food safe at home?**

8. **What purpose(s) do food additives serve?**

9. **What is the purpose of the Delaney Clause? What are the complications surrounding this food law?**

10. **List the most common food-preservation techniques.**

11. **What are scientists' two major concerns about genetically engineered crops?**

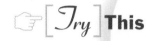

Bacterial Detective

What sources of bacteria do you encounter in your everyday activities? Here's an experiment to find out.

First, you'll need...
Cotton swabs
Six or more Petri dishes with agar
If you are unable to obtain a set of agar-filled Petri dishes from your school or local health department, you can make your own culture medium. Here's how:

- Add 2 teaspoons of unflavored gelatin (1 packet) and 2 teaspoons of sugar to $^2/_3$ cup of water.
- Bring the solution to a boil and stir for 1 minute until everything is dissolved. Pour $^1/_4$ inch of the solution into each Petri dish or other suitable container.

Then, using separate Petri dishes,

1. Pluck a hair and lay it in one Petri dish.
2. Sneeze or cough into another Petri dish.
3. Run a cotton swab around a nostril and carefully zigzag it across the agar in another Petri dish.
4. Run a cotton swab across a dampened kitchen sink sponge and carefully zigzag it across the agar in another Petri dish.
5. Run a cotton swab around a clean kitchen countertop and carefully zigzag it across the agar in another Petri dish.
6. Use the same procedure to collect additional samples from any other area in which bacteria may be present.
7. Finally, store the Petri dishes in a warm environment, at a constant temperature around 80°F. Check your specimens periodically. Within a week, you should see something growing!

Organic Foods

Organic foods are increasing in popularity. Are organic foods widely available in your neighborhood? What types of organic produce can you find? Go to either a natural food store or the local grocery store and look at the array of organic produce. Compare the prices of organic produce to nonorganic produce. Do you think the cost differences outweigh possible benefits? Compare the look of the organic and nonorganic produce. Do you see any differences? What other organic products can you find?

References

1 Mead PS, Slutsker L, Dietz V, et al. Food-related illness and death in the United States. *Emerg Infect Dis.* 1999;5:607–625.

2 US Environmental Protection Agency and US Departments of Health and Human Services and Agriculture. *Food Safety from Farm to Table: A National Food-Safety Initiative.* Washington, DC: 1997.

3 Position of the American Dietetic Association: Food and Water Safety. Am Diet Assoc. 1997;97:184–189.

4 Advance notice of proposed rulemaking: *Salmonella enteritidis* in eggs. *Federal Register.* May 19, 1998; 63:27502–27511.

5 US Food and Drug Administration Pesticide Program. *Residue Monitoring 1999.* 13th annual report. Washington, DC: Author; April 2000.

6 Ibid.

7 Ibid.

8 Food Quality Protection Act: Title III of Public Law 104–170; 1996.

9 Consumers Union. *Do you know what you're eating? An analysis of US Government data on pesticide residues in food.* Consumers Union of United States; Feb 1999. Yonkers, NY.

10 Ibid.

11 Greener greens? *Consumer Reports.* January, 1998:12–18.

12 US Department of Agriculture. Labeling and Marketing Information, National Organic Program Fact Sheet. Washington, DC; March 2000.

13 National Organic Program, Agricultural Marketing Service, USDA, June 2000.

14 Greener greens? Op. cit.

15 Greener greens? Op. cit.

16 National Organic Program, Op. cit. and US Department of Agriculture. Questions and answers about the National Organic Program proposed rule. Washington, DC: Author; Dec 1997.

17 Institute of Medicine. Committee on Drug Use in Food Animals. *The Use of Drugs in Food Animals: Benefits and Risks.* Washington, DC: National Academy Press; 1999.

18 US Food and Drug Administration. FDA Stops Distribution of Some Eggs and Catfish Because of Dioxin-Contaminated Animal Feed. www.cfsan.fda.gov/~lrd/hhsdiox.html. Accessed 11/1/00.

19 US Food and Drug Administration. *Foodborne Pathogenic Microorganisms and Natural Toxins Handbook.* Washington, DC: Author; 1992.

20 Segal M. Stalking the wild mushroom. *FDA Consumer.* October 1994:20–24.

21 US Food and Drug Administration. *Foodborne Pathogenic Microorganisms . . . .* Op. cit.

22 Food Allergy Network. Information. www.foodallergy.org/information.html. Accessed 11/1/2000.

23 US Environmental Protection Agency and US Departments of Health and Human Services and Agriculture. Op. cit.

24 Ibid.

25 Pathogen reduction: Hazard Analysis and Critical Control Point (HACCP) systems; final rule. *Federal Register.* July 25, 1996;61:38805–38989.

26 Hazard Analysis and Critical Control Point (HACCP) for the safe and sanitary processing and importing of juice. *Federal Register.* April 24, 1998;63:20449–20486.

27 US Department of Health and Human Services, Food and Drug Administration. *Food Code.* Washington, DC: Author; 1997.

28 Partnership for Food Safety Education. Fight Bac!: Four Simple Steps to Food Safety. www.fightbac.org. Accessed 11/1/00.

29 US Department of Agriculture. USDA Issues Final Rule on Safe Handling Labels for Meat and Poultry Products. Press release 0860.93; Oct. 8, 1993.

30 Food labeling: warning and notice statement: labeling of juice products; final rule. *Federal Register.* July 8, 1998;63:37029–37056.

31 Food labeling: safe handling statements: labeling of shell eggs: refrigeration of shell eggs held for retail distribution. *Federal Register.* July 6, 1999;64:36491–36516.

32 Wolf ID. Critical issues in food safety, 1991-2000. *Food Technol.* 1992;46:64–70.

33 Wood OB, Bruhn CM. Position of the American Dietetic Association: food irradiation. *J Am Diet Assoc.* 2000;100:246–253.

34 US Environmental Protection Agency and US Departments of Health and Human Services and Agriculture. Op. cit.

35 Wood OB, Bruhn CM. Op. cit.

36 Henkel J. Irradiation: a safe measure for safer food. *FDA Consumer.* May/June 1998.

37 Wood OB, Bruhn CM. Op. cit.

38 Pohlman A, Wood OB, Mason AC. Influence of audiovisuals and food samples on consumer acceptance of food irradiation. *Food Technol.* 1994;48(12):46–49.

39 Henkel J. Genetic engineering: fast forwarding to future foods. *FDA Consumer.* February 1998 update.

40 Overseeing biotech foods. *Genetic Engineering News.* 2000;20(10):1,37.

41 Nash, MJ. Grains of hope. *Time.* July 31, 2000;39–46.

42 Thompson, L. Are bioengineered foods safe? *FDA Consumer.* Jan/Feb 2000.

43 Gould F, Anderson A, Jones A, et al. Initial frequency of alleles for resistance to *Bacillus thuringiensis* toxins in field populations of *Heliothis virescens. Proc Natl Acad Sci.* 1997;94:3519–3523.

44 Kota M, Daniell H, Varma S, et al. Overexpression of the *Bacillus thuringiensis* (Bt) Cry2Aa2 protein in chloroplasts confers resistance to plants against susceptible and Bt-resistant insects. *Proc Natl Acad Sci.* 1999;96:1840–1845.

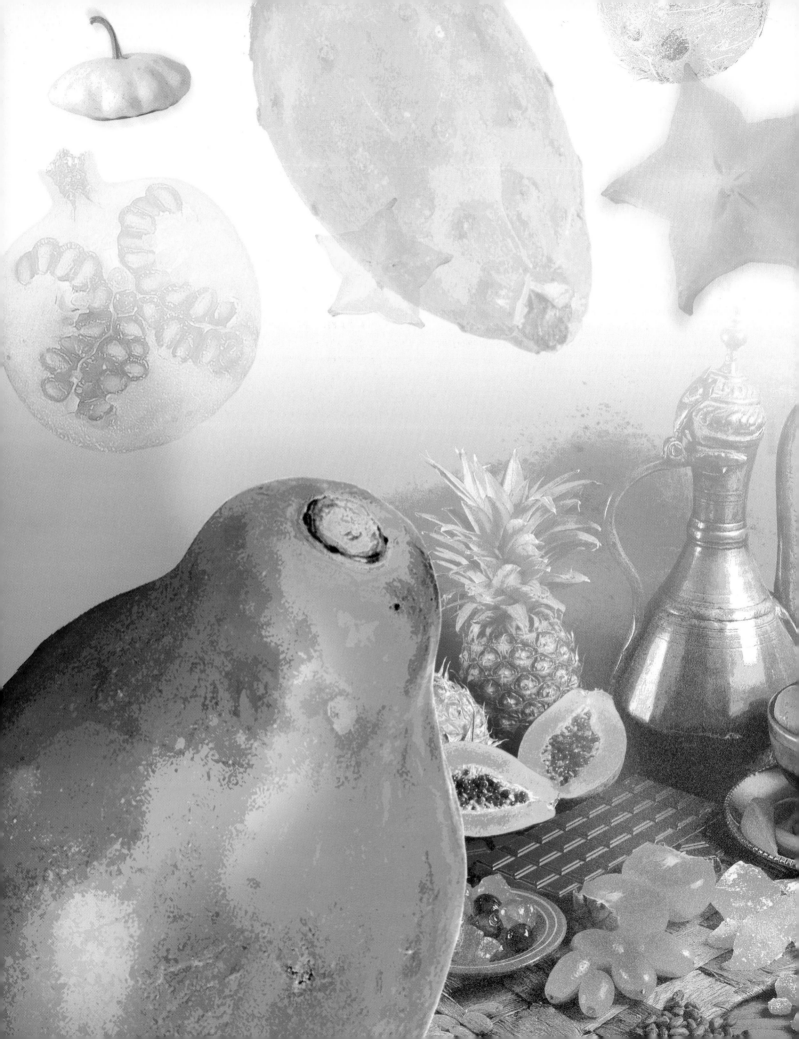

Chapter 18

World View of Nutrition

Think About It

1 Have you ever experienced hunger without being able to satisfy it within a day?
2 Have you seen evidence of hunger or malnutrition in your community?
3 What can you do to help eliminate hunger in North America?
4 How do you feel about the United States sending food to impoverished countries?

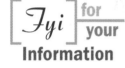

Fyi for your Information

This chapter's FYI boxes include practical information on the following topics:

- Hungry and Homeless
- AIDS and Malnutrition
- Tough Choices

The web site for this book offers many useful tools and is a great source for additional nutrition information for both students and instructors. Visit the site at **nutrition.jbpub.com** for information on the world view of nutrition. You'll find exercises that explore the following topics:

- The ADA and World Hunger
- U.S. Food Insecurity
- Individual Actions Count
- UNICEF

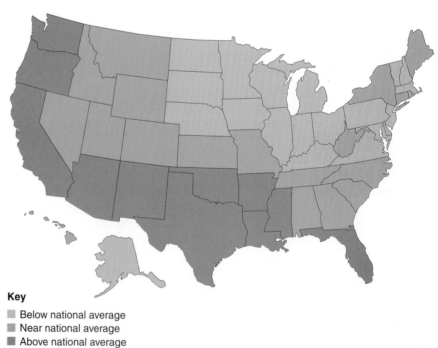

hunger The uneasy or painful sensation caused by a lack of food; the recurrent and involuntary lack of access to food that may produce malnutrition over time.

malnutrition Failure to achieve nutrient requirements, which can impair physical and/or mental health. It may result from consuming too little food or a shortage or imbalance of key nutrients.

*E*ach day on your way to class, you pass a soup kitchen. You look at the long line of men and women waiting to get their meals, and wonder what brought them to this point. You wonder how many similar soup lines exist in your community, and how many people need food assistance, but can't get it. If **hunger** exists in our rich country, what about people living in poor countries?

Almost 800 million people in the developing world do not have enough to eat. Another 34 million in industrialized and transitional countries chronically worry about having enough food.[1] And every day 35,000 people die, directly or indirectly, from **malnutrition**.[2]

In this chapter, we look at hunger and malnutrition. By *hunger* we don't mean that mildly empty feeling one gets before mealtime. We mean the inability, day after day, to satisfy basic nutrition needs, the gnawing emptiness that creates a constant focus on eating and how to obtain food. In contrast to the hunger dieters feel from cutting calories, this deprivation is involuntary and unwanted.

PREVALENCE OF FOOD INSECURITY

Key

- Below national average
- Near national average
- Above national average

Figure 18.1 **Prevalence of food insecurity.** The National Health and Nutrition Examination Survey (NHANES III) found that food insecurity is as common among the working poor as the unemployed. Food insecurity is more common in southern and western states. **Source:** Calculated by USDA Economic Research Service (ERS) based on Current Population Survey Food Security Supplement data, September 1996, April 1997, and August 1998.

Technically speaking *malnutrition* can be any kind of unhealthy nutritional status, including the result of imbalance and excess—obesity or toxicity from oversupplementation, for example. And although we touch on obesity as an emerging issue, even in developing countries, by and large in this chapter *malnutrition* means undernutrition resulting from hunger.

Along the spectrum of malnutrition and hunger is the less extreme condition of **food insecurity**, the ongoing worry about having enough to eat. At the opposite end of the spectrum is **food security**, access to nutritionally adequate and safe food. Most people in the industrialized world are food secure. Overabundance and obesity are the primary problems in these populations, but malnutrition is a serious problem among certain groups such as the homeless and urban poor.

Malnutrition in the United States

The Face of American Malnutrition

In the food-rich United States, food insecurity remains a problem.[3] (See **Figure 18.1.**) It is characterized by anxiety about having enough to eat and the worry about running out of food and having no money to purchase more. Some people actually go hungry in the United States: almost 10 million people, over a third of them children, lived in a household in which at least one person experienced hunger during 1998.[4]

Households that are struggling to meet basic food needs tend to follow a typical pattern as their plight worsens. First, adults worry about having enough food. Then, they stretch resources and juggle other necessities, with more of the budget going for fixed expenses than for food. The quality and variety of the diet declines. Next, the adults eat less and less often. And finally, as food becomes more limited, the children also eat less.

Surprisingly, there's more obesity among low-income, food-insecure groups than among those with higher incomes. But the quality of those low-income diets is typically poor, and with worsening food insecurity come progressively more disordered eating patterns. Patterns such as binge eating can become habitual and contribute to obesity.[5]

Among the food-insecure, intake of healthful foods and the micronutrients they contain are significantly reduced. Although unlikely to cause overt deficiency disease, the subtle effects of this suboptimal diet are serious and costly, showing up years later as chronic illness, or more immediately as reduced immune function. More illness, more medicines, more doctor visits and hospital stays, more missed days and poorer performance at school and work, poor pregnancy outcome, delayed growth and development—suboptimal nutrition contributes to them all.

Prevalence and Distribution

How much hunger and food insecurity exist in the United States? Until recently, data that could answer the question were mostly fragmentary or suggestive. Estimates were based on the percentage of the population living in poverty (see **Table 18.1**), with the assumption that they were at risk of undernutrition. Such estimates are somewhat flawed because being at risk does not necessarily mean that people *are* poorly nourished. Many people with limited financial resources manage to eat well. On the other hand,

food insecurity Limited or uncertain availability of nutritionally adequate and safe foods, or limited or uncertain ability to acquire acceptable foods in socially acceptable ways.

food security Access to enough food for an active, healthy life, including (1) the ready availability of nutritionally adequate and safe foods and (2) an assured ability to acquire acceptable foods in socially acceptable ways.

Food Recovery and Gleaning

*E*ach year more than 96 billion pounds of food produced in this country go to waste. Programs throughout the country are rescuing much of this wholesome food and distributing it to people in need. "Gleaning" is harvesting excess food from farms, orchards, and packing houses. Perishable items are also salvaged from wholesale and retail markets; fresh foods that are wholesome but will spoil before they can be sold are given to local food pantries and meal providers. Canned goods and other staples are collected from groceries, distributors, food processors, and individual homes. Even surplus food from restaurants, caterers, and other food services is collected by some charities for local food programs.

Think About It 1

Food Security Supplement Survey A federally funded survey that measures the prevalence and severity of food insecurity and hunger.

Personal Responsibility and Work Opportunity Reconciliation Act A 1996 federal welfare reform plan that dramatically changed the nation's welfare system into one that requires work in exchange for time-limited assistance. Also called the Welfare Reform Act.

under certain circumstances such as loss of a job, people who live well above the poverty line may be food insecure.

In 1995 the U.S. Census Bureau began tracking hunger with an annual **Food Security Supplement Survey**, which asks about food availability and hunger in the household (see **Table 18.2**). From 1996 through 1998, Americans in 9.7 percent of households worried about having enough to eat, and those in 3.5 percent of households also experienced hunger.[6] These findings were down slightly from findings of 1995.[7] The figures are consistent with those of NHANES III, in which 3.5 percent of households reported not having enough to eat *sometimes*, and 0.6 percent said they often did not have enough to eat.[8]

Both surveys found a strong, but not perfect, association with poverty and an interaction of economic and social factors. Food insecurity and hunger were highest in the inner city, in Hispanic and African American households, and in households with young children, those headed by women, and those headed by a person with limited education. (See **Figure 18.2A–D.**) Clearly then, to end food insecurity and hunger, nutrition programs must be accompanied by social and economic efforts.

The Working Poor

Employment does not guarantee that families always have enough to eat. NHANES III found that food insecurity is as common among the working poor as the unemployed. Since the 1996 **Personal Responsibility and Work Opportunity Reconciliation Act**, commonly called welfare reform, thousands have left the welfare roles for jobs. Often the pay is too little to lift households above poverty level,[9] and work-related expenses such as transportation or child care further depress family budgets. Low-paid workers may be unaware that they still qualify for food assistance programs. On the other hand, their work hours may preclude program participation.

Table 18.1 Poverty Guidelines: Income levels defined as poverty for a given household size

Size of Family Unit	48 Contiguous States and D.C.	Alaska	Hawaii
1	$8,350	$10,430	$9,590
2	11,250	14,060	12,930
3	14,150	17,690	16,270
4	17,050	21,320	19,610
5	19,950	24,950	22,950
6	22,850	28,580	26,290
7	25,750	32,210	29,630
8	28,650	35,840	32,970
For each additional person, add	2,900	3,630	3,340

Note: Despite the limits to the use of household income as a proxy for estimating food insecurity, poverty remains an intuitively reasonable indicator. In addition to food, income must cover housing, clothing, transportation, medical care, and other essentials.

Source: *Federal Register.* 2000;65(31):7555–7557.

The Isolated

People who live in remote rural areas can be far from food resources and lack access to transportation. Other people become isolated despite living in populated cities. Even though they live in a crowded neighborhood or apartment building, they are alone and are physically or mentally unable to obtain adequate food.

Elders

The infirmities of age, along with feelings of vulnerability, keep some elderly people homebound and lonely, conditions hardly conducive to a healthy appetite. Physical ailments may make cooking and eating difficult, while actually increasing nutrient needs. Elders often have small incomes with little prospect for improvement. Like others with limited resources, they cut food purchases to pay for other necessities. Although food assistance may be available, pride or shame may keep an older person from participating in such programs.[10]

The Homeless or Inadequately Housed

The homeless rely on soup kitchens and other public programs for much of their food. Some resort to handouts, and even forage through garbage. Many are mentally ill or substance abusers. The addict often has little interest in eating, and may sell available food to buy more drugs. Many other people live in welfare hotels, single-room-occupancy facilities, or rooming houses without storage or cooking facilities. Budget-stretching strategies such as buying food in bulk and carefully using leftovers are out of the question for these people; as the monthly budget dwindles, they often rely on fast-food meals and then soup kitchens.

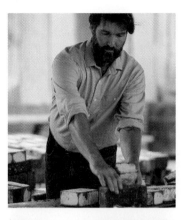
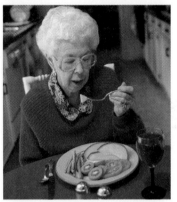
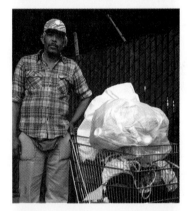
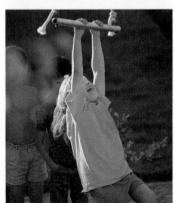

 Table 18.2 **Sample Questions from the Food Security Questionnaire**

Light Food Insecurity

"We worried whether our food would run out before we got money to buy more."
   Was that often, sometimes, or never true for you in the last 12 months?

"The food that we bought just didn't last and we didn't have money to get more."
   Was that often, sometimes, or never true for you in the last 12 months?

Moderate Food Insecurity

In the last 12 months did you or other adults in the household ever cut the size of your meals or skip meals because there wasn't enough money for food?

In the last 12 months, were you ever hungry but didn't eat because you couldn't afford enough food?

Severe Food Insecurity

In the last 12 months did you or other adults in the household ever not eat for a whole day because there wasn't enough money for food?

(For households with children) In the last 12 months did any of the children ever not eat for a whole day because there wasn't enough money for food?

Source: Nord M, Jemison K, Bickel G. Prevalence of Food Insecurity and Hunger, by State, 1996–1998. http://www.ers.usda.gov/epubs/pdf/fanrr2/fanrr2.pdf.

Figure 18.2 Americans most at risk for hunger include working poor, elders, homeless people, and children.

Food Research and Action Center (FRAC)
Founded in 1970 as a public interest law firm, FRAC is a nonprofit child advocacy group that works to improve public policies to eradicate hunger and undernutrition in the United States.

Special Supplemental Nutrition Program for Women, Infants, and Children (WIC) A USDA program that provides federal grants to states for supplemental foods, health-care referrals, and nutrition education for low-income pregnant, breastfeeding, and non-breastfeeding postpartum women, and to infants and children at nutritional risk.

Children

Perhaps no group is more vulnerable to hunger than the young. Growth and development are delayed in poorly nourished children. They get sick more often. It is harder for them to concentrate in school. Children are captives of their family circumstances; poverty and lack of nutritious food in the household are beyond a child's control. Approximately 4 million children under age 12 go hungry in the United States, and another 9.6 million are at risk of hunger.[11] These figures, based on the most comprehensive study of childhood hunger ever conducted in the United States, were estimated by the **Food Research and Action Center (FRAC)**, a nonprofit advocacy group that fights childhood hunger and undernutrition.

Attacking Hunger in America

Government efforts to fight hunger began during the Great Depression of the 1930s. From that modest beginning, federal efforts have grown to include at least 14 programs that address hunger (see **Table 18.3**). The School Lunch Program was created in 1946, after many young men had failed the physical requirements to be drafted to serve in World War II because of poor nutrition. The Food Stamp Program, begun on a small scale years earlier, was greatly expanded in the early 1970s following an exposé of hunger in Appalachia and the Mississippi Delta, and the television documentary "Hunger in America." The federal government initiated the **Special Supplemental Nutrition Program for Women, Infants, and Children (WIC)** in the 1970s as a response to concerns about maternal and child health. Other government programs have since been added to meet the special needs of the young, the elderly, the disadvantaged, and the disabled.

Nonprofit community agencies, charities, religious organizations, and similar groups, were organized during hard economic times in the 1980s to create a large network of food pantries, soup kitchens, and services for

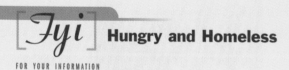

[*Fyi*] Hungry and Homeless

FOR YOUR INFORMATION

A shabbily dressed man slowly pushes a shopping cart along the sidewalk. It is laden with bottles and cans that he can redeem for cash. In front of a supermarket, a woman and child clutch a sign scrawled with the words "Hungry. Please help." On a street corner, a man confronts every passing car with a sign that says "Will work for food." When confronted by a homeless person, do you feel uncomfortable? Do you turn away? Or do you try to help?

Who are the homeless? Single men and families with children are the largest homeless groups. Roughly equal in size, they comprise about 80 percent of the homeless population. Single women (13 percent) and

unaccompanied minors (7 percent) account for the remainder. About 20 percent of the homeless are mentally ill—about the same number that are employed. Nearly one-third are substance abusers.[1]

Hunger in the homeless is caused by a number of interrelated factors including low-paying jobs, unemployment and employment-related problems, high housing costs, substance abuse, poverty or lack of income, and food stamp cuts. Family members—children and their parents—most frequently request emergency food assistance. Two-thirds of the adults requesting food assistance are employed.[2]

Complex challenges face the homeless,

who may sleep in the streets or in emergency shelters. The homeless get food from many sources—shelters, drop-in centers, fast-food restaurants, and garbage bins. Soup kitchens are a primary source of meals, yet negotiating this system to obtain adequate food can be a formidable and time-consuming task. Also, while homeless people often are eligible for food stamps, they are extremely limited in their ability to store and prepare food, and few restaurants are authorized to accept food stamps.

A major public health concern for homeless people is not only whether they are getting enough to eat but also the nutritional quality of their diet. This concern is complicated by

home-delivered meals. Most of the federal government's programs for direct distribution of food or meals operate at the local level through these networks. Both laypeople and professionals like dietitians work in these programs, either as volunteers or as staff, to fight hunger and malnutrition.

Food assistance programs have greatly reduced the prevalence of hunger, but not of food insecurity, which requires social and economic change. The following are among the federal government's most far-reaching programs against hunger.

Table 18.3 U.S. Programs That Address Food Insecurity and Hunger

Food Stamp Program

Nutrition Assistance Program for Puerto Rico

National School Lunch Program

School Breakfast Program

Child and Adult Care Food Program

Summer Food Service Program

Special Milk Program

Special Supplemental Nutrition Program for Women, Infants, and Children (WIC)

Commodity Supplemental Food Program

Food Distribution Program on Indian Reservations

Elderly Nutrition Program

Disaster Feeding Program

The Emergency Food Assistance Program (TEFAP)

Food Distribution Program for Charitable Institutions and Summer Camps

Source: Position of American Dietetic Association: Domestic food and nutrition security. *J Am Diet Assoc.* 1998;98:337–342.

the special needs of infants, children, and women, especially pregnant women. Diets of the homeless often are nutritionally inadequate. Studies of homeless women and children indicate that they consume less than half of the RDA for iron, zinc, magnesium, and folate daily.[3] Homeless adult males have diets low in calcium, zinc, B_6, and calories. Homeless adults consume less than 50 percent of the RDA for calcium. Poor diets put the homeless at an increased risk for illness and chronic conditions. Pregnant women, children, and people with compromised health status are particularly vulnerable.

Homeless families and individuals rely on emergency food assistance facilities not only during emergencies, but for extended periods. Unfortunately, these facilities are strained beyond their capacities—more than 40 percent cannot provide an adequate quantity of food.[4] Some shelters have resorted to rationing to extend their food resources to a greater number of people. Because of a lack of resources, over half may be forced to turn away people. Addressing hunger is a top priority. Once access to food is secure, a nutritionally adequate diet and dealing with health issues become reasonable.

1 The United States Conference of Mayors. December 1999. A Status Report on Hunger and Homelessness in America's Cities, 1999. http://www.usmayors.org/uscm/homeless/hunger99.pdf. Accessed 9/30/00.

2 Ibid.

3 Silliman K, Yamanoha M, Morrissey A. Evidence of nutritional risk in a population of homeless adults in rural Northern California. *J Am Diet Assoc.* 1998;98:908–910.

4 The United States Conference of Mayors. Op. cit.

Food Stamp Program A USDA program that helps single people and families with little or no income to buy food.

Electronic Benefits System (EBT) Electronic delivery of government benefits that relies on a single plastic card to access food benefits at point-of-sale locations.

National School Lunch Program A USDA program that provides nutritious lunches and the opportunity to practice skills learned in classroom nutrition education; enacted in 1946 to provide U.S. children at least one healthful meal every school day.

School Breakfast Program A USDA program that assists schools in providing a nutritious morning meal to children nationwide.

Child and Adult Care Food Program A federally funded program that reimburses approved family child care providers for USDA-approved foods served to pre-school children; also provides funds for meals and snacks served at after-school programs for school-age children and to adult day care centers serving chronically impaired adults or people over age 60.

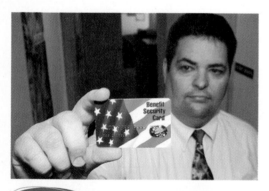

Figure 18.3 Electronic benefits transfer card.

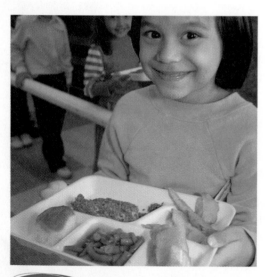

Figure 18.4 National school lunch program.

The Food Stamp Program

The **Food Stamp Program** is our main food security program. More than 18 million Americans received food stamps in 1999.[12] Income level of the household determines eligibility. For fiscal year 2000, the gross annual income for a family of four could not exceed $21,720.[13] The 1996 welfare reform reduced benefits per person, and made eligibility requirements stricter. It also toughened recertification for eligibility and put time limits on the benefits of able-bodied adults who did not work. All illegal immigrants and many legal immigrants were made ineligible for food stamps.

Actually the term *food stamp* is becoming a misnomer. Almost half of the people who receive benefits use **Electronic Benefits Transfer (EBT)** cards. (See **Figure 18.3**.) The card resembles and functions like a debit card. Each month the household's benefit amount is credited to the card, which is then used at participating groceries. Recipients can use food stamp benefits to purchase only food, and not nonfood items like paper goods, pet food, and alcohol. The benefit amount varies according to household size and income level, with some recipients getting as little as $10 per month. The average monthly individual benefit for 1999 was $73.[14]

Special Supplemental Nutrition Program for Women, Infants, and Children

The WIC program provides food to pregnant and breastfeeding women, infants, and preschoolers. In 1999 more than 7 million women and children received WIC benefits each month. To be eligible, the participant must be at nutritional risk and household income must be less than 185 percent of the poverty level. For fiscal year 2000, the gross annual income for a family of four could not exceed $31,543.[15]

Nutrition assessment and nutrition education are important components of the WIC program. Participants receive coupons, or "checks," for specific categories of healthful foods, and they "cash" them at participating groceries. Unlike food stamps, the amount of the WIC benefit varies with nutritional need, not income.

National School Lunch Program

The **National School Lunch Program** ensures that children in primary and secondary schools receive at least one healthy meal every school day (supplemented in many areas by the **School Breakfast Program**). For a family of four in fiscal 2000, the child's meals are free if the household income is less than $22,165; the meals are reduced in price if household income is less than $31,543.[16] The lunch must provide one-third or more of dietary requirements for key nutrients. The program operates in more than 96,000 public and nonprofit private schools and residential child care institutions. It provides nutritionally balanced, low-cost or free lunches to nearly 27 million children each school day.[17] (See **Figure 18.4**.)

Child and Adult Care Food Program

The **Child and Adult Care Food Program** provides funds for children's meals and snacks at nonprofit licensed child care centers, day care homes, after-school programs, and similar settings. Nutritious meals for elderly or disabled people are also funded at nonprofit facilities such as adult day care centers and recreation centers.

Key Concepts. *Overt malnutrition in the United States is uncommon. However, almost 10 percent of American households suffer food insecurity, and in more than 3 percent of American households someone has gone hungry. Food insecurity and hunger are strongly associated with poverty. Groups at risk include the working poor, the isolated, the homeless, children, and elders. A large network of individual volunteers, nonprofit agencies, and charities, together with major government programs such as Food Stamps, WIC, and School Lunch, have done much to reduce hunger. However, food insecurity, which continues among an unacceptably large number of people, must be overcome by social and economic improvements.*

World Health Organization (WHO) A global organization that directs and coordinates international health work. Its goal is the attainment by all peoples of the highest possible level of health defined as a state of complete physical, mental, and social well-being and not merely the absence of disease or infirmity.

Malnutrition in the Developing World

The numbers are staggering. In the developing world, 790 million people do not have enough to eat. Two out of five children are stunted by lack of food, one in three is underweight, and one in ten has significant wasting of muscle and fat tissue. The enormity of the problem can be overwhelming, until you learn that these statistics represent an improvement over former years. The proportion of undernourished people in developing countries has declined from 30 percent in 1979–1981, to 20 percent in 1990–1992, to 18 percent in 1995–1997—proof that progress is possible.[18]

But progress is much too slow and uneven in the 98 countries monitored by the **World Health Organization (WHO)**. In only 37 countries did the numbers of hungry people decline during the 1990s. In 27 other countries, the proportion of undernourished people actually increased.[19] (See **Figure 18.5**.)

Figure 18.5 **Global hunger.** Although the proportion of the world's population that is chronically undernourished has been decreasing over the last few decades, undernutrition is still widespread, particularly in certain regions. Furthermore, projections to the year 2010 suggest that there is little change in the absolute number of chronically undernourished people. **Source:** Food and Agriculture Organization of the United Nations; Luxembourg Income Study: First World Hunger, USDA; Second Harvest. WEBSITE http://www.fao.org/sd/eidirect/wfs/wfs1.htm.

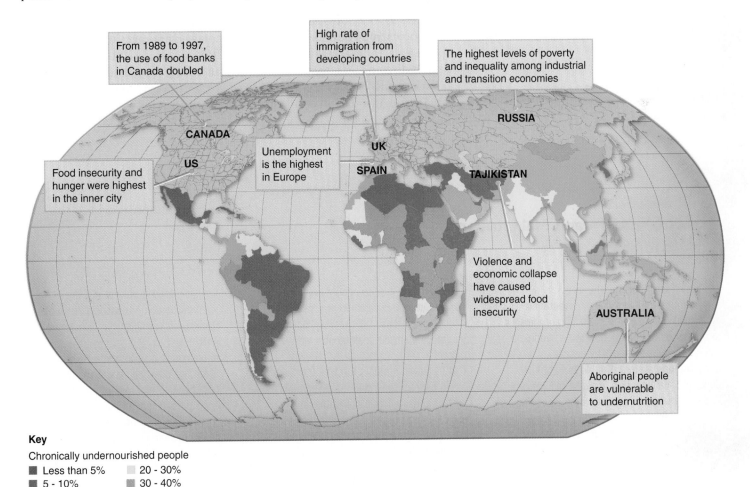

From 1989 to 1997, the use of food banks in Canada doubled

High rate of immigration from developing countries

The highest levels of poverty and inequality among industrial and transition economies

Food insecurity and hunger were highest in the inner city

Unemployment is the highest in Europe

Violence and economic collapse have caused widespread food insecurity

Aboriginal people are vulnerable to undernutrition

CANADA
US
UK
SPAIN
RUSSIA
TAJIKISTAN
AUSTRALIA

Key
Chronically undernourished people
- ■ Less than 5%
- ■ 5 - 10%
- ■ 10 - 20%
- ■ 20 - 30%
- ■ 30 - 40%
- ■ 40% and above
- ■ Comparable data not available

Food and Agriculture Organization (FAO) The largest autonomous UN agency; the FAO works to alleviate poverty and hunger by promoting agricultural development, improved nutrition, and the pursuit of food security

Think
About It

4

Where were you born?

*Y*our survival was greatly influenced by the location of your birth. Angola has the highest infant mortality rate (195 deaths per 1,000 live births), according to estimates for 2000. Other countries with high infant mortality rates include Sierra Leone (148 per 1,000), Afghanistan (149 per 1,000), and Liberia (134 per 1,000). At the other end of the spectrum is Finland (4 per 1,000). Canada (5 per 1,000) does better than the United States (7 per 1,000).

Hunger in the developing world is chronic. "It is debilitating. It blights the lives of all who are affected and undermines national economies and development processes where it is found on a large scale," says the **Food and Agriculture Organization** of the United Nations.[20] Although food shortages severe enough to cause endemic starvation or famine have lessened significantly, natural disasters, epidemics, economic or political upheaval, or war can quickly precipitate famine.[21]

Why Hunger?

Why, in a world of plenty, does hunger still exist? The causes are simple, but the solutions are tremendously complex; they require economic, political, and social change, as well as improvements in nutrition, food production, and environmental safeguards. As you study the critical nutrient deficiencies in the developing world, you will see that poverty, infection, poor sanitation, and social upheaval interact with nutrient shortages to bring about the deficiencies.

Social and Economic Factors

Poverty, overpopulation, and the migration to overcrowded cities are closely interrelated causes of hunger (**Figure 18.6**). Each situation worsens the effects of the others as they steadily drive a population toward malnutrition.

Poverty

Poverty is the most important underlying reason for chronic hunger. It limits access to food, obviously. It limits purchase of farming supplies to grow food, boats and equipment to fish, and storage equipment to prevent spoilage. It limits access to medical care. It compromises efforts at sanitation. It discourages education and the chance for personal advancement.

For nations, poverty means paralyzed economic development and too few jobs; inadequate investments in infrastructure and basic housing; and too few resources to train doctors, nutritionists, nurses, and other health-care workers.

AIDS and Malnutrition

FOR YOUR INFORMATION

Like other infections, HIV interacts with malnutrition in a vicious, devastating cycle. Left untreated, HIV infection progresses to the acquired immunodeficiency syndrome (AIDS). The virus attacks by destroying its victim's immune system. Unable to fight infections and malignancies, disease quickly depletes marginal nutrient stores, speeding the way to severe malnutrition and death. But malnutrition and HIV interact on several other levels, as well:

- Low vitamin A levels in pregnant women increase the rate of HIV transmission to their unborn babies.[1]

- HIV is transmitted to infants in breast milk; but in impoverished regions, substitutions for breast milk typically increase infantile diarrhea, malnutrition, and death.[2]
- AIDS leaves mothers too weak to feed and care for their children. Eventually AIDS turns children into orphans.
- AIDS disables parents so they cannot work to support and feed their families.
- Reduced levels of micronutrients in an HIV-infected person are associated with faster progression of HIV disease and AIDS.[3]

- Weight loss and muscle wasting in an infected person are associated with faster progression of HIV disease and AIDS.[4]
- Infections that accompany AIDS cause fever and diarrhea, worsening malnutrition. Nausea and loss of appetite also contribute to malnutrition.
- Severe protein-energy malnutrition (PEM) is characteristic of untreated AIDS, and frequently the ultimate cause of death.

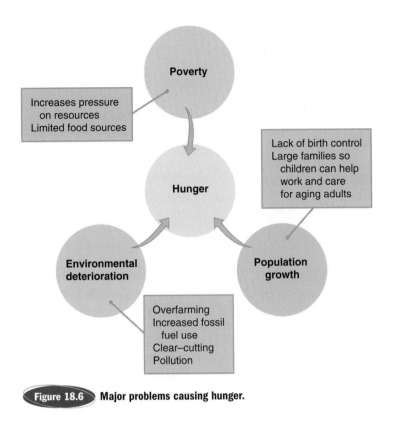

Poverty

Increases pressure
on resources
Limited food sources

Hunger

Lack of birth control
Large families so
children can help
work and care
for aging adults

Environmental
deterioration

Population
growth

Overfarming
Increased fossil
fuel use
Clear–cutting
Pollution

Figure 18.6 Major problems causing hunger.

Population Growth

Population growth in many regions is outstripping gains in food production, education, employment, health care, and economic progress. The burgeoning numbers stress limited environmental resources, contributing to environmental degradation and pollution. In rural areas where farmland is limited, each small parcel of family land is subdivided with each generation, until there is too little land to support each family.

As of June 2000, sub-Saharan Africa had 24.5 million people infected with HIV. Southeast Asia had 5.6 million people infected with HIV, and Latin America had 1.3 million.[5] Without treatment or a cure, these people are doomed to death, usually within 10 years of the initial infection. The fate of severe PEM in millions of people appears unavoidable. If we do not arrest the continued transmission of HIV, the number of PEM victims will climb even higher.

1 Semba RD, Miotti PG, Chiphangwi JD. Maternal vitamin A deficiency and mother-to-child transmission of HIV-1. *Lancet.* 1994;343:1593–1597.

2 Desclaux A, Taverne B, Alfieri C, et al. Socio-cultural obstacles in the prevention of HIV transmission through breast-milk in West Africa. Program and abstracts of the 13th International AIDS Conference; July 9–14, 2000; Durban, South Africa. Abstract MoOrD205.

3 Tang AM, Graham NMH, Kirby AJ, et al. Dietary micronutrient intake and risk of progression to acquired immunodeficiency syndrome (AIDS) in human immunodeficiency virus type-1 (HIV-1)-infected homosexual men. *Am J Epidem.* 1993;138:937–951.

4 Coodley GO, Loveless MO, Merrill TM. The HIV wasting syndrome: a review. *J Acq Immune Def Syndr.* 1994;7:681–694.

5 Joint United Nations Programme on HIV/AIDS. Report on the Global HIV/AIDS Epidemic. Geneva, Switzerland: UNAIDS; June 2000.

Quick Bites

Food Supply versus Food Safety

Sometimes obtaining food is more important than safety. Street-vended food is important in the diets of many urban populations, particularly the socially disadvantaged. Health authorities responsible for food safety should balance their risk management with food availability and hunger. Rigorous application of codes and regulations suited to larger and permanent food-service establishments may cause the disappearance of the street vendors with consequent aggravation of hunger and malnutrition. WHO encourages the development of regulations that empower vendors to take greater responsibility for the preparation of safe food.

Quick Bites

Rehydration Therapy for Diarrhea

Simple and inexpensive packets of carbohydrate and salts diluted with sterile water replace lost fluids and electrolytes. These packets are saving thousands of people each year.

You might think that poverty would pressure parents to limit family size, but ironically, poverty and sickness do just the reverse. Where child mortality rates are high, having many babies is a guarantee some children will survive. In countries that have no economic safeguards for disability, unemployment, or old age, parents consider their children a source of security and support in times of need. Many other factors contribute to large families, from ignorance of birth control methods to the attitude that big families reflect the father's masculinity. Some political groups also encourage high birth rates and fast population growth as a way to achieve political or military dominance.

To slow population growth, socioeconomic and cultural changes that make smaller family size acceptable, even desirable, must accompany access to birth control.

Urbanization

Urbanization is a worldwide trend. As rural lands become too crowded, or exhausted farmland no longer supports good crops, rural people migrate to the city in hopes of jobs and a better life. Unfortunately, in fast-growing cities, social disorder, sanitary conditions, and living standards may be much worse. Hunting, fishing, foraging, and gardening—sources of accessible food in the rural setting—are seldom an option in the city. Breastfeeding becomes impractical for many mothers who could nurse their babies while doing farm work, but cannot do so with jobs in the city.

Infection and Disease

Infection interacts with malnutrition, each making its victim more vulnerable to the other, each making the other worse, in a downward spiral. Nutrient deficiencies lower resistance to infections.[22] In turn, the fever of infection speeds depletion of calories and nutrients. Other symptoms (e.g., loss of appetite, weakness, nausea, and mouth lesions) limit ability to eat. Infectious diarrhea is especially dangerous, quickly wasting what few nutrients are consumed; infants and young children can die quickly from loss of electrolytes. Programs that prevent or control infection (e.g., immunizations, improvements in hygiene and sanitation, providing safe water, and access to medicine and medical care) all indirectly improve nutrition status.

Today, infection with the human immunodeficiency virus (HIV) provides a dramatic demonstration of the interaction between malnutrition and infection. Transmission of the virus from mother to fetus is greater when the mother is deficient in vitamin A.[23] The infection progresses fastest in people who are poorly nourished.[24] And severe loss of weight and muscle are hallmarks of the advanced disease, acquired immune deficiency syndrome (AIDS). As of June 2000, 34.3 million people were infected with HIV—more than 90 percent in the developing world and more than 24 million of them in sub-Saharan Africa.[25] A nutrition disaster is on the horizon.

Political Disruptions and Natural Disasters

Social upheavals and natural disasters such as floods and drought can leave famine in their wakes. The resulting displacement of populations and often inequitable food distribution usually lead to hunger and malnutrition.

War

Whereas poverty is the underlying cause of chronic mild to moderate malnutrition, war and its aftermath cause severe malnutrition and famine. War diverts limited financial resources from development efforts to expenditures for fighting and destruction. Men and women no longer farm, fish, or bring home a paycheck—they are in the army. Households become fatherless and sometimes motherless, often permanently. Crops and croplands are destroyed, along with irrigation systems, food-processing facilities, and transportation infrastructure, which may have taken decades to develop.

Refugees

Masses of refugees, many very young, old, infirm, and already weakened by chronic hunger, find themselves without the basic elements of sustenance. The resulting famine has become an all too common sight on the evening news. International relief agencies have learned to respond to these emergencies nimbly and with great determination, but logistic difficulties (e.g., mobilizing manpower, obtaining foods, transporting supplies, setting up feeding stations, etc.) may slow relief until it is too late for the sickest or weakest. Some refugee groups are inaccessible, hidden, or intentionally kept hungry as part of a political plan; emergency food may never reach many of them.

Sanctions

International sanctions and embargoes create food shortages, both directly and indirectly, by limiting access to agricultural supplies, fuel, and food-processing supplies. Some people argue that shortages created by embargoes hurt powerless people rather than government officials; others say that such actions are preferable to war.

Floods, Droughts, Mudslides, and Hurricanes

Many countries are not equipped to deal with food shortages and hunger from natural disasters. International relief agencies and other governments step in to help when possible. Some U.S. agencies involved are the USDA, the U.S. State Department through its Agency for International Development, and the Center for Disease Control and Prevention (CDC) through its Center for Communicable Diseases. These agencies offer both short-term, emergency efforts and long-term programs for repair and rebuilding.

Inequitable Food Distribution

Advances in agriculture have increased food production worldwide. Enough calories are now produced to supply the energy needs of every person on earth.[26] But distribution of these calories is uneven: among the continents, among nations, within nations, and even in families.

In some societies the father of the family may be wrongly perceived as having the greatest nutrition needs, and be given priority for the most nutritious, high-protein foods. In those societies, older boys would have second priority; pregnant and breastfeeding women, women in general, and small children would have the lowest priority. Nations may follow a similar pattern, ensuring that their soldiers or men of fighting age receive scarce foodstuffs.

Regional Trends

In sub-Saharan Africa, where the population is growing at an unprecedented rate of 3 percent per year, food production cannot keep pace; in fact, food availability per capita is declining.[27] Economic factors, violent regional conflicts, and the tremendous cost of the AIDS epidemic contribute to widespread, worsening hunger.

Among the former communist countries of Eastern Europe and Eurasia, abrupt economic transition and political upheaval have led to severe food

Quick Bites

Accidental Solution

Sometimes a solution to undernutrition is not planned. On October 9, 1998, the *Wall Street Journal* carried the headline, "In Guatemala, Organic Farms Sprout on Civil War Turf." During the country's 35-year civil war, local farmers abandoned their land. As the farmlands reverted to jungle and pesticides leached away, wild spices thrived. With the trend for "organic" spices, coffee, and natural dyes, the premium prices commanded by these new crops could be significant for the farmers' incomes.

Quick Bites

Emergency Management

Imagine a civil war in a developing country that displaces tens of thousands of people. What are the most important measures for preventing sickness and death among these refugees? Protection from violence heads the list, closely followed by adequate food rations, clean water and sanitation, diarrheal disease control, measles immunization, and maternal and child health care.

shortages, often worsened by violent conflicts. In Latin America, despite great progress, hunger remains in pockets of rural poverty and in inner-city slums.

There has been progress, however. Improved national economies have led to reduction in hunger in the Middle East. In the Asia-Pacific region, per capita food supplies have increased, in part a result of austere birth control measures in China as well as improved food production. However, even in nations that have achieved food sufficiency, there may remain regions of impoverishment or isolation that have food shortages.

Agriculture and Environment: A Tricky Balance

Advances in agriculture increase food supplies and reduce food costs. Because the economies of most developing countries are based on agriculture, improvements boost rural incomes and buying power, increase demand for agricultural labor, stimulate commerce among small vendors and food processors, and ultimately help a nation's economy.

Dramatic gains in agricultural productivity took place in the 1960s and 1970s with the development of new seed varieties, especially rice and corn. The seeds greatly increased crop yields. Expectations were so strong that these seeds would finally solve the world's food shortage that their development and use was dubbed the "Green Revolution." Despite its successes, the Green Revolution had limitations. The seeds required irrigation and heavy use of pesticides and fertilizers, which poor farmers could not afford. The farming techniques were sometimes hard on the environment. Gains from the Green Revolution have now about reached their limit, and if current trends continue, threaten to be lost to the population explosion.

Proponents of agricultural biotechnology see it as another step along the continuum of plant-breeding techniques and a promising tool to increase crop production. Some uses of biotechnology are well accepted, for example diagnostic kits that identify plants and insects by DNA and tissue culture for plant reproduction, a technique already in widespread commercial use. More controversial is the modification of plant genetic material. The

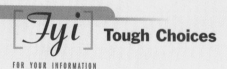

Tough Choices

FOR YOUR INFORMATION

Imagine you live in a poor village of a developing country. How would you make these choices?

- You've learned you must boil your drinking water to prevent diarrhea. But that means cutting young trees for firewood. You recently planted those trees to stop erosion. What do you do?

- You've recently given birth to your fourth child. Your husband was injured in an accident and is unable to work. But you can work at a nearby factory, and use

your pay to buy food and clothes for the older children. How would you feed the new baby?

- Your small herd of goats provides milk for your young children. You like the goats because they can survive in the rough, hilly countryside. But the goats are overgrazing the grasses on the hillside. What can you do?

- Insects have destroyed your crop. In the past, you burned fields after harvest to control insects, but you've learned that

"slash and burn" is bad for the land. You've thought about using a chemical pesticide, but it is too expensive. You could clear the jungle for another growing field. Do you have other choices? What should you do?

- You can grow either vegetables to feed your family or a "cash crop" to sell for export. The cash crop would help pay for medicine and other necessities. Which should you grow?

erance to adverse conditions, increase yield, and improve nutritional quality. Chapter 17, "Food Safety and Technology," describes the techniques and controversies surrounding this application of biotechnology.

At the other end of the technology spectrum is a renewed appreciation for and conservation of traditional seed varieties, those selected over the generations by local farmers, because they do well in local conditions. In developing countries, farmers typically save some of these seeds at each harvest to use the next planting season. The seeds grow well in the regions where they've evolved, whereas imported seeds, no matter how scientifically bred, often fail.

In addition to seed selection, strategies to optimize agriculture include irrigation, soil preparation, improved planting and harvest methods, erosion prevention, fertilizing, pest control, and flood control. The methods should be affordable, suitable for the level of local development, and protective of the environment. For example, where there is an abundant supply of willing farm laborers and gasoline is expensive, using heavy-duty farm machinery makes little sense. Other examples include mulching to conserve water and control weeds and manures (after composting to kill pathogens) to reduce the need for fertilizer.

Environmental Degradation

Environmental degradation is a growing concern in both the developing and the industrialized world. In developing countries, there is pressure for more land to support rapidly expanding populations of the poor. In industrialized countries, there is pressure for more land by the affluent, seeking more houses, larger properties, more recreation areas, and so on. Residents of the industrialized world consume vast amounts of resources (e.g., water, fuel, wood, paper, textiles, and food) without a thought, and often without making the small effort to conserve or recycle. Residents of the developing world consume much less per person, but the impact of their numbers is greater.

Environmental degradation has nutritional consequences because it threatens food production. Urbanization and the expansion of cities reduce farmlands to grow food. The pressure to supply food to growing populations leads to clear-cutting marginal land, eventually eroding hilly terrain, or quickly exhausting fragile rain forest soils. Overdependence on irrigation can drain water, eventually creating deserts. The destruction of vast areas of natural ground cover can lead to global climate changes. Overuse of pesticides and fertilizers pollutes waterways, destroying fish and seafood.

Key Concepts: *Despite gains in eradicating malnutrition, 18 percent of the people in the developing world continue to suffer from chronic hunger. Although world food supplies are adequate, factors including poverty, poor sanitation, urbanization, and inefficient food distribution allow hunger to continue. Infection, especially HIV/AIDS, rapid population growth, wars, and environmental degradation threaten to reverse hard-won gains.*

Malnutrition: Its Nature, Its Victims, and Its Eradication

Previous chapters discussed the diseases of nutritional deficiency. Most of these diseases exist throughout the developing world, but seldom in isolation. Typically the malnourished person has two or more co-existing deficiencies, each worsening the severity of the other. Keep the potential for this deadly synergy in mind as we discuss some of the major categories of malnutrition.

Quick Bites

Vaccine Veggies

Genetic engineers are experimenting with inserting vaccine molecules into plants. William Landridge, a molecular biologist at California's Loma Linda School of Medicine, has successfully added anti-cholera toxin genes to the potato. Potatoes are a dietary staple in Peru, Bolivia, and India where cholera causes dehydrating diarrhea and death. Every year, 2.2 million children die from dehydration due to diarrhea. Edible vaccines could overcome the problems of refrigeration and distribution that impede vaccination by injection. Next on the menu? Bananas and tomatoes may be even more effective vehicles than potatoes.

Quick Bites

Who produces the world's soybeans?

Before 1900, the soybean was rarely grown in the United States. Today, it is the largest American crop. The United States produces 75 percent of the world's soybeans.

iodine deficiency disorders (IDD) A wide range of disorders that affect growth and development due to iodine deficiency.

Protein-Energy Malnutrition

As you learned in Chapter 6, lack of protein and also energy can have devastating consequences, especially on the young. In kwashiorkor, the body and face swell with excess fluid, the hair turns wispy and red, and a terrible rash develops; without treatment, the person dies. Marasmus paints an even more dramatic picture of sunken eyes, shriveled limbs, and the skeleton's outlines clearly visible; it is as deadly as kwashiorkor.

Protein-energy malnutrition (see Chapter 6) is most often a condition of infants and children. Their fast growth creates high nutrient demands, leaving them especially vulnerable to inappropriate food distribution in the family, inappropriate infant and child feeding practices, and interactions of infection with malnutrition.[28] PEM typically develops after a child is weaned from the breast. Men in the household may have priority for nutritious food. In big families, the young child must also compete for food with many siblings.

In the developing world, breastfeeding is almost always essential to an infant's survival. Inappropriate bottle-feeding puts a baby at grave risk. Relative to income, formula is usually very expensive and is often diluted to make it "stretch." Contaminated water and lack of other hygienic requirements for bottle preparation cause diarrhea. The combination of diarrhea and nutritional deficiency from watered-down formula is often fatal.

A tremendous educational effort, including promotion of breastfeeding, has reduced the global prevalence and severity of infant and childhood PEM. The prevalence of PEM (as measured by low weight for age) has fallen from more than 37 percent in 1980 to less than 27 percent in 1999.[29] Severe PEM typified by kwashiorkor or marasmus has become more sporadic, occurring mainly as a result of war or natural disaster.

However, mild to moderate PEM continues to pose a grave problem in the developing world, putting children at risk of delayed growth, impaired psychological development, and the deadly interactions of disease and malnutrition. In fact, almost half of all deaths of children younger than 5 are still associated with PEM. Most of these deaths are from mild to moderate PEM interacting with other illness, rather than from severe malnutrition.[30] Moreover, with an epidemic of HIV infection raging in many developing countries, the return of widespread severe PEM threatens.

Iodine Deficiency Disorders

Iodine deficiency is the developing world's most important cause of preventable brain damage and impaired psychomotor development.[31] Its impairment of intellectual ability and work performance is potentially so widespread that **iodine deficiency disorders (IDD)** can actually slow a nation's social and economic development. (See **Figure 18.7**.)

Iodine deficiency is most devastating during pregnancy, causing spontaneous abortions, stillbirths, and birth defects including cretinism, a disease of mental retardation that is often severe. Deafness and spastic paralysis are likely to accompany the retardation. In regions of Africa where goitrogenic diets (typically, those high in "bitter" or cyanide-containing cassava) worsen the deficiency, dwarfism also occurs. Moreover, iodine deficiency is damaging at all ages, limiting mental development in infants and children, and producing apathy and marginal mental function in adults. Localized iodine deficiency affects not only the human population, but also the fertility and survival of livestock and thus can impede social and economic development.[32]

Iodine deficiency disorders are endemic throughout much of the devel-

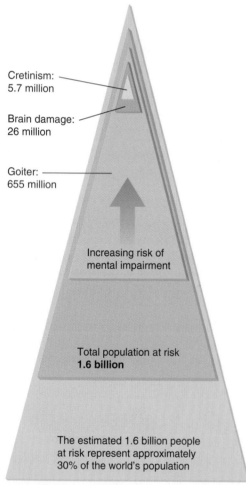

THE TOLL OF IODINE DEFICIENCY

Estimated impact of iodine deficiency worldwide. Even mild goiter (thyroid gland enlargement) is associated with some degree of mental impairment.

Cretinism: 5.7 million

Brain damage: 26 million

Goiter: 655 million

Increasing risk of mental impairment

Total population at risk **1.6 billion**

The estimated 1.6 billion people at risk represent approximately 30% of the world's population

The chart does not include an estimated yearly total of 60,000 miscarriages, stillbirths and neonatal deaths stemming from severe iodine deficiency in the mother during early pregnancy.

 Figure 18.7 **The toll of iodine deficiency.** Iodine deficiency remains the single greatest cause of preventable brain damage and mental retardation worldwide.
Source: © World Health Organization.

oping world where the soil is low in iodine, typically mountainous areas or areas far from the oceans. These areas are often isolated, impoverished, and insular. There is little consumption of imported food, a potential source of iodine. Iodine deficiency has been identified in 130 countries on all continents. According to the World Health Organization, there are currently 16 million people with cretinism in the developing world, and more than 49 million people are affected by lesser degrees of IDD-related brain damage.

Disturbing though these figures may be, great strides have been made in IDD prevention, mainly through iodizing salt. Countries with salt iodization programs have increased from 46 in 1990 to 93 in 1999; more than two-thirds of households in IDD-affected countries now use iodized salt.[33] The result is a dramatic improvement of iodine status in countries that have had salt iodization programs in place for 5 years or more. The cost is merely five cents per person per year.

Vitamin A Deficiency

Vitamin A deficiency is the leading cause of preventable childhood blindness. It is the leading cause of needless visual impairment in women and children. It also predisposes its victims to infection, and it worsens existing infections.

Vitamin A deficiency is most damaging to infants, children, and pregnant or lactating women. Among children in the developing world, 250,000 to 500,000 children each year become blind as a result of xeropthalmia; about half of them will die within a year of their blindness. Currently, some three million children under 5 years of age have signs of xeropthalmia.[34] **Table 18.4** gives WHO's estimates, by region, of the numbers of children younger than 5 who have vitamin A deficiency.

Another 140 million to 250 million children have subclinical vitamin A deficiency, often co-existing with marginal PEM. The vitamin deficiency predisposes infants and children to diarrheal diseases, which in turn worsen the child's nutritional status, leading to severe PEM. Common childhood infections, most notably measles, are much more serious in vitamin A-deficient children, with a much greater risk of death or permanent damage from complications.

In communities where vitamin A deficiency exists, pregnant and breastfeeding women often experience night blindness. Maternal death, poor pregnancy outcome, and failure to lactate are all increased with vitamin A deficiency. Vitamin A levels in the breast milk of these women are likely to be low, as well, putting their infants at later risk of deficiency.

Many countries are taking a multipronged approach to vitamin A deficiency that includes promotion of breastfeeding, fortification of foods, supplementation, and nutrition education. Foods like eggs, dairy foods, and liver are promoted as important for women and children; educational programs also encourage growing and eating fruits and vegetables high in beta-carotene. However, dietary change can be difficult and slow. The best sources of vitamin A are often the most expensive or inaccessible. For absorption and conversion to vitamin A, beta-carotene requires dietary fat—another expensive item in many areas—and other factors not completely understood. Meanwhile, periodic single, large-dose vitamin A supplements, often given in tandem with maternal-child immunizations, are proving an effective short-term measure.

Biotechnology may have a significant impact on vitamin A deficiency. Scientists have developed new transgenic strains of rice that are rich in beta-carotene. When the transgenic rice plants are crossed with locally

Table 18.4 Estimated Number of Children under Age 5 with Clinical Vitamin A Deficiency

Africa Region	1,080,000
The Americas	60,000
Eastern Mediterranean Region	60,000
South-East Asia	1,300,000
Western Pacific Region	100,000

Source: World Health Organization. www.WHO.int/nut.

Quick Bites

Is breastfeeding always best?

An HIV-positive mother can transmit the virus to her baby though breast milk. HIV-positive women whose infants were spared HIV transmission during pregnancy face the dilemma of how to feed those babies. In developing countries, the WHO is working to prevent HIV transmission through breastfeeding while continuing to protect, promote, and support breastfeeding as the best way to feed babies of women who are HIV-negative and women who do not know their status. Unfortunately, alternatives such as formula feeding are expensive, risk food poisoning from mixing with contaminated water, and often carry a social stigma.

grown strains of rice, they become suited to a particular region's climate and growing conditions. Such crops may play a critical role in feeding the world's burgeoning population and alleviating widespread vitamin A deficiency.[35]

Iron-Deficiency Anemia

The World Health Organization estimates that worldwide, 39 percent of preschool-age children and 52 percent of pregnant women are anemic, and that 90 percent of these people live in developing countries. Fast growth in young children and reproductive blood loss in women make them especially vulnerable to low-iron diets. However, iron deficiency occurs in all age groups. Like deficiencies discussed previously, anemia impairs psychomotor development, work capacity, learning capacity, and resistance to disease. Anemia during pregnancy increases morbidity and mortality rates for mother and baby. For all groups of people, anemia can cause profound fatigue, and severe anemia causes death.

The anemias of the developing world demonstrate the interaction of multiple nutrient deficiencies, which in turn interact with infection, sanitation, and poverty. Supplying iron alone is seldom enough to correct the problem.

Iron-deficient diets are monotonous, high in starch and cereal grains. During digestion cereals may bind with the very limited iron the diet provides, preventing its absorption. Other blood-building nutrients such as vitamins B_6 and B_{12} and folate are in short supply as well.

Anemia-producing parasites are common in areas of iron deficiency, aggravating the effects of poor diet. Blood cells are destroyed by malarial infections. Intestinal malabsorption and intestinal bleeding are caused by amoebic dysentery and schistosomiasis, acquired when human waste contaminates the water that people drink or where people bathe, and by hookworm where human waste contaminates the fields where people walk barefoot. People debilitated by anemia may be too weak to build outhouses, too poor to buy shoes or fuel to boil water, or too apathetic to clear standing water where malaria-carrying mosquitoes breed. Moreover, more than likely, they do not understand the connection between sanitation, infection, and malnutrition. Added to this mix are excessive blood loss from repeated pregnancies, inherited blood disorders such as sickle cell disease, and chronic bacterial or viral infections such as HIV.

Efforts to increase intake of iron-rich foods have limited effectiveness because these foods are costly, and dietary improvements are likely to come too slowly. Supplementation targeted to women and children and fortification are now the mainstays of anemia prevention and treatment, along with public health programs attacking anemia's other causes. Unfortunately, overcoming poverty and improving sanitation are not as easy as taking an iron pill, and so the prevalence of iron-deficiency anemia has remained essentially unchanged over the years.[36]

Deficiencies of Other Micronutrients

Deficiencies of zinc and calcium often co-exist with other deficiencies, contributing to morbidity and mortality during periods of growth, and threatening immune function and skeletal health in people who survive to old age.

Selenium deficiency, although limited to only a few countries, has serious consequences. It occurs where the soil is selenium-poor, in distinct regional patterns in China and Russia. In China, where the deficiency is most severe, it causes Keshan disease, in which heart muscle is destroyed, and death follows. Keshan disease affects mainly women and children. The condition can be prevented by selenium supplementation or by fortification, as in programs undertaken in New Zealand where soil is also low in selenium.

The classical deficiency diseases beriberi, pellagra, and scurvy still occur among the world's poorest and most underprivileged people. Most often, however, these diseases strike the victims of war and political strife—the refugees. Since 1990, at least 11 outbreaks of beriberi or pellagra have been reported among refugee populations, primarily in Africa.[37] Diets based on milled cereals and starchy roots, all poor thiamin sources, predispose populations to beriberi. Corn-based diets low in niacin and tryptophan predispose to pellagra. The disruption of refugee life can easily tip the balance from marginal deficiency to overt deficiency disease.

Overweight and Obesity

In some developing countries, obesity exists right alongside undernutrition. Obesity is more likely in areas of economic advancement and urban areas, less so in rural populations. Its prevalence is rising rapidly in Latin America and the Caribbean, but obesity still is relatively uncommon in Asia and Africa.

The factors leading to obesity in poor communities are different from those in affluent societies. Cultural attitudes toward overweight may be more accepting, even admiring. Calorie-dense foods that have few other nutrients are often cheap, satisfying, convenient, and heavily promoted; some are foreign brands that have become affordable status symbols. With urbanization and modernization, trends that typically reduce physical activity, comes a reduction in caloric expenditure that can be dramatic. Malnutrition itself may actually play a role; there's evidence that malnutrition during fetal development and early childhood predisposes people to obesity in adulthood.[38]

Key Concepts: *The most critical nutritional deficiencies in today's developing world are protein, calories, iodine, vitamin A, and iron. There have been gains in reducing the severity and prevalence of protein-energy malnutrition, through breastfeeding promotion, nutrition education, and improvements in food supplies. Fortification and supplementation programs are effectively attacking iodine and vitamin A deficiencies but have had less success overcoming iron deficiency. All of the underlying causes of malnutrition must be addressed to reduce and eliminate these and other deficiencies.*

Quick Bites

Undernutrition Cannot Be Blamed for Everything

In all third-world populations, low weight- and height-for-age are common among preschool and school children, affecting 10 to 50 percent. Most experts attribute this shortfall to insufficiency of food. A study of African school children, however, found no significant difference between well-fed and underfed pupils on measures such as their class position, games aptitude, and interest in education. Among children of school age, one must be careful not to overrate the effects of undernutrition nor the health disadvantages from mild to moderate malnutrition.

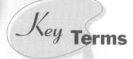

LEARNING *Portfolio* c h a p t e r 1 8

Key Terms

Study Points

➤ Hunger and malnutrition continue to be problems in both industrialized and developing countries.

➤ Although most people in the United States are food secure, malnutrition is a serious problem for the working poor, the rural poor, elders, the homeless, and children.

➤ According to the 1996–1998 Food Security Supplement Survey, almost 10 percent of American households worry about having enough to eat and over 3 percent experience hunger.

➤ The Food Stamp Program, the Special Supplemental Nutrition Program for Women, Infants, and Children (WIC), the National School Lunch and Breakfast Programs, and the Child and Adult Care Food Program are among the many federal programs that address hunger in the United States.

➤ Although the rates of malnutrition and hunger in the developing world declined in the last three decades of the twentieth century, progress is still too slow and uneven. It is estimated that 790 million people in the developing world do not have enough to eat.

➤ Social and economic factors, infection, disease, political disruptions, natural disasters, and inequitable food distribution all contribute to hunger in the developing world.

➤ Advances in agricultural practices have increased food supplies and reduced food costs in the developing world; however, the increase in production has led to environmental degradation as a result of urbanization, clear cutting, overirrigation, and soil erosion.

➤ Protein-energy malnutrition (PEM) refers to conditions, such as kwashiorkor and marasmus, that result from not having enough to eat.

➤ Infants and children are most likely to suffer from PEM. However, nutrition education efforts, including promotion of breastfeeding, have reduced the severity and prevalence of PEM.

➤ Iodine deficiency is the largest cause of preventable brain damage and impaired psychomotor development in the developing world. It can cause damage to people of all ages.

➤ Great strides have been made in preventing iodine deficiency disorders (IDD) through salt iodization programs. More than two-thirds of households in IDD-affected countries now use iodized salt.

➤ Vitamin A deficiency is the leading cause of preventable childhood blindness. It also makes its victims more vulnerable to infection, diarrheal diseases, and PEM.

➤ Pregnant and breastfeeding women with vitamin A deficiency are at increased risk of death, poor pregnancy outcomes, and lactation failure.

➤ Many countries are taking a multipronged approach to vitamin A deficiency that includes promotion of breastfeeding, fortification of foods, supplementation, and nutrition education.

➤ Unfortunately, the best sources of vitamin A are often expensive and inaccessible, but scientists have developed new transgenic strains of rice that are rich in beta-carotene and that may play a critical role in alleviating widespread vitamin A deficiency.

➤ The WHO estimates that world wide 39 percent of pre-school-age children and 52 percent of pregnant women are anemic, and that 90 percent of these people live in developing countries.

➤ The anemias of the developing world demonstrate the interaction of multiple nutrient deficiencies, which in turn interact with infection, poor sanitation, and poverty.

➤ Food fortification and iron supplementation targeted to women and children are the mainstays of anemia prevention and treatment, along with efforts to overcome poverty and improve sanitation.

➤ The classical deficiency diseases beriberi, pellagra, and scurvy still occur among the worlds' poorest and most underprivileged people.

➤ In some developing countries, obesity exists right alongside undernutrition.

Study Questions

1. What's the difference between food insecurity and hunger?
2. What is food security?
3. List four common nutritional deficiencies worldwide.
4. List four causes of malnutrition worldwide.
5. List some of the organizations and programs fighting hunger and food insecurity in the United States.
6. What populations are at increased risk of nutritional deficiencies, and why?

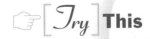

Try This

Try Giving Up Your Stove and Refrigerator

A homeless person has no kitchen facilities to store or prepare food. For one day, eat a balanced diet without resorting to cooking or using your refrigerator. Some of the foods you could have include:

> breads, bagels, tortillas, rolls
>
> cereals
>
> crackers
>
> milk—canned, evaporated, or aseptic packaging
>
> cheese—hard cheeses keep well
>
> pudding cups (single-serve, nonrefrigerated type)
>
> tuna/chicken—canned
>
> sardines, salmon—canned
>
> nuts, peanut butter
>
> beans—canned
>
> fruits and vegetables-fresh, canned, dried fruits

How satisfying did you find this eating pattern? What did you miss most? What would it be like to eat this way for an extended time?

Community Food Programs

The purpose of this exercise is to see how you can contribute to decreasing or eliminating food insecurity in your community. Look in the phone book (under "Food Programs" and "Human Services") to see what programs are available. Consider volunteering at your local food bank or another community program to help feed people who do not have the means to feed themselves.

References

1 The State of Food Insecurity in the World 1999. Food and Agriculture Organization of the United Nations. http://www.fao.org/NEWS/1999/img/SOFI99-E.PDF. Accessed 9/30/00.

2 Position of the American Dietetic Association: world hunger. *J Am Diet Assoc.* 95;1995:1160–1162.

3 Kendall A, Kennedy E. Position of the American Dietetic Association: domestic food and nutrition security. *J Am Diet Assoc.* 98;1998:337–342.

4 US Department of Agriculture. Office of Analysis, Nutrition and Evaluation, Food and Nutrition Service. Household Food Security in the United States 1995–1998. Advance Report. Alexandria, VA: Author; 2000.

5 Kendall A, Olson CM, Frongillo EA. Relationship of hunger and food insecurity to food availability and consumption. *J Am Diet Assoc.* 1996;96:1019–1024.

6 Nord M, Jemison K, Bickel G. Prevalence of Food Insecurity and Hunger, by State, 1996-1998. Food Assistance and Nutrition Research report 2 (FANRR-2). Alexandria, VA: USDA, Economic Research Service, Food and Nutrition Service; September 1999.

7 Hamilton WL, Cook JT, Thompson WW, et al. Household Food Security in the United States in 1995. Executive Summary. Alexandria, VA: USDA, Office of Analysis and Evaluation, Food and Consumer Service; 1997.

8 Alaimo K, Briefel RR, Frongillo EA, Olson C. Food insufficiency exists in the United States: results for the third National Health and Nutrition Examination Survey (NHANES III). *Am J Pub Health.* 1998;88:419–426.

9 Schlesinger JM. Working full time is no longer enough. *Wall Street Journal.* June 29, 2000:A2, 12.

10 Wellman NS, Weddle DO, Kranz S, Brain CT. Elder insecurities: poverty, hunger, and malnutrition. *J Am Diet Assoc.* 1997;97(suppl):S120–S122.

11 Food Research and Action Center. Hunger in the U.S. http://www.frac.org/html/hunger_in_the_us/hunger_index.html. Accessed 9/30/00.

12 USDA Food and Nutrition Service Online. National Level Annual Summary: Participation and costs 1969–1999. Data as of September 25, 2000. http://www.fns.usda.gov/pd/fssummar.htm. Accessed 9/30/00.

13 USDA. Food Stamps Income, Resources, and Benefits. October 1999. http://www.fns.usda.gov/fsp/fsResBenEli.htm. Accessed 9/30/00.

14 USDA Food and Nutrition Service Online. Op. cit.

15 USDA Food and Nutrition Service Online. WIC Frequently Asked Questions. http://www.fns.usda.gov/wic/MENU/FAQ/FAQ.HTM#1. Accessed 9/30/00.

16 USDA Food and Nutrition Service Online. School Programs: Income Eligibility Guidelines. http://www.fns.usda.gov/cnd/Lunch/Governance/Notices/00-01ieg.htm. Accessed 9/30/00.

17 USDA Food and Nutrition Service Online. School Lunch Program. http://www.fns.usda.gov/cnd/Lunch/Default.htm. Accessed 9/30/00.

18 Food and Agriculture Organization of the United Nations. The State of Food Insecurity in the World 1999. http://www.fao.org/NEWS/1999/img/SOFI99-E.PDF. Accessed 9/30/00.

19 Ibid.

20 Food and Agriculture Organization of the United Nations. Undernourishment around the World. www.FAO.org/focus/e/sofi/under-e.htm. Accessed 9/30/00.

21 Uvin P. The state of world hunger. In: Uvin P, ed. *The Hunger Report 1993.* Newark, NJ: Gordon and Breach Science Publishers; 1994.

22 Mata LJ, Urrutia JJ, Albertazzi C. Influence of recurrent infections on nutrition and growth of children in Guatemala. *Am J Clin Nutr.* 1972;25:1267–1275.

23 Semba RD, Miotti PG, Chipangwi JD, et al. Maternal vitamin A deficiency and mother-to-child transmission of HIV-1. *Lancet.* 1994;343:1593–1597.

24 Tang AM, Graham NMH, Kirby AJ, et al. Dietary micronutrient intake and risk of progression to acquired immunodeficiency syndrome (AIDS) in human immunodeficiency virus type 1 (HIV-1)-infected homosexual men. *Am J Epidem.* 1993;138:937–951.

25 Joint United Nations Programme on HIV/AIDS. Report on the Global HIV/AIDS Epidemic. Geneva, Switzerland: UNAIDS; June 2000.

26 Position of the American Dietetic Association: world hunger. Op. cit.

27 Ibid.

28 Keusch GT, Scrimshaw NS. Selective primary health care: strategies for control of disease in the developing world. XXIII. Control of infection to reduce the percentile of infantile and childhood malnutrition. *Rev Infect Dis.* 1986;8:273–287.

29 World Health Organization Nutrition for Health and Development. "Malnutrition—The Global Picture." www.who.int/nut/. Accessed 9/30/00.

30 World Health Organization. Nutrition for Health and Development Activities and Outputs. www.who.int/nut/. Accessed 9/30/00.

31 Ibid.

32 Stanbury JB. Iodine deficiency and the iodine deficiency disorders. In: Ziegler EE, Filer LJ, eds. *Present Knowledge in Nutrition.* 7th ed. Washington, DC: International Life Science Institute; 1996.

33 World Health Organization. Nutrition for Health and Development Activities and Outputs. Op. cit.

34 Ibid.

35 Nash M. Grains of Hope. *Time.* 156:5(July 31, 2000):38–46.

36 World Health Organization. Nutrition for Health and Development Activities and Outputs. Op. cit.

37 Ibid.

38 Pena M, Bacallao J. Obesity and Poverty: A New Public Health Challenge. PAHO scientific publication 576. Geneva, Switzerland: World Health Organization; 2000.

Appendices

APPENDIX A Food Composition Tables

Beverage and Beverage Mixes, p. A-1; Breakfast Cereals, p. A-4; Condiments, Sauces and Gravies, p. A-6; Dairy Products and Substitutes, p. A-8; Desserts, p. A-14; Eggs, Substitutes, and Egg Dishes, p. A-22; Fast Foods/Restaurants, p. A-22; Fats, Oils, Margarines, Shortenings, and Substitutes, p. A-30; Fish, Seafood, and Shellfish, p. A-34; Fruits, p. A-36; Grains and Grain Products, p. A-40; Infant Foods, p. A-48; Juices: Fruit, Vegetable, Blends, p. A-50; Meals, Entrees, and Mixed Dishes, p. A-50; Meats, p. A-56; Meat Substitutes, Tofu, Vegetarian Foods, p. A-60; Nuts, Seeds, and Products, p. A-62; Poultry, p. A-64; Salad Dressings, Dips, and Mayonnaise, p. A-66; Salads, p. A-68; Sandwiches, p. A-68; Snack Foods: Chips, Pretzels, Popcorn, p. A-70; Soups, Stews and Chilis, p. A-70; Spices, Flavors, and Seasonings and Miscellaneous Baking Products, p. A-72; Sweets, Sugars, Candy, p. A-74; Vegetables and Legumes, p. A-76

ERA CODE	FOOD DESCRIPTION	AMT	UNIT	WT (g)	WTR (g)	CAL (kcal)	PROT (g)	CARB (g)	FIBR (g)	FAT (g)	SATF (g)	MONO (g)	POLY (g)
Beverage and Beverage Mixes													
Alcoholic Beverages													
22500	Beer	1.5	cup	356.4	329	146	1	9	1	0	0	0	0
22512	Beer-Light	1.5	cup	29.5	28	8	<1	<1	0	0	0	0	0
20276	Beer-Non-Alcoholic	1.5	cup	355.5		58	<1	12	0	0	0	0	0
22519	Coffee Liqueur, 53 proof	1.5	fl oz	52.2	16	175	<1	24	0	<1	<0.1	0.1	0.1
22521	De Menthe Liqueur 72 proof	1.5	fl oz	50.4	14	187	0	21	0	<1	<0.1	<0.1	0.1
22543	Gin-Rum-Vodka-Whiskey, 100prf	1.5	fl oz	41.7	24	123	0	0	0	0	0	0	0
22514	Gin-Rum-Vodka-Whiskey, 80prf	1.5	fl oz	41.7	28	96	0	0	0	0	0	0	0
22516	Gin-Rum-Vodka-Whiskey, 86prf	1.5	fl oz	41.7	27	104	0	<1	0	0	0	0	0
22542	Gin-Rum-Vodka-Whiskey, 94prf	1.5	fl oz	41.7	25	115	0	0	0	0	0	0	0
22601	Sangria Wine Drink	0.5	cup	118	102	79	<1	11	<1	<1	0	0	<0.1
22509	Sherry-Dry	0.5	cup	117	104	82	<1	2	0	0	0	0	0
22518	Wine-Dessert, Dry	0.5	cup	118	94	149	<1	5	0	0	0	0	0
22507	Wine-Dessert, Sweet	0.5	cup	118	86	181	<1	14	0	0	0	0	0
20077	Wine-Light-Non Alcoholic	0.5	cup	116	114	7	1	1	0	0	0	0	0
20076	Wine-Non Alcoholic	0.5	cup	116	114	7	1	1	0	0	0	0	0
22501	Wine-Red	0.5	cup	118	104	85	<1	2	0	0	0	0	0
22502	Wine-Rosé	0.5	cup	118	105	84	<1	2	0	0	0	0	0
22504	Wine-White, Medium	0.5	cup	118	106	80	<1	1	0	0	0	0	0
Carbonated Drinks													
20006	Club Soda	1.5	cup	355	355	0	0	0	0	0	0	0	0
20054	Cola, Caffeine Free	1.5	cup	360		160	0	41	0	0	0	0	0
20030	Cola, Diet	1.5	cup	355	354	4	<1	<1	0	0	0	0	0
20056	Cola, Diet, Caffeine Free	1.5	cup	360		0	0	0	0	0	0	0	0
20005	Cola, Regular	1.5	cup	372	333	153	0	39	0	0	0	0	0
20028	Cream Soda	1.5	cup	371	321	185	0	49	0	0	0	0	0
20189	Creme Soda, Diet	1.5	cup	360		0	0	0	0	0	0	0	0
20007	Diet Soda, Assorted Flavors	1.5	cup	355	354	0	0	<1	0	0	0	0	0
20027	Dr. Pepper Type Soda	1.5	cup	368	329	151	0	38	0	<1	0.3	0	0
20008	Ginger Ale	1.5	cup	366	334	124	0	32	0	0	0	0	0
20031	Grape Soda	1.5	cup	372	330	160	0	42	0	0	0	0	0
20032	Lemon-Lime Soda	1.5	cup	368	330	147	0	38	0	0	0	0	0
20029	Orange Soda	1.5	cup	372	326	178	0	46	0	0	0	0	0
20009	Root Beer	1.5	cup	370	330	151	0	39	0	0	0	0	0
Coffee and Substitutes													
20012	Coffee, Brewed	1	cup	237	235	5	<1	1	0	<1	<0.1	0	<0.1
20065	Coffee-Decaf, Brewed	1	cup	240	238	5	<1	1	0	0	<0.1	0	<0.1

< = Trace amount present   Blank = Not available

ERA, EatRight Analysis CD-ROM; **AMT,** amount; **WT,** weight; **WTR,** water; **CAL,** calories; **PROT,** protein; **CARB,** carbohydrate; **FIBR,** fiber; **FAT,** fat; **SATF,** saturated fat; **MONO,** monosaturated fat; **POLY,** polyunsaturated fat; **CHOL,** cholesterol; **V,** vitamin; **THI,** thiamin; **RIB,** riboflavin; **NIA,** niacin; **FOL,** folate; **CALC,** calcium; **PHOS,** phosphate; **SOD,** sodium; **POT,** potassium; **MAG,** magnesium

CHOL (mg)	V-A (RE)	THI (mg)	RIB (mg)	NIA (mg)	V-B6 (mg)	FOL (µg)	V-B12 (µg)	V-C (mg)	V-E (mg)	CALC (mg)	PHOS (mg)	SOD (mg)	POT (mg)	MAG (mg)	IRON (mg)	ZINC (mg)
0	0	<0.1	0.1	1.6	0.2	12	0.1	0	0	18	43	18	89	21	0.1	0.1
0	0	<0.1	<0.1	0.1	<0.1	1	<0.1	0	0	1	4	1	5	1	<0.1	<0.1
0							0					3				
0	0	<0.1	<0.1	0.1	0	0	0	0	0	1	3	4	16	2	<0.1	<0.1
0	0	0	0	<0.1	0	0	0	0	0	0	0	3	0	0	<0.1	<0.1
0	0	<0.1	<0.1	<0.1	0	0	0	0	0	0	2	<1	1	0	<0.1	<0.1
0	0	<0.1	<0.1	<0.1	0	0	0	0	0	0	2	<1	1	0	<0.1	<0.1
0	0	<0.1	<0.1	<0.1	0	0	0	0	0	0	2	<1	1	0	<0.1	<0.1
0	0	<0.1	<0.1	<0.1	0	0	0	0	0	0	2	<1	1	0	<0.1	<0.1
0	2	<0.1	<0.1	0.1	<0.1	3	0	5	<0.1	5	5	8	42	4	0.1	0.1
0	0	<0.1	<0.1	0.1	<0.1	1	<0.1	0	0	9	16	9	104	12	0.5	0.1
0	0	<0.1	<0.1	0.2	0	<1	0	0	0	9	11	11	109	11	0.3	0.1
0	0	<0.1	<0.1	0.2	0	<1	0	0	0	9	11	11	109	11	0.3	0.1
0	0	0	<0.1	0.1	<0.1	1	0	0	0	10	17	8	102	12	0.5	0.1
0	0	0	<0.1	0.1	<0.1	1	0	0	0	10	17	8	102	12	0.5	0.1
0	0	<0.1	<0.1	0.1	<0.1	2	<0.1	0	0	9	17	6	132	15	0.5	0.1
0	0	<0.1	<0.1	0.1	<0.1	1	<0.1	0	0	9	18	6	117	12	0.4	0.1
0	0	<0.1	<0.1	0.1	<0.1	<1	0	0	0	11	17	6	94	12	0.4	0.1
0	0	0	0	0	0	0	0	0	0	18	0	75	7	4	<0.1	0.3
0							0				49	45	0			
0	0	<0.1	0.1	0	0	0	0	0	0	14	32	21	0	4	0.1	0.3
0							0				49	55	54			
0	0	0	0	0	0	0	0	0	0	11	45	15	4	4	0.1	<0.1
0	0	0	0	0	0	0	0	0	0	19	0	44	4	4	0.2	0.3
0							0				0	55	0			
0	0	0	0	0	0	0	0	0	0	14	39	57	7	4	0.1	0.2
0	0	0	0	0	0	0	0	0	0	11	41	37	4	0	0.1	0.1
0	0	0	0	0	0	0	0	0	0	11	0	26	4	4	0.6	0.2
0	0	0	0	0	0	0	0	0	0	11	0	56	4	4	0.3	0.3
0	0	0	0	<0.1	0	0	0	0	0	7	0	41	4	4	0.3	0.2
0	0	0	0	0	0	0	0	0	0	19	45	45	7	4	0.2	0.4
0	0	0	0	0	0	0	0	0	0	18	0	48	4	4	0.2	0.3
0	0	0	0	0.5	0	<1	0	0	0	5	2	5	128	12	0.1	<0.1
0	0	0	0	0.5	0	<1	0	0	0	5	2	5	130	12	0.1	<0.1

ERA, EatRight Analysis CD-ROM; AMT, amount; WT, weight; WTR, water; CAL, calories; PROT, protein; CARB, carbohydrate;
FIBR, fiber; FAT, fat; SATF, saturated fat; MONO, monosaturated fat; POLY, polyunsaturated fat

ERA CODE	FOOD DESCRIPTION	AMT	UNIT	WT (g)	WTR (g)	CAL (kcal)	PROT (g)	CARB (g)	FIBR (g)	FAT (g)	SATF (g)	MONO (g)	POLY (g)
Beverage and Beverage Mixes (continued)													
Coffee and Substitutes (continued)													
20044	Cappucino, Prep from Mix	0.75	cup	192	178	61	<1	11	0	2	1.8	0.1	<0.1
20048	Postum Coffee Substitute	1	cup	240	237	12	<1	2	0	<1	<0.1	<0.1	0.1
20093	Coffee+Chicory, Inst, Prep	1	cup	179	177	7	<1	1	0	<1	<0.1	0	<0.1
20023	Coffee, Prep from Instant	1	cup	238.4	236	5	<1	1	0	0	0	0	0
20091	Coffee-Decaf, Inst, Prep	1	cup	179	177	4	<1	1	0	<1	<0.1	0	<0.1
20063	Espresso Coffee	1	cup	240	235	22	<1	4	0	<1	0.2	0	0.2
20064	Espresso Coffee-Decaf	1	cup	240	235	22	<1	4	0	<1	0.2	0	0.2
20108	French Coffee-Mix+Water	0.75	cup	189	178	57	1	7	0	3	2.9	0.2	0.1
22517	French Van Coffee, Prep from Mix	1	ea	14	<1	65	<1	10	<1	3	0.6		
20109	Mocha Coffee, Prep from Mix	0.75	cup	188	177	51	1	8	<1	2	1.6	0.1	<0.1
Dairy Mixes and Drinks													
73	Cocoa-Prep From Mix	0.75	cup	209	178	119	2	24	1	3	1.8	1	0.1
21	Cocoa, Prep w/Whole Milk	1	cup	250	202	192	10	29	2	6	3.6	1.7	0.2
46	Cocoa-SugarFree, Prep from Mix	0.75	cup	192	177	48	4	8	<1	<1	0.2	0.1	<0.1
27	Instant Breakfast+Skim Milk	1	cup	282		216	16	36	<1	1	0.7	0.3	<0.1
101	Instant Breakfast+1% Milk	1	cup	281		233	15	36	<1	3	2	0.9	0.1
26	Instant Breakfast+2% Milk	1	cup	281		252	15	36	<1	5	3.3	1.5	0.2
25	Instant Breakfast+Whole Milk	1	cup	281		280	15	36	<1	9	5.4	2.5	0.3
41	Nestle's Quik-Strawberry+Milk	1	cup	266	215	234	8	33	0	8	5.1	2.4	0.3
38	Ovaltine Drink-Choc Flavor	1	cup	265	215	225	9	29	<1	9	5.5	2.6	0.4
62006	SlimFast Straw Pwdr Scoop	1	ea	28	1	100	5	20	2	1			
62652	UltraSlimFast Choc Pwdr Scoop	1	ea	33	2	120	5	22	5	1	0		
Fruit Flavored Drinks													
20421	All Sport Drink, Fruit Punch	1	cup	240		53	0	15	0	0	0	0	0
20314	Crystal Light Drink, Citrus	1	cup	238.4		5	0	0	0	0	0	0	0
20052	Five Alive Citrus Drink	1	cup	248	218	114	1	29	0	<1	0	0	<0.1
20024	Fruit Punch Drink, Canned	1	cup	248	218	116	0	30	<1	<1	<0.1	<0.1	<0.1
20035	Fruit Punch Drink, Prep from Frzn	1	cup	247	218	114	0	29	<1	<1	<0.1	<0.1	<0.1
20648	Gatorade	1	cup	240.9	225	60	0	15	0	0	0	0	0
20101	Grape Drink-Canned	1	cup	250	221	112	<1	29	0	<1	<0.1	0	<0.1
20158	Hi-C Fruit Punch	1	cup	250.1		130	0	34	0	0	0	0	0
20016	Koolade, Dry+Sugar+Water	1	cup	262	237	97	0	25	0	<1	<0.1	<0.1	<0.1
20017	Koolade-SugarFree, Dry+Water	1	cup	240	228	43	0	11	0	0	0	0	0
20000	Lemonade, Prep from Frozen	1	cup	248	221	99	<1	26	<1	<1	<0.1	<0.1	<0.1
20045	Lemonade, Prep from Mix	1	cup	266	237	112	0	29	0	<1	<0.1	<0.1	<0.1
20047	Lemonade-LoCal, Prep from Mix	1	cup	237	235	5	0	1	0	0	0	0	0
20002	Limeade, Prep from Frozen	1	cup	247	220	101	0	27	<1	<1	<0.1	<0.1	<0.1
20004	Orange Drink, Prep from Mix	1	cup	248	218	114	0	29	0	0	<0.1	<0.1	<0.1
20025	Pineapple Orange Drink, Canned	1	cup	250	217	125	3	30	<1	0	0	0	0
20117	Pink Lemonade, Prep from Frzn	1	cup	247	220	99	<1	26	0	<1	<0.1	<0.1	<0.1
20070	Sunny Delight Orange Ade	1	cup	248	216	126	0	32	<1	<1	<0.1	<0.1	<0.1
62020	UltraSlimFast Fruit Pwdr w/OJ	1	cup	279		200	11	44	6	<1			

< = Trace amount present   Blank = Not available

CHOL, cholesterol; V, vitamin; THI, thiamin; RIB, riboflavin; NIA, niacin; FOL, folate;
CALC, calcium; PHOS, phosphate; SOD, sodium; POT, potassium; MAG, magnesium

CHOL (mg)	V-A (RE)	THI (mg)	RIB (mg)	NIA (mg)	V-B6 (mg)	FOL (µg)	V-B12 (µg)	V-C (mg)	V-E (mg)	CALC (mg)	PHOS (mg)	SOD (mg)	POT (mg)	MAG (mg)	IRON (mg)	ZINC (mg)
0	0	<0.1	<0.1	0.3	0	0	0	0	0.1	8	27	104	119	10	0.2	0.1
0	0	<0.1	<0.1	0.5	<0.1	1	0	0	0	7	17	10	58	10	0.1	0.1
0	0	0	<0.1	0.4	0	0	0	0	0	5	5	11	61	5	0.1	0.1
0	0	0	0	0.7	0	0	0	0	0	7	7	7	86	10	0.1	0.1
0	0	0	<0.1	0.5	0	0	0	0	0	5	5	5	63	7	0.1	0.1
0	0	<0.1	0.4	12.5	<0.1	2	0	<1	0	5	17	34	276	192	0.3	0.1
0	0	<0.1	0.4	12.5	<0.1	2	0	<1	0	5	17	34	276	192	0.3	0.1
0	0	0	<0.1	0.7	0	0	0	0	0	8	42	30	136	2	<0.1	<0.1
0	0							0		2	28	56	76		<0.1	
0	0	<0.1	<0.1	0.3	0	0	0	0	<0.1	8	28	36	118	9	0.2	0.2
0	150	0.2	0.2	2	<0.1	0	0.4	6	0.1	104	111	207	405	23	1.8	0.3
20	138	0.1	0.4	0.4	0.1	15	0.9	2	0.3	315	292	128	500	70	1.1	1.5
2	<1	<0.1	0.2	0.2	<0.1	2	0.3	0	0.1	90	134	173	405	33	0.7	0.6
9	703	0.4	0.4	5.5	0.5	118	1.6	31	7.5	407	406	268	755	112	4.8	4.1
14	698	0.4	0.5	5.5	0.5	118	1.5	31	7.6	406	393	266	731	118	4.9	4.1
23	693	0.4	0.5	5.5	0.5	118	1.5	31	7.5	401	390	264	726	118	4.9	4.1
38	630	0.4	0.5	5.5	0.5	118	1.5	31	7.5	396	385	262	719	117	4.9	4.1
32	74	0.1	0.4	0.2	0.1	12	0.9	2	0.3	293	229	128	370	32	0.2	0.9
34	901	0.7	1.3	10.9	1	32	0.9	34	0.3	384	313	244	620	53	3.8	1.2
5	75	0.4	0.2	7	0.6	100	1.2	18	10.1	150	100	130	210	100	6.3	4.5
5	225	0.4	0.2	10	0.6	100	2.1	27	20.1	150	100	140	200	100	6.3	4.5
0	0							0	0	0	7	37	37		0	
0	0							0	6	0		0	45		0	
0	10	<0.1	<0.1	0.4	<0.1	5	0	67	0	22	25	7	278	15	2.8	0.1
0	3	0.1	0.1	0.1	0	3	0	73	0	20	2	55	62	5	0.5	0.3
0	2	<0.1	<0.1	0.1	<0.1	2	0	108	0	10	2	10	32	5	0.2	0.1
0	0	<0.1	0	0	0	0	0	0	0	0	22	96	26	2	0.1	<0.1
0	<1	<0.1	<0.1	0.1	<0.1	1	0	85	0	8	2	15	12	5	0.4	0.3
0							0	100				30				
0	0	0	<0.1	<0.1	0	<1	0	31	0	42	52	37	3	3	0.1	0.1
0	2	<0.1	<0.1	<0.1	0	5	0	78	0	17	5	50	50	5	0.6	0.3
0	5	<0.1	0.1	<0.1	<0.1	5	0	10	0	7	5	7	37	5	0.4	0.1
0	0	0	<0.1	0	0	0	0	34	0	29	3	19	3	3	0.1	0.1
0	0	0	0	0	0	<1	0	6	0	50	24	7	0	2	0.1	0.1
0	0	<0.1	<0.1	0.1	0	2	0	7	0	7	2	5	32	2	0.1	<0.1
0	550	<0.1	<0.1	0	0	143	0	121	0	62	37	12	50	2	0.2	0.1
0	132	0.1	<0.1	0.5	0.1	27	0	56	0	12	10	8	115	15	0.7	0.2
0	<1	<0.1	0.1	<0.1	<0.1	5	0	10	0	7	5	7	37	5	0.4	0.1
0	5	<0.1	<0.1	0.1	<0.1	5	0	85	0	15	2	40	45	5	0.7	0.2
	250	0.5	0.6	7	0.7	140	2.1	60		400	400	30	590	140	6.3	5.2

ERA, EatRight Analysis CD-ROM; **AMT**, amount; **WT**, weight; **WTR**, water; **CAL**, calories; **PROT**, protein; **CARB**, carbohydrate; **FIBR**, fiber; **FAT**, fat; **SATF**, saturated fat; **MONO**, monosaturated fat; **POLY**, polyunsaturated fat

ERA CODE	FOOD DESCRIPTION	AMT	UNIT	WT (g)	WTR (g)	CAL (kcal)	PROT (g)	CARB (g)	FIBR (g)	FAT (g)	SATF (g)	MONO (g)	POLY (g)
Beverage and Beverage Mixes (continued)													
Teas													
20118	Camomile Tea, Brewed	1	cup	237	236	2	0	<1	0	<1	<0.1	<0.1	<0.1
20036	Herbal Tea, Brewed	0.75	cup	178	177	2	0	<1	0	<1	<0.1	<0.1	<0.1
20014	Tea, Brewed	1	cup	237	236	2	0	1	0	<1	<0.1	<0.1	<0.1
20020	Tea, Prep from Instant	1	cup	237	236	2	<1	<1	0	0	0	0	0
20079	Tea-Decaf-LoCal, Prep from Frzn	1	cup	245	243	6	<1	2	0	<1	<0.1	<0.1	<0.1
20038	Tea-Lemon, Prep from Instant	1	cup	238	236	5	<1	1	0	<1	0	0	<0.1
20040	Tea-Lemon-LoCal, Prep from Inst	1	cup	237	235	5	<1	1	0	<1	0	0	<0.1
20022	Tea-Sweet, Prep from Instant	1	cup	259	236	88	<1	22	0	<1	<0.1	<0.1	<0.1
Water													
20050	Bottled Water-Perrier	1	cup	237	237	0	0	0	0	0	0	0	0
20051	Bottled Water-PolandSprings	1	cup	237	237	0	0	0	0	0	0	0	0
20010	Tonic / Quinine Water	1	cup	244	222	83	0	21	0	0	0	0	0
20121	Tonic Water-SugFree	1	ea	355	354	0	0	<1	0	0	0	0	0
20041	Water	1	cup	237	237	0	0	0	0	0	0	0	0
Breakfast Cereals													
Cereals, Hot, Cooked													
40094	Corn Grits-White, Cooked	1	cup	242	206	145	3	31	<1	<1	0.1	0.1	0.2
40093	Corn Grits-White-Enr, Cooked	1	cup	242	206	145	3	31	<1	<1	0.1	0.1	0.2
40078	Cream of Rice Cereal, Cooked	1	cup	244	214	127	2	28	<1	<1	0.1	0.1	0.1
40014	Malt O Meal-Pl/Choc, Cooked	1	cup	240	210	122	4	26	1	<1	0.1	0.1	<0.1
40015	Maypo Cereal, Cooked	0.75	cup	180	149	128	4	24	4	2	0.3	0.5	0.7
40138	Multigrain Cereal, Cooked	1	cup	246	194	202	7	40	4	2	0.3	0.5	1.1
40000	Oatmeal-Cooked-No Salt	1	cup	234	200	145	6	25	4	2	0.4	0.7	0.9
40072	Oatmeal-Instant-Pkt-Prepared	1	ea	177	151	104	4	18	3	2	0.3	0.6	0.7
40075	Oatmeal-Inst-Flavored-Pkt-Prep	1	ea	155	116	153	4	31	3	2	0.4	0.6	0.7
40088	Ralston Cereal-Cooked	1	cup	253	218	134	6	28	6	1	0.1	0.1	0.4
40002	Rolled Wheat-Cooked	1	cup	240	201	149	5	33	4	1	0.1	0.1	0.5
40016	Roman Meal Cereal-Cooked	0.75	cup	181	150	110	5	25	6	1	0.1	0.1	0.3
40080	Wheatena Cereal-Cooked	1	cup	243	208	136	5	29	7	1	0.2	0.2	0.6
Cereals, Ready To Eat													
40063	100% Natural Cereal	1	cup	104	3	462	11	71	8	17	7.4	7.4	2.2
40003	All-Bran Cereal	0.75	cup	32		119	4	24	3	2	0.3	0.5	0.6
40246	AlphaBits Cereal-Frosted	1	cup	32	<1	130	3	27	1	1	0.3		
40123	Amaranth Flakes Cereal	1	cup	38	1	134	4	27	4	4	0.8	1.2	1.6
40029	Bran Buds Cereal	0.33	cup	30	1	83	3	24	12	1	0.1	0.2	0.4
40031	C.W. Post Cereal+Raisins	1	cup	103	4	446	9	74	14	15	11	1.7	1.4
40030	C.W. Post Cereal-Plain	1	cup	97	2	421	9	73	7	13	1.7	6	4.7
40032	Cap'n Crunch Cereal	1	cup	37	1	147	2	32	1	2	0.5	0.4	0.3
40037	Cocoa Pebbles Cereal	1	cup	33	1	129	1	29	1	1	0.4	0.6	0.2
40036	Corn Bran Cereal	1	cup	36	1	120	2	30	6	1	0.3	0.3	0.4
40039	CornFlakes-Honey Crisp Cereal	0.75	cup	30		112	2	27	1	<1	<0.1	0.1	0.1
40040	Crispy Wheat`n Raisins Cereal	1	cup	43	3	150	3	35	3	1	0.1	0.1	0.1
40043	Frosted Mini-Wheats Cereal	1	cup	55	3	186	5	45	6	1	0.2	0.1	0.6
40025	Frosted Flakes Cereal	0.75	cup	31	1	116	1	28	1	<1	<0.1	0.1	0.1

< = Trace amount present　　　　　　　　Blank = Not available

CHOL, cholesterol; **V,** vitamin; **THI,** thiamin; **RIB,** riboflavin; **NIA,** niacin; **FOL,** folate;
CALC, calcium; **PHOS,** phosphate; **SOD,** sodium; **POT,** potassium; **MAG,** magnesium

CHOL (mg)	V-A (RE)	THI (mg)	RIB (mg)	NIA (mg)	V-B6 (mg)	FOL (μg)	V-B12 (μg)	V-C (mg)	V-E (mg)	CALC (mg)	PHOS (mg)	SOD (mg)	POT (mg)	MAG (mg)	IRON (mg)	ZINC (mg)
0	5	<0.1	<0.1	0	0	1	0	0	0.2	5	0	2	21	2	0.2	0.1
0	0	<0.1	<0.1	0	0	1	0	0	0	4	0	2	16	2	0.1	0.1
0	0	0	<0.1	0	0	12	0	0	0	0	2	7	88	7	<0.1	<0.1
0	0	0	<0.1	0.1	<0.1	1	0	0	0	5	2	7	47	5	<0.1	0.1
0	0	0	<0.1	0	0	13	0	0	0	<1	2	7	90	7	<0.1	<0.1
0	0	0	<0.1	0.1	<0.1	1	0	0	0	5	2	14	50	5	<0.1	0.1
0	0	0	<0.1	0.1	<0.1	5	0	0	0	5	2	24	40	5	0.1	0.1
0	0	0	<0.1	0.1	<0.1	10	0	0	0	5	3	8	49	5	0.1	0.1
0	0	0	0	0	0	0	0	0	0	33	0	2	0	0	0	0
0	0	0	0	0	0	0	0	0	0	2	0	2	0	2	<0.1	0
0	0	0	0	0	0	0	0	0	0	2	0	10	0	0	<0.1	0.2
0	0	0	0	0	0	0	0	0	0	14	39	57	7	4	0.1	0.2
0	0	0	0	0	0	0	0	0	0	5	0	7	0	2	<0.1	0.1
0	0	<0.1	<0.1	0.5	0.1	2	0	0	0.1	0	29	0	53	10	0.5	0.2
0	0	0.2	0.1	2	0.1	75	0	0	0.1	0	29	0	53	10	1.5	0.2
0	0	0	0	1	0.1	7	0	0	<0.1	7	41	2	49	7	0.5	0.4
0	0	0.5	0.2	5.8	<0.1	5	0	0	0.3	5	24	2	31	5	9.6	0.2
0	527	0.5	0.5	7	0.7	7	2.2	22	1.3	94	185	7	158	38	6.3	1.1
0	116	0.4	0.5	4.4	0.5	17	0	0	3.4	69	184	2	138	66	5.4	0.9
0	5	0.3	<0.1	0.3	<0.1	9	0	0	0.2	19	178	2	131	56	1.6	1.1
0	453	0.5	0.3	5.5	0.7	97	0	0	0.7	163	133	285	99	42	6.3	1.1
0	302	0.3	0.3	4	0.4	81	0	0	0.2	105	132	234	112	39	3.9	0.9
0	0	0.2	0.2	2	0.1	18	0.1	0	0.3	13	147	5	154	58	1.6	1.4
0	0	0.2	0.1	2.1	0.2	26	0	0	2.2	17	166	0	170	53	1.5	1.2
0	0	0.2	0.1	2.3	0.1	18	0	0	0.7	22	161	2	226	81	1.6	1.3
0	0	<0.1	<0.1	1.3	<0.1	17	0	0	0.9	10	146	5	187	49	1.4	1.7
1	1	0.4	0.2	1.8	0.2	26	0.1	<1	2.2	100	322	28	456	109	3.1	2.5
0	5	0.1	0.1	0.6	<0.1	13	0	0	0.7	21	147	202	157	46	1.3	1
0	225	0.4	0.4	5	0.5	100	1.5	0		10	67	212	62	25	2.7	1.5
0	3	<0.1	<0.1	1	<0.1	4	0	1	3.2	6	126	13	134	10	0.7	0.1
0	225	0.4	0.4	5	0.5	90	0	15	0.5	20	166	200	270	83	4.5	6.4
<1	1363	1.3	1.5	18.1	1.9	364	5.5	0	0.7	50	232	161	260	74	16.4	1.6
<1	1284	1.3	1.5	17.1	1.7	342	5.1	0	0.7	47	224	167	198	67	15.4	1.6
0	5	0.5	0.6	6.9	0.7	137	0	0	0.2	7	39	286	47	13	6.2	5.1
0	330	0.4	0.5	5.5	0.5	110	0	13	0.3	9	55	133	71	18	4.9	4.1
0	5	0.1	0.6	6.7	0.7	134	0	0	0.2	27	48	338	75	19	10.1	5
0	75	0.4	0.4	5	0.5	100	0	15	<0.1	<1	14	261	27	5	4.5	0.1
0	293	0.3	0.3	3.9	0.4	78	0	0	0.4	54	110	223	180	33	3.5	0.8
0	0	0.4	0.4	5.4	0.5	110	1.6	0	0.5	20	160	2	183	56	15.4	1.6
0	225	0.4	0.4	5	0.5	100	0	15	<0.1	1	17	281	34	8	4.7	0.1

ERA, EatRight Analysis CD-ROM; **AMT**, amount; **WT**, weight; **WTR**, water; **CAL**, calories; **PROT**, protein; **CARB**, carbohydrate; **FIBR**, fiber; **FAT**, fat; **SATF**, saturated fat; **MONO**, monosaturated fat; **POLY**, polyunsaturated fat

ERA CODE	FOOD DESCRIPTION	AMT	UNIT	WT (g)	WTR (g)	CAL (kcal)	PROT (g)	CARB (g)	FIBR (g)	FAT (g)	SATF (g)	MONO (g)	POLY (g)
Breakfast Cereals (continued)													
Cereals, Ready To Eat (continued)													
40038	Fruitangy Ohs Cereal	1	cup	31	1	122	2	27	1	1	0.3	0.5	0.3
40245	Golden Crisp Cereal	0.75	cup	27	1	107	1	25	0	<1	0.1		
13343	Granola-LowFat	0.5	cup	53		210	5	40	3	3	1		
40045	Granola-LowFat w/Raisins	0.66	cup	55		213	5	44	3	3	0.8	1.3	0.6
40009	Granola-Oats-Honey-Raisin	0.5	cup	51		225	5	34	3	9	3.6	3.8	1.1
40265	GrapeNut Flakes Cereal	0.75	cup	29	1	106	3	24	3	1	0.2	0.2	0.5
40129	Heartwise Cereal	1	cup	39	1	113	4	31	9	1	0.2	0.2	0.4
40052	Honey Bran Cereal	1	cup	35	1	119	3	29	4	1	0.3	0.1	0.3
40051	Honey Nut Cheerios Cereal	1	cup	33	1	126	3	27	2	1	0.2	0.5	0.2
40134	Just Right Cereal	1	cup	43	1	160	3	36	2	1	0.1	0.2	0.8
40053	Kashi GoodFrendz Cereal	0.75	cup	30		90	3	24	8	1			
5014	Kashi Medly Cereal	0.5	cup	30		100	4	20	2	1			
40054	King Vitamin Cereal	1	cup	21	<1	81	2	18	1	1	0.2	0.3	0.2
40010	Kix Cereal	1.5	cup	28.35	1	108	2	24	1	1	0.2	0.1	<0.1
40011	Life Cereal	1	cup	44	2	167	4	35	3	2	0.3	0.6	0.8
40124	Mueslix Five Grain Cereal	1	cup	82	7	289	6	63	6	5	0.7	2	1.8
40275	Post Bran'ola Raisin Cereal	0.5	cup	55		200	4	44	5	3	0.5		
40018	Puffed Rice Cereal	1	cup	14	1	54	1	12	<1	<1	<0.1	<0.1	<0.1
40023	Puffed Wheat Cereal	1	cup	12	<1	44	2	9	1	<1	<0.1	<0.1	0.1
40066	Quisp Cereal	1	cup	30	1	121	1	26	1	2	0.5	0.4	0.2
40393	Raisin Nut Bran Cereal	1	cup	55	2	209	5	41	5	4	0.7	1.9	0.5
40017	Rice Krispies Cereal	1	cup	28	1	111	2	25	<1	<1	<0.1	<0.1	<0.1
40062	Shredded Wheat-Lg Biscuit	1	ea	23.6	1	85	3	19	2	<1	0.1	0.1	0.2
40022	Shredded Wheat-Sm Biscuit	0.75	cup	32	2	114	4	26	3	1	0.1	0.1	0.3
40068	Sugar Smacks Cereal	0.75	cup	27	1	103	2	24	1	1	0.3	0.1	0.2
40070	Tasteeos Cereal	1	cup	24	1	94	3	19	3	1	0.2	0.2	0.2
40024	Toasted Oat Cereal	1	cup	30		114	3	23	2	2	0.3	0.5	0.4
40021	Total Wheat Cereal	0.75	cup	30	1	105	3	24	3	1	0.2	0.1	0.1
Condiments, Sauces and Gravies													
Condiments													
27000	Catsup/Ketchup	1	cup	245	163	255	4	67	3	1	0.1	0.1	0.4
27001	Catsup/Ketchup-Packet	1	ea	6	4	6	<1	2	<1	<1	<0.1	<0.1	<0.1
27012	Dill Pickle	1	ea	65	60	12	<1	3	1	<1	<0.1	<0.1	0.1
27013	Dill Pickle-Slices	10	pce	60	55	11	<1	2	1	<1	<0.1	<0.1	<0.1
27004	Horseradish-Prepared	1	tsp	5	4	2	<1	1	<1	<1	<0.1	<0.1	<0.1
27009	Olives-Large-Ripe-Pitted	10	ea	44	35	51	<1	3	1	5	0.6	3.5	0.4
27042	Olives-Green-Stuffed	10	ea	40	32	41	1	1	<1	4	0.6	3.2	0.4
27016	Pickle-Sweet-Medium	1	ea	35	23	41	<1	11	<1	<1	<0.1	<0.1	<0.1
435	Mustard-Yellow-Prepared	1	cup	250	204	165	10	19	8	8	0.4	5.4	1.5
Gravies													
53023	Beef Gravy-Canned	1	cup	233	204	123	9	11	1	5	2.7	2.2	0.2
53006	Beef Gravy-Homemade	1	cup	270	231	213	5	15	1	15	3.8	6.9	4.1
53027	Brown Gravy-Dry Mix+Water	1	cup	258	237	75	2	13	<1	2	0.8	0.7	0.1

< = Trace amount present   Blank = Not available

CHOL, cholesterol; **V,** vitamin; **THI,** thiamin; **RIB,** riboflavin; **NIA,** niacin; **FOL,** folate;
CALC, calcium; **PHOS,** phosphate; **SOD,** sodium; **POT,** potassium; **MAG,** magnesium

CHOL (mg)	V-A (RE)	THI (mg)	RIB (mg)	NIA (mg)	V-B6 (mg)	FOL (μg)	V-B12 (μg)	V-C (mg)	V-E (mg)	CALC (mg)	PHOS (mg)	SOD (mg)	POT (mg)	MAG (mg)	IRON (mg)	ZINC (mg)
0	311	0.4	0.4	5.2	0.5	104	0	12	0.3	3	55	152	59	18	4.7	3.9
0	225	0.4	0.4	5	0.5	100	1.5	0		4	37	40	34	16	1.8	1.5
0	200							0		20		50			1.8	
1	2	0.2	0.1	1	0.1	13	0	<1	0.3	33	130	145	189	44	1.4	1
1	1	0.1	0.1	0.8	0.1	14	0.1	<1	0.5	59	152	19	250	49	1.2	1
0	225	0.4	0.4	5	0.5	100	1.5	0	0.1	11	88	140	99	30	8.1	1.2
0	310	0.5	0.6	7	0.7	136	2	0	<0.1	30	154	168	265	55	6.2	2.1
0	463	0.5	0.5	6.2	0.6	23	1.9	19	0.8	16	132	202	150	46	5.6	0.9
0	248	0.4	0.5	5.5	0.6	110	0	16	0.3	22	113	285	94	32	4.9	4.1
0	294	0.3	0.3	3.9	0.4	80	1.2	0	1.8	11	83	264	95	27	12.7	0.7
0	0	<0.1	<0.1	1.2	0.1	7		0		0	102	70	119		0.4	
0	0	0.1	0.1	1.1	0.1	7		0		0	84	50	108		0.4	
0	212	0.3	0.3	3.5	0.4	71	1.1	8	6.7	3	54	176	58	18	5.9	2.7
0	355	0.4	0.4	4.7	0.5	94	0	14	0.1	41	40	249	39	9	7.7	3.5
0	2	0.6	0.6	7.3	0.7	147	0	0	0.2	134	186	240	109	43	12.3	5.5
0	747	0.7	0.8	9.8	1	197	3.3	1	8.9	67	215	107	369	82	8.9	7.5
0	375	0.4	0.4	5	0.5	100	1.5	0		0	100	220	220	40	4.5	1.5
0	0	0.1	<0.1	0.9	0	1	0	0	<0.1	1	17	1	16	4	0.4	0.2
0	<1	<0.1	<0.1	1.4	<0.1	4	0.1	0	0.1	3	40	1	44	16	0.6	0.4
0	4	0.4	0.5	5.7	0.6	113	0	0	0.2	6	47	216	40	15	5.1	4.2
0	0	0.4	0.4	5	0.5	100	0	0	2	74	163	246	218	54	4.5	1.1
0	371	0.5	0.6	6.9	0.7	138	0.1	15	0.1	5	31	206	27	12	0.7	0.5
0	0	0.1	0.1	1.1	0.1	12	0	0	0.1	10	86	<1	77	40	0.7	0.6
0	0	0.1	0.1	1.7	0.1	16	0	0	0.5	12	113	3	116	42	1.4	1.1
0	225	0.4	0.4	5	0.5	100	0	15	0.1	3	40	51	42	16	1.8	0.4
0	318	0.3	0.4	4.2	0.4	85	1.3	13	0.2	11	96	183	71	26	6.9	0.7
0	102	0.4	0.4	5.1	0.5	103	0	12	0.8	12	116	284	87	29	8.5	4.4
0	375	1.5	1.7	20.1	2	400	7.7	60	23.5	258	211	199	97	32	18	15
0	250	0.2	0.2	3.3	0.4	37	0	37	3.6	47	96	2905	1178	54	1.7	0.6
0	6	<0.1	<0.1	0.1	<0.1	1	0	1	0.1	1	2	71	29	1	<0.1	<0.1
0	21	<0.1	<0.1	<0.1	<0.1	1	0	1	0.1	6	14	833	75	7	0.3	0.1
0	20	<0.1	<0.1	<0.1	<0.1	1	0	1	0.1	5	13	769	70	7	0.3	0.1
0	0	0	<0.1	<0.1	<0.1	3	0	1	0	3	2	16	12	1	<0.1	<0.1
0	18	<0.1	0	<0.1	<0.1	0	0	<1	1.3	39	1	384	4	2	1.5	0.1
0	25	0	<0.1	<0.1	<0.1	1	0	5	1.1	21	7	826	28	8	0.6	0.1
0	5	<0.1	<0.1	0.1	<0.1	<1	0	<1	0.1	1	4	329	11	1	0.2	<0.1
7	0	0.1	0.1	1.5	<0.1	5	0.2	0	0.6	14	70	1304	189	5	1.6	2.3
5	300	<0.1	0.1	1.2	<0.1	5	0.3	0	0.4	54	78	1558	294	5	1.3	2.2
3	0	<0.1	0.1	0.8	0	0	0	0	0.3	67	44	1075	57	10	0.2	0.3

ERA, EatRight Analysis CD-ROM; **AMT,** amount; **WT,** weight; **WTR,** water; **CAL,** calories; **PROT,** protein; **CARB,** carbohydrate;
FIBR, fiber; **FAT,** fat; **SATF,** saturated fat; **MONO,** monosaturated fat; **POLY,** polyunsaturated fat

ERA CODE	FOOD DESCRIPTION	AMT	UNIT	WT (g)	WTR (g)	CAL (kcal)	PROT (g)	CARB (g)	FIBR (g)	FAT (g)	SATF (g)	MONO (g)	POLY (g)
Condiments, Sauces and Gravies (continued)													
Gravies (continued)													
53022	Chicken Gravy-Canned	1	cup	238	203	188	5	13	1	14	3.4	6.1	3.6
53028	Chicken Gravy-Dry+Water	1	cup	260	238	83	3	14	<1	2	0.5	0.9	0.4
53005	Chicken Gravy-Homemade	1	cup	260	221	194	12	13	1	10	2.8	4.3	2.6
53026	Mushroom Gravy-Canned	1	cup	238	212	119	3	13	1	6	1	2.8	2.4
53039	Mushroom Gravy-Dry+Water	1	cup	258	237	70	2	14	1	1	0.5	0.3	<0.1
53033	Turkey Gravy-Canned	1	cup	238	211	121	6	12	1	5	1.5	2.1	1.2
53045	Turkey Gravy-Dry+Water	1	cup	261	237	86	3	15	1	2	0.5	0.8	0.4
Sauces													
53388	Alfredo Sauce-DiGiorno	0.25	cup	62		230	4	2	0	22	10		
53396	Alfredo Sauce-LowFat-DiGiorno	0.25	cup	69		170	5	16	0	10	6		
53000	Barbecue Sauce	1	cup	250	202	188	4	32	3	4	0.7	1.9	1.7
53015	Cheese Sauce	0.5	cup	101	64	221	10	9	<1	16	9.3	4.9	2.2
53016	Curry Sauce	0.5	cup	115	102	74	3	3	<1	6	1	2.6	1.7
53103	Enchilada Sauce-Green	1	cup	250	217	187	4	13	4	14	8.1	3.9	1.2
53102	Enchilada Sauce-Red	1	cup	250	205	321	3	10	2	31	16.7	10.1	2.8
53351	Hoisin Sauce	2	Tbs	34		70	1	14	0	2	0		
53110	Hollandaise Sauce-Mix+Water	1	cup	259.2	217	238	5	14	1	20	11.6	5.9	0.9
53098	Horseradish Sauce	1	Tbs	14	10	30	<1	1	<1	3	1.8	0.8	0.1
7563	Miso Sauce	1	cup	248	141	389	13	73	6	7	1	1.5	3.8
53106	Pesto Sauce	1	cup	232	48	1240	45	16	7	114	30.5	69.6	8
53466	Salsa Ready-to-Serve	1	cup	259	234	73	3	16	4	1	0.1	0.1	0.3
53002	Soy Sauce	1	Tbs	16	11	9	1	1	<1	<1	0	<0.1	<0.1
53267	Soy Sauce-Lite	1	Tbs	18	13	15	1	2	0	<1	0		
53011	Spaghetti Sauce w/Meat-Canned	1	cup	250	212	178	7	19	4	8	1.8	3.3	1.8
53010	Spaghetti Sauce w/Meat-Recipe	1	cup	248	189	287	16	21	4	17	4.5	6.2	4.3
53014	Spaghetti Sauce+Mushroom-Can	0.75	cup	185	155	162	2	19	2	4	0.6	2.3	1.2
53008	Spaghetti/Marinara Sauce	1	cup	250	217	142	4	21	4	5	0.7	2.2	1.8
53001	Szechuan Sauce	1	cup	250	202	188	4	32	3	4	0.7	1.9	1.7
53085	Tabasco Sauce/Pepper Sauce	1	Tbs	15.6	15	2	<1	<1	<1	<1	<0.1	<0.1	<0.1
53415	Tartar Sauce-NonFat-Kraft	2	Tbs	32		25	0	5	<1	0	0	0	0
53004	Teriyaki Sauce	1	Tbs	18	12	15	1	3	<1	0	0	0	0
53025	White Sauce-Dry Mix+Milk	1	cup	264	215	240	10	21	<1	13	6.4	4.7	1.7
53007	White Sauce-Recipe	1	cup	250	192	355	9	20	<1	27	7.8	9.1	8.8
53099	Worcestershire Sauce	1	cup	272	190	182	0	45	0	0	0	0	0
Dairy Products and Substitutes													
Creams and Substitutes													
501	Cream-Coffee/Table	1	cup	240	177	469	6	9	0	46	28.8	13.4	1.7
500	Cream-Half & Half	1	cup	242	195	315	7	10	0	28	17.3	8	1
502	Cream-Heavy Whipping-Liq	1	cup	238	137	820	5	7	0	88	54.8	25.4	3.3
503	Cream-Hvy Whipping-Whipped	2	cup	239	138	824	5	7	0	88	55	25.5	3.3
511	Cream-Light Whipping-Liq	1	cup	239	152	699	5	7	0	74	46.2	21.7	2.1
527	Cream-Medium Fat-25%	1	cup	239	164	583	6	8	0	60	37.3	17.2	2.2
540	Cremora NonDairy Creamer	1	tsp	2	<1	12	<1	1	0	1	0.7	<0.1	0

< = Trace amount present   Blank = Not available

CHOL, cholesterol; **V**, vitamin; **THI**, thiamin; **RIB**, riboflavin; **NIA**, niacin; **FOL**, folate;
CALC, calcium; **PHOS**, phosphate; **SOD**, sodium; **POT**, potassium; **MAG**, magnesium

CHOL (mg)	V-A (RE)	THI (mg)	RIB (mg)	NIA (mg)	V-B6 (mg)	FOL (μg)	V-B12 (μg)	V-C (mg)	V-E (mg)	CALC (mg)	PHOS (mg)	SOD (mg)	POT (mg)	MAG (mg)	IRON (mg)	ZINC (mg)
5	264	<0.1	0.1	1.1	<0.1	5	0.2	0	0.4	48	69	1373	259	5	1.1	1.9
3	0	0.1	0.1	0.8	<0.1	3	0.2	3	0.1	39	47	1133	62	10	0.3	0.3
110	653	0.1	0.4	3.2	0.1	98	4.7	1	0.6	31	124	1365	302	9	3.1	2.9
0	0	0.1	0.1	1.6	<0.1	29	0	0	0.2	17	36	1356	252	5	1.6	1.7
0	0	0.1	0.1	0.8	<0.1	3	0.2	2	<0.1	49	44	1400	57	8	0.3	0.3
5	0	<0.1	0.2	3.1	<0.1	5	0.2	0	0.1	10	69	1373	259	5	1.7	1.9
3	0	0.1	0.1	1	<0.1	3	0.3	2	0.1	50	50	1495	65	10	0.3	0.3
45	80	0	0.1	0				0		100	100	550	75	0	0	
30	80	0	0.1	0				0		150	100	600	80	8	0	
0	218	0.1	0.1	2.2	0.2	10	0	18	2.8	48	50	2037	435	45	2.2	0.5
36	167	0.1	0.2	0.5	<0.1	10	0.4	1	1.2	267	202	515	126	17	0.6	1.1
0	61	<0.1	0.1	1.6	<0.1	3	0.1	<1	1	9	38	392	104	3	0.5	0.1
43	156	0.1	0.2	2.9	0.2	13	0.1	23	0.9	77	118	30	540	41	1.2	0.6
91	349	0.1	0.1	0.7	0.1	17	0.1	20	1.6	55	76	36	336	20	0.6	0.3
0	0							0		0		500			0	
52	220	0.1	0.2	0.1	0.5	21	0.8	<1	0.6	124	127	1565	124	8	0.9	0.8
6	27	<0.1	<0.1	<0.1	<0.1	2	<0.1	<1	0.1	16	12	10	20	2	<0.1	<0.1
0	10	0.1	0.3	1	0.2	37	0	0	<0.1	77	173	4061	208	53	3.2	3.7
80	336	0.1	0.4	1.6	0.3	58	1.4	18	11.3	1762	908	1904	726	126	8.5	4.3
0	155	0.1	0.1	2.1	0.3	41	0	36	1.6	78	67	1124	552	34	2.5	0.6
0	0	<0.1	<0.1	0.4	<0.1	3	0	0	0	3	20	871	64	7	0.3	0.1
0	0							0		3		505			0.1	
15	176	0.1	0.1	3.5	0.3	25	0.5	19	3	54	104	982	742	43	2.1	1.3
46	487	0.2	0.3	6	0.5	30	1.4	37	5.3	59	173	868	1098	62	3.5	3.4
0	362	0.1	0.1	1.4	0.2	19	0	14	2.9	22	45	744	500	22	1.5	0.5
0	95	0.1	0.1	2.7	0.3	25	0	20	3.1	55	80	1030	738	42	1.8	0.4
0	218	0.1	0.1	2.2	0.2	10	0	18	2.8	48	50	2037	435	45	2.2	0.5
<1	65	<0.1	<0.1	0.1	<0.1	<1	9.4	<1	0.1	4	3	92	20	1	0.4	<0.1
0	0							0		0		210	15		0	
0	0	<0.1	<0.1	0.2	<0.1	4	0	0	0	4	28	690	40	11	0.3	<0.1
34	92	0.1	0.4	0.5	0.1	16	1.1	3	10	425	256	797	444	264	0.3	0.5
29	310	0.2	0.4	1	0.1	14	0.8	2	3.4	260	216	368	343	32	0.7	0.9
0	30	0.2	0.4	1.9	0	0	0	35	0	291	163	2665	2176	35	14.4	0.5
159	437	0.1	0.4	0.1	0.1	6	0.5	2	0.4	231	192	95	292	21	0.1	0.6
89	259	0.1	0.4	0.2	0.1	6	0.8	2	0.3	254	230	98	314	25	0.2	1.2
326	1001	0.1	0.3	0.1	0.1	9	0.4	1	1.5	154	148	89	179	17	0.1	0.5
328	1006	0.1	0.3	0.1	0.1	9	0.4	1	1.5	154	149	90	180	17	0.1	0.5
265	705	0.1	0.3	0.1	0.1	9	0.5	1	1.4	166	146	82	231	17	0.1	0.6
209	554	0.1	0.3	0.1	0.1	5	0.5	2	1.4	216	169	88	275	20	0.1	0.6
0	<1		0									6				

ERA, EatRight Analysis CD-ROM; **AMT**, amount; **WT**, weight; **WTR**, water; **CAL**, calories; **PROT**, protein; **CARB**, carbohydrate; **FIBR**, fiber; **FAT**, fat; **SATF**, saturated fat; **MONO**, monosaturated fat; **POLY**, polyunsaturated fat

ERA CODE	FOOD DESCRIPTION	AMT	UNIT	WT (g)	WTR (g)	CAL (kcal)	PROT (g)	CARB (g)	FIBR (g)	FAT (g)	SATF (g)	MONO (g)	POLY (g)
Dairy Products and Substitutes (continued)													
Creams and Substitutes (continued)													
517	Mocha Mix Creamer	1	Tbs	14.2		19	<1	1	0	2	0.3	0	0.7
504	Sour Cream-Cultured	1	cup	230	163	493	7	10	0	48	30	13.9	1.8
505	Sour Cream-Imitation	1	cup	230	164	479	6	15	0	45	40.9	1.4	0.1
515	Sour Cream-LowCal	1	Tbs	15	12	20	<1	1	0	2	1.1	0.5	0.1
526	Whip Topping-LowCal, from mix	1	cup	80	66	42	1	8	0	5	2.5	1.1	0.9
Milks and Non-Dairy Milks													
7	Buttermilk-Cultured-Skim	1	cup	245	221	99	8	12	0	2	1.3	0.6	0.1
19	Chocolate Milk-1% Fat	1	cup	250	211	158	8	26	1	2	1.5	0.8	0.1
18	Chocolate Milk-2% Fat	1	cup	250	209	179	8	26	1	5	3.1	1.5	0.2
59	Chocolate Milk-NonFat	1	cup	250	211	144	9	27	1	1	0.7	0.3	<0.1
20	Chocolate Milk-Whole	1	cup	250	206	208	8	26	2	8	5.3	2.5	0.3
98	Eggnog-2% Fat	1	cup	254	215	191	12	17	0	8	3.7	2.7	0.7
17	Eggnog-Whole Milk	1	cup	254	189	342	10	34	0	19	11.3	5.7	0.9
80	Evaporated Milk-2% Fat	1	cup	252	196	232	19	28	0	5	3.1	1.4	0.2
10	Evaporated Milk-Skim	1	cup	256	203	199	19	29	0	1	0.3	0.2	<0.1
23	Goat Milk	1	cup	244	212	168	9	11	0	10	6.5	2.7	0.4
54	Lactose Reduced Milk-1% Fat	1	cup	246	222	103	8	12	0	3	1.6	0.8	0.1
56	Lactose Reduced Milk-NonFat	1	cup	245	222	86	8	12	0	<1	0.3	0.1	<0.1
4	Milk-1% Fat	1	cup	244	220	102	8	12	0	3	1.6	0.7	0.1
2	Milk-2% Fat	1	cup	244	218	121	8	12	0	5	2.9	1.4	0.2
6	Milk-NonFat	1	cup	245	222	86	8	12	0	<1	0.3	0.1	<0.1
1	Milk-Whole-3.3% Fat	1	cup	244	215	150	8	11	0	8	5.1	2.4	0.3
57	Nonfat Dry Milk Powder+Water	1	cup	245	223	82	8	12	0	<1	0.1	<0.1	<0.1
20033	Soy Milk	1	cup	245	228	81	7	4	3	5	0.5	0.8	2
7801	Soy Milk Bev-Carob (Eden)	1	cup	244		150	6	23	0	4	0.5		
7775	Soy Milk Bev-Vanilla (VitaSoy)	1	cup	228.3		190	7	27		6	1	1	3
11	Sweetened Condensed Milk	1	cup	306	83	982	24	166	0	27	16.8	7.4	1
82	Vitamite Imitation Milk	1	cup	244	220	112	4	13	0	5	0.6	1.2	2.9
Natural Cheeses													
1029	Asiago Cheese-Shredded	1	cup	108	40	406	31	4	0	30	19.2	7.9	1
1003	Blue Cheese	1	cup	135	57	477	29	3	0	39	25.2	10.5	1.1
1037	Brick Cheese-Shredded	1	cup	113	46	419	26	3	0	34	21.2	9.7	0.9
1004	Brie Cheese-Sliced	1	cup	144	70	480	30	1	0	40	25.1	11.5	1.2
1006	Camembert Cheese	1	cup	246	127	737	49	1	0	60	37.5	17.3	1.8
1227	Cheddar Cheese-FatFree (Lifetime)	0.25	cup	31	18	44	9	1	0	0	0	0	0
1423	Cheddar Cheese-LowFat	0.25	cup	31	15	89	10	1	0	5	3.3		
1091	Cheddar Cheese-LowFat-LowSod	1	cup	113	73	195	27	2	0	8	5	2.3	0.2
1105	Cheddar Cheese-LowSod	1	cup	113	44	450	28	2	0	37	23.5	10.4	1.1
1008	Cheddar Cheese-Shredded	1	cup	113	42	455	28	1	0	37	23.8	10.6	1.1
1010	Colby Cheese-Shredded	1	cup	113	43	445	27	3	0	36	22.8	10.5	1.1
1047	Cottage Cheese-1% Lowfat	1	cup	226	186	164	28	6	0	2	1.5	0.7	0.1
1014	Cottage Cheese-2% lowfat	1	cup	226	179	203	31	8	0	4	2.8	1.2	0.1
1013	Cottage Cheese-Crm-Lg Curd	1	cup	225	178	232	28	6	0	10	6.4	2.9	0.3
1012	Cottage Cheese-Crm-Sm Curd	1	cup	210	166	217	26	6	0	9	6	2.7	0.3

< = Trace amount present   Blank = Not available

CHOL, cholesterol; **V**, vitamin; **THI**, thiamin; **RIB**, riboflavin; **NIA**, niacin; **FOL**, folate;
CALC, calcium; **PHOS**, phosphate; **SOD**, sodium; **POT**, potassium; **MAG**, magnesium

CHOL (mg)	V-A (RE)	THI (mg)	RIB (mg)	NIA (mg)	V-B6 (mg)	FOL (μg)	V-B12 (μg)	V-C (mg)	V-E (mg)	CALC (mg)	PHOS (mg)	SOD (mg)	POT (mg)	MAG (mg)	IRON (mg)	ZINC (mg)
0										1	8	7	20	0		
102	448	0.1	0.3	0.2	<0.1	25	0.7	2	1.5	268	195	122	331	26	0.1	0.6
0	0	0	0	0	0	0	0	0	0.3	6	102	235	369	15	0.9	2.7
6	17	<0.1	<0.1	<0.1	<0.1	2	<0.1	<1	0.1	16	14	6	19	2	<0.1	0.1
0	0	0	0	0	0	0	0	0	<0.1	2	24	85	21	1	<0.1	<0.1
9	20	0.1	0.4	0.1	0.1	12	0.5	2	0.2	285	218	257	371	27	0.1	1
7	148	0.1	0.4	0.3	0.1	12	0.9	2	0.1	287	256	152	426	33	0.6	1
17	142	0.1	0.4	0.3	0.1	12	0.8	2	1.5	284	254	150	422	33	0.6	1
4	142	0.1	0.3	0.3	0.1	14	0.9	2	0.1	292	265	121	486	45	0.7	1.2
30	72	0.1	0.4	0.3	0.1	12	0.8	2	0.2	280	251	149	417	33	0.6	1
194	197	0.1	0.6	0.2	0.1	30	1.2	2	0.6	270	270	155	368	32	0.7	1.3
149	203	0.1	0.5	0.3	0.1	2	1.1	4	0.6	330	278	138	420	47	0.5	1.2
20	331	0.1	0.8	0.4	0.1	21	0.6	3	0.1	717	482	285	821	67	0.7	2.2
9	300	0.1	0.8	0.4	0.1	22	0.6	3	0.2	741	499	294	849	69	0.7	2.3
28	137	0.1	0.3	0.7	0.1	1	0.2	3	0.2	326	270	122	499	34	0.1	0.7
10	145	0.1	0.4	0.2	0.1	13	0.9	2	0.1	302	237	124	384	34	0.1	1
4	149	0.1	0.3	0.2	0.1	13	0.9	2	0.1	302	247	126	406	28	0.1	1
10	144	0.1	0.4	0.2	0.1	12	0.9	2	0.1	300	235	123	381	34	0.1	1
18	139	0.1	0.4	0.2	0.1	12	0.9	2	0.2	297	232	122	377	33	0.1	1
4	149	0.1	0.3	0.2	0.1	13	0.9	2	0.1	302	247	126	406	28	0.1	1
33	76	0.1	0.4	0.2	0.1	12	0.9	2	0.2	291	228	120	370	33	0.1	0.9
4	162	0.1	0.4	0.2	0.1	11	0.9	1	<0.1	284	224	132	388	29	0.1	1.1
0	7	0.4	0.2	0.4	0.1	4	0	0	<0.1	10	120	29	345	47	1.4	0.6
0	0	0.9	0.1	1.2	0.1	40		0		60	100	105	330	40	1.8	0.6
0		0.2	0.2							80		130	210		0.7	
104	248	0.3	1.3	0.6	0.2	34	1.4	8	0.7	868	775	389	1136	78	0.6	2.9
0	149	0	0	0.2	0	0	0	0	0	200	244	134	366	2	0.2	0.2
99	273	<0.1	0.4	0.1	0.1	7	1.8	0	0.5	1037	653	281	120	39	0.2	4.2
102	308	<0.1	0.5	1.4	0.2	49	1.6	0	0.9	712	523	1883	346	31	0.4	3.6
107	341	<0.1	0.4	0.1	0.1	23	1.4	0	0.6	761	510	632	153	27	0.5	2.9
144	262	0.1	0.7	0.5	0.3	94	2.4	0	0.9	265	271	906	219	29	0.7	3.4
177	620	0.1	1.2	1.5	0.6	153	3.2	0	1.6	953	853	2070	459	49	0.8	5.9
3	95									443		244				
17	95							1		277		105			0.4	
24	70	<0.1	<0.1	0.1	0.1	20	0.9	0	0.2	794	547	24	126	31	0.8	3.5
113	325	<0.1	0.4	0.1	0.1	20	0.9	0	0.4	794	547	24	126	31	0.8	3.5
118	314	<0.1	0.4	0.1	0.1	21	0.9	0	0.4	815	579	701	111	31	0.8	3.5
107	311	<0.1	0.4	0.1	0.1	21	0.9	0	0.4	774	516	683	143	29	0.9	3.5
10	25	<0.1	0.4	0.3	0.2	28	1.4	0	1.5	138	302	918	193	12	0.3	0.9
19	45	0.1	0.4	0.3	0.2	30	1.6	0	0.1	155	340	918	217	14	0.4	0.9
34	108	<0.1	0.4	0.3	0.2	27	1.4	0	1.4	135	296	911	190	12	0.3	0.8
31	101	<0.1	0.3	0.3	0.1	26	1.3	0	1.3	126	277	850	177	11	0.3	0.8

ERA, EatRight Analysis CD-ROM; **AMT,** amount; **WT,** weight; **WTR,** water; **CAL,** calories; **PROT,** protein; **CARB,** carbohydrate; **FIBR,** fiber; **FAT,** fat; **SATF,** saturated fat; **MONO,** monosaturated fat; **POLY,** polyunsaturated fat

ERA CODE	FOOD DESCRIPTION	AMT	UNIT	WT (g)	WTR (g)	CAL (kcal)	PROT (g)	CARB (g)	FIBR (g)	FAT (g)	SATF (g)	MONO (g)	POLY (g)
Dairy Products and Substitutes (continued)													
Natural Cheeses (continued)													
1015	Cream Cheese	1	cup	232	125	810	18	6	0	81	51	22.8	2.9
1115	Cream Cheese-FatFree	2	Tbs	33		30	5	2	0	0	0	0	0
1098	Cream Cheese-LowFat	1	Tbs	15	10	35	2	1	0	3	1.7	0.7	0.1
1083	Cream Cheese-Soft	2	Tbs	30		100	2	1	0	10	7		
1050	Edam Cheese	1	cup	132	55	471	33	2	0	37	23.2	10.7	0.9
1016	Feta Cheese-Shredded	1	cup	150	83	395	21	6	0	32	22.4	6.9	0.9
1052	Fontina Cheese-Shredded	1	cup	108	41	420	28	2	0	34	20.7	9.4	1.8
1078	Goat Cheese-hard	1	oz	28.35	8	128	9	1	0	10	7	2.3	0.2
1080	Goat Cheese-soft type	1	cup	246	149	659	46	2	0	52	35.8	11.8	1.2
1054	Gouda Cheese	1	cup	132	55	470	33	3	0	36	23.2	10.2	0.9
1074	Gruyere Cheese-Shredded	1	cup	108	36	446	32	<1	0	35	20.4	10.8	1.9
1038	Havarti Cheese-Diced	1	cup	132	54	490	31	4	0	39	24.8	11.3	1
1223	Jack Cheese-FatFree (Lifetime)	1	cup	124	72	177	35	4	0	0	0	0	0
1017	Monterey Jack Cheese-Shredded	1	cup	113	46	422	28	1	0	34	21.5	9.9	1
1056	Mozzarella Cheese-Whole-Shred	1	cup	113	61	318	22	3	0	24	14.9	7.4	0.9
1058	Mozzarella-PartSkim-Shredded	1	cup	113	61	287	27	3	0	18	11.4	5.1	0.5
1021	Muenster Cheese-Shredded	1	cup	113	47	416	26	1	0	34	21.6	9.8	0.7
1060	Neufchatel Cheese	1	cup	232	144	603	23	7	0	54	34.3	15.7	1.5
1075	Parmesan Cheese-Grated	1	cup	100		456	42	4	0	30	19.1	8.7	0.7
1112	Parmesan Cheese-Shredded	1	Tbs	5	1	21	2	<1	0	1	0.9	0.4	<0.1
1062	Port du Salut Cheese-Shredded	1	cup	113	51	397	27	1	0	32	18.9	10.6	0.8
1023	Provolone Cheese-Diced	1	cup	132	54	464	34	3	0	35	22.5	9.8	1
1024	Ricotta Cheese-Part Skim	1	cup	246	183	340	28	13	0	19	12.1	5.7	0.6
1064	Ricotta Cheese-Whole Milk	1	cup	246	176	428	28	7	0	32	20.4	8.9	0.9
1066	Romano Cheese-Grated	1	cup	100		387	32	4	0	27	17.1	7.8	0.6
1026	Roquefort Cheese-Crumbled	1	cup	135	53	498	29	3	0	41	26	11.4	1.8
1059	String Cheese Stick	1	ea	28.35	15	72	7	1	0	5	2.9	1.3	0.1
1428	Swiss Cheese-LowFat	0.25	cup	31	13	100	9	1	0	7	4.4		
1027	Swiss Cheese-Shredded	1	cup	108	40	406	31	4	0	30	19.2	7.9	1
Processed Cheese and Cheese Substitutes													
1001	American Cheese Food	1	oz	28.35	12	94	6	2	0	7	4.4	2	0.2
1000	American Processed Cheese	1	pce	21	8	79	5	<1	0	7	4.1	1.9	0.2
1002	Cheez Whiz/Cheese Spread	1	cup	244	116	709	40	21	0	52	32.5	15.2	1.5
1081	Kraft Free Singles Cheese	1	pce	19		30	4	3	0	0	0	0	0
1069	Pimento Proc Cheese-Shred	1	cup	113	44	424	25	2	0	35	22.2	10.1	1.1
1071	Swiss Cheese Food-Slice	1	pce	21	9	68	5	1	0	5	3.3	1.4	0.1
1272	Velveeta Cheese Spread	1	oz	28	13	85	5	3	0	6	4		
1094	Velveeta-LowFat-LowSod	1	pce	34	21	61	8	1	0	2	1.5	0.7	0.1
1420	White American Cheese-FatFree	0.25	cup	31	19	27	5	1	0	0	0	0	0
Yogurt													
7546	Tofu Yogurt	1	cup	262	203	254	9	43	1	5	0.7	1	2.7
2428	Yogurt-Custard Type-Berry	6	oz	170		180	7	30		4			
2014	Yogurt-LowFat-Coffee/Vanilla	1	cup	245	194	209	12	34	0	3	2	0.8	0.1

< = Trace amount present   Blank = Not available

CHOL, cholesterol; **V,** vitamin; **THI,** thiamin; **RIB,** riboflavin; **NIA,** niacin; **FOL,** folate;
CALC, calcium; **PHOS,** phosphate; **SOD,** sodium; **POT,** potassium; **MAG,** magnesium

CHOL (mg)	V-A (RE)	THI (mg)	RIB (mg)	NIA (mg)	V-B6 (mg)	FOL (µg)	V-B12 (µg)	V-C (mg)	V-E (mg)	CALC (mg)	PHOS (mg)	SOD (mg)	POT (mg)	MAG (mg)	IRON (mg)	ZINC (mg)
254	886	<0.1	0.5	0.2	0.1	31	1	0	2.2	185	242	686	277	15	2.8	1.3
2	143		0.3				0.1	0		100	150	160	65	0	0	0.3
8	33	<0.1	<0.1	<0.1	<0.1	3	0.1	0	0.1	17	22	44	25	1	0.3	0.1
30	86	<0.1					0	0		20	20	100	40	0	0	0
118	334	<0.1	0.5	0.1	0.1	21	2	0	1	965	707	1273	248	39	0.6	4.9
134	192	0.2	1.3	1.5	0.6	48	2.5	0	<0.1	739	506	1674	93	29	1	4.3
125	313	<0.1	0.2	0.2	0.1	6	1.8	0	0.4	594	374	864	69	15	0.2	3.8
30	135	<0.1	0.3	0.7	<0.1	1	<0.1	0	0.2	254	207	98	14	15	0.5	0.4
113	696	0.2	0.9	1.1	0.6	30	0.5	0	1.1	344	630	905	64	39	4.7	2.3
150	230	<0.1	0.4	0.1	0.1	28	2	0	0.5	924	721	1081	159	38	0.3	5.1
119	325	0.1	0.3	0.1	0.1	11	1.7	0	0.4	1091	654	363	87	39	0.2	4.2
125	399	<0.1	0.5	0.2	0.1	27	1.7	0	0.7	889	595	739	179	32	0.6	3.4
13	380									1771		974				
100	286	<0.1	0.4	0.1	0.1	21	0.9	0	0.4	843	502	606	91	31	0.8	3.4
89	272	<0.1	0.3	0.1	0.1	8	0.7	0	0.7	584	419	422	76	21	0.2	2.5
65	200	<0.1	0.3	0.1	0.1	10	0.9	0	0.7	730	523	526	95	26	0.2	3.1
108	357	<0.1	0.4	0.1	0.1	14	1.7	0	0.5	810	528	709	152	31	0.5	3.2
176	696	<0.1	0.5	0.3	0.1	26	0.6	0	2.2	175	316	927	265	18	0.6	1.2
79	173	<0.1	0.4	0.3	0.1	8	1.4	0	0.8	1375	807	1861	107	51	0.9	3.2
4	9	<0.1	<0.1	<0.1	<0.1	<1	0.1	0	<0.1	63	37	85	5	3	<0.1	0.2
139	420	<0.1	0.3	0.1	0.1	21	1.7	0	0.6	734	407	603	153	27	0.5	2.9
91	348	<0.1	0.4	0.2	0.1	14	1.9	0	0.5	998	655	1155	182	36	0.7	4.3
76	278	0.1	0.5	0.2	<0.1	32	0.7	0	1.6	669	449	307	308	36	1.1	3.3
124	330	<0.1	0.5	0.3	0.1	30	0.8	0	1.6	509	389	207	257	28	0.9	2.9
104	141	<0.1	0.4	0.1	0.1	7	1.1	0	0.7	1063	760	1200	86	41	0.8	2.6
122	404	0.1	0.8	1	0.2	66	0.9	0	2.7	893	529	2442	122	40	0.8	2.8
16	50	<0.1	0.1	<0.1	<0.1	2	0.2	0	0.2	183	131	132	24	7	0.1	0.8
22	95							1		277		39			0.4	
99	273	<0.1	0.4	0.1	0.1	7	1.8	0	0.5	1037	653	281	120	39	0.2	4.2
18	57	<0.1	0.1	<0.1	<0.1	2	0.4	0	0.2	141	113	274	103	8	0.2	0.9
20	61	<0.1	0.1	<0.1	<0.1	2	0.1	0	0.1	129	156	300	34	5	0.1	0.6
135	461	0.1	1.1	0.3	0.3	17	1	0	1.7	1371	1737	3282	590	70	0.8	6.3
2	86		0.1					0	0	150	714	290	55		0	
106	364	<0.1	0.4	0.1	0.1	9	0.8	3	0.5	694	840	1613	183	25	0.5	3.4
17	51	<0.1	0.1	<0.1	<0.1	1	0.5	0	0.1	152	110	326	60	6	0.1	0.7
22	89	0.1						<1		130	242	420	94		0.1	0.5
12	22	<0.1	0.1	<0.1	<0.1	3	0.3	0	0.2	232	281	2	61	8	0.1	1.1
5	62							1		164		459			0.4	
0	8	0.2	0.1	0.6	0.1	16	0	7	0.8	309	100	92	123	105	2.8	0.8
15	21	0.1	0.3				0.4			200	150	95	310			
12	32	0.1	0.5	0.3	0.1	26	1.3	2	0.1	420	330	161	537	40	0.2	2

ERA, EatRight Analysis CD-ROM; **AMT,** amount; **WT,** weight; **WTR,** water; **CAL,** calories; **PROT,** protein; **CARB,** carbohydrate; **FIBR,** fiber; **FAT,** fat; **SATF,** saturated fat; **MONO,** monosaturated fat; **POLY,** polyunsaturated fat

ERA CODE	FOOD DESCRIPTION	AMT	UNIT	WT (g)	WTR (g)	CAL (kcal)	PROT (g)	CARB (g)	FIBR (g)	FAT (g)	SATF (g)	MONO (g)	POLY (g)
Dairy Products and Substitutes (continued)													
Yogurt (continued)													
2001	Yogurt-LowFat-Fruit	1	cup	245	182	250	11	47	0	3	1.7	0.7	0.1
2000	Yogurt-LowFat-Plain	1	cup	245	208	155	13	17	0	4	2.5	1	0.1
2034	Yogurt-Nonfat-LowCal Sweetener	1	cup	241	208	122	11	19	1	<1	0.2	0.1	<0.1
2012	Yogurt-NonFat-Plain	1	cup	245	209	137	14	19	0	<1	0.3	0.1	<0.1
2099	Yogurt-NonFat-Vanilla/Coffee	1	cup	245	187	223	13	43	0	<1	0.3	0.1	<0.1
2013	Yogurt-Whole Milk-Plain	1	cup	245	215	150	9	11	0	8	5.1	2.2	0.2
Desserts													
Cakes													
46004	Angelfood Cake	1	pce	28.35	9	73	2	16	<1	<1	<0.1	<0.1	0.1
46098	Applesauce Cake-No Icing	1	pce	87	20	313	3	52	2	12	2.4	5	3.5
46103	Banana Cake-No Icing	1	pce	87	29	262	3	46	1	8	1.6	3.6	2.1
46010	Carrot Cake-CreamChz Icing	1	pce	111	23	484	5	52	1	29	5.4	7.2	15.1
49001	Cheesecake-Mix-Prepared	1	pce	99	44	271	5	35	2	13	6.6	4.5	0.8
49004	Cheesecake (pce=1/12)	1	pce	80	36	257	4	20	<1	18	7.9	6.9	1.3
49017	Cheesecake-Chocolate	1	pce	128	37	505	8	49	2	32	15.5	11.3	3.6
46115	Choc Sponge Cake-No Icing	1	pce	66	20	197	5	36	1	4	1.4	1.5	0.5
46013	Chocolate Cake+Choc Icing	1	pce	64	15	235	3	35	2	10	3.1	5.6	1.2
46118	Chocolate Cake+Van Icing	1	pce	103		358	4	58	1	14	3.6	6.4	3.2
46093	Coffee Cake-Cinn+Crumb Top	1	pce	63	14	263	4	29	1	15	3.7	8.2	2
46097	Coffee Cake-Fruit	1	pce	50	16	156	3	26	1	5	1.2	2.8	0.7
46106	Date Pudding Cake	1	pce	42	14	131	2	19	1	6	3	1.9	0.3
45562	Funnel Cake-6 inch diam	1	pce	90	38	278	7	29	1	14	2.7	4.4	6.3
46066	German Choc CakeMix-Prep+Ic	1	pce	111	30	404	4	55	2	21	5.3	8.7	5.5
46000	Gingerbread Cake-Homemade	1	pce	74	21	263	3	36	1	12	3	5.3	3.1
42209	Hoecake-1/8th Pone	1	pce	61	31	129	2	24	2	3	0.6	1.2	1.1
46109	Ice Cream Cake Roll (pce=1/10)	1	pce	34	13	101	1	14	<1	5	2.1	1.8	0.8
46111	Lemon Cake+Icing-2 Layer	1	pce	109	24	385	3	71	1	11	1.9	4.8	3.4
46070	Pineapple Upside Down Cake	1	pce	115	37	367	4	58	1	14	3.4	6	3.8
46107	Plum Pudding Cake	1	pce	42	14	131	2	19	1	6	3	1.9	0.3
46016	Pound Cake w/Butter	1	pce	28.35	7	110	2	14	<1	6	3.3	1.7	0.3
46077	Shortcake Biscuit-Recipe	1	ea	65	18	225	4	32	1	9	2.5	3.9	2.4
46011	Snack Cake/Choc+Filling	1	ea	50	10	188	2	30	<1	7	1.4	2.8	2.6
46116	Spice Cake w/Icing	1	pce	109	29	368	5	62	1	12	3.2	5.9	1.9
46078	Sponge Cake-Recipe	1	pce	63	19	187	5	36	<1	3	0.8	1	0.4
46008	Twinkie Snack Cake	1	ea	42.5	9	155	1	27	<1	5	1.1	1.7	1.4
46017	White Cake w/White Icing	1	pce	71	14	266	2	45	1	10	4.3	3.8	1
46007	White Cake w/Choc Icing	1	pce	100		364	3	64	1	12	5.2	3.6	1.8
46012	Yellow Cake w/Choc Icing	1	pce	64	14	242	2	35	1	11	3	6.1	1.4
Cookies, Brownies and Bars													
47073	Almond Cookie	2	ea	20	1	103	2	10	1	6	1	3.4	1.6
47000	Brownie+Nuts+Icing-Commerc	1	ea	61	8	247	3	39	1	10	2.6	5.5	1.4
47019	Brownie-FudgeNut-Recipe	1	ea	24	3	112	1	12	1	7	1.8	2.6	2.3
47005	Butter Cookie-Thin	5	ea	25	1	117	2	17	<1	5	2.8	1.4	0.2

< = Trace amount present   Blank = Not available

CHOL, cholesterol; **V,** vitamin; **THI,** thiamin; **RIB,** riboflavin; **NIA,** niacin; **FOL,** folate;
CALC, calcium; **PHOS,** phosphate; **SOD,** sodium; **POT,** potassium; **MAG,** magnesium

CHOL (mg)	V-A (RE)	THI (mg)	RIB (mg)	NIA (mg)	V-B6 (mg)	FOL (µg)	V-B12 (µg)	V-C (mg)	V-E (mg)	CALC (mg)	PHOS (mg)	SOD (mg)	POT (mg)	MAG (mg)	IRON (mg)	ZINC (mg)
10	27	0.1	0.4	0.2	0.1	23	1.1	2	0.1	372	292	143	476	36	0.2	1.8
15	39	0.1	0.5	0.3	0.1	27	1.4	2	0.1	447	352	172	573	43	0.2	2.2
3	6	0.1	0.4	0.5	0.1	32	1.1	26	0.2	370	291	139	550	41	0.6	1.8
4	5	0.1	0.6	0.3	0.1	30	1.5	2	<0.1	488	383	187	624	47	0.2	2.4
4	4	0.1	0.5	0.3	0.1	27	1.3	2	<0.1	436	343	168	559	42	0.2	2.1
31	74	0.1	0.3	0.2	0.1	18	0.9	1	0.2	296	232	114	379	28	0.1	1.4
0	0	<0.1	0.1	0.2	<0.1	10	<0.1	0	<0.1	40	9	212	26	3	0.1	<0.1
22	10	0.1	0.1	1.1	0.1	6	<0.1	1	1.6	17	45	141	144	11	1.4	0.2
32	83	0.1	0.2	1.2	0.2	11	0.1	3	1.2	26	50	181	168	15	1.1	0.3
60	426	0.2	0.2	1.1	0.1	13	0.1	1	11.3	28	79	273	124	20	1.4	0.5
29	98	0.1	0.3	0.5	0.1	30	0.3	<1	1.1	170	232	376	209	19	0.5	0.5
44	117	<0.1	0.2	0.2	<0.1	14	0.1	<1	2.2	41	74	166	72	9	0.5	0.4
118	296	0.2	0.3	1.3	0.1	14	0.2	<1	2	71	144	239	189	37	2.2	0.9
138	62	0.1	0.2	0.7	0.1	14	0.3	1	0.4	21	89	42	98	20	1.7	0.6
27	16	<0.1	0.1	0.4	<0.1	11	0.1	<1	4.7	28	78	214	128	22	1.4	0.4
35	102	0.1	0.1	0.6	<0.1	7	0.1	0		71	147	404	168	22	2.1	0.4
20	21	0.1	0.1	1.1	<0.1	38	0.1	<1	2.2	34	68	221	77	14	1.2	0.5
4	10	<0.1	0.1	1.3	<0.1	24	<0.1	<1	0.4	22	59	192	45	8	1.2	0.3
15	10	0.1	0.1	0.5	0.1	3	0.1	<1	0.2	46	36	66	199	23	1	0.2
63	58	0.2	0.3	1.9	0.1	14	0.2	<1	2.4	128	137	116	155	18	1.9	0.6
53	23	0.1	0.1	1.1	<0.1	4	0.1	0	1.2	53	173	368	151	19	1.2	0.5
24	10	0.1	0.1	1.3	0.1	24	<0.1	<1	6.9	53	40	242	325	52	2.1	0.3
0	0	0.1	0.1	1	0.1	5	0	0	0.4	70	98	132	87	39	1.2	0.6
15	22	<0.1	0.1	0.3	<0.1	2	0.1	<1	0.3	42	40	45	57	9	0.5	0.2
34	62	0.1	0.1	0.7	<0.1	6	0.1	1	1.6	67	154	359	53	6	0.8	0.2
25	75	0.2	0.2	1.4	<0.1	30	0.1	1	2.1	138	94	367	129	15	1.7	0.4
15	10	0.1	0.1	0.5	0.1	3	0.1	<1	0.2	46	36	66	199	23	1	0.2
63	44	<0.1	0.1	0.4	<0.1	12	0.1	0	0.2	10	39	113	34	3	0.4	0.1
2	12	0.2	0.2	1.7	<0.1	34	<0.1	<1	1.3	133	93	329	69	10	1.7	0.3
8	2	0.1	0.1	1.2	<0.1	14	<0.1	0	1.7	36	46	212	61	20	1.7	0.3
50	39	0.1	0.2	1.1	<0.1	9	0.1	<1	2.2	76	209	281	136	13	1.5	0.4
107	49	0.1	0.2	0.8	<0.1	25	0.2	0	0.3	26	63	144	89	6	1	0.4
7	2	0.1	0.1	0.5	<0.1	12	<0.1	<1	0.9	19	79	155	37	3	0.5	0.1
6	23	0.1	0.1	0.6	<0.1	4	<0.1	<1	1.3	34	46	166	41	4	0.6	0.1
18	58	0.1	0.1	0.4	<0.1	3	0.1	<1	1	78	132	308	72	5	0.7	0.2
35	21	0.1	0.1	0.8	<0.1	14	0.1	0	1.9	24	103	216	114	19	1.3	0.4
9	41	0.1	0.1	0.5	<0.1	4	<0.1	<1	1.6	15	35	47	44	15	0.5	0.2
10	4	0.2	0.1	1	<0.1	13	<0.1	0	1.3	18	62	190	91	19	1.4	0.4
18	48	<0.1	<0.1	0.2	<0.1	7	<0.1	<1	0.7	14	32	82	42	13	0.4	0.2
29	42	0.1	0.1	0.8	<0.1	10	0.1	0	0.1	7	26	88	28	3	0.6	0.1

ERA, EatRight Analysis CD-ROM; **AMT**, amount; **WT**, weight; **WTR**, water; **CAL**, calories; **PROT**, protein; **CARB**, carbohydrate; **FIBR**, fiber; **FAT**, fat; **SATF**, saturated fat; **MONO**, monosaturated fat; **POLY**, polyunsaturated fat

ERA CODE	FOOD DESCRIPTION	AMT	UNIT	WT (g)	WTR (g)	CAL (kcal)	PROT (g)	CARB (g)	FIBR (g)	FAT (g)	SATF (g)	MONO (g)	POLY (g)
Desserts (continued)													
Cookies, Brownies and Bars (continued)													
47075	Butterscotch Brownie	1	ea	34	4	152	2	20	<1	8	1.4	3.3	2.5
47032	Choc Chip Cookie-Commerc	1	ea	10	<1	45	1	7	<1	2	0.4	0.6	0.5
47035	Choc Chip Cookie-Mix-Prep	1	ea	16	1	79	1	10	<1	4	1.3	2.1	0.4
47002	Choc Chip Cookie-Recipe-Marg	1	ea	16	1	78	1	9	<1	5	1.3	1.7	1.3
47041	Chocolate Wafer Cookie	2	ea	12	1	52	1	9	<1	2	0.5	0.6	0.5
47042	Coconut Macaroons-Recipe	1	ea	24	3	97	1	17	<1	3	2.7	0.1	<0.1
47012	Fig Bar Cookie	1	ea	16	3	56	1	11	1	1	0.2	0.5	0.4
47043	Fortune Cookie	1	ea	8	1	30	<1	7	<1	<1	0.1	0.1	<0.1
47376	Fruit Cookie-NoFat (Archway)	1	ea	28		90	2	21	0	0	0	0	0
47045	Gingersnap Cookie	1	ea	7	<1	29	<1	5	<1	1	0.2	0.4	0.1
47009	Lady Finger Cookie	4	ea	44	9	161	5	26	<1	4	1.5	1.8	0.7
47078	Lemon Bar Cookie	1	ea	16	2	69	1	10	<1	3	0.6	1.4	0.8
47046	Marshmallow Cookie-ChocDip	1	ea	13	1	55	1	9	<1	2	0.6	1.2	0.3
47109	Molasses Cookie	1	ea	15	1	64	1	11	<1	2	0.5	1.1	0.3
47171	Nilla Wafer Cookie (Nabisco)	8	ea	32		140	1	24	<1	5	1	1.5	0
47054	Oatmeal Cookie-Homemade	1	ea	15	1	67	1	10	<1	3	0.5	1.1	0.8
47051	Oatmeal Cookie-Mix-Prep	1	ea	16	1	74	1	10	1	3	0.8	1.7	0.4
47496	Oatmeal Raisin Cookie (Archway)	1	ea	26	3	107	1	17	1	4	0.8	1.3	0.3
47010	Peanut Butter Cookie-Homemade	1	ea	20	1	95	2	12	<1	5	0.9	2.2	1.4
47062	Pecan Shortbread Cookie	1	ea	14	<1	76	1	8	<1	5	1.1	2.6	0.6
23171	Rice Krispies Bar	1	ea	28	4	107	1	20	<1	3	0.6	1.3	0.8
47038	Sandw Cookie-Choc-ChocDip	1	ea	17	<1	82	1	11	1	4	1.3	2.5	0.5
47006	Sandwich Cookie-all types	4	ea	40	1	189	2	28	1	8	1.5	3.4	2.9
47180	Sandwich Cookie-Oreo	3	ea	33		160	2	23	1	7	1.5	3	0.5
47059	Sandwich Cookie-Peanut Butter	1	ea	14	<1	67	1	9	<1	3	0.7	1.6	0.5
47071	Sandwich Cookie-Vanilla	1	ea	10	<1	48	<1	7	<1	2	0.3	0.8	0.8
47007	Shortbread Cookie	4	ea	32	1	161	2	21	1	8	2	4.3	1
47153	Snackwell DevFd Cookie-Svg	1	ea	16	3	49	1	12	<1	<1	0.1	<0.1	<0.1
47160	Snackwell VanSanCookie-Svg	2	ea	26	1	109	1	21	1	2	0.5	0.8	0.2
47164	Snackwell ChocSanCookie-Svg	3	ea	33	1	135	2	26	1	3	0.8	1	0.2
47011	Snickerdoodle Cookie	1	ea	20	4	81	1	12	<1	3	2.1	1	0.2
47064	Sugar Cookie	1	ea	15	1	72	1	10	<1	3	0.8	1.8	0.4
47068	Sugar Cookie-Made w/Marg	1	ea	14	1	66	1	8	<1	3	0.7	1.4	1
47069	Sugar Wafers-Creme Filled	1	ea	9	<1	46	<1	6	<1	2	0.3	0.9	0.8
Dessert Toppings													
23069	Butterscotch Topping	2	Tbs	41	13	103	1	27	<1	<1	<0.1	<0.1	0
23070	Caramel Topping	2	Tbs	41	13	103	1	27	<1	<1	<0.1	<0.1	0
23013	Chocolate Syrup-thin	1	cup	300	93	837	6	195	5	3	1.6	0.9	0.1
509	Dessert Topping/DreamWhip	1	cup	80	53	151	3	13	0	10	8.5	0.7	0.2
508	FrznDessertTopping/Cool Whip	1	cup	75	38	239	1	17	0	19	16.3	1.2	0.4
23014	Hot Fudge Chocolate Topping	1	cup	340	74	1190	16	214	10	30	13.5	13.1	0.9
23071	Marshmallow Creme Topping	2	Tbs	38	8	122	<1	30	<1	<1	<0.1	<0.1	<0.1
23162	Nuts in Syrup Topping	2	Tbs	41	8	167	2	22	1	9	0.8	2	5.6
510	Whipped Cream-Pressurized	1	cup	60	37	154	2	7	0	13	8.3	3.8	0.5

< = Trace amount present   Blank = Not available

CHOL, cholesterol; **V**, vitamin; **THI**, thiamin; **RIB**, riboflavin; **NIA**, niacin; **FOL**, folate;
CALC, calcium; **PHOS**, phosphate; **SOD**, sodium; **POT**, potassium; **MAG**, magnesium

CHOL (mg)	V-A (RE)	THI (mg)	RIB (mg)	NIA (mg)	V-B6 (mg)	FOL (μg)	V-B12 (μg)	V-C (mg)	V-E (mg)	CALC (mg)	PHOS (mg)	SOD (mg)	POT (mg)	MAG (mg)	IRON (mg)	ZINC (mg)
21	67	0.1	0.1	0.5	<0.1	5	<0.1	<1	1	24	31	90	72	10	0.8	0.2
0	<1	<0.1	<0.1	0.3	<0.1	7	0	0	0.2	2	8	38	12	3	0.3	0.1
7	3	<0.1	<0.1	0.3	<0.1	1	<0.1	0	0.4	8	15	47	34	6	0.3	0.1
5	26	<0.1	<0.1	0.2	<0.1	5	<0.1	<1	0.5	6	16	58	36	9	0.4	0.1
<1	<1	<0.1	<0.1	0.3	<0.1	6	<0.1	0	0.2	4	16	70	25	6	0.5	0.1
0	0	<0.1	<0.1	<0.1	<0.1	1	<0.1	0	0.1	2	10	59	37	5	0.2	0.2
0	1	<0.1	<0.1	0.3	<0.1	4	<0.1	<1	0.2	10	10	56	33	4	0.5	0.1
<1	<1	<0.1	<0.1	0.1	<0.1	4	0	0	<0.1	1	3	22	3	1	0.1	<0.1
0	0								0	<0.1	0		95		0.4	
0	<1	<0.1	<0.1	0.2	<0.1	5	0	0	0.1	5	6	46	24	3	0.4	<0.1
161	73	0.1	0.2	0.9	0.1	34	0.3	2	0.6	21	76	65	50	5	1.6	0.5
12	32	<0.1	<0.1	0.2	<0.1	2	<0.1	1	0.4	7	12	42	11	1	0.2	0.1
0	<1	<0.1	<0.1	0.1	<0.1	2	<0.1	<1	0.3	6	13	22	24	5	0.3	0.1
0	0	0.1	<0.1	0.5	<0.1	11	0	0	0.3	11	14	69	52	8	1	0.1
2										20		100	30		1.1	
5	27	<0.1	<0.1	0.2	<0.1	5	<0.1	<1	0.4	16	25	90	27	6	0.4	0.1
7	3	<0.1	<0.1	0.2	<0.1	2	<0.1	<1	0.4	5	28	75	30	8	0.4	0.1
3	1	0.1	<0.1	0.4				0		8		98	60		0.6	
6	31	<0.1	<0.1	0.7	<0.1	11	<0.1	<1	2.5	8	23	104	46	8	0.4	0.2
5	<1	<0.1	<0.1	0.3	<0.1	9	<0.1	0	0.5	4	12	39	10	3	0.3	0.1
0	85	0.1	0.1	1.3	0.1	28	<0.1	4	0.4	2	12	123	12	4	0.5	0.1
0	<1	<0.1	<0.1	0.2	<0.1	3	<0.1	0	0.6	6	15	55	41	7	0.5	0.1
0	<1	<0.1	0.1	0.8	<0.1	17	<0.1	0	1.7	10	39	242	70	18	1.6	0.3
0												220	60		0.7	
0	<1	<0.1	<0.1	0.5	<0.1	6	<0.1	<1	0.5	7	26	52	27	7	0.4	0.1
0	0	<0.1	<0.1	0.3	<0.1	6	0	0	0.4	3	8	35	9	1	0.2	<0.1
6	4	0.1	0.1	1.1	<0.1	19	<0.1	0	1	11	35	146	32	5	0.9	0.2
0	<1	<0.1	<0.1	0.2	<0.1	3	<0.1	<1	0	5	11	28	18	4	0.4	0.1
<1	<1	<0.1	0.1	0.7	<0.1		<0.1	0		17	36	95	28	5	0.6	0.2
<1	<1	<0.1	0.1	0.7	<0.1		<0.1	0		18	67	253	53	16	0.9	0.2
9	32	0.1	<0.1	0.4	<0.1	2	<0.1	<1	0.2	8	10	74	24	2	0.5	0.1
8	4	<0.1	<0.1	0.4	<0.1	7	<0.1	<1	0.4	3	12	54	9	2	0.3	0.1
4	35	<0.1	<0.1	0.3	<0.1	7	<0.1	<1	0.5	10	13	69	11	2	0.3	0.1
0	0	<0.1	<0.1	0.2	<0.1	4	0	0	0.4	2	5	13	5	1	0.2	<0.1
<1	11	<0.1	<0.1	<0.1	<0.1	1	<0.1	<1	0	22	19	143	34	3	0.1	0.1
<1	11	<0.1	<0.1	<0.1	<0.1	1	<0.1	<1	0	22	19	143	34	3	0.1	0.1
0	9	<0.1	0.2	1	<0.1	12	0	1	3	42	387	216	672	195	6.3	2.2
8	39	<0.1	0.1	<0.1	<0.1	3	0.2	1	0.1	72	69	53	120	8	<0.1	0.2
0	64	0	0	0	0	0	0	0	0.1	5	6	19	14	1	0.1	<0.1
7	14	0.2	0.8	1	0.2	14	0.7	1	9.9	275	459	1176	1230	173	4.4	2.3
0	<1	0	0	<0.1	0	<1	0	0	0	1	3	19	2	1	0.1	<0.1
0	2	0.1	<0.1	0.2	0.1	9	0	<1	0.4	16	46	17	86	26	0.4	0.4
46	124	<0.1	<0.1	<0.1	<0.1	2	0.2	0	0.4	61	54	78	88	6	<0.1	0.2

ERA, EatRight Analysis CD-ROM; **AMT**, amount; **WT**, weight; **WTR**, water; **CAL**, calories; **PROT**, protein; **CARB**, carbohydrate; **FIBR**, fiber; **FAT**, fat; **SATF**, saturated fat; **MONO**, monosaturated fat; **POLY**, polyunsaturated fat

ERA CODE	FOOD DESCRIPTION	AMT	UNIT	WT (g)	WTR (g)	CAL (kcal)	PROT (g)	CARB (g)	FIBR (g)	FAT (g)	SATF (g)	MONO (g)	POLY (g)
Desserts (continued)													
Doughnuts													
45505	Cake Doughnut	1	ea	47	10	198	2	23	1	11	1.7	4.4	3.7
45524	Cake Doughnut-Choc Icing	1	ea	43	6	204	2	21	1	13	3.5	7.5	1.6
45508	Chocolate Eclair+Custard	1	ea	100		262	6	24	1	16	4.1	6.5	3.9
45509	Cream Puff+Custard	1	ea	130	70	335	9	30	1	20	4.8	8.5	5.4
45563	Cream Filled Yeast Doughnut	1	ea	85	32	307	5	26	1	21	4.6	10.3	2.6
45527	French Cruller Doughnut	1	ea	41	7	169	1	24	<1	8	1.9	4.3	0.9
45507	Jelly Filled Doughnut	1	ea	85	30	289	5	33	1	16	4.1	8.7	2
45559	Mexican Crueller	1	ea	26	6	116	1	12	<1	7	2	4.1	0.9
45560	Oriental Doughnut/Okinawan	1	ea	18	3	76	1	10	<1	4	0.9	2	0.4
45506	Yeast Doughnut-Plain	1	ea	60	15	242	4	27	1	14	3.5	7.7	1.7
Frozen Desserts													
2070	Banana Split w/WhipCream	1	ea	425	217	1088	15	124	1	65	37.5	18.7	5.3
23174	Frozen Fruit Juice Bar	1	ea	77	60	63	1	16	0	<1	<0.1	0	<0.1
2043	Frozen Yogurt Bar-Choc Coat	1	ea	41	21	109	1	12	<1	7	5.3	0.8	0.2
2035	Frozen Yogurt-Choc-Soft	0.5	cup	72	46	115	3	18	2	4	2.6	1.3	0.2
2071	Frozen Yogurt-LowFat-Choc	1	cup	193	134	219	10	42	3	4	2.4	1.1	0.1
2075	Frozen Yogurt-LowFat-Van/Fruit	1	cup	193	143	203	9	37	0	3	1.7	0.7	0.1
2039	Frozen Yogurt-NonFat-Choc	1	cup	193	135	207	11	43	3	2	1	0.5	0.1
2079	Frozen Yogurt-NonFat-Van/Fruit	1	cup	193	143	191	10	38	0	<1	0.2	0.1	<0.1
2064	Frozen Yogurt-Vanilla	0.5	cup	72	47	114	3	17	0	4	2.5	1.1	0.2
23094	Frozen Juice Bar w/Cream	1	ea	65	43	86	1	19	<1	1	0.8	0.4	0.1
2032	Hot Fudge Sundae	1	ea	158	94	284	6	48	0	9	5	2.3	0.8
2055	Ice Cream Bar-Choc-Dove	1	ea	101	38	339	3	36	2	23	13.8	7.2	0.7
2028	Ice Cream Bar-Creamsicle	1	ea	66	44	91	2	18	<1	2	1.2	0.6	0.1
2029	Ice Cream Bar-Drumstick	1	ea	60	29	159	3	18	1	9	4.4	3.1	1
2030	Ice Cream Bar-Fudgesicle	1	ea	73	48	104	3	18	1	3	2.1	1	0.1
2084	Ice Cream Bar-Health	1	ea	68	33	206	2	17	<1	15	11.6	2.3	0.4
2089	Ice Cream Sandwich-Chipwich	1	ea	59	28	144	3	22	1	6	3.2	1.7	0.4
2087	Ice Cream Sandwich	1	ea	59	28	144	3	22	1	6	3.2	1.7	0.4
2050	Ice Cream-Hard-Choc	0.5	cup	66	37	142	3	19	1	7	4.5	2.1	0.3
2008	Ice Cream-Soft-French Vanilla	0.5	cup	86	51	185	4	19	0	11	6.4	3	0.4
2063	Ice Cream-Strawberry	0.5	cup	66	40	127	2	18	<1	6	3.4	1.6	0.2
2004	Ice Cream-Vanilla	0.5	cup	66	40	133	2	16	0	7	4.5	2.1	0.3
2006	Ice Cream-Vanilla-Rich	0.5	cup	74	42	178	3	17	0	12	7.4	3.4	0.4
2057	Ice Milk-Chocolate	1	cup	131	86	189	6	34	1	4	2.6	1.2	0.2
2009	Ice Milk-Hard-Vanilla	0.5	cup	66	45	92	3	15	0	3	1.7	0.8	0.1
23051	Ice Slushy	1	cup	193	129	247	1	63	0	0	0	0	0
2216	Ice Cream-ChChipCookDo-Rich	0.5	cup	106		270	4	30	0	17	9		
2105	Ice Cream-Cookies&Crm-LowFat	0.5	cup	71		120	3	21	1	2	1	1	0
49013	Ice Cream Cone-Cake/Wafer	1	ea	4	<1	17	<1	3	<1	<1	<0.1	0.1	0.1
49014	Ice Cream Cone-Sugar/Rolled	1	ea	10	<1	40	1	8	<1	<1	0.1	0.1	0.1
2020	Milkshake-Chocolate	1	cup	166	119	211	6	34	1	6	3.8	1.8	0.2
2011	Orange Sherbet	0.5	cup	99	65	137	1	30	0	2	1.1	0.5	0.1
70308	OrangeSorbet+VanIceCrm-Rich	0.5	cup	106		190	2	24	0	9	5		

< = Trace amount present   Blank = Not available

CHOL, cholesterol; **V**, vitamin; **THI**, thiamin; **RIB**, riboflavin; **NIA**, niacin; **FOL**, folate;
CALC, calcium; **PHOS**, phosphate; **SOD**, sodium; **POT**, potassium; **MAG**, magnesium

CHOL (mg)	V-A (RE)	THI (mg)	RIB (mg)	NIA (mg)	V-B6 (mg)	FOL (µg)	V-B12 (µg)	V-C (mg)	V-E (mg)	CALC (mg)	PHOS (mg)	SOD (mg)	POT (mg)	MAG (mg)	IRON (mg)	ZINC (mg)
17	8	0.1	0.1	0.9	<0.1	22	0.1	<1	1.9	21	126	257	60	9	0.9	0.3
26	5	0.1	<0.1	0.6	<0.1	12	0.1	<1	1.9	15	87	184	84	17	1.1	0.3
127	191	0.1	0.3	0.8	0.1	28	0.3	<1	2.1	63	107	337	117	15	1.2	0.6
174	259	0.2	0.4	1.1	0.1	36	0.5	<1	2.9	86	142	443	150	16	1.5	0.8
20	16	0.3	0.1	1.9	0.1	54	0.1	0	2.3	21	65	263	68	17	1.6	0.7
5	1	0.1	0.1	0.9	<0.1	14	<0.1	0	1	11	50	141	32	5	1	0.1
22	14	0.3	0.1	1.8	0.1	53	0.2	0	2.1	21	72	249	67	17	1.5	0.6
2	6	<0.1	<0.1	0.4	<0.1	1	<0.1	0	1	2	8	7	8	2	0.3	0.1
13	7	<0.1	0.1	0.4	<0.1	2	<0.1	<1	0.5	24	22	38	15	2	0.4	0.1
4	2	0.2	0.1	1.7	<0.1	26	0.1	<1	2.4	26	56	205	65	13	1.2	0.5
204	531	0.1	0.9	0.5	0.2	19	1.4	2	0.5	466	484	360	783	92	1.6	2.7
0	2	<0.1	<0.1	0.1	<0.1	5	0	7	0	4	5	3	41	3	0.1	<0.1
1	18	<0.1	0.1	0.1	<0.1	2	0.1	<1	<0.1	46	43	28	74	6	0.1	0.2
4	31	<0.1	0.2	0.2	0.1	8	0.2	<1	0.1	106	100	71	188	19	0.9	0.4
10	25	0.1	0.4	0.4	0.1	21	0.9	1	0.1	300	300	113	621	75	1.7	2.1
10	27	0.1	0.4	0.2	0.1	19	0.9	1	0.1	307	241	118	393	29	0.1	1.5
3	3	0.1	0.4	0.4	0.1	22	1	1	<0.1	326	321	123	655	78	1.7	2.2
3	3	0.1	0.4	0.2	0.1	20	1	1	<0.1	334	263	129	428	32	0.2	1.6
1	41	<0.1	0.2	0.2	0.1	4	0.2	1	<0.1	103	93	63	152	10	0.2	0.3
5	8	<0.1	0.1	0.1	<0.1	3	0.1	8	<0.1	29	5	20	64	2	0.1	<0.1
21	57	0.1	0.3	1.1	0.1	9	0.6	2	0.7	207	228	182	395	33	0.6	0.9
38	95	<0.1	0.2	0.3	<0.1	2	0.2	<1	0.7	74	139	56	260	63	1.1	1.1
6	20	<0.1	0.1	0.1	<0.1	3	0.3	2	<0.1	62	48	43	99	7	0.1	0.3
21	55	<0.1	0.1	0.9	<0.1	8	0.2	<1	0.4	66	82	44	145	21	0.4	0.7
10	33	<0.1	0.2	0.1	<0.1	5	0.5	1	<0.1	101	98	60	221	24	0.5	0.5
24	63	<0.1	0.1	0.1	<0.1	3	0.2	<1	<0.1	70	62	43	126	11	0.2	0.4
20	53	<0.1	0.1	0.2	<0.1	5	0.2	<1	0.1	60	64	36	122	13	0.3	0.4
20	53	<0.1	0.1	0.2	<0.1	5	0.2	<1	0.1	60	64	36	122	13	0.3	0.4
22	79	<0.1	0.1	0.1	<0.1	11	0.2	<1	1.1	72	71	50	164	19	0.6	0.4
78	132	<0.1	0.2	0.1	<0.1	8	0.4	1	0.3	113	100	52	152	10	0.2	0.4
19	51	<0.1	0.2	0.1	<0.1	8	0.2	5	0.2	79	66	40	124	9	0.1	0.2
29	77	<0.1	0.2	0.1	<0.1	3	0.3	<1	0	84	69	53	131	9	0.1	0.5
45	136	<0.1	0.1	0.1	<0.1	4	0.3	1	0	87	70	41	118	8	<0.1	0.3
12	35	0.1	0.2	0.2	0.1	8	0.6	1	0.1	189	156	82	310	26	0.3	0.8
9	31	<0.1	0.2	0.1	<0.1	4	0.4	1	0	92	72	56	139	10	0.1	0.3
0	0	<0.1	0	<0.1	<0.1	0	0	2	0	4	2	42	6	2	0.3	<0.1
80	150								1	100		95			1.1	
5	40	<0.1	0.2						0	100	141	90	254			
0	0	<0.1	<0.1	0.2	<0.1	4	0	0	0.1	1	4	6	4	1	0.1	<0.1
0	0	0.1	<0.1	0.5	<0.1	8	0	0	0.1	4	10	32	14	3	0.4	0.1
22	38	0.1	0.4	0.3	0.1	6	0.6	1	0.4	188	169	161	332	28	0.5	0.7
6	14	<0.1	0.1	0.1	<0.1	5	0.2	3	0.1	53	40	46	95	8	0.1	0.5
60	60	<0.1	0.1	0.9				9		80	64	45	114		0	

ERA, EatRight Analysis CD-ROM; **AMT**, amount; **WT**, weight; **WTR**, water; **CAL**, calories; **PROT**, protein; **CARB**, carbohydrate; **FIBR**, fiber; **FAT**, fat; **SATF**, saturated fat; **MONO**, monosaturated fat; **POLY**, polyunsaturated fat

ERA CODE	FOOD DESCRIPTION	AMT	UNIT	WT (g)	WTR (g)	CAL (kcal)	PROT (g)	CARB (g)	FIBR (g)	FAT (g)	SATF (g)	MONO (g)	POLY (g)
Desserts (continued)													
Frozen Desserts (continued)													
23050	Popsicle/Ice Pops-Double	1	ea	128	102	92	0	24	0	0	0	0	0
2026	Pudding Pop-Chocolate	1	ea	47	30	72	2	12	<1	2	2.1	0	0
2027	Pudding Pop-Vanilla	1	ea	47	30	75	2	13	0	2	2.1	0	0
2066	Sorbet-Citrus	1	cup	200	152	184	1	46	<1	0	0	0	0
2065	Sorbet-Fruit	1	cup	200	157	164	2	40	0	<1	0	0	0.1
Fruit Desserts													
49031	Apple Crisp	0.5	cup	141	87	230	3	46	2	5	1	2.2	1.6
49006	Apple Dumpling	1	ea	151	78	357	2	53	2	16	3.6	8.2	3.4
49015	Apple Strudel	1	pce	71	31	194	2	29	2	8	1.5	2.3	3.8
49002	Cherry Cobbler-3x3in pce	1	pce	129	85	198	2	34	1	6	1.2	2.8	1.9
49018	Fruit Filled Blintz	1	ea	70	44	124	4	17	<1	4	1.3	1.8	0.9
49008	Peach Cobbler-3x3in piece	1	pce	130	84	204	2	36	2	6	1.2	2.8	1.9
Gelatin Desserts													
23052	Gelatin/Jello-Prepared	0.5	cup	135	114	80	2	19	0	0	0	0	0
23156	Gelatin/Jello Dessert w/Fruit	0.5	cup	106	86	73	1	18	1	<1	0.1	<0.1	0.1
23093	Gelatin/Jello-SugFree-Prepared	0.5	cup	117	115	8	1	1	0	0	0	0	0
Pastries and Sweet Rolls													
45515	Apple Fritter	1	ea	24	9	87	1	8	<1	6	1.2	2.4	1.6
45550	Apple Turnover	1	ea	82	27	290	3	37	1	15	3	6.5	4.6
45516	Baklava-2x2x2.5 in piece	1	pce	78	19	336	5	29	2	23	9.3	8.1	4.2
45523	Cheese Croissant	1	ea	57	12	236	5	27	1	12	6.1	3.7	1.4
45552	Cherry Turnover	1	ea	78	32	240	3	31	1	12	2.4	5.2	3.7
45557	Chinese Pastry	1	oz	28	13	67	1	13	<1	2	0.2	0.5	0.8
42166	Cinnamon Roll-Bkd-Frosted	1	ea	30	7	109	2	17	1	4	1	2.2	0.5
45555	Guava Turnover	1	ea	78	34	234	2	28	3	13	2.5	5.5	3.9
42188	Jelly Filled Sweet Roll	1	ea	55	13	202	3	29	1	8	2.2	4.7	1.1
48057	Lemon Meringue Tart	1	ea	117	58	301	4	41	1	14	2.9	5.9	3.9
42094	Pan Dulce w/Topping	1	ea	79	17	291	5	48	1	9	1.8	4	2.5
45540	Popover-Mix-Prepared	1	ea	33	18	67	3	10	<1	1	0.4	0.6	0.2
45504	Poptart-Fruit Filled	1	ea	52	6	204	2	37	1	5	0.8	2.2	2
45604	Poptart-Fruit Filled-Frosted	1	ea	52	6	205	2	37	1	6	1	3.2	1.3
Pies													
48151	Apple Pie	1	pce	126		350	2	41	2	21	4	6	0.5
70557	Boston Cream Pie	1	pce	106		240	3	48	1	4	1.5	1.7	0.8
48153	Cherry Pie	1	pce	120		340	3	45	1	22	4	7	0.5
48154	Chocolate Crème Pie	1	pce	124		280	4	36	1	14	4	4	0
48155	Lemon Meringue Pie	1	pce	119		250	2	41	<1	9	2	3	0
48058	Pecan Pie-Single-Bama Pie	1	ea	85	14	363	4	46	2	20	2.8	10.4	5.3
48156	Pumpkin Pie	1	pce	121		260	3	34	1	13	3	4	0
Puddings and Custards													
2617	Bread Pudding+Raisins	0.5	cup	126	79	212	7	31	1	7	2.9	2.7	1.2

< = Trace amount present   Blank = Not available

CHOL, cholesterol; **V,** vitamin; **THI,** thiamin; **RIB,** riboflavin; **NIA,** niacin; **FOL,** folate;
CALC, calcium; **PHOS,** phosphate; **SOD,** sodium; **POT,** potassium; **MAG,** magnesium

CHOL (mg)	V-A (RE)	THI (mg)	RIB (mg)	NIA (mg)	V-B6 (mg)	FOL (μg)	V-B12 (μg)	V-C (mg)	V-E (mg)	CALC (mg)	PHOS (mg)	SOD (mg)	POT (mg)	MAG (mg)	IRON (mg)	ZINC (mg)
0	0	0	0	0	0	0	0	0	0	0	0	15	5	1	0	<0.1
1	16	<0.1	0.1	0.1	<0.1	1	0.3	<1	<0.1	66	53	78	105	10	0.2	0.2
1	24	<0.1	0.1	<0.1	<0.1	2	0.2	<1	<0.1	61	47	50	65	5	<0.1	0.2
0	54	<0.1	0.1	0.3	<0.1	44	0	51	0.1	18	26	16	200	16	0.9	<0.1
0	6	<0.1	<0.1	0.3	0.1	12	0	19	0	10	12	8	106	8	0.4	0.1
0	44	0.1	0.1	1.1	0.1	7	0	3		39	35	257	137	10	1.1	0.2
0	93	0.1	0.1	0.8	0.1	6	<0.1	5	5.9	50	38	302	212	17	1.3	0.2
4	6	<0.1	<0.1	0.2	<0.1	10	0.2	1	2.2	11	23	191	106	6	0.3	0.1
1	135	0.1	0.1	0.8	0.1	9	<0.1	2	1.3	28	34	294	133	9	1.8	0.2
53	73	0.1	0.1	0.4	<0.1	8	0.2	1	0.5	35	59	93	78	7	0.8	0.3
1	105	0.1	0.1	1.2	<0.1	6	<0.1	3	1.5	24	40	291	159	10	0.9	0.2
0	0	0	<0.1	<0.1	<0.1	0	0	0	0	3	30	57	1	1	<0.1	<0.1
0	3	<0.1	<0.1	0.2	0.1	4	0	4	0.1	5	22	30	110	7	0.1	0.1
0	0	0	<0.1	<0.1	<0.1	0	0	0	0	2	32	56	0	1	<0.1	<0.1
20	13	<0.1	0.1	0.3	<0.1	3	0.1	<1	0.7	13	22	10	34	3	0.3	0.1
0	3	0.2	0.1	1.5	<0.1	5	0	1	1.9	6	33	4	56	7	1.3	0.2
36	124	0.2	0.2	1.4	<0.1	11	<0.1	1	2	33	93	292	144	35	1.7	0.5
32	112	0.3	0.2	1.2	<0.1	42	0.2	<1	0.6	30	74	316	75	14	1.2	0.5
0	26	0.1	0.1	1.2	<0.1	6	0	1	1.6	8	28	8	59	7	1.6	0.2
0	<1	<0.1	<0.1	0.3	<0.1	1	0	0	0.3	6	15	3	25	7	0.2	0.1
0	<1	0.1	0.1	1.1	<0.1	16	<0.1	<1	0.5	10	104	250	19	4	0.8	0.1
<1	32	0.1	0.1	1.5	0.1	6	<0.1	48	2	13	33	13	120	9	1.1	0.2
34	33	0.2	0.1	1.2	0.1	12	0.1	1	1.5	39	43	196	86	10	0.9	0.3
69	31	0.1	0.2	1.1	<0.1	10	0.1	3	1.7	13	52	23	50	7	1.2	0.3
26	67	0.2	0.2	2	<0.1	19	0.1	<1	1.2	13	56	75	57	9	1.8	0.3
37	16	0.1	0.1	0.4	<0.1	6	0.1	<1	0.4	9	30	143	25	5	0.6	0.2
0	150	0.2	0.2	2	0.2	34	<0.1	<1	10.1	14	58	218	58	9	1.8	0.3
0	100	0.2	0.2	2	0.2	52	0	0	0	11	46	211	44	8	1.8	0.6
0								1				220	75		1.1	
4	7	<0.1	0.1	0.3	0.1			1		43		240	105		0.5	
0								1				220	90		1.4	
45	20									80		300	130		1.1	
35												180	25		0.7	
38	19	0.2	0.2	1.2	<0.1	11	0.1	<1	1.7	14	80	54	90	25	1.4	1
55	200							2		60		210	180		1.4	
83	82	0.1	0.3	0.8	0.1	16	0.3	1	5.1	144	137	291	282	24	1.4	0.7

ERA, EatRight Analysis CD-ROM; **AMT,** amount; **WT,** weight; **WTR,** water; **CAL,** calories; **PROT,** protein; **CARB,** carbohydrate; **FIBR,** fiber; **FAT,** fat; **SATF,** saturated fat; **MONO,** monosaturated fat; **POLY,** polyunsaturated fat

ERA CODE	FOOD DESCRIPTION	AMT	UNIT	WT (g)	WTR (g)	CAL (kcal)	PROT (g)	CARB (g)	FIBR (g)	FAT (g)	SATF (g)	MONO (g)	POLY (g)
Desserts (continued)													
Puddings and Custards (continued)													
2613	Egg Custard-Mix+Whl Milk	0.5	cup	133	97	162	5	23	0	5	3	1.7	0.3
2625	Flan CarmCustardMix+WhMlk	0.5	cup	133	99	150	4	25	<1	4	2.5	1.2	0.2
2628	Pudding-Instant+2%Milk	0.5	cup	147	110	153	4	29	0	2	1.5	0.7	0.2
2605	Pudding-Instant+Whole Milk	0.5	cup	147	108	163	5	28	1	5	2.7	1.4	0.3
2614	Pudding-LowCal (D-Zerta)	0.5	cup	130	110	81	4	12	0	2	1	0.5	0.1
2636	Pudding-RegMix+2% Milk	0.5	cup	142	105	150	5	28	<1	3	1.8	0.8	0.1
2604	Pudding-RegMix+Whole Milk	0.5	cup	142	106	158	5	26	1	5	3	1.4	0.2
48044	Pumpkin Pie Mix-Canned	1	cup	270	193	281	3	71	22	<1	0.2	<0.1	<0.1
2653	Tapioca Pudding+2% Milk	0.5	cup	141	105	147	4	28	0	2	1.5	0.7	0.1
Eggs, Substitutes, and Egg Dishes													
19539	Deviled Egg-1/2+Filling	1	ea	31	22	63	4	<1	0	5	1.2	1.7	1.5
19581	Egg Beaters-Egg Substitute	0.25	cup	61		30	6	1	0	0	0	0	0
19522	Egg White-Cooked	1	ea	33.4	29	17	4	<1	0	0	0	0	0
19507	Egg White-Raw-Fresh	1	cup	243	213	122	26	3	0	0	0	0	0
19506	Egg White-Raw-Fresh-Large	1	ea	33.4	29	17	4	<1	0	0	0	0	0
19523	Egg Yolk-Cooked	1	ea	16.6	8	59	3	<1	0	5	1.6	1.9	0.7
19508	Egg Yolk-Raw-Fresh-Large	1	ea	16.6	8	59	3	<1	0	5	1.6	1.9	0.7
19511	Egg-Hard Boiled-Chopped	1	cup	136	101	211	17	2	0	14	4.4	5.5	1.9
19510	Egg-Hard Cooked/Boiled	1	ea	50	37	78	6	1	0	5	1.6	2	0.7
19509	Egg-Large-Fried in Marg	1	ea	46	32	92	6	1	0	7	1.9	2.7	1.3
19517	Egg-Poached-Large	1	ea	50	38	74	6	1	0	5	1.5	1.9	0.7
19516	Egg-Scrambled+Milk+Marg	1	ea	61	45	101	7	1	0	7	2.2	2.9	1.3
19500	Egg-Whole-Raw-Fresh-Large	1	cup	243	183	362	30	3	0	24	7.5	9.3	3.3
19535	Omelet-1Egg+Cheese & Ham	1	ea	78	52	156	11	2	0	11	4.5	4.4	1.4
19543	Omelet-1Egg+Mushroom	1	ea	69	54	88	6	2	<1	6	1.8	2.4	1
19537	Omelet-3Egg+On+Pep+Tom Ms	1	ea	145	116	178	8	6	1	14	3.4	5.9	3
19534	Omelet-Plain (1 Lrg Egg)	1	ea	61	46	93	6	1	0	7	1.9	2.8	1.3
Fast Foods/Restaurants													
Arby's													
6432	Arby's Curly Fries	3.5	oz	99		337	4	43		18	7.4	7.6	1.5
69045	Arby's Q Sandwich	1	ea	190		389	18	48		15	5.4	6.3	3.5
53256	Arby's Sauce	0.5	oz	14		15	<1	3		<1	0	0.1	0.1
69056	Beef'nCheddar Sandwich	1	ea	194		508	25	43		26	7.7	12	6.8
57015	Cheddar Fries-Serving	5	oz	142		399	6	46		22	9	10	1.7
69046	Grill Chicken Deluxe Sandwich	1	ea	230		430	24	42		20	3.5	5.1	4.4
69048	Italian Sub Sandwich	1	ea	297		671	34	47		39	12.8	15.7	8.5
69051	Roast Beef Sandwich-Lt-Deluxe	1	ea	182		294	18	33		10	3.4	4.6	2
69052	Roast Chick Sandwich-Lt-Deluxe	1	ea	195		276	24	33		7	1.7	2.9	2.5
69055	Phily Beef'nSwiss Sandwich	1	ea	197		467	24	38		25	9.6	10.6	5.1
56336	Roast Beef Sandwich-Reg	1	ea	155		383	22	35	1	18	6.9	7.9	3.4
56337	Roast Beef Sandwich-Jr	1	ea	89		233	12	23	<1	11	3.8	4.8	2.3
69049	Roast Beef Sub Sandwich	1	ea	305		623	38	47		32	11.5	13	6.8
69042	Roast Chicken Club Sandwich	1	ea	238		503	30	37		27	6.9	9.8	10.4

< = Trace amount present   Blank = Not available

CHOL, cholesterol; **V**, vitamin; **THI**, thiamin; **RIB**, riboflavin; **NIA**, niacin; **FOL**, folate;
CALC, calcium; **PHOS**, phosphate; **SOD**, sodium; **POT**, potassium; **MAG**, magnesium

CHOL (mg)	V-A (RE)	THI (mg)	RIB (mg)	NIA (mg)	V-B6 (mg)	FOL (μg)	V-B12 (μg)	V-C (mg)	V-E (mg)	CALC (mg)	PHOS (mg)	SOD (mg)	POT (mg)	MAG (mg)	IRON (mg)	ZINC (mg)
81	44	0.1	0.3	0.2	0.1	11	0.6	1	0.1	194	174	198	283	25	0.3	0.7
16	35	<0.1	0.2	0.1	<0.1	5	0.3	1	0.1	150	114	65	192	16	0.1	0.5
9	66	<0.1	0.2	0.1	0.1	6	0.4	1	0.1	150	318	435	192	18	0.1	0.5
16	31	<0.1	0.2	0.1	0.1	6	0.4	1	0.1	150	351	417	244	26	0.4	0.6
7	71	<0.1	0.2	0.1	<0.1	5	0.4	1	0.1	152	212	302	195	17	0.1	0.5
10	68	<0.1	0.2	0.2	0.1	6	0.4	1	0.1	160	138	149	240	30	0.5	0.7
17	37	<0.1	0.2	0.1	0.1	6	0.4	1	0.1	158	132	146	231	21	0.5	0.6
0	2241	<0.1	0.3	1	0.4	94	0	9	2.2	100	122	562	373	43	2.9	0.7
8	69	<0.1	0.2	0.1	0.1	6	0.4	1	0.1	149	117	172	189	17	0.1	0.5
122	50	<0.1	0.1	<0.1	<0.1	13	0.3	0	0.6	15	50	50	37	3	0.3	0.3
0	60		0.9		0.1	32	0.6	0	0.8	20		125	85		1.1	0.6
0	0	<0.1	0.1	<0.1	<0.1	1	0.1	0	0	2	4	55	48	4	<0.1	<0.1
0	0	<0.1	1.1	0.2	<0.1	7	0.5	0	0	15	32	398	347	27	0.1	<0.1
0	0	<0.1	0.2	<0.1	<0.1	1	0.1	0	0	2	4	55	48	4	<0.1	<0.1
213	97	<0.1	0.1	<0.1	0.1	18	0.4	0	0.5	23	81	7	16	1	0.6	0.5
213	97	<0.1	0.1	<0.1	0.1	24	0.5	0	0.5	23	81	7	16	1	0.6	0.5
577	228	0.1	0.7	0.1	0.2	60	1.5	0	1.4	68	234	169	171	14	1.6	1.4
212	84	<0.1	0.3	<0.1	0.1	22	0.6	0	0.5	25	86	62	63	5	0.6	0.5
211	114	<0.1	0.2	<0.1	0.1	17	0.4	0	0.8	25	89	162	61	5	0.7	0.5
212	95	<0.1	0.2	<0.1	0.1	18	0.4	0	0.5	24	88	140	60	5	0.7	0.6
215	119	<0.1	0.3	<0.1	0.1	18	0.5	<1	0.8	43	104	171	84	7	0.7	0.6
1032	464	0.2	1.2	0.2	0.3	114	2.4	0	2.6	119	432	306	294	24	3.5	2.7
198	133	0.1	0.3	0.6	0.1	17	0.6	<1	0.8	113	179	372	145	12	0.8	1.2
177	102	<0.1	0.2	0.3	0.1	17	0.4	<1	0.7	42	100	147	97	9	0.7	0.6
220	211	0.1	0.4	0.8	0.2	30	0.5	19	2	60	142	170	269	16	1.2	0.8
214	114	<0.1	0.2	<0.1	0.1	18	0.4	0	0.8	26	90	165	62	5	0.7	0.6
0	0	0.1	0.1	2			0			20		167	724		1.4	0.6
29		0.3	0.4	9.2						70		1268	456		9.2	0.6
0												113	28		0.4	
52		0.4	0.6	9.8				1		150		1166	321		6.1	3
9		0.1	0.1	2			0			80		443	742		1.4	0.9
44	80	0.3	0.3	13.6				8		70		901	659		2.5	
69	100	0.9	0.5	8.2				11		410		2062	565		4.3	
42	40	0.3	0.5	8.4				8		130		826	392		4.5	
33	40	0.4	0.7	9.4				7		130		326	392		2.9	
53		0.3	0.5	8.8				19		290		1144	409		4.1	3.8
43	0	0.3	0.5	11	0.2	14		1		60	120	936	422	16	4.9	3.8
22		0.2	0.3	6.6	0.1	7				40	60	519	201	8	2.7	1.5
73	100	0.6	0.7	10.1				9		410		1847	708		7.7	
46		0.5	0.7	10.6				8		180		1143	534		2.9	2.2

ERA, EatRight Analysis CD-ROM; **AMT,** amount; **WT,** weight; **WTR,** water; **CAL,** calories; **PROT,** protein; **CARB,** carbohydrate; **FIBR,** fiber; **FAT,** fat; **SATF,** saturated fat; **MONO,** monosaturated fat; **POLY,** polyunsaturated fat

ERA CODE	FOOD DESCRIPTION	AMT	UNIT	WT (g)	WTR (g)	CAL (kcal)	PROT (g)	CARB (g)	FIBR (g)	FAT (g)	SATF (g)	MONO (g)	POLY (g)
Fast Foods/Restaurants (continued)													
Arby's (continued)													
69050	Tuna Sub Sandwich	1	ea	284		663	74	50		37	8.2	11.8	17
69044	Turkey Sub Sandwich	1	ea	277		486	33	46		19	5.3	6	7
Burger King													
57002	BK Broiler Chicken Sandwich	1	ea	248		550	30	41	2	29	6		
56360	Chicken Sandwich	1	ea	229		710	26	54	2	43	9		
57001	Double Cheeseburger	1	ea	210		600	41	28	1	36	17		
56362	Ocean Catch Fish Filet	1	ea	255		700	26	56	3	41	6		
56363	Onion Rings-Serving	1	ea	124		310	4	41	6	14	2	8	4
57000	Whopper Jr Sandwich+Cheese	1	ea	177		460	23	29	2	28	10		
56999	Whopper Jr Sandwich	1	ea	164		420	21	29	2	24	8		
56354	Whopper Sandwich	1	ea	270		640	27	45	3	39	11		
56355	Whopper Sandwich+Cheese	1	ea	294		730	33	46	3	46	16		
Dairy Queen													
2131	Banana Split	1	ea	369		510	8	96	3	12	8		
2132	Blizzard-Heath Flavor	1	ea	404		820	14	119	1	33	20		
2227	Blizzard-Strawberry-Regular	1	ea	383		570	12	95	1	16	11		
2239	Breeze-Health-Regular	1	ea	404		710	15	123	1	18	11		
2237	Breeze-Strawberry-Regular	1	ea	383		460	13	99	1	1	1	0	0
2133	Buster Bar	1	ea	149		450	10	41	2	28	12		
2222	Cone-Chocolate-Regular	1	ea	213		360	9	56	0	11	8		
2135	Dilly Bar	1	ea	85		210	3	21	0	13	7	3	3
2136	Dipped Cone-Regular	1	ea	234		510	9	63	1	25	13		
69027	Double Bacon Cheeseburger	1	ea	269		670	40	29	2	43	19		
13236	Hot Dog-Super-1/4lb	1	ea	198		590	20	41		38	16	16	4
56374	Hotdog	1	ea	99		240	9	19	1	14	5		
56375	Hotdog+Cheese	1	ea	113		290	12	20	1	18	8	8	2
2141	Hot Fudge Brownie Delight	1	ea	305		710	11	102	1	29	14	12	2
2051	Ice Cream-Chocolate-Soft	1	cup	173	100	355	6	48	1	17	10.3	4.8	0.6
2145	Malt-Regular-Vanilla	1	ea	418		610	13	106	<1	14	8	2	2
2147	Mr. Misty-Regular	1	ea	330		250	0	63	0	0	0	0	0
2151	Peanut Buster Parfait	1	ea	305		730	16	99	2	31	17		
2224	Shake-Chocolate-Regular	1	ea	539		770	17	130	0	20	13		
56371	Single Cheeseburger	1	ea	152		340	20	29	2	17	8		
56368	Single Hamburger	1	ea	138		290	17	29	2	12	5	6	1
2154	Sundae-Chocolate-Regular	1	ea	241		410	8	73	0	10	6		
Dominos Pizza													
57025	Pepperoni Pizza-Deep Dish	2	pce	218	94	622	26	63	3	29	11.3		
57016	Pepperoni Pizza-Hand Tossed	2	pce	159.4	72	406	18	50	3	15	6.5		
57019	Pepperoni Pizza-Thin Crust	2	pce	156.7	69	447	20	40	2	23	9.2		
57028	Saus Mushrm Pizza Deep Dish	2	pce	235.7	110	618	26	66	4	28	10.8		
57029	Veggie Pizza-Deep Dish	2	pce	235.7	117	576	24	65	4	25	9.2		
57017	Veggie Pizza-Hand Tossed	2	pce	176	95	360	15	52	3	10	4.6		
57023	Veggie Pizza-Thin Crust	2	pce	178.7	99	386	17	43	3	17	6.4		

< = Trace amount present   Blank = Not available

CHOL, cholesterol; **V**, vitamin; **THI**, thiamin; **RIB**, riboflavin; **NIA**, niacin; **FOL**, folate; **CALC**, calcium; **PHOS**, phosphate; **SOD**, sodium; **POT**, potassium; **MAG**, magnesium

CHOL (mg)	V-A (RE)	THI (mg)	RIB (mg)	NIA (mg)	V-B6 (mg)	FOL (µg)	V-B12 (µg)	V-C (mg)	V-E (mg)	CALC (mg)	PHOS (mg)	SOD (mg)	POT (mg)	MAG (mg)	IRON (mg)	ZINC (mg)
43	100	0.6	0.7	14.2				9		410		1847	708		7.7	
51	20	13.2	0.5	18.8						400		2033	500		4.7	
80	60							6		60		480			5.4	
60	0							0		100		1400			3.6	
135	80							0		200		1060			4.5	
90	20							1		60		980			2.7	
0	0					0		0		100		810			1.4	
75	80							5		150		770			3.6	
60	40							5		60		530			3.6	
90	100	0.3	0.4	7	0.3			9		80		870			4.5	
115	150	0.3	0.5	7	0.3			9		250		1350			4.5	
30	200	0.2	0.3	0.4	0.2			15		250	40	180	860		1.8	
60	300	0.2	0.8					1		450	450	580	730		1.8	
50	300	0.2	0.7					9		450	350	260	700		1.8	
20	20	0.1	0.8					2		450	479	580	575		2.7	
10	0	0.1	0.7					9		450	378	270	530		2.7	
15	80	0.1	0.2	3	0.1			0		150	250	280	400		1.1	
30	200	0.1	0.4					1		250	300	180	525		1.8	
10	60	<0.1	0.1		0.1			0		100	80	75	170		0.4	
30	150	0.1	0.4	0.2	0.1			2		300	225	200	435		1.8	
135	40	0.4	0.5	7.7				4		600	389	1210	467		2.7	
60		0.4	0.3	5						100	150	1360	340		2.7	
25	20	0.2	0.1	2				4		60	60	730	170		1.8	
40	60	0.2	0.2	2				4		150	150	950	180		1.8	
35	80	0.2	0.7	0.3	0.2			1		300	600	340	510		5.4	
43	147	0.1	0.3	0.2	0.1	9	0.6	1	0.5	206	184	89	384	37	0.7	1
45	80	0.1	0.6	0.8	0.2			<1		400	350	230	570		1.4	
0	0	0	0		0			2		0		10			0	
35	150	0.2	0.5	3	0.2			1		300	450	400	660		1.8	
70	400	0.2	0.8	1.1				2		600	543	420	814		2.7	
55	60	0.3	0.3	3.9				4		150	243	850	263		3.6	
45	40	0.3	0.2	3.9				4		60	145	630	252		2.7	
30	150	0.1	0.3	0.4	0.2			0		250	204	210	394		1.4	
44	155							3		456		1382			5	
32	94							3		282		1179			4.3	
43	116							4		428		1276			1.9	
43	158							4		460		1355			5.2	
32	160							13		460		1232			5.2	
19	99							13		286		1028			4.4	
26	123							17		433		1076			2	

ERA, EatRight Analysis CD-ROM; **AMT**, amount; **WT**, weight; **WTR**, water; **CAL**, calories; **PROT**, protein; **CARB**, carbohydrate; **FIBR**, fiber; **FAT**, fat; **SATF**, saturated fat; **MONO**, monosaturated fat; **POLY**, polyunsaturated fat

ERA CODE	FOOD DESCRIPTION	AMT	UNIT	WT (g)	WTR (g)	CAL (kcal)	PROT (g)	CARB (g)	FIBR (g)	FAT (g)	SATF (g)	MONO (g)	POLY (g)
Fast Foods/Restaurants (continued)													
Generic Fast Food													
56606	Croissant+Egg & Cheese	1	ea	127	58	368	13	24		25	14.1	7.5	1.4
5463	Hashbrown Potatoes-Svg	0.5	cup	72	43	151	2	16		9	4.3	3.9	0.5
56667	Hotdog+Chili	1	ea	114	54	296	14	31		13	4.9	6.6	1.2
66004	Hotdog/Frankfurter & Bun	1	ea	98	53	242	10	18		15	5.1	6.9	1.7
56639	Nachos-Chips+Cheese	7	pce	113	46	346	9	36		19	7.8	8	2.2
6176	Onion Rings-Serving	8.5	pce	83	31	276	4	31		16	7	6.7	0.7
Hardees													
56407	Big Country Breakfast+Bacon	1	ea	217		740	25	81		43	13	22	8
56411	Biscuit 'n Gravy	1	ea	221		510	10	55		28	9	14	5
2247	Cool Twist Cone-Van/Choc	1	ea	118		180	4	34		2	0.7	1.3	0
2158	Cool Twist Sundae-HotFudge	1	ea	156		290	7	51		6	3	1.6	0.2
69061	Frisco Hamburger	1	ea	242		760	36	43		50	18		
56420	Hot Ham 'n Cheese Sandwich	1	ea	201		530	18	49		30	9		
56417	Mushroom & Swiss Burger	1	ea	203		520	30	37		27	13	12	2
56418	Roast Beef Sandwich-Regular	1	ea	124		270	15	28		11	5	4	2
2250	Shake-Peach	1	ea	345		390	10	77		4	3		
Jack in the Box													
69032	Bacon Cheeseburger	1	ea	242		710	35	41	0	45	15	15.7	8.7
1215	Beef Teriyaki Bowl	1	ea	440		640	28	124	7	3	1		
56430	Breakfast Jack Sandwich	1	ea	121		300	18	30	0	12	4.8	4.8	2.4
56441	Chicken Fajita Pita	1	ea	189		290	24	29	3	8	3	3.6	1.4
69035	Chicken Sandwich	1	ea	160		400	20	38	0	18	4		
69063	Chicken Caesar Pita Sandwich	1	ea	237		520	27	44	4	26	6		
90094	Cinnamon Churritos-Svg	1	ea	75		330	3	34	3	21	5		
69036	Country Fried Steak Sandwich	1	ea	153		450	14	42	0	25	7		
69033	Grilled Sourdough Burger	1	ea	223		670	32	39	0	43	16	17.8	7.9
56436	Jumbo Jack Burger	1	ea	229		560	26	41	0	32	10	13	8
56437	Jumbo Jack Burger+Cheese	1	ea	242		610	29	41	0	36	12	15	9
69064	Monterey Roast Beef Sandwich	1	ea	238		540	30	40	3	30	9		
69040	Sourdough Breakfast Sandwich	1	ea	147		380	21	31	0	20	7		
KFC													
15169	Chicken Breast-ExtraCrispy	1	ea	168		470	39	17	1	28	8	16.7	3.3
15163	Chicken Breast-Original	1	ea	153		400	29	16	1	24	6	14.4	3.6
15170	Chicken Leg-ExtraCrispy	1	ea	67		195	15	7	1	12	3	7.4	1.6
15165	Chicken Leg-Original	1	ea	61		140	13	4	0	9	2	5.3	1.7
15177	Hot Wings-Pieces	6	pce	135		471	27	18	2	33	8		
15184	Hot&Spicy Chicken Drumstick	1	ea	64		175	13	9	1	10	3		
15187	Hot&Spicy Chicken Wing	1	ea	55		210	10	9	1	15	4		
Long John Silvers													
15199	Chicken Plank-2 pce	1	ea	112		240	16	22		12	3.2	8.4	0.2
56459	Clam Dinner	1	ea	361		990	24	114		52	10.9	31.3	9.9

< = Trace amount present   Blank = Not available

CHOL, cholesterol; **V,** vitamin; **THI,** thiamin; **RIB,** riboflavin; **NIA,** niacin; **FOL,** folate;
CALC, calcium; **PHOS,** phosphate; **SOD,** sodium; **POT,** potassium; **MAG,** magnesium

CHOL (mg)	V-A (RE)	THI (mg)	RIB (mg)	NIA (mg)	V-B6 (mg)	FOL (μg)	V-B12 (μg)	V-C (mg)	V-E (mg)	CALC (mg)	PHOS (mg)	SOD (mg)	POT (mg)	MAG (mg)	IRON (mg)	ZINC (mg)
216	255	0.2	0.4	1.5	0.1	47	0.8	<1		244	348	551	174	22	2.2	1.8
9	2	0.1	<0.1	1.1	0.2	8	<0.1	5	0.1	7	69	290	267	16	0.5	0.2
51	6	0.2	0.4	3.7	<0.1	73	0.3	3		19	192	480	166	10	3.3	0.8
44	0	0.2	0.3	3.6	<0.1	48	0.5	<1	0.3	24	97	670	143	13	2.3	2
18	92	0.2	0.4	1.5	0.2	10	0.8	1		272	276	816	172	55	1.3	1.8
14	1	0.1	0.1	0.9	0.1	55	0.1	1	0.3	73	86	430	129	16	0.8	0.3
305										166		1800	530		5	
15										150		1500	210		2	
10										123		120	180		2	
20										152		310	173		0.4	
70												1280				
65										288		1710	300		3	
45										294		890	370		5	
25										105		780	260		4	
25												290				
110	80	0.2	0.5	8.8	0.4			9		250		1240	540		5.4	
25	1000							6		150		930	430		4.5	
185	80	0.5	0.4	3				9		200		890	220		2.7	
35	100	0.8	0.2	6				6		250		700	430		2.7	
45	40							0		150		1290	180		1.8	
55	80							2		250		1050	490		2.7	
20	0							0		20		200	170		5.4	
35	20							5		60		890	270		2.7	
110	150	0.6	0.5	8	0.3			6		200		1140	510		4.5	
65	40	0.4	0.3	1.8				6		100		700	450		4.5	
80	60	0.4	0.4	1.6				6		200		780	460		5.4	
75	80							5		300		1270	500		3.6	
235	150							9		250		1120	260		3.6	
	160	20							1		20		874			1.1
135	20							1		40		1116			1.1	
77	20							1		20		375			0.7	
75	20							1		20		422			0.7	
150	20							1		40		1230			1.4	
77	20							1		20		360			0.7	
55	20							1		20		350			0.7	
30		0.2	0.3	7								790	320		1.1	0.6
75	40	0.8	0.4	12				12		200		1830	910		4.5	3

ERA, EatRight Analysis CD-ROM; **AMT,** amount; **WT,** weight; **WTR,** water; **CAL,** calories; **PROT,** protein; **CARB,** carbohydrate; **FIBR,** fiber; **FAT,** fat; **SATF,** saturated fat; **MONO,** monosaturated fat; **POLY,** polyunsaturated fat

ERA CODE	FOOD DESCRIPTION	AMT	UNIT	WT (g)	WTR (g)	CAL (kcal)	PROT (g)	CARB (g)	FIBR (g)	FAT (g)	SATF (g)	MONO (g)	POLY (g)
Fast Foods/Restaurants (continued)													
Long John Silvers (continued)													
56462	Fish & More	1	ea	407		890	31	92		48	10.1	28.5	9.5
69030	Fish Sandwich Batter Dip	1	ea	159		340	18	40		13	3.1	8.9	1
57009	Fish-Shrimp-Chicken Dinner	1	ea	513		1160	45	113		65	14.2	40.3	9.6
57010	Fish-Shrimp-Clams Dinner	1	ea	512		1240	44	123		70	15.2	44.2	9.9
56467	Fish+Fries-2pce-Batter Dip	1	ea	261		610	27	52		37	7.9	23.5	5.3
57004	Fish+LemCrumb Dinner-2pce	1	ea	334		330	24	46		5	0.9	1.6	1.2
57003	Fish+LemCrumb Dinner-3pce	1	ea	493		610	39	86		13	2.2	3.9	5.3
56461	Fish-Batter Fried-Serving	1	ea	88		180	12	12		11	2.7	8.1	0.2
15198	Lt Herb Chicken-alaCarte	1	ea	100		120	22			4	1.2	1.7	1.1
27110	Malt Vinegar-Serving	1	ea	8		1	0	0	0				
19118	Seafood Gumbo w/Cod	1	ea	198		120	9	4		8	2.1	3.2	2.6
McDonalds													
69010	Big Mac Sandwich	1	ea	216		560	26	45	3	31	10		
42332	Biscuit+Biscuit Spread	1	ea	84		290	5	34	1	15	3		
56675	Breakfast Burrito	1	ea	117		320	13	23	2	20	7		
69009	Cheeseburger	1	ea	121		320	15	35	2	13	6		
15174	Chicken McNuggets	1	ea	71		190	12	10	0	11	2.5		
42335	Danish-Apple	1	ea	105		360	5	51	1	16	5		
69005	Egg McMuffin	1	ea	136		290	17	27	1	12	4.5		
42064	English Muffin+Butter	1	ea	63	21	189	5	30	2	6	2.4	1.5	1.3
69013	Filet-O-Fish Sandwich	1	ea	156		450	16	42	2	25	4.5		
2166	Frozen Yogurt Cone-Vanilla	1	ea	90		150	4	23	0	4	3		
4732	Grill Chick Dlxe Sand w/oMayo	1	ea	205		300	27	38	4	5	1		
69008	Hamburger	1	ea	107		260	13	34	2	9	3.5		
4730	Hamburger-Deluxe-w/Bacon	1	ea	247		590	32	39	4	34	12		
6155	Hashbrown Potatoes	1	ea	53		130	1	14	1	8	1.5		
45069	Hotcakes+Marg+Syrup	1	ea	228		610	9	104	2	18	3.5		
47147	McDonaldland Cookies	1	ea	42		180	3	32	1	5	1		
69011	Quarter Pounder	1	ea	172		420	23	37	2	21	8		
69012	Quarter Pounder+Cheese	1	ea	200		530	28	38	2	30	13		
69006	Sausage McMuffin	1	ea	112		360	13	26	1	23	8		
19579	Scrambled Eggs-1 svg	1	ea	102		160	13	1	0	11	3.5		
2167	Shake-LowFat-Choc	1	ea	294.6		360	11	60	1	9	6		
2168	Shake-LowFat-Strawberrry	1	ea	294		360	11	60	0	9	6		
2169	Shake-LowFat-Vanilla	1	ea	293.4		360	11	59	0	9	6		
Pizza Hut													
56481	Cheese Pizza-Pan Style	1	pce	108		261	12	28	2	11	5	3.4	1.7
56490	Pepperoni Pizza-Hand Tossed	1	pce	103.8		238	12	29	2	8	4		
56482	Pepperoni Pizza-Pan Style	1	pce	103.8		265	11	28	2	12	4	5	1.9
56493	Pepperoni Pizza-Pers Pan	1	ea	255.2		637	27	69	5	28	10	11.8	4.5
56483	Supreme Pizza-Pan Style	1	pce	136.4		311	15	28	3	15	6	6	2.1
56494	Supreme Pizza-Pers Pan	1	ea	327.4		722	33	70	6	34	12	14.8	5.6
56487	Supreme Pizza-Thin/Crispy	1	pce	115.9		257	14	21	2	13	5		

< = Trace amount present   Blank = Not available

CHOL, cholesterol; **V**, vitamin; **THI**, thiamin; **RIB**, riboflavin; **NIA**, niacin; **FOL**, folate;
CALC, calcium; **PHOS**, phosphate; **SOD**, sodium; **POT**, potassium; **MAG**, magnesium

CHOL (mg)	V-A (RE)	THI (mg)	RIB (mg)	NIA (mg)	V-B6 (mg)	FOL (μg)	V-B12 (μg)	V-C (mg)	V-E (mg)	CALC (mg)	PHOS (mg)	SOD (mg)	POT (mg)	MAG (mg)	IRON (mg)	ZINC (mg)
75	40	0.5	0.5	12				9		200		1790	1230		3.6	2.2
30		0.4	0.3	6				1		80		890	370		3.6	1.5
135	40	0.8	0.7	16				9		200		2590	1450		4.5	3.8
140	40	0.9	0.7	16				9		200		2630	1390		5.4	3.8
60		0.4	0.3	8				9		40		1480	900		1.8	1.2
75	1000	0.3	0.3	14				18		80		640	440		1.8	0.9
125	700	0.8	0.6	24				6		200		1420	990		5.4	2.2
30		0.2	0.2	3								490	260		0.4	0.3
60		0.1	0.3									570	270		0.7	0.6
												15	10			
25	200	0.2	0.2	3						100		740	310		1.8	1.5
85	60	0.5	0.4	6.1	0.3	49	2.3	4	1	250	267	1070	455	46	4.5	4.8
0	2	0.3	0.3	2.5	<0.1	5		0	0.9	60	390	780	116	10	1.8	0.3
195	100							9		150		600			1.8	
40	60	0.3	0.3	3.8	0.1	24	1.2	2	0.5	200	176	820	279	27	2.7	2.6
40	0	0.1	0.1	5	0.2		0.2	0	0.9	9	194	340	204	17	0.7	0.7
40	100	0.3	0.2	2				1		80	0	290	113		1.1	
235	100	0.5	0.4	3.3	0.1	33	0.7	1	0.8	200	268	790	197	23	2.7	1.5
13	33	0.3	0.3	2.6	<0.1	57	<0.1	1	0.1	103	85	386	69	13	1.6	0.4
50	40	0.3	0.2	2.8	0.1	32	0.6	0	1.6	150	197	870	286	34	1.8	0.8
20	60							1		100		75			0.4	
50	40							5		60		930			2.7	
30	22	0.3	0.3	3.8	0.1	21	1	2	0.2	150	111	580	258	24	2.7	2.2
100	100							6		150		1150			4.5	
0	0	0.1	<0.1	0.9	0.1	8	0	2	0.6	7	51	330	212	11	0.4	0.2
25	80	0.2	0.3	1.9	0.1	<1	0.3	<1	1.2	150	516	680	292	28	1.1	0.5
0	0	0.2	0.1	1.5	<0.1			0	0.7	20	52	190	46	8	1.8	0.3
70	20	0.4	0.3	6.8	0.2	28	2.6	2	0.4	150	208	820	408	34	4.5	4.7
95	100	0.4	0.4	6.8	0.3	33	2.9	2	0.8	300		1290			4.5	
45	40	0.6	0.3	3.8	0.1	16	0.5	0	0.7	200	156	740	191	22	1.8	1.5
425	135	0.1	0.5	0.1	0.1	44	1.1	0	0.9	40	172	170	126	10	1.1	1.1
40	73	0.1	0.5	0.4	0.1			1		350	354	250	542		0.7	
40	73	0.1	0.5	0.4	0.1			6		350	329	180	542		0.7	
40	73	0.1	0.5	0.3				1		350	327	250	534		0.4	
25	105	0.3	0.3	2.7	0.1			4		144		501	168	32	1.5	2.2
24	93	0.4	0.3	3.8				6		101		689	305	42	1.6	3
24	95	0.3	0.2	2.7	0.1	0		4		103		569	199	28	1.6	2.1
55	233	0.6	0.7	8.2	0.2			10		250		1340	407	60	4	3.8
30	98	0.4	0.4	3.2	0.2			5		117		764	310	41	2.3	3
66	240	0.7	0.8	9.9	0.4			14		276		1760	604	74	5.2	4.7
31	99	0.3	0.3	3.1				6		119		795	315	39	1.8	2.7

ERA, EatRight Analysis CD-ROM; **AMT,** amount; **WT,** weight; **WTR,** water; **CAL,** calories; **PROT,** protein; **CARB,** carbohydrate; **FIBR,** fiber; **FAT,** fat; **SATF,** saturated fat; **MONO,** monosaturated fat; **POLY,** polyunsaturated fat

ERA CODE	FOOD DESCRIPTION	AMT	UNIT	WT (g)	WTR (g)	CAL (kcal)	PROT (g)	CARB (g)	FIBR (g)	FAT (g)	SATF (g)	MONO (g)	POLY (g)
Fast Foods/Restaurants (continued)													
Subway													
52127	Chicken Taco Salad	1	ea	370		250	18	15	2	14	5		
69117	Club Sandwich (6-inch)	1	ea	246		297	21	40	3	5	1		
52120	Cold Cut Salad	1	ea	330		191	13	11	1	11	3		
69123	Italian Sandwich (6-inch)	1	ea	232		467	20	38	3	24	9		
69129	Meatball Sandwich (6-inch)	1	ea	260		404	18	44	3	16	6		
52121	Pizza Salad	1	ea	335		277	12	13	2	20	8		
52116	Seafood/Crab Salad	1	ea	331		161	13	11	2	8	1		
52118	Tuna Salad	1	ea	331		205	12	11	1	13	2		
69107	Tuna Sandwich (6-inch)	1	ea	178		279	11	38	2	9	2		
69109	Veggie Sandwich (6-inch)	1	ea	175		222	9	38	3	3	0		
Taco Bell													
56691	7 Layer Burrito	1	ea	283		530	16	66	13	23	7		
56690	Big Beef Burrito Supreme	1	ea	298		520	24	54	11	23	10		
56688	Chicken Burrito	1	ea	171		345	17	41		13	5		
56689	Chicken Soft Taco	1	ea	121		200	14	21	2	7	2.5		
45585	Cinnamon Twists-1 svg	1	ea	28		140	1	19	0	6	0		
56531	Mexican Pizza	1	ea	220		570	21	42	8	35	10		
56534	Nachos Bellgrande-1 svg	1	ea	312		770	21	84	17	39	11		
56684	Nachos Supreme-1 svg	1	ea	198		450	14	45	9	24	8		
56536	Pintos+Cheese+Red Sauce	1	ea	120		190	9	18	10	9	4		
56526	Soft Taco Supreme	1	ea	142		260	12	23	3	14	7		
56693	Steak Soft Taco	1	ea	128		230	15	20	2	10	2.5		
56524	Taco	1	ea	78		180	9	12	3	10	4		
56692	Taco Supreme	1	ea	113		220	10	14	3	14	7		
Taco Time													
56540	Crispy Bean Burrito	1	ea	164.2	77	427	15	53	9	18	5		
56541	Crispy Meat Burrito	1	ea	162.8	58	552	34	39	7	30	10		
56553	Mexi-Fries-Serving	1	ea	114.2	67	266	3	27		17			
56546	Natural Super Taco	1	ea	312.4	186	609	40	58	14	26	12.6		
56544	Soft Combo Burrito	1	ea	272		617	39	66	18	23	10		
Wendy's													
56571	Bacon Cheeseburger	1	ea	166		380	20	34	2	19	7	10.2	1.4
56574	Big Classic Burger+Cheese	1	ea	282		580	34	46	3	30	12		
2177	Frosty Dairy Dessert-Med	1	ea	298		440	11	73	0	11	7		
69059	Grilled Chicken Sandwich	1	ea	189		310	27	35	2	8	1.5		
69058	Junior Cheeseburger Deluxe	1	ea	180		360	18	36	3	17	6		
69057	Junior Hamburger	1	ea	118		270	15	34	2	10	3.5		
56566	Single Burger-Deluxe	1	ea	219		420	25	37	3	20	7		
Fats, Oils, Margarines, Shortenings, and Substitutes													
Fat Substitutes													
8133	Butter Buds	1	Tbs	5	<1	19	<1	4	0	<1	<0.1	<0.1	<0.1
8002	Pam CkingSpray-BtrFlav-1/3sec	1	ea	0.266		2	<1	<1		<1	<0.1		

< = Trace amount present   Blank = Not available

CHOL, cholesterol; **V,** vitamin; **THI,** thiamin; **RIB,** riboflavin; **NIA,** niacin; **FOL,** folate;
CALC, calcium; **PHOS,** phosphate; **SOD,** sodium; **POT,** potassium; **MAG,** magnesium

CHOL (mg)	V-A (RE)	THI (mg)	RIB (mg)	NIA (mg)	V-B6 (mg)	FOL (µg)	V-B12 (µg)	V-C (mg)	V-E (mg)	CALC (mg)	PHOS (mg)	SOD (mg)	POT (mg)	MAG (mg)	IRON (mg)	ZINC (mg)
52	361							35		115		990			3	
26	120							15		29		1341			4	
64	282							33		46		1127			2	
57	169							15		40		1592			4	
33	142							16		32		1035			4	
50	390							33		100		1336			2	
32	284							32		25		599			2	
32	298							32		29		654			2	
16	126							14		26		583			3	
0	120							15		25		582			3	
25	300							6		200		1280			3.6	
55	600							5		150		1520			2.7	
57	440							1		140		854			2.5	
35	60							1		80		540			0.7	
0	40	0.1	<0.1	0.6	<0.1			0		0		190	22		0.4	
45	400	0.3	0.3	2.9	1.1	59		5		250		1040	403	79	3.6	5.3
35	150	0.1	0.4	2.4				4		200		1310	733		3.6	
30	100							4		150		810			2.7	
15	250	0.1	0.1	0.4	0.2	64	0	0		150		650	360	103	1.8	2
35	150							4		100		590			1.8	
25	40							0		80		1020			1.4	
25	100	0.1	0.1	1.2	0.1			0		80		330	159		1.1	
35	150							0		100		350			1.1	
12	24	0.4	0.2	2.2	0.4	14				158	238	453	382		4.4	2.2
58	60	0.3	0.4	5.5	0.4	74		2		197	276	1000	506		4.4	4.4
0	0	0.1	<0.1	0.9			0	3		11	40	798	277		0.9	
80	118	0.5	0.5	5.5	0.6	82		6		331	457	889	827		7.7	5.5
63	96	0.5	0.5	5.3	0.6	75		5		292	418	1343	760		7.5	5.3
60	80	0.3	0.3	6.4	0.3	28	2	6		170	334	850	375	38	3.4	5.9
100	150	0.4	1.5	6				15		250		1460	578		5.4	
50	200	0.1	0.6	0.4	0.2	23	1.1	0		410	328	239	714	60	1.4	1.3
65	40							6		100		790			2.7	
50	100							6		180		890			3.4	
30	20							1		110		610			3.1	
70	60	0.4	0.3	5.8				6		130		920	468		4.7	
<1	0	0	0	0	0	0	0	0	0	1	<1	60	<1	0	0.1	0
	0												0			

ERA, EatRight Analysis CD-ROM; **AMT**, amount; **WT**, weight; **WTR**, water; **CAL**, calories; **PROT**, protein; **CARB**, carbohydrate; **FIBR**, fiber; **FAT**, fat; **SATF**, saturated fat; **MONO**, monosaturated fat; **POLY**, polyunsaturated fat

ERA CODE	FOOD DESCRIPTION	AMT	UNIT	WT (g)	WTR (g)	CAL (kcal)	PROT (g)	CARB (g)	FIBR (g)	FAT (g)	SATF (g)	MONO (g)	POLY (g)
Fats, Oils, Margarines, Shortenings, and Substitutes (continued)													
Fats, Oils, Spreads													
8004	Beef Fat/Tallow-Drippings	1	cup	205	0	1849	0	0	0	205	102	85.7	8.2
8826	Benecol Spread-Serving	1	ea	8		27	0	0		3	0.4	0.9	1.7
8825	Benecol Spread-Tablespoon	1	Tbs	14		48	0	0		5	0.7	1.6	3
8031	Butter Oil/Ghee	1	cup	205	<1	1795	1	0	0	204	126.9	58.9	7.6
8001	Butter-Pat	1	ea	5	1	36	<1	<1	0	4	2.5	1.2	0.2
8000	Butter-Regular-Salted-Cup	1	cup	227	36	1627	2	<1	0	184	114.8	54.5	6.8
8000	Butter-Regular-Salted-Tbsp	1	Tbs	14.19	2	102	<1	<1	0	12	7.2	3.4	0.4
8025	Butter-Unsalted-Cup	1	cup	227	41	1627	2	<1	0	184	114.6	53.2	6.8
8025	Butter-Unsalted-Tablespoon	1	Tbs	14.19	3	102	<1	<1	0	12	7.2	3.3	0.4
8142	Butter-Whipped	1	cup	151	24	1082	1	<1	0	122	76.2	35.4	4.5
8084	Canola Oil-Cup	1	cup	218	0	1927	0	0	0	218	15.5	128.4	64.5
8084	Canola Oil-Tablespoon	1	Tbs	13.6	0	120	0	0	0	14	1	8	4
8005	Chicken Fat	1	cup	205	<1	1845	0	0	0	204	61.1	91.6	42.8
8037	Coconut Oil-Cup	1	cup	218	0	1879	0	0	0	218	188.5	12.6	3.9
8037	Coconut Oil-Tablespoon	1	Tbs	13.6	0	117	0	0	0	14	11.8	0.8	0.2
8067	Cod Liver Oil (Fish Oil)	1	Tbs	13.6	0	123	0	0	0	14	3.1	6.4	3.1
8009	Corn Oil-Cup	1	cup	218	0	1927	0	0	0	218	27.7	52.8	127.9
8009	Corn Oil-Tablespoon	1	Tbs	13.6	0	120	0	0	0	14	1.7	3.3	8
8081	Cottonseed Oil-Cup	1	cup	218	0	1927	0	0	0	218	56.5	38.8	113.1
8081	Cottonseed Oil-Tablespoon	1	Tbs	13.6	0	120	0	0	0	14	3.5	2.4	7.1
8012	Crisco/Wesson Oil-Cup	1	cup	218	0	1923	0	0	0	218	31.3	50.7	126
8012	Crisco/Wesson Oil-Tablespoon	1	Tbs	13.6	0	120	0	0	0	14	2	3.2	7.9
8179	Margarine-Hard-Stick-Cup	1	cup	225.6	35	1621	2	2	0	182	29.5	84.8	59.1
8179	Margarine-Hard-Stick-Tbsp	1	Tbs	14.1	2	101	<1	<1	0	11	1.8	5.3	3.7
8165	Margarine-Liquid	1	Tbs	14.2	2	102	<1	0	0	11	1.9	4	5.1
8168	Margarine-Soft-Tub	1	Tbs	14.1	2	101	<1	<1	0	11	1.9	5.1	3.8
8134	Margarine-Unsalted-Cup	1	cup	225.6	42	1610	1	1	0	181	33.8	82.8	56.4
8134	Margarine-Unsalted-Tablespoon	1	Tbs	14.1	3	101	<1	<1	0	11	2.1	5.2	3.5
8008	Olive Oil-Cup	1	cup	216	0	1909	0	0	0	216	29.2	159.1	18.1
8008	Olive Oil-Tablespoon	1	Tbs	13.6	0	119	0	0	0	14	1.8	9.9	1.1
8083	Palm Kernel Oil-Cup	1	cup	218	0	1879	0	0	0	218	177.6	24.9	3.5
8083	Palm Kernel Oil-Tablespoon	1	Tbs	13.6	0	117	0	0	0	14	11.1	1.5	0.2
8082	Palm Oil-Cup	1	cup	218	0	1927	0	0	0	218	107.4	80.7	20.3
8082	Palm Oil-Tablespoon	1	Tbs	13.6	0	120	0	0	0	14	6.7	5	1.3
8026	Peanut Oil-Cup	1	cup	216	0	1909	0	0	0	216	36.5	99.8	69.1
8026	Peanut Oil-Tablespoon	1	Tbs	13.6	0	119	0	0	0	14	2.3	6.2	4.3
8010	Safflower Oil-Cup	1	cup	218	0	1927	0	0	0	218	13.5	31.3	162.6
8010	Safflower Oil-Tablespoon	1	Tbs	13.6	0	120	0	0	0	14	0.9	2	10.2
8027	Sesame Oil-Cup	1	cup	218	0	1927	0	0	0	218	31	86.5	90.9
8027	Sesame Oil-Tablespoon	1	Tbs	13.6	0	120	0	0	0	14	1.9	5.4	5.7
8176	Shedd's Spread-Tub	1	Tbs	14.5	8	60	<1	<1	0	6	0.8	2.4	2.4
8007	Shortening (Crisco)	1	cup	205	0	1812	0	0	0	205	51.2	91.2	53.5
8028	Soybean+Cottonseed Oil-Cup	1	cup	218	0	1927	0	0	0	218	39.2	64.3	104.8
8028	Soybean+Cottonseed Oil-Tbsp	1	Tbs	13.6	0	120	0	0	0	14	2.5	4	6.6

< = Trace amount present   Blank = Not available

CHOL, cholesterol; **V**, vitamin; **THI**, thiamin; **RIB**, riboflavin; **NIA**, niacin; **FOL**, folate;
CALC, calcium; **PHOS**, phosphate; **SOD**, sodium; **POT**, potassium; **MAG**, magnesium

CHOL (mg)	V-A (RE)	THI (mg)	RIB (mg)	NIA (mg)	V-B6 (mg)	FOL (µg)	V-B12 (µg)	V-C (mg)	V-E (mg)	CALC (mg)	PHOS (mg)	SOD (mg)	POT (mg)	MAG (mg)	IRON (mg)	ZINC (mg)
223	0	0	0	0	0	0	0	0	6.2	0	0	<1	<1	0	0	0
0	50								0.8							
0	88								1.4							
525	1896	<0.1	<0.1	<0.1	<0.1	<1	<0.1	0	6.2	8	6	3	10	1	<0.1	<0.1
11	38	0	<0.1	<0.1	0	<1	<0.1	0	0.1	1	1	41	1	<1	<0.1	<0.1
497	1711	<0.1	0.1	0.1	<0.1	7	0.3	0	3.6	54	52	1875	59	5	0.4	0.1
31	107	<0.1	<0.1	<0.1	<0.1	<1	<0.1	0	0.2	3	3	117	4	<1	<0.1	<0.1
497	1711	<0.1	0.1	0.1	<0.1	6	0.3	0	3.6	53	52	25	59	5	0.4	0.1
31	107	<0.1	<0.1	<0.1	<0.1	<1	<0.1	0	0.2	3	3	2	4	<1	<0.1	<0.1
330	1138	<0.1	0.1	0.1	<0.1	4	0.2	0	2.4	35	34	1248	39	3	0.2	0.1
0	0	0	0	0	0	0	0	0	45.8	0	0	0	0	0	0	0
0	0	0	0	0	0	0	0	0	2.9	0	0	0	0	0	0	0
174	0	0	0	0	0	0	0	0	6.2	0	0	0	0	0	0	0
0	0	0	0	0	0	0	0	0	0.6	0	0	0	0	0	0.1	0
0	0	0	0	0	0	0	0	0	<0.1	0	0	0	0	0		0
78	4080	0	0	0	0	0	0	0	3	0	0	0	0	0	0	0
0	0	0	0	0	0	0	0	0	181.3	0	0	0	0	0	0	0
0	0	0	0	0	0	0	0	0	11.3	0	0	0	0	0	0	0
0	0	0	0	0	0	0	0	0	142.1	0	0	0	0	0	0	0
0	0	0	0	0	0	0	0	0	8.9	0	0	0	0	0	0	0
0	0	0	0	0	0	0	0	0	203.8	<1	1	0	0	<1	<0.1	0
0	0	0	0	0	0	0	0	0	12.7			0	0			0
0	1802	0	<0.1	<0.1	0	3	0.2	<1	34.9	67	52	2128	96	6	0	
0	113	0	<0.1	<0.1	0	<1	<0.1	<1	2.2	4	3	133	6	<1	0	
0	113	<0.1	<0.1	<0.1	<0.1	<1	<0.1	<1	10.6	9	7	111	13	1	0	0
0	113	0	<0.1	0	0	<1	<0.1	<1	5.8	4	3	152	5	<1	0	0
0	1802	0	<0.1	0	0	2	0.1	<1	106	39	30	5	56	3	0	0
0	113	0	<0.1	0	0	<1	<0.1	<1	6.6	2	2	<1	3	<1	0	0
0	0	0	0	0	0	0	0	0	27.2	<1	3	<1	0	<1	0.8	0.1
0	0	0	0	0	0	0	0	0	1.7							
0	0	0	0	0	0	0	0	0	13.5	0	0	0	0	0	0	0
0	0	0	0	0	0	0	0	0	0.8	0	0	0	0	0	0	0
0	0	0	0	0	0	0	0	0	83.7	0	<1	0	0	0	<0.1	0
0	0	0	0	0	0	0	0	0	5.2	0	<1	0	0	0	<0.1	0
0	0	0	0	0	0	0	0	0	54	<1	0	<1	<1	<1	0.1	<0.1
0	0	0	0	0	0	0	0	0	3.4	<1	0	<1	<1	<1	<0.1	<0.1
0	0	0	0	0	0	0	0	0	93.9	0	0	0	0	0	0	0
0	0	0	0	0	0	0	0	0	5.9	0	0	0	0	0	0	0
0	0	0	0	0	0	0	0	0	63.4	0	0	0	0	0	0	0
0	0	0	0	0	0	0	0	0	4	0	0	0	0	0	0	0
0	144	0	<0.1	<0.1	0	<1	<0.1	<1	1.4	3	2	110	4	<1	0	0
0	0	0	0	0	0	0	0	0	201.5	0	0	0	0	0	0	0
0	0	0	0	0	0	0	0	0	216.2	0	0	0	0	0	0	0
0	0	0	0	0	0	0	0	0	13.5	0	0	0	0	0	0	0

ERA, EatRight Analysis CD-ROM; **AMT**, amount; **WT**, weight; **WTR**, water; **CAL**, calories; **PROT**, protein; **CARB**, carbohydrate; **FIBR**, fiber; **FAT**, fat; **SATF**, saturated fat; **MONO**, monosaturated fat; **POLY**, polyunsaturated fat

ERA CODE	FOOD DESCRIPTION	AMT	UNIT	WT (g)	WTR (g)	CAL (kcal)	PROT (g)	CARB (g)	FIBR (g)	FAT (g)	SATF (g)	MONO (g)	POLY (g)
Fats, Oils, Margarines, Shortenings, and Substitutes (continued)													
Fats, Oils, Spreads (continued)													
8132	Touch of Butter Spread-Tub	1	Tbs	14.2	5	77	<1	0	0	9	2	4.4	1.9
8085	Walnut Oil-Cup	1	cup	218	0	1927	0	0	0	218	19.8	49.7	137.9
8085	Walnut Oil-Tablespoon	1	Tbs	13.6	0	120	0	0	0	14	1.2	3.1	8.6
8011	Wesson Sunlite/Sunflr Oil-Cup	1	cup	218	0	1927	0	0	0	218	22.5	42.5	143.2
8011	Wesson Sunlite/Sunflr Oil-Tbsp	1	Tbs	13.6	0	120	0	0	0	14	0.2	2.7	8.9
8038	Wheat Germ Oil-Cup	1	cup		0	1923	0	0	0	218	40.9	32.8	134.3
8038	Wheat Germ Oil-Tablespoon	1	Tbs	13.6	0	120	0	0	0	14	2.6	2.1	8.4
Fish, Seafood, and Shellfish													
19086	Abalone-Cooked	2	oz	56.7	28	119	19	7	0	1	0.2	0.1	0.1
17124	Anchovies+Oil-Canned	5	ea	20	10	42	6	0	0	2	0.4	0.8	0.5
17128	Catfish-Steamed/Poached	1	cup	132	91	223	26	0	0	13	2.9	5.9	2.6
17034	Caviar-Granular-Black/Red	1	Tbs	16	8	40	4	1	0	3	0.6	0.7	1.2
19049	Clams-Baked/Broiled-Small	15	ea	150	109	210	23	5	0	11	1.9	4.4	2.9
19002	Clams-Canned-Drained	1	cup	160	102	237	41	8	0	3	0.3	0.3	0.9
17000	Cod-Batter Fried	4	pce	64	43	111	11	4	<1	5	1	2	1.7
17001	Cod-Steamed/Poached	1	cup	132	101	135	30	0	0	1	0.1	0.1	0.4
19420	Crab Cakes-Blue Crab	1	ea	60	43	93	12	<1	0	5	0.9	1.7	1.4
19036	Crab Leg-Alaska King-Boiled	1	ea	134	104	130	26	0	0	2	0.2	0.2	0.7
19052	Crab-Baked/Broiled	1	cup	118	87	163	22	<1	0	8	1.3	3	2.3
19038	Crayfish/Crawdads-Steam/Boiled	3	oz	85	67	70	14	0	0	1	0.2	0.2	0.3
17003	Fish Patty/FrozenSq-Heated	1	ea	57	26	155	9	14	0	7	1.8	2.9	1.8
17002	Fish Sticks-Frozen-Heated	1	ea	28	13	76	4	7	0	3	0.9	1.4	0.9
17040	Fried Fish Cakes-Frzn-Heated	1	ea	85	45	230	8	15	1	15	5.9	3.4	3.4
17103	Gefiltefish-Sweet-Commercial	1	pce	42	34	35	4	3	0	1	0.2	0.3	0.1
17071	Grouper Fillet-Bkd/Brld	1	ea	202	148	238	50	0	0	3	0.6	0.5	0.8
17090	Haddock Fillet-Bkd/Brld	1	ea	150	111	168	36	0	0	1	0.2	0.2	0.5
17047	Herring Fillet-Baked/Broiled	1	ea	143	92	290	33	0	0	17	3.7	6.8	3.9
17012	Herring-Pickled	1	pce	20	11	52	3	2	0	4	0.5	2.4	0.3
19057	Lobster-Baked/Broiled-Pieces	1	cup	145	108	169	29	2	0	4	2.4	1.3	0.3
19044	Mussels-Steamed/Boiled	3	oz	85	52	146	20	6	0	4	0.7	0.9	1
19048	Octopus-Cooked-Moist	3	oz	85	51	139	25	4	0	2	0.4	0.3	0.4
19025	Octopus-Raw	3	oz	85	68	70	13	2	0	1	0.2	0.1	0.2
17121	Orange Roughy-Baked/Broiled	3	oz	85	59	76	16	0	0	1	<0.1	0.5	<0.1
19027	Oysters-Eastern-Boiled/Steamed	6	ea	42	30	58	6	3	0	2	0.6	0.3	0.8
19009	Oysters-Eastern-Breaded-Fried	6	ea	88	57	173	8	10	<1	11	2.8	4.1	2.9
19026	Oysters-Eastern-Raw	1	cup	248	211	169	17	10	0	6	1.9	0.8	2.4
19012	Prawns/Lrg Shrimp-Steamed	4	ea	22	17	22	5	0	0	<1	0.1	<0.1	0.1
18807	Salmon Croquette	1	ea	63	38	137	9	7	1	8	1.9	3.4	2.4
17123	Salmon Fillet-Baked/Broiled	1	ea	308	184	560	78	0	0	25	3.9	8.3	10
17059	Salmon-Canned-Drained-Cup	1	cup	150	103	230	31	0	0	11	2.5	4.7	2.8
17060	Sardines+Oil-Can-Drained	1	ea	12	7	25	3	0	0	1	0.2	0.5	0.6
19061	Scallops-Baked/Broiled	4	ea	100		134	20	3	0	4	0.7	1.5	1.2
19070	Scallops-Battered-Fried	10	ea	80	45	185	14	11	<1	9	1.9	3.8	2.7
17086	Sea Bass Fillet-Baked/Broiled	1	ea	101	73	125	24	0	0	3	0.7	0.5	1

< = Trace amount present   Blank = Not available

CHOL, cholesterol; **V,** vitamin; **THI,** thiamin; **RIB,** riboflavin; **NIA,** niacin; **FOL,** folate;
CALC, calcium; **PHOS,** phosphate; **SOD,** sodium; **POT,** potassium; **MAG,** magnesium

CHOL (mg)	V-A (RE)	THI (mg)	RIB (mg)	NIA (mg)	V-B6 (mg)	FOL (µg)	V-B12 (µg)	V-C (mg)	V-E (mg)	CALC (mg)	PHOS (mg)	SOD (mg)	POT (mg)	MAG (mg)	IRON (mg)	ZINC (mg)
1	113	<0.1	<0.1	<0.1	0	<1	<0.1	<1	1.2	3	2	140	4	<1	0	0
0	0	0	0	0	0	0	0	0	70	0	0	0	0	0	0	0
0	0	0	0	0	0	0	0	0	4.4	0	0	0	0	0	0	0
0	0	0	0	0	0	0	0	0	138.6	0	0	0	0	0	0	0
0	0	0	0	0	0	0	0	0	8.7	0	0	0	0	0	0	0
0	0	0	0	0	0	0	0	0	418.7	0	0	0	0	0	0	0
0	0	0	0	0	0	0	0	0	26.2	0	0	0	0	0	0	0
96	2	0.2	0.1	1.3	0.1	4	0.5	2	4.5	33	151	290	198	46	3.3	0.9
17	4	<0.1	0.1	4	<0.1	2	0.2	0	1	46	50	734	109	14	0.9	0.5
78	21	0.5	0.1	3.2	0.2	13	3.5	1	2	15	300	79	419	34	0.8	1.2
94	90	<0.1	0.1	<0.1	0.1	8	3.2	0	1.1	44	57	240	29	48	1.9	0.2
60	223	0.1	0.3	3	0.1	27	82.9	22	3.1	84	301	202	559	16	24.7	2.4
107	274	0.2	0.7	5.4	0.2	46	158.2	35	3	147	541	179	1004	29	44.7	4.4
32	6	<0.1	0.1	1.5	0.2	6	0.5	1	0.8	19	116	58	245	16	0.5	0.3
61	11	<0.1	0.1	2.9	0.5	9	1.3	4	0.4	12	258	105	565	36	0.4	0.7
90	49	0.1	<0.1	1.7	0.1	32	3.6	2	0.9	63	128	198	194	20	0.6	2.5
71	12	0.1	0.1	1.8	0.2	68	15.4	10	1.2	79	375	1436	351	84	1	10.2
111	57	0.1	0.1	3.7	0.2	56	8.1	4	1.9	118	230	375	363	37	1	4.7
113	13	<0.1	0.1	1.9	0.1	37	1.8	1	1.3	51	230	80	252	28	0.7	1.5
64	18	0.1	0.1	1.2	<0.1	10	1	0	0.8	11	103	332	149	14	0.4	0.4
31	9	<0.1	<0.1	0.6	<0.1	5	0.5	0	0.4	6	51	163	73	7	0.2	0.2
22	17	<0.1	0.1	1.4	<0.1	10	0.9	0	0.9	9	142	150	296	15	0.3	0.3
13	11	<0.1	<0.1	0.4	<0.1	1	0.4	<1	0.1	10	31	220	38	4	1	0.3
95	101	0.2	<0.1	0.8	0.7	21	1.4	0	1.3	42	289	107	960	75	2.3	1
111	28	0.1	0.1	6.9	0.5	20	2.1	0	1.8	63	362	130	598	75	2	0.7
110	44	0.2	0.4	5.9	0.5	16	18.8	1	1.9	106	433	164	599	59	2	1.8
3	52	<0.1	<0.1	0.7	<0.1	<1	0.9	0	0.3	15	18	174	14	2	0.2	0.1
111	70	<0.1	0.1	1.5	0.1	16	4.4	0	1.5	87	261	570	496	49	0.6	4.1
48	77	0.3	0.4	2.5	0.1	64	20.4	12	1.2	28	242	314	228	31	5.7	2.3
82	69	<0.1	0.1	3.2	0.6	20	30.6	7	2	90	237	391	536	51	8.1	2.9
41	38	<0.1	<0.1	1.8	0.3	14	17	4	1	45	158	196	298	26	4.5	1.4
22	20	0.1	0.2	3.1	0.3	7	2	0	0.5	32	218	69	327	32	0.2	0.8
44	23	0.1	0.1	1	<0.1	6	14.7	3	0.7	38	85	177	118	40	5	76.3
71	79	0.1	0.2	1.5	0.1	27	13.8	3	2	55	140	367	215	51	6.1	76.7
131	74	0.2	0.2	3.4	0.2	25	48.3	9	2.1	112	335	523	387	116	16.5	225.2
43	15	<0.1	<0.1	0.6	<0.1	1	0.3	<1	0.2	9	30	49	40	7	0.7	0.3
30	14	<0.1	0.1	2.9	0.2	10	1.2	2	1.3	95	145	266	203	17	0.5	0.5
219	40	0.8	1.5	31	2.9	89	9.4	0	3.9	46	788	172	1934	114	3.2	2.5
66	80	<0.1	0.3	8.2	0.4	15	0.4	0	2.4	358	489	807	566	44	1.6	1.5
17	8	<0.1	<0.1	0.6	<0.1	1	1.1	0	<0.1	46	59	61	48	5	0.3	0.2
40	46	<0.1	0.1	1.3	0.2	18	1.8	3	1.7	30	266	231	392	68	0.4	1.2
66	29	0.1	0.1	1.4	0.1	14	1	2	1.8	35	184	171	253	44	1	0.9
54	65	0.1	0.2	1.9	0.5	6	0.3	0	0.6	13	250	88	331	54	0.4	0.5

ERA, EatRight Analysis CD-ROM; AMT, amount; WT, weight; WTR, water; CAL, calories; PROT, protein; CARB, carbohydrate; FIBR, fiber; FAT, fat; SATF, saturated fat; MONO, monosaturated fat; POLY, polyunsaturated fat

ERA CODE	FOOD DESCRIPTION	AMT	UNIT	WT (g)	WTR (g)	CAL (kcal)	PROT (g)	CARB (g)	FIBR (g)	FAT (g)	SATF (g)	MONO (g)	POLY (g)
Fish, Seafood, and Shellfish (continued)													
19013	Shrimp-Small-Boiled/Steamed	10	ea	40	31	40	8	0	0	<1	0.1	0.1	0.2
19000	Small Clams-Steamed/Boiled	20	ea	190	121	281	49	10	0	4	0.4	0.3	1
17022	Snapper Fillet-Baked/Broiled	1	ea	170	120	218	45	0	0	3	0.6	0.5	1
17004	Sole/Flounder-Fillet-Bread/Fried	1	ea	81	48	179	16	7	<1	9	2	3.8	2.7
17068	Sole/Flounder-Fillet-Broiled	1	ea	127	93	148	31	0	0	2	0.5	0.3	0.8
19068	Squid/Calamari-Baked	1	cup	140	99	194	26	5	0	7	1.4	2.2	2.1
17080	Surimi	3	oz	85	65	84	13	6	0	1	0.2	0.1	0.4
17066	Swordfish Broiled/Baked	1	pce	106	73	164	27	0	0	5	1.5	2.1	1.3
17101	Tuna-Bluefin-Baked/Broiled	3	oz	85	50	156	25	0	0	5	1.4	1.7	1.6
17025	Tuna-Lt-Oil-Can-Drnd-Cup	1	cup	146	87	289	43	0	0	12	2.2	4.3	4.2
17027	Tuna-Lt-Wat-Cnd-Drnd-Cup	1	cup	154	115	179	39	0	0	1	0.4	0.2	0.5
19040	Whelk-Steamed/Boiled	3	oz	85	27	234	41	13	0	1	0.1	<0.1	<0.1
17145	Whiting-Baked/Broiled	1	cup	132	99	153	31	0	0	2	0.5	0.6	0.8
Fruits													
3005	Apple Rings-Dried	10	ea	64	20	156	1	42	6	<1	<0.1	<0.1	0.1
3000	Apple+Peel-Medium	1	ea	138	116	81	<1	21	4	<1	0.1	<0.1	0.1
3308	Apple-Baked-Unsweetened	1	ea	161	133	102	<1	26	5	1	0.1	<0.1	0.2
3003	Apple-Peeled-Medium	1	ea	128	108	73	<1	19	2	<1	0.1	<0.1	0.1
3147	Applesauce-Canned-Sweet	1	cup	255	203	194	<1	51	3	<1	0.1	<0.1	0.1
3006	Applesauce-Canned-Unsweet	1	cup	244	216	105	<1	28	3	<1	<0.1	<0.1	<0.1
3013	Apricot Halves-Dried-Each	1	ea	3.5	1	8	<1	2	<1	<1	<0.1	<0.1	<0.1
3151	Apricots+Juice-Can	1	cup	244	211	117	2	30	4	<1	<0.1	<0.1	<0.1
3157	Apricots-Fresh-Pitted	1	ea	35	30	17	<1	4	1	<1	<0.1	0.1	<0.1
3016	Avocado-Fresh	1	ea	201	149	324	4	15	10	31	4.9	19.3	3.9
3307	Banana Chips	1	cup	92	4	477	2	54	7	31	26.6	1.8	0.6
3020	Banana-Fresh	1	ea	118	88	108	1	28	3	1	0.2	<0.1	0.1
3024	Blackberries-Fresh	1	cup	144	123	75	1	18	8	1	<0.1	0.1	0.3
3028	Blackberries-Frozen	1	cup	151	124	97	2	24	8	1	<0.1	0.1	0.4
3029	Blueberries-Fresh	1	cup	145	123	81	1	20	4	1	<0.1	0.1	0.2
3031	Blueberries-Frozen	1	cup	155	134	79	1	19	4	1	0.1	0.1	0.4
3231	Blueberries-Fz-Sweet-Thaw	1	cup	230	178	186	1	50	5	<1	<0.1	<0.1	0.1
3239	Breadfruit	1	cup	220	155	227	2	60	11	1	0.1	0.1	0.1
3076	Cantaloupe Melon	1	ea	552	496	193	5	46	4	2	0.4	<0.1	0.6
3075	Cantaloupe Melon-Cubes	1	cup	160	144	56	1	13	1	<1	0.1	<0.1	0.2
3240	Carambola/Starfruit-Fresh	1	ea	127	115	42	1	10	3	<1	<0.1	<0.1	0.2
3079	Casaba/Crenshaw Melon	1	ea	1640	1508	426	15	102	13	2	0.4	<0.1	0.6
3078	Casaba/Crenshaw Melon-Cubes	1	cup	170	156	44	2	11	1	<1	<0.1	<0.1	0.1
3039	Cranberries-Fresh	1	cup	95	82	47	<1	12	4	<1	<0.1	<0.1	0.1
3040	Cranberry Sauce-Strained	1	cup	277	168	418	1	108	3	<1	<0.1	0.1	0.2
3043	Dates-Chopped	1	cup	178	40	490	4	131	13	1	0.3	0.3	0.1
3044	Dates-Whole-Each	10	ea	83	19	228	2	61	6	<1	0.2	0.1	<0.1
3162	Dried Figs	1	ea	19	5	48	1	12	2	<1	<0.1	<0.1	0.1
3271	Feijoa Fruit-Raw	1	ea	50	43	24	1	5	2	<1	0.1	<0.1	0.2
3160	Figs-Medium-Fresh	1	ea	50	40	37	<1	10	2	<1	<0.1	<0.1	0.1
3045	Fruit Cocktail+HeavySyrup	1	cup	248	199	181	1	47	2	<1	<0.1	<0.1	0.1

< = Trace amount present   Blank = Not available

CHOL, cholesterol; **V,** vitamin; **THI,** thiamin; **RIB,** riboflavin; **NIA,** niacin; **FOL,** folate; **CALC,** calcium; **PHOS,** phosphate; **SOD,** sodium; **POT,** potassium; **MAG,** magnesium

CHOL (mg)	V-A (RE)	THI (mg)	RIB (mg)	NIA (mg)	V-B6 (mg)	FOL (μg)	V-B12 (μg)	V-C (mg)	V-E (mg)	CALC (mg)	PHOS (mg)	SOD (mg)	POT (mg)	MAG (mg)	IRON (mg)	ZINC (mg)
78	26	<0.1	<0.1	1	0.1	1	0.6	1	0.3	16	55	90	73	14	1.2	0.6
127	325	0.3	0.8	6.4	0.2	55	187.8	42	3.7	175	642	213	1193	34	53.1	5.2
80	60	0.1	<0.1	0.6	0.8	10	5.9	3	1.4	68	342	97	887	63	0.4	0.7
55	15	0.1	0.1	2.8	0.2	9	1.1	1	2.2	38	164	148	306	29	0.9	0.5
86	14	0.1	0.1	2.8	0.3	12	3.2	0	2.9	23	367	133	437	74	0.4	0.8
395	57	<0.1	0.6	3.5	0.1	8	2.1	8	2.7	56	376	124	420	56	1.2	2.6
26	17	<0.1	<0.1	0.2	<0.1	1	1.4	0	0.2	8	240	122	95	37	0.2	0.3
53	43	<0.1	0.1	12.5	0.4	2	2.1	1	0.7	6	357	122	391	36	1.1	1.6
42	643	0.2	0.3	9	0.4	2	9.2	0	1.1	8	277	42	274	54	1.1	0.7
26	34	0.1	0.2	18.1	0.2	8	3.2	0	1.8	19	454	517	302	45	2	1.3
46	26	<0.1	0.1	20.5	0.5	6	4.6	0	0.8	17	251	520	365	42	2.4	1.2
110	42	<0.1	0.2	1.7	0.6	10	15.4	6	0.2	96	240	350	590	146	8.6	2.8
111	45	0.1	0.1	2.2	0.2	20	3.4	0	0.5	82	376	174	573	36	0.6	0.7
0	0	0	0.1	0.6	0.1	0	0	2	0.7	9	24	56	288	10	0.9	0.1
0	7	<0.1	<0.1	0.1	0.1	4	0	8	0.9	10	10	0	159	7	0.2	0.1
0	7	<0.1	<0.1	0.1	0.1	3	0	8	0.6	12	12	0	179	9	0.3	0.1
0	5	<0.1	<0.1	0.1	0.1	1	0	5	0.1	5	9	0	145	4	0.1	0.1
0	3	<0.1	0.1	0.5	0.1	2	0	4	2.3	10	18	8	156	8	0.9	0.1
0	7	<0.1	0.1	0.5	0.1	1	0	3	0.6	7	17	5	183	7	0.3	0.1
0	25	0	<0.1	0.1	<0.1	<1	0	<1	0.1	2	4	<1	48	2	0.2	<0.1
0	412	<0.1	<0.1	0.8	0.1	4	0	12	2.2	29	49	10	403	24	0.7	0.3
0	91	<0.1	<0.1	0.2	<0.1	3	0	4	0.3	5	7	<1	104	3	0.2	0.1
0	123	0.2	0.2	3.9	0.6	124	0	16	4.6	22	82	20	1203	78	2	0.8
0	7	0.1	<0.1	0.7	0.2	13	0	6	5	17	52	6	493	70	1.1	0.7
0	9	0.1	0.1	0.6	0.7	23	0	11	0.4	7	24	1	467	34	0.4	0.2
0	23	<0.1	0.1	0.6	0.1	49	0	30	1	46	30	0	282	29	0.8	0.4
0	17	<0.1	0.1	1.8	0.1	51	0	5	1.1	44	45	2	211	33	1.2	0.4
0	14	0.1	0.1	0.5	0.1	9	0	19	2.7	9	14	9	129	7	0.2	0.2
0	12	<0.1	0.1	0.8	0.1	10	0	4	3.1	12	17	2	84	8	0.3	0.1
0	9	<0.1	0.1	0.6	0.1	15	0	2	4.6	14	16	2	138	5	0.9	0.1
0	9	0.2	0.1	2	0.2	31	0	64	2.5	37	66	4	1078	55	1.2	0.3
0	1777	0.2	0.1	3.2	0.6	94	0	233	1.7	61	94	50	1705	61	1.2	0.9
0	515	0.1	<0.1	0.9	0.2	27	0	68	0.5	18	27	14	494	18	0.3	0.3
0	62	<0.1	<0.1	0.5	0.1	18	0	27	0.5	5	20	3	207	11	0.3	0.1
0	49	1	0.3	6.6	2	279	0	262	2.5	82	115	197	3444	131	6.6	2.6
0	5	0.1	<0.1	0.7	0.2	29	0	27	0.3	8	12	20	357	14	0.7	0.3
0	5	<0.1	<0.1	0.1	0.1	2	0	13	0.9	7	9	1	67	5	0.2	0.1
0	6	<0.1	0.1	0.3	<0.1	3	0	6	0.4	11	17	80	72	8	0.6	0.1
0	9	0.2	0.2	3.9	0.3	22	0	0	0.2	57	71	5	1160	62	2	0.5
0	4	0.1	0.1	1.8	0.2	10	0	0	0.1	27	33	2	541	29	1	0.2
0	2	<0.1	<0.1	0.1	<0.1	1	0	<1	0	27	13	2	135	11	0.4	0.1
0	0	<0.1	<0.1	0.1	<0.1	19	0	10		8	10	2	78	4	<0.1	<0.1
0	7	<0.1	<0.1	0.2	0.1	3	0	1	0.4	18	7	<1	116	8	0.2	0.1
0	50	<0.1	<0.1	0.9	0.1	6	0	5	2.1	15	27	15	218	12	0.7	0.2

ERA, EatRight Analysis CD-ROM; **AMT,** amount; **WT,** weight; **WTR,** water; **CAL,** calories; **PROT,** protein; **CARB,** carbohydrate; **FIBR,** fiber; **FAT,** fat; **SATF,** saturated fat; **MONO,** monosaturated fat; **POLY,** polyunsaturated fat

ERA CODE	FOOD DESCRIPTION	AMT	UNIT	WT (g)	WTR (g)	CAL (kcal)	PROT (g)	CARB (g)	FIBR (g)	FAT (g)	SATF (g)	MONO (g)	POLY (g)
Fruits (continued)													
3163	Fruit Cocktail+LiteSyrup	1	cup	242	204	138	1	36	2	<1	<0.1	<0.1	0.1
3164	Fruit Cocktail-Juice Pack	1	cup	237	207	109	1	28	2	<1	<0.1	<0.1	<0.1
3313	Fruit Cocktail-Water Pack	1	cup	237	215	76	1	20	2	<1	<0.1	<0.1	<0.1
3048	Grapefruit-Fresh-Pieces	1	cup	230	209	74	1	19	3	<1	<0.1	<0.1	0.1
3047	Grapefruit-Fresh-White	0.5	ea	118	107	39	1	10	1	<1	<0.1	<0.1	<0.1
3060	Grapes-Concord	1	cup	92	75	62	1	16	1	<1	0.1	<0.1	0.1
3057	Grapes-Red-Cup	1	cup	160	129	114	1	28	2	1	0.3	<0.1	0.3
3054	Grapes-White-Seedless-Cup	1	cup	160	129	114	1	28	2	1	0.3	<0.1	0.3
3207	Guava-Fresh	1	ea	90	77	46	1	11	5	1	0.2	<0.1	0.2
3081	Honeydew Melon (1/10th)	1	pce	160	143	56	1	15	1	<1	<0.1	<0.1	0.1
3080	Honeydew Melon-Cubes	1	cup	170	152	60	1	16	1	<1	<0.1	<0.1	0.1
3065	Kiwifruit	1	ea	76	63	46	1	11	3	<1	<0.1	<0.1	0.2
3066	Lemon-Fresh-Peeled	1	ea	58	52	17	1	5	2	<1	<0.1	<0.1	0.1
3071	Lime-Fresh-Peeled	1	ea	67	59	20	<1	7	2	<1	<0.1	<0.1	<0.1
3257	Lychees	1	ea	9.6	8	6	<1	2	<1	<1	<0.1	<0.1	<0.1
3221	Mango-Fresh-Whole	1	ea	207	169	134	1	35	4	1	0.1	0.2	0.1
3215	Nectarine-Fresh	1	ea	136	117	67	1	16	2	1	0.1	0.2	0.3
3082	Orange-Fresh-Medium	1	ea	131	114	62	1	15	3	<1	<0.1	<0.1	<0.1
3083	Orange-Fresh-Sections-Cup	1	cup	180	156	85	2	21	4	<1	<0.1	<0.1	<0.1
3089	Oranges-Mandarin-Canned	1	cup	249	223	92	2	24	2	<1	<0.1	<0.1	<0.1
3171	Papaya-Fresh	1	ea	304	270	118	2	30	5	<1	0.1	0.1	0.1
3098	Peaches-Canned+Heavy Syrup	1	cup	262	208	194	1	52	3	<1	<0.1	0.1	0.1
3173	Peaches-Canned+Light Syrup	1	cup	251	213	136	1	37	3	<1	<0.1	<0.1	<0.1
3096	Peach-Fresh-Medium	1	ea	98	86	42	1	11	2	<1	<0.1	<0.1	<0.1
3103	Pears-Bartlett-Fresh-Med	1	ea	166	139	98	1	25	4	1	<0.1	0.1	0.2
3107	Pears-Canned+Heavy Syrup	1	cup	266	214	197	1	51	4	<1	<0.1	0.1	0.1
3179	Pears-Canned+Juice	1	cup	248	214	124	1	32	4	<1	<0.1	<0.1	<0.1
3177	Pears-Canned+Light Syrup	1	cup	251	212	143	<1	38	4	<1	<0.1	<0.1	<0.1
3115	Pineapple-Canned+HeavySyrup	1	ea	49	39	38	<1	10	<1	<1	<0.1	<0.1	<0.1
3183	Pineapple-Canned+Juice	1	cup	250	209	150	1	39	2	<1	<0.1	<0.1	0.1
3181	Pineapple-Canned+Light Syrup	1	cup	252	216	131	1	34	2	<1	<0.1	<0.1	0.1
3113	Pineapple-Fresh-Slices	1	pce	84	73	41	<1	10	1	<1	<0.1	<0.1	0.1
5632	Plantain-Fried-Ripe	1	cup	169	81	425	2	61	4	22	3	6.8	11.5
3121	Plum-Medium-Fresh	1	ea	66	56	36	1	9	1	<1	<0.1	0.3	0.1
3126	Prunes-Dried	10	ea	84	27	201	2	53	6	<1	<0.1	0.3	0.1
3129	Raisins-Seedless-Packed	1	cup	165	25	495	5	130	7	1	0.2	<0.1	0.2
3130	Raisins-Seedless-Unpacked	1	cup	145	22	435	5	115	6	1	0.2	<0.1	0.2
3131	Raspberries-Fresh	1	cup	123	106	60	1	14	8	1	<0.1	0.1	0.4
3235	Raspberries-Frozen-Sweet	1	cup	250	182	258	2	65	11	<1	<0.1	<0.1	0.2
3133	Rhubarb-Fzn-Cooked+Sugar	1	cup	240	163	278	1	75	5	<1	<0.1	<0.1	0.1
3209	Rhubarb-Raw-Diced	1	cup	122	114	26	1	6	2	<1	0.1	<0.1	0.1
3664	Starfruit-Raw-Cube-Cup	1	cup	137	124	45	1	11	4	<1	<0.1	<0.1	0.3
3236	Strawberries-Frzn/Sweet/Thaw	1	cup	255	187	245	1	66	5	<1	<0.1	<0.1	0.2
3136	Strawberries-Medium Size	1	ea	12	11	4	<1	1	<1	<1	<0.1	<0.1	<0.1
3135	Strawberries-Sliced-Cup	1	cup	166	152	50	1	12	4	1	<0.1	0.1	0.3
3037	Sweet Cherries-Fresh-Cup	1	cup	145	117	104	2	24	3	1	0.3	0.4	0.4

< = Trace amount present   Blank = Not available

CHOL, cholesterol; **V,** vitamin; **THI,** thiamin; **RIB,** riboflavin; **NIA,** niacin; **FOL,** folate;
CALC, calcium; **PHOS,** phosphate; **SOD,** sodium; **POT,** potassium; **MAG,** magnesium

CHOL (mg)	V-A (RE)	THI (mg)	RIB (mg)	NIA (mg)	V-B6 (mg)	FOL (µg)	V-B12 (µg)	V-C (mg)	V-E (mg)	CALC (mg)	PHOS (mg)	SOD (mg)	POT (mg)	MAG (mg)	IRON (mg)	ZINC (mg)
0	51	<0.1	<0.1	0.9	0.1	7	0	5	2.1	15	27	15	215	12	0.7	0.2
0	73	<0.1	<0.1	1	0.1	6	0	6	2.1	19	33	9	225	17	0.5	0.2
0	59	<0.1	<0.1	0.9	0.1	6	0	5	0.7	12	26	9	223	17	0.6	0.2
0	28	0.1	<0.1	0.6	0.1	23	0	79	0.6	28	18	0	320	18	0.2	0.2
0	1	<0.1	<0.1	0.3	0.1	12	0	39	0.3	14	9	0	175	11	0.1	0.1
0	9	0.1	0.1	0.3	0.1	4	0	4	0.3	13	9	2	176	5	0.3	<0.1
0	11	0.1	0.1	0.5	0.2	6	0	17	1.1	18	21	3	296	10	0.4	0.1
0	11	0.1	0.1	0.5	0.2	6	0	17	1.1	18	21	3	296	10	0.4	0.1
0	71	<0.1	<0.1	1.1	0.1	13	0	165	1	18	22	3	256	9	0.3	0.2
0	6	0.1	<0.1	1	0.1	10	0	40	0.2	10	16	16	434	11	0.1	0.1
0	7	0.1	<0.1	1	0.1	10	0	42	0.3	10	17	17	461	12	0.1	0.1
0	14	<0.1	<0.1	0.4	0.1	29	0	74	0.9	20	30	4	252	23	0.3	0.1
0	2	<0.1	<0.1	0.1	<0.1	6	0	31	0.5	15	9	1	80	5	0.3	<0.1
0	1	<0.1	<0.1	0.1	<0.1	5	0	19	0.2	22	12	1	68	4	0.4	0.1
0	0	<0.1	<0.1	0.1	<0.1	1	0	7	0.1	<1	3	<1	16	1	<0.1	<0.1
0	805	0.1	0.1	1.2	0.3	29	0	57	2.3	21	23	4	323	19	0.3	0.1
0	101	<0.1	0.1	1.3	<0.1	5	0	7	1.2	7	22	0	288	11	0.2	0.1
0	28	0.1	0.1	0.4	0.1	40	0	70	0.3	52	18	0	237	13	0.1	0.1
0	38	0.2	0.1	0.5	0.1	55	0	96	0.4	72	25	0	326	18	0.2	0.1
0	212	0.2	0.1	1.1	0.1	11	0	85	1.2	27	25	12	331	27	0.7	1.3
0	85	0.1	0.1	1	0.1	116	0	188	3.4	73	15	9	781	30	0.3	0.2
0	86	<0.1	0.1	1.6	<0.1	8	0	7	2.6	8	29	16	241	13	0.7	0.2
0	88	<0.1	0.1	1.5	<0.1	8	0	6	2.2	8	28	13	243	13	0.9	0.2
0	53	<0.1	<0.1	1	<0.1	3	0	6	1	5	12	0	193	7	0.1	0.1
0	3	<0.1	0.1	0.2	<0.1	12	0	7	0.8	18	18	0	208	10	0.4	0.2
0	0	<0.1	0.1	0.6	<0.1	3	0	3	1.3	13	19	13	173	11	0.6	0.2
0	2	<0.1	<0.1	0.5	<0.1	3	0	4	1.2	22	30	10	238	17	0.7	0.2
0	0	<0.1	<0.1	0.4	<0.1	3	0	2	1.3	13	18	13	166	10	0.7	0.2
0	<1	<0.1	<0.1	0.1	<0.1	2	0	4	<0.1	7	3	<1	51	8	0.2	0.1
0	10	0.2	<0.1	0.7	0.2	12	0	24	0.2	35	15	2	305	35	0.7	0.2
0	3	0.2	0.1	0.7	0.2	12	0	19	0.3	35	18	3	265	40	1	0.3
0	2	0.1	<0.1	0.4	0.1	9	0	13	0.1	6	6	1	95	12	0.3	0.1
0	162	0.1	0.1	1.2	0.5	21	0	25	4.7	5	65	8	858	71	1.1	0.3
0	21	<0.1	0.1	0.3	0.1	1	0	6	0.6	3	7	0	114	5	0.1	0.1
0	167	0.1	0.1	1.6	0.2	3	0	3	2.1	43	66	3	626	38	2.1	0.4
0	2	0.3	0.1	1.3	0.4	5	0	5	1.2	81	160	20	1239	54	3.4	0.4
0	1	0.2	0.1	1.2	0.4	5	0	5	1	71	141	17	1088	48	3	0.4
0	16	<0.1	0.1	1.1	0.1	32	0	31	0.6	27	15	0	187	22	0.7	0.6
0	15	<0.1	0.1	0.6	0.1	65	0	41	1.1	38	42	2	285	32	1.6	0.4
0	17	<0.1	0.1	0.5	<0.1	13	0	8	0.5	348	19	2	230	29	0.5	0.2
0	12	<0.1	<0.1	0.4	<0.1	9	0	10	0.2	105	17	5	351	15	0.3	0.1
0	67	<0.1	<0.1	0.6	0.1	19	0	29	0.5	5	22	3	223	12	0.4	0.2
0	5	<0.1	0.1	1	0.1	38	0	106	0.4	28	33	8	250	18	1.5	0.2
0	<1	<0.1	<0.1	<0.1	<0.1	2	0	7	<0.1	2	2	<1	20	1	<0.1	<0.1
0	5	<0.1	0.1	0.4	0.1	29	0	94	0.4	23	32	2	276	17	0.6	0.2
0	30	0.1	0.1	0.6	0.1	6	0	10	1.3	22	28	0	325	16	0.6	0.1

ERA, EatRight Analysis CD-ROM; **AMT,** amount; **WT,** weight; **WTR,** water; **CAL,** calories; **PROT,** protein; **CARB,** carbohydrate; **FIBR,** fiber; **FAT,** fat; **SATF,** saturated fat; **MONO,** monosaturated fat; **POLY,** polyunsaturated fat

ERA CODE	FOOD DESCRIPTION	AMT	UNIT	WT (g)	WTR (g)	CAL (kcal)	PROT (g)	CARB (g)	FIBR (g)	FAT (g)	SATF (g)	MONO (g)	POLY (g)
Fruits (continued)													
3158	Sweet Cherries-Frozen	1	cup	259	196	230	3	58	5	<1	0.1	0.1	0.1
3087	Tangelo-Medium	1	ea	95	82	45	1	11	2	<1	<0.1	<0.1	<0.1
3138	Tangerine-Fresh	1	ea	84	74	37	1	9	2	<1	<0.1	<0.1	<0.1
3142	Watermelon-Fresh Pieces	1	cup	152	139	49	1	11	1	1	0.1	0.2	0.2
Grains and Grain Products													
Bagels													
42100	Bagel-Cinnamon Raisin	1	ea	71	23	194	7	39	2	1	0.2	0.1	0.5
42041	Bagel-Egg-3.5 inch diam	1	ea	71	23	197	8	38	2	1	0.3	0.3	0.5
42103	Bagel-Oat Bran	1	ea	71	23	181	8	38	3	1	0.1	0.2	0.3
42000	Bagel-Plain-3.5in diam	1	ea	71	23	195	7	38	2	1	0.2	0.1	0.5
42092	Bagel-Whole Wheat	1	ea	55	16	145	6	31	5	1	0.1	0.1	0.3
Biscuits													
42206	Biscuit-Cheese-2 in diam	1	ea	30	8	113	3	13	<1	6	1.7	2.3	1.4
42110	Biscuit-LowFat Dough-Baked	1	ea	21	6	63	2	12	<1	1	0.3	0.6	0.2
42002	Biscuit-Mix-Enr+Milk-Baked	1	ea	57	16	191	4	28	1	7	1.6	2.4	2.5
42001	Biscuit-Recipe	1	ea	60	17	212	4	27	1	10	2.6	4.2	2.5
42205	Biscuit-Whole Wheat-3inch	1	ea	63	18	198	6	30	5	7	1.7	3	2.2
42203	Crumpet-3.75 inch	1	ea	45	24	80	3	17	1	<1	0.1	<0.1	0.2
42071	Scone	1	ea	42	12	150	4	19	1	6	2	2.6	1.3
42072	Scone-Whole Wheat	1	ea	42	11	144	5	18	3	7	2.1	2.6	1.4
Breads and Rolls													
42171	Armenian Bread	1	pce	20	7	54	2	10	1	1	0.2	0.2	0.3
42039	Banana Bread-Recipe w/Marg	1	pce	60	18	196	3	33	1	6	1.3	2.7	1.9
42052	Boston Brown Bread-Canned	1	pce	45	21	88	2	19	2	1	0.1	0.1	0.3
42090	Challah/Egg Bread	1	pce	40	14	115	4	19	1	2	0.6	0.9	0.4
42115	Cornbread-Dry Mix-Prep	1	ea	60	19	188	4	29	1	6	1.6	3.1	0.7
42116	Cornbread-Recipe w/2%Milk	1	pce	65	25	173	4	28	2	5	1	1.2	2.1
42042	Cracked Wheat Bread-Slice	1	pce	25	9	65	2	12	1	1	0.2	0.5	0.2
42015	Croissant-4.5x4x2 inch	1	ea	57	13	231	5	26	1	12	6.6	3.1	0.6
42173	Cuban/Spanish/Portug Bread	1	pce	20	7	55	2	10	1	1	0.1	0.2	0.1
42157	Dinner Roll/Bun	1	ea	28	9	84	2	14	1	2	0.5	1	0.3
42160	Dinner Roll/Bun-Wheat	1	ea	36	13	98	3	17	1	2	0.5	1.1	0.4
42169	Dinner Roll—Bran	1	ea	28	10	76	3	14	1	2	0.2	0.6	0.6
42091	Egg Bread/Challah-Toasted	1	pce	37	10	116	4	19	1	2	0.6	1.1	0.4
42043	French/Vienna Bread	1	pce	25	9	68	2	13	1	1	0.2	0.3	0.2
42368	Garlic Bread-Frozen	1	pce	47		160	5	14	1	10	3	4	1.5
42184	Garlic Roll	1	ea	35	11	105	3	18	1	3	0.6	1.3	0.4
42020	Hamburger Bun	1	ea	43	15	123	4	22	1	2	0.5	0.4	1.1
42022	Hard Roll-White	1	ea	57	18	167	6	30	1	2	0.3	0.6	1
42021	Hotdog/Frankfurter Bun	1	ea	40	14	114	3	20	1	2	0.5	0.3	1
49012	Hush Puppies-Recipe	1	ea	22	6	74	2	10	1	3	0.5	0.7	1.6
42118	Indian Fry Bread	1	pce	90	24	296	6	48	2	9	2.1	3.6	2.3
42046	Italian Bread	1	pce	30	11	81	3	15	1	1	0.3	0.2	0.4
42185	Mexican Bolillo Roll	1	ea	117	43	307	10	61	2	2	0.4	0.2	0.6

< = Trace amount present   Blank = Not available

CHOL, cholesterol; **V**, vitamin; **THI**, thiamin; **RIB**, riboflavin; **NIA**, niacin; **FOL**, folate;
CALC, calcium; **PHOS**, phosphate; **SOD**, sodium; **POT**, potassium; **MAG**, magnesium

CHOL (mg)	V-A (RE)	THI (mg)	RIB (mg)	NIA (mg)	V-B6 (mg)	FOL (µg)	V-B12 (µg)	V-C (mg)	V-E (mg)	CALC (mg)	PHOS (mg)	SOD (mg)	POT (mg)	MAG (mg)	IRON (mg)	ZINC (mg)
0	49	0.1	0.1	0.5	0.1	11	0	3	0.3	31	41	3	515	26	0.9	0.1
0	20	0.1	<0.1	0.3	0.1	29	0	51	0.2	38	13	0	172	10	0.1	0.1
0	77	0.1	<0.1	0.1	0.1	17	0	26	0.3	12	8	1	132	10	0.1	0.2
0	56	0.1	<0.1	0.3	0.2	3	0	15	0.2	12	14	3	176	17	0.3	0.1
0	0	0.3	0.2	2.2	<0.1	64	0	<1	0.1	13	71	229	105	20	2.7	0.8
17	23	0.4	0.2	2.4	0.1	62	0.1	<1	1.9	9	60	358	48	18	2.8	0.5
0	<1	0.2	0.2	2.1	<0.1	58	0	<1	0.2	9	78	360	82	22	2.2	0.6
0	0	0.4	0.2	3.2	<0.1	62	0	0	1.9	53	68	379	72	21	2.5	0.6
0	0	0.2	0.1	2.9	0.2	33	0	<1	0.5	16	159	296	190	58	1.8	1.3
4	16	0.1	0.1	0.8	<0.1	3	0.1	<1	0.6	91	68	150	46	6	0.8	0.3
0	0	0.1	<0.1	0.7	<0.1	14	0	0	0.2	4	98	305	39	4	0.6	0.1
2	15	0.2	0.2	1.7	<0.1	30	0.1	<1	1.6	105	268	544	107	14	1.2	0.3
2	14	0.2	0.2	1.8	<0.1	37	<0.1	<1	2.7	141	98	348	73	11	1.7	0.3
2	14	0.1	0.1	2.2	0.1	13	0.1	<1	1.3	155	199	210	200	57	1.7	1.2
0	0	0.1	<0.1	0.4	<0.1	4	0	0	<0.1	50	72	324	37	7	0.4	0.2
49	69	0.1	0.2	1.2	<0.1	8	0.1	<1	0.7	80	74	171	49	7	1.3	0.3
0	71	0.1	0.1	1.3	0.1	11	0.1	<1	0.9	86	126	174	114	33	1.1	0.8
0	0	0.1	0.1	0.9	<0.1	6	0	0	0.1	16	21	117	22	5	0.6	0.2
26	72	0.1	0.1	0.9	0.1	20	0.1	1	1.1	13	35	181	80	8	0.8	0.2
<1	5	<0.1	0.1	0.5	<0.1	5	<0.1	0	0.3	32	50	284	143	28	0.9	0.2
20	9	0.2	0.2	1.9	<0.1	42	<0.1	0	0.3	37	42	197	46	8	1.2	0.3
37	26	0.1	0.2	1.2	0.1	33	0.1	<1	0.7	44	226	467	77	12	1.1	0.4
26	35	0.2	0.2	1.5	0.1	42	0.1	<1	0.6	162	110	428	96	16	1.6	0.4
0	0	0.1	0.1	0.9	0.1	15	<0.1	0	0.2	11	38	134	44	13	0.7	0.3
38	106	0.2	0.1	1.2	<0.1	35	0.1	<1	0.5	21	60	424	67	9	1.2	0.4
0	0	0.1	0.1	0.9	<0.1	6	0	0	<0.1	9	21	122	23	5	0.5	0.2
<1	0	0.1	0.1	1.1	<0.1	27	<0.1	<1	0.2	33	32	146	37	6	0.9	0.2
0	0	0.2	0.1	1.5	<0.1	18	0	0	0.4	63	37	122	41	13	1.3	0.3
0	<1	0.1	0.1	1.1	<0.1	18	0	<1	0.2	6	55	1	53	14	0.9	0.3
21	9	0.1	0.2	1.8	<0.1	33	<0.1	0	0.3	38	43	200	47	8	1.2	0.3
0	0	0.1	0.1	1.2	<0.1	24	0	0	0.1	19	26	152	28	7	0.6	0.2
30	0	0.2	0.1	1.6				0		0		250			3.6	
<1	0	0.2	0.1	1.4	<0.1	10	<0.1	<1	0.3	42	41	181	47	8	1.1	0.3
0	0	0.1	0.1	1.7	<0.1	41	<0.1	<1	0.7	60	38	241	61	9	1.4	0.3
0	0	0.3	0.2	2.4	<0.1	54	0	0	0.2	54	57	310	62	15	1.9	0.5
0	0	0.2	0.1	1.6	<0.1	38	<0.1	<1	0.6	56	35	224	56	8	1.3	0.2
10	9	0.1	0.1	0.6	<0.1	16	<0.1	<1	0.5	61	42	147	32	5	0.7	0.1
0	0	0.4	0.3	3.3	<0.1	67	0	0	1.7	210	141	626	67	14	3.2	0.4
0	0	0.1	0.1	1.3	<0.1	28	0	0	0.1	23	31	175	33	8	0.9	0.3
1	4	0.7	0.5	6.6	<0.1	41	<0.1	<1	0.1	14	90	7	98	22	3.8	0.8

ERA, EatRight Analysis CD-ROM; **AMT,** amount; **WT,** weight; **WTR,** water; **CAL,** calories; **PROT,** protein; **CARB,** carbohydrate; **FIBR,** fiber; **FAT,** fat; **SATF,** saturated fat; **MONO,** monosaturated fat; **POLY,** polyunsaturated fat

ERA CODE	FOOD DESCRIPTION	AMT	UNIT	WT (g)	WTR (g)	CAL (kcal)	PROT (g)	CARB (g)	FIBR (g)	FAT (g)	SATF (g)	MONO (g)	POLY (g)
Grains and Grain Products (continued)													
Breads and Rolls (continued)													
42047	Mixed Grain Bread-Slice	1	pce	26	10	65	3	12	2	1	0.2	0.4	0.2
42097	Multigrain Bread-LowCal	1	pce	23	10	46	2	10	3	1	0.1	0.1	0.3
42190	Pannetone-Italian Sweetbread	1	pce	27	8	87	2	15	1	2	1.2	0.7	0.2
42007	Pita Pocket Bread-White	1	ea	60	19	165	5	33	1	1	0.1	0.1	0.3
42080	Pita Pocket Bread-Whole Wheat	1	ea	64	20	170	6	35	5	2	0.3	0.2	0.7
42454	Pretzel-Soft	1	ea	138		390	12	84	3	1	0		
42456	Pretzel-Soft-Whole Wheat	1	ea	140		390	13	82	8	2	0		
42006	Pumpernickel Bread-Slice	1	pce	26	10	65	2	12	2	1	0.1	0.2	0.3
42051	Raisin Bread	1	pce	26	9	71	2	14	1	1	0.3	0.6	0.2
42005	Rye Bread	1	pce	32	12	83	3	15	2	1	0.2	0.4	0.3
42045	Sourdough Bread-Med Slice	1	pce	25	9	68	2	13	1	1	0.2	0.3	0.2
42034	Submarine Roll/Hoagie	1	ea	135	46	386	11	68	4	7	1.6	3.4	1.2
42013	Wheat Berry Bread	1	pce	25	9	65	2	12	1	1	0.2	0.4	0.2
42136	Wheat Bran Bread	1	pce	36	14	89	3	17	1	1	0.3	0.6	0.2
42012	Wheat Bread	1	pce	25	9	65	2	12	1	1	0.2	0.4	0.2
42095	Wheat Bread-LowCal	1	pce	23	10	46	2	10	3	1	0.1	0.1	0.2
42216	White Bread	1	pce	30	11	80	2	15	1	1	0.2	0.2	0.6
42084	White Bread-LowCal	1	pce	23	10	48	2	10	2	1	0.1	0.2	0.1
42014	Whole Wheat Bread	1	pce	28	11	69	3	13	2	1	0.3	0.5	0.3
42057	Whole Wheat Roll	1	ea	28.35	9	75	2	14	2	1	0.2	0.3	0.6
Bread Crumbs, Croutons, Stuffing													
42004	Bread Crumbs-Dry-Grated	1	cup	108	7	427	14	78	3	6	1.3	2.6	1.2
42144	Bread Crumbs-Seasoned-Dry	1	cup	120	7	440	17	84	5	3	0.9	1.2	0.8
42016	Croutons	1	cup	30	2	122	4	22	2	2	0.5	0.9	0.4
42148	Croutons-Seasoned	1	cup	40	1	186	4	25	2	7	2.1	3.8	0.9
42037	Stuffing Mix-Bread-Prep	0.5	cup	100		178	3	22	3	9	1.7	3.8	2.6
42147	Stuffing Mix-Cornbread-Prep	0.5	cup	100		179	3	22	3	9	1.8	3.9	2.7
Crackers													
43562	100% StoneWheat Crackers	3	ea	12	<1	53	1	8	1	2	0.4	1.1	0.3
43555	BetterCheddCrackers-LowSod	3	ea	3.9	<1	20	<1	2	<1	1	0.4	0.4	0.2
139	Butter Crackers (Club)	2	ea	8	<1	40	1	5	<1	2	0.3	0.9	0.8
43500	Cheese Crackers-Cheez-its	10	ea	10	<1	50	1	6	<1	3	0.9	1.2	0.2
43501	Cheese Crackers-PnutButter Filled	6	ea	42	2	202	5	24	1	10	2.3	4.9	2
43527	Graham Cracker-Chocolate	1	ea	14	<1	68	1	9	<1	3	1.9	1.1	0.1
43502	Graham Cracker-Plain	2	ea	14	1	59	1	11	<1	1	0.2	0.6	0.5
43534	Matzoh Crackers-Plain	1	ea	28.35	1	112	3	24	1	<1	0.1	<0.1	0.2
43509	Melba Toast-Plain	1	pce	5	<1	20	1	4	<1	<1	<0.1	<0.1	0.1
43507	Oyster Crackers	1	ea	1	<1	4	<1	1	<1	<1	<0.1	0.1	<0.1
43505	Oyster Crackers-crushed	1	cup	70	3	304	6	50	2	8	2.1	4.5	1.2
43543	Round Crackers (Ritz)	10	ea	30	1	151	2	18	<1	8	1.1	3.2	2.9
43541	Rye Crackers-Cheese Filled	6	ea	42	2	202	4	26	2	9	2.5	5.1	1.2
43532	Rye Crispbread	1	ea	10	1	37	1	8	2	<1	<0.1	<0.1	0.1
43506	Saltine Crackers	4	ea	12	<1	52	1	9	<1	1	0.4	0.8	0.2
43586	Saltine Crackers-UnsaltedTops	2	ea	6		25	1	4	0	<1	0	0	0

< = Trace amount present   Blank = Not available

CHOL, cholesterol; **V,** vitamin; **THI,** thiamin; **RIB,** riboflavin; **NIA,** niacin; **FOL,** folate;
CALC, calcium; **PHOS,** phosphate; **SOD,** sodium; **POT,** potassium; **MAG,** magnesium

CHOL (mg)	V-A (RE)	THI (mg)	RIB (mg)	NIA (mg)	V-B6 (mg)	FOL (µg)	V-B12 (µg)	V-C (mg)	V-E (mg)	CALC (mg)	PHOS (mg)	SOD (mg)	POT (mg)	MAG (mg)	IRON (mg)	ZINC (mg)
0	0	0.1	0.1	1.1	0.1	21	<0.1	<1	0.3	24	46	127	53	14	0.9	0.3
2	0	0.1	0.1	0.9	<0.1	14	0	0	<0.1	18	57	117	40	20	0.6	0.5
19	23	0.1	0.1	1	<0.1	19	0.1	<1	0.1	16	40	28	54	5	0.8	0.2
0	0	0.4	0.2	2.8	<0.1	57	0	0	0.4	52	58	322	72	16	1.6	0.5
0	0	0.2	0.1	1.8	0.2	22	0	0	0.6	10	115	340	109	44	2	1
0	0									40		1100			2.7	
0	0									40		1290			2.7	
0	0	0.1	0.1	0.8	<0.1	21	0	0	0.1	18	46	174	54	14	0.7	0.4
0	0	0.1	0.1	0.9	<0.1	23	0	<1	0.2	17	28	101	59	7	0.8	0.2
0	<1	0.1	0.1	1.2	<0.1	28	0	<1	0.2	23	40	211	53	13	0.9	0.4
0	0	0.1	0.1	1.2	<0.1	24	0	0	0.1	19	26	152	28	7	0.6	0.2
0	0	0.7	0.4	5.3	0.1	36	<0.1	0	0.6	188	119	756	190	27	4.3	0.8
0	0	0.1	0.1	1	<0.1	19	0	0	0.1	26	38	132	50	12	0.8	0.3
0	0	0.1	0.1	1.6	0.1	25	0	0	0.2	27	67	175	82	29	1.1	0.5
0	0	0.1	0.1	1	<0.1	19	0	0	0.1	26	38	132	50	12	0.8	0.3
0	0	0.1	0.1	0.9	<0.1	16	0	<1	<0.1	18	23	118	28	9	0.7	0.3
<1	0	0.1	0.1	1.2	<0.1	28	<0.1	0	0.1	32	28	161	36	7	0.9	0.2
0	<1	0.1	0.1	0.8	<0.1	22	0.1	<1	<0.1	22	28	104	17	5	0.7	0.3
0	0	0.1	0.1	1.1	0.1	14	<0.1	0	0.3	20	64	148	71	24	0.9	0.5
0	0	0.1	<0.1	1	0.1	9	0	0	0.4	30	64	136	77	24	0.7	0.6
0	<1	0.8	0.5	7.4	0.1	118	<0.1	0	1	245	159	931	239	50	6.6	1.3
1	2	0.2	0.2	3.3	0.2	131	<0.1	<1	0.2	119	160	3180	324	46	3.8	1.1
0	0	0.2	0.1	1.6	<0.1	40	0	0	0.2	23	34	209	37	9	1.2	0.3
3	4	0.2	0.2	1.9	<0.1	35	0.1	0	0.9	38	56	495	72	17	1.1	0.4
0	81	0.1	0.1	1.5	<0.1	101	<0.1	0	1.4	32	42	543	74	12	1.1	0.3
0	85	0.1	0.1	1.2	<0.1	97	<0.1	1	1.4	26	34	455	62	13	0.9	0.2
0	0	<0.1	<0.1	0.5	<0.1	3	0	0	0.5	6	35	79	36	12	0.4	0.3
1	1	<0.1	<0.1	0.2	<0.1	1	<0.1	0	<0.1	6	9	18	4	1	0.2	<0.1
0	0	<0.1	<0.1	0.3	<0.1	6	0	0	0.4	10	18	68	11	2	0.3	0.1
1	3	0.1	<0.1	0.5	0.1	8	<0.1	0	0.3	15	22	100	14	4	0.5	0.1
2	14	0.2	0.1	2.7	0.6	37	<0.1	<1	1.9	33	136	417	103	24	1.2	0.5
0	<1	<0.1	<0.1	0.3	<0.1	2	0	0	0.2	8	19	41	29	8	0.5	0.1
0	0	<0.1	<0.1	0.6	<0.1	8	0	0	0.3	3	15	85	19	4	0.5	0.1
0	0	0.1	0.1	1.1	<0.1	33	0	0	0.1	4	25	1	32	7	0.9	0.2
0	0	<0.1	<0.1	0.2	<0.1	6	0	0	<0.1	5	10	41	10	3	0.2	0.1
0	0	<0.1	<0.1	0.1	0	1	0	0	<0.1	1	1	13	1	<1	0.1	<0.1
0	0	0.4	0.3	3.7	<0.1	87	0	0	1.2	83	74	911	90	19	3.8	0.5
0	0	0.1	0.1	1.2	<0.1	23	0	0	1.4	36	68	254	40	8	1.1	0.2
4	16	0.3	0.2	1.5	<0.1	34	0.1	<1	0.8	93	142	438	144	16	1	0.3
0	0	<0.1	<0.1	0.1	<0.1	5	0	0	0.1	3	27	26	32	8	0.2	0.2
0	0	0.1	0.1	0.6	<0.1	15	0	0	0.2	14	13	156	15	3	0.6	0.1
0									0.1		50		5		0.4	

ERA, EatRight Analysis CD-ROM; AMT, amount; WT, weight; WTR, water; CAL, calories; PROT, protein; CARB, carbohydrate; FIBR, fiber; FAT, fat; SATF, saturated fat; MONO, monosaturated fat; POLY, polyunsaturated fat

ERA CODE	FOOD DESCRIPTION	AMT	UNIT	WT (g)	WTR (g)	CAL (kcal)	PROT (g)	CARB (g)	FIBR (g)	FAT (g)	SATF (g)	MONO (g)	POLY (g)
Grains and Grain Products (continued)													
Crackers (continued)													
43561	Saltines-Whole Wheat	3	ea	9	<1	39	1	6	1	1	0.3	0.7	0.2
43593	SnackWell FatFree WheatCrckr	7	ea	15	<1	60	2	12	1	<1	0.1	0.1	0.1
43595	SnackWell LowFatGoldenCrackr	1	ea	14	<1	58	1	11	<1	1	0.2	0.3	0.1
43508	Triscuits Whole Wheat Cracker	2	ea	8	<1	35	1	5	1	1	0.3	0.5	0.5
43547	Wheat Crackers	5	ea	10	<1	47	1	6	<1	2	0.5	1.1	0.3
43548	Wheat Crackers-Cheese Filled	6	ea	42	1	209	4	24	1	10	1.7	4.3	3.8
43564	Wheat Crackers-Thin	4	ea	8	<1	38	1	5	<1	2	0.3	0.9	0.2
43549	Wheat Crackers-PnutBtr Filled	1	ea	7	<1	35	1	4	<1	2	0.3	0.8	0.6
43554	WheatThin Crackers-LowSod	5	ea	10	<1	46	1	7	<1	2	0.6	0.7	0.4
Flours, Cooked Grains													
38030	All Purpose White Flour-Enrich	1	cup	125	15	455	13	95	3	1	0.2	0.1	0.5
38003	Barley-Pearled-Cooked	1	cup	157	108	193	4	44	6	1	0.1	0.1	0.3
38001	Barley-Whole-Cooked	1	cup	200	130	270	7	59	14	2	0.4	0.3	1.2
38171	Bread Flour-Enriched	0.25	cup	31		100	4	22	1	0	0	0	0
38028	Bulgar Wheat-Cooked	1	cup	182	142	151	6	34	8	<1	0.1	0.1	0.2
38039	Cake Flour-Baked Value	1	cup	109	14	394	9	85	2	1	0.1	0.1	0.4
38041	Cornmeal-Enrich-BakedValue	1	cup	138	16	505	12	107	10	2	0.3	0.6	1
30000	Cornstarch	1	Tbs	8	1	30	<1	7	<1	<1	0	<0.1	<0.1
38076	Couscous-Cooked	1	cup	157	114	176	6	36	2	<1	<0.1	<0.1	0.1
38044	Light Rye Flour-BakedValue	1	cup	102	9	374	9	82	15	1	0.1	0.2	0.6
38052	Millet-Cooked	0.5	cup	120	86	143	4	28	2	1	0.2	0.2	0.6
38078	Oat Bran-Cooked	1	cup	219	184	88	7	25	6	2	0.4	0.6	0.7
38064	Oat Bran-Dry	1	cup	94	6	231	16	62	14	7	1.2	2.2	2.6
38043	Rolled Oats-Baked Value	1	cup	80	7	307	13	54	8	5	0.9	1.6	1.8
38008	Rolled Oats-Dry	1	cup	81	7	311	13	54	9	5	0.9	1.6	1.9
38024	Wheat Bran-Crude	0.5	cup	29	3	63	5	19	12	1	0.2	0.2	0.6
38055	Wheat Germ-HoneyCrunch	1	cup	113	4	420	30	66	12	9	1.5	1.2	5.5
38026	Wheat Germ-Toasted	1	cup	113	6	432	33	56	15	12	2.1	1.7	7.5
38318	Wheat Flour-Unbleach-All Purpose	1	cup	125	15	455	13	95	3	1	0.2	0.1	0.5
38037	White Flour-Enr-Baked	1	cup	125	15	455	13	95	4	1	0.2	0.1	0.5
38032	Whole Wheat Flour	1	cup	120	12	407	16	87	15	2	0.4	0.3	0.9
38040	Whole Wheat Flour-Baked	1	cup	120	12	407	16	87	15	2	0.4	0.3	0.9
Granola and Cereal Bars, Diet and Energy Bars													
62729	Balance Bar-BananaCoconut	1	ea	50		190	14	21	1	6	3		
53227	Cereal Bar-Nutrigrain-MixBerry	100	g	100		370	4	73	2	8	1.5	5	1.1
23100	Granola Bar-Almond-Hard	1	ea	23.6	1	117	2	15	1	6	3	1.8	0.9
23105	Granola Bar-Choc Chip-Soft	1	ea	42.5	2	178	3	29	2	7	4.3	1.5	0.8
23108	Granola Bar-PeanutButter-Soft	1	ea	23.6	2	100	2	15	1	4	0.9	1.6	1
23059	Granola Bar-Plain-Hard	1	ea	24.5	1	115	2	16	1	5	0.6	1.1	3
23097	Granola Bar-Raisin-Soft	1	ea	42.5	3	190	3	28	2	8	4.1	1.2	1.4
23104	Granola Bar-Soft	1	ea	28.35	2	126	2	19	1	5	2.1	1.1	1.5
23065	Kudos Bar-Nutty Fudge	1	ea	28.35		120	1	20	1	4	2		
62206	Power Bar	1	ea	65		230	10	45	3	2			
62640	SlimFast NutriBar-DutchChoc	1	ea	34	3	140	5	20	2	5	2	1.5	1

< = Trace amount present   Blank = Not available

CHOL, cholesterol; **V,** vitamin; **THI,** thiamin; **RIB,** riboflavin; **NIA,** niacin; **FOL,** folate;
CALC, calcium; **PHOS,** phosphate; **SOD,** sodium; **POT,** potassium; **MAG,** magnesium

CHOL (mg)	V-A (RE)	THI (mg)	RIB (mg)	NIA (mg)	V-B6 (mg)	FOL (μg)	V-B12 (μg)	V-C (mg)	V-E (mg)	CALC (mg)	PHOS (mg)	SOD (mg)	POT (mg)	MAG (mg)	IRON (mg)	ZINC (mg)
0	0	<0.1	<0.1	0.5	<0.1	2	0	0	0.2	2	17	93	19	6	0.4	0.1
<1	<1	<0.1	0.1	0.7	<0.1			<0.1	0	28	61	169	43	7	0.6	0.2
<1	<1	0.1	0.1	0.7	<0.1			<0.1	<1	28	51	144	15	3	0.6	0.1
0	0	<0.1	<0.1	0.4	<0.1	2	0	0	0.3	4	24	53	24	8	0.2	0.2
0	0	0.1	<0.1	0.5	<0.1	4	0	0	0.4	5	22	80	18	6	0.4	0.2
3	4	0.2	0.2	1.3	0.1	27	0.1	1	0.3	86	160	383	128	23	1.1	0.4
0	0	<0.1	<0.1	0.4	<0.1	1	0	0	0.3	4	18	64	15	5	0.4	0.1
0	0	<0.1	<0.1	0.4	<0.1	5	0	0	<0.1	12	24	56	21	3	0.2	0.1
0	2	<0.1	<0.1	0.5	<0.1	3	0	0	0.1	3	19	25	22	5	0.4	0.1
0	0	1	0.6	7.4	0.1	192	0	0	1.7	19	135	2	134	28	5.8	0.9
0	2	0.1	0.1	3.2	0.2	25	0	0	0.3	17	85	5	146	35	2.1	1.3
0	0	0.2	0.1	2.8	0.2	16	0	0	3.1	26	230	1	230	44	2.1	1.6
0	0	0.2	0.1	1.6		40		0		0		0			1.4	
0	0	0.1	0.1	1.8	0.2	33	0	0	0.5	18	73	9	124	58	1.7	1
0	0	0.8	0.4	6.7	<0.1	118	0	0	0.2	15	93	2	114	17	8	0.7
0	57	0.8	0.5	6.3	0.3	181	0	0	3	7	116	4	224	55	5.7	1
0	0	0	0	0	0	0	0	0	0	<1	1	1	<1	<1	<0.1	<0.1
0	0	0.1	<0.1	1.5	0.1	24	0	0	<0.1	13	35	8	91	13	0.6	0.4
0	0	0.3	0.1	0.7	0.2	16	0	0	0.9	21	198	2	238	71	1.8	1.8
0	0	0.1	0.1	1.6	0.1	23	0	0	0.7	4	120	2	74	53	0.8	1.1
0	0	0.3	0.1	0.3	0.1	13	0	0	0.5	22	261	2	201	88	1.9	1.2
0	0	1.1	0.2	0.9	0.2	49	0	0	2	55	690	4	532	221	5.1	2.9
0	8	0.5	0.1	0.6	0.1	18	0	0	0.9	42	379	3	280	118	3.4	2.5
0	8	0.6	0.1	0.6	0.1	26	0	0	0.6	42	384	3	284	120	3.4	2.5
0	0	0.2	0.2	3.9	0.4	23	0	0	2.6	21	294	1	343	177	3.1	2.1
0	11	1.5	0.8	5.3	0.6	376	0	0	31	56	1142	12	1089	307	9.1	15.7
0	0	1.9	0.9	6.3	1.1	398	0	7	33.6	51	1294	5	1070	362	10.3	18.8
0	0	1	0.6	7.4	0.1	192	0	0	1.7	19	135	2	134	28	5.8	0.9
0	0	0.8	0.6	6.6	0.1	135	0	0	1.7	19	135	2	134	28	5.8	0.9
0	0	0.5	0.3	7.6	0.4	53	0	0	2.8	41	415	6	486	166	4.7	3.5
0	0	0.4	0.2	6.9	0.4	37	0	0	2.8	41	415	6	486	166	4.7	3.5
5	500	0.5	0.6	4	0.6	80	1.8	60	42	200	200	150	105	16	3.6	5.2
0	405	1	1.1	13.5	1.4	108	0	0	0	39	98	297	188	26	4.9	4.1
0	1	0.1	<0.1	0.1	<0.1	3	0	0	0.4	8	54	60	64	19	0.6	0.4
<1	2	0.1	0.1	0.4	<0.1	9	0.1	0	0.4	40	98	116	144	33	1.1	0.6
<1	<1	0.1	<0.1	0.7	<0.1	8	<0.1	0	0.3	21	59	97	69	20	0.5	0.4
0	4	0.1	<0.1	0.4	<0.1	6	0	<1	0.3	15	68	72	82	24	0.7	0.5
<1	0	0.1	0.1	0.5	<0.1	9	0.1	0	0.5	43	94	120	154	31	1	0.6
<1	0	0.1	<0.1	0.1	<0.1	7	0.1	0	0.3	30	65	79	92	21	0.7	0.4
0	20							1		200		75		8	0.4	
0		1.5	1.7	20	2	400	6	60		300	350	110	150	140	5.4	5.2
	375	0.4	0.4	5	0.4	40	1.5	15	5	40	40	80	150	16	4.5	3.7

ERA, EatRight Analysis CD-ROM; AMT, amount; WT, weight; WTR, water; CAL, calories; PROT, protein; CARB, carbohydrate; FIBR, fiber; FAT, fat; SATF, saturated fat; MONO, monosaturated fat; POLY, polyunsaturated fat

ERA CODE	FOOD DESCRIPTION	AMT	UNIT	WT (g)	WTR (g)	CAL (kcal)	PROT (g)	CARB (g)	FIBR (g)	FAT (g)	SATF (g)	MONO (g)	POLY (g)
Grains and Grain Products (continued)													
Granola and Cereal Bars, Diet and Energy Bars (continued)													
62205	Tiger Sport Bar	1	ea	65.2		230	11	40	4	2			
62643	UltrSlmFstBar-ChwyCarmlCrnch	1	ea	28.35	2	110	0	20	2	3	2.5		
62641	UltrSlmFstBar-PntCarmlCrnch	1	ea	28.35	2	120	1	22	1	3	1.7	0.9	0.4
Muffins													
44520	Blueberry Muffin-made w/2% Milk	1	ea	57	23	162	4	23	1	6	1.2	1.5	3.1
44528	Bran Muffin-made w/2% Milk	1	ea	57	20	161	4	24	2	7	1.3	1.7	3.6
44530	Chocolate Chip Muffin	1	ea	58	19	188	4	27	1	7	2.4	2.9	1.6
44524	Corn Muffin-made w/2%Milk	1	ea	57	19	180	4	25	2	7	1.3	1.7	3.5
42059	English Muffin	1	ea	57	24	134	4	26	2	1	0.1	0.2	0.5
42082	English Muffin-100% Wheat	1	ea	66	30	134	6	27	4	1	0.2	0.3	0.6
42214	English Muffin-Cheese	1	ea	63	26	153	5	28	2	2	0.8	0.5	0.6
42060	English Muffin-Sourdough	1	ea	56	24	132	4	26	2	1	0.1	0.2	0.5
44515	Muffin-Plain-made w/2% Milk	1	ea	57	21	169	4	24	2	6	1.2	1.6	3.3
44514	Oat Bran Muffin	1	ea	57	20	154	4	28	3	4	0.6	1	2.4
42017	Popover-Recipe-Whole Milk	1	ea	40	22	90	3	11	<1	3	1.1	1	1
44522	Toasted Muffin-Corn	1	ea	33	8	114	2	19	1	4	0.6	0.9	2.1
44518	Toaster Muffin-Blueberry	1	ea	33	10	103	2	18	1	3	0.5	0.7	1.8
44531	Whole Wheat Muffin	1	ea	47	16	140	4	20	2	6	1.3	2.3	1.6
44536	Zucchini Muffin w/Nuts	1	ea	58	16	219	3	27	1	11	1.5	3.4	5.3
Pancakes, French Toast, and Waffles													
45006	Crepe-Pancake-No Filling	1	ea	102	58	230	9	22	1	11	3.2	4.6	2.6
42156	French Toast-Rec w/2%Milk	1	pce	65	36	149	5	16	1	7	1.8	2.9	1.7
45023	Pancake-Blueberry-Recipe	1	ea	38	20	84	2	11	<1	3	0.8	0.9	1.6
45025	Pancake-Buttermilk-Recipe	1	ea	38	20	86	3	11	<1	4	0.7	0.9	1.7
45044	Pancake-Chinese	1	ea	28	14	58	1	13	<1	<1	<0.1	<0.1	<0.1
45067	Pancake-Frozen-Heated-6in	1	ea	73	33	167	4	32	1	2	0.6	0.9	0.7
45002	Pancake-Mix-Prepared	1	ea	38	20	74	2	14	<1	1	0.2	0.3	0.3
45001	Pancake-Plain-Recipe	1	ea	38	20	86	2	11	1	4	0.8	0.9	1.7
45008	Pancake-Whole Wheat	1	ea	44	23	92	4	13	1	3	0.8	0.8	1.1
45036	Rye Pancakes-4 inch	1	ea	21	7	63	1	10	1	2	0.5	0.9	0.6
45035	Sourdough Pancakes-4 inch	1	ea	21	11	46	1	7	<1	1	0.3	0.4	0.6
45038	Waffle-Blueberry-Round	1	ea	75	35	178	4	28	2	5	0.9	2.1	1.8
45093	Waffle-Buttermilk-Eggo	1	ea	39		110	2	15	0	4	0.8		
45005	Waffle-Frozen-Toasted	1	ea	33	14	87	2	13	1	3	0.5	1.1	0.9
45003	Waffles-From Recipe	1	ea	75	32	218	6	25	1	11	2.1	2.6	5.1
45017	Waffle-Whole Grain-Frozen	1	ea	39	17	105	4	13	1	4	1.2	1.8	1.1
Pasta													
38048	Chow Mein Noodles-Dry	1	cup	45	<1	237	4	26	2	14	2	3.5	7.8
38047	Egg Noodles-Enr-Cooked	1	cup	160	110	213	8	40	2	2	0.5	0.7	0.7
38103	Lasagna-Noodles-Cooked	2	ea	110	73	155	5	31	1	1	0.1	0.1	0.3
38119	Linguini Noodles-Cooked	1	cup	140	92	197	7	40	2	1	0.1	0.1	0.4
38102	Macaroni-Enriched-Cooked	1	cup	140	92	197	7	40	2	1	0.1	0.1	0.4
38150	Noodle Roni-Prepared	1	cup	165	111	247	8	40	2	6	1.2	2.5	1.7

< = Trace amount present   Blank = Not available

CHOL, cholesterol; **V,** vitamin; **THI,** thiamin; **RIB,** riboflavin; **NIA,** niacin; **FOL,** folate;
CALC, calcium; **PHOS,** phosphate; **SOD,** sodium; **POT,** potassium; **MAG,** magnesium

CHOL (mg)	V-A (RE)	THI (mg)	RIB (mg)	NIA (mg)	V-B6 (mg)	FOL (µg)	V-B12 (µg)	V-C (mg)	V-E (mg)	CALC (mg)	PHOS (mg)	SOD (mg)	POT (mg)	MAG (mg)	IRON (mg)	ZINC (mg)
	50	1.5	1.7	20	2	400	6	60	20	350	400	100	280	140	4.5	
5	225	<0.1	0.3	3	0.3	60	0.9	60	20.1	250	150	45			2.7	0.6
5	15	0.2	0.3	3	0.3	60	0.9	6	3	150	150	35			2.7	0.6
21	22	0.2	0.2	1.3	<0.1	27	0.1	1	1	108	83	251	70	9	1.3	0.3
19	142	0.2	0.3	2.3	0.2	30	0.1	4	1.3	106	162	335	181	44	2.4	1.6
23	21	0.2	0.2	1.4	<0.1	7	0.1	<1	0.7	91	87	117	92	16	1.5	0.4
24	29	0.2	0.2	1.4	0.1	35	0.1	<1	1	148	101	333	83	13	1.5	0.3
0	0	0.3	0.2	2.2	<0.1	46	<0.1	0	0.8	99	76	264	75	12	1.4	0.4
0	0	0.2	0.1	2.2	0.1	32	0	0	0.5	175	186	420	139	47	1.6	1.1
3	9	0.3	0.2	2.3	<0.1	23	<0.1	<1	0.1	127	96	297	82	13	1.5	0.5
0	0	0.2	0.2	2.2	<0.1	45	<0.1	0	0.8	97	74	260	73	12	1.4	0.4
22	23	0.2	0.2	1.3	<0.1	29	0.1	<1	1	114	87	266	69	10	1.4	0.3
0	0	0.1	0.1	0.2	0.1	30	<0.1	0	1.2	36	214	224	289	89	2.4	1
47	28	0.1	0.1	0.7	<0.1	7	0.1	<1	0.2	37	56	82	64	7	0.8	0.3
4	7	0.1	0.1	0.8	<0.1	19	<0.1	0	0.5	6	50	142	30	5	0.5	0.1
2	22	0.1	0.1	0.7	<0.1	18	<0.1	0	0.6	4	19	158	27	4	0.2	0.1
20	18	0.1	0.1	1.2	0.1	9	0.1	<1	0.9	102	122	140	119	31	1	0.7
38	22	0.1	0.1	1	<0.1	9	0.1	1	2	39	48	113	66	8	1.2	0.3
161	99	0.2	0.4	1.3	0.1	19	0.5	<1	1.3	94	148	77	162	17	1.6	0.8
75	86	0.1	0.2	1.1	<0.1	28	0.2	<1	0.7	65	76	311	87	11	1.1	0.4
21	19	0.1	0.1	0.6	<0.1	14	0.1	1	0.4	78	57	156	52	6	0.7	0.2
22	11	0.1	0.1	0.6	<0.1	14	0.1	<1	0.5	60	53	198	55	6	0.6	0.2
0	0	<0.1	<0.1	0.3	<0.1	1	0	0	<0.1	5	18	1	18	4	0.1	0.2
7	21	0.3	0.3	2.9	0.1	36	0.1	<1	0.5	45	272	372	53	10	2.5	0.5
5	3	0.1	0.1	0.6	<0.1	14	0.1	<1	0.4	48	127	239	66	8	0.6	0.1
22	21	0.1	0.1	0.6	<0.1	14	0.1	<1	0.4	83	60	167	50	6	0.7	0.2
27	28	0.1	0.2	1	<0.1	13	0.1	<1	1.3	110	164	252	123	20	1.4	0.5
8	4	<0.1	<0.1	0.3	<0.1	2	<0.1	<1	0.3	22	25	58	97	15	0.5	0.2
8	4	0.1	0.1	0.6	<0.1	7	<0.1	0	0.3	3	16	53	17	3	0.5	0.1
15	235	0.3	0.3	2.9	0.6	23	1.6	2	0.7	150	271	506	96	15	2.9	0.4
12	150	0.2	0.2	2	0.2	40	0.6	0		20		240	32		1.8	
8	120	0.1	0.2	1.5	0.3	15	0.8	0	0.3	77	139	260	42	7	1.5	0.2
52	49	0.2	0.3	1.6	<0.1	34	0.2	<1	2.2	191	142	383	119	14	1.7	0.5
37	30	0.1	0.1	0.8	<0.1	7	0.2	<1	0.6	102	95	132	90	16	0.8	0.4
0	4	0.3	0.2	2.7	<0.1	40	0	0	9	9	72	198	54	23	2.1	0.6
53	10	0.3	0.1	2.4	0.1	102	0.1	0	0.1	19	110	11	45	30	2.5	1
0	0	0.2	0.1	1.8	<0.1	77	0	0	<0.1	8	59	1	34	20	1.5	0.6
0	0	0.3	0.1	2.3	<0.1	98	0	0	0.1	10	76	1	43	25	2	0.7
0	0	0.3	0.1	2.3	<0.1	98	0	0	<0.1	10	76	1	43	25	2	0.7
53	47	0.3	0.1	2.4	0.1	11	0.1	<1	0.6	21	112	56	47	31	2.5	1

ERA, EatRight Analysis CD-ROM; **AMT**, amount; **WT**, weight; **WTR**, water; **CAL**, calories; **PROT**, protein; **CARB**, carbohydrate; **FIBR**, fiber; **FAT**, fat; **SATF**, saturated fat; **MONO**, monosaturated fat; **POLY**, polyunsaturated fat

ERA CODE	FOOD DESCRIPTION	AMT	UNIT	WT (g)	WTR (g)	CAL (kcal)	PROT (g)	CARB (g)	FIBR (g)	FAT (g)	SATF (g)	MONO (g)	POLY (g)
Grains and Grain Products (continued)													
Pasta (continued)													
57319	Noodles&Sce-Romanoff (Lipton)	0.66	cup	65		260	9	41	2	7	3.5		
57323	Pasta&Sc-CreamBrocc (Lipton)	0.66	cup	69		260	8	45	1	6	2.5		
38092	Pasta/Noodles-Fresh-Cooked	2	oz	57	39	75	3	14	1	1	0.1	0.1	0.2
38067	Ramen Noodles-Cooked	1	cup	227	195	154	3	20	1	7	1.7	1.2	3.3
38147	Rice Noodles-Cooked	1	cup	160	127	135	<1	33	<1	<1	<0.1	<0.1	<0.1
38104	Rotini Noodles-Cooked	1	cup	140	92	197	7	40	2	1	0.1	0.1	0.4
38109	Shells Pasta-Jumbo—Cooked	2	ea	46	30	65	2	13	1	<1	<0.1	<0.1	0.1
38105	Shells Pasta-Small-Cooked	1	cup	115	76	162	5	33	1	1	0.1	0.1	0.3
38113	Shells Pasta-WhlWheat-Cooked	1	cup	140	94	174	7	37	4	1	0.1	0.1	0.3
38118	Spaghetti Noodles-Enr-Cooked	1	cup	140	92	197	7	40	2	1	0.1	0.1	0.4
38121	SpagNoodles-Enr-Ckd+Salt	1	cup	140	92	197	7	40	2	1	0.1	0.1	0.4
38066	SpagNoodles-Spinach-Cooked	1	cup	140	95	182	6	37	5	1	0.1	0.1	0.4
38060	SpagNoodles-WhlWheat-Cooked	1	cup	140	94	174	7	37	6	1	0.1	0.1	0.3
56129	Spinach Tortellini	1	cup	122	75	232	12	25	1	9	3.3	3.4	1.3
Rice													
38010	Brown Rice-Long Grain-Cooked	1	cup	195	142	216	5	45	4	2	0.4	0.6	0.6
38082	Brown Rice-Med Grain-Cooked	0.5	cup	97.5	71	109	2	23	2	1	0.2	0.3	0.3
38145	Fried Rice-Meatless	1	cup	166	112	271	5	34	1	12	1.8	3.2	6.7
38083	Glutinous Sticky Rice-Ckd	1	cup	174	133	169	4	37	2	<1	0.1	0.1	0.1
56316	Rice Pilaf	1	cup	206	149	261	4	45	1	7	1.3	3.2	1.9
57360	Rice&Sauce-Oriental (Lipton)	0.5	cup	59		230	6	46	1	1	0		
57337	Rice&Sauce-Original (Lipton)	0.5	cup	63		250	7	51	2	1	0		
57355	Rice-Saute-HerbButr (Lipton)	0.5	cup	60		240	6	42	1	5	2		
57341	Rice-Saute-Oriental (Lipton)	0.5	cup	61		240	6	43	1	4	1.5		
56131	Spanish Rice	1	cup	243	190	216	5	42	3	4	0.6	1.5	1.4
38013	White Rice-LongGrain-Cooked	1	cup	158	108	205	4	44	1	<1	0.1	0.1	0.1
38019	White Rice-LongGrain-Inst-Ckd	1	cup	165	126	162	3	35	1	<1	0.1	0.1	0.1
38097	White Rice-MedGrain-Cooked	1	cup	186	128	242	4	53	1	<1	0.1	0.1	0.1
38021	Wild Rice-Cooked	1	cup	164	121	166	7	35	3	1	0.1	0.1	0.3
Tortillas and Taco/Tostada Shells													
42027	Taco Shell-Corn	1	ea	13.6	1	64	1	8	1	3	0.5	1.3	1.2
42023	Tortilla-Corn-Enr-Reg-6 inch	1	ea	26	11	58	1	12	1	1	0.1	0.2	0.3
42011	Edible Bowl-Corn-6.25 inch	1	ea	44		165	5	25	0	5	3		
42025	Tortilla-Flour-8 inch	1	ea	72	19	234	6	40	2	5	1.3	2.7	0.8
42079	Tortilla-Whole Wheat	1	ea	35	11	73	3	20	2	<1	0.1	0.1	0.2
Infant Foods													
60616	BabyFd Cereal-Rice+MixFruit	1	Tbs	15	12	12	<1	3	<1	<1	<0.1	<0.1	<0.1
60491	Beef Stew-Toddler	1	Tbs	16	14	8	1	1	<1	<1	0.1	0.1	<0.1
60660	BabyFd Vegetable+Beef	1	Tbs	16	14	10	<1	1	<1	<1	0.1	0.1	<0.1
60638	BabyFd Turkey Meat Sticks	10	ea	100		182	14	1	<1	14	4.1	4.7	3.6
60500	BabyFd Carrots	1	Tbs	14	13	4	<1	1	<1	<1	<0.1	<0.1	<0.1
60632	BabyFd Sweet Potatoes	1	Tbs	14	12	8	<1	2	<1	<1	<0.1	0	<0.1
60309	Similac Infant Formula	0.46	cup	114		100	3	10		5			

< = Trace amount present   Blank = Not available

CHOL, cholesterol; **V,** vitamin; **THI,** thiamin; **RIB,** riboflavin; **NIA,** niacin; **FOL,** folate; **CALC,** calcium; **PHOS,** phosphate; **SOD,** sodium; **POT,** potassium; **MAG,** magnesium

CHOL (mg)	V-A (RE)	THI (mg)	RIB (mg)	NIA (mg)	V-B6 (mg)	FOL (μg)	V-B12 (μg)	V-C (mg)	V-E (mg)	CALC (mg)	PHOS (mg)	SOD (mg)	POT (mg)	MAG (mg)	IRON (mg)	ZINC (mg)
70	20							0		60		920			2.7	
10	20							0		40		840			2.7	
19	3	0.1	0.1	0.6	<0.1	36	0.1	0	0.1	3	36	3	14	10	0.6	0.3
<1	2	<0.1	<0.1	0.3	<0.1	3	<0.1	<1	2.3	13	24	802	49	10	0.4	0.2
0	0	<0.1	0	0.1	<0.1	<1	0	0	<0.1	11	11	7	3	2	0.7	0.2
0	0	0.3	0.1	2.3	<0.1	98	0	0	<0.1	10	76	1	43	25	2	0.7
0	0	0.1	<0.1	0.8	<0.1	32	0	0	<0.1	3	25	<1	14	8	0.6	0.2
0	0	0.2	0.1	1.9	<0.1	80	0	0	<0.1	8	62	1	36	21	1.6	0.6
0	0	0.2	0.1	1	0.1	7	0	0	0.1	21	125	4	62	42	1.5	1.1
0	0	0.3	0.1	2.3	<0.1	98	0	0	0.1	10	76	1	43	25	2	0.7
0	0	0.3	0.1	2.3	<0.1	98	0	0	0.4	10	76	140	43	25	2	0.7
0	21	0.1	0.1	2.1	0.1	17	0	0	0.1	42	151	20	81	87	1.5	1.5
0	0	0.2	0.1	1	0.1	7	0	0	1.2	21	125	4	62	42	1.5	1.1
158	183	0.2	0.4	1.8	0.1	35	0.5	1	0.9	143	168	252	138	24	2.4	1
0	0	0.2	<0.1	3	0.3	8	0	0	1.4	20	162	10	84	84	0.8	1.2
0	0	0.1	<0.1	1.3	0.1	4	0	0	0.6	10	75	1	77	43	0.5	0.6
43	21	0.2	0.1	2.2	0.1	22	0.1	4	2.5	28	89	261	128	23	1.9	0.9
0	0	<0.1	<0.1	0.5	<0.1	2	0	0	0.2	3	14	9	17	9	0.2	0.7
0	64	0.3	<0.1	2.5	0.1	8	<0.1	1	1.1	25	76	151	111	19	2.3	0.8
2	0							0		0		750			1.8	
0	0							1		20		890			1.8	
2	0							0		0		870			1.1	
0	0							1		0		910			1.1	
0	115	0.2	0.1	3	0.3	20	0	37	1.4	77	90	295	537	39	2.4	0.9
0	0	0.3	<0.1	2.3	0.1	92	0	0	0.3	16	68	2	55	19	1.9	0.8
0	0	0.1	0.1	1.5	<0.1	68	0	0	0.2	13	23	5	7	8	1	0.4
0	0	0.3	<0.1	3.4	0.1	108	0	0	0.3	6	69	0	54	24	2.8	0.8
0	0	0.1	0.1	2.1	0.2	43	0	0	0.5	5	134	5	166	52	1	2.2
0	5	<0.1	<0.1	0.2	0.1	1	0	0	0.4	22	34	50	24	14	0.3	0.2
0	0	<0.1	<0.1	0.4	0.1	30	0	0	0.3	46	82	42	40	17	0.4	0.2
0	0	0.2	0.1			114			0				52			
0	0	0.4	0.2	2.6	<0.1	89	0	0	1.3	90	89	344	94	19	2.4	0.5
0	0	0.1	<0.1	0.9	0.1	8	0	0	0.4	10	82	171	82	26	0.7	0.5
0	<1	<0.1	<0.1	0.3	<0.1	<1	<0.1	1	<0.1	2	3	2	8	1	0.4	<0.1
2	40	<0.1	<0.1	0.2	<0.1	1	0.1	<1	<0.1	1	7	55	23	2	0.1	0.1
1	41	<0.1	<0.1	0.1	<0.1	1	<0.1	<1	<0.1	2	6	12	20	2	0.1	0.1
65	6	<0.1	0.2	1.8	0.1	11	1	2	0.4	72	103	483	91	16	1.2	1.8
0	165	<0.1	<0.1	0.1	<0.1	2	0	1	0.1	3	3	7	28	2	0.1	<0.1
0	93	<0.1	<0.1	0.1	<0.1	1	0	1	0.1	2	3	3	34	2	0.1	<0.1
	90	0.1	0.2	1	0.1	15	0.2	9	2	90	70	34	132	7	0.2	0.8

ERA, EatRight Analysis CD-ROM; **AMT**, amount; **WT**, weight; **WTR**, water; **CAL**, calories; **PROT**, protein; **CARB**, carbohydrate; **FIBR**, fiber; **FAT**, fat; **SATF**, saturated fat; **MONO**, monosaturated fat; **POLY**, polyunsaturated fat

ERA CODE	FOOD DESCRIPTION	AMT	UNIT	WT (g)	WTR (g)	CAL (kcal)	PROT (g)	CARB (g)	FIBR (g)	FAT (g)	SATF (g)	MONO (g)	POLY (g)
Juices: Fruit, Vegetable, Blends													
3008	Apple Juice-Canned/Bottled	1	cup	248	218	116	<1	29	<1	<1	<0.1	<0.1	0.1
3010	Apple Juice-FrznConc+Water	1	cup	239	210	112	<1	28	<1	<1	<0.1	<0.1	0.1
3015	Apricot Nectar-Canned	1	cup	251	213	140	1	36	2	<1	<0.1	0.1	<0.1
5226	Carrot Juice-Canned	1	cup	236	210	94	2	22	2	<1	0.1	<0.1	0.2
20042	Clam and Tomato Juice	1	cup	242	211	116	1	26	<1	3	0.1	<0.1	<0.1
3042	Cranberry Juice Cocktail	1	cup	253	216	144	0	36	<1	<1	<0.1	<0.1	0.1
3276	CranberryJce Cocktail-LowCal	1	cup	237	226	45	0	11	0	0	0	0	0
3062	Grape Juice-Canned/Bottled	1	cup	253	213	154	1	38	<1	<1	0.1	<0.1	0.1
3064	Grape Juice-FrznConc+Water	1	cup	250	217	128	<1	32	<1	<1	0.1	<0.1	0.1
3052	Grapefruit Juice-Canned	1	cup	247	222	94	1	22	<1	<1	<0.1	<0.1	0.1
3053	Grapefruit Juice-FrznConc+Water	1	cup	247	220	101	1	24	<1	<1	<0.1	<0.1	0.1
3304	Guava Nectar	1	cup	250	211	149	<1	38	2	<1	0.1	<0.1	0.1
3069	Lemon Juice-Bottled	1	cup	244	226	51	1	16	1	1	0.1	<0.1	0.2
3073	Lime Juice-bottled	1	cup	246	228	52	1	16	1	1	0.1	0.1	0.2
3303	Mango Nectar	1	cup	250	211	146	1	38	2	<1	0.1	0.1	0.1
3046	Orange Juice+Calcium	1	cup	247.2		110	2	26	0	0	0	0	0
3092	Orange Juice-Chilled	1	cup	249	220	110	2	25	<1	1	0.1	0.1	0.2
3090	Orange Juice-Fresh	1	cup	248	219	112	2	26	<1	<1	0.1	0.1	0.1
3091	Orange Juice-FrznConc+Water	1	cup	249	219	112	2	27	<1	<1	<0.1	<0.1	<0.1
3226	Orange Strawberry Banana Juice	1	cup	247.2		110	1	27	0	0	0	0	0
3095	Papaya Nectar-Canned	1	cup	250	212	142	<1	36	2	<1	0.1	0.1	0.1
3120	Pineapple Juice-Canned-Unswt	1	cup	250	214	140	1	34	<1	<1	<0.1	<0.1	0.1
3128	Prune Juice-Bottled	1	cup	256	208	182	2	45	3	<1	<0.1	0.1	<0.1
3102	Tangerine Orange Juice	1	cup	247.2		110	2	25	0	0	0	0	0
5397	Tomato Juice-Canned-LowSod	1	cup	243	228	41	2	10	2	<1	<0.1	<0.1	0.1
5188	Tomato Juice-Canned-Regular	1	cup	243	228	41	2	10	1	<1	<0.1	<0.1	0.1
20080	V-8 Juice-LowSodium	1	cup	242	226	46	2	11	2	<1	<0.1	<0.1	0.1
Meals, Entrees, and Mixed Dishes													
Canned Meals, Entrees, and Dishes													
7040	Baked Beans w/Pork-Canned	1	cup	253	181	268	13	51	14	4	1.5	1.7	0.5
7037	Baked Beans-Homemade	1	cup	253	165	382	14	54	14	13	4.9	5.4	1.9
7038	Baked Beans-Vegetarian-Cnd	0.5	cup	127	92	118	6	26	6	1	0.1	<0.1	0.2
56092	Chicken Chow Mein-Canned	1	cup	250	222	95	6	18	2	1	0	0.1	0.8
7004	Pork & Beans+TomatoSc-Can	1	cup	253	184	248	13	49	12	3	1	1.1	0.3
56096	Spaghetti+Sauce+Cheese-Can	1	cup	250	200	190	6	38	2	2	0	0.4	0.5
Frozen Meals, Entrees, and Dishes													
16234	Beef Pot Pie-Banquet	1	ea	198		330	9	38	3	15	7		
70734	Beef Pot Pie-Swansons	1	ea	198		415	11	41	2	23	9		
11094	Beef Pot Roast-LeanCuisine	1	ea	255		206	17	22	4	5	1.3	2.3	0.8
11118	Beef Pot Roast Din-HealthyChoice	1	ea	312		300	20	41	8	6	2		
56737	Cheese Cannelloni-LeanCuisine	1	ea	259		270	21	28	3	8	3.5	1.5	0.5
56901	Cheese Ravioli-LeanCuisine	1	ea	241		250	12	32	4	8	3	2	1
15964	Chicken Chow Mein+Rice-LnCuis	1	ea	255		210	13	28	2	5	1	2	1
15967	Chicken Parmesan-LeanCuisine	1	ea	308		220	22	22	5	5	1.5	1.5	1

< = Trace amount present   Blank = Not available

CHOL, cholesterol; **V,** vitamin; **THI,** thiamin; **RIB,** riboflavin; **NIA,** niacin; **FOL,** folate;
CALC, calcium; **PHOS,** phosphate; **SOD,** sodium; **POT,** potassium; **MAG,** magnesium

CHOL (mg)	V-A (RE)	THI (mg)	RIB (mg)	NIA (mg)	V-B6 (mg)	FOL (µg)	V-B12 (µg)	V-C (mg)	V-E (mg)	CALC (mg)	PHOS (mg)	SOD (mg)	POT (mg)	MAG (mg)	IRON (mg)	ZINC (mg)
0	<1	0.1	<0.1	0.2	0.1	<1	0	2	<0.1	17	17	7	295	7	0.9	0.1
0	0	<0.1	<0.1	0.1	0.1	1	0	1	<0.1	14	17	17	301	12	0.6	0.1
0	331	<0.1	<0.1	0.7	0.1	3	0	2	0.7	18	23	8	286	13	1	0.2
0	2584	0.2	0.1	0.9	0.5	9	0	20	1	57	99	68	689	33	1.1	0.4
0	53	0.1	0.1	0.5	0.2	38	73.9	10	1.2	29	188	874	217	53	1.4	2.6
0	1	<0.1	<0.1	0.1	<0.1	1	0	90	0	8	5	5	46	5	0.4	0.2
0	1	<0.1	<0.1	0.1	<0.1	<1	0	76	0	21	2	7	52	5	0.1	<0.1
0	3	0.1	0.1	0.7	0.2	7	0	<1	0	23	28	8	334	25	0.6	0.1
0	2	<0.1	0.1	0.3	0.1	3	0	60	0.1	10	10	5	52	10	0.2	0.1
0	2	0.1	<0.1	0.6	<0.1	26	0	72	0.4	17	27	2	378	25	0.5	0.2
0	2	0.1	0.1	0.5	0.1	9	0	83	0.4	20	35	2	336	27	0.3	0.1
0	21	<0.1	<0.1	0.4	<0.1	3	0	47	0.4	11	10	7	93	5	0.2	0.1
0	5	0.1	<0.1	0.5	0.1	25	0	61	0.5	27	22	51	249	20	0.3	0.1
0	5	0.1	<0.1	0.4	0.1	19	0	16	0.2	30	25	39	184	17	0.6	0.1
0	292	<0.1	0.1	0.5	0.1	7	0	19	1.1	12	11	6	141	10	0.2	0.1
0	0	0.2		0.8	0.1	60		108	0	350		0	450		0	
0	20	0.3	0.1	0.7	0.1	45	0	82	0.5	25	27	2	473	27	0.4	0.1
0	50	0.2	0.1	1	0.1	75	0	124	0.5	27	42	2	496	27	0.5	0.1
0	20	0.2	<0.1	0.5	0.1	109	0	97	0.5	22	40	2	473	25	0.2	0.1
0	0	0		0	0	0		6	0	20		5	380		0	
0	28	<0.1	<0.1	0.4	<0.1	5	0	8	0.1	25	0	12	78	8	0.9	0.4
0	1	0.1	0.1	0.6	0.2	58	0	27	0.1	42	20	2	335	32	0.6	0.3
0	1	<0.1	0.2	2	0.6	1	0	10	0.4	31	64	10	706	36	3	0.5
0	0	0.2		0.8	0.1	60		27	0	20		0	450		0	
0	136	0.1	0.1	1.6	0.3	48	0	44	2.2	22	46	24	535	27	1.4	0.3
0	136	0.1	0.1	1.6	0.3	48	0	44	2.2	22	46	877	535	27	1.4	0.3
0	283	0.1	0.1	1.8	0.3	51	0	67	0.8	27	41	653	467	27	1	0.5
18	46	0.1	0.1	1.1	0.2	92	0	5	1	134	273	1047	782	86	4.3	3.7
13	0	0.3	0.1	1	0.2	122	0	3	1.3	154	276	1067	906	109	5	1.8
0	22	0.2	0.1	0.5	0.2	30	0	4	0.7	64	132	504	376	41	0.4	1.8
8	28	0.1	0.1	1	0.1	12	0.1	12	0.9	45	85	725	418	14	1.2	1.3
18	30	0.1	0.1	1.3	0.2	57	0	8	1.5	142	296	1113	759	89	8.3	14.8
8	120	0.3	0.3	4.5	0.1	6	0	10	2.1	40	88	955	302	21	2.8	1.1
25	150							0		20		1000			1.1	
25	150							0		20		740			1.8	
38	195											495				
40	250							18		20		600			1.8	
30	60	0.1	0.3	1.6	0.1	<1	0	12		350		500	400	36	1.1	1.6
55	150	0.1	0.3	1.2	0.2	48	0.3	6		200	168	500	400	42	1.1	1.5
35	20	0.2	0.2	5				6		20		510	300	30	0.4	1.1
50	150	0.2	0.3	7				6		100		530	820	59	1.4	1.3

ERA, EatRight Analysis CD-ROM; **AMT,** amount; **WT,** weight; **WTR,** water; **CAL,** calories; **PROT,** protein; **CARB,** carbohydrate; **FIBR,** fiber; **FAT,** fat; **SATF,** saturated fat; **MONO,** monosaturated fat; **POLY,** polyunsaturated fat

ERA CODE	FOOD DESCRIPTION	AMT	UNIT	WT (g)	WTR (g)	CAL (kcal)	PROT (g)	CARB (g)	FIBR (g)	FAT (g)	SATF (g)	MONO (g)	POLY (g)
Meals, Entrees, and Mixed Dishes (continued)												
Frozen Meals, Entrees, and Dishes (continued)												
16260	ChickenBroc Alfredo-HealthyChce	1	ea	326		300	25	34	2	7	3		
82034	ChickenEnchiladaDin-HlthyChce	1	ea	320		298	13	46	4	7	3.1	2.6	1
16252	ChickenFettucAlfred-HealthyChce	1	ea	241		280	25	30	4	7	2.5		
83000	Egg Roll-Chicken-ChunKing	6	pce	106		210	6	30	3	7	1.5		
83001	Egg Roll-Shrimp-ChunKing	6	pce	106		190	5	29	3	6	1		
56740	Lasagna w/Meat Sauce-LnCuisne	1	ea	291		270	19	34	5	6	2.5	1.5	0.5
56731	Lasagna-Zucchini-LeanCuisine	1	ea	312		240	17	33	4	4	1.5	2	0.5
18825	Lemon Pepper Fish Din-HlthyChc	1	ea	303		320	14	50	5	7	2		
66047	Macaroni & Cheese-HealthyChce	1	ea	255		240	12	36	3	5	2.5		
81080	Manicotti-3 Cheese HealthyChce	1	ea	312		300	15	40	5	9	3		
11093	Meatloaf-LeanCuisine	1	ea	266		270	21	24	4	10	4	2.5	0.5
70767	MexicanStyleDinner-HungryMan	1	ea	567		690	26	87	13	27	9		
56739	Rigatoni-LeanCuisine	1	ea	255		180	10	25	4	4	1.5	0.5	0.5
11063	Salisbury Steak Dinner-Swansons	1	ea	312		340	16	35	6	15	6		
56732	Spaghetti w/Meatballs-LnCuisine	1	ea	269	201	298	18	40	5	8	2.1	2.7	1.3
56076	Spinach Souffle	1	cup	136	100	219	11	3	3	18	7.1	6.8	3.1
56738	Stuffed Cabbage-LeanCuisine	1	ea	269		199	12	26	6	6	1.7	2.4	0.7
16928	Turkey Pot Pie-Banquet	1	ea	198		370	10	38	3	20	8		
Homemade and Generic Meals, Entrees, and Dishes												
15907	Almond Chicken	1	cup	242	186	280	22	16	3	15	1.9	6.1	5.6
10081	Beef Cube Steak-Flour Fried	1	ea	165	79	460	44	18	1	22	6.2	8.2	5.8
11008	Beef Stroganoff	1	cup	256	183	408	26	16	1	27	10.6	7.9	6.3
66025	Burrito-Bean	2	ea	217	114	447	14	71	8	13	6.9	4.7	1.2
56629	Burrito-Bean+Cheese	2	ea	186	100	378	15	55		12	6.8	2.5	1.8
66024	Burrito-Beef	2	ea	220	109	524	27	59	2	21	10.4	7.4	0.9
15930	Cashew Chicken	1	cup	162	88	431	29	11	2	31	5.2	13.9	9.7
56075	Cheese Souffle-Recipe	1	cup	112	79	196	12	6	<1	14	5.6	4.8	2.8
56213	Chicken Helper-ChickenDumplng	1	cup	244	175	372	26	22	1	19	5.1	7.8	4.6
15927	Chicken Parmigiana	1	pce	182	120	320	28	16	1	16	5.3	4.9	4
56112	Chilis Rellenos	1	ea	143	84	365	17	8	1	30	12.5	9	6.7
56634	Chimichanga-Beef	1	ea	174	88	424	20	43	2	20	8.5	8.1	1.1
56121	Chimichanga-Beef & Bean	1	ea	118	73	241	8	21	3	14	2.9	6	4.3
56243	Chop Suey-Beef-No Noodles	1	cup	220	166	271	22	12	3	15	3.7	6.5	3.5
56248	Chop Suey-Pork-No Noodles	1	cup	220	165	286	22	12	3	17	4.2	7.8	3.4
57618	Chow Mein, Pork, w/Noodles	1	cup	220	136	448	22	31	4	27	4.8	7.7	12.8
57619	Chow Mein-Beef w/o Noodles	1	cup	220	166	271	22	12	3	15	3.7	6.5	3.5
57622	Chow Mein-Chicken w/o Noodles	1	cup	220	179	193	20	10	2	8	1.7	2.8	3
57621	Chow Mein-Pork w/o Noodles	1	cup	220	165	286	22	12	3	17	4.2	7.8	3.4
56132	Egg Foo Yung Patty	1	ea	86	67	113	6	3	1	8	2	3.4	2.1
57524	Egg Roll, w/Meat	1	ea	64	43	113	5	9	1	6	1.4	3	1.3
56060	Enchilada-Chicken	1	ea	121.9		195	13	16	2	9	3.6	2.6	2.1
56124	Fajita-Beef	1	ea	223	144	399	23	36	3	18	5.5	7.6	3.5
56123	Fajita-Chicken	1	ea	223	145	363	20	44	5	12	2.2	5.5	3.1
56119	Flauta-Beef	1	ea	113	57	354	14	13	2	28	4.8	11.8	9.4

< = Trace amount present   Blank = Not available

CHOL, cholesterol; **V,** vitamin; **THI,** thiamin; **RIB,** riboflavin; **NIA,** niacin; **FOL,** folate;
CALC, calcium; **PHOS,** phosphate; **SOD,** sodium; **POT,** potassium; **MAG,** magnesium

CHOL (mg)	V-A (RE)	THI (mg)	RIB (mg)	NIA (mg)	V-B6 (mg)	FOL (µg)	V-B12 (µg)	V-C (mg)	V-E (mg)	CALC (mg)	PHOS (mg)	SOD (mg)	POT (mg)	MAG (mg)	IRON (mg)	ZINC (mg)
50	20							12		100		530			1.8	
38	154							18		134	237	563	384		0.8	
35	0							2		100		600			1.1	
10	3	0.1	0.1	0.7				1		20	90	260	120		0.4	
10	20	0.1	<0.1	0.4				4		20	50	360	80		0.4	
25	100	0.2	0.3	3	0.3			12		150		560	620	44	1.8	2.9
15	100	0.5	0.3	2				18		200		470	570	62	1.1	2.1
30	100							30		20		480			1.1	
20	0							0		200		600			1.1	
35	150							0		250		550			1.8	
55	60							1		80		530	520		1.8	
35	300							36		300		2170			3.6	
20	200	0.2	0.3	4				6		100		560	520	44	1.4	2.9
30	1000							6		80		920			2.7	
5	0									94		465			2.4	
184	674	0.1	0.3	0.5	0.1	80	1.4	3	1.2	230	231	763	201	38	1.3	1.3
24	0							53		105		412				
45	150							0		40		850			1.1	
40	37	0.1	0.2	9.5	0.4	26	0.3	7	3.8	69	252	526	549	60	2	1.6
125	5	0.3	0.5	7	0.7	17	4.7	<1	1.7	80	380	316	652	54	6.4	8.4
85	99	0.2	0.4	4.5	0.3	20	2.6	2	2.4	92	308	677	556	40	3.6	4.9
4	33	0.6	0.6	4.1	0.3	87	1.1	2	2	113	98	985	653	87	4.5	1.5
28	238	0.2	0.7	3.6	0.2	74	0.9	2		214	180	1166	497	80	2.3	1.6
64	29	0.2	0.9	6.4	0.3	130	2	1	2.3	84	174	1491	739	81	6.1	4.7
64	58	0.2	0.1	13.2	0.6	43	0.3	8	3.9	49	263	907	428	63	2	1.5
194	167	0.1	0.4	0.3	0.1	23	0.8	<1	1.3	209	200	298	146	16	0.8	1
89	52	0.2	0.3	9.3	0.3	11	0.3	2	0.9	128	261	244	297	35	2.5	1.9
137	146	0.2	0.3	8.5	0.4	17	0.4	9	2.4	198	317	641	471	45	2.3	2.4
168	250	0.1	0.4	0.9	0.3	29	0.5	113	4.7	398	307	522	386	36	1.7	2
9	16	0.5	0.6	5.8	0.3	84	1.5	5		63	124	910	586	63	4.5	5
17	40	0.1	0.1	2.3	0.2	16	0.5	11	2.5	48	99	230	323	28	2	1.5
50	116	0.2	0.2	4.2	0.4	42	2	23	2	38	238	924	556	42	2.9	3.5
56	118	0.6	0.3	4.8	0.4	40	0.5	24	2	48	227	926	527	40	1.9	2.4
48	19	0.8	0.4	6.2	0.4	42	0.4	20	2.7	45	249	848	489	53	3.3	2.6
50	116	0.2	0.2	4.2	0.4	42	2	23	2	38	238	924	556	42	2.9	3.5
50	14	0.1	0.2	6.9	0.4	50	0.2	10	1	36	185	651	415	35	1.7	1.6
56	118	0.6	0.3	4.8	0.4	40	0.5	24	2	48	227	926	527	40	1.9	2.4
185	86	<0.1	0.3	0.4	0.1	30	0.4	5	1.2	31	93	317	117	12	1	0.7
37	16	0.2	0.1	1.3	0.1	10	0.1	2	0.8	15	57	274	124	10	0.8	0.5
36	110	0.1	0.1	3.1	0.2	15	0.2	16	2.7	162	216	312	203	34	1	1.3
45	43	0.4	0.3	5.4	0.4	23	2.1	27	1.7	84	238	316	479	38	3.8	3.5
39	65	0.4	0.3	6.1	0.4	42	0.1	37	1.7	101	188	343	534	48	3.3	1.6
37	21	0.1	0.1	1.9	0.2	10	1.2	19	4.7	51	179	68	313	28	1.9	3.4

ERA, EatRight Analysis CD-ROM; **AMT,** amount; **WT,** weight; **WTR,** water; **CAL,** calories; **PROT,** protein; **CARB,** carbohydrate; **FIBR,** fiber; **FAT,** fat; **SATF,** saturated fat; **MONO,** monosaturated fat; **POLY,** polyunsaturated fat

ERA CODE	FOOD DESCRIPTION	AMT	UNIT	WT (g)	WTR (g)	CAL (kcal)	PROT (g)	CARB (g)	FIBR (g)	FAT (g)	SATF (g)	MONO (g)	POLY (g)
Meals, Entrees, and Mixed Dishes (continued)													
Homemade and Generic Meals, Entrees, and Dishes (continued)													
56120	Flauta-Chicken	1	ea	113	62	330	13	12	2	26	4.2	10.7	9.3
56232	Greek Meat Pie-8 inch	1	ea	417	247	947	34	73	5	57	13.5	25.6	14.2
56242	Gumbo w/Rice	1	cup	244	203	193	14	17	2	8	1.6	2.6	2.7
56153	Hamburger Helper-Beef+Tom	1	cup	249	185	275	29	24	2	7	2.3	2.9	0.6
56310	Hamburger Helper-Mac+Cheese	1	cup	243	173	340	28	22	1	15	7.7	5.1	0.7
56150	Hash-Roast Beef	1	cup	190	131	312	21	21	2	16	4.9	5.7	3.3
56239	Jambalaya-Shrimp	1	cup	243	176	310	27	28	1	9	1.8	3.8	2.8
56296	Knish-Meat	1	ea	50	19	175	7	13	1	11	2.6	4.9	2.3
56294	Knish-Potato	1	ea	61	22	215	5	21	1	12	2.6	5.8	3.3
13900	Lamb Curry	1	cup	236	188	256	28	3	1	14	3.9	4.9	3.4
56108	Lasagna w/Meat-Recipe	1	pce	245	164	392	23	40	3	16	8	5.2	0.8
18800	Lobster Newburg	1	cup	244	150	611	30	11	<1	50	29.6	14.7	2.3
56082	Macaroni+Cheese-Recipe	1	cup	200	116	430	17	40	1	22	8.9	8.8	3.6
56250	Moo Goo Gai Pan	1	cup	216	168	272	15	12	3	19	3.8	6.7	7
56080	Moussaka-Lamb/Eggplant	1	cup	250	204	237	16	13	4	13	4.6	5.4	1.9
19403	Oysters Rockefeller	1	cup	224	165	301	16	21	3	17	7.7	5.7	2.4
56234	Pork Chop Suey+Noodles	1	cup	220	136	448	22	31	4	27	4.8	7.7	12.8
56292	Pork Dumpling-Fried	1	ea	100		341	13	25	1	21	4.8	9.1	5.7
56288	Pork Egg Foo Yung-Patty	1	ea	86	65	124	8	4	1	8	2.1	3	2.3
56122	Quesadilla	1	ea	54	19	183	6	18	1	10	3.5	3.4	2.2
56098	Quiche Lorraine 1/8 Pie	1	pce	176	93	526	15	25	1	41	18.9	14.3	5.2
56128	Ravioli-Cheese+TomSce-Svg	1	ea	250	180	341	15	38	2	15	6.4	5	1.9
56303	Ravioli-Meat w/Tomato Sauce	2	ea	70	48	110	6	10	1	5	1.7	2.1	0.5
57517	Shrimp Creole w/Rice	1	cup	243	176	310	27	28	1	9	1.8	3.8	2.8
57523	Spring Roll-Fresh	1	ea	64	43	113	5	9	1	6	1.4	3	1.3
56291	Spring Roll-Meat	1	ea	64	43	113	5	9	1	6	1.4	3	1.3
56236	Stuffed Grape Leaves-Lamb	1	ea	21	12	56	2	2	1	4	1.1	2.5	0.5
56074	Stuffed Green Pepper	1	ea	172		229	11	20	2	11	5	4.9	0.5
56244	Sukiyaki	1	cup	162	126	172	19	7	1	8	2.9	3.1	0.7
56315	Sushi+Egg-Seaweed Rolled	1	cup	166	124	202	9	22	<1	8	2.2	3.2	1.6
56313	Sushi+Fish+Vegetables	1	cup	166	109	232	9	47	2	1	0.2	0.2	0.2
56314	Sushi+Veg-Seaweed Rolled	1	cup	166	118	194	4	43	1	<1	0.1	0.1	0.1
56312	Sushi-No Fish+Vegetables	1	cup	166	106	240	5	53	2	<1	0.1	0.1	0.1
56311	Sushi-No Fish-No Veges	1	cup	145	82	256	5	57	1	<1	0.1	0.1	0.1
56235	Sweet & Sour Pork+Rice	1	cup	244	182	270	13	40	1	6	1.6	2.4	1.7
56061	Taco-Chicken	1	ea	77.3		173	15	9	1	8	3.2	3.1	1.4
56113	Tamale-Meat	1	ea	70	45	134	6	11	1	7	2.6	3.1	1
56130	Tortellini-Meat	1	cup	190	115	373	24	33	1	15	5.4	5.7	2.1
56645	Tostada-Beef+Cheese	1	ea	163	101	314	19	23		16	10.4	3.3	1
56089	Tuna Noodle Casserole	1	cup	202	151	237	17	25	1	7	1.9	1.5	3.2
11902	Veal Scallopini	1	pce	96	57	238	18	1	<1	17	4.8	7.4	3.2
Pizza													
56996	Cheese Sausage-BagelBites	4	pce	88		200	10	24	3	7	2.5		
57166	Deluxe Pizza-Kraft Piece	1	pce	125	65	298	14	27	2	15	6.5		

< = Trace amount present   Blank = Not available

CHOL, cholesterol; V, vitamin; THI, thiamin; RIB, riboflavin; NIA, niacin; FOL, folate;
CALC, calcium; PHOS, phosphate; SOD, sodium; POT, potassium; MAG, magnesium

CHOL (mg)	V-A (RE)	THI (mg)	RIB (mg)	NIA (mg)	V-B6 (mg)	FOL (µg)	V-B12 (µg)	V-C (mg)	V-E (mg)	CALC (mg)	PHOS (mg)	SOD (mg)	POT (mg)	MAG (mg)	IRON (mg)	ZINC (mg)
35	26	0.1	0.1	3.1	0.2	8	0.1	18	4.4	50	140	71	268	27	0.9	1.1
66	829	0.7	0.6	8.8	0.5	42	2.4	15	6.5	45	355	1032	751	62	6.5	4.7
40	63	0.2	0.2	4.5	0.2	46	2.4	14	1.4	71	152	542	446	40	2.6	15.2
86	98	0.3	0.3	5.6	0.5	19	2.7	13	1.6	26	289	666	740	55	4	4.5
92	70	0.2	0.3	4	0.3	16	2	0	0.3	188	335	736	348	36	3.4	4.6
57	<1	0.2	0.2	3.7	0.5	16	1.8	7	1.2	19	204	470	587	36	2.5	5
181	133	0.3	0.1	4.8	0.2	12	1.2	17	2.3	104	300	370	439	64	4.4	1.7
52	89	0.1	0.2	1.5	<0.1	8	0.3	<1	1.2	12	61	107	88	8	1.2	1
59	130	0.2	0.2	1.5	0.1	10	0.1	1	1.7	16	60	140	96	10	1.3	0.4
89	2	0.1	0.3	8.1	0.2	28	2.9	1	1.2	36	284	323	496	40	3	6.6
58	158	0.2	0.3	4.2	0.2	20	1	14	1.2	270	299	391	460	50	3.1	3.3
369	523	0.1	0.4	1.6	0.2	32	4	1	2	241	398	647	607	55	1.2	4.1
42	234	0.2	0.4	1.8	0.1	10	0.3	1	3.5	362	322	1086	240	37	1.8	1.2
35	142	0.2	0.3	4.4	0.3	42	0.3	34	3.7	130	199	304	488	34	1.7	1.6
97	105	0.2	0.3	4.1	0.2	45	1.4	6	0.9	68	179	432	557	40	1.8	2.6
87	805	0.4	0.4	4	0.3	122	21	27	2.2	195	254	708	583	115	10.3	97.9
48	19	0.8	0.4	6.2	0.4	42	0.4	20	2.7	45	249	848	489	53	3.3	2.6
27	11	0.5	0.3	3.6	0.2	9	0.3	<1	2.3	33	131	86	198	18	1.8	1.1
167	86	0.1	0.2	0.8	0.1	22	0.4	3	1.1	27	105	131	157	12	0.8	0.9
13	41	0.1	0.1	1.1	<0.1	6	0.1	15	1	132	107	230	77	13	1.2	0.6
221	279	0.3	0.5	2	0.1	19	0.6	1	2	231	261	221	239	24	1.9	1.5
162	236	0.3	0.4	2.9	0.2	30	0.4	9	2.1	172	220	574	405	33	3.1	1.5
48	49	0.1	0.1	1.7	0.1	8	0.5	2	0.7	20	62	50	148	11	1.2	1
181	133	0.3	0.1	4.8	0.2	12	1.2	17	2.3	104	300	370	439	64	4.4	1.7
37	16	0.2	0.1	1.3	0.1	10	0.1	2	0.8	15	57	274	124	10	0.8	0.5
37	16	0.2	0.1	1.3	0.1	10	0.1	2	0.8	15	57	274	124	10	0.8	0.5
5	145	<0.1	<0.1	0.6	<0.1	6	0.1	2	0.5	22	19	14	41	8	0.4	0.3
34	44	0.1	0.1	2.7	0.3	17	0.7	55	0.7	16	85	201	232	20	1.8	2.3
148	256	0.1	0.4	3.1	0.4	61	1.5	5	0.7	62	204	675	463	47	3.2	3.6
224	145	0.1	0.3	1.4	0.1	30	0.5	2	0.9	45	140	562	136	19	1.7	1
11	136	0.3	0.1	3	0.2	15	0.3	4	0.6	25	109	93	218	27	2.3	0.8
0	66	0.2	<0.1	2	0.1	11	0	3	0.1	22	64	5	106	21	1.6	0.7
0	152	0.3	0.1	2.6	0.1	16	0	4	0.2	25	84	88	169	24	2.6	0.9
0	0	0.3	<0.1	2.7	0.1	4	0	0	0.1	20	71	6	78	18	2.7	0.7
28	23	0.5	0.2	3.8	0.4	10	0.3	14	0.8	28	142	618	311	35	2	1.5
45	39	0.1	0.1	4.2	0.2	16	0.2	1	0.8	94	153	106	166	28	1	1.3
19	14	0.2	0.1	2.5	0.1	4	0.2	1	0.3	24	67	84	140	21	1.4	0.9
240	134	0.5	0.6	4.5	0.2	29	0.9	<1	1.1	178	290	437	231	28	3.1	2.2
41	96	0.1	0.6	3.1	0.2	75	1.2	3		217	179	896	572	64	2.9	3.7
41	13	0.2	0.1	7.8	0.2	10	1.5	1	1.2	34	155	772	182	31	2.3	1.2
65	101	<0.1	0.2	5.1	0.2	12	0.9	1	1.7	54	172	278	253	19	1	2.8
15	80							12		100		500	140		0.7	
28	93							8		233		597			1.3	

ERA, EatRight Analysis CD-ROM; **AMT,** amount; **WT,** weight; **WTR,** water; **CAL,** calories; **PROT,** protein; **CARB,** carbohydrate; **FIBR,** fiber; **FAT,** fat; **SATF,** saturated fat; **MONO,** monosaturated fat; **POLY,** polyunsaturated fat

ERA CODE	FOOD DESCRIPTION	AMT	UNIT	WT (g)	WTR (g)	CAL (kcal)	PROT (g)	CARB (g)	FIBR (g)	FAT (g)	SATF (g)	MONO (g)	POLY (g)
Meals, Entrees, and Mixed Dishes (continued)													
Pizza (continued)													
56733	FrBread Cheese Pizza-LnCuisine	1	ea	145	73	298	19	41	3	7	3.4	1.3	0.4
56736	FrBread Deluxe Pizza-LnCuisine	1	ea	174		330	23	45	5	6	2.5	2	1
56735	FrBread Pepperoni Pizza-LnCuisn	1	ea	149		330	20	46	4	7	3	2.5	1
57215	Supreme Pizza-Light-Kraft	1	ea	640		1252	116	139	9	42	16.2		
Meats													
Beef													
10051	Beef Jerky-Large Piece	1	ea	19.8	5	81	7	2	<1	5	2.1	2.2	0.2
10008	Corned Beef-Canned	1	cup	140	81	350	38	0	0	21	8.7	8.3	0.9
10036	Corned Beef-Cooked-Lean	1	pce	42	25	105	8	<1	0	8	2.7	3.9	0.3
10060	Filet Mignon Steak-Broiled-Lean	1	ea	156	94	329	44	0	0	16	5.8	5.9	0.6
10724	Ground Beef-Lean-Broiled	3	oz	85	45	238	24	0	0	15	5.9	6.6	0.6
10463	Ground Beef-Reg-Broiled	3	oz	85	44	248	23	0	0	17	6.5	7.2	0.6
10722	Ground Beef-XLean-Broiled	3	oz	85	46	225	24	0	0	13	5.3	5.9	0.5
10021	London Broil-Broiled-Lean	3	oz	85	52	176	23	0	0	9	3.7	3.5	0.3
11018	Meat Loaf-Beef Only	1	pce	108	67	231	18	7	<1	14	4.9	6.1	0.7
10028	Porterhouse Steak-Broiled-Ln	1	ea	170	102	366	44	0	0	20	6.9	8.9	0.6
10024	Rib Eye Steak-Broiled-Lean	3	oz	85	50	191	24	0	0	10	4	4.2	0.3
10016	Round-PotRoasted-Lean+Fat	1	pce	42	22	116	12	0	0	7	2.7	3.1	0.3
40067	Salisbury Steak-Flame Brld	1	ea	72	42	160	16	3	1	10	3.9	4.2	0.4
10624	Short Ribs-Braised	3	oz	85	30	400	18	0	0	36	15.1	16	1.3
10005	Sirloin Steak-Broiled-Lean	1	ea	156	96	315	47	0	0	12	4.9	5.3	0.5
10050	Stew Meat-Cooked-Lean Only	1	cup	140	79	330	44	0	0	16	6	6.9	0.5
10064	Strip Steak-Broiled-Lean	1	ea	241	144	499	69	0	0	23	8.7	9.1	0.7
10007	TBone Steak-Broiled-Lean	1	ea	184	113	377	49	0	0	18	6.6	8.3	0.6
Game Meats													
14008	Beefalo Meat-Roasted	3	oz	85	52	160	26	0	0	5	2.3	2.3	0.2
14009	Bison/Buffalo Meat-Roasted	3	oz	85	57	122	24	0	0	2	0.8	0.8	0.2
14013	Deer/Venison-Roasted	3	oz	85	55	134	26	0	0	3	1.1	0.7	0.5
14014	Elk Meat-Roasted	3	oz	85	56	124	26	0	0	2	0.6	0.4	0.3
14029	Frog Legs-Steamed	2	ea	100		106	24	0	0	<1	0.1	0.1	0.1
14004	Rabbit-Roasted	3.5	oz	100		197	29	0	0	8	2.4	2.2	1.6
14030	Turtle Meat-Cooked	1	cup	140	96	220	33	<1	0	9	1.8	4.1	2.6
14032	Venison Steak-Fried	1	ea	85	53	147	28	0	0	3	1.2	0.9	0.6
Goat													
13530	Goat Meat-Boiled	1	oz	28.35	19	41	8	0	0	1	0.3	0.4	0.1
14016	Goat Ribs-Cooked	1	ea	46	31	66	12	0	0	1	0.4	0.6	0.1
Lamb													
13524	Ground Lamb-Broiled	3	oz	85	47	240	21	0	0	17	6.9	7.1	1.2
13522	Kabob Meat-Broiled-Lean	2	oz	56.7	36	105	16	0	0	4	1.5	1.7	0.4
13513	Loin Chop Broiled-Lean	1	ea	46	28	99	14	0	0	4	1.6	2	0.3
13523	Stew Meat-Braised-Lean	3	oz	85	48	190	29	0	0	7	2.7	3	0.7
13501	Leg of Lamb-Roasted-Lean	3	oz	85	54	162	24	0	0	7	2.3	2.9	0.4

< = Trace amount present   Blank = Not available

CHOL, cholesterol; **V,** vitamin; **THI,** thiamin; **RIB,** riboflavin; **NIA,** niacin; **FOL,** folate; **CALC,** calcium; **PHOS,** phosphate; **SOD,** sodium; **POT,** potassium; **MAG,** magnesium

CHOL (mg)	V-A (RE)	THI (mg)	RIB (mg)	NIA (mg)	V-B6 (mg)	FOL (µg)	V-B12 (µg)	V-C (mg)	V-E (mg)	CALC (mg)	PHOS (mg)	SOD (mg)	POT (mg)	MAG (mg)	IRON (mg)	ZINC (mg)
17	51							5		384		341	315		3.1	
30	100							6		250		560	380		3.6	
25	100							6		250		590	350		3.6	
93	928							28		1855		3292			8.3	
10	0	<0.1	<0.1	0.3	<0.1	27	0.2	0	0.1	4	81	438	118	10	1.1	1.6
120	0	<0.1	0.2	3.4	0.2	13	2.3	0	1.1	17	155	1408	190	20	2.9	5
41	0	<0.1	0.1	1.3	0.1	3	0.7	0	0.1	3	52	476	61	5	0.8	1.9
131	0	0.2	0.5	6.1	0.7	11	4	0	0.2	11	371	98	654	47	5.6	8.7
86	0	0.1	0.2	5.1	0.3	9	2.3	0	0.2	10	155	76	297	20	2.1	5.3
86	0	<0.1	0.2	5.5	0.3	8	2.8	0	0.2	10	162	79	278	19	2.3	4.9
84	0	0.1	0.3	5	0.3	9	2.2	0	0.2	8	162	70	314	21	2.4	5.5
57	0	0.1	0.2	4.3	0.3	7	2.8	0	0.1	6	201	71	352	20	2.2	4.1
90	20	0.1	0.3	4	0.1	12	1.7	1	0.1	43	161	133	295	22	2	3.7
117	0	0.2	0.4	7.9	0.7	14	3.9	0	0.2	12	359	117	624	46	5.3	9
68	0	0.1	0.2	4.1	0.3	7	2.8	0	0.1	11	177	59	335	23	2.2	5.9
40	0	<0.1	0.1	1.6	0.1	4	1	0	0.2	3	103	21	118	9	1.3	2.1
42	18	0.1	0.1	2.6	0.3	6	1.6	2	0.1	29	232	500	259	26	2	4.5
80	0	<0.1	0.1	2.1	0.2	4	2.2	0	0.2	10	138	42	190	13	2	4.1
139	0	0.2	0.5	6.7	0.7	16	4.4	0	0.6	17	381	103	629	50	5.2	10.2
143	0	0.1	0.4	4.5	0.4	11	3.7	0	0.2	14	346	94	388	33	5	12.3
183	0	0.2	0.5	12.9	1	19	4.8	0	0.3	19	525	164	954	65	6	12.6
108	0	0.2	0.5	8.5	0.7	15	4.2	0	0.5	11	396	131	696	52	5.8	9.8
49	0	<0.1	0.1	4.2	0.3	15	2.2	8	0.2	20	212	70	390	<1	2.6	5.4
70	0	0.1	0.2	3.2	0.3	7	2.4	0	0.1	7	178	48	307	22	2.9	3.1
95	0	0.2	0.5	5.7	0.3	4	2.7	0	0.2	6	192	46	285	20	3.8	2.3
62	0	0.2	0.7	4.9	0.2	3	5.5	0	<0.1	4	153	52	279	20	3.1	2.7
72	20	0.2	0.3	1.6	0.2	16	0.5	0	1.4	26	160	84	372	29	2	1.4
82	0	0.1	0.2	8.4	0.5	11	8.3	0	0.9	19	263	47	383	21	2.3	2.3
82	126	0.2	0.2	1.7	0.2	21	1.5	<1	2.1	197	299	209	383	33	2.3	1.6
103	0	0.1	0.6	5.8	0.2	5	5.3	0	0.2	5	207	52	307	24	4.1	2.5
21	0	<0.1	0.2	1.1	0	1	0.3	0	<0.1	5	57	24	115	0	1.1	1.5
34	0	<0.1	0.3	1.8	0	2	0.5	0	<0.1	8	92	40	186	0	1.7	2.4
82	0	0.1	0.2	5.7	0.1	16	2.2	0	0.2	19	171	69	288	20	1.5	4
51	0	0.1	0.2	3.7	0.1	13	1.7	0	0.1	7	127	43	190	18	1.3	3.3
44	0	0.1	0.1	3.2	0.1	11	1.2	0	0.1	9	104	39	173	13	0.9	1.9
92	0	0.1	0.2	5.1	0.1	18	2.3	0	0.2	13	174	60	221	24	2.4	5.6
76	0	0.1	0.2	5.4	0.1	20	2.2	0	0.2	7	175	58	287	22	1.8	4.2

ERA, EatRight Analysis CD-ROM; **AMT**, amount; **WT**, weight; **WTR**, water; **CAL**, calories; **PROT**, protein; **CARB**, carbohydrate; **FIBR**, fiber; **FAT**, fat; **SATF**, saturated fat; **MONO**, monosaturated fat; **POLY**, polyunsaturated fat

ERA CODE	FOOD DESCRIPTION	AMT	UNIT	WT (g)	WTR (g)	CAL (kcal)	PROT (g)	CARB (g)	FIBR (g)	FAT (g)	SATF (g)	MONO (g)	POLY (g)
Meats (continued)													
Lunchmeats and Sausages													
13006	Bologna-Beef & Pork	1	pce	28.4	15	90	3	1	0	8	3	3.8	0.7
13007	Bologna-Turkey	1	pce	28.4	18	57	4	<1	0	4	1.4	1.4	1.2
13079	Bratwurst Sausage Link-Cooked	1	ea	85	48	256	12	2	0	22	7.9	10.4	2.3
13066	Braunschweiger Sausage	2	pce	57	27	205	8	2	0	18	6.2	8.5	2.1
13052	Breakfast Sausage-Turkey	1	pce	28.4	17	65	6	0	0	5	1.6	1.8	1.2
13070	Chorizo Sausage-Link	1	ea	60	19	273	14	1	0	23	8.6	11	2.1
56668	Corndog (hotdog+coating)	1	ea	175	82	460	17	56		19	5.2	9.1	3.5
13034	Ham Salad Spread	1	Tbs	15	9	32	1	2	0	2	0.8	1.1	0.4
13250	Hot Dog-Beef-Fat Free	1	ea	50		39	7	3	0	<1	0.1	0.1	<0.1
13009	Hotdog-Beef & Pork	1	ea	57	31	182	6	1	0	17	6.1	7.8	1.6
13008	Hotdog-Beef-2oz	1	ea	57	31	180	7	1	0	16	6.9	7.8	0.8
13012	Hotdog-Turkey	1	ea	45	28	102	6	1	0	8	2.7	2.5	2.2
13015	Italian Pork Sausage Link-Ckd	1	ea	67	33	216	13	1	0	17	6.1	8	2.2
13043	Kielbasa Sausage	1	pce	26	14	81	3	1	0	7	2.6	3.4	0.8
13019	Liverwurst-Pork	1	pce	18	9	59	3	<1	0	5	1.9	2.4	0.5
13020	Pastrami-Turkey	2	pce	57	40	80	10	1	0	4	1	1.2	0.9
13021	Pepperoni Sausage	4	pce	22	6	109	5	1	0	10	3.5	4.6	1
13051	Pickle & Pimento Loaf	2	pce	57	33	149	7	3	0	12	4.5	5.5	1.5
13022	Polish Sausage-Pork	1	ea	227	121	740	32	4	0	65	23.4	30.7	7
13023	Salami-Beef-Cooked	1	pce	23	13	60	3	1	0	5	2.1	2.2	0.2
13026	Salami-Dry-Beef & Pork	2	pce	20	7	84	5	1	0	7	2.4	3.4	0.6
10035	Sizzlean Formed Bacon-Cooked	3	pce	34	9	153	11	<1	0	12	4.9	5.7	0.5
13105	Spam-Canned	1	pce	28.35	14	95	4	1	<1	9			
13328	Turkey Lunchmeat-Roasted	1	oz	28.35	21	28	5	1	0	1	0.1	0.2	0.1
13112	Turkey Breast-Smkd-FatFree	1	pce	28		23	4	1	0	<1	0.1	0.1	<0.1
Pork and Ham													
12000	Bacon-Regular-Cooked	3	pce	19	2	109	6	<1	0	9	3.3	4.5	1.1
12002	Canadian Bacon-Grilled	2	pce	46.5	29	86	11	1	0	4	1.3	1.9	0.4
12225	Ham-Canned-Unheated-XLean	1	cup	140	100	202	25	0	0	10	3.4	5	1.1
12006	Ham-Whole-Rstd-Lean Only	1	cup	140	92	220	35	0	0	8	2.6	3.5	0.9
12082	Pork Chop-Breaded-Baked	1	ea	80	44	184	21	5	<1	8	2.9	3.7	0.9
12086	Pork Chop-Smoked-Lean	1	ea	67	43	114	17	0	0	5	1.6	2.2	0.5
12236	Pork Country Rib-Lean-Rstd	3	oz	85	49	210	23	0	0	13	4.5	5.5	0.9
12035	Pork Loin Chop-Broiled-Lean	1	ea	79	48	166	23	0	0	8	2.9	3.5	0.6
12031	Pork Loin-Roasted Slice	1	ea	89	51	221	24	0	0	13	4.8	5.8	1.1
12098	Spareribs-Braised-Lean	3	oz	85	51	199	22	0	0	12	4.2	5	0.9
Veal													
11900	Breaded Veal Patty-Fried	1	ea	79	41	212	16	7	<1	13	4.4	5.9	1.2
11530	Ground Veal-Broiled	3	oz	85	57	146	21	0	0	6	2.6	2.4	0.5
11514	Veal Chop-Med-Fried-Lean	1	ea	85	52	156	28	0	0	4	1.1	1.4	0.3
11527	Veal Sirloin-Roasted	3	oz	85	53	172	21	0	0	9	3.8	3.5	0.6
11517	Veal Loin Cutlet-Brsd-Lean+Fat	1	ea	80	42	227	24	0	0	14	5.4	5.4	0.9
11519	Veal Rib-Roasted-Lean+Fat	3	oz	85	51	194	20	0	0	12	4.6	4.6	0.8

< = Trace amount present   Blank = Not available

CHOL, cholesterol; **V**, vitamin; **THI**, thiamin; **RIB**, riboflavin; **NIA**, niacin; **FOL**, folate; **CALC**, calcium; **PHOS**, phosphate; **SOD**, sodium; **POT**, potassium; **MAG**, magnesium

CHOL (mg)	V-A (RE)	THI (mg)	RIB (mg)	NIA (mg)	V-B6 (mg)	FOL (μg)	V-B12 (μg)	V-C (mg)	V-E (mg)	CALC (mg)	PHOS (mg)	SOD (mg)	POT (mg)	MAG (mg)	IRON (mg)	ZINC (mg)
16	0	<0.1	<0.1	0.7	0.1	1	0.4	0	0.1	3	26	289	51	3	0.4	0.6
28	0	<0.1	<0.1	1	0.1	2	0.1	0	0.2	24	37	249	57	4	0.4	0.5
51	0	0.4	0.2	2.7	0.2	2	0.8	1	0.2	37	127	473	180	13	1.1	2
89	2405	0.1	0.9	4.8	0.2	25	11.4	0	0.2	5	96	652	113	6	5.3	1.6
23	0	<0.1	0.1	1.4	0.1	1	0.5	0	0.2	5	52	191	76	6	0.5	1
53	0	0.4	0.2	3.1	0.3	1	1.2	0	0.1	5	90	741	239	11	1	2
79	37	0.3	0.7	4.2	0.1	103	0.4	0	0.7	102	166	973	262	18	6.2	1.3
6	0	0.1	<0.1	0.3	<0.1	<1	0.1	0	0.7	1	18	137	22	2	0.1	0.2
15	0							0		10	64	464	234	10	1	1.2
28	0	0.1	0.1	1.5	0.1	2	0.7	0	0.2	6	49	638	95	6	0.7	1
35	0	<0.1	0.1	1.4	0.1	2	0.9	0	0.2	11	50	585	95	2	0.8	1.2
48	0	<0.1	0.1	1.9	0.1	4	0.1	0	0.3	48	60	642	81	6	0.8	1.4
52	0	0.4	0.2	2.8	0.2	3	0.9	1	0.2	16	114	618	204	12	1	1.6
17	0	0.1	0.1	0.7	<0.1	1	0.4	0	0.1	11	38	280	70	4	0.4	0.5
28	1494	<0.1	0.2	0.8	<0.1	5	2.4	0	0.1	5	41	155	31	2	1.2	0.4
31	0	<0.1	0.1	2	0.2	3	0.1	0	0.4	5	114	596	148	8	0.9	1.2
17	0	0.1	0.1	1.1	0.1	1	0.6	0	0.1	2	26	449	76	4	0.3	0.6
21	4	0.2	0.1	1.2	0.1	3	0.7	0	0.1	54	80	792	194	10	0.6	0.8
159	0	1.1	0.3	7.8	0.4	5	2.2	2	0.6	27	309	1988	538	32	3.3	4.4
15	0	<0.1	<0.1	0.7	<0.1	<1	0.7	0	0.2	2	26	270	52	3	0.5	0.5
16	0	0.1	0.1	1	0.1	<1	0.4	0	0.1	2	28	372	76	3	0.3	0.6
40	0	<0.1	0.1	2.2	0.1	3	1.2	0	0.1	3	80	766	140	9	1.1	2.2
16	5	<0.1	0.1	0.9						2		445	54	3	0.4	0.7
11	0							0		2	71	313	63	6	0.3	0.3
10	0							0		3	69	300	61	8	0.2	0.2
16	0	0.1	0.1	1.4	0.1	1	0.3	0	0.1	2	64	303	92	5	0.3	0.6
27	0	0.4	0.1	3.2	0.2	2	0.4	0	0.2	5	138	719	181	10	0.4	0.8
53	0	1.2	0.3	6.4	0.6	8	1.1	0	0.7	8	290	1786	468	22	1.3	2.6
77	0	1	0.4	7	0.7	6	1	0	0.4	10	318	1857	442	31	1.3	3.6
57	1	0.7	0.3	3.9	0.4	5	0.5	1	0.4	17	197	333	331	22	0.8	1.8
32	0	0.5	0.2	3.2	0.2	3	0.7	0	0.2	7	163	825	196	11	0.7	2
79	2	0.5	0.3	4	0.4	4	0.7	<1	0.4	25	188	25	297	20	1.1	3.2
62	2	0.7	0.3	4.1	0.4	5	0.6	1	0.3	13	200	51	346	23	0.7	2
73	3	0.9	0.3	5	0.5	5	0.6	1	0.3	17	215	53	363	23	0.9	2.1
73	2	0.5	0.2	3.5	0.3	3	0.6	1	0.4	21	143	54	293	15	1.2	3.4
80	8	0.1	0.2	5.9	0.3	11	0.7	0	1	35	153	142	227	20	1.1	2
88	0	0.1	0.2	6.8	0.3	9	1.1	0	0.2	14	184	71	286	20	0.8	3.3
91	0	0.1	0.3	10.7	0.4	14	1.3	0	0.4	6	246	65	376	27	0.7	2.9
87	0	0.1	0.3	7.5	0.3	13	1.2	0	0.4	11	190	71	298	22	0.8	2.8
94	0	<0.1	0.2	7.2	0.2	11	1	0	0.9	22	176	64	224	19	0.9	2.9
94	0	<0.1	0.2	5.9	0.2	11	1.2	0	0.8	9	167	78	251	19	0.8	3.5

ERA, EatRight Analysis CD-ROM; **AMT,** amount; **WT,** weight; **WTR,** water; **CAL,** calories; **PROT,** protein; **CARB,** carbohydrate; **FIBR,** fiber; **FAT,** fat; **SATF,** saturated fat; **MONO,** monosaturated fat; **POLY,** polyunsaturated fat

ERA CODE	FOOD DESCRIPTION	AMT	UNIT	WT (g)	WTR (g)	CAL (kcal)	PROT (g)	CARB (g)	FIBR (g)	FAT (g)	SATF (g)	MONO (g)	POLY (g)
Meats (continued)													
Variety Meats and By-Products													
10015	Beef Heart-Simmered	3	oz	85	54	149	24	<1	0	5	1.4	1.1	1.2
10010	Beef Liver-Fried	3	oz	85	47	184	23	7	0	7	2.3	1.4	1.5
10019	Beef Tripe-Pickled	1	oz	28.4	25	18	3	0	0	<1	0.1	0.1	<0.1
15025	Chicken Gizzards-Simmered	1	cup	145	98	222	39	2	0	5	1.5	1.3	1.5
15005	Chicken Livers-Simmered	7	ea	140	96	220	34	1	0	8	2.6	1.9	1.3
16048	Smoked GooseLiver Pate-Cnd	1	Tbs	13	5	60	1	1	0	6	1.9	3.3	0.1
Meat Substitutes, Tofu, Vegetarian Foods													
Generic													
7518	Firm Tofu-Raw	1	cup	252	211	194	20	7	1	11	1.6	2.5	6.3
7503	Miso (soybean)	1	cup	275	114	566	32	77	15	17	2.4	3.7	9.4
7508	Natto-Soybean-Fermented	1	cup	175	96	371	31	25	9	19	2.8	4.3	10.9
7718	Soy Burger-BlackBean&Salsa	1	ea	142		200	19	20	3	4	1.5		
7564	Tempeh	1	cup	166	99	320	31	16	9	18	3.7	5	6.4
8835	Tofu Franks/Wiener-Each	1	ea	38		45	9	5	2	0	0	0	0
7520	Tofu-Fried	1	pce	13	7	35	2	1	1	3	0.4	0.6	1.5
7500	Tofu-Regular	1	cup	248	216	151	16	4	<1	9	1.3	2	5.2
7511	Vegetarian Breakfast Links	1	ea	25	13	64	5	2	1	5	0.7	1.1	2.3
7512	Vegetarian Breakfast Patty	1	ea	38	19	97	7	4	1	7	1.1	1.7	3.5
7548	Vegetarian Chicken-BreadFried	1	pce	57	40	97	6	3	3	7	1	1.6	3.9
7549	Vegetarian Fish Sticks	2	ea	57	26	165	13	5	3	10	1.6	2.5	5.3
7550	Vegetarian Frankfurter	1	ea	51	30	102	10	4	2	5	0.8	1.2	2.6
7551	Vegetarian Luncheon Meat	1	pce	67	31	188	17	6	3	11	1.7	2.6	5.6
7561	Vegetarian Meat Patties	1	ea	71	41	142	15	6	3	6	1	1.6	3.3
7552	Vegetarian Meatballs	7	ea	70	41	140	15	6	3	6	1	1.5	3.3
7554	Vegetarian Soyburger	1	ea	71	41	142	15	6	3	6	1	1.6	3.3
Green Giant													
7673	HarvestBurger-Italian-Frozen	1	ea	90		140	17	8	5	4	1.5	0.5	0.5
7674	HarvestBurger-Original-Frozen	1	ea	90	58	137	18	7	6	4	1	2.1	0.3
Lightlife Foods													
8169	Vegetarian Baloney-Pce	1	pce	14.33	10	20	3	1	0	1	0.3		
8173	Vegetarian Ham-Country-Piece	1	pce	14.33	10	17	3	1	0	0	0	0	0
8159	Vegetarian Italian Sausage-Lean	1	ea	40		60	5	5	0	2	1		
8166	Vegetarian Sausage-Lean-Bfast	1	ea	35		60	4	4	0	3	1		
Loma Linda													
7727	Vege ChickenNugget Frozen	5	pce	85	40	244	12	13	5	16	2.5	4	8.8
7666	Vege SandwichSpread-Canned	1	ea	55	38	85	4	7	3	4	0.9	2.1	1.4
Morningstar Farms													
7726	Black Bean Burger	1	ea	78	47	115	12	15	5	1	0.2	0.2	0.4
7752	Breakfast Strip-Frozen	2	pce	16	7	56	2	2	1	4	0.7	1.1	2.6
7724	Deli Franks	1	ea	45	23	112	10	4	3	6	0.9	2	3.3
7665	Vege Chicken Patties-Frozen	1	ea	71		177	7	15	2	10	1.3	2.6	5.9

< = Trace amount present   Blank = Not available

CHOL, cholesterol; V, vitamin; THI, thiamin; RIB, riboflavin; NIA, niacin; FOL, folate;
CALC, calcium; PHOS, phosphate; SOD, sodium; POT, potassium; MAG, magnesium

CHOL (mg)	V-A (RE)	THI (mg)	RIB (mg)	NIA (mg)	V-B6 (mg)	FOL (μg)	V-B12 (μg)	V-C (mg)	V-E (mg)	CALC (mg)	PHOS (mg)	SOD (mg)	POT (mg)	MAG (mg)	IRON (mg)	ZINC (mg)
164	0	0.1	1.3	3.5	0.2	2	12.1	1	0.6	5	212	54	198	21	6.4	2.7
410	9119	0.2	3.5	12.3	1.2	187	95	20	1.4	9	392	90	309	20	5.3	4.6
19	0	0	<0.1	0.5	<0.1	<1	0.3	0	<0.1	36	24	13	5	2	0.5	0.5
281	81	<0.1	0.4	5.8	0.2	77	2.8	2	2.3	14	225	97	260	29	6	6.4
883	6878	0.2	2.4	6.2	0.8	1078	27.1	22	2.4	20	437	71	196	29	11.9	6.1
20	130	<0.1	<0.1	0.3	<0.1	8	1.2	<1	0.2	9	26	91	18	2	0.7	0.1
0	2	0.2	0.3	<0.1	0.2	83	0	1	0.1	408	370	20	444	116	3.7	2.5
0	25	0.3	0.7	2.4	0.6	91	0	0	<0.1	182	421	10029	451	116	7.5	9.1
0	0	0.3	0.3	0	0.2	14	0	23	<0.1	380	304	12	1275	201	15.1	5.3
0												660				
0	0	0.1	0.6	4.4	0.4	40	0.1	0	<0.1	184	442	15	684	134	4.5	1.9
0	0	0.2					0.6	0		20		240	90		1.1	
0	0	<0.1	<0.1	<0.1	<0.1	3	0	0	<0.1	48	37	2	19	8	0.6	0.3
0	2	0.1	0.1	1.3	0.1	109	0	<1	8.4	275	228	20	298	67	2.8	1.6
0	16	0.6	0.1	2.8	0.2	6	0	0	0.5	16	56	222	58	9	0.9	0.4
0	24	0.9	0.2	4.3	0.3	10	0	0	0.8	24	86	337	88	14	1.4	0.6
0	0	0.4	0.3	2.7	0.3	32	1.2	0	1.1	13	140	228	171	7	1	0.4
0	0	0.6	0.5	6.8	0.9	58	2.4	0	2.3	54	256	279	342	13	1.1	0.8
0	0	0.6	0.6	8.2	0.5	40	1.2	0	1	17	175	219	76	9	0.9	0.6
0	0	0.6	0.4	7.4	0.7	67	1.7	0	2	27	296	576	188	15	1.5	1.1
0	0	0.6	0.4	7.1	0.9	55	1.7	0	1.2	21	244	390	128	13	1.5	1.3
0	0	0.6	0.4	7	0.8	55	1.7	0	1.2	20	241	385	126	13	1.5	1.3
0	0	0.6	0.4	7.1	0.9	55	1.7	0	1.2	21	244	390	128	13	1.5	1.3
0	0	0.3	0.1	4	0.3		1.5	0		80		370			2.7	6.8
0	0	0.3	0.2	6.3	0.4	22	0	0	1.6	102	225	411	432	70	3.9	8.1
0	0							1		7		80			0.2	
0	0							<1		0		100			1.8	
0	0							2		20		160			1.1	
0	0							2		20		130			0.9	
2	0	0.7	0.3	2.9	0.4		4.5	0		40	172	709	153		1.4	0.4
1	10	0.3	0.3	1.8	0.5		3.6	0		20	73	255	139		1.3	0.4
1	14	8.1	0.1	0	0.2		0.1	0	0.4	56	150	499	269	44	1.8	0.9
<1	0	0.8	<0.1	0.6	0.1		0.4	0		7	48	220	15		0.3	0.1
<1	0	0.1	<0.1	0	<0.1		<0.1	0	1.3	17	42	431	50	4	0.6	0.4
1	0	2.2	0.2	1.5	0.1		0.9	0		11	106	536	163		1	0.3

ERA, EatRight Analysis CD-ROM; **AMT**, amount; **WT**, weight; **WTR**, water; **CAL**, calories; **PROT**, protein; **CARB**, carbohydrate; **FIBR**, fiber; **FAT**, fat; **SATF**, saturated fat; **MONO**, monosaturated fat; **POLY**, polyunsaturated fat

ERA CODE	FOOD DESCRIPTION	AMT	UNIT	WT (g)	WTR (g)	CAL (kcal)	PROT (g)	CARB (g)	FIBR (g)	FAT (g)	SATF (g)	MONO (g)	POLY (g)
Meat Substitutes, Tofu, Vegetarian Foods (continued)													
Morningstar Farms (continued)													
7722	Vege Patties	1	ea	67	40	119	11	10	4	4	0.5	1.1	2.2
7746	Vegetarian Grillers	1	ea	64	35	139	14	5	3	7	1.7	2.2	3
Natural Touch													
7792	Black Bean Burger	1	ea	78	46	123	13	15	5	1	0.2	0.3	0.5
7758	Lentil Rice Loaf	1	pce	90	57	166	8	14	4	9	2.6	1.7	4.3
7669	Nine Bean Loaf	1	ea	85	55	147	8	13	6	7	1.2	2.4	3.4
7670	Vegan Burger	1	ea	85	61	91	14	8	4	1	0.1	0.3	0.2
Worthington Foods													
8127	Vegetarian Frank/Wiener-Jumbo	1	ea	76		80	16	4	1	0	0	0	0
7634	Vegetarian Beef-Frozen	3	pce	55	32	113	9	4	3	7	1.2	2.7	2.6
7732	Vegetarian Burger	0.25	cup	55	39	60	9	2	1	2	0.3	0.5	1.1
7636	Vegetarian Chicken-Frozen	2	pce	57	39	86	10	1	1	5	0.8	1.2	2.6
7610	Vegetarian Choplets-Canned	2	pce	92	66	93	17	3	2	2	0.9	0.3	0.3
7607	Vegetarian CountryStew-Frozen	1	cup	240	195	208	13	20	5	9	1.6	2.3	4.8
7639	Vegetarian Cutlets-Canned	1	pce	61	43	66	11	3	2	1	0.5	0.4	0.2
7632	Vegetarian Egg Rolls-Frozen	1	ea	85		181	6	20	2	8	1.7	4.5	2.3
7642	Vegetarian Fillets-Frozen	2	pce	85	48	183	16	8	4	10	1.9	3.5	4.3
7734	Vegetarian Leanies-Frozen	1	pce	40	22	106	7	2	1	8	1.3	2.9	3.5
7618	Vegetarian Salami-Frozen	3	pce	57	32	130	12	2	2	8	0.9	1.4	5.8
7624	Vegetarian Tuno-Frozen	1	ea	55	39	83	6	2	1	5	0.9	1.3	3.2
7626	Vegetarian Veelets-Frozen	1	ea	85		171	15	10	5	8	1.5	2.5	3.9
Nuts, Seeds, and Products													
4548	Almonds-Blanched-Sliced	1	cup	105	5	610	23	21	11	53	4.1	33.9	12.6
4503	Almonds-Slivered/Pkd Measure	1	cup	108	6	624	23	21	13	55	4.2	34.7	13.2
4566	Almonds-Toasted-Whole	1	oz	28.35	1	167	6	6	3	14	1.4	9.4	3
4525	Black Walnuts-Chopped	1	cup	125	5	759	30	15	6	71	4.5	15.9	46.9
4519	Cashews-Dry Roasted+Salt	1	cup	137	2	786	21	45	4	63	12.5	37.4	10.7
4621	Cashews-Dry Roast-No Salt	1	cup	137	2	786	21	45	4	63	12.5	37.4	10.7
4596	Cashews-Oil Roasted	1	cup	130	5	749	21	37	5	63	12.4	36.9	10.6
4622	Cashews-Oil Roast-No Salt	1	cup	130	5	749	21	37	5	63	12.4	36.9	10.6
4538	Chestnuts-Roasted	1	cup	143	58	350	5	76	7	3	0.6	1.1	1.2
4649	Coconut Cream-Canned	1	cup	296	211	568	8	25	7	52	46.5	2.2	0.6
4528	Coconut Milk-Raw	1	cup	240	162	552	5	13	5	57	50.7	2.4	0.6
4511	Coconut-Dried-Sweet-Shred	1	cup	93	12	466	3	44	4	33	29.3	1.4	0.4
4510	Coconut-Dried-Unsweet	1	cup	78	2	515	5	19	13	50	44.6	2.1	0.6
4508	Coconut-Raw Piece-2.5x2in	1	pce	45	21	159	1	7	4	15	13.4	0.6	0.2
4556	English Walnuts-Chopped	1	cup	120	5	785	18	16	8	78	7.4	10.7	56.6
4557	English Walnuts-Halves	1	cup	100		654	15	14	7	65	6.1	8.9	47.2
4514	Filberts/Hazelnuts-Chopped	1	cup	115	6	722	17	19	11	70	5.1	52.5	9.1
4513	Filberts/Hazelnuts-Whole	1	cup	135	7	848	20	23	13	82	6	61.7	10.7
4587	Macadamia Nuts-Oil Roasted	1	cup	134	2	962	10	17	12	102	15.4	80.9	1.8
4533	Mixed Nuts+Pnuts-Oil Roast	1	cup	142	3	876	24	30	14	80	12.4	45	18.9

< = Trace amount present   Blank = Not available

CHOL, cholesterol; V, vitamin; THI, thiamin; RIB, riboflavin; NIA, niacin; FOL, folate;
CALC, calcium; PHOS, phosphate; SOD, sodium; POT, potassium; MAG, magnesium

CHOL (mg)	V-A (RE)	THI (mg)	RIB (mg)	NIA (mg)	V-B6 (mg)	FOL (µg)	V-B12 (µg)	V-C (mg)	V-E (mg)	CALC (mg)	PHOS (mg)	SOD (mg)	POT (mg)	MAG (mg)	IRON (mg)	ZINC (mg)
1	77	6.5	0.1	0	0	29	0	0	1	48	124	382	180	29	1.2	0.6
2	0	11.7	0.2	3	0.4		4.9	0		43	111	256	127		1.2	0.5
1	15							0		76	156	323	228		1.9	1
2	78	0.1	0.1	0	<0.1		0.1	0		21	202	366	161		1.2	1
2	151	0.1	0.1	0				1		27	180	319	187		0.6	0.9
0	0	0.3	0.6	4.1	0.2	246	0	0	<0.1	87	181	382	434	16	2.9	0.7
0	0							1		40		590			0.7	
0	0	0.9	0.3	6.5	0.6		4	0		4	92	624	44		2.6	0.2
0	0	0.1	0.1	2	0.2		1.1	0		4	56	269	25		1.7	0.4
1	0	0.3	0.1	1.2	0.2		0.9	0		12	113	374	276		2.1	0.3
0	0	<0.1	0.1	0	0.1		0	0		6	75	500	40		0.4	0.7
2	216	1.8	0.3	4.2	0.9		3.7	0		51	187	826	270		5.1	1
0	0	<0.1	<0.1	0	<0.1		0	0		4	50	340	29		0.2	0.4
1	0	1.2	0.2	0	<0.1		0.1	0		15	93	384	96		0.6	0.3
2	0	0.7	0.1	1	0.4		2.7	0		15	183	749	132		2.1	0.9
1	0	0.2	0.1	1	0.2		0.8	0		25	93	425	43		0.9	0.2
2	0	0.8	0.1	1.1	0.3		0.6	0		26	67	930	93		1.4	0.3
<1	0	0.1	<0.1	1.2	0.3		2	0		20	88	287	34		1.2	0.4
1	0	1.8	0.2	1.6	0.3		3	0		36		388	121		0.5	0.6
0	1	0.2	0.6	3.8	0.1	32	0	0	26.2	227	504	29	721	289	3.9	3.3
0	1	0.3	0.9	4.2	0.1	31	0	0	28.3	268	512	1	786	297	4.6	3.6
0	0	<0.1	0.2	0.8	<0.1	18	0	<1	6.7	80	156	3	219	86	1.4	1.4
0	38	0.3	0.1	0.9	0.7	82	0	4	3.3	72	580	1	655	252	3.8	4.3
0	0	0.3	0.3	1.9	0.3	95	0	0	15.1	62	671	877	774	356	8.2	7.7
0	0	0.3	0.3	1.9	0.3	95	0	0	10.2	62	671	22	774	356	8.2	7.7
0	0	0.6	0.2	2.3	0.3	88	0	0	14.3	53	554	814	689	332	5.3	6.2
0	0	0.6	0.2	2.3	0.3	88	0	0	10.4	53	554	22	689	332	5.3	6.2
0	3	0.3	0.2	1.9	0.7	100	0	37	1.7	41	153	3	846	47	1.3	0.8
0	0	0.1	0.1	0.1	0.1	42	0	5	2.2	3	65	148	299	50	1.5	1.8
0	0	0.1	0	1.8	0.1	39	0	7	1.8	38	240	36	631	89	3.9	1.6
0	0	<0.1	<0.1	0.4	0.3	8	0	1	1.3	14	100	244	313	46	1.8	1.7
0	0	<0.1	0.1	0.5	0.2	7	0	1	1.1	20	161	29	424	70	2.6	1.6
0	0	<0.1	<0.1	0.2	<0.1	12	0	1	0.3	6	51	9	160	14	1.1	0.5
0	5	0.4	0.2	2.3	0.6	118	0	2	3.5	125	415	2	529	190	3.5	3.7
0	4	0.3	0.2	1.9	0.5	98	0	1	2.9	104	346	2	441	158	2.9	3.1
0	5	0.7	0.1	2.1	0.6	130	0	7	17.5	131	334	0	782	187	5.4	2.8
0	5	0.9	0.2	2.4	0.8	152	0	8	20.5	154	392	0	918	220	6.3	3.3
0	1	0.3	0.1	2.7	0.3	21	0	0	19	60	268	348	441	157	2.4	1.5
0	3	0.7	0.3	7.2	0.3	118	0	1	17	153	659	16	825	334	4.6	7.2

ERA, EatRight Analysis CD-ROM; **AMT,** amount; **WT,** weight; **WTR,** water; **CAL,** calories; **PROT,** protein; **CARB,** carbohydrate; **FIBR,** fiber; **FAT,** fat; **SATF,** saturated fat; **MONO,** monosaturated fat; **POLY,** polyunsaturated fat

ERA CODE	FOOD DESCRIPTION	AMT	UNIT	WT (g)	WTR (g)	CAL (kcal)	PROT (g)	CARB (g)	FIBR (g)	FAT (g)	SATF (g)	MONO (g)	POLY (g)
Nuts, Seeds, and Products (continued)													
4594	Mixed Nuts-NoPnts-Oil Roast	1	cup	144	5	886	22	32	8	81	13.1	47.7	16.5
4668	Peanut Butter-Natural	2	Tbs	32	<1	187	8	7	2	16	2.2	7.9	5
4626	Peanut Butter-Smooth-Salted	2	Tbs	32	<1	188	8	7	2	16	3.1	7.5	4.5
4576	Peanut Butter-Chunky-NoSalt	2	Tbs	32	<1	188	8	7	2	16	3.1	7.5	4.5
4590	Peanuts-Dry Roasted w/Salt	1	oz	28.35	<1	166	7	6	2	14	2	7	4.4
4542	Peanuts-Oil Roasted-Unsalted	1	cup	133	3	773	35	25	9	66	9.1	32.5	20.7
4578	Pecans-Dried Halves	1	cup	108	4	746	10	15	10	78	6.7	44	23.3
4577	Pecans-Dried-Chopped	1	cup	119	4	822	11	16	11	86	7.3	48.5	25.7
4554	Pine Nuts/Pinon-Dried	10	ea	1	<1	6	<1	<1	<1	1	0.1	0.2	0.3
4520	Pistachio Nuts-Dried	1	cup	128	5	705	26	37	13	55	6.8	29	16.7
4564	Pumpkin Seeds-Roasted+Salt	1	cup	64	3	285	12	34	3	12	2.3	3.9	5.7
4523	Sesame Seeds-Whole-Dried	1	cup	144	7	825	26	34	17	72	10	27	31.4
4545	Sunflower Seeds-Dry	1	cup	144	8	821	33	27	15	71	7.5	13.6	47.1
4552	Sunflower Seeds-Oil Roasted	1	cup	135	4	830	29	20	9	78	8.1	14.8	51.2
4532	Tahini (Sesame Butter)	1	Tbs	15	<1	91	3	3	1	8	1.2	3.2	3.7
Poultry													
Chicken													
15016	Boned Chicken+Broth-Canned	1	ea	142	97	234	31	0	0	11	3.1	4.5	2.5
15003	Chicken Breast+Skin-Flour Fried	1	ea	196	111	435	62	3	<1	17	4.8	6.9	3.8
15001	Chicken Breast+Skin-Roastd	1	ea	196	122	386	58	0	0	15	4.3	5.9	3.3
15057	Chicken Breast-NoSkin-Fried	1	ea	172	104	322	58	1	0	8	2.2	3	1.8
15004	Chicken Breast-NoSkin-Roasted	1	ea	172	112	284	53	0	0	6	1.7	2.1	1.3
15042	Chicken Drumstick-Fried	1	ea	42	26	82	12	0	0	3	0.9	1.2	0.8
15008	Chicken Drumstick-Roasted	1	ea	52	33	112	14	0	0	6	1.6	2.2	1.3
15035	Chicken Drumstk-NoSkin-Roast	1	ea	44	29	76	12	0	0	2	0.7	0.8	0.6
15028	Chicken Meat-All-Fried	1	cup	140	81	307	43	2	<1	13	3.4	4.7	3
15000	Chicken Meat-All-Roasted	1	cup	140	89	266	40	0	0	10	2.9	3.7	2.4
15006	Chicken Meat-All-Stewed	1	cup	140	94	248	38	0	0	9	2.6	3.3	2.2
15902	Chicken Patty-Breaded-Cooked	1	ea	75	37	213	12	11	<1	13	4.1	6.4	1.7
15009	Chicken Thigh+Skin-Flour Fried	1	ea	62	34	162	17	2	<1	9	2.5	3.6	2.1
15010	Chicken Thigh+Skin-Roasted	1	ea	62	37	153	16	0	0	10	2.7	3.8	2.1
15011	Chicken Thigh-NoSkin-Fried	1	ea	52	31	113	15	1	0	5	1.4	2	1.3
15012	Chicken Thigh-NoSkin-Roast	1	ea	52	33	109	13	0	0	6	1.6	2.2	1.3
15002	Chicken Wing+Skin-Roasted	1	ea	34	19	99	9	0	0	7	1.9	2.6	1.4
15029	Chicken Wing-Flour Fried	1	ea	32	16	103	8	1	<1	7	1.9	2.8	1.6
15027	Chicken-Dark Meat-Roasted	1	cup	140	88	287	38	0	0	14	3.7	5	3.2
15032	Chicken-Light Meat-Roasted	1	cup	140	91	242	43	0	0	6	1.8	2.2	1.4
15903	Chicken Wings-Buffalo/Spicy	1	pce	16	9	49	4	<1	<1	3	0.9	1.3	0.9
Turkey													
16003	Ground Turkey-Patty-Cooked	1	ea	82	49	193	22	0	0	11	2.8	4	2.6
16040	Tom Turkey-NoSkin-Roasted	1	cup	140	91	235	41	0	0	7	2.2	1.4	1.9
16002	Turkey Dark Meat-Roasted	1	cup	140	88	262	40	0	0	10	3.4	2.3	3
16000	Turkey Meat-All-Roasted	1	cup	140	91	238	41	0	0	7	2.3	1.4	2
16001	Turkey White Meat-Roasted	1	cup	140	96	196	42	0	0	2	0.5	0.3	0.4

< = Trace amount present   Blank = Not available

CHOL, cholesterol; **V**, vitamin; **THI**, thiamin; **RIB**, riboflavin; **NIA**, niacin; **FOL**, folate;
CALC, calcium; **PHOS**, phosphate; **SOD**, sodium; **POT**, potassium; **MAG**, magnesium

CHOL (mg)	V-A (RE)	THI (mg)	RIB (mg)	NIA (mg)	V-B6 (mg)	FOL (μg)	V-B12 (μg)	V-C (mg)	V-E (mg)	CALC (mg)	PHOS (mg)	SOD (mg)	POT (mg)	MAG (mg)	IRON (mg)	ZINC (mg)
0	3	0.7	0.7	2.8	0.3	81	0	1	17.3	153	646	16	783	361	3.7	6.7
0	0	0.1	<0.1	4.3	0.1	46	0	0	2.4	17	114	2	210	56	0.7	1.1
0	0	<0.1	<0.1	4.4	0.1	29	0	0	2.4	13	101	156	239	51	0.6	0.9
0	0	<0.1	<0.1	4.4	0.1	29	0	0	3.2	13	101	5	239	51	0.6	0.9
0	0	0.1	<0.1	3.8	0.1	41	0	0	2.8	15	101	230	186	50	0.6	0.9
0	0	0.3	0.1	19	0.3	167	0	0	9.9	117	688	8	907	246	2.4	8.8
0	8	0.7	0.1	1.3	0.2	24	0	1	4	76	299	0	443	131	2.7	4.9
0	9	0.8	0.2	1.4	0.2	26	0	1	4.4	83	330	0	488	144	3	5.4
0	<1	<0.1	<0.1	<0.1	<0.1	1	0	<1	0.1	<1	<1	1	6	2	<0.1	<0.1
0	71	1.1	0.2	1.7	2.2	65	0	6	5.9	137	627	1	1250	155	5.5	2.8
0	4	<0.1	<0.1	0.2	<0.1	6	0	<1	2.5	35	59	368	588	168	2.1	6.6
0	1	1.1	0.4	6.5	1.1	139	0	0	3.3	1404	906	16	674	505	21	11.2
0	7	3.3	0.4	6.5	1.1	327	0	2	72.4	167	1015	4	992	510	9.7	7.3
0	7	0.4	0.4	5.6	1.1	316	0	2	67.9	76	1537	814	652	171	9	7
0	1	0.2	<0.1	0.8	<0.1	15	0	0	0.3	21	118	<1	69	53	1	1.6
88	48	<0.1	0.2	9	0.5	6	0.4	3	0.6	20	158	714	196	17	2.2	2
174	29	0.2	0.3	26.9	1.1	12	0.7	0	1.4	31	457	149	508	59	2.3	2.2
165	53	0.1	0.2	24.9	1.1	8	0.6	0	1.1	27	419	139	480	53	2.1	2
156	12	0.1	0.2	25.4	1.1	7	0.6	0	0.7	28	423	136	475	53	2	1.9
146	10	0.1	0.2	23.6	1	7	0.6	0	0.7	26	392	127	440	50	1.8	1.7
39	8	<0.1	0.1	2.6	0.2	4	0.1	0	0.2	5	78	40	104	10	0.6	1.4
47	16	<0.1	0.1	3.1	0.2	4	0.2	0	0.3	6	91	47	119	12	0.7	1.5
41	8	<0.1	0.1	2.7	0.2	4	0.1	0	0.3	5	81	42	108	11	0.6	1.4
132	25	0.1	0.3	13.5	0.7	10	0.5	0	0.6	24	287	127	360	38	1.9	3.1
125	22	0.1	0.2	12.8	0.7	8	0.5	0	0.8	21	273	120	340	35	1.7	2.9
116	21	0.1	0.2	8.6	0.4	8	0.3	0	0.7	20	210	98	252	29	1.6	2.8
45	22	0.1	0.1	5	0.2	8	0.2	<1	1.5	12	150	399	184	15	0.9	0.8
60	18	0.1	0.2	4.3	0.2	7	0.2	0	0.7	9	116	55	147	16	0.9	1.6
58	30	<0.1	0.1	3.9	0.2	4	0.2	0	0.7	7	108	52	138	14	0.8	1.5
53	11	<0.1	0.1	3.7	0.2	5	0.2	0	0.4	7	103	49	135	14	0.8	1.5
49	10	<0.1	0.1	3.4	0.2	4	0.2	0	0.4	6	95	46	124	12	0.7	1.3
29	16	<0.1	<0.1	2.3	0.1	1	0.1	0	0.5	5	51	28	63	6	0.4	0.6
26	12	<0.1	<0.1	2.1	0.1	2	0.1	0	0.5	5	48	25	57	6	0.4	0.6
130	31	0.1	0.3	9.2	0.5	11	0.4	0	1	21	251	130	336	32	1.9	3.9
119	13	0.1	0.2	17.4	0.8	6	0.5	0	0.5	21	302	108	346	38	1.5	1.7
13	9	<0.1	<0.1	1	0.1	<1	<0.1	<1	0.1	2	24	13	29	3	0.2	0.3
84	0	<0.1	0.1	4	0.3	6	0.3	0	0.3	20	161	88	221	20	1.6	2.3
108	0	0.1	0.3	7.4	0.7	11	0.5	0	0.6	35	300	104	421	36	2.5	4.4
119	0	0.1	0.3	5.1	0.5	13	0.5	0	1.2	45	286	111	406	34	3.3	6.2
106	0	0.1	0.3	7.6	0.6	10	0.5	0	0.6	35	298	98	417	36	2.5	4.3
120	0	0.1	0.2	9.7	0.8	8	0.5	0	0.1	21	302	78	388	39	2.2	2.9

ERA, EatRight Analysis CD-ROM; **AMT,** amount; **WT,** weight; **WTR,** water; **CAL,** calories; **PROT,** protein; **CARB,** carbohydrate; **FIBR,** fiber; **FAT,** fat; **SATF,** saturated fat; **MONO,** monosaturated fat; **POLY,** polyunsaturated fat

ERA CODE	FOOD DESCRIPTION	AMT	UNIT	WT (g)	WTR (g)	CAL (kcal)	PROT (g)	CARB (g)	FIBR (g)	FAT (g)	SATF (g)	MONO (g)	POLY (g)
Poultry (continued)													
Turkey (continued)													
16276	TurkeyChunk White-Cnd-Water	0.25	cup	62		90	16	4	1	2	0.5		
Duck, Emu, Ostrich and Other													
15069	Cornish Game Hen-Roasted	1	ea	306	180	796	68	0	0	56	15.4	24.5	11
14001	Duck+Skin-Domestic-Roasted	1	cup	140	73	472	27	0	0	40	13.5	18.1	5.1
14000	Duck-Meat Only-Roasted	1	ea	442	284	888	104	0	0	50	18.4	16.4	6.3
16289	Emu Thigh-Raw	3	oz	85		79	17			1			
14002	Goose Meat-NoSkin-Roasted	1	ea	1182	676	2813	342	0	0	150	53.9	51.3	18.2
14003	Goose+Skin-Domestic-Roast	0.5	ea	774	402	2360	195	0	0	170	53.2	79.3	19.5
16332	Ostrich-Tenderloin-Ckd	1	oz	28.35	19	38	7	0	0	1	0.3	0.4	0.3
Salad Dressings, Dips, and Mayonnaise													
Dips													
7083	Jalapeno Pepper Bean Dip	1	cup	262	180	376	16	49	18	14	1.9	3.4	8.2
8136	Sour Cream Dip-Cup Meas	1	cup	243	160	536	9	20	2	48	29.5	14.2	1.9
Mayonnaise													
8046	Mayonnaise	1	Tbs	13.8	2	99	<1	<1	0	11	1.6	3.1	5.7
8069	Mayonnaise-FatFree	1	Tbs	16	13	11	<1	2	<1	<1	0.1		
8032	Mayonnaise-Imitation	1	Tbs	15	9	35	<1	2	0	3	0.5	0.7	1.6
8033	Mayonnaise-LowCal	1	Tbs	15	9	35	<1	2	0	3	0.5	0.7	1.6
8148	Mayonnaise-LowCal-LowSod	1	Tbs	14	9	32	<1	2	0	3	0.5	0.6	1.5
8021	Miracle Whip	1	Tbs	14.7	6	57	<1	4	0	5	0.7	1.3	2.6
8122	Miracle Whip-Light	1	Tbs	14	8	36	<1	3	0	3	0.4	0.6	1.5
Salad Dressings-Lower Calorie/Fat/Sodium/Cholest													
8023	1000 Island Dressing-LowCal	1	Tbs	15.31	11	24	<1	2	<1	2	0.2	0.4	0.9
286	Benecol French Dressing	1	Tbs	15		65	0	3	0	6	1		
287	Benecol Ranch Dressing	1	Tbs	14.5		65	0	2	0	6	1		
8498	Catalina Dressing-FatFree	1	Tbs	17.5		22	0	6	<1	0	0	0	0
8017	Dijon Vinaigrette-Lite	1	Tbs	15	12	16	<1	1	<1	1	0.2	0.3	0.9
8499	French Dressing-FatFree	1	Tbs	17.5		20	0	6	<1	0	0	0	0
8014	French Dressing-LowCal	1	Tbs	16.25	11	22	<1	4	0	8	0.1	0.2	0.6
8504	Honey Dijon Dressing-FatFree	1	Tbs	17.5		25	<1	6	<1	0	0	0	0
8491	Italian Dressing-FatFree	1	Tbs	16.5	13	10	<1	2	<1	<1	0.1		
8016	Italian Dressing-LowCal	1	Tbs	15	12	16	<1	1	<1	1	0.2	0.3	0.9
8493	Ranch Dressing-FatFree	1	Tbs	17.5	11	24	<1	5	<1	<1	<0.1		
Salad Dressings-Regular													
8024	1000 Island Dressing	1	Tbs	15.625	7	59	<1	2	0	6	0.9	1.3	3.1
8013	Blue Cheese Dressing	1	Tbs	15.31	5	77	1	1	0	8	1.5	1.9	4.3
8066	Caesar Salad Dressing	1	Tbs	11.5	4	53	1	<1	<1	5	0.9	3.6	0.5
8015	French Dressing	1	Tbs	15.6	6	67	<1	3	0	6	1.5	1.2	3.4
8124	Honey Mustard Dressing	1	Tbs	15.6	5	51	<1	7	<1	3	0.3	0.9	1.4
8020	Italian Dressing	1	Tbs	14.7	6	69	<1	1	0	7	1	1.6	4.1
8035	Oil & Vinegar Dressing	1	Tbs	16	8	72	0	<1	0	8	1.5	2.4	3.9

< = Trace amount present   Blank = Not available

CHOL, cholesterol; **V,** vitamin; **THI,** thiamin; **RIB,** riboflavin; **NIA,** niacin; **FOL,** folate;
CALC, calcium; **PHOS,** phosphate; **SOD,** sodium; **POT,** potassium; **MAG,** magnesium

CHOL (mg)	V-A (RE)	THI (mg)	RIB (mg)	NIA (mg)	V-B6 (mg)	FOL (µg)	V-B12 (µg)	V-C (mg)	V-E (mg)	CALC (mg)	PHOS (mg)	SOD (mg)	POT (mg)	MAG (mg)	IRON (mg)	ZINC (mg)
35	0							0	0			220			0	
401	98	0.2	0.6	18	0.9	6	0.9	2	0.8	40	447	196	750	55	2.8	4.6
118	88	0.2	0.4	6.8	0.3	8	0.4	0	1.8	15	218	83	286	22	3.8	2.6
393	102	1.1	2.1	22.5	1.1	44	1.8	0	7.7	53	897	287	1113	88	11.9	11.5
42															4.2	
1134	142	1.1	4.6	48.2	5.6	142	5.8	0	33	165	3652	898	4586	296	33.9	37.5
704	162	0.6	2.5	32.3	2.9	15	3.2	0	20	101	2089	542	2546	170	21.9	20.3
27												20			0.8	
0	78	0.3	0.1	0.9	0.3	188	0	37	3.1	86	283	12	793	101	3.9	1.8
100	437	0.1	0.4	1.1	0.1	27	0.7	2	1.5	288	252	1820	449	37	0.4	0.7
8	12	0	0	0	0.1	1	<0.1	0	8	2	4	78	5	<1	0.1	<0.1
2	3							0	0.5	1	4	120	8		<0.1	
4	0	0	0	0	0	0	0	0	2.7	<1	<1	75	2	<1	0	<0.1
4	0	0	0	0	0	0	0	0	2.7	<1	<1	75	2	<1	0	<0.1
3	1	0	<0.1	0	0	<1	<0.1	0	0.5	0	0	15	1	0	0	<0.1
4	12	<0.1	<0.1	<0.1	<0.1	1	<0.1	0	4.4	2	4	104	1	<1	<0.1	<0.1
4	9	<0.1	<0.1	0	<0.1	1	<0.1	0	0.6	2	4	99	1	<1	<0.1	<0.1
2	15	<0.1	<0.1	<0.1	<0.1	1	<0.1	0	0.2	2	3	153	17	<1	0.1	<0.1
0	0							0		0		85			0	
0	0							0		0		125			0	
0	75							0		0		180	30		0	
1	0	0	0	0	0	0	0	0	1.4	<1	1	118	2	0	<0.1	<0.1
0	75							0		0		150	20		0	
0	21	0	0	0	0	0	0	0	0.8	2	2	128	13	0	0.1	<0.1
0	0							0		0		165	25		0.2	
<1	5							<1		7	34	215	19		<0.1	
1	0	0	0	0	0	0	0	0	1.4	<1	1	118	2	0	<0.1	<0.1
<1	<1							<1		5	14	177	15		<0.1	
4	15	<0.1	<0.1	<0.1	<0.1	1	<0.1	0	0.2	2	2	109	18	<1	0.1	<0.1
3	10	<0.1	<0.1	<0.1	<0.1	1	0.4	<1	7.5	12	11	168	6	0	<0.1	<0.1
12	6	<0.1	<0.1	0.5	<0.1	2	0.1	1	0.7	22	19	198	20	3	0.2	0.1
0	20	<0.1	<0.1	0	<0.1	1	<0.1	0	5.9	2	2	214	12	0	0.1	<0.1
0	0	<0.1	<0.1	<0.1	<0.1	<1	0	<1	0.6	3	3	37	10	2	0.1	0.1
0	4	<0.1	<0.1	0	<0.1	1	<0.1	0	1.5	1	1	116	2	<1	<0.1	<0.1
0	0	0	0	0	0	0	0	0	8.3	0	0	<1	1	0	0	0

ERA, EatRight Analysis CD-ROM; **AMT,** amount; **WT,** weight; **WTR,** water; **CAL,** calories; **PROT,** protein; **CARB,** carbohydrate; **FIBR,** fiber; **FAT,** fat; **SATF,** saturated fat; **MONO,** monosaturated fat; **POLY,** polyunsaturated fat

ERA CODE	FOOD DESCRIPTION	AMT	UNIT	WT (g)	WTR (g)	CAL (kcal)	PROT (g)	CARB (g)	FIBR (g)	FAT (g)	SATF (g)	MONO (g)	POLY (g)
Salad Dressings, Dips, and Mayonnaise (continued)													
Salad Dressings-Regular (continued)													
8022	Russian Dressing	1	Tbs	15.31	5	76	<1	2	0	8	1.1	1.8	4.5
8019	Vinegarette Dressing	1	Tbs	14.7	6	69	<1	1	0	7	1	1.6	4.1
8123	Yogurt Dressing	1	Tbs	15.4	13	11	<1	1	<1	1	0.3	0.2	0.1
Salads													
56109	Carrot Raisin Salad	1	cup	175	101	405	3	42	4	28	4	7.8	14.5
56628	Chef Style Salad	1.5	cup	326	269	267	26	5		16	8.2	5.2	1.4
56002	Chicken Salad w/Celery	0.5	cup	78	41	268	11	1	<1	25	3.1	4.5	15.8
56253	Crab Salad	1	cup	208	153	282	27	11	1	14	2	3.5	7.1
5638	Cucumber Salad w/Vinegar	1	cup	159	145	48	1	12	1	<1	<0.1	<0.1	0.1
56003	Egg Salad	1	cup	183	105	584	17	3	0	56	10.5	17.4	23.9
5637	Mixed Salad Greens/Lettuce	1	cup	55	52	9	1	2	1	<1	<0.1	<0.1	0.1
56005	Potato Salad+Mayo+Eggs	1	cup	250	190	358	7	28	3	20	3.6	6.2	9.3
56257	Seafood Salad	1	cup	208	152	328	26	5	1	23	3.2	16	2.4
56256	Shrimp Salad	1	cup	182	131	282	27	6	1	17	2.6	4.5	8.4
5537	Spinach Salad-No Dressing	1	cup	74	51	108	5	11	2	5	1.4	2.2	0.7
56916	Tabbouleh/Tabbuli	1	cup	160	124	199	3	16	4	15	2	10.8	1.4
56643	Taco Salad	1.5	cup	198	143	279	13	24		15	6.8	5.2	1.7
56118	Three Bean Salad	1	cup	150	121	140	4	15	5	8	1.1	1.7	4.4
5677	Tossed Green Salad	0.75	cup	104	98	19	1	4	1	<1	<0.1	<0.1	0.1
56007	Tuna Salad	1	cup	205	129	383	33	19	0	19	3.2	5.9	8.4
56006	Waldorf Salad	1	cup	137	79	408	4	13	2	40	4.2	7.3	27
Sandwiches													
10047	Beef Sand Steak-Steak Ums	1	ea	41	24	104	10	0	0	7	2.6	2.9	0.2
56008	BLT Sandwich-Firm White	1	ea	133		336	11	32	2	18	4.5	6.1	6.1
56281	Bologna Sandwich	1	ea	83	34	256	7	26	1	13	4.1	6.3	2.1
56016	Chicken Salad San-FirmWhite	1	ea	118.8		397	12	35	2	23	3.7	6	12
57519	Chicken Fajita w/Cheese on Pita	1	ea	207	142	311	22	28	2	12	4.5	3.4	3.3
56020	Corned Beef+Swiss on Rye	1	ea	156		420	28	22	<1	26	9.4	7.4	6.3
56024	Egg Salad Sandwich on White	1	ea	125.6		409	11	35	2	25	4.4	6.8	12
66011	Fish Sandwich+Cheese+TartarSc	1	ea	183	83	523	21	48	<1	29	8.1	8.9	9.4
56268	French Dip Sandwich AuJus	1	ea	193	118	363	25	34	2	13	4.7	5.8	0.9
69017	Grilled Chicken Sandwich	1	ea	113		210	18	24	2	5	2		
56012	Grilled Cheese Sandw on White	1	ea	127.8		428	19	34	1	24	13.1	7.5	2
56272	Gyro Sandwich	1	ea	105	67	170	12	21	1	4	1.5	1.4	0.4
56033	Ham & Swiss on Rye Sandwich	1	ea	149.5		338	22	22	<1	19	6.5	5.1	6
56066	Ham Salad Sandwich on Wheat	1	ea	130.6		356	11	35	3	20	4.5	6.8	7.4
56031	Ham Sandwich on Wheat	1	ea	156.3		329	22	28	3	14	2.7	4.4	6
56267	Pastrami Sandwich	1	ea	134	71	331	14	27	2	18	6.2	8.7	1
56038	Patty Melt Sandwich on Rye	1	ea	181.9		561	37	22	3	37	13.2	11.7	8.4
56040	Peanut Butter & Jelly on White	1	ea	101		351	12	47	3	15	3.1	6.7	3.9
56266	Reuben Sandwich-Grilled	1	ea	181	97	464	21	30	3	29	9.9	9.7	6.7
56046	Roast Beef Sandwich on Wheat	1	ea	155.8		397	29	32	3	17	3.2	4.3	8.3
56671	Submarine Sandwich w/Coldcuts	1	ea	228	132	456	22	51	2	19	6.8	8.2	2.3

< = Trace amount present   Blank = Not available

CHOL, cholesterol; **V,** vitamin; **THI,** thiamin; **RIB,** riboflavin; **NIA,** niacin; **FOL,** folate;
CALC, calcium; **PHOS,** phosphate; **SOD,** sodium; **POT,** potassium; **MAG,** magnesium

CHOL (mg)	V-A (RE)	THI (mg)	RIB (mg)	NIA (mg)	V-B6 (mg)	FOL (μg)	V-B12 (μg)	V-C (mg)	V-E (mg)	CALC (mg)	PHOS (mg)	SOD (mg)	POT (mg)	MAG (mg)	IRON (mg)	ZINC (mg)
3	32	<0.1	<0.1	0.1	<0.1	2	<0.1	1	7.3	3	6	133	24	<1	0.1	0.1
0	4	<0.1	<0.1	0	<0.1	1	<0.1	0	1.5	1	1	116	2	<1	<0.1	<0.1
2	4	<0.1	<0.1	<0.1	<0.1	1	<0.1	<1	<0.1	15	12	6	22	2	<0.1	0.1
20	2889	0.2	0.1	1.3	0.4	18	0.1	11	20.5	53	92	235	630	28	1.5	0.4
140	137	0.4	0.4	6	0.4	101	0.8	16		235	401	743	401	49	2	3.1
48	31	<0.1	0.1	3.3	0.3	8	0.2	1	6.3	16	80	200	138	11	0.6	0.8
142	37	0.2	0.1	4.5	0.3	79	9.8	7	2.8	157	292	700	536	49	1.5	5.7
0	20	<0.1	<0.1	0.2	0.1	16	0	6	0.1	19	29	3	206	21	0.5	0.2
581	262	0.1	0.7	0.1	0.5	61	1.6	0	7.7	74	238	464	181	13	1.8	1.4
0	150	<0.1	0.1	0.2	<0.1	64	0	9	0.4	30	18	14	174	13	0.7	0.2
170	82	0.2	0.2	2.2	0.4	17	0	25	19	48	130	1322	635	38	1.6	0.8
132	51	0.1	0.1	2.4	0.2	31	1.8	12	4	92	283	352	503	54	2	3.3
206	42	0.1	0.1	3.3	0.3	15	1.3	6	3.4	87	280	392	366	52	3.4	1.5
77	176	0.1	0.3	1.7	0.1	60	0.2	7	0.9	46	83	227	242	27	1.5	0.6
0	69	0.1	0.1	1.1	0.1	31	0	28	2.2	29	64	799	246	36	1.2	0.5
44	77	0.1	0.4	2.5	0.2	83	0.6	4		192	142	762	416	51	2.3	2.7
0	20	0.1	0.1	0.4	<0.1	56	<0.1	4	1.7	35	76	520	246	27	1.5	0.6
0	209	0.1	<0.1	0.4	0.1	36	0	11	0.4	14	24	11	201	11	0.5	0.2
27	55	0.1	0.1	13.7	0.2	16	2.5	5	21.9	35	365	824	365	39	2	1.1
21	39	0.1	<0.1	0.4	0.4	27	0.1	6	27.6	43	84	236	270	39	0.9	0.6
33	0	<0.1	0.1	1.9	0.1	4	0.8	0	0.1	3	66	29	128	9	1	2.2
22	31	0.4	0.2	3.5	0.1	37	0.3	12	6.1	67	133	630	252	22	2.2	1
16	37	0.3	0.2	2.7	0.1	19	0.4	<1	0.8	60	74	598	112	15	2	0.9
33	24	0.3	0.2	4	0.2	29	0.1	1	14.8	76	114	498	158	20	2.3	0.9
51	102	0.3	0.3	5.1	0.3	35	0.4	33	1.5	187	221	784	372	37	2.1	2
82	81	0.2	0.3	2.7	0.2	19	1.7	1	7.3	268	272	1392	225	28	3.1	3.6
157	76	0.3	0.3	2.3	0.2	41	0.4	0	10.8	87	134	566	133	18	2.4	0.8
68	97	0.5	0.4	4.2	0.1	92	1.1	3	1.8	185	311	939	353	37	3.5	1.2
54	0	0.4	0.4	5.9	0.2	25	2	0	0.4	104	212	616	380	32	4.2	5.1
20	0								0	60		420	220		1.4	
56	212	0.3	0.4	2.2	0.1	28	0.4	<1	2.5	414	491	1182	174	27	2.1	2.1
34	11	0.2	0.2	3.1	0.1	18	0.9	4	0.3	46	116	272	209	21	1.9	2.3
57	79	0.7	0.4	4.1	0.3	16	1.2	15	6.8	257	327	1597	343	29	2.2	2.6
29	8	0.5	0.2	3.7	0.2	25	0.5	4	9.2	69	166	933	215	33	2.4	1.3
45	8	1	0.3	6.5	0.5	27	0.7	22	6.5	72	277	1634	422	43	2.7	2.3
51	3	0.3	0.3	4.8	0.1	21	1	2	0.3	68	135	1334	243	23	2.6	2.7
113	123	0.3	0.5	6.1	0.3	25	2.4	<1	10.4	221	327	701	391	36	4.2	7.1
2	<1	0.3	0.2	5.3	0.1	40	0	<1	1.1	60	141	293	245	56	2.3	1.1
82	94	0.2	0.4	3.4	0.2	37	1.3	4	0.8	299	291	1348	261	39	2.9	4
43	12	0.3	0.3	6.8	0.4	34	2.2	12	9.1	72	232	1605	484	42	4.3	4
36	80	1	0.8	5.5	0.1	87	1.1	12		189	287	1650	394	68	2.5	2.6

ERA, EatRight Analysis CD-ROM; **AMT,** amount; **WT,** weight; **WTR,** water; **CAL,** calories; **PROT,** protein; **CARB,** carbohydrate; **FIBR,** fiber; **FAT,** fat; **SATF,** saturated fat; **MONO,** monosaturated fat; **POLY,** polyunsaturated fat

ERA CODE	FOOD DESCRIPTION	AMT	UNIT	WT (g)	WTR (g)	CAL (kcal)	PROT (g)	CARB (g)	FIBR (g)	FAT (g)	SATF (g)	MONO (g)	POLY (g)
Sandwiches (continued)													
56047	Tuna Salad Sandwich on White	1	ea	131		356	15	40	2	15	2.4	3.8	7.9
56053	Turkey Sandwich-Whole Wheat	1	ea	168.8		364	26	33	4	15	2.3	3.5	8.4
56103	Turkey Ham Sandwich on Rye	1	ea	149.5		280	21	20	<1	14	2.5	2.8	6.9
56059	Turkey Ham+Cheese on Wheat	1	ea	156.3		396	23	28	3	22	8.2	5.3	6.8
Snack Foods-Chips, Pretzels, Popcorn													
44061	Bagel Chips	5	pce	70	2	298	6	52	4	7	1.3	2.1	3.4
44029	Bugles Corn Chips-Plain	2	oz	56.7	1	289	3	36	1	15	12.9	1	0.4
44001	Cheetos Cheese Puffs	1	cup	20	<1	111	2	11	<1	7	1.3	4.1	1
44032	Chex Party Mix	1	cup	42.5	1	181	5	28	2	7	2.3	3.9	1.1
44033	Combos Pretzels w/Cheese	10	pce	30	1	139	3	20		5			
44002	Corn Chips (Fritos)	1	cup	26	<1	140	2	15	1	9	1.2	2.5	4.3
44031	Cornnuts-Toasted Corn Nuggets	10	pce	18	<1	79	2	13	1	3	0.5	1.3	0.6
44037	Cracker Jacks Snack	1	cup	42.5	1	170	3	34	2	3	0.4	1.2	1.4
44004	Dorito Chips-Nacho Flavor	1	cup	26	<1	129	2	16	1	7	1.3	3.9	0.9
44012	Popcorn-Air Popped-Plain	1	cup	8	<1	31	1	6	1	<1	<0.1	0.1	0.2
44014	Popcorn-Caramel Corn	1	cup	35.2	1	152	1	28	2	5	1.3	1	1.6
44038	Popcorn-Cheese	1	cup	11	<1	58	1	6	1	4	0.7	1.1	1.7
44013	Popcorn-Cooked in Oil+Salt	1	cup	11	<1	55	1	6	1	3	0.5	0.9	1.5
44006	Potato Chips	10	pce	20	<1	107	1	11	1	7	2.2	2	2.4
44040	Potato Chips-BBQ	20	pce	26	<1	128	2	14	1	8	2.1	1.7	4.3
44043	Potato Chips-Light	20	pce	40	<1	188	3	27	2	8	1.7	1.9	4.4
44015	Pretzels-Dutch Twist	10	pce	60	2	229	5	48	2	2	0.4	0.8	0.7
44017	Rice Cake-CarmelCorn-Mini	1	ea	3.2	<1	13	<1	3	<1	<1	0.1	<0.1	<0.1
44016	Rice Cake-Plain-Regular Size	1	ea	9		35	1	7	<1	<1	0.1	0.1	0.1
44064	Rice Cake-Unsalted	2	ea	18	1	70	1	15	1	1	0.1	0.2	0.2
44266	Tortilla Chips-Low Fat	13	pce	28		110	2	24	2	1	0	0.3	0.7
44267	Tortilla Chips-No Salt	13	pce	28		110	3	24	2	1	0		
44054	Tortilla Chips-Nacho-LowFat	10	ea	16	<1	71	1	11	1	2	0.5	1.4	0.3
44058	Trail Mix-Regular	1	cup	150	14	693	21	67	8	44	8.3	18.8	14.5
44085	Trail Mix-Regular-Unsalted	1	cup	150	14	693	21	67	8	44	8.3	18.8	14.5
44060	Trail Mix-Tropical	1	cup	140	13	570	9	92	9	24	11.9	3.5	7.2
Soups, Stews and Chilis													
50000	Bean+Bacon Soup w/Water	1	cup	253	213	172	8	23	9	6	1.5	2.2	1.8
50001	Beef Broth/Bouillon-Prepared	1	cup	240	234	17	3	<1	0	1	0.3	0.2	<0.1
50183	Beef Broth-Canned-LowSodium	1	cup	240	230	38	5	1	0	1	0.4	0.7	0.3
50033	Beef Broth-Cube+Water	1	cup	241	236	7	1	1	0	<1	0.1	0.1	0
50003	Beef Noodle Soup+Water	1	cup	244	224	83	5	9	1	3	1.1	1.2	0.5
50066	Beef Soup-Chunky-Prepared	1	cup	240	200	170	12	20	1	5	2.5	2.1	0.2
50060	Black Bean Soup+Water	1	cup	247	216	116	6	20	4	2	0.4	0.5	0.5
50204	Bouillabaise Soup/Chowder	1	cup	227	177	241	34	5	1	9	2	3.9	1.5
50071	Cheese Soup+Milk	1	cup	251	207	231	9	16	1	15	9.1	4.1	0.5
50004	Chicken Broth-Can+Water	1	cup	244	234	39	5	1	0	1	0.4	0.6	0.3
50035	Chicken Broth-Cube+Water	1	cup	243	237	12	1	2	0	<1	0.1	0.1	0.1
50005	Chicken Noodle Soup+Water	1	cup	241	222	75	4	9	1	2	0.6	1.1	0.6

< = Trace amount present   Blank = Not available

CHOL, cholesterol; **V**, vitamin; **THI**, thiamin; **RIB**, riboflavin; **NIA**, niacin; **FOL**, folate;
CALC, calcium; **PHOS**, phosphate; **SOD**, sodium; **POT**, potassium; **MAG**, magnesium

CHOL (mg)	V-A (RE)	THI (mg)	RIB (mg)	NIA (mg)	V-B6 (mg)	FOL (μg)	V-B12 (μg)	V-C (mg)	V-E (mg)	CALC (mg)	PHOS (mg)	SOD (mg)	POT (mg)	MAG (mg)	IRON (mg)	ZINC (mg)
15	22	0.3	0.2	5.8	0.1	29	0.7	1	11.9	76	167	605	180	25	2.5	0.7
43	12	0.3	0.2	9.8	0.5	39	1.8	0	9.7	59	359	1664	418	77	2.7	2.3
55	8	0.2	0.3	4.3	0.3	17	0.3	<1	7	51	213	1182	341	25	4.1	3
64	90	0.3	0.4	4.4	0.3	30	0.4	0	6.6	246	411	1389	354	44	3.7	3.2
0	0	0.1	0.1	1.6	0.2	46	0	<1	1.7	9	145	419	167	39	1.4	0.9
0	18	0.2	0.1	0.8	<0.1	2	0	0	1.1	2	25	579	46	6	1.4	0.1
1	7	0.1	0.1	0.6	<0.1	24	<0.1	<1	1	12	22	210	33	4	0.5	0.1
0	6	0.7	0.2	7.2	0.7	0	5.3	20	0.1	15	79	432	114	27	10.5	0.9
2	2	0.1	0.2	1	<0.1	2	<0.1	0	0.1	59	43	335	39	7	0.3	0.2
0	2	<0.1	<0.1	0.3	0.1	5	0	0	1.6	33	48	164	37	20	0.3	0.3
0	0	<0.1	<0.1	0.3	<0.1	0	0	0	0.2	2	50	99	50	20	0.3	0.3
0	3	<0.1	0.1	0.8	0.1	7	0	0	0.6	28	54	125	151	34	1.7	0.5
1	11	<0.1	<0.1	0.4	0.1	4	<0.1	<1	1	38	63	184	56	21	0.4	0.3
0	2	<0.1	<0.1	0.2	<0.1	2	0	0	<0.1	1	24	<1	24	10	0.2	0.3
2	4	<0.1	<0.1	0.8	<0.1	1	<0.1	0	0.4	15	29	73	38	12	0.6	0.2
1	5	<0.1	<0.1	0.2	<0.1	1	0.1	<1	<0.1	12	40	98	29	10	0.2	0.2
0	2	<0.1	<0.1	0.2	<0.1	2	0	<1	<0.1	1	28	97	25	12	0.3	0.3
0	0	<0.1	<0.1	0.8	0.1	9	0	6	1.3	5	33	119	255	13	0.3	0.2
0	6	0.1	0.1	1.2	0.2	22	0	9	1.3	13	48	195	328	20	0.5	0.2
0	0	0.1	0.1	2.8	0.3	11	0	10	1.2	8	77	197	698	36	0.5	<0.1
0	0	0.3	0.4	3.2	0.1	103	0	0	0.5	22	68	1029	88	21	2.6	0.5
<1	1	<0.1	<0.1	0.1	<0.1	1	0	<1	<0.1	1	6	14	6	3	<0.1	<0.1
0	0	<0.1	<0.1	0.6	0.1	2	0	0	<0.1	1	33	14	25	14	0.1	2
0	1	<0.1	<0.1	1.4	<0.1	4	0	0	<0.1	2	65	5	52	24	0.3	0.5
0	0	<0.1	<0.1	0.4				0		37	80	200	85		0.4	0
0													0			
<1	7	<0.1	<0.1	0.1	<0.1	4	0	<1	0.1	25	51	160	44	16	0.3	
0	3	0.7	0.3	7.1	0.4	106	0	2	5.3	117	518	344	1027	237	4.6	4.8
0	3	0.7	0.3	7.1	0.4	106	0	2	5.3	117	518	15	1027	237	4.6	4.8
0	7	0.6	0.2	2.1	0.5	59	0	11	3.1	80	260	14	993	134	3.7	1.6
3	89	0.1	<0.1	0.6	<0.1	32	0.1	2	0.1	81	132	951	402	46	2	1
0	0	<0.1	0.1	1.9	<0.1	5	0.2	0	0	14	31	782	130	5	0.4	0
0	0	0	0.1	3.3	<0.1	5	0.2	0	<0.1	10	72	72	206	2	0.5	0.2
0	1	<0.1	<0.1	0.2	0	2	0	0	<0.1	2	12	1156	19	2	0.1	<0.1
5	63	0.1	0.1	1.1	<0.1	20	0.2	<1	<0.1	15	46	952	100	5	1.1	1.5
14	262	0.1	0.2	2.7	0.1	13	0.6	7	0.2	31	120	866	336	5	2.3	2.6
0	49	0.1	0.1	0.5	0.1	25	<0.1	1	0.1	44	106	1197	274	42	2.1	1.4
90	89	0.2	0.2	5	0.4	28	10.4	12	2	83	340	416	732	74	3.9	1.9
48	148	0.1	0.3	0.5	0.1	10	0.4	1	0.3	289	251	1019	341	20	0.8	0.7
0	0	<0.1	0.1	3.3	<0.1	5	0.2	0	<0.1	10	73	776	210	2	0.5	0.2
0	5	<0.1	<0.1	0.2	0	2	<0.1	0	<0.1	12	12	792	24	2	0.1	<0.1
7	72	0.1	0.1	1.4	<0.1	22	0.1	<1	0.1	17	36	1106	55	5	0.8	0.4

ERA, EatRight Analysis CD-ROM; **AMT**, amount; **WT**, weight; **WTR**, water; **CAL**, calories; **PROT**, protein; **CARB**, carbohydrate; **FIBR**, fiber; **FAT**, fat; **SATF**, saturated fat; **MONO**, monosaturated fat; **POLY**, polyunsaturated fat

ERA CODE	FOOD DESCRIPTION	AMT	UNIT	WT (g)	WTR (g)	CAL (kcal)	PROT (g)	CARB (g)	FIBR (g)	FAT (g)	SATF (g)	MONO (g)	POLY (g)
Soups, Stews and Chilis (continued)													
50037	Chicken Noodle Soup-Dry+Water	1	cup	252	237	58	2	9	<1	1	0.3	0.5	0.4
50020	Chicken Rice Soup+Water	1	cup	241	226	60	4	7	1	2	0.5	0.9	0.4
56001	Chili+Beans-Canned	1	cup	256	193	287	15	30	11	14	6	6	0.9
50007	Chili Beef Soup+Water	1	cup	250	212	170	7	21	10	7	3.3	2.8	0.3
7557	Chili-Vegetarian	1	cup	214	138	282	38	30	10	4	0.6	1.3	1.8
50008	Clam Chowder-NewEng+Milk	1	cup	248	211	164	9	17	1	7	3	2.3	1.1
50093	Clam Chowder-Manhattan-Prep	1	cup	240	206	134	7	19	3	3	2.1	1	0.1
50098	Consommé+Gelatin+Water	1	cup	241	232	29	5	2	0	0	0	0	0
50213	Crab Bisque Soup	1	cup	248	202	236	20	12	<1	12	3.4	4.7	2.7
50011	Cream Mushroom Soup+Milk	1	cup	248	210	203	6	15	<1	14	5.1	3	4.6
50049	Cream Mushroom Soup+Water	1	cup	244	220	129	2	9	<1	9	2.4	1.7	4.2
50189	Cream of Broccoli Soup	1	cup	237	197	206	9	17	2	12	4	5.1	2.5
50006	Cream of Chicken Soup+Milk	1	cup	248	210	191	7	15	<1	11	4.6	4.5	1.6
50018	Cream of Chicken Soup+Water	1	cup	244	221	117	3	9	<1	7	2.1	3.3	1.5
50026	Cream Potato Soup+Milk	1	cup	248	215	149	6	17	<1	6	3.8	1.7	0.6
50190	Egg Drop Soup	1	cup	244	229	73	8	1	0	4	1.1	1.5	0.6
50103	Gazpacho Soup-Prepared	1	cup	244	229	46	7	4	<1	<1	<0.1	<0.1	0.1
50182	Hot & Sour Soup	1	cup	244	211	162	15	5	1	8	2.7	3.4	1.2
50105	Lentil & Ham Soup-Prepared	1	cup	248	213	139	9	20	2	3	1.1	1.3	0.3
50214	Lobster Bisque Soup	1	cup	248	199	252	20	13	<1	13	4.2	5.5	2.7
50009	Minestrone Soup+Water	1	cup	241	220	82	4	11	1	3	0.6	0.7	1.1
50040	Onion Soup-Dry Mix+Water	1	cup	246	237	27	1	5	1	1	0.1	0.3	0.1
50024	Oyster Stew+Milk	1	cup	245	218	135	6	10	0	8	5	2.1	0.3
50025	Split Pea+Ham Soup+Water	1	cup	253	207	190	10	28	2	4	1.8	1.8	0.6
50209	Sweet & Sour Soup	1	cup	244	222	72	3	14	2	1	0.3	0.3	0.1
50012	Tomato Soup+Milk	1	cup	248	210	161	6	22	3	6	2.9	1.6	1.1
50028	Tomato Soup+Water	1	cup	244	220	85	2	17	<1	2	0.4	0.4	1
50186	Vege Soup-LowSod+Water	1	cup	241	220	78	3	15	3	1	0.2	0.2	0.5
50144	Vegetable Soup-Chunky-Prep	1	cup	240	210	122	4	19	1	4	0.6	1.6	1.4
50013	Vegetarian Vege Soup+Water	1	cup	241	222	72	2	12	<1	2	0.3	0.8	0.7
50027	Vichyssoise Soup	1	cup	248	215	149	6	17	<1	6	3.8	1.7	0.6
50181	Wonton Soup	1	cup	241	203	182	14	14	1	7	2.3	3	1
Spices, Flavors, and Seasonings and Miscellaneous Baking Products													
23010	Baking Chocolate-Square	1	ea	28.4	<1	148	3	8	4	16	9.2	5.2	0.5
28004	Baking Powder	1	tsp	4.6	<1	2	0	1	<1	0	0	0	0
28003	Baking Soda	1	tsp	4.6	<1	0	0	0	0	0	0	0	0
26001	Basil-Dried	1	Tbs	4.5	<1	11	1	3	2	<1	<0.1	<0.1	0.1
26040	Celery Seed	1	Tbs	6.5	<1	25	1	3	1	2	0.1	1	0.2
26002	Chili Powder	1	Tbs	7.5	1	24	1	4	3	1	0.2	0.3	0.6
23012	Chocolate Chips-Semisweet	1	cup	168	1	805	7	106	10	50	29.8	16.7	1.6
26003	Cinnamon	1	Tbs	6.8	1	18	<1	5	4	<1	<0.1	<0.1	<0.1
28200	Cocoa Powder	1	cup	86	3	197	17	47	29	12	6.9	3.9	0.4
26038	Coriander/Cilantro-Fresh	0.25	cup	4	4	1	<1	<1	<1	<1	0	<0.1	<0.1
26004	Curry Powder	1	Tbs	6.3	1	20	1	4	2	1	0.1	0.3	0.2
26021	Dill Weed-Dried	1	Tbs	3.1	<1	8	1	2	<1	<1	<0.1	0.1	<0.1

< = Trace amount present   Blank = Not available

CHOL, cholesterol; **V,** vitamin; **THI,** thiamin; **RIB,** riboflavin; **NIA,** niacin; **FOL,** folate;
CALC, calcium; **PHOS,** phosphate; **SOD,** sodium; **POT,** potassium; **MAG,** magnesium

CHOL (mg)	V-A (RE)	THI (mg)	RIB (mg)	NIA (mg)	V-B6 (mg)	FOL (μg)	V-B12 (μg)	V-C (mg)	V-E (mg)	CALC (mg)	PHOS (mg)	SOD (mg)	POT (mg)	MAG (mg)	IRON (mg)	ZINC (mg)
10	5	0.2	0.1	1.1	<0.1	18	0.1	0	0.1	5	30	577	33	8	0.5	0.2
7	65	<0.1	<0.1	1.1	<0.1	1	0.1	<1	0.1	17	22	814	101	0	0.7	0.3
44	87	0.1	0.3	0.9	0.3	58	0	4	1.9	120	394	1336	934	115	8.8	5.1
12	150	0.1	0.1	1.1	0.2	18	0.3	4	1.4	42	148	1035	525	30	2.1	1.4
0	148	0.2	0.1	2.4	0.3	164	0	11	2.5	107	435	709	730	71	8.8	2.5
22	40	0.1	0.2	1	0.1	10	10.2	3	0.1	186	156	992	300	22	1.5	0.8
14	329	0.1	0.1	1.8	0.3	9	7.9	12	0.1	67	84	1000	384	19	2.6	1.7
0	0	<0.1	<0.1	0.7	<0.1	3	0	1	<0.1	10	31	636	154	0	0.5	0.4
85	145	0.2	0.3	2.9	0.2	47	5.8	5	2	253	299	584	490	46	1	3.7
20	37	0.1	0.3	0.9	0.1	10	0.5	2	1.3	178	156	918	270	20	0.6	0.6
2	0	<0.1	0.1	0.7	<0.1	5	<0.1	1	1.2	46	49	881	100	5	0.5	0.6
15	258	0.1	0.4	0.8	0.2	40	0.4	48	2.4	256	222	204	481	41	0.9	1
27	94	0.1	0.3	0.9	0.1	8	0.5	1	0.2	181	151	1046	273	17	0.7	0.7
10	56	<0.1	0.1	0.8	<0.1	2	0.1	<1	0.2	34	37	986	88	2	0.6	0.6
22	67	0.1	0.2	0.6	0.1	9	0.5	1	0.1	166	161	1061	322	17	0.5	0.7
103	41	<0.1	0.2	3	0.1	15	0.5	0	0.3	21	108	728	220	5	0.8	0.5
0	261	<0.1	<0.1	0.9	0.1	10	0	7	0.5	24	37	739	224	7	1	0.2
34	2	0.3	0.3	5	0.2	13	0.4	1	0.1	29	188	1010	384	29	1.9	1.5
7	35	0.2	0.1	1.4	0.2	50	0.3	4	0.2	42	184	1319	357	22	2.7	0.7
63	196	0.1	0.4	1	0.1	17	2.6	2	2.1	275	310	450	548	50	0.5	2.7
2	234	0.1	<0.1	0.9	0.1	36	0	1	0.1	34	55	911	313	7	0.9	0.7
0	0	<0.1	0.1	0.5	0	1	0	<1	0.1	12	30	849	64	5	0.1	0.1
32	44	0.1	0.2	0.3	0.1	10	2.6	4	0.5	167	162	1041	235	20	1.1	10.3
8	46	0.1	0.1	1.5	0.1	3	0.3	2	0.2	23	212	1006	400	48	2.3	1.3
5	31	0.1	0.1	0.9	0.1	16	<0.1	17	0.5	27	43	1291	227	15	0.6	0.3
17	109	0.1	0.2	1.5	0.2	21	0.4	68	2.6	159	149	744	449	22	1.8	0.3
0	68	0.1	0.1	1.4	0.1	15	0	66	2.5	12	34	695	264	7	1.8	0.2
0	301	0.1	0.1	1.9	0.2	17	0	1	1.9	27	54	468	522	31	0.8	0.5
0	588	0.1	0.1	1.2	0.2	17	0	6	0.6	55	72	1010	396	7	1.6	3.1
0	301	0.1	<0.1	0.9	0.1	11	0	1	0.8	22	34	822	210	7	1.1	0.5
22	67	0.1	0.2	0.6	0.1	9	0.5	1	0.1	166	161	1061	322	17	0.5	0.7
53	99	0.4	0.3	4.6	0.2	19	0.4	3	0.4	31	152	543	316	21	1.8	1.1
0	3	<0.1	<0.1	0.3	<0.1	2	0	0	1.7	21	118	4	236	88	1.8	1.1
0	0	0	0	0	0	0	0	0	0	270	101	488	1	1	0.5	0
0	0	0	0	0	0	0	0	0	0	0	0	1258	0	0	0	0
0	42	<0.1	<0.1	0.3	0.1	12	0	3	0.1	95	22	2	154	19	1.9	0.3
0	<1	<0.1	<0.1	0.2	<0.1	1	0	1	0.1	115	36	10	91	29	2.9	0.4
0	262	<0.1	0.1	0.6	0.1	8	0	5	0.1	21	23	76	144	13	1.1	0.2
0	4	0.1	0.2	0.7	0.1	5	0	0	10.1	54	222	18	613	193	5.3	2.7
0	2	<0.1	<0.1	0.1	<0.1	2	0	2	0	84	4	2	34	4	2.6	0.1
0	2	0.1	0.2	1.9	0.1	28	0	0	1.9	110	631	18	1310	429	11.9	5.9
0	11	<0.1	<0.1	<0.1	<0.1	<1	0	<1	0.1	4	1	1	22	1	0.1	<0.1
0	6	<0.1	<0.1	0.2	<0.1	10	0	1	<0.1	30	22	3	97	16	1.9	0.3
0	18	<0.1	<0.1	0.1	<0.1		0	2		55	17	6	102	14	1.5	0.1

ERA, EatRight Analysis CD-ROM; **AMT**, amount; **WT**, weight; **WTR**, water; **CAL**, calories; **PROT**, protein; **CARB**, carbohydrate; **FIBR**, fiber; **FAT**, fat; **SATF**, saturated fat; **MONO**, monosaturated fat; **POLY**, polyunsaturated fat

ERA CODE	FOOD DESCRIPTION	AMT	UNIT	WT (g)	WTR (g)	CAL (kcal)	PROT (g)	CARB (g)	FIBR (g)	FAT (g)	SATF (g)	MONO (g)	POLY (g)
Spices, Flavors, and Seasonings and Miscellaneous Baking Products (continued)												
26007	Garlic Powder	1	Tbs	8.4	1	28	1	6	1	<1	<0.1	<0.1	<0.1
26023	Ginger-Ground	1	Tbs	5.4	1	19	<1	4	1	<1	0.1	0.1	0.1
26008	Onion Powder	1	Tbs	6.5	<1	23	1	5	<1	<1	<0.1	<0.1	<0.1
26009	Oregano-Ground	1	Tbs	4.5	<1	14	<1	3	2	<1	0.1	<0.1	0.2
26010	Paprika	1	Tbs	6.9	1	20	1	4	1	1	0.1	0.1	0.6
26016	Pepper-Black	1	Tbs	6.4	1	16	1	4	2	<1	0.1	0.1	0.1
26037	Pepper-White	1	Tbs	7.1	1	21	1	5	2	<1	<0.1	0.1	<0.1
26031	Sage-Ground	1	Tbs	2	<1	6	<1	1	1	<1	0.1	<0.1	<0.1
26014	Salt	1	Tbs	18	<1	0	0	0	0	0	0	0	0
26091	Salt Substitute (Morton)	0.25	tsp	1.1	<1	1	<1	<1		<1			
26048	Salt-Light (Morton)	0.25	tsp	1.4	0	<1	0	<1		0	0	0	0
28002	Yeast-Brewer's	1	Tbs	8	<1	23	3	3	3	<1	<0.1	<0.1	0
28000	Yeast-Dry-Active-Baker's	1	tsp	4	<1	12	2	2	1	<1	<0.1	0.1	0
Sweets, Sugars, Candy												
Candies and Confections, Gum												
23049	Almond Joy Candy Bar	1	ea	49	5	229	2	29	2	13	8.5	3.2	0.7
23110	Baby Ruth Candy Bar	1	ea	60	3	289	4	39	2	13	7.1	3.7	1.9
23226	Breathsaver Mints-Spearmint	1	pce	2		10	0	0	0	0	0	0	0
23066	Butterfinger Candy Bar	1	ea	61	1	293	8	40	1	11	6.3	3.4	1.7
23015	Caramel-Plain/Chocolate	1	pce	10.1	1	39	<1	8	<1	1	0.7	0.1	<0.1
23082	Chewing Gum	1	pce	3	<1	10	0	3	0	<1	<0.1	<0.1	<0.1
23083	Chewing Gum-Sugarless	1	pce	4	<1	11	0	4	0	<1	<0.1	<0.1	<0.1
23063	Chocolate Candy Kisses	6	pce	28.4	<1	145	2	17	1	9	5.2	2.8	0.3
23021	Chocolate Coated Peanuts	1	cup	149	3	773	20	74	7	50	21.8	19.2	6.5
23022	Chocolate Covered Raisins	1	cup	190	21	741	8	130	8	28	16.7	9	1
23053	Divinity Candy-Homemade	1	pce	11	1	38	<1	10	0	0	0	0	0
23036	English Toffee Candy Bar	1	ea	39	1	217	2	23	1	13	8.5	4.3	0.5
23024	Fondant Candy	1	pce	16	1	57	0	15	0	0	0	0	0
23025	Fudge-Chocolate	1	pce	17	2	65	<1	14	<1	1	0.9	0.4	0.1
23026	Fudge-Chocolate-Nuts	1	pce	19	1	81	1	14	<1	3	1.1	0.8	1
23029	Gumdrops Candy-Small	10	pce	36	<1	139	0	36	0	0	0	0	0
23030	Gummy Bears Candy	10	pce	22	<1	85	0	22	0	0	0	0	0
23031	Hard Candy, All Flavors	1	pce	6	<1	24	0	6	0	<1	0	0	0
23033	Jelly Beans Candy	10	pce	11	1	40	0	10	0	<1	<0.1	<0.1	<0.1
23048	M&M's Peanut Choc Candy	10	pce	20	<1	103	2	12	1	5	2.1	2.2	0.8
23046	M&M's Plain Choc Candy	10	pce	7	<1	34	<1	5	<1	1	0.9	0.5	<0.1
23064	Marshmallow Creme	2	Tbs	12		40	0	10	0	0	0	0	0
23007	Marshmallows	1	ea	7.2	1	23	<1	6	<1	<1	<0.1	<0.1	<0.1
23018	Milk Choc Bar+Almonds	1	ea	41	1	216	4	22	3	14	7	5.5	0.9
23019	Milk Choc Bar+Peanuts	1	ea	28.4		157	5	11	2	12	3.4	5.1	2.6
23058	Milk Choc Bar+RiceCereal	1	ea	40	1	198	3	25	1	11	6.4	3.5	0.3
23016	Milk Chocolate Candy Bar	1	ea	44	1	226	3	26	1	14	8.1	4.4	0.5
23038	Milky Way Candy Bar	1	ea	60	4	254	3	43	1	10	4.7	3.6	0.4
23081	Peanut Brittle-Homemade	1	cup	147	3	666	11	102	3	28	7.4	12.5	6.9
23138	Praline Candy-Homemade	1	pce	39	4	177	1	24	1	9	0.7	5.9	2.4

< = Trace amount present   Blank = Not available

CHOL, cholesterol; **V,** vitamin; **THI,** thiamin; **RIB,** riboflavin; **NIA,** niacin; **FOL,** folate;
CALC, calcium; **PHOS,** phosphate; **SOD,** sodium; **POT,** potassium; **MAG,** magnesium

CHOL (mg)	V-A (RE)	THI (mg)	RIB (mg)	NIA (mg)	V-B6 (mg)	FOL (μg)	V-B12 (μg)	V-C (mg)	V-E (mg)	CALC (mg)	PHOS (mg)	SOD (mg)	POT (mg)	MAG (mg)	IRON (mg)	ZINC (mg)
0	0	<0.1	<0.1	0.1	0.2	<1	0	2	<0.1	7	35	2	92	5	0.2	0.2
0	1	<0.1	<0.1	0.3	0.1	2	0	<1	<0.1	6	8	2	72	10	0.6	0.3
0	0	<0.1	<0.1	<0.1	0.1	11	0	1	<0.1	24	22	3	61	8	0.2	0.2
0	31	<0.1	<0.1	0.3	0.1	12	0	2	0.1	71	9	1	75	12	2	0.2
0	418	<0.1	0.1	1.1	0.1	7	0	5	0.6	12	24	2	162	13	1.6	0.3
0	1	<0.1	<0.1	0.1	<0.1	1	0	1	0.1	28	11	3	81	12	1.8	0.1
0	0	<0.1	<0.1	<0.1	<0.1	1	0	1	0.2	19	12	<1	5	6	1	0.1
0	12	<0.1	<0.1	0.1	<0.1	5	0	1	<0.1	33	2	<1	21	9	0.6	0.1
0	0	0	0	0	0	0	0	0	0	4	0	6976	1	<1	0.1	<0.1
							0					<1	476			
							0			1		273	364	1		
0	0	1.2	0.3	3	0.4	313	<0.1	0		17	140	10	151	18	1.4	0.6
0	<1	0.1	0.2	1.6	0.1	94	0	<1	0.2	3	52	2	80	4	0.7	0.3
2	2	<0.1	0.1	0.2	<0.1		0.1	<1	1.2	30	69	72	120	32	0.7	0.4
2	0	0.1	0.1	1.7	<0.1	19	<0.1	0	1.1	25	91	136	238	48	0.1	0.8
0												0	0			
1	0	0.1	<0.1	1.5	<0.1	16	<0.1	0	1	16	80	121	232	48	0.5	0.7
1	1	<0.1	<0.1	<0.1	<0.1	1	0	<1	<0.1	14	12	25	22	2	<0.1	<0.1
0	0	0	0	0	0	0	0	0	0	0	0	<1	<1	0	0	0
0	0	0	0	0	0	0	0	0	0	1	0	<1	0	0	0	0
6	16	<0.1	0.1	0.1	<0.1	2	0.1	<1	0.4	54	61	23	109	17	0.4	0.4
13	0	0.2	0.3	6.3	0.3	12	0.4	0	14.5	155	316	61	748	140	2	2.9
6	13	0.2	0.3	0.8	0.2	10	0.3	<1	4	163	272	68	977	86	3.2	1.5
0	<1	0	<0.1	<0.1	0	0	<0.1	0		<1	<1	5	2	<1	<0.1	<0.1
20	27	<0.1	0.1	<0.1	<0.1		0.1	<1	3.7	51	58	108	93	13	0.2	0.3
0	<1	0	<0.1	0	0	0	0	0	0	<1	<1	6	3	<1	<0.1	<0.1
2	8	<0.1	<0.1	<0.1	<0.1	<1	<0.1	<1	<0.1	7	10	11	18	4	0.1	0.1
3	9	<0.1	<0.1	<0.1	<0.1	2	<0.1	<1	0.5	10	18	11	30	9	0.1	0.1
0	0	0	0	0	0	0	0	0	0	1	<1	16	2	<1	0.1	0
0	0	0	0	0	0	0	0	0	0	1	<1	10	1	<1	0.1	0
0	0	0	0	0	0	0	0	0	0	<1	<1	2	<1	<1	<0.1	0
0	0	0	0	0	0	0	0	0	0	<1	<1	3	4	<1	0.1	<0.1
2	5	<0.1	<0.1	0.7	<0.1	7	<0.1	<1	1	20	46	10	69	15	0.2	0.5
1	4	<0.1	<0.1	<0.1	<0.1	<1	<0.1	<1	0.2	7	10	4	19	3	0.1	0.1
0	0							0	0	0		10	0	0		
0	<1	0	0	<0.1	0	<1	0	0	0	<1	1	3	<1	<1	<0.1	<0.1
8	6	<0.1	0.2	0.3	<0.1	5	0.1	<1	3.7	92	108	30	182	37	0.7	0.5
3	6	0.1	0.1	2.1	<0.1	24	<0.1	0	2.2	33	83	11	152	35	0.5	0.7
8	4	<0.1	0.1	0.2	<0.1	4	0.1	<1	1.6	68	77	58	137	20	0.3	0.4
10	24	<0.1	0.1	0.1	<0.1	4	0.2	<1	2.2	84	95	36	169	26	0.6	0.6
8	19	<0.1	0.1	0.2	<0.1	6	0.2	1	1	78	86	144	145	20	0.5	0.4
19	69	0.3	0.1	5.1	0.2	103	<0.1	0	2.4	44	163	664	306	74	2	1.4
0	2	0.1	<0.1	0.1	<0.1	5	0	<1	0.6	12	43	24	82	20	0.5	0.8

ERA, EatRight Analysis CD-ROM; **AMT,** amount; **WT,** weight; **WTR,** water; **CAL,** calories; **PROT,** protein; **CARB,** carbohydrate; **FIBR,** fiber; **FAT,** fat; **SATF,** saturated fat; **MONO,** monosaturated fat; **POLY,** polyunsaturated fat

ERA CODE	FOOD DESCRIPTION	AMT	UNIT	WT (g)	WTR (g)	CAL (kcal)	PROT (g)	CARB (g)	FIBR (g)	FAT (g)	SATF (g)	MONO (g)	POLY (g)
Sweets, Sugars, Candy (continued)													
Candies and Confections, Gum (continued)													
23043	Reese's Peanut Butter Cup	1	ea	50	1	270	5	27	2	16	5.6	6.6	2.8
23143	Skittles Bite Size Candy	10	pce	10.7	<1	43	<1	10	0	<1	0.1	0.3	<0.1
23040	Snickers Candy Bar	1	ea	57	3	273	5	34	1	14	5.1	6	2.8
23144	Starburst Fruit Candy	1	pce	5	<1	20	<1	4	0	<1	0.1	0.2	0.2
23147	Taffy Candy-Homemade	1	pce	15	1	56	<1	14	0	<1	0.3	0.1	<0.1
23075	Three Muskateers CandyBar	1	ea	60	3	250	2	46	1	8	3.9	2.6	0.3
23173	Toffee Candy-Homemade	1	pce	12	<1	65	<1	8	0	4	2.4	1.1	0.1
23117	Tootsie Roll Candy-BiteSize	7	ea	35	3	126	1	31	<1	1	0.2	0.4	0.3
23154	Twizzlers-Small Pkg	1	ea	71	12	237	2	55	1	1	0.3		
23089	Yogurt Covered Raisins	1	cup	191	19	750	8	139	5	22	19.5	0.4	0.6
23152	York Peppermint Patty-Large	1	ea	42	4	165	1	34	1	3	1.8	1	0.1
Jams and Jellies													
23000	Apple Butter	1	Tbs	18	10	31	<1	8	<1	0	0	0	0
23054	Jam/Preserves	1	Tbs	20	6	56	<1	14	<1	<1	<0.1	<0.1	0
23003	Jelly	1	Tbs	19	6	54	<1	13	<1	<1	<0.1	<0.1	<0.1
23278	Fruit Spread-LowCal-Strawberry	1	Tbs	20		20	0	5	0	0	0	0	0
23005	Marmalade-Orange	1	Tbs	20	7	49	<1	13	<1	0	0	0	0
23165	Jelly-Reduced Sugar	1	Tbs	18.8	10	34	<1	9	<1	<1	<0.1	0	<0.1
Sugars and Syrups													
25010	Corn Syrup-Dark	1	cup	328	75	925	0	251	0	0	0	0	0
25000	Corn Syrup-Light	1	cup	328	75	925	0	251	0	0	0	0	0
25001	Honey-Strained/Extracted	1	cup	339	58	1030	1	279	1	0	0	0	0
25002	Maple Syrup	1	Tbs	20	6	52	0	13	0	<1	<0.1	<0.1	<0.1
25004	Molasses-Blackstrap Cane	1	cup	328	94	771	0	199	0	0	0	0	0
23042	Pancake Syrup	1	Tbs	20	5	57	0	15	0	0	0	0	0
23091	Pancake Syrup-Lite	1	Tbs	18	10	29	0	8	0	0	0	0	0
23172	Pancake Syrup-Reduced Cal	1	Tbs	15	8	25	0	7	0	0	0	0	0
25005	Sugar-Brown	1	cup	220	4	827	0	214	0	0	0	0	0
25071	Sugar-Raw	1	cup	195	3	733	0	190	0	0	0	0	0
25006	Sugar-White-Granulated	1	cup	200	0	774	0	200	0	0	0	0	0
25009	Sugar-White-Powdered	1	cup	120	<1	467	0	119	0	<1	<0.1	<0.1	0.1
Vegetables and Legumes													
5314	Acorn Squash-Baked	1	cup	205	170	115	2	30	9	<1	0.1	<0.1	0.1
5010	Alfalfa Sprouts	0.5	cup	16.5	15	5	1	1	<1	<1	<0.1	<0.1	0.1
5191	Artichoke Hearts-Marinated-Cnd	2	pce	28		25	1	3	1	2	0		
5000	Artichoke-Globe-Cooked	1	ea	120	101	60	4	13	6	<1	<0.1	<0.1	0.1
6033	Arugula-Chopped-Raw	0.5	cup	10	9	2	<1	<1	<1	<1	<0.1	<0.1	<0.1
5842	Asparagus-Canned+Liq-LowSod	0.5	cup	122	115	18	2	3	1	<1	0.1	<0.1	0.1
5007	Asparagus-Spears-Canned	1	pce	18	17	3	<1	<1	<1	<1	<0.1	<0.1	0.1
5004	Asparagus-Spears-Cooked	4	ea	60	55	14	2	3	1	<1	<0.1	<0.1	0.1
5401	Bamboo Shoots-Canned Slices	1	cup	131	124	25	2	4	2	1	0.1	<0.1	0.2
5249	Bamboo Shoots-Cooked Slices	1	cup	120	115	14	2	2	1	<1	0.1	<0.1	0.1
5250	Bamboo Shoots-Whole-Boiled	1	ea	144	138	17	2	3	1	<1	0.1	<0.1	0.1

< = Trace amount present   Blank = Not available

CHOL, cholesterol; **V**, vitamin; **THI**, thiamin; **RIB**, riboflavin; **NIA**, niacin; **FOL**, folate; **CALC**, calcium; **PHOS**, phosphate; **SOD**, sodium; **POT**, potassium; **MAG**, magnesium

CHOL (mg)	V-A (RE)	THI (mg)	RIB (mg)	NIA (mg)	V-B6 (mg)	FOL (µg)	V-B12 (µg)	V-C (mg)	V-E (mg)	CALC (mg)	PHOS (mg)	SOD (mg)	POT (mg)	MAG (mg)	IRON (mg)	ZINC (mg)
2	10	0.1	0.1	2.3	0.1	28	0.1	<1	3.9	39	102	158	176	44	0.6	0.9
0	0	0	<0.1	<0.1	0	0	0	7	<0.1	0	<1	2	1	<1	<0.1	<0.1
7	22	0.1	0.1	2.4	0.1	23	0.1	<1	2.3	54	126	152	185	41	0.4	1.3
0	0	0	0	0	0	0	0	3	0.1	<1	<1	3	<1	<1	<0.1	0
1	5	0	<0.1	<0.1	0	0	<0.1	0	0.1	<1	<1	13	1	<1	<0.1	<0.1
7	14	<0.1	0.1	0.1	<0.1	0	0.1	<1	0.4	50	55	116	80	17	0.4	0.3
13	38	<0.1	<0.1	<0.1	<0.1	<1	<0.1	<1	0.2	4	4	22	6	<1	<0.1	<0.1
0	1	<0.1	<0.1	<0.1	<0.1	<1	<0.1	<1	0.1	9	14	28	36	11	0.1	0.2
0	0	<0.1	<0.1	0.1	<0.1		0	0		5	220	175	45	4	0.2	0.1
1	2	0.2	0.3	1.5	0.3	17	0.6	4	2.6	214	249	85	1061	46	2.5	0.9
<1	<1	<0.1	<0.1	0.4	<0.1			<0.1	0	6	40	10	54	26	0.4	0.3
0	2	<0.1	<0.1	<0.1	<0.1	<1	0	<1	<0.1	3	2	1	16	1	0.1	<0.1
0	<1	0	<0.1	<0.1	<0.1	7	0	2	0	4	2	6	15	1	0.1	<0.1
0	<1	0	<0.1	<0.1	<0.1	<1	0	<1	0	2	1	5	12	1	<0.1	<0.1
0	0							0		0		20	25		0	
0	1	<0.1	<0.1	<0.1	<0.1	7	0	1	0	8	1	11	7	<1	<0.1	<0.1
0	<1	<0.1	<0.1	<0.1	<0.1	<1	0	0	<0.1	1	1	<1	13	1	<0.1	<0.1
0	0	<0.1	<0.1	0.1	<0.1	0	0	0	0	59	36	508	144	26	1.2	0.1
0	0	<0.1	<0.1	0.1	<0.1	0	0	0	0	10	7	397	13	7	0.2	0.1
0	0	0	0.1	0.4	0.1	7	0	2	0	20	14	14	176	7	1.4	0.7
0	0	<0.1	<0.1	<0.1	0	0	0	0	0	13	<1	2	41	3	0.2	0.8
0	0	0.1	0.2	3.5	2.3	3	0	0	0	2820	131	180	8173	705	57.4	3.3
0	0	<0.1	<0.1	<0.1	0	0	0	0	0	<1	2	17	<1	<1	<0.1	<0.1
0	0	<0.1	<0.1	<0.1	0	0	0	0	0	2	1	37	6	1	0.3	<0.1
0	0	<0.1	<0.1	<0.1	0	0	0	0	0	<1	6	30	<1	0	<0.1	<0.1
0	0	<0.1	<0.1	0.2	0.1	2	0	0	0	187	48	86	761	64	4.2	0.4
0	0	<0.1	<0.1	0.2	0.1	2	0	0	0	166	43	76	675	57	3.7	0.4
0	0	0	<0.1	0	0	0	0	0	0	2	4	2	4	0	0.1	0.1
0	0	0	0	0	0	0	0	0	0	1	2	1	2	0	0.1	<0.1
0	88	0.3	<0.1	1.8	0.4	38	0	22	1.4	90	92	8	896	88	1.9	0.3
0	3	<0.1	<0.1	0.1	<0.1	6	0	1	<0.1	5	12	1	13	4	0.2	0.2
0	0							10		0		105			0	
0	22	0.1	0.1	1.2	0.1	61	0	12	0.2	54	103	114	425	72	1.5	0.6
0	24	<0.1	<0.1	<0.1	<0.1	10	0	2	<0.1	16	5	3	37	5	0.1	<0.1
0	65	0.1	0.1	1	0.1	104	0	20	0.2	18	46	32	210	11	0.7	0.6
0	10	<0.1	<0.1	0.2	<0.1	17	0	3	0.2	3	8	52	31	2	0.3	0.1
0	32	0.1	0.1	0.6	0.1	88	0	6	0.6	12	32	7	96	6	0.4	0.3
0	1	<0.1	<0.1	0.2	0.2	4	0	1	0.5	10	33	9	105	5	0.4	0.9
0	0	<0.1	0.1	0.4	0.1	3	0	0	0.8	14	24	5	640	4	0.3	0.6
0	0	<0.1	0.1	0.4	0.1	3	0	0	1	17	29	6	768	4	0.3	0.7

ERA, EatRight Analysis CD-ROM; **AMT,** amount; **WT,** weight; **WTR,** water; **CAL,** calories; **PROT,** protein; **CARB,** carbohydrate; **FIBR,** fiber; **FAT,** fat; **SATF,** saturated fat; **MONO,** monosaturated fat; **POLY,** polyunsaturated fat

ERA CODE	FOOD DESCRIPTION	AMT	UNIT	WT (g)	WTR (g)	CAL (kcal)	PROT (g)	CARB (g)	FIBR (g)	FAT (g)	SATF (g)	MONO (g)	POLY (g)
Vegetables and Legumes (continued)													
7084	Bean Cake	1	ea	32	7	130	2	16	1	7	1	2.9	2.6
5319	Beans-Baby Limas-Boiled	0.5	cup	85	57	104	6	20	5	<1	0.1	<0.1	0.1
7058	Beans-Baby Limas-Dry-Boiled	0.5	cup	91	61	115	7	21	7	<1	0.1	<0.1	0.2
7012	Beans-Black-Dry-Ckd	1	cup	172	113	227	15	41	15	1	0.2	0.1	0.4
7021	Beans-Great Northern-Boiled	1	cup	177	122	209	15	37	12	1	0.2	<0.1	0.3
5231	Beans-Green-Cannd+Liq-LowSod	1	cup	240	227	36	2	8	4	<1	0.1	<0.1	0.1
5015	Beans-Green-Canned-Drained	1	cup	135	126	27	2	6	3	<1	<0.1	<0.1	0.1
5011	Beans-Green-Fresh-Boiled	0.5	cup	62.5	56	22	1	5	2	<1	<0.1	<0.1	0.1
5013	Beans-Green-Frozen-Boiled	1	cup	135	123	38	2	9	4	<1	0.1	<0.1	0.1
7087	Beans-Kidney-Canned+Liquid	0.5	cup	128	100	104	7	19	4	<1	0.1	<0.1	0.2
7022	Beans-Navy-Dry-Cooked	1	cup	182	115	258	16	48	12	1	0.3	0.1	0.4
7051	Beans-Pinto-Canned+Liquid	0.5	cup	120	93	103	6	18	6	1	0.2	0.2	0.3
7013	Beans-Pinto-Dry-Cooked	1	cup	171	110	234	14	44	15	1	0.2	0.2	0.3
7047	Beans-Red Kidney-Boiled	1	cup	177	118	225	15	40	13	1	0.1	0.1	0.5
7135	Beans-Red Kidney-Canned-Drain	1	cup	256	176	302	19	55	23	1			
5022	Beets-Fresh-Diced-Cooked	0.5	cup	85	74	37	1	8	2	<1	<0.1	<0.1	0.1
5310	Beets-Pickled-Slices	1	cup	227	186	148	2	37	6	<1	<0.1	<0.1	0.1
5311	Beets-Whole-Pickled	1	ea	50	41	32	<1	8	1	<1	<0.1	<0.1	<0.1
5679	Broccoflower-Cooked	1	cup	156	140	50	5	10	5	<1	0.1	<0.1	0.1
5678	Broccoflower-Raw	1	cup	100		32	3	6	3	<1	<0.1	<0.1	0.1
5653	Broccoli Pieces-Steamed	1	cup	156	141	44	5	8	5	1	0.1	<0.1	0.3
5029	Broccoli Spear-Cooked	1	ea	180	163	50	5	9	5	1	0.1	<0.1	0.3
5028	Broccoli-Pieces-Boiled	0.5	cup	78	71	22	2	4	2	<1	<0.1	<0.1	0.1
5030	Broccoli-Pieces-Frozen-Cooked	1	cup	184	167	52	6	10	6	<1	<0.1	<0.1	0.1
5026	Broccoli-Raw-Chopped	1	cup	88	80	25	3	5	3	<1	<0.1	<0.1	0.1
5033	Brussels Sprouts-Cooked	1	cup	156	136	61	4	14	4	1	0.2	0.1	0.4
5035	Brussels Sprouts-Frozen-Cooked	1	cup	155	134	65	6	13	6	1	0.1	<0.1	0.3
5237	Cabbage-Bok Choy-Boiled	1	cup	170	162	20	3	3	3	<1	<0.1	<0.1	0.1
5041	Cabbage-Bok Choy-Raw	1	cup	70	67	9	1	2	1	<1	<0.1	<0.1	0.1
5671	Cabbage-Chinese-Steamed	1	cup	170	162	22	3	4	2	<1	<0.1	<0.1	0.2
5038	Cabbage-Cooked	1	cup	150	140	33	2	7	3	1	0.1	<0.1	0.3
5040	Cabbage-Pe Tsai-Raw-Pieces	1	cup	76	72	12	1	2	2	<1	<0.1	<0.1	0.1
5235	Cabbage-Pe-Tsai-Boiled	1	cup	119	113	17	2	3	3	<1	<0.1	<0.1	0.1
5036	Cabbage-Raw-Shredded	1	cup	70	64	18	1	4	2	<1	<0.1	<0.1	0.1
5042	Cabbage-Red-Raw	1	cup	70	64	19	1	4	1	<1	<0.1	<0.1	0.1
5046	Carrot-Raw-Grated	0.5	cup	55	48	24	1	6	2	<1	<0.1	<0.1	<0.1
5045	Carrot-Raw-Whole	1	ea	72	63	31	1	7	2	<1	<0.1	<0.1	0.1
5439	Carrots-Baby-Raw-2.75inch	1	ea	10	9	4	<1	1	<1	<1	<0.1	<0.1	<0.1
5047	Carrots-Cooked	0.5	cup	78	68	35	1	8	3	<1	<0.1	<0.1	0.1
5358	Carrots-Frozen-Cooked	0.5	cup	73	66	26	1	6	3	<1	<0.1	<0.1	<0.1
5625	Cassava/Yuca Blanca-Cooked	1	cup	137	81	221	2	53	2	<1	0.1	0.1	0.1
5052	Cauliflower Flowerets-Boiled	3	ea	54	50	12	1	2	1	<1	<0.1	<0.1	0.1
5053	Cauliflower-Frozen-Cooked	1	cup	180	169	34	3	7	5	<1	0.1	<0.1	0.2
5049	Cauliflower-Raw-Cup	0.5	cup	50	46	12	1	3	1	<1	<0.1	<0.1	<0.1
5054	Celery-Raw-Chopped	0.5	cup	60	57	10	<1	2	1	<1	<0.1	<0.1	<0.1
5055	Celery-Raw-Large Outer Stalk	1	ea	40	38	6	<1	1	1	<1	<0.1	<0.1	<0.1

< = Trace amount present   Blank = Not available

CHOL, cholesterol; **V,** vitamin; **THI,** thiamin; **RIB,** riboflavin; **NIA,** niacin; **FOL,** folate; **CALC,** calcium; **PHOS,** phosphate; **SOD,** sodium; **POT,** potassium; **MAG,** magnesium

CHOL (mg)	V-A (RE)	THI (mg)	RIB (mg)	NIA (mg)	V-B6 (mg)	FOL (µg)	V-B12 (µg)	V-C (mg)	V-E (mg)	CALC (mg)	PHOS (mg)	SOD (mg)	POT (mg)	MAG (mg)	IRON (mg)	ZINC (mg)
0	0	0.1	<0.1	0.5	<0.1	9	0	0	1.2	3	21	1	58	6	0.7	0.2
0	31	0.1	0.1	0.9	0.2	22	0	9	1.4	27	110	14	484	63	2.1	0.7
0	0	0.1	0.1	0.6	0.1	136	0	0	0.2	26	116	3	365	48	2.2	0.9
0	2	0.4	0.1	0.9	0.1	256	0	0	1	46	241	2	611	120	3.6	1.9
0	<1	0.3	0.1	1.2	0.2	181	0	2	1.9	120	292	4	692	88	3.8	1.6
0	77	0.1	0.1	0.5	0.1	44	0	8	0.3	58	46	34	221	31	2.2	0.5
0	47	<0.1	0.1	0.3	<0.1	43	0	6	0.2	35	26	354	147	18	1.2	0.4
0	42	<0.1	0.1	0.4	<0.1	21	0	6	0.1	29	24	2	187	16	0.8	0.2
0	54	<0.1	0.1	0.5	0.1	31	0	6	0.2	66	42	12	170	32	1.2	0.6
0	0	0.1	0.1	0.6	0.1	63	0	2	0.3	35	134	444	329	40	1.6	0.7
0	<1	0.4	0.1	1	0.3	255	0	2	2.1	127	286	2	670	107	4.5	1.9
0	3	0.1	0.1	0.3	0.1	72	0	1	1.1	52	110	353	292	32	1.8	0.8
0	<1	0.3	0.2	0.7	0.3	294	0	4	1.6	82	274	3	800	94	4.5	1.8
0	0	0.3	0.1	1	0.2	229	0	2	0.1	50	251	4	713	80	5.2	1.9
0	1	0.4	0.3	1.6	0.1	179	0				333			99		2
0	3	<0.1	<0.1	0.3	0.1	68	0	3	0.3	14	32	65	259	20	0.7	0.3
0	2	<0.1	0.1	0.6	0.1	60	0	5	0.3	25	39	599	336	34	0.9	0.6
0	<1	<0.1	<0.1	0.1	<0.1	13	0	1	0.1	6	8	132	74	8	0.2	0.1
0	11	0.1	0.1	1.2	0.3	76	0	98	0.5	50	100	36	502	31	1.1	0.8
0	7	0.1	0.1	0.8	0.2	57	0	74	0.3	32	64	23	322	20	0.1	0.5
0	228	0.1	0.2	0.9	0.2	94	0	123	0.7	75	103	42	505	39	1.4	0.6
0	250	0.1	0.2	1	0.3	90	0	134	3	83	106	47	526	43	1.5	0.7
0	108	<0.1	0.1	0.4	0.1	39	0	58	1.3	36	46	20	228	19	0.7	0.3
0	348	0.1	0.1	0.8	0.2	104	0	74	3	94	101	44	331	37	1.1	0.6
0	136	0.1	0.1	0.6	0.1	62	0	82	1.5	42	58	24	286	22	0.8	0.4
0	112	0.2	0.1	0.9	0.3	94	0	97	1.3	56	87	33	494	31	1.9	0.5
0	91	0.2	0.2	0.8	0.4	157	0	71	1.3	37	84	36	504	37	1.1	0.6
0	437	0.1	0.1	0.7	0.3	69	0	44	0.2	158	49	58	631	19	1.8	0.3
0	210	<0.1	<0.1	0.3	0.1	46	0	32	0.1	74	26	46	176	13	0.6	0.1
0	15	0.1	0.1	0.8	0.3	95	0	5	0.2	178	63	110	427	32	1.4	0.3
0	20	0.1	0.1	0.4	0.2	30	0	30	2.5	46	22	12	146	12	0.3	0.1
0	91	<0.1	<0.1	0.3	0.2	60	0	21	0.1	59	22	7	181	10	0.2	0.2
0	115	0.1	0.1	0.6	0.2	64	0	19	0.2	38	46	11	268	12	0.4	0.2
0	9	<0.1	<0.1	0.2	0.1	30	0	23	1.2	33	16	13	172	10	0.4	0.1
0	3	<0.1	<0.1	0.2	0.1	14	0	40	1.2	36	29	8	144	10	0.3	0.1
0	1547	0.1	<0.1	0.5	0.1	8	0	5	0.3	15	24	19	178	8	0.3	0.1
0	2025	0.1	<0.1	0.7	0.1	10	0	7	0.4	19	32	25	232	11	0.4	0.1
0	150	<0.1	<0.1	0.1	<0.1	3	0	1	<0.1	2	4	4	28	1	0.1	<0.1
0	1914	<0.1	<0.1	0.4	0.2	11	0	2	0.4	24	23	51	177	10	0.5	0.2
0	1292	<0.1	<0.1	0.3	0.1	8	0	2	0.7	20	19	43	115	7	0.3	0.2
0	2	0.1	0.1	1.1	0.1	24	0	19	0.3	21	34	18	338	28	0.4	0.4
0	1	<0.1	<0.1	0.2	0.1	24	0	24	<0.1	9	17	8	77	5	0.2	0.1
0	4	0.1	0.1	0.6	0.2	74	0	56	0.1	31	43	32	250	16	0.7	0.2
0	1	<0.1	<0.1	0.3	0.1	28	0	23	<0.1	11	22	15	152	8	0.2	0.1
0	8	<0.1	<0.1	0.2	0.1	17	0	4	0.4	24	15	52	172	7	0.2	0.1
0	5	<0.1	<0.1	0.1	<0.1	11	0	3	0.3	16	10	35	115	4	0.2	0.1

ERA, EatRight Analysis CD-ROM; **AMT,** amount; **WT,** weight; **WTR,** water; **CAL,** calories; **PROT,** protein; **CARB,** carbohydrate; **FIBR,** fiber; **FAT,** fat; **SATF,** saturated fat; **MONO,** monosaturated fat; **POLY,** polyunsaturated fat

ERA CODE	FOOD DESCRIPTION	AMT	UNIT	WT (g)	WTR (g)	CAL (kcal)	PROT (g)	CARB (g)	FIBR (g)	FAT (g)	SATF (g)	MONO (g)	POLY (g)
Vegetables and Legumes (continued)													
5399	Chili Peppers-Hot Green-Raw	0.5	cup	75	66	30	2	7	1	<1	<0.1	<0.1	0.1
5288	Chili Peppers-Red-Raw Pieces	0.5	cup	75	66	30	2	7	1	<1	<0.1	<0.1	0.1
5061	Collard Greens-Boiled	1	cup	190	174	49	4	9	5	1	0.1	<0.1	0.3
5062	Collard Greens-Frozen-Boiled	1	cup	170	150	61	5	12	5	1	0.1	<0.1	0.4
5515	Corn w/Red Pepper-Mexican	1	cup	227	176	170	5	41	5	1	0.2	0.4	0.6
5201	Corn-Canned+Liquid	0.5	cup	128	104	82	2	20	2	1	0.1	0.2	0.3
5066	Corn-Canned-Drained	0.5	cup	82	63	66	2	15	2	1	0.1	0.2	0.4
5364	Corn On Cob-Small-Frozen-Ckd	1	ea	63	46	59	2	14	2	<1	0.1	0.1	0.2
5380	Corn On Cob-Yellow-Med-Boiled	1	ea	77	54	83	3	19	2	1	0.2	0.3	0.5
5560	Corn-White-Boiled	1	ea	77	54	83	3	19	2	1	0.2	0.3	0.5
5562	Corn-White-Canned+Liquid	0.5	cup	128	104	82	2	20	1	1	0.1	0.2	0.3
5563	Corn-White-Canned-Drained	0.5	cup	82	63	66	2	15	2	1	0.1	0.2	0.4
5393	Corn-White-Frozen-Cooked	0.5	cup	82	63	66	2	16	2	<1	0.1	0.1	0.2
5379	Corn-Yellow-Boiled	0.5	cup	82	57	89	3	21	2	1	0.2	0.3	0.5
5065	Corn-Yellow-Frozen-Boiled	0.5	cup	82	63	66	2	16	2	<1	0.1	0.1	0.2
5068	Creamed Corn-Canned	0.5	cup	128	101	92	2	23	2	1	0.1	0.2	0.3
5071	Cucumber-Raw-Pieces w/Peel	0.5	cup	52	50	7	<1	1	<1	<1	<0.1	<0.1	<0.1
5070	Cucumber-Whole-8 inch	1	ea	301	289	39	2	8	2	<1	0.1	<0.1	0.2
5673	Eggplant Pieces-Steamed	1	cup	96	88	25	1	6	2	<1	<0.1	<0.1	<0.1
5674	Eggplant Pieces-Stir Fried	1	cup	96	88	25	1	6	2	<1	<0.1	<0.1	<0.1
5202	Escarole/Curly Endive	1	cup	50	47	8	1	2	2	<1	<0.1	<0.1	<0.1
7055	Fava/Broadbeans-Canned+Liq	0.5	cup	128	103	91	7	16	5	<1	<0.1	0.1	0.1
7027	Fava/Broadbeans-Dry-Cooked	1	cup	170	122	187	13	33	9	1	0.1	0.1	0.3
5139	French Fries-Frozen-Heated	10	pce	50	18	166	2	20	2	9	3	5.7	0.7
5460	French Fries-Veg Oil-Serving	1	ea	115	41	393	5	46	4	21	4.4	12.2	3.6
5536	Fried Green Tomatoes	1	ea	144	97	284	5	19	1	22	4.6	9.4	6.4
56638	Frijoles+Cheese	1	cup	167	115	225	11	29		8	4.1	2.6	0.7
7088	Garbanzo Beans/Chickpeas+Liq	0.5	cup	120	84	143	6	27	5	1	0.1	0.3	0.6
7001	Garbanzo Beans/Chickpeas-Ckd	1	cup	164	99	269	15	45	12	4	0.4	1	1.9
26005	Garlic Cloves-Fresh	4	ea	12	7	18	1	4	<1	<1	<0.1	<0.1	<0.1
5140	HashBrown Potatoes-Frzn-Ckd	1	cup	156	88	340	5	44	3	18	7	8	2.1
5141	HashBrowns-Frozen-FriedPatty	1	ea	29	16	63	1	8	1	3	1.3	1.5	0.4
5640	Hominy-Cooked	1	cup	165	136	119	2	24	4	1	0.2	0.4	0.7
38077	Hominy-White-Canned	1	cup	165	136	119	2	24	4	1	0.2	0.4	0.7
5470	Hominy-Yellow-Canned	1	cup	160	132	115	2	23	4	1	0.2	0.4	0.6
7081	Hummous/Hummus	1	cup	246	160	421	12	50	13	21	3.1	8.7	7.8
5293	Jalapeno Peppers-Chop-Can	0.5	cup	68	60	18	1	3	2	1	0.1	<0.1	0.3
6099	Jalapeno Peppers-Raw	1	ea	45	40	11	<1	2		<1			
6208	Japanese StirFry Veg (Birdseye)	0.5	cup	116	106	35	2	7	2	<1	<0.1		
5224	Jicama	1	cup	120	108	46	1	11	6	<1	<0.1	<0.1	0.1
5075	Kale-Cooked	1	cup	130	118	36	2	7	3	1	0.1	<0.1	0.2
5206	Leeks-Raw	1	ea	89	74	54	1	13	2	<1	<0.1	<0.1	0.1
7086	Lentil Loaf-3/4 in slice	1	pce	47	29	83	4	10	3	4	0.4	0.9	2.1
7006	Lentils-Cooked	1	cup	198	138	230	18	40	16	1	0.1	0.1	0.3
5080	Lettuce-Butterhead-Chopped	1	cup	56	54	7	1	1	1	<1	<0.1	<0.1	0.1
5083	Lettuce-Iceberg-Chopped	1	cup	55	53	7	1	1	1	<1	<0.1	<0.1	0.1

< = Trace amount present   Blank = Not available

CHOL, cholesterol; **V,** vitamin; **THI,** thiamin; **RIB,** riboflavin; **NIA,** niacin; **FOL,** folate; **CALC,** calcium; **PHOS,** phosphate; **SOD,** sodium; **POT,** potassium; **MAG,** magnesium

CHOL (mg)	V-A (RE)	THI (mg)	RIB (mg)	NIA (mg)	V-B6 (mg)	FOL (µg)	V-B12 (µg)	V-C (mg)	V-E (mg)	CALC (mg)	PHOS (mg)	SOD (mg)	POT (mg)	MAG (mg)	IRON (mg)	ZINC (mg)
0	58	0.1	0.1	0.7	0.2	18	0	182	0.5	14	34	5	255	19	0.9	0.2
0	806	0.1	0.1	0.7	0.2	18	0	182	0.5	14	34	5	255	19	0.9	0.2
0	595	0.1	0.2	1.1	0.2	177	0	35	1.7	226	49	17	494	32	0.9	0.8
0	1016	0.1	0.2	1.1	0.2	129	0	45	0.9	357	46	85	427	51	1.9	0.5
0	52	<0.1	0.2	2.2	0.2	77	0	20	2.5	11	141	788	347	57	1.8	0.8
0	19	<0.1	0.1	1.2	<0.1	49	0	7	0.2	5	65	273	210	20	0.5	0.5
0	13	<0.1	0.1	1	<0.1	40	0	7	0.1	4	53	175	160	16	0.7	0.3
0	13	0.1	<0.1	1	0.1	19	0	3	0.2	2	47	3	158	18	0.4	0.4
0	17	0.2	0.1	1.2	<0.1	36	0	5	0.4	2	79	13	192	25	0.5	0.4
0	0	0.2	0.1	1.2	<0.1	36	0	5	0.1	2	79	13	192	25	0.5	0.4
0	0	<0.1	0.1	1.2	<0.1	49	0	7	0.4	5	65	15	210	20	0.5	0.5
0	0	<0.1	0.1	1	<0.1	40	0	7	0.1	4	53	265	160	16	0.7	0.3
0	0	0.1	0.1	1.1	0.1	25	0	3	0.1	3	47	4	120	16	0.3	0.3
0	18	0.2	0.1	1.3	<0.1	38	0	5	0.4	2	84	14	204	26	0.5	0.4
0	18	0.1	0.1	1.1	0.1	25	0	3	0.1	3	47	4	120	16	0.3	0.3
0	13	<0.1	0.1	1.2	0.1	57	0	6	0.4	4	65	365	172	22	0.5	0.7
0	11	<0.1	<0.1	0.1	<0.1	7	0	3	0.1	7	10	1	75	6	0.1	0.1
0	63	0.1	0.1	0.7	0.1	39	0	16	0.8	42	60	6	433	33	0.8	0.6
0	6	0.1	<0.1	0.5	0.1	18	0	1	0.1	7	21	3	208	11	0.3	0.1
0	6	0.1	<0.1	0.5	0.1	18	0	1	0.1	7	21	3	208	11	0.3	0.1
0	102	<0.1	<0.1	0.2	<0.1	71	0	3	0.2	26	14	11	157	8	0.4	0.4
0	1	<0.1	0.1	1.2	0.1	42	0	2	0.1	33	101	580	310	41	1.3	0.8
0	3	0.2	0.2	1.2	0.1	177	0	1	0.2	61	212	8	456	73	2.5	1.7
0	0	<0.1	<0.1	1.3	0.1	11	0	3	0.3	6	48	306	270	12	0.8	0.2
0	0	0.1	<0.1	3.3	0.4	44	0	13	1.4	16	148	228	792	45	0.9	0.5
41	82	0.2	0.2	1.4	0.1	13	0.1	21	3	101	102	134	254	17	1.5	0.4
37	70	0.1	0.3	1.5	0.2	112	0.7	2		189	175	882	604	85	2.2	1.7
0	2	<0.1	<0.1	0.2	0.6	80	0	5	0.2	38	108	359	206	35	1.6	1.3
0	5	0.2	0.1	0.9	0.2	282	0	2	1.9	80	276	11	477	79	4.7	2.5
0	0	<0.1	<0.1	0.1	0.1	<1	0	4	<0.1	22	18	2	48	3	0.2	0.1
0	0	0.2	<0.1	3.8	0.2	10	0	10	0.3	23	112	53	680	27	2.4	0.5
0	0	<0.1	<0.1	0.7	<0.1	2	0	2	0.1	4	21	10	126	5	0.4	0.1
0	0	<0.1	<0.1	0.1	<0.1	2	0	0	0.1	16	58	346	15	26	1	1.7
0	0	<0.1	<0.1	0.1	<0.1	2	0	0	0.1	16	58	346	15	26	1	1.7
0	18	<0.1	<0.1	0.1	<0.1	2	0	0	0.2	16	56	336	14	26	1	1.7
0	5	0.2	0.1	1	1	146	0	19	2.5	123	276	600	428	71	3.9	2.7
0	116	<0.1	<0.1	0.3	0.1	10	0	7	0.5	16	12	1136	131	10	1.3	0.2
	30						0	53	0.4			2	2			
0	74	0.1	0.1	0.9	0.1	35	0	32		31	42	439	191	15	0.7	
0	2	<0.1	<0.1	0.2	0.1	14	0	24	0.5	14	22	5	180	14	0.7	0.2
0	962	0.1	0.1	0.6	0.2	17	0	53	1.1	94	36	30	296	23	1.2	0.3
0	9	0.1	<0.1	0.4	0.2	57	0	11	0.8	53	31	18	160	25	1.9	0.1
0	<1	0.1	<0.1	0.7	0.1	61	0	1	2.2	18	88	44	156	27	1.5	0.6
0	2	0.3	0.1	2.1	0.4	358	0	3	1.2	38	356	4	731	71	6.6	2.5
0	54	<0.1	<0.1	0.2	<0.1	41	0	4	0.4	18	13	3	144	7	0.2	0.1
0	18	<0.1	<0.1	0.1	<0.1	31	0	2	0.4	10	11	5	87	5	0.3	0.1

ERA, EatRight Analysis CD-ROM; **AMT,** amount; **WT,** weight; **WTR,** water; **CAL,** calories; **PROT,** protein; **CARB,** carbohydrate; **FIBR,** fiber; **FAT,** fat; **SATF,** saturated fat; **MONO,** monosaturated fat; **POLY,** polyunsaturated fat

ERA CODE	FOOD DESCRIPTION	AMT	UNIT	WT (g)	WTR (g)	CAL (kcal)	PROT (g)	CARB (g)	FIBR (g)	FAT (g)	SATF (g)	MONO (g)	POLY (g)
Vegetables and Legumes (continued)													
5084	Lettuce-Iceberg-Leaf	1	pce	15	14	2	<1	<1	<1	<1	<0.1	<0.1	<0.1
5086	Lettuce-Looseleaf-Chopped	1	cup	56	53	10	1	2	1	<1	<0.1	<0.1	0.1
5087	Lettuce-Looseleaf-Leaf	1	pce	10	9	2	<1	<1	<1	<1	<0.1	<0.1	<0.1
5305	Mixed Vegetable-Canned-Drain	1	cup	163	142	77	4	15	5	<1	0.1	<0.1	0.2
5516	Mixed Vegetables-Cnd-LowSod	1	cup	182	164	66	3	13	6	<1	0.1	<0.1	0.2
5187	Mixed Vegetables-Frzn-Cooked	1	cup	182	151	107	5	24	8	<1	0.1	<0.1	0.1
5021	Mung Bean Sprouts-Boiled	1	cup	124	116	26	3	5	1	<1	<0.1	<0.1	<0.1
5197	Mung Bean Sprouts-Canned	1	cup	125	120	15	2	3	1	<1	<0.1	<0.1	<0.1
5092	Mushroom Pieces-Boiled	0.5	cup	78	71	21	2	4	2	<1	<0.1	<0.1	0.1
5094	Mushroom Pieces-Canned	0.5	cup	78	71	19	1	4	2	<1	<0.1	<0.1	0.1
5090	Mushroom Slices-Raw	0.5	cup	35	32	9	1	1	<1	<1	<0.1	<0.1	<0.1
5514	Mushroom-Batter Fried	5	ea	70	44	156	2	11	1	12	1.5	3.6	6
5091	Mushroom-Raw-Whole	1	ea	23	21	6	1	1	<1	<1	<0.1	<0.1	<0.1
5096	Mustard Greens-Boiled	1	cup	140	132	21	3	3	3	<1	<0.1	0.2	0.1
5098	Okra Pods-Boiled	8	ea	85	76	27	2	6	2	<1	<0.1	<0.1	<0.1
5100	Okra Pods-Frozen-Boiled	0.5	cup	92	84	26	2	5	3	<1	0.1	<0.1	0.1
5099	Okra Slices-Boiled	0.5	cup	80	72	26	1	6	2	<1	<0.1	<0.1	<0.1
5644	Okra-Batter Fried	1	cup	92	62	175	2	14	2	12	1.7	3.1	7.1
5190	Onion Rings-Frozen-Heated	2	ea	20	6	81	1	8	<1	5	1.7	2.2	1
5106	Onion Slices-Raw	1	pce	38	34	14	<1	3	1	<1	<0.1	<0.1	<0.1
5104	Onion-Raw-Medium-Whole	1	ea	110	99	42	1	9	2	<1	<0.1	<0.1	0.1
5108	Onions-Boiled	0.5	cup	105	92	46	1	11	1	<1	<0.1	<0.1	0.1
5101	Onions-Chopped-Raw	1	cup	160	143	61	2	14	3	<1	<0.1	<0.1	0.1
26012	Parsley-Fresh-Chopped	0.5	cup	30	26	11	1	2	1	<1	<0.1	0.1	<0.1
5212	Parsnips-Boiled	1	cup	156	121	126	2	30	6	<1	0.1	0.2	0.1
5281	Peas+Carrots-Canned+Liquid	1	cup	255	225	97	6	22	5	1	0.1	0.1	0.3
5123	Peas+Carrots-Frozen-Boiled	0.5	cup	80	69	38	2	8	2	<1	0.1	<0.1	0.2
7016	Peas-Cowpea/Blackeye-Canned	1	cup	240	191	185	11	33	8	1	0.3	0.1	0.6
7018	Peas-Cowpea/Blackeye-Dry-Boil	1	cup	172	120	200	13	36	11	1	0.2	0.1	0.4
5117	Peas-Green-Boiled	1	cup	160	124	134	9	25	9	<1	0.1	<0.1	0.2
5214	Peas-Green-Canned+Liquid	0.5	cup	124	106	66	4	12	4	<1	0.1	<0.1	0.2
5267	Peas-Green-LowSod-Cnd+Liq	0.5	cup	124	106	66	4	12	4	<1	0.1	<0.1	0.2
5118	Peas-Greens-Frozen-Boiled	0.5	cup	80	64	62	4	11	4	<1	<0.1	<0.1	0.1
5124	Pepper-Sweet Green-Fresh	1	cup	149	137	40	1	10	3	<1	<0.1	<0.1	0.2
5126	Pepper-Sweet Green-Cooked	0.5	cup	68	62	19	1	5	1	<1	<0.1	<0.1	0.1
5125	Pepper-Sweet Green-Whole	1	ea	74	68	20	1	5	1	<1	<0.1	<0.1	0.1
5128	Pepper-Sweet Red- Raw-Chpd	1	cup	149	137	40	1	10	3	<1	<0.1	<0.1	0.2
5441	Pepper-Sweet Yellow-Large	1	ea	186	171	50	2	12	2	<1	0.1	<0.1	0.2
5622	Pickled Vegetables	1	cup	163	149	44	2	10	3	<1	<0.1	<0.1	0.1
5227	Pimento-Canned	1	Tbs	12	11	3	<1	1	<1	<1	<0.1	<0.1	<0.1
5228	Pimento Slices-Canned	20	pce	20	19	5	<1	1	<1	<1	<0.1	<0.1	<0.1
5352	Potato Pieces-Canned	0.5	cup	90	76	54	1	12	2	<1	<0.1	<0.1	0.1
5339	Potato Skin-Oven Baked	1	ea	58	27	115	2	27	5	<1	<0.1	<0.1	<0.1
5130	Potato-Baked-Flesh-Medium	0.5	cup	61	46	57	1	13	1	<1	<0.1	<0.1	<0.1
5947	Potato-Baked-Salted w/Skin	1	ea	202	144	220	5	51	5	<1	0.1	<0.1	0.1
5276	Potatoes-Au Gratin from Mix	1	cup	245	194	228	6	31	2	10	6.3	2.9	0.3

< = Trace amount present   Blank = Not available

CHOL, cholesterol; **V,** vitamin; **THI,** thiamin; **RIB,** riboflavin; **NIA,** niacin; **FOL,** folate; **CALC,** calcium; **PHOS,** phosphate; **SOD,** sodium; **POT,** potassium; **MAG,** magnesium

CHOL (mg)	V-A (RE)	THI (mg)	RIB (mg)	NIA (mg)	V-B6 (mg)	FOL (µg)	V-B12 (µg)	V-C (mg)	V-E (mg)	CALC (mg)	PHOS (mg)	SOD (mg)	POT (mg)	MAG (mg)	IRON (mg)	ZINC (mg)
0	5	<0.1	<0.1	<0.1	<0.1	8	0	1	0.1	3	3	1	24	1	0.1	<0.1
0	106	<0.1	<0.1	0.2	<0.1	28	0	10	0.6	38	14	5	148	6	0.8	0.2
0	19	<0.1	<0.1	<0.1	<0.1	5	0	2	0.1	7	2	1	26	1	0.1	<0.1
0	1898	0.1	0.1	0.9	0.1	38	0	8	1	44	68	243	474	26	1.7	0.7
0	924	0.1	0.1	0.9	0.1	33	0	7	0.4	38	67	47	251	27	1.2	0.9
0	779	0.1	0.2	1.5	0.1	35	0	6	0.8	46	93	64	308	40	1.5	0.9
0	1	0.1	0.1	1	0.1	36	0	14	0.1	15	35	12	125	17	0.8	0.6
0	2	<0.1	0.1	0.3	<0.1	12	0	<1	0.1	18	40	175	34	11	0.5	0.3
0	0	0.1	0.2	3.5	0.1	14	0	3	0.2	5	68	2	278	9	1.4	0.7
0	0	0.1	<0.1	1.2	<0.1	10	0	0	0.2	9	51	332	101	12	0.6	0.6
0	0	<0.1	0.1	1.4	<0.1	4	<0.1	1	0.1	2	36	1	130	4	0.4	0.3
2	6	0.1	0.3	2.3	<0.1	8	<0.1	1	2.3	15	119	112	154	7	1.2	0.4
0	0	<0.1	0.1	0.9	<0.1	3	<0.1	1	0.1	1	24	1	85	2	0.2	0.2
0	424	0.1	0.1	0.6	0.1	103	0	35	3	104	57	22	283	21	1	0.2
0	49	0.1	<0.1	0.7	0.2	39	0	14	0.6	54	48	4	274	48	0.4	0.5
0	47	0.1	0.1	0.7	<0.1	134	0	11	0.6	88	42	3	215	47	0.6	0.6
0	46	0.1	<0.1	0.7	0.1	37	0	13	0.6	50	45	4	258	46	0.4	0.4
2	39	0.2	0.1	1.4	0.1	38	<0.1	10	3	61	122	122	190	36	1.3	0.5
0	5	0.1	<0.1	0.7	<0.1	13	0	<1	1.3	6	16	75	26	4	0.3	0.1
0	0	<0.1	<0.1	0.1	<0.1	7	0	2	0.1	8	13	1	60	4	0.1	0.1
0	0	<0.1	<0.1	0.2	0.1	21	0	7	0.3	22	36	3	173	11	0.2	0.2
0	0	<0.1	<0.1	0.2	0.1	16	0	5	0.4	23	37	3	174	12	0.3	0.2
0	0	0.1	<0.1	0.2	0.2	30	0	10	0.5	32	53	5	251	16	0.4	0.3
0	156	<0.1	<0.1	0.4	<0.1	46	0	40	0.5	41	17	17	166	15	1.9	0.3
0	0	0.1	0.1	1.1	0.1	91	0	20	1.6	58	108	16	572	45	0.9	0.4
0	1471	0.2	0.1	1.5	0.2	47	0	17	1.4	59	117	663	255	36	1.9	1.5
0	621	0.2	0.1	0.9	0.1	21	0	6	0.9	18	39	54	126	13	0.8	0.4
0	2	0.2	0.2	0.8	0.1	123	0	6	0.2	48	168	718	413	67	2.3	1.7
0	3	0.3	0.1	0.9	0.2	358	0	1	0.5	41	268	7	478	91	4.3	2.2
0	96	0.4	0.2	3.2	0.3	101	0	23	0.8	43	187	5	434	62	2.5	1.9
0	47	0.1	0.1	1	0.1	35	0	12	0.3	22	66	310	124	21	1.3	0.9
0	47	0.1	0.1	1	0.1	35	0	12	0.8	22	66	11	124	21	1.3	0.9
0	54	0.2	0.1	1.2	0.1	47	0	8	0.4	19	72	70	134	23	1.3	0.8
0	94	0.1	<0.1	0.8	0.4	33	0	133	1	13	28	3	264	15	0.7	0.2
0	40	<0.1	<0.1	0.3	0.2	11	0	51	0.5	6	12	1	113	7	0.3	0.1
0	47	<0.1	<0.1	0.4	0.2	16	0	66	0.5	7	14	1	131	7	0.3	0.1
0	849	0.1	<0.1	0.8	0.4	33	0	283	1.1	13	28	3	264	15	0.7	0.2
0	45	0.1	<0.1	1.7	0.3	48	0	341	1.3	20	45	4	394	22	0.9	0.3
0	1128	0.1	0.1	0.8	0.2	27	0	56	0.5	32	45	332	348	19	0.7	0.3
0	32	<0.1	<0.1	0.1	<0.1	1	0	10	0.1	1	2	2	19	1	0.2	<0.1
0	53	<0.1	<0.1	0.1	<0.1	1	0	17	0.1	1	3	3	32	1	0.3	<0.1
0	0	0.1	<0.1	0.8	0.2	6	0	5	0.1	4	25	197	206	13	1.1	0.3
0	0	0.1	0.1	1.8	0.4	13	0	8	<0.1	20	59	12	332	25	4.1	0.3
0	0	0.1	<0.1	0.9	0.2	6	0	8	<0.1	3	30	3	238	15	0.2	0.2
0	0	0.2	0.1	3.3	0.7	22	0	26	0.1	20	115	493	844	55	2.7	0.6
37	76	<0.1	0.2	2.3	0.1	16	0	8	2.9	203	233	1075	536	37	0.8	0.6

ERA, EatRight Analysis CD-ROM; **AMT**, amount; **WT**, weight; **WTR**, water; **CAL**, calories; **PROT**, protein; **CARB**, carbohydrate; **FIBR**, fiber; **FAT**, fat; **SATF**, saturated fat; **MONO**, monosaturated fat; **POLY**, polyunsaturated fat

ERA CODE	FOOD DESCRIPTION	AMT	UNIT	WT (g)	WTR (g)	CAL (kcal)	PROT (g)	CARB (g)	FIBR (g)	FAT (g)	SATF (g)	MONO (g)	POLY (g)
Vegetables and Legumes (continued)													
5569	Potatoes-Mashed w/Milk+Butter	1	cup	210	160	223	4	35	4	9	5.8	2.5	0.3
5464	Potatoes-Mashed-Flakes-Prep	1	cup	210	160	237	4	32	5	12	7.2	3.3	0.5
5269	Potatoes-O'Brien-Frozen-Cooked	1	cup	194	120	396	4	42	3	26	6.4	11.3	6.7
5271	Potatoes-Scalloped from Mix	1	cup	245	194	228	5	31	3	11	6.4	3	0.5
5136	Potato-Peeled-Boiled-Pieces	0.5	cup	78	60	67	1	16	1	<1	<0.1	<0.1	<0.1
5451	Radicchio-Raw-Shredded	0.5	cup	20	19	5	<1	1	<1	<1	<0.1	<0.1	<0.1
5144	Radish-Red-Slices	0.5	cup	58	55	12	<1	2	1	<1	<0.1	<0.1	<0.1
5143	Radish-Red-Whole	10	ea	45	43	9	<1	2	1	<1	<0.1	<0.1	<0.1
5238	Red Cabbage-Boiled	0.5	cup	75	70	16	1	3	2	<1	<0.1	<0.1	0.1
7024	Refried Beans/Frijoles-Canned	1	cup	252	191	237	14	39	13	3	1.2	1.4	0.4
5088	Romaine Lettuce-Chopped	1	cup	56	53	8	1	1	1	<1	<0.1	<0.1	0.1
5969	Rutabaga-Mashed-w/Salt	0.5	cup	120	107	47	2	10	2	<1	<0.1	<0.1	0.1
5145	Sauerkraut-Canned+Liquid	1	cup	236	218	45	2	10	6	<1	0.1	<0.1	0.1
5531	Sauerkraut-Canned-LowSod	1	cup	142	131	27	1	6	4	<1	<0.1	<0.1	0.1
5270	Scalloped Potatoes-recipe	1	cup	245	198	211	7	26	5	9	3.4	3.3	1.8
5427	Shallots-Raw-Chopped	1	Tbs	10	8	7	<1	2	<1	<1	<0.1	<0.1	<0.1
5385	Shiitake Mushrooms-Boiled Pieces	1	cup	145	121	80	2	21	3	<1	0.1	0.1	<0.1
5122	Snow Pea Pods-Boiled	1	cup	160	142	67	5	11	4	<1	0.1	<0.1	0.2
5296	Snow Pea Pods-Frozen-Boiled	0.5	cup	80	69	42	3	7	2	<1	0.1	<0.1	0.1
7015	Soybeans-Dry-Cooked	1	cup	172	108	298	29	17	10	15	2.2	3.4	8.7
5147	Spinach-Boiled	1	cup	180	164	41	5	7	4	<1	0.1	<0.1	0.2
5146	Spinach-Raw-Chopped	1	cup	30	27	7	1	1	1	<1	<0.1	<0.1	<0.1
7020	Split Peas-Cooked	1	cup	196	136	231	16	41	16	1	0.1	0.2	0.3
5114	Spring/Green Onion-Pieces	0.5	cup	50	45	16	1	4	1	<1	<0.1	<0.1	<0.1
5317	Squash-Butternut-Baked	1	cup	205	180	82	2	22	6	<1	<0.1	<0.1	0.1
5453	Squash-Hubbard-Baked	1	cup	240	204	120	6	26	6	1	0.3	0.1	0.6
5455	Squash-Spaghetti-Boiled	1	cup	155	143	42	1	10	2	<1	0.1	<0.1	0.2
5152	Squash-Summer-Boiled	1	cup	180	169	36	2	8	3	1	0.1	<0.1	0.2
5303	Squash-Winter-Baked	1	cup	205	182	80	2	18	6	1	0.3	0.1	0.5
5251	Succotash-Boiled	1	cup	192	131	221	10	47	9	2	0.3	0.3	0.7
5154	Succotash-Frozen-Boiled	1	cup	170	126	158	7	34	7	2	0.3	0.3	0.7
5601	Succotash-Whole Corn-Canned	1	cup	255	209	161	7	36	7	1	0.2	0.2	0.6
5155	Sweet Potato-Baked+Skin	1	ea	114	83	117	2	28	3	<1	<0.1	<0.1	0.1
5166	Sweet Potatoes-Candied	1	pce	105	70	144	1	29	3	3	1.4	0.7	0.2
5059	Swiss Chard-Boiled	1	cup	175	162	35	3	7	4	<1	<0.1	<0.1	<0.1
5302	Taro Slices-Cooked	1	cup	132	84	187	1	46	7	<1	<0.1	<0.1	0.1
5266	Tater Tots-Frozen-Heated	10	ea	79	42	175	3	24	3	8	4	3.4	0.6
5476	Tomato Puree-Canned	1	cup	250	219	100	4	24	5	<1	0.1	0.1	0.2
5178	Tomatoes-Boiled-Cup Measure	1	cup	240	221	65	3	14	2	1	0.1	0.2	0.4
5179	Tomatoes-Canned	1	cup	240	225	46	2	10	2	<1	<0.1	<0.1	0.1
5171	Tomatoes-Cherry	1	ea	17	16	4	<1	1	<1	<1	<0.1	<0.1	<0.1
5170	Tomatoes-Fresh-Chopped	1	cup	180	169	38	2	8	2	1	0.1	0.1	0.2
5474	Tomatoes-Stewed-Cnd-LowSod	1	cup	255	232	71	2	17	3	<1	<0.1	0.1	0.1
5446	Tomatoes-Sun Dried	1	cup	54	8	139	8	30	7	2	0.2	0.3	0.6
5169	Tomato-Fresh-Medium	1	ea	123	115	26	1	6	1	<1	0.1	0.1	0.2
5173	Tomato-Fresh-Slices	2	pce	40	38	8	<1	2	<1	<1	<0.1	<0.1	0.1

< = Trace amount present   Blank = Not available

CHOL, cholesterol; **V,** vitamin; **THI,** thiamin; **RIB,** riboflavin; **NIA,** niacin; **FOL,** folate;
CALC, calcium; **PHOS,** phosphate; **SOD,** sodium; **POT,** potassium; **MAG,** magnesium

CHOL (mg)	V-A (RE)	THI (mg)	RIB (mg)	NIA (mg)	V-B6 (mg)	FOL (μg)	V-B12 (μg)	V-C (mg)	V-E (mg)	CALC (mg)	PHOS (mg)	SOD (mg)	POT (mg)	MAG (mg)	IRON (mg)	ZINC (mg)
25	42	0.2	0.1	2.3	0.5	17	0	13	0.6	55	97	620	607	38	0.5	0.6
29	44	0.2	0.1	1.4	<0.1	16	0.2	20	1.5	103	118	697	489	38	0.5	0.4
0	37	0.1	0.3	2.8	0.7	24	0	20	0.4	39	180	83	918	66	1.9	1.1
27	51	<0.1	0.1	2.5	0.1	23	0	8	0.4	88	137	835	497	34	0.9	0.6
0	0	0.1	<0.1	1	0.2	7	0	6	<0.1	6	31	4	256	16	0.2	0.2
0	1	<0.1	<0.1	0.1	<0.1	12	0	2	0.5	4	8	4	60	3	0.1	0.1
0	1	<0.1	<0.1	0.2	<0.1	16	0	13	0	12	10	14	134	5	0.2	0.2
0	<1	<0.1	<0.1	0.1	<0.1	12	0	10	0	9	8	11	104	4	0.1	0.1
0	2	<0.1	<0.1	0.2	0.1	9	0	26	0.1	28	22	6	105	8	0.3	0.1
20	0	0.1	<0.1	0.8	0.4	28	0	15	0	88	217	753	673	83	4.2	2.9
0	146	0.1	0.1	0.3	<0.1	76	0	13	0.4	20	25	4	162	3	0.6	0.1
0	67	0.1	<0.1	0.9	0.1	18	0	23	0.2	58	67	305	391	28	0.6	0.4
0	5	<0.1	0.1	0.3	0.3	56	0	35	4	71	47	1559	401	31	3.5	0.4
0	3	<0.1	<0.1	0.2	0.1	34	0	21	0.1	43	28	437	241	18	2.1	0.3
15	47	0.2	0.2	2.6	0.4	27	0	26	0.8	140	154	821	926	47	1.4	1
0	12	<0.1	<0.1	<0.1	<0.1	3	0	1	<0.1	4	6	1	33	2	0.1	<0.1
0	0	0.1	0.2	2.2	0.2	30	0	<1	0.2	4	42	6	170	20	0.6	1.9
0	21	0.2	0.1	0.9	0.2	47	0	77	4.7	67	88	6	384	42	3.2	0.6
0	14	0.1	0.1	0.4	0.1	28	0	18	2.3	47	46	4	174	22	1.9	0.4
0	2	0.3	0.5	0.7	0.4	93	0	3	3.4	175	421	2	886	148	8.8	2
0	1474	0.2	0.4	0.9	0.4	262	0	18	3.6	245	101	126	839	157	6.4	1.4
0	202	<0.1	0.1	0.2	0.1	58	0	8	0.8	30	15	24	167	24	0.8	0.2
0	2	0.4	0.1	1.7	0.1	127	0	1	1.5	27	194	4	710	71	2.5	2
0	20	<0.1	<0.1	0.3	<0.1	32	0	9	0.2	36	18	8	138	10	0.7	0.2
0	1435	0.1	<0.1	2	0.3	39	0	31	1.4	84	55	8	582	59	1.2	0.3
0	1449	0.2	0.1	1.3	0.4	39	0	23	0.3	41	55	19	859	53	1.1	0.4
0	17	0.1	<0.1	1.3	0.2	12	0	5	0.2	33	22	28	181	17	0.5	0.3
0	52	0.1	0.1	0.9	0.1	36	0	10	0.3	49	70	2	346	43	0.6	0.7
0	730	0.2	<0.1	1.4	0.1	57	0	20	0.2	29	41	2	896	16	0.7	0.5
0	56	0.3	0.2	2.5	0.2	63	0	16	2.2	33	225	33	787	102	2.9	1.2
0	39	0.1	0.1	2.2	0.2	56	0	10	1.7	26	119	76	450	39	1.5	0.8
0	38	0.1	0.1	1.6	0.1	81	0	12	2.4	28	140	564	416	48	1.4	1.3
0	2487	0.1	0.1	0.7	0.3	26	0	28	0.3	32	63	11	397	23	0.5	0.3
8	440	<0.1	<0.1	0.4	<0.1	12	0	7	4	27	27	74	198	12	1.2	0.2
0	550	0.1	0.2	0.6	0.1	15	0	32	3.3	102	58	313	961	150	4	0.6
0	0	0.1	<0.1	0.7	0.4	25	0	7	0.6	24	100	20	639	40	0.9	0.4
0	2	0.2	0.1	1.7	0.2	13	0	5	0.1	24	38	589	300	15	1.2	0.2
0	320	0.2	0.1	4.3	0.4	28	0	26	6.3	42	100	998	1065	60	3.1	0.6
0	178	0.2	0.1	1.8	0.2	31	0	55	2.8	14	74	26	670	34	1.3	0.3
0	144	0.1	0.1	1.8	0.2	19	0	34	1.6	72	46	355	530	29	1.3	0.4
0	11	<0.1	<0.1	0.1	<0.1	3	0	3	0.2	1	4	2	38	2	0.1	<0.1
0	112	0.1	0.1	1.1	0.1	27	0	34	1.7	9	43	16	400	20	0.8	0.2
0	138	0.1	0.1	1.8	<0.1	14	0	29	1	84	51	564	607	31	1.9	0.4
0	47	0.3	0.3	4.9	0.2	37	0	21	<0.1	59	192	1131	1850	105	4.9	1.1
0	76	0.1	0.1	0.8	0.1	18	0	23	1.1	6	30	11	273	14	0.6	0.1
0	25	<0.1	<0.1	0.3	<0.1	6	0	8	0.4	2	10	4	89	4	0.2	<0.1

ERA, EatRight Analysis CD-ROM; **AMT,** amount; **WT,** weight; **WTR,** water; **CAL,** calories; **PROT,** protein; **CARB,** carbohydrate; **FIBR,** fiber; **FAT,** fat; **SATF,** saturated fat; **MONO,** monosaturated fat; **POLY,** polyunsaturated fat

ERA CODE	FOOD DESCRIPTION	AMT	UNIT	WT (g)	WTR (g)	CAL (kcal)	PROT (g)	CARB (g)	FIBR (g)	FAT (g)	SATF (g)	MONO (g)	POLY (g)
Vegetables and Legumes (continued)													
5174	Tomato-Fresh-Wedge	1	pce	31	29	7	<1	1	<1	<1	<0.1	<0.1	<0.1
5172	Tomato-Italian/Plum-Fresh	1	ea	62	58	13	1	3	1	<1	<0.1	<0.1	0.1
5183	Turnip Cubes-Boiled	0.5	cup	78	73	16	1	4	2	<1	<0.1	<0.1	<0.1
5185	Turnip Greens-Boiled	1	cup	144	134	29	2	6	5	<1	0.1	<0.1	0.1
5186	Turnip Greens-Frozen-Boiled	0.5	cup	82	74	25	3	4	3	<1	0.1	<0.1	0.1
7490	Wasabi Radish-Cooked	1	cup	147	140	25	1	5	2	<1	0.1	0.1	0.2
5387	Water Chestnuts-Canned-Slices	0.5	cup	70	60	35	1	9	2	<1	<0.1	0	<0.1
5223	Watercress Sprigs-Fresh	10	ea	25	24	3	1	<1	<1	<1	<0.1	<0.1	<0.1
5222	Watercress-Fresh	0.5	cup	17	16	2	<1	<1	<1	<1	<0.1	<0.1	<0.1
7053	White Beans-Boiled	1	cup	179	113	249	17	45	11	1	0.2	0.1	0.3
5553	Yams-Orange+Syrup-Canned	1	cup	228	176	203	2	48	6	<1	0.1	<0.1	0.2
5160	Yams-Orange-Peeled-Boiled	1	cup	328	239	344	5	80	6	1	0.2	<0.1	0.4
5667	Zucchini Slices-Steamed	1	cup	180	172	25	2	5	2	<1	0.1	<0.1	0.1
5327	Zucchini Squash-Boiled	1	cup	180	170	29	1	7	3	<1	<0.1	<0.1	<0.1
5326	Zucchini Squash-Raw	1	cup	130	124	18	2	4	2	<1	<0.1	<0.1	0.1

< = Trace amount present   Blank = Not available

CHOL, cholesterol; **V,** vitamin; **THI,** thiamin; **RIB,** riboflavin; **NIA,** niacin; **FOL,** folate;
CALC, calcium; **PHOS,** phosphate; **SOD,** sodium; **POT,** potassium; **MAG,** magnesium

CHOL (mg)	V-A (RE)	THI (mg)	RIB (mg)	NIA (mg)	V-B6 (mg)	FOL (μg)	V-B12 (μg)	V-C (mg)	V-E (mg)	CALC (mg)	PHOS (mg)	SOD (mg)	POT (mg)	MAG (mg)	IRON (mg)	ZINC (mg)
0	19	<0.1	<0.1	0.2	<0.1	5	0	6	0.3	2	7	3	69	3	0.1	<0.1
0	38	<0.1	<0.1	0.4	<0.1	9	0	12	0.6	3	15	6	138	7	0.3	0.1
0	0	<0.1	<0.1	0.2	0.1	7	0	9	<0.1	17	15	39	105	6	0.2	0.2
0	792	0.1	0.1	0.6	0.3	170	0	39	2.5	197	42	42	292	32	1.2	0.2
0	654	<0.1	0.1	0.4	0.1	32	0	18	2.4	125	28	12	184	21	1.6	0.3
0	0	0	<0.1	0.2	0.1	26	0	22	0	25	35	19	419	13	0.2	0.2
0	0	<0.1	<0.1	0.3	0.1	4	0	1	0.3	3	13	6	83	4	0.6	0.3
0	118	<0.1	<0.1	0.1	<0.1	2	0	11	0.2	30	15	10	82	5	0.1	<0.1
0	80	<0.1	<0.1	<0.1	<0.1	2	0	7	0.2	20	10	7	56	4	<0.1	<0.1
0	0	0.2	0.1	0.2	0.2	144	0	0	0.4	161	202	11	1004	113	6.6	2.5
0	1304	0.1	0.1	1	0.1	15	0	24	0.5	34	62	100	422	30	1.8	0.4
0	5592	0.2	0.5	2.1	0.8	36	0	56	0.9	69	89	43	604	33	1.8	0.9
0	58	0.1	0.1	0.7	0.1	34	0	14	0.2	27	58	5	446	40	0.8	0.4
0	43	0.1	0.1	0.8	0.1	30	0	8	0.3	23	72	5	455	40	0.6	0.3
0	44	0.1	<0.1	0.5	0.1	29	0	12	0.5	20	42	4	322	29	0.5	0.3

Starch List

Cereals, grains, pasta, breads, crackers, snacks, starchy vegetables, and cooked dried beans, peas, and lentils are starches. In general, one starch is:

- 1/2 cup of cereal, grain, pasta, or starchy vegetable,
- 1 ounce of a bread product, such as 1 slice of bread,
- 3/4 to 1 ounce of most snack foods. (Some snack foods may also have added fat.)

One starch exchange equals

15 grams carbohydrate,

3 grams protein,

0–1 grams fat,

and 80 calories.

Bread

Bagel	1/2 (1 oz)
Bread, reduced-calorie	2 slices (1 1/2 oz)
Bread, white, whole-wheat, pumpernickel, rye	1 slice (1 oz)
Bread sticks, crisp, 4 in. long x 1/2 in.	2 (2/3 oz)
English muffin	1/2
Hot dog or hamburger bun	1/2 (1 oz)
Pita, 6 in. across	1/2
Roll, plain, small	1 (1 oz)
Raisin bread, unfrosted	1 slice (1 oz)
Tortilla, corn, 6 in. across	1
Tortilla, flour, 7–8 in. across	1
Waffle, 4 1/2 in. square, reduced-fat	1

Cereals And Grains

Bran cereals	1/2 cup
Bulgur	1/2 cup
Cereals	1/2 cup
Cereals, unsweetened, ready-to-eat	3/4 cup
Cornmeal (dry)	3 Tbsp
Couscous	1/3 cup
Flour (dry)	3 Tbsp
Granola, low-fat	1/4 cup
Grape-Nuts	1/4 cup
Grits	1/2 cup
Kasha	1/2 cup
Millet	1/4 cup
Muesli	1/4 cup
Oats	1/2 cup
Pasta	1/2 cup
Puffed cereal	1 1/2 cups

Rice milk	1/2 cup
Rice, white or brown	1/3 cup
Shredded Wheat	1/2 cup
Sugar-frosted cereal	1/2 cup
Wheat germ	3 Tbsp

Starchy Vegetables

Baked beans	1/3 cup
Corn	1/2 cup
Corn on cob, medium	1 (5 oz)
Mixed vegetables with corn, peas, or pasta	1 cup
Peas, green	1/2 cup
Plantain	1/2 cup
Potato, baked or boiled	1 small (3 oz)
Potato, mashed	1/2 cup
Squash, winter (acorn, butternut)	1 cup
Yam, sweet potato, plain	1/2 cup

Crackers And Snacks

Animal crackers	8
Graham crackers, 2 1/2 in. square	3
Matzoh	3/4 oz
Melba toast	4 slices
Oyster crackers	24
Popcorn (popped, no fat added or low-fat microwave)	3 cups
Pretzels	3/4 oz
Rice cakes, 4 in. across	2
Saltine-type crackers	6
Snack chips, fat-free (tortilla, potato)	15–20 (3/4 oz)
Whole-wheat crackers, no fat added	2–5 (3/4 oz)

Dried Beans, Peas, And Lentils

(Count as 1 starch exchange, plus 1 very lean meat exchange.)

Beans and peas (garbanzo, pinto, kidney, white, split, black-eyed)	1/2 cup
Lima beans	2/3 cup
Lentils	1/2 cup
Miso ✎	3 Tbsp

Starchy Foods Prepared With Fat

(Count as 1 starch exchange, plus 1 fat exchange.)

Biscuit, 2 1/2 in. across	1
Chow mein noodles	1/2 cup
Cornbread, 2 in. cube	1 (2 oz)
Crackers, round butter type	6
Croutons	1 cup
French-fried potatoes	16–25 (3 oz)
Granola	1/4 cup

✎ = 400 mg or more of sodium per serving.

Muffin, small . . . . 1 (1 1/2 oz)
Pancake, 4 in. across 2
Popcorn, microwave . . . . 3 cups
Sandwich crackers, cheese or peanut butter filling 3
Stuffing, bread (prepared) . . . . 1/3 cup
Taco shell, 6 in. across 2
Waffle, 4 1/2 in. square 1
Whole-wheat crackers, fat added . . . . 4–6 (1 oz)

Fruit List

Fresh, frozen, canned, and dried fruits and fruit juices are on this list. In general, one fruit exchange is:

- 1 small to medium fresh fruit,
- 1/2 cup of canned or fresh fruit or fruit juice,
- 1/4 cup of dried fruit.

One fruit exchange equals

15 grams carbohydrate and

60 calories.

The weight includes skin, core, seeds, and rind.

Fruit

Apple, unpeeled, small . . . . 1 (4 oz)
Applesauce, unsweetened . . . . 1/2 cup
Apples, dried . . . . 4 rings
Apricots, fresh . . . . 4 whole (5 1/2 oz)
Apricots, dried . . . . 8 halves
Apricots, canned . . . . 1/2 cup
Banana, small . . . . 1 (4 oz)
Blackberries . . . . 3/4 cup
Blueberries . . . . 3/4 cup
Cantaloupe, small . . . . 1/3 melon (11 oz) or 1 cup cubes
Cherries, sweet, fresh . . . . 12 (3 oz)
Cherries, sweet, canned . . . . 1/2 cup
Dates 3
Figs, fresh . . . . 1 1/2 large or 2 medium (3 1/2 oz)
Figs, dried 1 1/2
Fruit cocktail . . . . 1/2 cup
Grapefruit, large . . . . 1/2 (11 oz)
Grapefruit sections, canned . . . . 3/4 cup
Grapes, small . . . . 17 (3 oz)
Honeydew melon . . . . 1 slice (10 oz) or 1 cup cubes
Kiwi . . . . 1 (3 1/2 oz)
Mandarin oranges, canned . . . . 3/4 cup
Mango, small . . . . 1/2 fruit (5 1/2 oz) or 1/2 cup
Nectarine, small . . . . 1 (5 oz)
Orange, small . . . . 1 (6 1/2 oz)
Papaya . . . . 1/2 fruit (8 oz) or 1 cup cubes
Peach, medium, fresh . . . . 1 (6 oz)
Peaches, canned . . . . 1/2 cup
Pear, large, fresh . . . . 1/2 (4 oz)

Pears, canned . . . . 1/2 cup
Pineapple, fresh . . . . 3/4 cup
Pineapple, canned . . . . 1/2 cup
Plums, small . . . . 2 (5 oz)
Plums, canned . . . . 1/2 cup
Prunes, dried 3
Raisins . . . . 2 Tbsp
Raspberries . . . . 1 cup
Strawberries . . . . 1 1/4 cup whole berries
Tangerines, small . . . . 2 (8 oz)
Watermelon . . . . 1 slice (13 1/2 oz) or 1 1/4 cup cubes

Fruit Juice

Apple juice/cider . . . . 1/2 cup
Cranberry juice cocktail . . . . 1/3 cup
Cranberry juice cocktail, reduced-calorie . . . . 1 cup
Fruit juice blends, 100% juice . . . . 1/3 cup
Grape juice . . . . 1/3 cup
Grapefruit juice . . . . 1/2 cup
Orange juice . . . . 1/2 cup
Pineapple juice . . . . 1/2 cup
Prune juice . . . . 1/3 cup

Milk List

Different types of milk and milk products are on this list. Cheeses are on the Meat list and cream and other dairy fats are on the Fat list. Based on the amount of fat they contain, milks are divided into skim/very low-fat milk, low-fat milk, and whole milk. One choice of these includes:

	Carbohydrate (grams)	Protein (grams)	Fat (grams)	Calories
Skim/very low-fat	12	8	0–3	90
Low-fat	12	8	5	120
Whole	12	8	8	150

One milk exchange equals

12 grams carbohydrate and

8 grams protein.

Skim And Very Low-fat Milk

(0–3 grams fat per serving)

Skim milk . . . . 1 cup
1/2% milk . . . . 1 cup
1% milk . . . . 1 cup
Nonfat or low-fat buttermilk . . . . 1 cup
Evaporated skim milk . . . . 1/2 cup
Nonfat dry milk . . . . 1/3 cup dry
Plain nonfat yogurt . . . . 3/4 cup
Nonfat or low-fat fruit-flavored yogurt sweetened with aspartame or with a non-nutritive sweetener . . . . 1 cup

Low-fat

(5 grams fat per serving)

2% milk	1 cup
Plain low-fat yogurt	3/4 cup
Sweet acidophilus milk	1 cup

Whole Milk

(8 grams fat per serving)

Whole milk	1 cup
Evaporated whole milk	1/2 cup
Goat's milk	1 cup
Kefir	1 cup

Other Carbohydrates List

Substitute food choices from this list for a starch, fruit, or milk choice on your meal plan. Some choices will also count as one or more fat choices.

One exchange equals

15 grams carbohydrate,

or 1 starch,

or 1 fruit,

or 1 milk.

Food	Serving Size	Exchanges Per Serving
Angel food cake, unfrosted	1/12th cake	2 carbohydrates
Brownie, small, unfrosted	2 in. square	1 carbohydrate, 1 fat
Cake, unfrosted	2 in. square	1 carbohydrate, 1 fat
Cake, frosted	2 in. square	2 carbohydrates, 1 fat
Cookie, fat-free	2 small	1 carbohydrate
Cookie or sandwich cookie with creme filling	2 small	1 carbohydrate, 1 fat
Cupcake, frosted	1 small	2 carbohydrates, 1 fat
Cranberry sauce, jellied	1/4 cup	2 carbohydrates
Doughnut, plain cake	1 medium (1 1/2 oz)	1 1/2 carbohydrates, 2 fats
Doughnut, glazed	3 3/4 in. across (2 oz)	2 carbohydrates, 2 fats
Fruit juice bars, frozen, 100% juice	1 bar (3 oz)	1 carbohydrate
Fruit snacks, chewy (pureed fruit concentrate)	1 roll (3/4 oz)	1 carbohydrate
Fruit spreads, 100% fruit	1 Tbsp	1 carbohydrate
Gelatin, regular	1/2 cup	1 carbohydrate
Gingersnaps	3	1 carbohydrate
Granola bar	1 bar	1 carbohydrate, 1 fat
Granola bar, fat-free	1 bar	2 carbohydrates
Hummus	1/3 cup	1 carbohydrate, 1 fat
Ice cream	1/2 cup	1 carbohydrate, 2 fats
Ice cream, light	1/2 cup	1 carbohydrate, 1 fat
Ice cream, fat-free, no sugar added	1/2 cup	1 carbohydrate
Jam or jelly, regular	1 Tbsp	1 carbohydrate
Mlik, chocolate, whole	1 cup	2 carbohydrates, 1 fat
Pie, fruit, 2 crusts	1/6 pie	3 carbohydrates, 2 fats
Pie, pumpkin or custard	1/8 pie	1 carbohydrate, 2 fats
Potato chips	12–18 (1 oz)	1 carbohydrate, 2 fats
Pudding, regular (made with low-fat milk)	1/2 cup	2 carbohydrates
Pudding, sugar-free (made with low-fat milk)	1/2 cup	1 carbohydrate
Salad dressing, fat-free ◆	1/4 cup	1 carbohydrate
Sherbet, sorbet	1/2 cup	2 carbohydrates
Spaghetti or pasta sauce, canned ◆	1/2 cup	1 carbohydrate, 1 fat
Sweet roll or Danish	1 (2 1/2 oz)	2 1/2 carbohydrates, 2 fats

◆ = *400 mg or more of sodium per serving.*

Syrup, light.................................	2 Tbsp...........	1 carbohydrate
Syrup, regular...............................	1 Tbsp...........	1 carbohydrate
Syrup, regular...............................	1/4 cup..........	4 carboydrates
Tortilla chips...............................	6–12 (1 oz)......	1 carbohydrate, 2 fats
Yogurt, frozen, low-fat, fat-free	1/3 cup..........	1 carbohydrate, 0–1 fat
Yogurt, frozen, fat-free, no sugar added.....	1/2 cup..........	1 carbohydrate
Yogurt, low-fat with fruit...................	1 cup	3 carbohydrates, 0–1 fat
Vanilla wafers..............................	5	1 carbohydrate, 1 fat

Vegetable List

Vegetables that contain small amounts of carbohydrates and calories are on this list. In general, one vegetable exchange is:

- 1/2 cup of cooked vegetables or vegetable juice,
- 1 cup of raw vegetables.

One vegetable exchange equals

5 grams carbohydrate,

2 grams protein,

0 grams fat, and

25 calories.

Artichoke
Artichoke hearts
Asparagus
Beans (green, wax, Italian)
Bean sprouts
Beets
Broccoli
Brussels sprouts
Cabbage
Carrots
Cauliflower
Celery
Cucumber
Eggplant
Green onions or scallions
Greens (collard, kale, mustard, turnip)
Kohlrabi
Leeks
Mixed vegetables (without corn, peas, or pasta)
Mushrooms
Okra
Onions
Pea pods
Peppers (all varieties)
Radishes
Salad greens (endive, escarole, lettuce, romaine, spinach)
Sauerkraut ◥

Spinach
Summer squash
Tomato
Tomatoes, canned
Tomato sauce ◥
Tomato/vegetable juice ◥
Turnips
Water chestnuts
Watercress
Zucchini

Meat And Meat Substitutes List

Meat and meat substitutes that contain both protein and fat are on this list. In general, one meat exchange is:

- 1 oz meat, fish, poultry, or cheese,
- 1/2 cup dried beans.

Based on the amount of fat they contain, meats are divided into very lean, lean, medium-fat, and high-fat lists. One ounce (one exchange) of each of these includes:

	Carbohydrate (grams)	Protein (grams)	Fat (grams)	Calories
Very lean	0	7	0–1	35
Lean	0	7	3	55
Medium-fat	0	7	5	75
High-fat	0	7	8	100

Very Lean Meat And Substitutes List

One exchange equals

0 grams carbohydrate,

7 grams protein,

0–1 grams fat,

and 35 calories.

One very lean meat exchange is equal to any one of the following items.

Poultry: Chicken or turkey (white meat, no skin), Cornish hen (no skin) .... 1 oz

Fish: Fresh or frozen cod, flounder, haddock, halibut, trout; tuna fresh
or canned in water . . . . 1 oz

Shellfish: Clams, crab, lobster, scallops, shrimp, imitation
shellfish . . . . 1 oz

Game: Duck or pheasant (no skin), venison, buffalo, ostrich. . . . 1 oz

Cheese with 1 gram or less fat per ounce:

Nonfat or low-fat cottage cheese . . . . 1/4 cup

Fat-free cheese . . . . 1 oz

Other: Processed sandwich meats with 1 gram or less fat per ounce,
such as deli thin, shaved meats, chipped beef ✎ ,
turkey ham. . . . . 1 oz

Egg whites 2

Egg substitutes, plain . . . . 1/4 cup

Hot dogs with 1 gram or less fat per ounce ✎ . . . . 1 oz

Kidney (high in cholesterol) . . . . 1 oz

Sausage with 1 gram or less fat per ounce . . . . 1 oz

Count as one very lean meat and one starch exchange:

Dried beans, peas, lentils (cooked) . . . . 1/2 cup

Lean Meat And Substitutes List

One exchange equals

0 grams carbohydrate,

7 grams protein,

3 grams fat,

and 55 calories.

One lean meat exchange is equal to any one of the following items.

Beef: USDA Select or Choice grades of lean beef trimmed of fat, such
as round, sirloin, and flank steak; tenderloin; roast (rib, chuck,
rump); steak (T-bone, porterhouse, cubed), ground round . . . 1 oz

Pork: Lean pork, such as fresh ham; canned, cured, or boiled ham;
Canadian bacon ✎ ; tenderloin, center loin chop. . . . . 1 oz

Lamb: Roast, chop, leg . . . . 1 oz

Veal: Lean chop, roast. . . . . 1 oz

Poultry: Chicken, turkey (dark meat, no skin), chicken white meat (with
skin), domestic duck or goose (well-drained of fat, no skin) . . 1 oz

Fish:

Herring (uncreamed or smoked) . . . . 1 oz

Oysters . . . . 6 medium

Salmon (fresh or canned), catfish. 1 oz

Sardines (canned) . . . . 2 medium

Tuna (canned in oil, drained) . . . . 1 oz

Game: Goose (no skin), rabbit. . . . . 1 oz

Cheese:

4.5%-fat cottage cheese . . . . 1/4 cup

Grated Parmesan . . . . 2 Tbsp

Cheeses with 3 grams or less fat per ounce . . . . 1 oz

Other:

Hot dogs with 3 grams or less fat per ounce ✎ . . . . . . 1 1/2 oz

Processed sandwich meat with 3 grams or less fat per ounce, such
as turkey pastrami or kielbasa . . . . 1 oz

Liver, heart (high in cholesterol) . . . . 1 oz

Medium-Fat Meat And Substitutes List

One exchange equals

0 grams carbohydrate,

7 grams protein,

5 grams fat,

and 75 calories.

One medium-fat meat exchange is equal to any one of the
following items.

Beef: Most beef products fall into this category (ground beef, meat-
loaf, corned beef, short ribs, Prime grades of meat trimmed of fat,
such as prime rib). . . . . 1 oz

Pork: Top loin, chop, Boston butt, cutlet . . . . 1 oz

Lamb: Rib roast, ground . . . . 1 oz

Veal: Cutlet (ground or cubed, unbreaded) . . . . 1 oz

Poultry: Chicken dark meat (with skin), ground turkey or ground
chicken, fried chicken (with skin) . . . . 1 oz

Fish: Any fried fish product . . . . 1 oz

Cheese: With 5 grams or less fat per ounce

Feta. . . . . 1 oz

Mozzarella . . . . 1 oz

Ricotta . . . . 1/4 cup (2 oz)

Other:

Egg (high in cholesterol, limit to 3 per week) 1

Sausage with 5 grams or less fat per ounce . . . . 1 oz

Soy milk. . . . . 1 cup

Tempeh . . . . 1/4 cup

Tofu . . . . 4 oz or 1/2 cup

High-Fat Meat And Substitutes List

One exchange equals

0 grams carbohydrate,

7 grams protein,

8 grams fat,

and 100 calories.

Remember these items are high in saturated fat, cholesterol,
and calories and may raise blood cholesterol levels if eaten
on a regular basis. One high-fat meat exchange is equal to
any one of the following items.

Pork: Spareribs, ground pork, pork sausage. . . . . 1 oz

Cheese: All regular cheeses, such as American ✎ , cheddar,
Monterey Jack, Swiss. . . . . 1 oz

Other: Processed sandwich meats with 8 grams or less fat per ounce,
such as bologna, pimento loaf, salami . . . . 1 oz

✎ = 400 mg or more of sodium per serving.

Sausage, such as bratwurst, Italian, knockwurst, Polish, smoked . . . . 1 oz
Hot dog (turkey or chicken) ✎ 1 (10/lb)
Bacon . . . . 3 slices (20 slices/lb)

Count as one high-fat meat plus one fat exchange:
Hot dog (beef, pork, or combination) ✎ 1 (10/lb)
Peanut butter (contains unsaturated fat) . . . . 2 Tbsp

Fat List

Fats are divided into three groups, based on the main type of fat they contain: monounsaturated, polyunsaturated, and saturated. Small amounts of monounsaturated and polyunsaturated fats in the foods we eat are linked with good health benefits. Saturated fats are linked with heart disease and cancer. In general, one fat exchange is:

- 1 teaspoon of regular margarine or vegetable oil,
- 1 tablespoon of regular salad dressings.

Monounsaturated Fats List
One fat exchange equals

5 grams fat and
45 calories.

Avocado, medium . . . . 1/8 (1 oz)
Oil (canola, olive, peanut) . . . . 1 tsp
Olives: ripe (black) . . . . 8 large
green, stuffed ✎ . . . . 10 large
Nuts
almonds, cashews . . . . 6 nuts
mixed (50% peanuts) . . . . 6 nuts
peanuts . . . . 10 nuts
pecans . . . . 4 halves
Peanut butter, smooth or crunchy . . . . 2 tsp
Sesame seeds . . . . 1 Tbsp
Tahini paste . . . . 2 tsp

Polyunsaturated Fats List
One fat exchange equals

5 grams fat and
45 calories.

Margarine: stick, tub, or squeeze . . . . 1 tsp
lower-fat (30% to 50% vegetable oil) . . . . 1 Tbsp
Mayonnaise: regular . . . . 1 tsp
reduced-fat . . . . 1 Tbsp
Nuts, walnuts, English . . . . 4 halves
Oil (corn, safflower, soybean) . . . . 1 tsp
Salad dressing: regular ✎ . . . . 1 Tbsp
reduced-fat . . . . 2 Tbsp

Miracle Whip Salad Dressing®: regular . . . . 2 tsp
reduced-fat . . . . 1 Tbsp
Seeds: pumpkin, sunflower . . . . 1 Tbsp

Saturated Fats List*
One fat exchange equals

5 grams of fat
and 45 calories.

Bacon, cooked . . . . 1 slice (20 slices/lb)
Bacon, grease . . . . 1 tsp
Butter: stick . . . . 1 tsp
whipped . . . . 2 tsp
reduced-fat . . . . 1 Tbsp
Chitterlings, boiled . . . . 2 Tbsp (1/2 oz)
Coconut, sweetened, shredded . . . . 2 Tbsp
Cream, half and half . . . . 2 Tbsp
Cream cheese: regular . . . . 1 Tbsp (1/2 oz)
reduced-fat . . . . 2 Tbsp (1 oz)
Fatback or salt pork, see below†
Shortening or lard . . . . 1 tsp
Sour cream: regular . . . . 2 Tbsp
reduced-fat . . . . 3 Tbsp

Free Foods List

A *free food* is any food or drink that contains less than 20 calories or less than 5 grams of carbohydrate per serving. Foods with a serving size listed should be limited to three servings per day. Foods listed without a serving size can be eaten as often as you like.

Fat-free Or Reduced-fat Foods

Cream cheese, fat-free . . . . 1 Tbsp
Creamers, nondairy, liquid . . . . 1 Tbsp
Creamers, nondairy, powdered . . . . 2 tsp
Mayonnaise, fat-free . . . . 1 Tbsp
Mayonnaise, reduced-fat . . . . 1 tsp
Margarine, fat-free . . . . 4 Tbsp
Margarine, reduced-fat . . . . 1 tsp
Miracle Whip®, nonfat . . . . 1 Tbsp
Miracle Whip®, reduced-fat . . . . 1 tsp
Nonstick cooking spray
Salad dressing, fat-free . . . . 1 Tbsp
Salad dressing, fat-free, Italian . . . . 2 Tbsp
Salsa . . . . 1/4 cup
Sour cream, fat-free, reduced-fat . . . . 1 Tbsp
Whipped topping, regular or light . . . . 2 Tbsp

†Use a piece 1 in. × 1 in. × 1/4 in. if you plan to eat the fatback cooked with vegetables. Use a piece 2 in × 1 in. × 1/2 in. when eating only the vegetables with the fatback removed.

*Saturated fats can raise blood cholesterol levels.

Sugar-free Or Low-sugar Foods

Candy, hard, sugar-free . . . . 1 candy
Gelatin dessert, sugar-free
Gelatin, unflavored
Gum, sugar-free
Jam or jelly, low-sugar or light . . . . 2 tsp
Sugar substitutes†
Syrup, sugar-free . . . . 2 Tbsp

†Sugar substitutes, alternatives, or replacements that are approved by the Food and Drug Administration (FDA) are safe to use. Common brand names include:

Equal® (aspartame)
Sprinkle Sweet® (saccharin)
Sweet One® (acesulfame K)
Sweet-10® (saccharin)
Sugar Twin® (saccharin)
Sweet 'n Low® (saccharin)

Drinks

Bouillon, broth, consommé ▲
Bouillon or broth, low-sodium
Carbonated or mineral water
Cocoa powder, unsweetened . . . . 1 Tbsp
Coffee
Club soda
Diet soft drinks, sugar-free

Drink mixes, sugar-free
Tea
Tonic water, sugar-free

Condiments

Catsup . . . . 1 Tbsp
Horseradish
Lemon juice
Lime juice
Mustard
Pickles, dill ▲ . . . . 1 1/2 large
Soy sauce, regular or light ▲
Taco sauce . . . . 1 Tbsp
Vinegar

Seasonings

Be careful with seasonings that contain sodium or are salts, such as garlic or celery salt, and lemon pepper.
Flavoring extracts
Garlic
Herbs, fresh or dried
Pimento
Spices
Tabasco® or hot pepper sauce
Wine, used in cooking
Worcestershire sauce

Combination Foods List

Many of the foods we eat are mixed together in various combinations. These combination foods do not fit into any one exchange list. This is a list of exchanges for some typical combination foods.

Food Entrees	Serving Size	Exchanges Per Serving
Tuna noodle casserole, lasagna, spaghetti with meatballs, chili with beans, macaroni and cheese ▲	1 cup (8 oz)	2 carbohydrates, 2 medium-fat meats
Chow mein (without noodes or rice)	2 cups (16 oz)	1 carbohydrate, 2 lean meats
Pizza, cheese, thin crust ▲	1/4 of 10 in. (5 oz)	2 carbohydrates, 2 medium-fat meats, 1 fat
Pizza, meat topping, thin crust ▲	1/4 of 10 in. (5 oz)	2 carbohydrates, 2 medium-fat meats, 2 fats
Pot pie ▲	1 (7 oz)	2 carbohydrates, 1 medium-fat meat, 4 fats
Frozen Entrees		
Salisbury steak with gravy, mashed potato ▲	1 (11 oz)	2 carbohydrates, 3 medium-fat meats, 3–4 fats
Turkey with gravy, mashed potato, dressing ▲	1 (11 oz)	2 carbohydrates, 2 medium-fat meats, 2 fats
Entree with less than 300 calories ▲	1 (8 oz)	2 carbohydrates, 3 lean meats
Soups		
Bean ▲	1 cup	1 carbohydrate, 1 very lean meat
Cream (made with water) ▲	1 cup (8 oz)	1 carbohydrate, 1 fat
Split pea (made with water) ▲	1/2 cup (4 oz)	1 carbohydrate
Tomato (made with water) ▲	1 cup (8 oz)	1 carbohydrate
Vegetable beef, chicken noodle, or other broth-type ▲	1 cup (8 oz)	1 carbohydrate

▲ = 400 mg or more of sodium per serving.

Fast Foods*

Food	Serving Size	Exchanges Per Serving
Burritos with beef ✎	2	4 carbohydrates, 2 medium-fat meats, 2 fats
Chicken nuggets ✎	6	1 carbohydrate, 2 medium-fat meats, 1 fat
Chicken breast and wing, breaded and fried ✎	1 each	1 carbohydrate, 4 medium-fat meats, 2 fats
Fish sandwich/tartar sauce ✎	1	3 carbohydrates, 1 medium-fat meat, 3 fats
French fries, thin	20–25	2 carbohydrates, 2 fats
Hamburger, regular	1	2 carbohydrates, 2 medium-fat meats
Hamburger, large ✎	1	2 carbohydrates, 3 medium-fat meats, 1 fat
Hot dog with bun ✎	1	1 carbohydrate, 1 high-fat meat, 1 fat
Individual pan pizza ✎	1	5 carbohydrates, 3 medium-fat meats, 3 fats
Soft-serve cone	1 medium	2 carbohydrates, 1 fat
Submarine sandwich ✎	1 sub (6 in.)	3 carbohydrates, 1 vegetable, 2 medium-fat meats, 1 fat
Taco, hard shell ✎	1 (6 oz)	2 carbohydrates, 2 medium-fat meats, 2 fats
Taco, soft shell ✎	1 (3 oz)	1 carbohydrate, 1 medium-fat meat, 1 fat

*Ask at your fast-food restaurant for nutrition information about your favorite fast foods.

Source: *Exchange Lists for Meal Planning. The American Diabetes Association, Alexandria, VA and The American Dietetics Association, Chicago, IL. 1995.*

APPENDIX C | Nutrition and Health for Canadians

- ➤ Recommended Nutrient Intakes for Canadians
- ➤ Food Labels
- ➤ Nutrition Recommendations for Canadians
- ➤ Food Guide
- ➤ The Canadian Food Guide
- ➤ Canada's Physical Activity Guide to Healthy Active Living

Recommended Nutrient Intakes for Canadians

Chapter 2 introduced the various dietary standards used in the United States such as the Food Guide Pyramid and the Recommended Daily Allowances (RDAs). Canada also has similar recommendations such as Canada's Food Guide and the Recommended Nutrient Intakes (RNI) for Canadians, which were issued by Health and Welfare Canada in 1990 (Tables C-1 and C-2).

Just as the 1989 RDAs are being replaced by the Dietary Reference Intakes (DRI) in the US, the 1990 RNI is also being replaced by the DRI. Recommendations from the DRI reports are presented on the inside front covers of this text. For nutrients that do not yet have new values, the RNI will continue to serve health professionals in Canada.

Table C-1 Recommended Nutrient Intakes for Canadians, 1990

Age	Sex	Weight (kg)	Protein (g/day)[a]	Vitamins						
				Vitamin A (RE/day)[b]	Vitamin E (mg/day)[c]	Vitamin C (mg/day)[d]	Iron (mg/day)	Iodine (μg/day)	Zinc (mg/day)
Infants (months)									
0–4	Both	6	12[e]	400	3	20	0.3[f]	30	2[g]
5–12	Both	9	12	400	3	20	7	40	3
Children (years)									
1	Both	11	13	400	3	20	6	55	4
2–3	Both	14	16	400	4	20	6	65	4
4–6	Both	18	19	500	5	25	8	85	5
7–9	M	25	26	700	7	25	8	110	7
	F	25	26	700	6	25	8	95	7
10–12	M	34	34	800	8	25	8	125	9
	F	36	36	800	7	25	8	110	9
13–15	M	50	49	900	9	30	10	160	12
	F	48	46	800	7	30	13	160	9
16–18	M	62	58	1000	10	40	10	160	12
	F	53	47	800	7	30	12	160	9
Adults (years)									
19–24	M	71	61	1000	10	40	9	160	12
	F	58	50	800	7	30	13	160	9
25–49	M	74	64	1000	9	40	9	160	12
	F	59	51	800	6	30	13[h]	160	9
50–74	M	73	63	1000	7	40	9	160	12
	F	63	54	800	6	30	8	160	9
75+	M	69	59	1000	6	40	9	160	12
	F	64	55	800	5	30	8	160	9
Pregnancy (additional amount needed)									
1st trimester			5	0	2	0	0	25	6
2nd trimester			20	0	2	10	5	25	6
3rd trimester			24	0	2	10	10	25	6
Lactation (additional amount needed)			20	400	3	25	0	50	6

NOTE: Recommended intakes of energy and of certain nutrients are not listed in this table because of the nature of the variables upon which they are based. The figures for energy are estimates of average requirements for expected patterns of activity (see Table C-2). For nutrients not shown, the following amounts are recommended based on at least 2000 kcalories per day and body weights as given: thiamin, 0.4 milligram per 1000 kcalories (0.48 milligram/5000 kilojoules); riboflavin, 0.5 milligram per 1000 kcalories (0.6 milligram/5000 kilojoules); niacin, 7.2 niacin equivalents per 1000 kcalories (8.6 niacin equivalents/5000 kilojoules); vitamin B$_6$, 15 micrograms, as pyridoxine, per gram of protein. Recommended intakes during periods of growth are taken as appropriate for individuals representative of the midpoint in each age group. All recommended intakes are designed to cover individual variations in essentially all of a healthy population subsisting upon a variety of common foods available in Canada.

Source: Health and Welfare Canada, *Nutrition Recommendations: The Report of the Scientific Review Committee* (Ottawa: Canadian Government Publishing Centre, 1990), Table 20, p. 204.

[a]The primary units are expressed per kilogram of body weight. The figures shown here are examples.

[b]One retinol equivalent (RE) corresponds to the biological activity of 1 microgram of retinol, 6 micrograms of beta-carotene, or 12 micrograms of other carotenes.

[c]Expressed as δ-α-tocopherol equivalents, relative to which β- and γ-tocopherol and α-tocotrienol have activities of 0.5, 0.1, and 0.3, respectively.

[d]Cigarette smokers should increase intake by 50 percent.

[e]The assumption is made that the protein is from breast milk or has the same biological value as breast milk and that, between 3 and 9 months, adjustment for the quality of the protein is made.

[f]Based on the assumption that breast milk is the source of iron.

[g]Based on the assumption that breast milk is the source of zinc.

[h]After menopause, the recommended intake is 8 milligrams per day.

Table C-2 Average Energy Requirements for Canadians

Age	Sex	Average Height (cm)	Average Weight (kg)	Requirements[a] (kcal/kg)[b]	(MJ/kg)[b]	(kcal/day)	(MJ/day)	(kcal/cm)	(MJ/cm)
Infants (months)									
0–2	Both	55	4.5	120–100	0.50–0.42	500	2.0	9	0.04
3–5	Both	63	7.0	100–95	0.42–0.40	700	2.8	11	0.05
6–8	Both	69	8.5	95–97	0.40–0.41	800	3.4	11.5	0.05
9–11	Both	73	9.5	97–99	0.41	950	3.8	12.5	0.05
Children and Adults (years)									
1	Both	82	11	101	0.42	1100	4.8	13.5	0.06
2–3	Both	95	14	94	0.39	1300	5.6	13.5	0.06
4–6	Both	107	18	100	0.42	1800	7.6	17	0.07
7–9	M	126	25	88	0.37	2200	9.2	17.5	0.07
	F	125	25	76	0.30	1900	8.0	15	0.06
10–12	M	141	34	73	0.30	2500	10.4	17.5	0.07
	F	143	36	61	0.25	2200	9.2	15.5	0.06
13–15	M	159	50	57	0.24	2800	12.0	17.5	0.07
	F	157	48	46	0.19	2200	9.2	14	0.06
16–18	M	172	62	51	0.21	3200	13.2	18.5	0.08
	F	160	53	40	0.17	2100	8.8	13	0.05
19–24	M	175	71	42	0.18	3000	12.6		
	F	160	58	36	0.15	2100	8.8		
25–49	M	172	74	36	0.15	2700	11.3		
	F	160	59	32	0.13	1900	8.0		
50–74	M	170	73	31	0.13	2300	9.7		
	F	158	63	29	0.12	1800	7.6		
75+	M	168	69	29	0.12	2000	8.4		
	F	155	64	23	0.10	1500	6.3		

[a]Requirements can be expected to vary within a range of ±30 percent.

[b]First and last figures are averages at the beginning and end of the three-month period.

Source: Health and Welfare Canada, *Nutrition Recommendations: The Report of the Scientific Review Committee* (Ottawa: Canadian Government Publishing Centre, 1990), Tables 5 and 6, pp. 25, 27.

INGREDIENTS: Fructose Syrup (from Grapes, Corn and Pears), Oat Bran, Maltodextrin (Complex Carbohydrate), Modified Milk Ingredients (Milk Protein with Lactose removed), Brown Rice, Almond Butter, Natural Berry Flavours, Carmine, Citric Acid, **VITAMINS AND MIERALS:** Dicalcium phosphate, Potassium bicarbonate, Ascorbic acid, Magnesium carbonate, Alpha tocopherol (vit. E), Zinc gluconate, Ferrous fumarate, Salt, Potassium iodide, Beta carotene (vit. A), Copper gluconate, Manganese sulfate, Calcium pantothenate, Pyridoxine hydrochloride (vit. B_6), Riboflavin (vit B_2), Niacin, Thiamin hydrochloride (vit. B_1), Cholecalciferol (vit. D), Folic acid, Biotin, Cyanocobalamin (vit. B_{12}).

INGRÉDIENTS: Sirop de fructose (de Raisin, de Maïs et de Poire), Son d'avione, Maltodextrine (glucide complexe), Substances latières modifiées (protéines du lait, lactose enlevé), Riz brun, Beurre d'amande, Arômes naturels de baie, Carmin, Acide citrique, **VITAMINES ET MINERAUX:** Phosphate bicalcique, Bicarbonate de potassium, Acide ascorbique, Carbonate de magnésium, Alpha tocophérol (vit. E), Gluconate de zinc Fumarate ferreux, Sel, Iodure de potassium, Bêta-carotène (vit. A), Gluconate de cuivre, Sulfate de manganèse, Pantothénate de calcium, Chlorhydrate de pyridoxine (vit. B_6) Riboflavine (vit. B_2), Niacine, Chlorhydrate de thiamine (vit B_1) Cholécalciférol (vit D), Acide folique, Biotine, Cyanocobalamine (vit B_{12}).

Nutrition Information Nutritionelle
per 65 g serving (1 bar) / par portion de 65 g (1 barre)

Energy/Énergie	**225 cal**
	940 kJ
Protein/Protéines	**11 g**
Fat/Matières grasses	**3.0 g**
polyunsaturates/polyinsaturés	1.0 g
linoleic acid/acide linoléque	0.8 g
monounsaturates/monoinsaturés	1.5 g
saturates/saturés	0.5 g
cholesterol/cholestérol	0 g
Carbohydrate/Glucides	**42 g**
dietary fibre/fibres alimentaires	3.0 g
Sodium	**250 mg**
Potassium	**375 mg**

Percentage of Canadian Recommended Daily Intake
Pourcentage de L'apport Quotidien Recommandé

Vitamin A/Vitamine A	13%	Pantothenate/Pantothénate	36%
Vitamin D/Vitamine D	13%	Calcium	36%
Vitamin E/Vitamine E	47%	Phosphorus/Phosphore	28%
Vitamin C/Vitamine C	25%	Magnesium/Magnésium	60%
Thiamine	57%	Iron/Fer	50%
Riboflavin/Riboflavine	53%	Zinc	55%
Niacin/Niacine	43%	Iodine/Iode	43%
Vitamin B_6/Vitamine B_6	55%	Biotin/Biotine	0.02 mg
Folacin/Folacine	45%	Copper/Cuivre	1.0 mg
Vitamin B_{12}/Vitamine B_{12}	75%	Manganese/Manganèse	1.0 mg

Figure C.1 How to read a food label.

Food Labels

Consumers should use food labels to gain information about the foods that they wish to purchase. The sample below demonstrates the reading of a food label.

Ingredients List must be included by law and must list all of the ingredients used in the product. Ingredients are listed in the order of the amount used. The amount is based on the weight of an ingredient rather than its volume.

Serving Size tells you the size of the serving for which the nutrition information is given. If you eat more or less than this amount, remember that the Calories and the content of other nutrients like fat and sodium increase or decrease as well!

Energy is the Calories (Cal) per serving. Energy is also given in kilojoules (kJ).

Fat shows the total amount of fat in food. This product gives the content of various kinds of fat. To choose lower fat foods, the most useful information is the grams of total fat.

Carbohydrate includes the content of sugars, starch and fibre. Sometimes you get the complete breakdown of carbohydrate. In this example you get a breakdown of fibre only.

Sodium is a measure of the amount of salt in a food.

Percentage of Recommended Daily Intake is the way in which vitamins and minerals are listed.

Nutrition Claims are used to highlight a key nutrition feature of a food. These are often put on the front of a package label in big, bold type such as "High in Fibre" or "Preservative Free." When a claim is made about any nutrient, detailed nutrition information on that nutrient must also be given somewhere on the package label.

Nutrition Recommendations for Canadians

- *The Canadian diet should provide energy consistent with the maintenance of body weight within the recommended range.* Physical activity should be appropriate to circumstances and capabilities. Both longevity and the incidence of a number of chronic diseases are associated adversely with body weights above or below the recommended range. There is, thus, a health benefit to controlling weight, but a possible downside to control by energy intake alone. Physical activity should also play a role. While the importance of maintaining some activity throughout life can be stressed, it is not possible to specify a level of physical activity appropriate for the whole population. As a general guideline it is desirable that adults, for as long as possible, maintain an activity level that permits an energy intake of at least 1800 kcal or 7.6 MJ/day while keeping weight within the recommended range.

- *The Canadian diet should include essential nutrients in amounts recommended.* One of the reasons for including physical activity as a desirable element in weight control is the increasing difficulty in meeting the recommended nutrient intake (RNI) as energy intake falls below 1800 kcal or 7.6 MJ/day. While it is important that the diet provide the recommended amounts of nutrients, it should be understood that no evidence was found that intakes in excess of the RNIs confer any health benefit. There is no general need for supplements except for vitamin D for infants and folic acid during pregnancy. Vitamin D supplementation might be required for elderly persons not exposed to the sun, and iron for pregnant women with low iron stores. It should be noted that while the habitual intake of certain nutrients, for example, protein and vitamin C, greatly exceeds the RNI, there is no reason to suggest that present intakes can be reduced.

- *The Canadian diet should include no more than 30% of energy as fat (33 g/1000 kcal or 39 g/5000 kJ) and no more than 10% as saturated fat (11 g/1000 kcal or 13 g/5000 kJ).* Diets high in fat have been associated with a high incidence of heart disease and certain types of cancer and a reduction in total fat intake is an important way to reduce the intake of saturated fat. The evidence linking saturated fat intake with elevated blood cholesterol and the risk of heart disease is among the most persuasive of all diet/disease relationships and was an important factor in establishing the recommended dietary pattern. Dietary cholesterol, though not as influential in affecting levels of blood cholesterol, is not without importance. A reduction in cholesterol intake normally will accompany a reduction in total fat and saturated fat. The recommendation to reduce total fat intake does not apply to children under the age of two years.

- *The Canadian diet should provide 55% of energy as carbohydrate (138 g/1000 kcal or 165 g/5000 kJ) from a variety of sources.* Sources selected should provide complex carbohydrates, a variety of dietary fibre and β-carotene. Carbohydrate is the preferred replacement for fat as a source of energy since protein intake already exceeds requirements. There are a number of reasons why the increased carbohydrate calories should be in the form of complex carbohydrates. Diets high in complex carbohydrates have been associated with a lower incidence of heart disease and cancer, and are sources of dietary fibre and of β-carotene.

- *The sodium content of the Canadian diet should be reduced.* The present food supply provides sodium in an amount greatly exceeding requirements. While there is insufficient evidence to support a quantitative recommendation, potential benefit would be expected from a reduction in current sodium intake. Consumers are encouraged to reduce the use of salt (sodium chloride) in cooking and at the table, but individual efforts will be relatively ineffective unless the food industry makes a determined effort to reduce the sodium content of processed and prepared food. A diet rich in fruits and vegetables will ensure an adequate intake of potassium.

- *The Canadian diet should include no more than 5% of total energy as alcohol, or two drinks daily, whichever is less.* There are many reasons to limit the use of alcohol. From the nutritional point of view, alcohol dilutes the nutrient density of the diet and can undermine the consumption of RNIs. The deleterious influence of alcohol on blood pressure provides more urgent reason for moderation. During pregnancy it is prudent to abstain from alcoholic beverages because a safe intake is not known with certainty.

- *The Canadian diet should contain no more caffeine than the equivalent of four regular cups of coffee per day.* This is a prudent measure in view of the increased risk for cardiovascular disease associated with high intakes of caffeine.

- *Community water supplies containing less than 1 mg/litre should be fluoridated to that level.* Fluoridation of community water supplies has proven to be a safe, effective and economical method of improving dental health.

From: Nutrition Recommendations . . . A Call for Action Summary Report of the Scientific Review Committee and the Communications/ Implementation Committee, 1992, 1989.

Food Guide

What is the Food Guide Based on?

"Canada's Food Guide to Healthy Eating" is based on these guidelines from Health Canada:

Canada's Guidelines for Healthy Eating

1. Enjoy a VARIETY of foods.
2. Emphasize cereals, breads, other grain products, vegetables and fruit.
3. Choose lower-fat dairy products, leaner meats and food prepared with little or no fat.
4. Achieve and maintain a healthy body weight by enjoying regular physical activity and healthy eating.
5. Limit salt, alcohol and caffeine.

What does the Food Guide tell you?

The rainbow side of the Food Guide gives you advice on how to choose foods.

'Enjoy a variety of foods from each group every day.'

Try something new! Explore the rainbow of foods that make up the 4 food groups. Enjoy foods with different tastes, textures and colours.

The 4 food groups provide you with the nutrients you need to be healthy. You need foods from each group because each group gives you different nutrients. You also need to choose different foods from within each food group to get all the nutrients your body needs. Look at the chart on the next page for the key nutrients each food group offers.

'Choose lower-fat foods more often.'

Everyone needs some fat in their diet, but most people eat too much fat. Eating more breads, cereals, grains, vegetables, fruit, peas, beans and lentils will help you cut down on fat. You can also choose lower-fat dairy products and leaner meats, poultry and fish.

Each of the 4 food groups includes foods that contain fat. Eat lower-fat foods from each group every day. Choose smaller amounts of higher-fat foods. If you do, you'll be able to enjoy the foods you love and eat well at the same time.

Tips to Reduce Fat

- Spread less butter or margarine on bread, buns or bagels.
- Have salads with less dressing or with a lower-fat dressing.
- Try vegetables without butter, margarine or rich sauces.
- Try skim, partly-skim or reduced-fat milk products in recipes.
- Choose meat, poultry or fish that are baked, broiled or microwaved. Serve with light broth or herbs.
- Have fried or deep-fried foods less often.
- Have snacks such as chips and chocolate bars less often

'Choose whole grain and enriched products more often.'

Whole grain products such as whole wheat, oats, barley or rye are suggested because they are high in starch and fibre. Enriched foods are recommended because they have some vitamins and minerals added back to them. Treat yourself to multi-grain breads, pumpernickel bagels, enriched pasta, brown rice, ready-to-eat bran cereals or oatmeal.

'Choose dark green and orange vegetables and orange fruit more often.'

These foods are higher than other vegetables and fruit in certain key nutrients like vitamin A and folacin. Go for salads, broccoli, spinach, squash, sweet potatoes, carrots, cantaloupes or orange juice.

'Choose lower-fat milk products more often.'

Lower-fat milk products have less fat and Calories, yet still provide the high quality protein and calcium essential to healthy eating. Whether it's milk, yogourt, cheese or milk powder, choose the lower-fat option. Look at labels and choose products with a lower % M.F. (Milk Fat) or % B.F. (Butter Fat). Then you can have the refreshing taste of milk products with less fat.

'Choose leaner meats, poultry, and fish, as well as dried peas, beans and lentils more often.'

Many leaner meats, poultry, fish and seafood choices are available to help you reduce your fat intake without losing important nutrients. Be sure to trim visible fat. Try baking, broiling, roasting or microwaving instead of frying, and drain off extra fat after cooking. To lower your fat while increasing your intake of starch and fibre, choose foods like baked beans, split pea soup or lentil casserole.

* For more information on Canada's Food Guide to Healthy Eating go to http://www.hc-sc.gc.ca/hppb/nutrition/pube/foodguid/foodguide.html.

The Canadian Food Guide

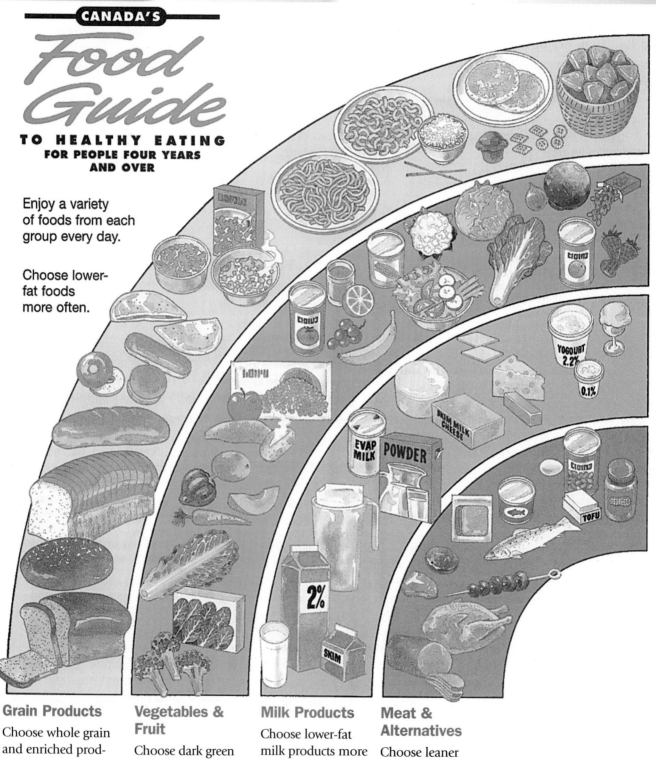

CANADA'S Food Guide

TO HEALTHY EATING
FOR PEOPLE FOUR YEARS AND OVER

Enjoy a variety of foods from each group every day.

Choose lower-fat foods more often.

Grain Products
Choose whole grain and enriched products more often.

Vegetables & Fruit
Choose dark green and orange vegetables and orange fruit more often.

Milk Products
Choose lower-fat milk products more often.

Meat & Alternatives
Choose leaner meats, poultry and fish, as well as dried peas, beans and lentils more often.

Figure C.2

Grain Products
5–12
SERVINGS PER DAY

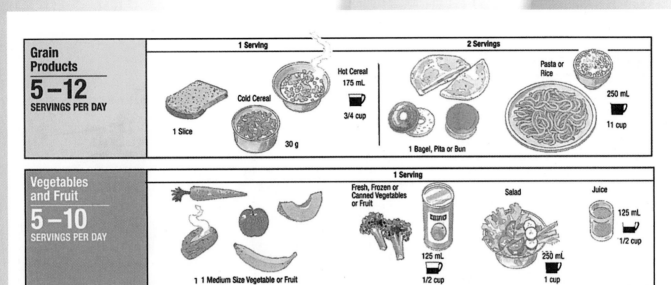

1 Serving

2 Servings

Hot Cereal
175 mL
3/4 cup

Cold Cereal

1 Slice

30 g

Pasta or Rice
250 mL
11 cup

1 Bagel, Pita or Bun

Vegetables and Fruit
5–10
SERVINGS PER DAY

1 Serving

Fresh, Frozen or Canned Vegetables or Fruit
125 mL
1/2 cup

Salad
250 mL
1 cup

Juice
125 mL
1/2 cup

1 1 Medium Size Vegetable or Fruit

Milk Products
SERVINGS PER DAY
Children 4–9 years: 2–3
Youth 10–16 years: 3–4
Adults: 2–4
Pregnant and Breast-feeding Women 3–4

1 Servings

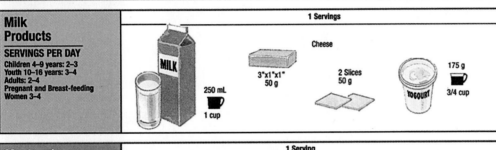

MILK
250 mL
1 cup

Cheese

3"x1"x1"
50 g

2 Slices
50 g

YOGOURT
175 g
3/4 cup

Other Foods

Taste and enjoyment can also come from other foods and beverages that are not part of the 4 food groups. Some of these foods are higher in fat or Calories, so use these foods in moderation.

Meat and Alternatives
2–3
SERVINGS PER DAY

1 Serving

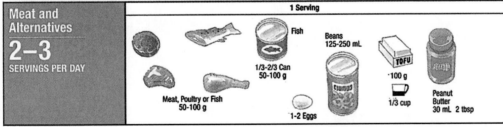

Fish
1/3-2/3 Can
50-100 g

Meat, Poultry or Fish
50-100 g

1-2 Eggs

Beans
125-250 mL

TOFU
100 g
1/3 cup

Peanut Butter
30 mL 2 tbsp

Canada's Physical Activity Guide to Healthy Active Living

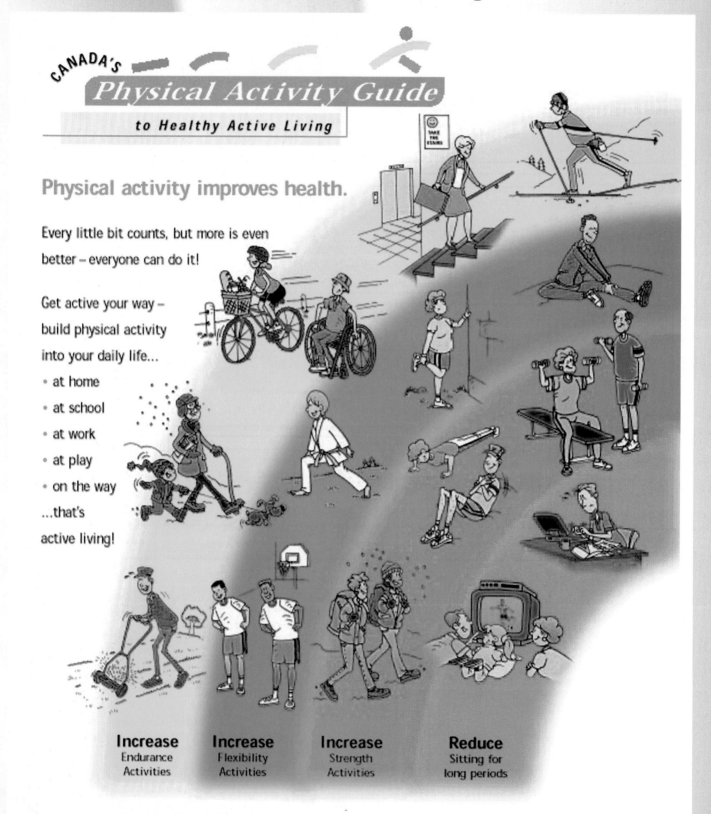

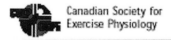

Figure C.3

Choose a variety of activities from these three groups:

Endurance

4-7 days a week
Continuous activities for your heart, lungs and circulatory system.

Flexibility

4-7 days a week
Gentle reaching, bending and stretching activities to keep your muscles relaxed and joints mobile.

Strength

2-4 days a week
Activities against resistance to strengthen muscles and bones and improve posture.

Starting slowly is very safe for most people. Not sure? Consult your health professional.

For a copy of the *Guide Handbook* and more information:
1-888-334-9769, or **www.paguide.com**

Eating well is also important. Follow *Canada's Food Guide to Healthy Eating* to make wise food choices.

Get Active Your Way, Every Day—For Life!

Scientists say accumulate 60 minutes of physical activity every day to stay healthy or improve your health. As you progress to moderate activities you can cut down to 30 minutes, 4 days a week. Add-up your activities in periods of at least 10 minutes each. Start slowly... and build up.

Time needed depends on effort

Very Light Effort	Light Effort *60 minutes*	Moderate Effort *30-60 minutes*	Vigorous Effort *20-30 minutes*	Maximum Effort
• Strolling	• Light walking	• Brisk walking	• Aerobics	• Sprinting
• Dusting	• Volleyball	• Biking	• Jogging	• Racing
	• Easy gardening	• Raking leaves	• Hockey	
	• Stretching	• Swimming	• Basketball	
		• Dancing	• Fast swimming	
		• Water aerobics	• Fast dancing	

Range needed to stay healthy

You Can Do It – Getting started is easier than you think

Physical activity doesn't have to be very hard. Build physical activities into your daily routine.

- Walk whenever you can – get off the bus early, use the stairs instead of the elevator.
- Reduce inactivity for long periods, like watching TV.
- Get up from the couch and stretch and bend for a few minutes every hour.
- Play actively with your kids.
- Choose to walk, wheel or cycle for short trips.

- Start with a 10 minute walk – gradually increase the time.
- Find out about walking and cycling paths nearby and use them.
- Observe a physical activity class to see if you want to try it.
- Try one class to start – you don't have to make a long-term commitment.
- Do the activities you are doing now, more often.

Benefits of regular activity:

- better health
- improved fitness
- better posture and balance
- better self-esteem
- weight control
- stronger muscles and bones
- feeling more energetic
- relaxation and reduced stress
- continued independent living in later life

Health risks of inactivity:

- premature death
- heart disease
- obesity
- high blood pressure
- adult-onset diabetes
- osteoporosis
- stroke
- depression
- colon cancer

  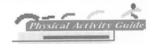

Canada's Physical Activity Guide to Healthy Active Living

Canada's Physical Activity Guide to Healthy Active Living is a Guide to help you make wise choices about physical activity. Choices that will improve your health, help prevent disease, and allow you to get the most out of life.

The Guide provides a rainbow of physical activities that can help you have more energy, move more easily, and get stronger. It tells you how much activity you should strive for and how to get started. It also lists the many benefits of physical activity and the health risks of inactivity.

For more information on Canada's Physical Activity Guide to Healthy Active Living go to http://www.hc-sc.gc.ca/hppb/paguide/main.html

Foods	Phytochemicals	Possible Benefits
Berries blueberries, strawberries, raspberries, blackberries, currants, etc.	Anthocyanidins, ellagic acid	Both act as antioxidants, thus as anti-cancer substances that may help protect cells. Ellagic acid has more than one anti-cancer activity. Anthocyanidins may also protect against heart disease. Berries are also rich in soluble fiber, which may help reduce cholesterol.
Chili Peppers	Capsaicin, which gives peppers their heat	Little is known about potential health benefits; capsaicin may be an antioxidant or otherwise interfere with cancer development. May help prevent blood clotting. Chili peppers are also rich in vitamin C.
Citrus Fruits oranges, grapefruit, lemons, limes, etc.	Flavanones such as hesperitin; coumarins; D-limonene (a monoterpene); carotenoids; flavonoids such as tangeretin and nobiletin	D-limonene, in citrus skin, can leach into the juice and may detoxify cancer promoters. Carotenoids may also fight cancer. Flavonoids act as antioxidants and may inhibit blood clotting. These fruits are also rich in vitamin C (a powerful antioxidant), other nutrients, and fiber.
Cruciferous Vegetables broccoli, broccoli sprouts, Brussels sprouts, kale, cabbage, cauliflower, etc.	Indoles; isothiocyanates such as sulphoraphane; carotenoids such as beta carotene	Long classified as anti-cancer foods. Sulforaphane may neutralize cancer-causing chemicals that damage cells; also interferes with tumor growth. Broccoli sprouts are particularly rich in the substances that convert into sulphoraphane. Indoles act to make estrogen less potent and thus may reduce the risk of breast cancer. These vegetables are also good sources of folic acid (a B vitamin), vitamin C, fiber, and carotenoids—all cancer fighters.
Flax seeds, flour	Lignans	Lignans are converted to a form of estrogen in the body and are thought to have some protective effect against cancer. Lignans are not found in flaxseed oil.
Garlic Family garlic, onions, shallots, leeks, chives, scallions	Allylic sulfides, other sulfur compounds, flavonoids such as quercetin	Adds flavor and zest to other good foods. May work against carcinogens and tumors in many ways, lowering risk of colon, stomach, and other cancers. May also benefit the heart. No certainty that cooked onions and garlic work as well as raw. Supplements are unproven and not recommended.
Herbs and Spices rosemary, sage, thyme, oregano, ginger, cumin, etc.	Carnasol, phenols, curcumin, gingerols, terpenoids, etc.	Major benefit: adding flavor and zest to other good foods. May act as antioxidants and anti-cancer agents, even in small amounts.
Legumes lima, kidney, navy, and other beans, lentils, etc.	Isoflavonoids, phytic acid, saponins, phytosterols	Anti-cancer activity; protection against heart disease. Phytosterols may protect against colon cancer. Beans contain folic acid (a B vitamin) and other nutrients, as well as soluble fiber, which may reduce blood cholesterol.
Nuts cashews, almonds, chestnuts, walnuts, etc.	Ellagic acid, saponins	Potential benefits to the heart may come from these chemicals or from the beneficial fats (poly- and monounsaturated) in nuts. High in calories and fat, nuts should be consumed in moderation.

Foods	Phytochemicals	Possible Benefits
Orange and Yellow Fruits and Vegetables; Leafy Greens apricots, papaya, sweet potatoes, mangoes, carrots, spinach, corn, pumpkin, sweet peppers, etc.	Carotenoids such as beta carotene, lutein, zeaxanthin	Many anticancer functions; strengthen the immune system; protect the retina from harmful radiation, thus reducing risk of macular degeneration. These fruits and vegetables are also rich in vitmain C, other vitamins, minerals, and fiber.
Red Grapes, Red Wine	Flavonols such as quercetin; resverarol, anthocyanidins, ellagic acid	Resveratrol may prevent damage to cells and curb tumor growth, reduce risk of skin cancer, and have beneficial effects on blood cholesterol. Quercetin may benefit the heart. Anthocyanidins and ellagic acid are antioxidants. Grapes, grape juice, and wine have different compounds and thus may have different effects.
Soy (Also a Legume) tofu, soy milk, soybeans, soy protein, etc.	Isoflavonoids such as daidzein and genistein; lignans; saponins; phytosterols	Isoflavonoids and lignans are converted to a kind of estrogen in the body, and are thought to have some protective effect against cancer. Saponins and phytosterols also have anti-cancer activity. Different forms of soy have varying amounts of beneficial phytochemicals.
Tea green, black, oolong, but not herb tea	Flavonols such as catechins and epigallocatechin gallate (EGCG), plus other flavonoids	Tea, particularly green tea, may reduce the risk of many cancers, according to new research. Flavonols and other flavonoids in tea may combat cancer on several fronts. EGCG is a more powerful antioxidant than vitamin E; both neutralize cell-damaging free radicals. Catechins may protect arteries from plaque build-up. Some evidence suggests that flavonoids in tea may lower blood cholesterol.
Tomatoes	Carotenoids, chiefly lycopene (also found, in much smaller amounts, in red peppers, pink grapefruit, guava, watermelon)	High intake, especially of cooked or processed tomatoes, may reduce risk of prostate and other cancers. Lycopene may fight cancer in several ways, including lowering potency of testosterone. Tomatoes also contain vitamin C and other nutrients,
Whole Grains whole wheat, oats, barley, rye, brown rice, etc.	Saponins, terpenoids, phytic acid, ellagic acid, phytoestrogens	Saponins may neutralize cancer-causing substances in the intestine. Terpenoids and phytic acid may help reduce heart disease and cancer risk. Also rich in fiber, which helps lower blood cholesterol and may reduce colon cancer risk. Beneficial elements are concentrated in bran and germ; refined grains have little fiber and greatly reduced amounts of beneficial plant chemicals, even when enriched.

Source: Beyond vitamins: The new nutrition revolution. The wellness guide—a special insert. UC Berkeley Wellness Letter. *April 1999.*

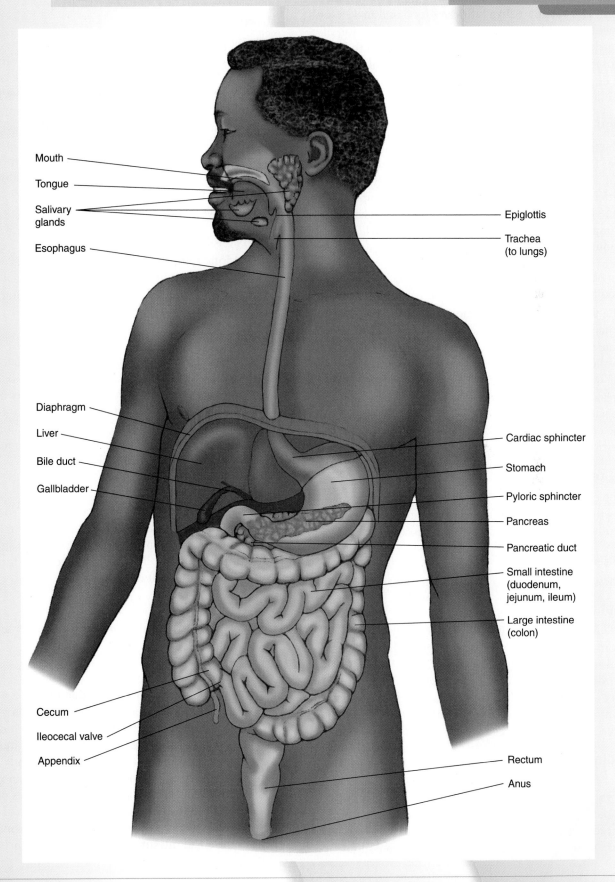

Mouth

Tongue

Salivary glands

Esophagus

Epiglottis

Trachea (to lungs)

Diaphragm

Liver

Bile duct

Gallbladder

Cardiac sphincter

Stomach

Pyloric sphincter

Pancreas

Pancreatic duct

Small intestine (duodenum, jejunum, ileum)

Large intestine (colon)

Cecum

Ileocecal valve

Appendix

Rectum

Anus

Mouth

- In the mouth, food is broken up by chewing with the teeth and tongue. Saliva lubricates food and makes swallowing easier. Salivary amylase begins the digestion of starch. The mouth warms or cools the food so that it is closer to body temperature. When the food bolus (a fairly liquid ball of food) is ready, swallowing is consciously initiated.

Tongue

- The tongue is a mobile mass of muscle that helps teeth tear food into pieces by forcing it against the bony palate. The tongue contains receptors for sweet, salty, sour and bitter tastes. Umami, a fifth taste elicited by monosodium glutamate, is a meaty, savory sensation. Flavor is a complex combination of taste, smells (the nose has about 6 million olfactory receptor cells), physical sensations (e.g., spicy foods) and food texture.

Salivary glands

- The three pairs of salivary glands produce saliva. The water in saliva helps dissolve food particles, facilitating taste sensations. The mucus in saliva lubricates food for swallowing and transport. Digestive enzymes begin breaking down foodstuffs. Salivary amylase begins the chemical breakdown of starches into simple sugars. Lingual lipase initiates the breakdown of fat. The mineral sodium and the enzyme lysozyme in the saliva act as disinfectants, destroying bacteria and microorganisms in food.

Epiglottis

- The epiglottis is a flap that acts as a valve during swallowing. It closes the entrance to the larynx and prevents food from entering the respiratory passages.

Trachea

- These tubes allow air to pass to and from the lungs.

Esophagus

- The esophagus is the tube that connects the mouth to the stomach. Wavelike muscle action (peristalsis) moves food through the esophagus to the stomach. The upper one-third of the muscles of the esophagus are under voluntary control, the middle third are a mixture of voluntarily controlled muscle and automatically controlled smooth muscle, while the lower third is smooth muscle alone.

Cardiac sphincter

- The cardiac sphincter is a muscular valve at the lower end of the esophagus. This control valve relaxes to allow food to pass into the stomach. When contracted, it prevents backflow (reflux) of stomach contents into the esophagus. Named for its proximity to the heart, a malfunction can cause painful esophageal reflux (heartburn) which can be so severe that it is mistaken for a heart attack.

Stomach

- The upper bag-like portion of the stomach acts as a hopper to receive and hold the food prior to delivery to the lower two-thirds. Three layers of smooth muscle surrounds this lower portion of the stomach. Muscular contractions churn the food, so the solids can ferment and mix with acids, fluid and protein-splitting enzymes. The result is a sticky semi-liquid, called chyme, that is gradually released into the duodenum (the first part of the small intestine). Stomach acid halts the digestion of starch, but the stomach also produces gastric lipase, an enzyme that begins the digestion of fat.

Pyloric sphincter

- The pyloric sphincter is a muscular valve that controls passage of chyme from the stomach to the small intestine. When contracted, it prevents backflow from the small intestine into the stomach.

Liver

- The liver is the body's chemical factory and detoxification center. It has many functions in controlling metabolism and deactivating hormones, drugs and toxins. It also produces bile—a mixture of bile salts, phospholipids, cholesterol, pigments, proteins and inorganic ions such as sodium. The detergent-like action of bile emulsifies fat, facilitating fat digestion.

Gallbladder

- The gallbladder stores and concentrates bile. The arrival of fatty food in the duodenum stimulates the release of the duodenal hormone CCK which signals the gallbladder to contract. The bile is then released into the duodenum, where it aids fat digestion.

Bile duct

- The bile duct carries bile from the gallbladder to the duodenum.

Pancreas

- The pancreas is a complex gland that produces a pancreatic juice rich in bicarbonate and enzymes. The pancreatic juice is released into the duodenum where it does its work. Pancreatic amylase breaks down starch into maltose. Lipase splits fats into monoglycerides, fatty acids and glycerol. The pancreatic proenzyme trypsinogen is converted to the enzyme trypsin. Trypsin splits polypeptides and proteins into amino-acids. Bicarbonate produced by the pancreas neutralizes the acid chyme that enters the small intestine. In addition, the pancreas produces insulin and glucagon—hormones that have important roles in regulating carbohydrate metabolism and blood sugar.

Pancreatic duct

• The pancreatic duct carries pancreatic juice from the pancreas to the duodenum.

Small intestine

• The small intestine is a tube approximately 10 feet long that is divided into three parts: the duodenum (the first 10 to 12 inches), the jejunum (about 4 feet), and the ileum (about 5 feet). Whereas the duodenum is mainly responsible for breaking down food, the jejunum and ileum primarily deal with the absorption of food. The duodenum secretes mucus, enzymes and hormones to aid digestion. Most digestion and absorption occurs in the small intestine. Intestinal cells secrete disaccharidases and peptidases to help complete carbohydrate and protein digestion. The intestinal lining is highly folded to increase its surface area and is richly supplied with vessels, which carry away absorbed nutrients in the blood and lymph. Undigested material is passed on to the large intestine.

Ileocecal valve (sphincter)

• The ileocecal valve is the sphincter at the lower end of the small intestine. When open, it permits food residue to move from the small intestine to the large intestine. When closed, it prevents backflow from the large intestine.

Large intestine

• The large intestine is made up of the appendix, cecum, colon, rectum and anus. The colon is about 2.5 inches in diameter and about 4 feet long. In the large intestine, bacteria break down dietary fiber and other undigested carbohydrates, releasing acids and gas. The large intestine absorbs water and minerals while dehydrating and processing the remaining undigested material into solid feces. The colon walls secrete a viscous mucus to help lubricate and mold the feces. This mucus also helps protect the colon wall from mechanical damage.

Appendix

• The appendix is a finger-like appendage attached to the cecum, the first part of the colon. The appendix has no known function.

Cecum

• The pouch-like beginning of the large intestine. The small intestine's ileum empties into the cecum.

Rectum

• The rectum stores waste prior to elimination.

Anus

• The anal sphincter holds the rectum closed. Either voluntary or involuntary control may open it to allow elimination.

APPENDIX F Biochemical Structures

> Nomenclature
> ATP/ADP/AMP
> Carbohydrates
> Amino Acids
> Fatty Acids
> Fat-Soluble Vitamins
> Water-Soluble Vitamins
> B Vitamins in Metabolic Pathways

Nomenclature

Prefixes

mono-	Means one subunit. For instance *mono*saccharide means a one-unit saccharide.
bi-, di-, and tri-	Mean two and three subunits bonded together to form a larger molecule.
poly-	Means many or a lot. A *poly*saccharide has many linked monosaccharide subunits.
oligo-	Means a structure with typically 3 to 10 subunits, but smaller than a polymer.

Suffixes

-ose	Sugars are named with *-ose* as a suffix They are subclassified with regard to the number of carbons i.e., 3 = triose, 4 = tetrose, 5 = pentose, 6 = hexose, 7 = heptose. The suffix *-ose*, refers to monosaccharides and disaccharides: sugars like gluc*ose*, fruct*ose*, sucr*ose* etc.
-ase	Many enzymes are named by attaching the suffix *-ase* to the substrate of the enzyme (the compound altered by enzymatic action). For instance a lipase cleaves a lipid substrate, a, disaccharidase cleaves a disaccharide, and a peptidase breaks the peptide bond between two amino acids.
-ol	Suffix for naming alcohols and phenols (e.g., ethan*ol*, glycer*ol*)
-ic, -ate, -oic, -oate	Suffixes for naming acids and acid salts.

Although the terms *lactic acid* and *lactate* often are used interchangeably, they are not identical chemical compounds. Lactic acid ($C_3H_6O_3$), as its name implies, is an acid. Lactate is any salt of lactic acid, for instance sodium lactate. When anaerobic glycolysis forms lactic acid, the acid quickly dissociates, releasing hydrogen (H^+) into solution. The lactate ion then immediately associates with sodium (Na^+) or potassium (K^+) to form a salt–sodium or potassium lactate. In substances such as pyruvate and lactate, the carboxyl group is COO^- (one oxygen has an available bond). In acids such as pyruvic acid and lactic acid, the carboxyl group is COOH (the available bond is filled with hydrogen). The suffixes -ic and -ate are used for the acid and salt forms of most carboxyl groups. For reasons of pronunciation, some carboxyl groups require the *-oic* or *-oate* suffixes, for instance butan*oic* acid, and its salt form butan*oate*.

-peptide	The suffix *peptide* refers to a molecule composed of 2 or more amino acids joined by peptide bonds. A di*peptide* is composed of 2 amino acids, a tri*peptide* of three, etc. A short string of amino acids is called a poly*peptide* and a long string is a protein.
-saccharide	The suffix *saccharide* refers to sugar. A poly*saccharide* for example is a large molecule composed of many sugar subunits. A polysaccharide may be composed of only one type of sugar (starch is made up of many glucose units) or of many different sugars. A lipopoly*saccharide*, for instance is made up of a variety of sugars bonded to a lipid.
hydrogen ion	Also known as a proton, this lone hydrogen has a positive charge (H^+). It has lost its electron and associates readily with negatively charged ions, like the hydroxyl ion (OH^-).
atomic hydrogen	A hydrogen atom with a single electron. This proton-electron combination is unstable and is a short-lived intermediate in some enzymatically catalyzed reactions. During oxidation-reduction reactions it is atomic hydrogen (hydrogen + electron), not hydrogen ions, (H^+) that is transferred.

Acids are substances that form hydrogen ions in solution. An acid dissociates to form a cation (H^+) and an anion (e.g., SO_4^-)

When the anion ends with the suffix *-ate* its acid name is simply the anion with suffix *-ic*, followed by the word *acid*. Here are some examples :

- H_2SO_4 - hydrogen sulf*ate* becomes sulfur*ic acid*
- H_3PO_4 - hydrogen phosph*ate* becomes phosphor*ic acid*
- HClO3 - hydrogen chlor*ate* becomes chlor*ic acid*

Functional Group	Structural Formula	Models
Hydroxyl	–OH	
Carbonyl	–C– ‖ O	
Carboxyl	–C⟨O, OH	
Amino	–N⟨H, H	
Sulfhydryl	–SH	
Phosphate	–O–P–OH (H above, O below double bond)	

Functional groups
These six functional groups are commonly involved in covalent and non-covalent binding to form molecules such as proteins and DNA.

ATP and Derivatives
ATP, ADP, and AMP

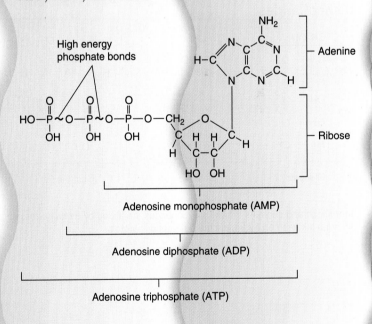

Carbohydrates

Monosaccharides

Glucose **Galactose** **Fructose**

The structures of glucose and galactose differ only by the location of the OH on carbon number 4.

Disaccharides

Glucose   Glucose
Maltose

Glucose   Galactose
Lactose

Glucose   Fructose
Sucrose

In maltose and sucrose, the monosaccharides are linked by alpha bonds. In lactose, a beta bond links galactose and glucose. The human digestive enzyme lactase can hydrolyse the beta bond in lactose.

Polysaccharides

Amylose
Starch molecule made of unbranched glucose chains.

Amylopectin
Starch molecule made of branched glucose chains. In amylopectin, the chain branches every thirty glucose units.
Glycogen is similar, but more highly branched (every ten glucose units).

Cellulose
Cellulose is a nearly straight chain of glucose units where the glucose molecules are linked by beta bonds.
Humans do not have the enzymes necessary to break the beta linkages in cellulose.

Amino Acids

Essential amino acids

Amino acids consist of a central carbon atom bonded to a carboxyl group, an amino group, a hydrogen and a side group. The shaded areas show the structure common to all amino acids.

Valine (Val)

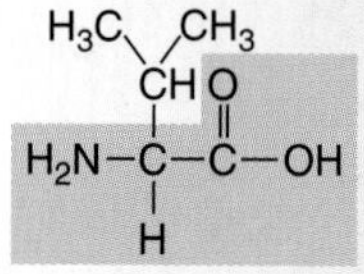

Leucine (Leu)

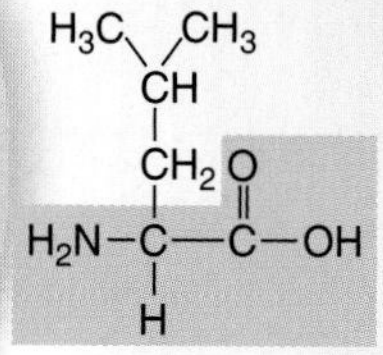

Isoleucine (Ile)

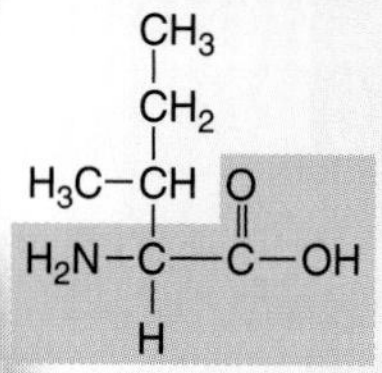

Threonine (Thr)

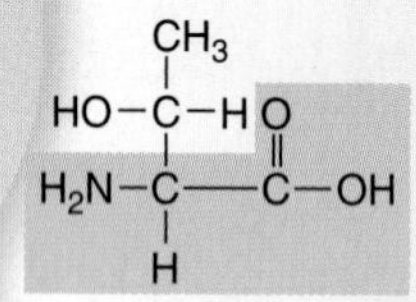

Lysine (Lys)

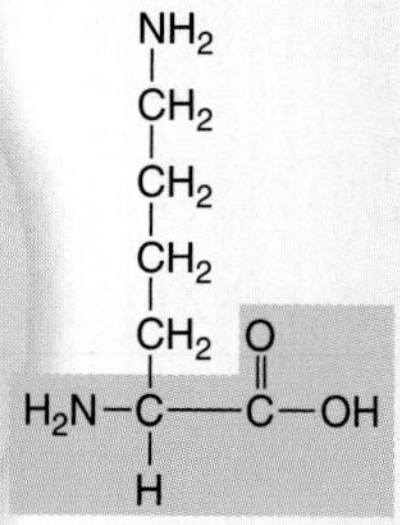

Histidine (His)

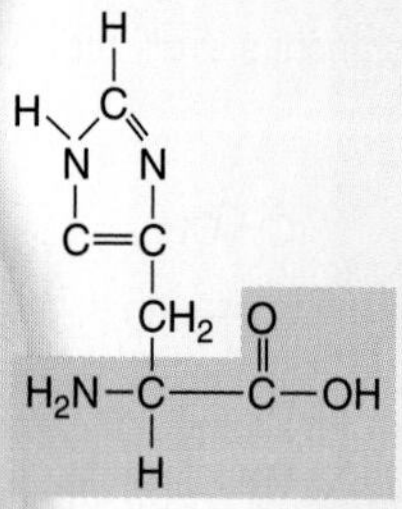

Phenylalanine (Phe)

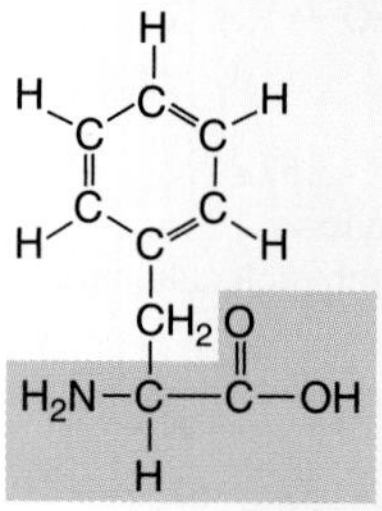

Tryptophan (Trp)

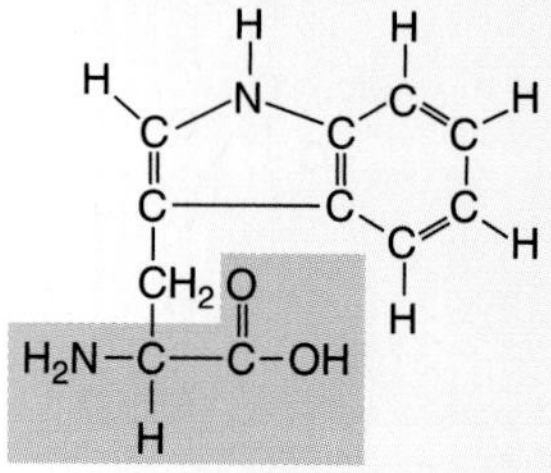

Methionine (Met)

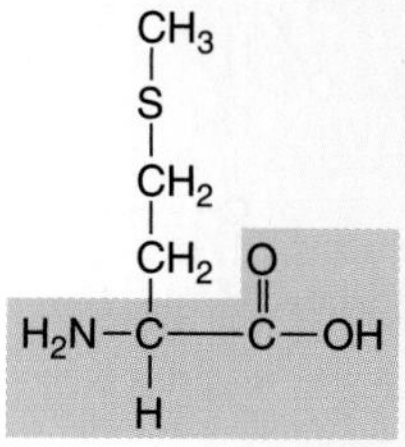

Nonessential amino acids

Glycine (Gly)

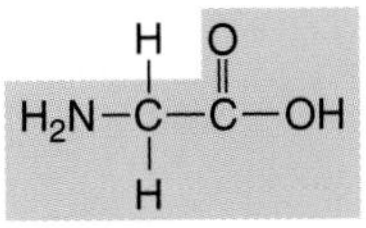

Alanine (Ala)

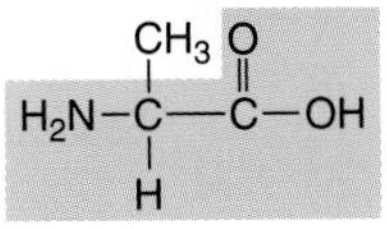

Serine (Ser)

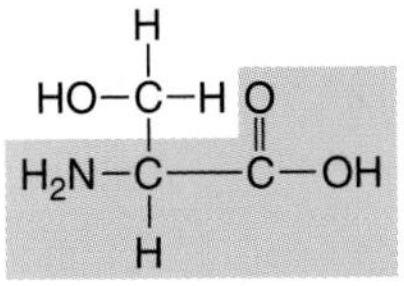

Aspartic acid (Asp)

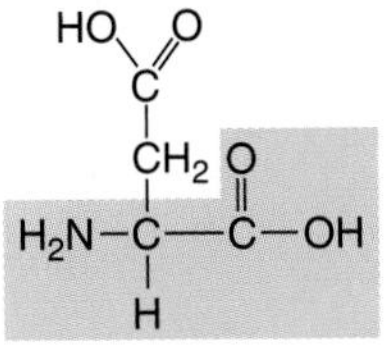

Glutamic acid (Glu)

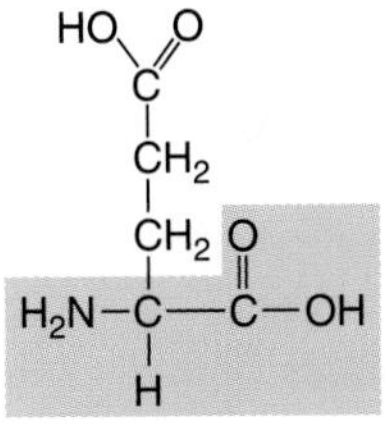

Asparagine (Asn)

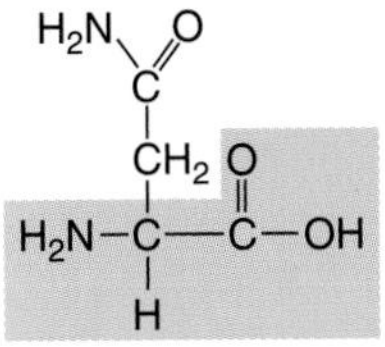

Glutamine (Gln)

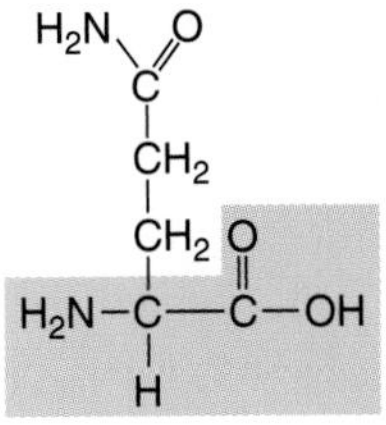

Arginine (Arg)

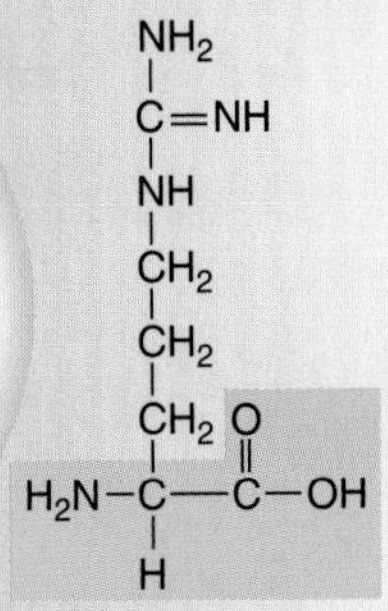

Tyrosine (Tyr)

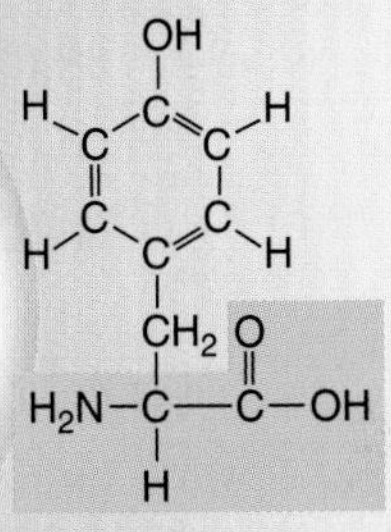

Cysteine (Cys)

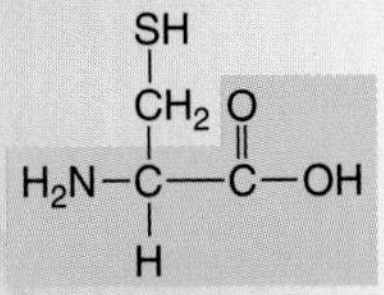

Proline (Pro)

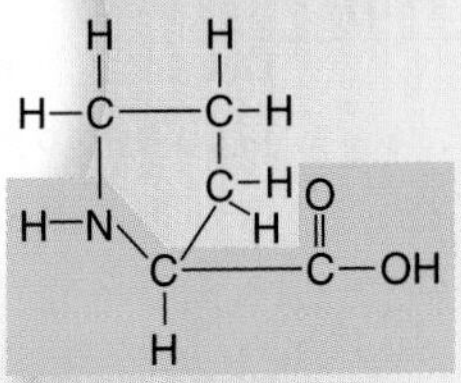

Proline is an imino acid. Its amino group has only one hydrogen and forms a ring.

Fatty Acids

Table F.1 Saturated Fatty Acids Found in Food

Saturated Fatty Acid	Chemical Formula	Number of Carbons	Major Food Sources
Butyric	$CH_3(CH_2)_2COOH$	4	Small amounts in butterfat
Caproic	$CH_3(CH_2)_4COOH$	6	Small amounts in butterfat
Caprylic	$CH_3(CH_2)_6COOH$	8	Small amounts in many fats, including butterfat. Especially found in oils of plant origin.
Capric	$CH_3(CH_2)_8COOH$	10	Small amounts in many fats, including butterfat. Especially found in oils of plant origin.
Lauric	$CH_3(CH_2)_{10}COOH$	12	Cinnamon, palm kernel, coconut oil, butter
Myristic	$CH_3(CH_2)_{12}COOH$	14	Nutmeg, palm kernel, coconut oil, butter
Palmitic	$CH_3(CH_2)_{14}COOH$	16	Common in all animal and plant fats
Stearic	$CH_3(CH_2)_{16}COOH$	18	Common in all animal and plant fats
Arachidic	$CH_3(CH_2)_{18}COOH$	20	Peanut oil
Behenic	$CH_3(CH_2)_{20}COOH$	22	Seeds
Lignoceric	$CH_3(CH_2)_{22}COOH$	24	Peanut oil

Table F.2 Unsaturated Fatty Acids Found in Food

Unsaturated Fatty Acid	Chemical Formula	Number of Carbons	Number of Double Bonds	Omega Notation*	Major Food Sources
Palmitoleic	$CH_3(CH_2)_5CH = CH(CH_2)_7COOH$	16	1	16:1ω7	Nearly all fats
Oleic	$CH_3(CH_2)_7CH = CH(CH_2)_7COOH$	18	1	18:1ω9	Perhaps the most common fatty acid in food
Linoleic	$CH_3(CH_2)_4(CH = CHCH_2)_2(CH_2)_6COOH$	18	2	18:2ω6	Corn, peanut, cottonseed, soybean, and several oils from other plants
Linolenic	$CH_3CH_2(CH = CHCH_2)_3(CH_2)_6COOH$	18	3	18:3ω3	Often in foods with linoleic acid, but particularly found in linseed oil
Arachidonic	$CH_3(CH_2)_4(CH = CHCH_2)_4(CH_2)_2COOH$	20	4	20:4ω6	Animal fats and peanut oil
Eicosapentanoic	$CH_3(CH_2)_3(CH = CHCH_2)_4(CH_2)_3COOH$	20	5	20:5ω3	Fish oils such as cod liver, mackerel and salmon
Docosahexanoic	$CH_3(CH_2)_2(CH = CHCH_2)_6COOH$	22	6	22:6ω3	Fish oils such as cod liver, mackerel and salmon

*Omega Notation = number of carbons: number of double bonds, the number following the omega symbol (ω) represents the location of the first double bond counting from the methyl (CH_3) end

Fat-Soluble Vitamins

Vitamin A and Beta-carotene

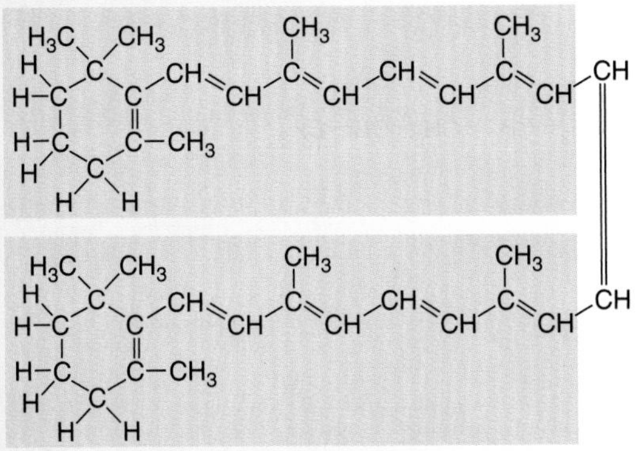

Vitamin A precursor: beta-carotene

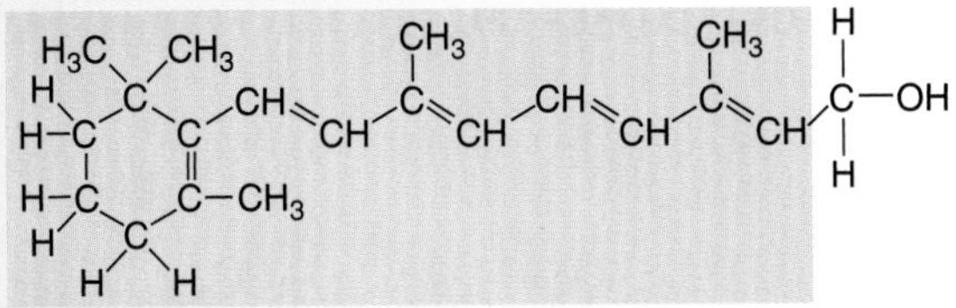

Vitamin A: retinol

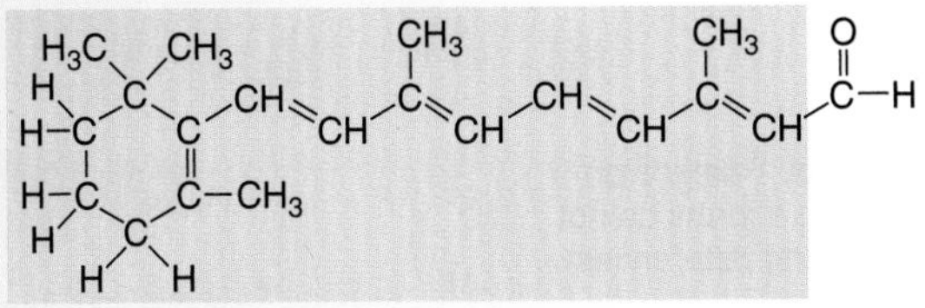

Vitamin A: retinal

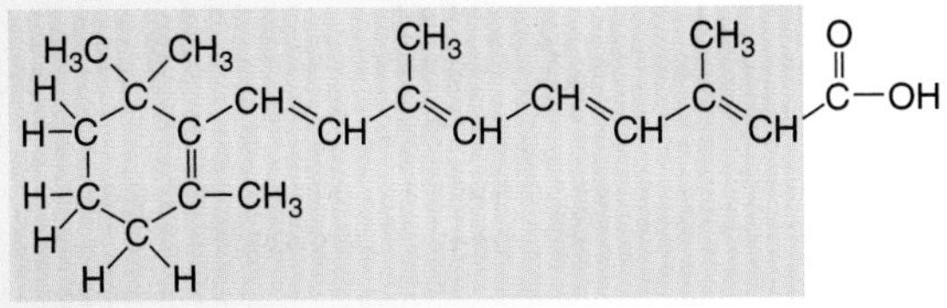

Vitamin A: retinoic acid

The shaded area highlights the structure common to all four molecules.

Vitamin D

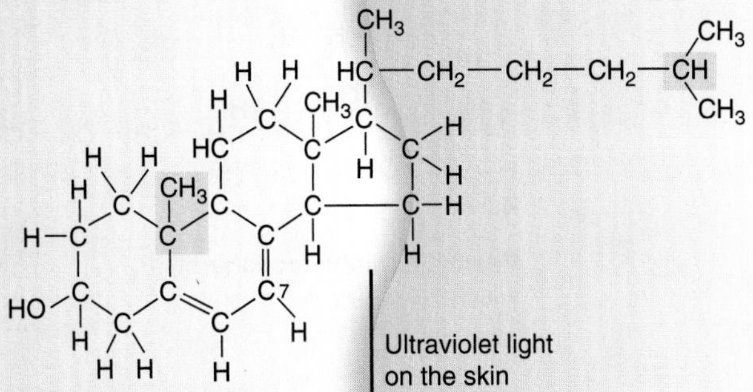

7–Dehydrocholesterol

Ultraviolet light on the skin

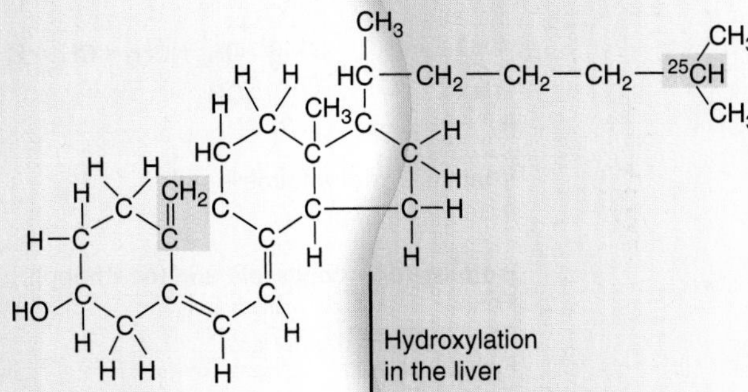

Cholecalciferol
(vitamin D₃)

Hydroxylation in the liver

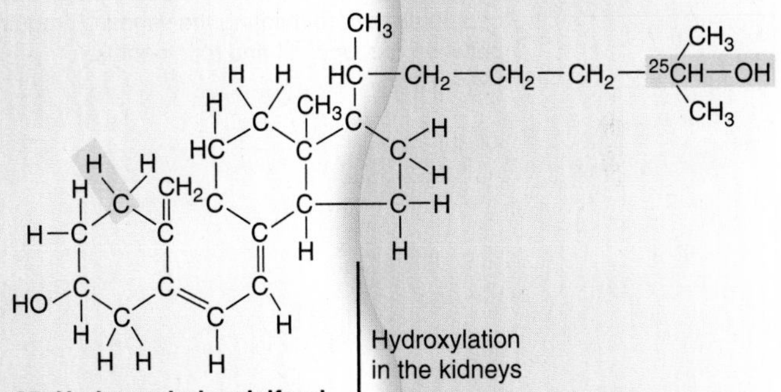

25–Hydroxycholecalciferol
(25–hydroxyvitamin D₃)

Hydroxylation in the kidneys

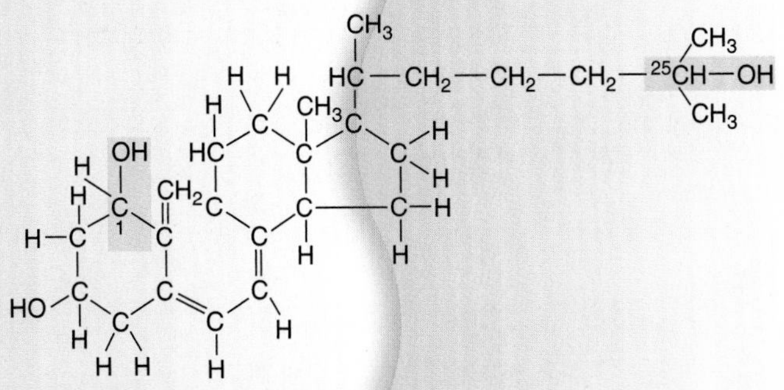

1, 25–Dihydroxycholecalciferol
(1, 25–dihydroxyvitamin D₃)
(calcitriol)

The shaded areas highlight the portion of the molecule that changes from stage to stage.

Vitamin E

Vitamin E (alpha-tocopherol)
4 isomers α, β, γ, δ

Vitamin E (alpha-tocotrienol)
4 isomers α, β, γ, δ

Isomers for tocopherols and tocotrienols
For α, $R_1 = CH_3$ $R_2 = CH_3$
For β, $R_1 = CH_3$ $R_2 = H$
For γ, $R_1 = H$ $R_2 = CH_3$
For δ, $R_1 = H$ $R_2 = H$

Vitamin E occurs in 8 forms but vitamin E activity is based on alpha-tocopherol. Humans do not convert β-, γ-, δ-tocopherols or the tocotrienols to alpha-tocopherol, so these forms do not contribute toward meeting the vitamin E requirement. The shading highlights the differences between tocopherols and tocotrienols.

Vitamin K

Menadione (vitamin K_3)
Synthetic form of Vitamin K

Phylloquinone (vitamin K_1)
Vitamin K naturally occurring in food

Menaquinone-n (vitamin K_2; n = 6, 7, or 9)
Vitamin K formed by bacteria in the large intestine

The shaded areas highlight the structure common to all three forms.

Water-Soluble Vitamins and Coenzymes

Thiamin and Coenzyme

Thiamin

Thiamin pyrophosphate (TPP)
Thiamin is part of the active coenzyme TPP. The shaded areas highlight the structure common to both molecules.

Water-Soluble Vitamins and Coenzymes (cont.)

Riboflavin and Coenzymes

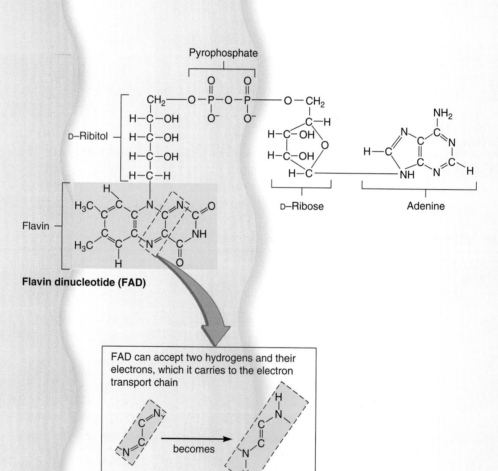

Riboflavin

Flavin mononucleotide (FMN)

Flavin dinucleotide (FAD)

FAD can accept two hydrogens and their electrons, which it carries to the electron transport chain

FAD (oxidized form) → becomes → FADH₂ (reduced form)

FAD and FADH₂

The flavin portion of these molecules is highlighted.

Niacin and Coenzymes

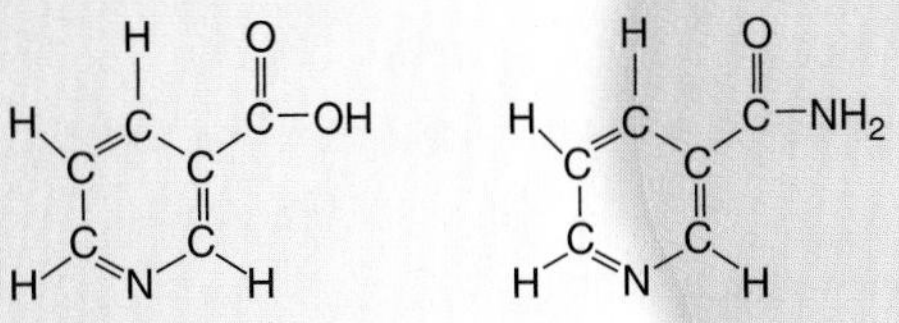

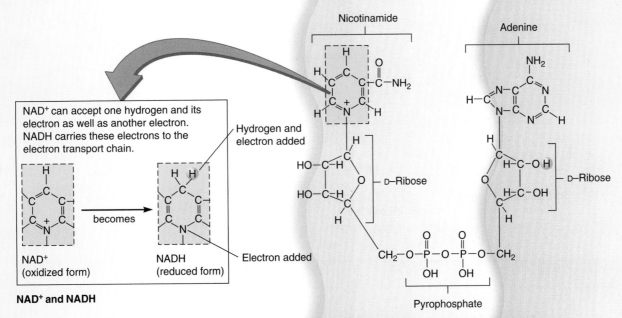

Nicotinic acid

Nicotinamide

Niacin (nicotinic acid and nicotinamide)

Nicotinamide

Adenine

NAD⁺ can accept one hydrogen and its electron as well as another electron. NADH carries these electrons to the electron transport chain.

Hydrogen and electron added

HO—C—H

HO—C—H

D–Ribose

H—C—O—H

H—C—OH

D–Ribose

becomes

NAD⁺
(oxidized form)

NADH
(reduced form)

Electron added

NAD⁺ and NADH

CH₂—O—P—O—P—O—CH₂

OH   OH

Pyrophosphate

Nicotinamide adenine dinucleotide (NAD⁺) and nicotinamide adenine dinucleotide phosphate (NADP⁺)
NADP⁺ is similar to NAD⁺ but the H attached to the O is replaced by a phosphate group.

Pantothenic Acid and Coenzyme A

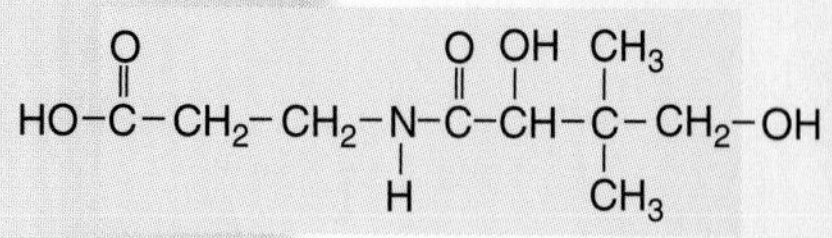

Pantothenic acid

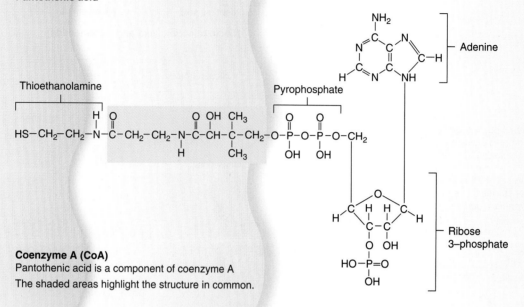

Coenzyme A (CoA)
Pantothenic acid is a component of coenzyme A
The shaded areas highlight the structure in common.

Biotin

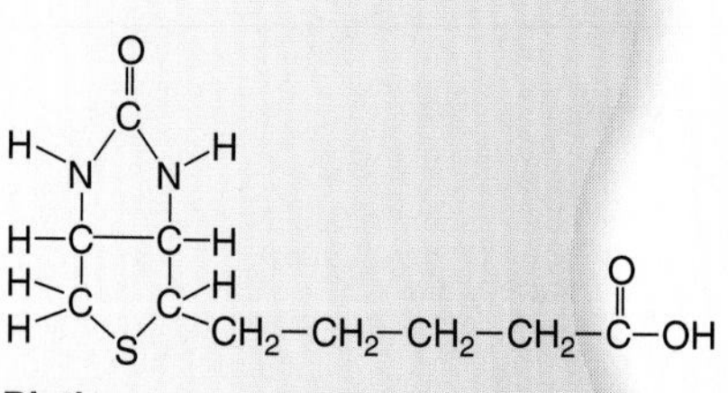

Biotin

Vitamin B$_6$ and Coenzymes

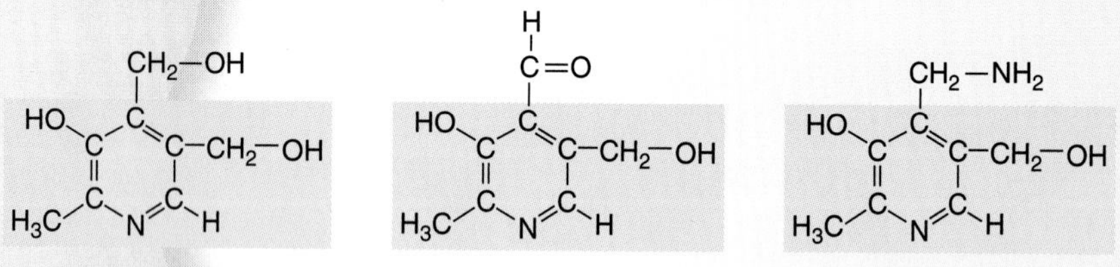

Pyridoxine

Pyridoxal

Pyridoxamine

Vitamin B$_6$ (pyridoxine, pyridoxal, and pyridoxamine)

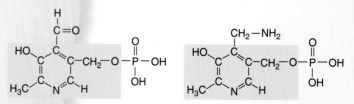

Pyridoxal phosphate (PLP)

Pyridoxamine phosphate (PMP)

Pyridoxal phosphate (PLP) and pyridoxamine phosphate (PMP) are the two
active coenzyme forms of vitamin B$_6$
The shaded areas highlight the structures in common.

Folate and Coenzyme

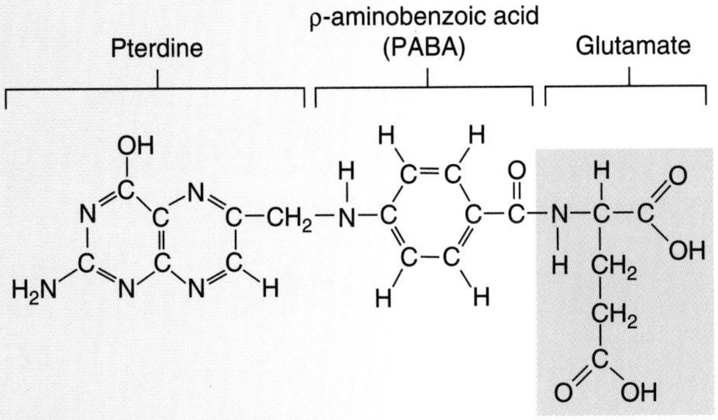

Folate

Folate contains at least one and up to 11 glutamates (see shaded area that contains a single glutamate). Folic acid contains only one glutamate.

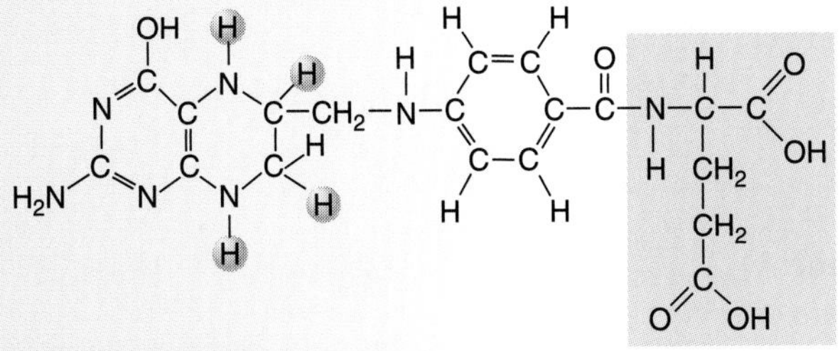

Tetrahydrofolic acid (THFA)

Adding 4 hydrogens to folate produces THFA, the active coenzyme form.

Vitamin B₁₂

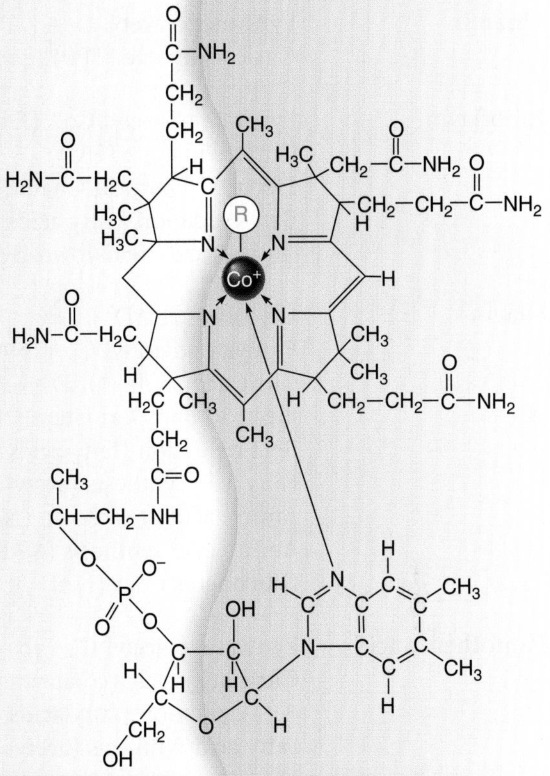

Vitamin B$_{12}$ (cobalamin)

R = CN in cyanocobalamin

R = OH in hydroxocobalamin

R = 5'–deoxyadenosyl in 5'–deoxyadenosylcobalamin

R = CH$_3$ in methylcobalamin

Arrows indicate that the free electron pairs of nitrogen are in close proximity to the positively charged cobalt.

Vitamin C

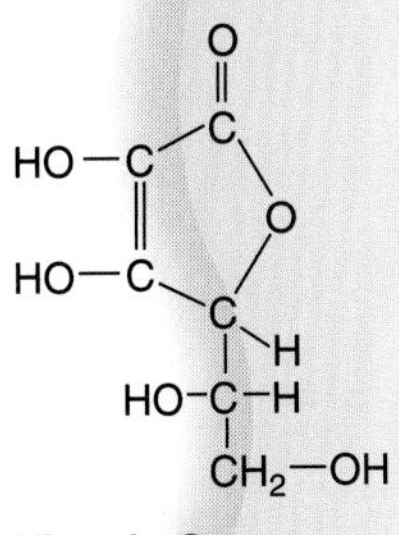

**Vitamin C
(Ascorbic acid)**

B vitamins in Major Metabolic Pathways

Thiamin	Pyruvate to acetyl CoA (TPP)
	Citric acid cycle (TPP)
Riboflavin	Pyruvate to acetyl CoA (FAD)
	Citric acid cycle (FAD)
	Electron Transport Chain (FAD, FMN)
	Beta-oxidation (fatty acids to acetyl CoA) (FAD)
	Amino acid breakdown (FAD)
Niacin	Glycolysis (NAD^+)
	Pyruvate to acetyl CoA (NAD^+)
	Citric acid cycle (NAD^+)
	Electron transport chain (NAD^+)
	Beta-oxidation (fatty acids to acetyl CoA) (NAD^+)
	Fatty acid synthesis (acetyl CoA to fatty acids) (NADPH)
	Amino acid breakdown (NAD^+)
	Amino acid synthesis (NAD^+, NADPH)
	Gluconeogenesis (NAD^+)
Pantothenic acid	Pyruvate to acetyl CoA (coenzyme A)
	Citric acid cycle (coenzyme A)
	Beta-oxidation (fatty acids to acetyl CoA) (coenzyme A)
	Fatty acid synthesis (acetyl CoA to fatty acids) (coenzyme A)
Biotin	Fatty acid synthesis (acetyl CoA to fatty acids) (biotin-enzyme)
	Gluconeogenesis (biotin-enzyme)
Vitamin B_6	Glycogen to Glucose (PLP)
	Amino acid breakdown (PLP)
	Amino acid synthesis (PLP)
Folate	Amino acid synthesis (THFA)
	Synthesis of some components of DNA and RNA (THFA)
Vitamin B_{12}	Amino acid breakdown (B_{12})
	Synthesis of some components of DNA and RNA (B_{12})

Major Metabolic Pathways APPENDIX G

- ➤ Glycolysis
- ➤ Citric Acid Cycle
- ➤ Electron Transport Chain
- ➤ Urea Cycle

Glycolysis

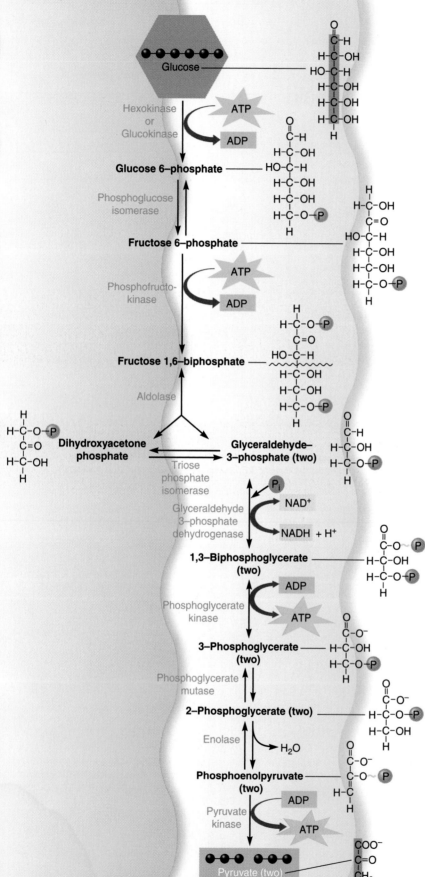

Glycolysis is the first step in metabolizing glucose and other monosaccharides for energy. Unlike the reaction that converts blood glucose to glucose 6-phosphate, the reaction that converts glucose from glycogen to glucose 6-phosphate does not require ATP. Thus the glycolysis of glucose from glycogen directly yields 3 ATP as compared to the 2 ATP from blood glucose. Additional ATP is produced from glycolytic NADH in the electron transport chain.

The reactions that convert fructose to fructose 6-phosphate require ATP so fructose produces the same amount of ATP as blood glucose. The same is true for galactose, which enters at glucose 6-phosphate.

Citric Acid Cycle

Electron Transport Chain

(site of oxidative phosphorylation)

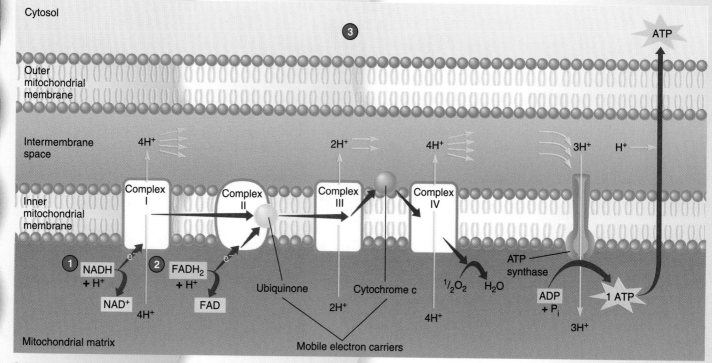

Complex I   NADH–Q reductase
Complex II   Succinate–Q reductase
Complex III Cytochrome reductase
Complex IV   Cytochrome oxidase

Complexes I, III, and IV are proton (H^+) pumps. Complex II does not pump protons.
The three proton pumps are linked by the mobile electron carriers ubiquinone and cytochrome c.

NADH

1 A pair of electrons from NADH enters the chain at complex I (NADH-Q reductase). The flow of electrons from NADH to ubiquinone leads to the pumping of 4 H^+ from the matrix to the intermembrane space. The flow of electrons from ubiquinone to cytochrome c through complex III (cytochrome reductase) pumps another 2 H^+ into the intermembrane space. As complex IV (cytochrome oxidase) catalyzes the transfer of electrons from cytochrome c to O_2, it pumps a another 4 H^+. (Complex IV actually uses 4 electrons to produce 2 H_2O from a single O_2.) The transit of the NADH electron pair through the electron transport chain pumps a total of 10 H^+ into the intermembrane space. Each 3 H^+ returning to the matrix through the ATP synthase produces 1 ATP. Another H^+ is consumed in transporting ATP from the matrix to the cytosol. Thus the two electrons from NADH produce about 2.5 ATP (10 pumped ÷ 4 = 2.5).

FADH$_2$

2 A pair of electrons from $FADH_2$ enter the chain at complex II (succinate-Q), which is the non-pumping complex. The flow of electrons from $FADH_2$ to ubiquinone does not pump any protons to the intermembrane space. The flow of electrons through complexes III and IV is the same as for NADH. Thus the transit of the two $FADH_2$ electrons through the electron transport chain pumps a total of 6 H^+ into the intermembrane space and produces about 1.5 ATP (6 ÷ 4 = 1.5).

Cytosolic NADH

3 Glycolysis forms NADH in the cytosol, but the outer mitochondrial membrane is impervious to NADH. How can NADH deliver its electrons to the electron transport chain? NADH transfers its pair of electrons to special carriers that can cross the mitochondrial membrane. One carrier, glycerol 3-phosphate, shuttles the electrons to the matrix and delivers them to FAD, thereby forming $FADH_2$. This $FADH_2$ delivers the electrons to the chain where they form 1.5 ATP.

In the heart and liver, malate shuttles the electrons from cytosolic NADH to the matrix. Malate crosses the mitochondrial membrane and delivers the electrons to NAD^+, thereby forming NADH inside the mitochondrion. This NADH delivers the electron pair to the chain where they form 2.5 ATP.

Depending on the carrier, cytosolic NADH may produce 1.5 or 2.5 ATP.

The Urea Cycle

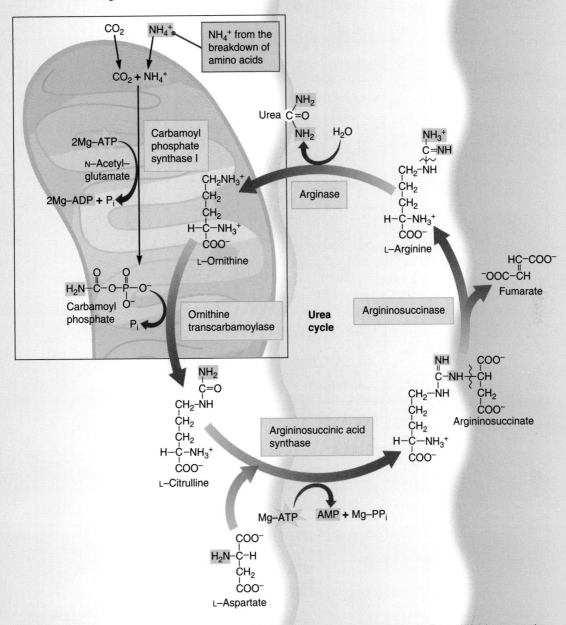

Some NH_4^+ from the breakdown of amino acids is used for biosynthesis of nitrogen compounds. Excess NH_4^+ is converted to urea and excreted.

APPENDIX H Calculations and Conversions

Energy from Food

grams carbohydrate $\times$ 4 kcal/g
grams protein $\times$ 4 kcal/g
grams fat $\times$ 9 kcal/g
grams alcohol $\times$ 7 kcal/g
total = energy from food

Example:

Carbohydrate	300 g $\times$ 4 kcal/g =	1,200 kcal
Protein	50 g $\times$ 4 kcal/g =	200 kcal
Fat	65 g $\times$ 9 kcal/g =	585 kcal
Alcohol	20 g $\times$ 7 kcal/g =	140 kcal
	TOTAL ENERGY	**2,125 kcal**

Calculating the percentage of calories for each:

Carbohydrate (1,200 kcal $\div$ 2,125 kcal) $\times$ 100 = 56.47%
Protein (200 kcal $\div$ 2,125 kcal) $\times$ 100 = 9.41%
Fat (585 kcal $\div$ 2,125 kcal) $\times$ 100 = 27.53%
Alcohol (140 kcal $\div$ 2,125 kcal) $\times$ 100 = 6.59%

Recommended Protein Intake for Adults

grams of recommended protein = weight in kilograms $\times$ 0.8 g/kg

Example:
A 70kg (154lb) person
grams of recommended protein = 70 kg $\times$ 0.8 g/kg = 56 grams protein, or
grams of recommended protein = (154 lb $\div$ 2.2) $\times$ 0.8 g/kg = 56 grams protein

Note: Endurance athletes involved in heavy training require 1.2 to 1.4 grams of protein per kilogram of body weight per day

Niacin Equivalents (NE)

Determining the amount of niacin from tryptophan:

NE = milligrams niacin
NE from tryptophan = grams excess protein $\div$ 6
NE = (grams dietary protein − protein RDA) $\div$ 6

Example: Assume dietary protein = 86 g and protein RDA = 56 g
NE = (86 g − 56 g) $\div$ 6
NE = 5

Dietary Folate Equivalents (DFE)

Dietary folate equivalents account for differences in the absorption of food folate, synthetic folic acid in dietary supplements, and folic acid added to fortified foods. Food in the stomach also affects bioavailability. Folic acid taken as a supplement when fasting is two times more bioavailable than food folate. Folic acid taken with food and folic acid in fortified foods is 1.7 times more bioavailable than food folate.

1 g DFE = 1 microgram of food folate
= 0.5 μg of folic acid supplement taken on an empty stomach
= 0.6 μg of folic acid supplement consumed with meals
= 0.6 μg of folic acid in fortified foods

1 μg folic acid as a fortificant = 1.7 μg DFE
1 μg folic acid as a supplement, fasting = 2.0 DFE

Example:

Food folate in cooked spinach	100 μg = 100 μg DFE
Ready to eat cereal fortified with folic acid	100 μg = 170 μg DFE
Supplemental folic acid taken without food	100 μg = 200 μg DFE

Estimating DFE from Daily Value
DFE = %DV $\times$ DV $\times$ bioavailability factor

Example:
Assume that a serving fortified breakfast cereal contains 10% of the Daily Value for folate
Daily Value = 400 μg folic acid

DFE = %DV $\times$ DV $\times$ bioavailability factor
DFE = 0.10 $\times$ 400 $\times$ 1.7
DFE = 68 μg which can be rounded to 70 μg

Retinol Activity Equivalents (RAE)

Retinol activity equivalents are a standardized measure of vitamin A activity that account for differences in the bioavailability of different sources of vitamin A. Of the provitamin A carotenoids, beta-carotene produces the most vitamin A.

1 RAE = 1 μg retinol
= 2 μg supplemental beta-carotene
= 12 μg dietary beta-carotene
= 24 μg dietary alpha-carotene or beta-crytoxanthin

Although outdated, many vitamin supplements still report vitamin A content as International Units (IU).

1 RAE = 3.33 IU as retinol
1 IU = 0.3 RAE

Vitamin D

Although outdated, many vitamin supplements still report vitamin D content as International Units (IU).

1 IU = 0.025 μg cholecalciferol
1 μg cholecalciferol = IU $\div$ 40

Example:
A vitamin supplement contains 100 IU vitamin D
μg cholecalciferol = 100 $\div$ 40 = 2.5

Tocopherol Equivalents (TE)

Although outdated, many vitamin supplements still report vitamin E content as International Units (IU) rather than tocopherol equivalents (TE). Two conversion factors are used to convert IU to TE. If the form of the supplement is "natural" or RRR-α-tocopherol (historically labeled as d-alpha-tocopherol), the conversion factor is 0.67 mg/IU. If the form of the supplement is *all rac*-α-tocopherol (historically labeled *dl*-α-tocopherol), the conversion factor is 0.45 mg/IU.

1 TE = 1 mg alpha-tocopherol

Examples:
A multivitamin supplement contains 30 IUs of *d*-α-tocopherol
TE = 30 $\times$ 0.67
TE = 20

A multivitamin supplement contains 30 IUs of *dl-α-*tocopherol
TE = 30 × 0.45
TE = 13.5

Estimating Energy Expenditure

Resting Energy Expenditure (REE)

<u>Harris-Benedict equations</u>
Adult men   REE = 66 + 13.7W + 5.0H − 6.8A
Adult women   REE = 655 + 9.6W + 1.8H − 4.7A
(W = weight in kilograms, H = height in centimeters, A = age)
Note: Harris-Benedict equations can overestimate resting energy expenditure, especially for obese people.

<u>Quick Estimate</u>
Adult men   REE = weight (kg) × 1.0 kcal/kg × 24 hours
               REE = weight (kg) × 1.0 x 24
For adult women: REE = weight (kg) × 0.9 kcal/kg × 24 hours
               REE = weight (kg) × 0.9 × 24

<u>Equation Table for Estimating REE (Most accurate method)</u>

Age (years)	REE Males	REE Females
0-3	(60.9*wt) − 54	(61.0*wt) − 51
3-10	(22.7*wt) + 495	(22.5*wt) + 499
10-18	(17.5*wt) + 651	(12.2*wt) + 746
18-30	(15.3*wt) + 679	(14.7*wt) + 496
30-60	(11.6*wt) + 879	(8.7*wt) + 829
>60	(13.5*wt) + 487	(10.5*wt) + 596

body weight is in kg and REE is kcal/day

Physical Activity

Physical activity energy expenditure = REE × table value

Physical Activity Energy Expenditure as percent of REE	Activity Level	Description
20-30%	Sedentary	Mostly resting with little or no activity
30-45%	Light	Occasional unplanned activity, e.g., going for a stroll
45-65%	Moderate	Daily planned activity, such as brisk walks
65-90%	Heavy	Daily workout routine requires several hours of continuous exercise
90-120%	Exceptional	Daily vigorous workouts for extended hours; training for competition

Thermic Effect of Food

thermic effect of food = (REE + physical activity) × 0.1

Total Energy Expenditure (TEE)

TEE = REE + physical activity + thermic effect of food
   See chapter 8 for examples using these calculations.

Body Mass Index (BMI)

U.S. Formula:

BMI = [Weight in pounds ÷ (Height in inches)^2] × 703

Example: A 154 pound man is 5 ft 8 inches tall
BMI = [154 ÷ (68 in × 68 in)] × 703
BMI = (154 ÷ 4,624) × 703
BMI = 23.42

Metric Formula:

BMI = Weight in kilograms ÷ [Height in meters]^2
or
BMI = [Weight in kilograms ÷ (Height in cm)^2] × 10,000

Example: A 70 kg man is 1.75 meters tall
BMI = 70 kg ÷ (1.75)^2
BMI = 70 ÷ 3.0625
BMI = 22.86

Metric Prefixes

giga-	G	1,000,000,000
mega-	M	1,000,000
kilo-	k	1,000
hecto-	h	100
deka-	da	10
deci-	d	0.1
centi-	c	0.01
milli-	m	0.001
micro-	μ	0.000001
nano-	n	0.000000001

Length: Metric and U.S. Equivalents

1 centimeter	0.3937 inch
1 decimeter	3.937 inches
1 foot	0.3048 meter
1 inch	2.54 centimeters
1 meter	39.37 inches
	1.094 yards
1 micron	0.001 millimeter
	0.00003937 inch
1 millimeter	0.03937 inch
1 yard	0.9144 meter

Capacities or Volumes

1 cup, measuring	8 fluid ounces
	1/2 liquid pint
1 gallon (U.S.)	231 cubic inches
	3.785 liters
	0.833 British gallon
	128 U.S. fluid ounces
1 gallon (British Imperial)	277.42 cubic inches
	1.201 U.S. gallons
	4.546 liters
	160 British fluid ounces

1 liter	1.057 liquid quarts
	0.908 dry quart
	61.024 cubic inches
1 milliliter	0.061 cubic inch
1 ounce, fluid or liquid (U.S.)	1.805 cubic inch
	29.574 milliliters
	1.041 British fluid ounces
1 pint, dry	33.600 cubic inches
	0.551 liter
1 pint, liquid	28.875 cubic inches
	0.473 liter
1 quart, dry (U.S.)	67.201 cubic inches
	1.101 liters
	0.969 British quart
1 quart, liquid (U.S.)	57.75 cubic inches
	0.946 liter
	0.833 British quart
1 quart (British)	69.354 cubic inches
	1.032 U.S. dry quarts
	1.201 U.S. liquid quarts
1 tablespoon, measuring	3 teaspoons
	1/2 fluid ounce
1 teaspoon, measuring	1/3 tablespoon
	1/6 fluid ounce
1 kilogram	2.205 pounds

1 microgram (μg- the Greek letter
mu in combination with the letter g) . . . . 0.000001 gram

Food Measurement Equivalents

16 tablespoons = 1 cup
12 tablespoons = 3/4 cup
10 tablespoons + 2 teaspoons = 2/3 cup
8 tablespoons = 1/2 cup
6 tablespoons = 3/8 cup
5 tablespoons + 1 teaspoon = 1/3 cup
4 tablespoons = 1/4 cup
2 tablespoons = 1/8 cup
2 tablespoons + 2 teaspoons = 1/6 cup
1 tablespoon = 1/16 cup
2 cups = 1 pint
2 pints = 1 quart
3 teaspoons = 1 tablespoon
48 teaspoons = 1 cup

Food Measurement Conversions: U.S. to Metric

Capacity

1/5 teaspoon	1 milliliter
1 teaspoon	5 milliliter
1 tablespoon	15 milliliter
1 fluid oz	30 milliliter
1/5 cup	47 milliliter

Weight

1 ounce	28 grams
1 pound	454 grams

1 cup	237 milliliter
2 cups (1 pint)	473 milliliter
4 cups (1 quart)	.95 liter
4 quarts (1 gal.)	3.8 liters

Food Measurement Conversions: Metric to U.S.

Capacity

1 milliliter	1/5 teaspoon
5 ml	1 teaspoon
15 ml	1 tablespoon
100 ml	3.4 fluid oz
240 ml	1 cup
1 liter	34 fluid oz
	4.2 cups
	2.1 pints
	1.06 quarts
	0.26 gallon

Weight

1 gram	0.035 ounce
100 grams	3.5 ounces
500 grams	1.10 pounds
1 kilogram	2.205 pounds
1 kilogram	35 oz

Conversion Factors

To change	To	Multiply by
centimeters	inches	.3937
centimeters	feet	.03281
cubic feet	cubic meters	.0283
cubic meters	cubic feet	35.3145
cubic meters	cubic yards	1.3079
cubic yards	cubic meters	.7646
feet	meters	.3048
gallons (U.S.)	liters	3.7853
grams	ounces avdp	.0353
grams	pounds	.002205
inches	millimeters	25.4000
inches	centimeters	2.5400
inches	meters	.0254
kilograms	pounds avdp or t	2.2046
liters	gallons (U.S.)	.2642
liters	pints (dry)	1.8162
liters	pints (liquid)	2.1134
liters	quarts (dry)	.9081
liters	quarts (liquid)	1.0567
meters	feet	3.2808
meters	yards	1.0936
millimeters	inches	.0394
ounces avdp.	grams	28.3495
ounces	pounds	.0625
ounces (troy)	ounces (avdp)	1.09714
pints (dry)	liters	.5506
pints (liquid)	liters	.4732
pounds ap or t	kilograms	.3782
pounds avdp	kilograms	.4536
pounds	ounces	16
quarts (dry)	liters	1.1012
quarts (liquid)	liters	.9463

Fahrenheit and Celsius (Centigrade) Scales

°Celsius	°Fahrenheit
−273.15	−459.67
−250	−418
−200	−328
−150	−238
−100	−148
−50	−58
−40	−40
−30	−22
−20	−4
−10	14
0	32
5	41
10	50
15	59
20	68
25	77
30	86
35	95
40	104
45	113
50	122
55	131

°Celsius	°Fahrenheit
60	140
65	149
70	158
75	167
80	176
85	185
90	194
95	203
100	212

Zero on the Fahrenheit scale represents the temperature produced by the mixing of equal weights of snow and common salt.

	°Fahrenheit	°Celsius
Boiling point of water	212°	100°
Freezing point of water	32°	0°
Normal body temperature	98.6°	37°
Comfortable room temperature	68-77°	20-25°
Absolute zero	−459.6°	−273.1°

Absolute zero is theoretically the lowest possible temperature, the point at which all molecular motion would cease.

To convert Fahrenheit to Celsius (Centigrade), subtract 32 and multiply by .6.

To convert Celsius (Centigrade) to Fahrenheit, multiply by 1.8 and add 32.

Growth Charts APPENDIX I

A complete set of growth charts is available on the Internet at www.cdc.gov/growthcharts. There are three sets, each with a different set of percentiles. Each set includes the following charts for girls and boys:

Weight-for-age percentiles: birth to 36 months

Length-for-age percentiles: birth to 36 months

Weight-for-length percentiles: birth to 36 months

Head circumference-for-age percentiles: birth to 36 months

Weight-for-age percentiles: 2 to 20 years

Stature-for-age percentiles: 2 to 20 years

Weight for stature percentiles

Body mass index-for-age percentiles: 2 to 20 years

2 to 20 years: Girls
Stature-for-age and Weight-for-age percentiles

NAME _____

RECORD # _____

Mother's Stature _____		Father's Stature _____		
Date	Age	Weight	Stature	BMI*

*To Calculate BMI: Weight (kg) ÷ Stature (cm) ÷ Stature (cm) x 10,000
or Weight (lb) ÷ Stature (in) ÷ Stature (in) x 703

AGE (YEARS)

12 13 14 15 16 17 18 19 20

AGE (YEARS)

STATURE

WEIGHT

97 90 75 50 25 10 3

SOURCE: Developed by the National Center for Health Statistics in collaboration with
the National Center for Chronic Disease Prevention and Health Promotion (2000).
http://www.cdc.gov/growthcharts

2 to 20 years: Boys
Stature-for-age and Weight-for-age percentiles

NAME _____

RECORD # _____

Mother's Stature _____		Father's Stature _____		
Date	Age	Weight	Stature	BMI*

*To Calculate BMI: Weight (kg) ÷ Stature (cm) ÷ Stature (cm) x 10,000
or Weight (lb) ÷ Stature (in) ÷ Stature (in) x 703

AGE (YEARS)

12 13 14 15 16 17 18 19 20

STATURE

in   cm

cm   in

AGE (YEARS)

2 3 4 5 6 7 8 9 10 11 12 13 14 15 16 17 18 19 20

WEIGHT

lb   kg

kg   lb

Stature percentiles: 97, 90, 75, 50, 25, 10, 3

Weight percentiles: 97, 90, 75, 50, 25, 10, 3

SOURCE: Developed by the National Center for Health Statistics in collaboration with
the National Center for Chronic Disease Prevention and Health Promotion (2000).
http://www.cdc.gov/growthcharts

Minimum Internal Cooking Temperatures

Fresh ground beef, veal, lamb, pork . . . . 160°F

Beef, veal, lamb-roasts, steaks, chops

Medium . . . . 160°F

Well done . . . . 170°F

Fresh pork-roasts, steaks, chops

Medium . . . . 160°F

Well done . . . . 170°F

Ham

Cook before eating . . . . 160°F

Fully cooked, to reheat . . . . 140°F

Poultry

Ground Chicken, Turkey . . . . 165°F

Whole Chicken, Turkey . . . . 180°F

Breasts, roasts . . . . 170°F

Thighs and wings . . . . Cook until juices run clear

Egg dishes, casseroles . . . . 160°F

Leftovers . . . . 165°F

Source: USDA Food Safety and Inspection Service

Cold Storage Chart

Since product dates aren't a guide for safe use of a product, consult this chart and follow these tips. These short but safe time limits will help keep refrigerated food (40 °F) from spoiling or becoming dangerous.

- Purchase the product before "sell-by" or expiration dates.
- Follow handling recommendations on product.
- Keep meat and poultry in its package until just before using.
- If freezing meat and poultry in its original package longer than 2 months, overwrap these packages with airtight heavy-duty foil, plastic wrap, or freezer paper, or place the package inside a plastic bag.

Because freezing (0 °F) keeps food safe indefinitely, recommended freezer storage times are for quality only.

Product	Refrigerator	Freezer
Eggs		
Fresh, in shell	3 weeks	Don't freeze
Raw yolks, whites	2 to 4 days	1 year
Hard cooked	1 week	Doesn't freeze well
Liquid pasteurized eggs or egg substitutes, opened	3 days	Don't freeze
unopened	10 days	1 year
Cooked egg dishes	3-4 days	Doesn't freeze well

Product	Refrigerator	Freezer
Dairy Products		
Swiss, brick, processed cheese	3-4 weeks	Can be frozen, but freezing affects texture and taste
Mayonnaise, commercial		
Refrigerate after opening	2 months	Don't freeze
TV Dinners, Frozen Casseroles		
Keep frozen until ready to heat	Keep frozen	3 to 4 months
Deli & Vacuum-Packed Products		
Store-prepared (or homemade) egg, chicken, tuna, ham, macaroni salads	3 to 5 days	Doesn't freeze well
Pre-stuffed pork & lamb chops, chicken breasts stuffed w/dressing	1 day	Doesn't freeze well
Store-cooked convenience meals	3 to 4 days	Doesn't freeze well
Commercial brand vacuum-packed dinners w/ USDA seal, unopened	2 weeks	Doesn't freeze well
Raw Hamburger, Ground & Stew Meat		
Hamburger & stew meats	1 to 2 days	3 to 4 months
Ground turkey, veal, pork, lamb & mixtures of them	1 to 2 days	3 to 4 months
Ham, Corned Beef		
Corned beef in pouch with pickling juices	5 to 7 days	Drained, 1 month
Ham, canned, labeled "Keep Refrigerated," unopened	6 to 9 months	Don't freeze
opened	3 to 5 days	1 to 2 months
Ham, fully cooked, whole	7 days	1 to 2 months
Ham, fully cooked, half	3 to 5 days	1 to 2 months
Ham, fully cooked, slices	3 to 4 days	1 to 2 months
Hot Dogs & Lunch Meats (in freezer wrap)		
Hot dogs, opened package	1 week	1 to 2 months
unopened package	2 weeks	1 to 2 months
Lunch meats, opened package	3 to 5 days	1 to 2 months
unopened package	2 weeks	1 to 2 months
Soups & Stews		
Vegetable or meat-added	3 to 4 days	2 to 3 months
Bacon & Sausage		
Bacon	7 days	1 month
Sausage, raw from pork, beef, chicken or turkey	1 to 2 days	1 to 2 months
Smoked breakfast links, patties	7 days	1 to 2 months
Summer sausage labeled "Keep Refrigerated," unopened	3 months	1 to 2 months
opened	3 weeks	1 to 2 months
Fresh Meat (Beef, Veal, Lamb & Pork)		
Steaks	3 to 5 days	6 to 12 months
Chops	3 to 5 days	4 to 6 months
Roasts	3 to 5 days	4 to 12 months
Variety meats (tongue, kidneys, liver, heart, chitterlings)	1 to 2 days	3 to 4 months

Product | Refrigerator | Freezer

Meat Leftovers

Product	Refrigerator	Freezer
Cooked meat and meat dishes	3 to 4 days	2 to 3 months
Gravy and meat broth	1 to 2 days	2 to 3 months

Fresh Poultry

Product	Refrigerator	Freezer
Chicken or turkey, whole	1 to 2 days	1 year
Chicken or turkey, parts	1 to 2 days	9 months
Giblets	1 to 2 days	3 to 4 months

Cooked Poultry, Leftover

Product	Refrigerator	Freezer
Fried chicken	3 to 4 days	4 months
Cooked poultry dishes	3 to 4 days	4 to 6 months
Pieces, plain	3 to 4 days	4 months
Pieces covered with broth, gravy	1 to 2 days	6 months
Chicken nuggets, patties	1 to 2 days	1 to 3 months

Fish

Product	Refrigerator	Freezer
Lean (such as cod)	1 to 2 days	up to 6 months
Fatty (such as blue, perch, salmon)	1 to 2 days	2-3 months

Source: Food Marketing Institute for fish and dairy products, USDA Food Safety and Inspection Service for all other foods.

Academic

www.mayohealth.org
Mayo Clinic nutrition information

www.navigator.tufts.edu
Tufts University Nutrition Navigator

Aging

www.aoa.dhhs.gov
Administration on Aging
330 Independence Avenue SW
Washington, DC 20201
(202) 619-0724

www.aarp.org
American Association of Retired Persons (AARP)
601 E Street NW
Washington, DC 20049
(202) 434-2277

www.americangeriatrics.org
American Geriatrics Society
770 Lexington Avenue
Suite 400
New York, NY 10021

www.aoa.dhhs.gov/naic
National Aging Information Center
330 Independence Avenue SW
Washington, DC 20201
(202) 619-7501

www.ncoa.org
National Council on Aging
1828 L Street NW
Washington, DC 20036

www.nih.gov/nia
National Institute on Aging
Public Information Office
31 Center Drive, MSC 2292
Bethesda, MD 20892
(301) 496-1752

www.nof.org
National Osteoporosis Foundation
1150 17th Street NW
Suite 500
Washington, DC 20036
(202) 223-2226

Alcohol & Drug Abuse

www.al-anon.alateen.org
Al-Anon/Alateen
1600 Corporate Landing Parkway
Virginia Beach, VA 23154-5617
(800) 356-9996

www.aa.org
Alcoholics Anonymous (AA)
General Services Office
475 Riverside Drive
New York, NY 10115
(212) 870-3400

www.wsoinc.com
Narcotics Anonymous (NA)
P.O. Box 9999
Van Nuys, CA 91409
(818) 773-9999; fax: (818) 700-0700

www.health.org
National Clearinghouse for Alcohol and Drug
Information (NCADI)
P.O. Box 2345
Rockville, MD 20847-2345
(800) 729-6686

www.ncadd.org
National Council on Alcoholism and Drug
Dependence (NCADD)
12 West 21st Street
New York, NY 10010
(800) 622-2255; (212) 206-6770; fax: (212) 645-1690

www.covesoft.com/csap.html
U.S. Center for Substance Abuse Prevention
1010 Wayne Avenue, Suite 850
Silver Spring, MD 20910
(301) 459-1591 ext. 244; fax: (301) 495-2919

Canadian Government—Federal

www.agr.ca
Agriculture and Agri-Food Canada
Public Information Request Services
Sir John Carling Building
930 Carling Avenue
Ottawa, Ontario K1A 0C5
(613) 759-1000; fax: (613) 759-6726

www.hc-sc.gc.ca/food-aliment/english/organization/nutrition.html
Bureau of Nutritional Sciences
Nutrition Research Division
Sir Fredrick G. Banting Research Center
Tunney's Pasture (2203C)
Ottawa, Ontario K1A 0L2
(613) 957-0919; fax: (613) 941-6182

www.hc-sc.gc.ca/food-aliment/english/organization/nutrition.html
Bureau of Nutritional Sciences
Nutrition Evaluation Division
Sir Fredrick G. Banting Research Center
Tunney's Pasture (2203A)
Ottawa, Ontario K1A 0L2
(613) 957-0352; fax: (613) 957-6636

Canadian Government—Federal (continued)

www.cfia-acia.agr.ca/
Canadian Food Inspection Agency
59 Camelot Drive
Nepean, Ontario K1A 0Y9
(613) 225-2342; fax: (613) 228-6653

www.cihi.ca
Canadian Institute for Health Information
377 Dalhousie Street
Suite 200
Ottawa, Ontario K1N 9N8
(613) 241-7860; fax: (613) 241-8120

www.cpha.ca
Canadian Public Health Association
400-1565 Carling Avenue
Ottawa, Ontario K1Z 8R1
(613) 725-3769; fax: (613) 725-9826

http://aceis.agr.ca/food/markets/nutraceu/enutrace.html
Functional Foods and Nutraceuticals
Food Bureau
597-930 Carling Avenue
Ottawa, ON K1A 0C5

www.hc-sc.gc.ca
Health Canada

www.nin.ca
National Institute of Nutrition
265 Carling Avenue, Suite 302
Ottawa, Ontario K1S 2E1
(613) 235-3355; fax: (613) 235-7032

Canadian Government—Provincial and Territorial

Consultant, Nutrition
Health and Wellness Promotion, Population Health,
Department of Health and Social Services, Government of the
Northwest Territories
Center Square Tower, 6th Floor
P.O. Box 1320
Yellowknife, NT X1A 2L9

Coordinator, Health Information
Resource Center
Department of Health and Social Services
1 Rochford Street, Box 2000
Charlottetown, PEI C1A 7N8

Director, Health Promotion
Department of Health, Government of Newfoundland
and Labrador
P.O. Box 8700
Confederation Building, West Block
St. John's, NF A1B 4J6

Director, Nutrition Services
Yukon Hospital Corporation
#5 Hospital Road
Whitehorse, YT Y1A 3H7

Executive Director
Health Programs
2nd Floor 800 Portage Avenue
Winnipeg, MB R3G 0P4

Health Promotion Unit
Population Health Branch
Saskatchewan Health
3475 Albert Street
Regina, SK S4S 6X6

Nutritionist
Preventive Services Branch
Ministry of Health
1520 Blanshard Street
Victoria, BC V8W 3C8
Population Health Strategies Branch
Alberta Health
23rd Floor, TELUS Plaza, North Tower
10025 Jasper Avenue
Edmonton, AB T5J 2N3

Project Manager, Public Health Management Services
Health and Community Services
P.O. Box 5100
520 King Street
Fredericton, NB E3B 5G8

Public Health Nutritionist
Central Health Region
201 Brownlow Avenue, Unit 4
Dartmouth, NS B3B 1W2

Responsables de la santé cardiovasculaire et de la nutrition
Ministère de la Santé et des Services sociaux, Service de la
Prévention
en Santé
3e étage, 1075, chemin Sainte-Foy
Quèbec, (Quèbec) G1S 2M1

Senior Consultant, Nutrition
Public Health Branch
Ministry of Health, 8th Floor
5700 Yonge St.
New York, Ontario M2M 4K5

Complementary & Alternative Nutrition

www.hc-sc.gc.ca/hpb/onhp/
171 Slater Street
9th Floor
Ottawa, ON K1P 5H7
(613) 946-1615

http://nccam.nih.gov/
National Center for Complementary and Alternative
Medicine, NIH

Consumer Organizations

www.diabetes.ca
Canadian Diabetes Association
15 Toronto Street
Suite 800
Toronto, ON M5C 2E3
(800) 226-8464, (416) 363-3373

www.cspinet.org
Center for Science in the Public Interest (CSPI)
1875 Conneticut Ave NW, Suite 300
Washington, DC 20009-5728
(202) 332-9110; fax: (202) 265-4954

www.choices.org
Choice in Dying, Inc.
1035 30th Street NW
Washington, DC 20007
(202) 338-9790; fax: (202) 338-0242

www.pueblo.gsa.gov
Consumer Information Center
Pueblo, CO 81009
(800) 688-9889; (888) 878-3256

www.consunion.org
Consumers Union of US, Inc.
101 Truman Avenue
Yonkers, NY 10703-1057
(914) 378-2000

www.ncahf.org
National Council against Health Fraud, Inc. (NCAHF)
P.O. Box 1276
Loma Linda, CA 92354
(909) 824-4690

www.quackwatch.com
Stephen Barrett, MD
P.O. Box 1747
Allentown, PA 18105
(610) 437-1795

Eating Disorders

www.aabainc.org
American Anorexia & Bulimia Association, Inc.
165 West 46th Street #1108
New York, NY 10036
(212) 575-6200

www.anred.com
Anorexia Nervosa and Related Eating Disorders (ANRED)
P.O. Box 5102
Eugene, OR 97405
(541) 344-1144

www.anad.org
National Association of Anorexia Nervosa and Associated
Disorders, Inc. (ANAD)
P.O. Box 7
Highland Park, IL 60035
(847) 831-3438; fax: (847) 433-4632

www.nedic.on.ca
National Eating Disorder Information Centre
200 Elizabeth Street, CW 1-211
Toronto, Ontario M5G 2C4
(416) 340-4156; fax: (416) 340-4736

Food Safety

www.foodsafetyalliance.org
Alliance for Food & Fiber
Food Safety Hotline
(800) 266-0200

www.cfsan.fda.gov
FDA Center for Food Safety and Applied Nutrition
200 C Street SW
Washington, DC 20204
(800) 332-4010

www.epa.gov/opptintr/lead/nlic.htm
National Lead Information Center
(800) 424-5323

www.ace.orst.edu/info/nptn
National Pesticide Telecommunications Network (NPTN)
Oregon State University
333 Weniger Hall
Corvallis, OR 97331-6502
(541) 737-6091

Seafood Safety Hotline
(800) 332-4010; (202) 205-4314

U.S. EPA Safe Drinking Water Hotline
(800) 426-4791

www.usda.gov/fsis
USDA Food Safety and Inspection Service
Food Safety Education Office
Room 1180-S
Washington, DC 20250
(202) 690-0351

USDA Meat and Poultry Hotline
(800) 535-4555

Infancy, Childhood & Adolescence

www.aap.org
American Academy of Pediatrics
141 Northwest Point Boulevard
Elk Grove Village, IL 60007-1098
(847) 434-4000; fax: (847) 434-8000

www.birthdefects,org
Association of Birth Defect Children, Inc.
930 Woodcock Road
Suite 225
Orlando, FL 32803
(407) 245-7035

www.cps.ca
Canadian Paediatric Society
100-2204 Walkley Road
Ottawa, ON K1G 4G8
(613) 526-9397; fax: (613) 526-3332

K-4 *Appendix K* INFORMATION RESOURCES

Infancy, Childhood & Adolescence (continued)

www.childrensfoundation.net
Children's Foundation
725 Fifteenth Street NW
Suite 505
Washington, DC 20005-2109
(202) 347-3300; fax: (202) 347-3382

www.KidsHealth.org
KidsHealth
The Nemours Foundation

www.nemch.org
National Center for Education in Maternal & Child Health
2000 15th Street North
Suite 701
Arlington, VA 22201-2617
(703) 524-7802

International Agencies

www.fao.org
Food and Agriculture Organization of the United Nations (FAO)
Liaison Office for North America
2175 K Street, Suite 300
Washington, DC 20437
(202) 653-2400

www.ificinfo.health.org
International Food Information Council Foundation
1100 Connecticut Avenue NW
Suite 430
Washington, DC 20036
(202) 296-6540

www.unicef.org
UNICEF
3 United Nations Plaza
New York, NY 10017
(212) 326-7000; fax: (212) 887-7465

www.who.org
World Health Organization (WHO)
Regional Office
525 23rd Street NW
Washington, DC 20037
(202) 974-3000; fax: (202) 974-3663

Pregnancy and Lactation

www.acog.org
American College of Obstetricians and Gynecologists
Resource Center
409 12th Street SW
Washington, DC 20024-2188
(202) 638-5577

www.lalecheleague.org
La Leche International, Inc.
1400 N. Meacham Road
Schaumburg, IL 60173-4048
(847) 519-7730

www.modimes.org
March of Dimes Birth Defects Foundation
1275 Mamaroneck Avenue
White Plains, NY 10605
(888) 663-4637

Professional Nutrition Organizations

ADA, The Nutrition Line
(800) 366-1655

www.eatright.org
American Dietetic Association (ADA)
216 West Jackson Boulevard
Suite 800
Chicago, IL 60606-6995
(800) 877-1600; fax: (312) 899-0040

www.faseb.org/ascn
American Society for Clinical Nutrition
9650 Rockville Pike
Bethesda, MD 20814-3998
(301) 530-7110; fax: (301) 571-1863

www.nutrition.org
American Society for Nutritional Sciences
9650 Rockville Pike
Suite 4500
Bethesda, MD 20815
(301) 530-7050; fax: (301) 571-1892

Canadian Dietetic Association
480 University Avenue
Suite 601
Toronto, ON M5G 1V2

Canadian Society for Nutritional Sciences
Department of Food and Nutrition
University of Manitoba
Winnipeg, Manitoba R3T 2N2

www.dietitians.ca
Dietitians of Canada
480 University Avenue, Suite 604
Toronto, Ontario M5G 1V2
(416) 596-0857; fax: (416) 596-0603

www.ilsi.org/hni.html
ILSI Human Nutrition Institute (HNI)
1126 Sixteenth Street NW
Washington, DC 20036
(202) 659-0524; fax: (202) 659-3617

www.ift.org
Institute of Food Technologists
221 N. LaSalle Street
Suite 300
Chicago, IL 60601-1291
(312) 782-8424; fax: (312) 782-8348

www.nas.edu
National Academy of Sciences/National Research
Council (NAS/NRC)
2101 Constitution Avenue NW
Washington, DC 20418
(202) 234-2000

www.stfx.ca/academic/human-nutrition/organization/one.html
Organization for Nutrition Education
Woodlawn Postal Outlet
P.O. Box 25
Guelph, ON N1H 8H6

www.sne.org
Society for Nutrition Education
1001 Connecticut Avenue, NW
Suite 528
Washington, DC 20036-5528
(202) 452-8534; fax: (202) 452-8536

Sports Nutrition

www.acsm.org
American College of Sports Medicine (ACSM)
401 W. Michigan Street
Indianapolis, IN 46202-3233
(317) 637-9200; fax: (317) 634-7817

www.acefitness.org
American Council on Exercise (ACE)
5820 Oberlin Drive
Suite 102
San Diego, CA 92121
(800) 529-8227

www.activeliving.canperd/index.html
Canadian Association for Health, Physical Education, Recreation, and Dance

www.csep.ca
Canadian Society for Exercise Physiology
185 Somerset St.
Suite 202
Ottawa, ON K2P 0J2
(613) 234-3755; fax: (613) 234-3565

www.indiana.edu/~preschal
President's Council on Physical Fitness and Sports
Humphrey Building, Room 738
200 Independence Avenue SW
Washington, DC 20201
(202) 690-9000; fax: (202) 690-5211

www.runnersworld.com/nutrition
Runners World
Rodale, Inc.
Emmaus, PA 18098
(610) 967-8809

www.smscc.ca
Sports Medicine and Science Council of Canada
1600 James Naismith Drive
Suite 306
Gloucester, Ontario K1B 5N4
(613) 748-5671; fax: (613) 748-5729

www.rssq.gouv.qc.ca
Sports Safety Board of Quebec

www.nutrifit.org
Sports, Cardiovascular and Wellness Nutritionists (SCAN)

www.ideafit.com
The International Association for Fitness Professionals (IDEA)
6190 Cornerstone Court East # 204
San Diego, CA 92121-3773
(800) 999-4332 ext 7; fax: (858) 535-8234

www.veggie.org/
Veggie Sports Association

www.wellweb.com/Nutrition_Fitness.htm
Wellness Web—Nutrition and Fitness
Mont Clare, PA (610) 525-1589

Supplements

www.odp.od.nih.gov/ods/databases/ibids.html
International Bibliographic Information on Dietary Supplements (IBIDS)

http://odp.od.nih.gov/ods/
Office of Dietary Supplements of the National, Institutes of Health

http://dietary-supplements.info.nih.gov
The Office of Dietary Supplements

Trade and Industry Organizations

www.aibonline.org
American Institute of Baking
1213 Bakers Way
P.O. Box 3999
Manhattan, KS 66505-3999
(800) 633-5137, (785) 537-4750; fax: (785) 537-1493

www.meatami.org
American Meat Institute
1700 North Moore Street
Suite 1600
Arlington, VA 22209
(703) 841-2400; fax: (703) 527-0938

www.beechnut.com
Beech-Nut Nutrition Company
100 S. 4th Street
St. Louis, MO 63102
(800) 233-2468

Trade and Industry Organizations (continued)

www.bestfoods.com
Best Foods
International Plaza
700 Sylvan Avenue
Englewood Cliffs, NJ 07632-9976
(201) 894-4000

www.gssiweb.com
Gatorade Sports Science Institute
617 West Main Street
Barrington, IL 60010
(800) 616-4774, (847) 304-2229

www.generalmills.com
General Mills, Inc.
Number One General Mills Boulevard
Minneapolis, MN 55426
(800) 328-6787

www.gerber.com
Gerber Products Co.
445 State Street
Fremont, MI 49413-0001
(800) 443-7237

www.heinz.com
H.J. Heinz Company
World Headquarters
P.O. Box 57
Pittsburgh, PA 15230-0057
(412) 456-5700

www.kellogs.com
Kellog Company
P.O. Box 3599
Battle Creek, MI 49016-3599
(616) 961-2000

www.kraftfoods.com
Kraft Foods
Consumer Response and Information Center
One Kraft Court
Glenview, IL 60025
(800) 323-0768

www.dairyinfo.com
National Dairy Council
10255 West Higgens Road
Suite 900
Rosemont, IL 60018-5616
(847) 803-2000

www.pillsbury.com
Pillsbury Company
2866 Pillsbury Center
Minneapolis, MN 55402
(800) 767-4466

www.pg.com/info
Procter and Gamble Company
One Procter and Gamble Plaza
Cincinnati, OH 45202
(513) 983-1100

www.sunkist.com
Sunkist Growers
Consumer Affairs, Fresh Fruit Division
14130 Riverside Drive
Sherman Oaks, CA 91423
(800) 248-7875

www.dannon.com
The Dannon Company
120 White Plains Road
Tarrytown, NY 10591-5536
(877) 326-6668

www.nutrasweet.com
The NutraSweet Company
P.O. Box 2986
Chicago, IL 60654-0986
(800) 323-5316

www.uffva.org
United Fresh Fruit and Vegetable Association
727 North Washington Street
Alexandria, VA 22314
(703) 836-3410

www.usarice.com
USA Rice Federation
4301 North Fairfax Drive
Suite 305
Arlington, VA 22203
(703) 351-8161

www.veris-online.org
VERIS Research Information Service
5325 S. 9th Avenue
LaGrange, IL 60525
(800) 554-1708; (612) 927-7104; fax: (612) 927-6406

Weight Management

http://nuts.uvm.edu/nusc/uww
Body Composition Tutorial

www.overeatersanonymous.org
Overeaters Anonymous (OA)
World Service Office
6075 Zenith Court NE
Rio Rancho, NM 87124
(505) 891-2664; fax: (505) 891-4320

www.shapeup.org
Shape Up America!
6707 Democracy Boulevard
Suite 306
Bethesda, MD 20817
(301) 493-5368

www.tops.org
TOPS (Take Off Pounds Sensibly)
4575 South Fifth Street
P.O. Box 07360
Milwaukee, WI 53207-0360
(800) 932-8677; (414) 482-4620

www.niddk.nih.gov/NutritionDocs.html
Weight Control Information Network

www.weightwatchers.com
Weight Watchers International
Consumer Affairs Department/IN
175 Crossways Park West
Woodbury, NY 11797
(516) 390-1400; fax: (516) 390-1632

World Hunger

www.bread.org
Bread for the World
1100 Wayne Avenue
Suite 1000
Silver Spring, MD 20910
(301) 608-2400

http://nutrition.tufts.edu/centers/hunger.shtml
Center on Hunger, Poverty and Nutrition Policy
Tufts University School of Medicine
11 Curtis Avenue
Medford, MA 02155
(617) 627-6223; fax: (617) 627-3688

www.freefromhunger.org
Freedom from Hunger
P.O. Box2000
1644 DaVinci Court
Davis, CA 95617
(530) 758-6200

www.oxfamamerica.org
Oxfam America
26 West Street
Boston, MA 02111-1206
(800) 776-9326; fax: (617) 728-2594

www.helwys.com/seedhome.htm
SEEDS Magazine
P.O. Box 6170
Waco, TX 76706
(254) 755-7745

www.worldwatch.org
Worldwatch Institute
1776 Massachusetts Avenue NW
Suite 800
Washington, DC 20036
(202) 452-1999

US Government

www.cdc.gov
Centers for Disease Control and Prevention
1600 Clifton Road
Atlanta, GA 30333
(800) 311-3435, (404) 639-3534

FDA Consumer Information Line
(301) 827-4420

www.cfsan.fda.gov
FDA Office of Food Labeling
HFS 150
200 C Street SW
Washington, DC 20204
(202) 205-4561; fax: (202) 205-4564

FDA Office of Plant and Dairy Foods and Beverages
HPS300
200 C Street SW
Washington, DC 20204
(202) 205-4064; fax: (202) 205-4422

FDA Office of Special Nutritionals
HFS450
200 C Street SW
Washington, DC 20204
(202) 205-4168; fax: (202) 205-5295

www.ftc.gov
Federal Trade Commission (FTC)
Public Reference Branch
(202) 326-2222

www.fda.gov
Food and Drug Administration (FDA)
Office of Consumer Affairs, HFE 1
Room 16-85
5600 Fishers Lane
Rockville, MD 20857
(301) 443-1544

www.nal.usda.gov/fnic
Food and Nutrition Information Center
National Agricultural Library, Room 304
10301 Baltimore Avenue
Beltsville, MD 20705-2351
(301) 504-5719; fax: (301) 504-6409

www.frac.org
Food Research Action Center (FRAC)
1875 Connecticut Avenue NW
Suite 540
Washington, DC 20009
(202) 986-2200; fax: (202) 986-2525

www.healthfinder.gov
Gateway for health and nutrition information

US Government (continued)

www.nidr.nih.gov
National Institute of Dental Research (NIDR)
National Institutes of Health
Bethesda, MD 20892-2190
(301) 496-4261

www.niddk.nih.gov
National Institute of Diabetes & Digestive & Kidney Diseases
Office of Communications and Public Liaison
NIDDK, NIH
31 Center Drive, MSC 2560
Bethesda, MD 20892-2560

www.nih.gov/health
National Institutes of Health search engine and free access to Medline and PubMed data bases

www.access.gpo.gov/su_docs
Superintendent of Documents
U.S. Government Printing Office
Washington, DC 20402
(202) 512-1071

www.usda.gov/fcs
U.S. Department of Agriculture (USDA)
14th Street SW and Independence Avenue
Washington, DC 20250
(202) 720-2791

www.os.dhhs.gov
U.S. Department of Health and Human Services
200 Independence Avenue SW
Washington, DC 20201
(202) 619-0257

www.epa.gov
U.S. Environmental Protection Agency (EPA)
401 Main Street SW
Washington, DC 20460
(202) 260-2090

www.pueblo.gsa.gov
U.S. General Services Organization Pueblo Colorado

www.hhs.gov/phs/
U.S. Public Health Service
Assistant Secretary of Health
Humphrey Building, Room 725-H
200 Independence Avenue SW
Washington, DC 20201
(202) 690-7694

www.usda.gov/fcs/cnpp.htm
USDA Center for Nutrition Policy and Promotion
1120 20th Street NW, Suite 200
North Lobby
Washington, DC 20036
(202) 208-2417

Study Question Answers

Chapter 1

1. Carbohydrate, protein, fat, vitamins, minerals, and water

3. Health beliefs are characterized by an individual's perception that he or she is susceptible to a disease and, if so, that action can be taken to prevent or delay its onset. Recommendations based on information about the links between dietary choices and the risk of disease are more likely to be heeded by people who feel susceptible to the disease. They see that dietary changes may lead to positive results.

5. Fat-soluble: vitamin A, vitamin D, vitamin E, and vitamin K
Water-soluble: vitamin C, thiamin (B_1), riboflavin (B_2), niacin (B_3), pyridoxine (B_6), cobalamin (B_{12}), folate, pantothenic acid, and biotin

7. An epidemiological study observes and compares how disease rates vary among different population groups and identifies conditions related to diseases or conditions within the populations. This enables researchers to identify associations between factors within the population and the particular disease being studied.

9. A placebo is an imitation treatment that looks the same as the experimental treatment (such as a sugar pill) but has no effect. The placebo is important for reducing bias because subjects do not know if they are receiving the intervention and are less inclined to alter their responses or report symptoms based on what they think should happen.

Chapter 2

1. The *Estimated Average Requirement* (EAR) is the nutrient intake level that is estimated to meet the needs of 50 percent of the individuals in an age and gender category.

The *Recommended Dietary Allowance* (RDA) is the daily intake level that meets the needs of most (97 to 98 percent) people in an age and gender category.

An *Adequate Intake* (AI) level is set when an RDA has not been established yet due to a lack of knowledge and need for more scientific research.

The *Tolerable Upper Intake Level* (UL) is the maximum daily intake level that is unlikely to pose health risks to almost all of the individuals in an age and gender category.

3. The exchange system divides foods into groups and assigns each food in a group a portion size comparable in calories and nutrients. A diet is planned by determining the number of servings from each exchange group that should be in each snack or meal. For example, the individual decides whether he or she will use the fruit "exchange" for ½ cup of orange juice or 1 small banana; each of the foods in a group can be *exchanged* for any other food in the same group.

Diabetics might use the exchange system because, if followed correctly, it can help them keep a consistent carbohydrate intake and keep their total calories in line with recommendations.

5. The % Daily Value reflects the amount of a nutrient in one serving of food compared to the amount recommended to be in a 2,000-kcalorie diet. For example, if a food label lists 20% DV for saturated fat, it means that one serving of this food contains 20% of the Daily Value for saturated fat. Because the DV for saturated fat is 20 grams (for a 2,000-kcal diet), this food would have 4 grams of saturated fat per serving (20% of 20 g = 4 g).

Chapter 3

1. Stomach contents have the lowest pH due to the stomach's production of hydrochloric acid. The pancreas secretes fluid that contains mostly water, bicarbonate, and digestive enzymes. In the small intestine, this basic solution secreted from the pancreas helps neutralize the acidic chyme entering from the stomach.

3. The small intestine.

5. Any three of the following:
   - The *salivary glands* produce saliva that moistens food, lubricating it for easy swallowing. Saliva contains enzymes that begin the process of chemical digestion.
   - The *pancreas* secretes digestive enzymes that help digest nutrients.
   - The *gallbladder* stores and concentrates bile from the liver.
   - The *liver* produces and secretes bile, which emulsifies fats in the small intestine thus aiding fat digestion.

7. Gastroesophageal reflux disease (GERD) occurs when the lower esophageal sphincter (LES) is weak or relaxes inappropriately, allowing the stomach's contents to flow back up into the esophagus. The acidic stomach contents irritate the esophageal lining, causing severe pain.

Chapter 4

1. Both starch and fiber are long chains of glucose molecules but we are unable to digest the bonds between the glucose units in fiber. Therefore, fiber moves through the small intestine undigested while starch is broken down into glucose and absorbed.

3. Carbohydrates provide energy (fuel) to the cells of the body. Consuming too little carbohydrate can result in the breakdown of body proteins that supply glucose and energy. Inadequate carbohydrate intake prevents fats from breaking down normally, and this results in ketosis.

5. The three groups at the bottom of the Food Guide Pyramid (all grains, fruits, and vegetables) contain the most carbohydrate-dense foods. Many foods in the dairy group also contribute quite a bit of carbohydrate. Legumes of the meat and meat alternatives group are rich in both

carbohydrates and protein. Sweets, of course, contain carbohydrates in the form of sugars.

7. Insulin is secreted in response to meal ingestion and its job is to lower blood glucose by increasing the uptake of glucose into cells. Glucagon is released in response to low blood glucose and is responsible for adding glucose to the blood from storage (from glycogen in liver and muscle tissue).

Chapter 5

1. Oils are triglycerides. Triglycerides contain a glycerol molecule and 3 fatty acids. These fatty acids can vary in three main ways: length, saturation, and omega number. An oil such as corn oil has more polyunsaturated fatty acids attached to glycerol than it does monounsaturated or saturated fatty acids. Therefore corn oil is known as a mostly polyunsaturated fat but like all oils it contains a mixture of fatty acids.

3. Triglycerides

5. Provide energy (9 kcals/g), provide a concentrated source of stored calories (triglycerides in fat cells), carry flavor in foods, pad and protect vital organs, provide thermal insulation (subcutaneous fat).

7.

	General Recommendations	Daily Value (for a 2,000-kcal diet)
Total fat	≤30% of total calories	65 g
Saturated fat	<10% of total calories	20 g
Polyunsaturated fat	10% of total calories	–
Monounsaturated fat	10–15% of total calories	–
Cholesterol	≤300 mg per day	≤300 mg

9. Linoleic acid and alpha-linolenic acid.

Chapter 6

1. Comprise muscles and organs; work as hormones, enzymes, and antibodies; help to regulate fluid and electrolyte balance; help to regulate acid-base balance; used as transporter molecules.

3. Nitrogen is part of the chemical structure of amino acids (proteins). Nitrogen is not in the chemical structure of carbohydrates and lipids. Nitrogen is part of the amino group, -NH_2.

5. Complementary proteins are two proteins that when combined, contain all of the essential amino acids in adequate amounts to support health. Examples include rice and beans, peanut butter on bread, corn bread and chili (beans).

7. Protein is used to make antibodies, which help fight infection. Without adequate dietary protein, synthesis of antibodies is impaired, and a person becomes more susceptible to infection.

9. Reduced blood cholesterol levels, reduced risk of some cancers, improved body weight, reduced blood pressure.

Chapter 7

1. ATP is the energy form usable by cells so it is called the universal energy currency. Most ATP is produced inside mitochondria; therefore mitochondria often are called the powerhouses of the cell.

3. NAD^+ and FAD^+ are the electron acceptors in the breakdown pathways. NADH and $FADH_2$ are the electron carrier forms. They carry these high-energy electrons to the electron transport chain where the electrons power the production of ATP.

5. Beta-oxidation, or fatty acid oxidation, is a step-by-step process that forms two-carbon molecules of acetyl CoA as it clips two carbon links from a fatty acid chain. It also produces NADH and $FADH_2$, which carry high-energy electrons to the electron transport chain for ATP production.

7. Ketone bodies refer to the three compounds (acetoacetate, acetone, and beta-hydroxybutyrate) made during incomplete fatty acid oxidation. Although some ketone bodies are always produced and used, they become a substantial alternative energy source when the body lacks carbohydrate and needs to fuel vital cells.

9. Gluconeogenesis is the making of "new" glucose. When the body has a low glucose supply, it can make glucose from the glycerol component of triglycerides and from some amino acids. Lipogenesis is the process of synthesizing long-chain fatty acids. Lipogenesis occurs when ATP is plentiful and building blocks are abundant. Precursors of fatty acid synthesis include ketogenic amino acids, alcohol, and fatty acids themselves.

Spotlight on Alcohol

1. A standard amount of beer, wine, and liquor has 12, 4–5, and 1½ ounces, respectively. This equals 15 grams of pure alcohol.

3. The liver is the chief organ for alcohol metabolism.

5. In alcohol metabolism NAD^+ is converted to NADH. When an excess amount of NADH is present it blocks (slows) the entry of acetyl CoA into the citric acid cycle. The acetyl CoA is diverted and used for fatty acid synthesis. The fat is stored in the liver since it is the organ responsible for alcohol metabolism.

7. Most health officials do not promote the consumption of alcohol. However, they do suggest that if alcohol is consumed it be done in moderation (no more than 2 drinks for males, 1 drink for females per day).

9. Among other things, alcohol can cause fetal alcohol syndrome. A safe lower limit for alcohol consumption during pregnancy is not currently known.

Chapter 8

1. Energy balance is the relationship between your energy intake and energy output. You are in energy equilibrium when your energy or caloric intake equals the amount of energy or calories you expend. People who maintain their weight over time are in energy equilibrium whether or not they are aware of their intake or expenditure. Positive energy balance (intake > output) results in weight gain while negative energy balance (intake < output) results in weight loss.

3. The metabolic rate of physical activity depends on the activity's duration, type (e.g., walking, running, or typing), and intensity. The longer you perform an activity, the greater its thermic effect. The more intense the activity, the greater its thermic effect. The greater use of large muscle groups (type of activity), the greater its thermic effect.

5. Genetic, physiological, metabolic, hormonal, sociocultural, environmental, behavioral, and psychological factors can all contribute to obesity.

7. Some health experts advocate replacing the goal of attaining a particular weight with the goal of *metabolic fitness,* which is the absence of metabolic or biochemical risk factors associated with obesity. Individuals are considered metabolically fit when their blood lipids are at safe levels and their blood pressure is normal. Four suggested goals for metabolic fitness, from most to least aggressive are to (1) significantly reduce the risk factors, (2) restore abnormal risk factors to normal ranges, (3) reverse the "high normal" or "borderline" factors, and (4) prevent risk factors in overweight individuals.

9. A balanced diet of moderate caloric intake, adequate exercise, cognitive-behavioral strategies for changing habits and behavior patterns, attention to balancing self-acceptance and the desire for change.

11. The term *underweight* applies to people who are 15 to 20 percent or more below the desirable weight for their height, or who have a BMI lower than 19.

Chapter 9

1. Vitamins A, D, E, and K are found in the fat and lipid components of food. Fat-soluble vitamins require bile for absorption and first travel in the lymphatic system (inside chylomicrons) before entering the bloodstream. Most fat-soluble vitamins are not readily excreted and are stored in the liver and adipose tissue.

3. Vitamin A is necessary for vision, reproduction, cell differentiation, immune function, and bone health.

5. Beta-carotene

7. Cholesterol

9. Vitamin K is necessary for the production of prothrombin, a protein that when activated is responsible for the formation of a solid clot.

Chapter 10

1. Thiamin functions in energy metabolism as the coenzyme thiamin pyrophosphate (TPP).

   Riboflavin functions in energy metabolism as the coenzymes flavin adenine dinucleotide (FAD) and flavin mononucleotide (FMN).

   Niacin functions in energy metabolism as the coenzymes nicotinamide adenine dinucleotide (NAD^+) and nicotinamide adenine dinucleotide phosphate ($NADP^+$).

   Biotin acts as a coenzyme critical to energy and amino acid metabolism, as well as fat and glycogen synthesis.

   Pantothenic acid functions in energy metabolism as part of coenzyme A.

   Vitamin B_6 functions in amino acid and fatty acid metabolism as the coenzymes pyridoxal phosphate (PLP) and pyridoxamine phosphate (PMP).

Folate functions in one-carbon transfer reactions in the synthesis of DNA and many other reactions.

Vitamin B_{12} promotes the growth and maintenance of the sheath that protects nerve fibers; activates the folate coenzyme, tetrahydrofolic acid (THFA).

Vitamin C, important in collagen synthesis, assists with absorption of iron, and is an antioxidant.

3. Thiamin – beriberi
   Riboflavin – ariboflavinosis
   Niacin – pellagra
   Biotin – no disease name, a deficiency causes hair loss, and loss of appetite
   Pantothenic acid – no disease name
   Folate – megaloblastic anemia
   Vitamin B_{12} – pernicious anemia
   Vitamin C – scurvy

5. The only water-soluble vitamins with demonstrated toxicity are niacin, vitamin B_6, and vitamin C. Excessive amounts of niacin can dilate the capillaries and cause tingling sensations. When this occurs, it is called a "niacin flush." Excessive amounts of vitamin B_6 can cause irreversible nerve degeneration, and excessive doses of vitamin C can cause diarrhea, nausea, and abdominal cramps.

Chapter 11

1. The physiological state of the body (i.e., is the body in a deficient or an overload state?) and the bioavailability of the mineral affect its absorption.

3. Aldosterone helps the kidney retain sodium, which in turn causes the body to hold on to more water. When the kidneys detect dehydration, they secrete renin. Renin then causes the formation of angiotensin, which leads to the release of aldosterone.

5. Because most foods contain ample amounts of sodium, there is no established RDA. The estimated minimum requirement of 500 milligrams per day for a healthy adult is much less than most Americans consume. The Daily Value for sodium is 2400 milligrams.

7. Calcium is important for blood clotting, nerve function, muscle contractions, and cell metabolism.

9. Alcoholics are at high risk of hypomagnesemia because their diet is poor and usually lacks magnesium. They tend to excrete magnesium in their urine in larger amounts than normal.

Chapter 12

1. Trace minerals differ from the major minerals in terms of their dietary requirements and their amounts in the body. The daily dietary recommendations for trace elements are less than 100 milligrams and the total amount of each trace element in the body is less than 5 grams.

3. Factors that can increase or decrease a mineral's bioavailability include:
   - the type of food the mineral is contained in,
   - the presence or absence of fibers and phytate,

- competition with other minerals,
- the acidity of the environment,
- a person's need for that mineral.

5. The initial stage of iron deficiency is iron depletion, which causes no physiological impairment. Measuring serum ferritin, which is proportional to body iron stores, assesses iron depletion.

   In the second stage of iron deficiency, there is a decrease in functional or transport iron. While hemoglobin and hematocrit remain in the normal range, other values begin to change as functional iron decreases. A new measure of this intermediate stage is the serum level of transferrin receptors (TfRs). As transport iron decreases and stores are depleted, TfR levels increase in proportion to the iron deficit. Other values used to detect this stage are transferrin saturation and protoporphyrin, the precursor of heme, which is elevated when the supply of iron is inadequate for heme synthesis.

   The third and most severe stage of iron deficiency is anemia and is characterized by decreased size and number of red blood cells, reduced hemoglobin and hematocrit, and pale red blood cells. This is referred to as microcytic hypochromic anemia. Symptoms include fatigue, pallor, breathlessness with exertion, decreased cold tolerance, behavioral changes, deficits in immune function, cognitive impairment, decreased work performance, and impaired growth.

7. The primary culprits in marginal zinc deficiency are increased needs, poor intake, poor absorption, and excessive losses. Diarrhea and chronic infections like pneumonia can cause excessive zinc excretion. These diseases are commonplace in developing countries where zinc deficiency may be widespread.

9. Iodine is an essential component of the two thyroid hormones triiodothyronine (T3) and thyroxine (T4). Although T3 is the active form of thyroid hormone, T4 is more prevalent in the body.

   Thyroid hormones regulate body temperature, basal metabolic rate, reproduction, and growth.

   Three selenium-dependent enzymes help convert T4 to the more active T3 form.

11. Wilson's disease is a genetic disorder of copper transport that is characterized by impaired excretion and toxic accumulation of copper in the liver, kidney, and eye. The prevalence of Wilson's disease (1 in 30,000) is higher than that of Menkes' syndrome. Patients with Wilson's disease frequently appear healthy until adolescence or early adulthood. Without treatment, patients develop serious liver and neurologic problems.

    Menkes' syndrome is a genetic copper deficiency resulting from a failure to absorb copper from the intestinal tract. The incidence is extremely rare (1 in 200,000). Menkes' syndrome results in neurological degeneration, peculiar kinky hair, and poor growth.

13. Fluoride decreases the demineralization of tooth enamel by organic acids that eat away the enamel. Fluoride also accelerates the subsequent remineralization. Fluoride also inhibits bacterial activity in dental plaques.

Chapter 13

1. *Smooth muscles* line blood vessel walls, bronchial tubes in the lungs, and most organs. Because smooth muscle is not under your conscious control, it also is called involuntary muscle. *Cardiac muscle* is the heart muscle and provides most of the heart's structure. *Skeletal muscles* attach to your skeleton. They are under conscious control and cause physical movements.

3. The anaerobic energy systems are the ATP-CP and lactic acid system (anaerobic glycolysis). The aerobic energy system is the oxygen energy system and includes the oxidative pathways of the citric acid cycle and electron transport chain.

   During the first few minutes of any activity, anaerobic metabolism provides most of the energy. As the duration of activity increases, but intensity remains low to moderate, aerobic metabolism takes over. High-intensity exercises performed for a short duration, such as sprinting and weight lifting, are primarily fueled anaerobically. Exercises performed at a lower intensity for a longer duration, such as long-distance running, cycling, walking, and swimming, are fueled primarily by the aerobic system.

5. Carbohydrate loading is a process by which athletes manipulate their carbohydrate intake and exercise regimen to maximize glycogen storage in their muscles. Carbo loading involves a gradual increase in daily carbohydrate intake up to 70 percent of total calories, along with a decrease in exercise intensity and duration. The glycogen content of exercised muscles has been shown to increase by 2 to 2.5 times in athletes who adhere to this protocol.

   Carbo loading can make a difference in endurance events of 60 to 90 consecutive minutes or more, such as long distance swimming, cross-country skiing, soccer, marathons, triathlons, and long distance cycling. It has been shown to extend the length of time athletes can exercise at a higher intensity.

7. Calcium, iron, zinc, and copper (any three).

9. Ergogenic aids are supplements that have been touted to increase athletic strength and/or endurance performance. There are several supplements marketed as ergogenic aids but most do not have research studies to back up their claims. Some like pyruvate, MCT (medium-chain triglyceride) oil, ginseng, CoQ$_{10}$, chromium, and creatine have both supportive and nonsupportive research. More research is necessary.

Spotlight on Eating Disorders

1. Social (i.e., societal pressure to be thin); psychological (i.e., peer and family relationships); biological (i.e., neurotransmitter/chemical balance).

3. The first goal of treatment is to stabilize the patient's physical condition. The second is to convert the patient, who is typically reluctant, into a willing participant in the treatment plan. A combination of hospitalization, psychotherapy, and pharmacotherapy is often necessary. Most experts doubt that patients with anorexia can be cured but research suggests that with intensive therapy, most patients can increase their weight. However, they may struggle all their lives with a moderate to severe preoccupation with food and body weight, poor social relationships, and depression. The earlier a patient begins treatment, the better the prognosis.

5. During a binge, people with bulimia typically consume massive quantities of highly palatable "forbidden" foods, like pastry, ice cream, and candy. This gorging typically takes place in secret and over a relatively short time span (1 to 2 hrs). Afterward, feeling physically ill from the overconsumption, sufferers use a variety of techniques to rid themselves of the food. These purging behaviors include vomiting and the use of emetics and laxatives. In addition to or instead of purging, they may follow a binge with a period of very strict fasting and increased exercise.

7. The female athlete triad comprises three separate but related conditions that occur in a small proportion of females who regularly exercise strenuously: (1) disordered eating, (2) amenorrhea, and (3) osteoporosis. The practice of disordered eating is associated with menstrual irregularities and subsequent bone loss, which may place such females at risk for premature osteoporosis.

Chapter 14

1. The three main components of preconception care are risk assessment, health promotion, and intervention. Risk assessment includes checking a woman's weight, vitamin and mineral status (including her intake of folate), and health habits (e.g., smoking, exercise, alcohol consumption). Health promotion includes providing educational materials regarding appropriate dietary and lifestyle changes, and intervention can include prescription of vitamin/mineral supplements or treatment of existing health conditions.

3. Physiological changes during pregnancy include an increase in total body fluid and blood volume; an increase in the size of the breast tissue, uterus, and adipose stores; and a reduction in the motility of the GI tract.

5. It recommends an additional serving from the Milk, Yogurt, and Cheese group during pregnancy. Instead of the usual two to three servings from the dairy foods, it recommends three to four during pregnancy. An additional serving of fruit, vegetable, and grain will meet the calorie recommendations for pregnancy and supply important vitamins and minerals.

7. Nausea, vomiting, heartburn, constipation, hemorrhoids.

9. The RDA for energy during lactation is 500 kcalories per day more than the RDA for nonpregnant women. To ensure adequate milk production and avoid nutrient deficiencies, a nursing mother should consume at least 1,800 kcalories a day. Chronically eating less than 1,500 kcalories a day may decrease milk volume to a level that cannot support infant growth and development. Also, losing more than 0.5 kilogram (1.1 lb) per week can reduce milk production.

11. Benefits to the infant begin with the antibodies in colostrum, including immunoglobulin A (IgA), the first line of defense against most infectious agents. Another beneficial biochemical in human milk is bifidus factor. This factor fosters the growth of the bacteria *Lactobacillus bifidus,* which in turn prevents the growth of harmful bacteria.

   Whey proteins, the major type of protein in human milk, are much easier to digest than casein, the major type of protein in cow's milk.

   Breast milk has higher amounts of cholesterol than infant formula does, which may be necessary to help an infant regulate its own cholesterol synthesis. In addition, docosahexaenoic acid (DHA) is found in breast milk and missing from most infant formulas. DHA is one of the two major omega-3 fatty acids and one of the most prevalent fats in the human brain and retina. Research suggests that DHA is beneficial to infant brain development.

Chapter 15

1. It is normal for infants to lose weight just after being born. In fact, they may lose up to 6 percent of their weight. This does not necessarily mean that an infant is at nutritional risk. Infants typically regain their birth weight within 2 weeks.

3. Babies need approximately 1.5 ml of water per kcal consumed. Breast-fed and formula-fed infants do not need supplemental water; the breast milk and properly mixed formula provide enough water for adequate hydration until significant amounts of solid foods have been added to the diet.

5. Solid foods (anything other than breast milk or infant formula) should be introduced no earlier than 4 to 6 months of age. Then, new foods should be introduced one at a time to check for any allergies or intolerances. Most parents begin with infant rice cereal, mixed to a thin consistency with water, breast milk, or infant formula. After the infant is eating cereal several times a day, strained fruits and vegetables are introduced.

7. Iron, possibly zinc, vitamins D and E (if parents follow a low fat diet).

9. Chronic nutrition problems that can affect children include obesity, lead toxicity, and early onset of indicators of heart disease. Infants and toddlers should not be given low-fat, high-fiber diets; when children reach the age of 3, dietary changes consistent with the *Dietary Guidelines for Americans* can gradually be made. Regular physical activity and limited sedentary activity such as television viewing are important factors in reducing obesity and chronic disease risk.

11. As at earlier ages, calcium, iron, and vitamin A are the nutrients that often are lacking in adolescent diets. Other nutritional concerns include obesity and eating disorders.

Chapter 16

1. Changes in body composition (decreased lean tissue); changes in vitamin status/absorption; slower GI tract movement; decreased immune function; sensory changes; decreased saliva production; changes in teeth/gums; subtle swallowing problems; changes in appetite (usually decreased); decreased liver and kidney function.

3. Vitamin E, vitamin D, folate, magnesium, calcium, zinc.

5. Older adults are at higher risk of vitamin D deficiency than younger adults. Because they typically are exposed to less sunlight, older people have less opportunity to produce vitamin D from sunlight, and the efficiency of vitamin D synthesis is reduced. Elders often do not consume enough dairy products, which are good sources of vitamin D.

7. Excess supplementation with certain vitamins or minerals may cause toxicity. Supplements: nutrients, herbals, or others, may interact with medications the person is already taking. These interactions may enhance or limit the effectiveness of the medication; both of these are undesirable outcomes.

9. Collards, spinach, and other leafy greens that are high in carotenoids may protect against the development of macular degeneration.

11. Meals on Wheels, Elderly Nutrition Program (ENP), Food Stamps.

Spotlight on Complementary and Alternative Nutrition

1. The growth of complementary and alternative medicine is due to many factors including more widespread acceptance, changes in regulations, and scientific validation of many therapies. Many individuals see these therapies as more cost effective, more natural, and more environmentally friendly than Western medicine.

3. DSHEA defines *dietary supplement* as "any product intended to supplement the diet," and it requires the word *supplement* be clearly printed on the label.

5. It is an example of a nutrient-content claim. Other types of claims can be made when appropriate: health claims, nutrition-support claims, and structure-function claims.

7. This represents a possible conflict of interest that could compromise objectivity and, therefore, the care their patients receive.

Chapter 17

1. Some types of pathogenic bacteria can directly infect a person who consumes contaminated food. Others may produce a toxin that can cause foodborne illness.

3. The following suggestions by the Consumers Union will help you limit your intake of pesticides:
   - Wash and peel produce.
   - Eat a wide variety of fruits and vegetables.

5. The most common food allergens are milk, eggs, peanuts, tree nuts, fish, soy, and wheat. The symptoms of food allergies include gastrointestinal problems, skin irritation, respiratory difficulties, shock, and death.

7. Some of the most important things to do when trying to keep a kitchen safe from pathogenic microorganisms include:
   - Make sure hands and kitchen surfaces are thoroughly clean.
   - Keep raw meats and poultry separate from other raw foods to avoid cross-contamination.
   - Use proper temperatures while cooking.
   - Chill food properly.

9. The Delaney Clause prohibits the use of any food additive shown to cause cancer in animals or humans. Critics charge that the Delaney Clause, combined with modern detection techniques, has created a situation where even very pure foods can be shown to be contaminated with traces of a carcinogen. Proponents say that any risk for cancer, even if minimal, is still too high.

11. The main concerns scientists have regarding genetically engineered crops are (1) the possibilities of producing new allergens since engineered crops may produce a novel protein and (2) the environmental effects of engineered crops.

Chapter 18

1. Food insecurity is the worry that one does not have the resources to obtain adequate food. Hunger is the physical sensation of unease or pain caused by a lack of food. Food insecurity can exist with or without hunger.

3. vitamin A, iodine, iron, protein and energy

5. Food Stamp Program, National School Lunch Program, School Breakfast Program, Child and Adult Care Food Program, The Food Research and Action Center (FRAC), Special Supplemental Nutrition Program for Women, Infants, and Children (WIC)

Index/Glossary

Key terms in the text appear here in **bold** followed by the definition.

ABC model of behavior A behavioral model that includes the external and internal events that precede and follow the behavior. The "A" stands for antecedents, the events that precede the behavior ("B"), which are followed by consequences ("C") that positively or negatively reinforce the behavior, 312

ABCDs of nutrition assessment Nutrition assessment components: *A*nthropometric measurements, *B*iochemical tests, *C*linical observations, and *D*ietary intake, 57

Abdominal cramps, 392

Absorption, cellular, 213, 221

Absorption The movement of substances into or across tissues; in particular, the passage of nutrients and other substances into the walls of the gastrointestinal tract and then into the bloodstream

  aging effect, 620

  and alcohol, 76, 262-63, 275-76

  of carbohydrates, 110-11

  of carotenoids, 342

  of cholesterol, 153

  energy extraction, 221

  in large intestine, 82

  of lipids, 155-56, 157, 173

  of minerals, 391, 413

    calcium, 424, 620

    iron, 446-48, 620

    phosphorous, 426-27

    zinc, 454-55, 457

  pregnancy effect, 554

  of proteins, 192-93, 213

  in small intestine, 66, 70, 71-3, 80-81

  and sports drinks, 406

  in stomach, 76

  of vitamins, 329-30, 357, 391, 434, 620

Accutane, 340

Acesulfame K ay-see-SUL-fame An artificial sweetener that is 200 times sweeter than common table sugar (sucrose). Because it is not digested and absorbed by the body, acesulfame contributes no calories to the diet and yields no energy when consumed, 125

Acetaldehyde A toxic intermediate compound (CH$_3$CHO) formed by the action of enzyme systems during the metabolism of alcohol, 262-63

Acetoacetate, 242

Acetaminophen, 264

Acetone, 242, 251

Acetyl CoA A key intermediate in the metabolic breakdown of carbohydrates, fatty acids, and amino acids. It consists of a two-carbon acetate group linked to coenzyme A, which is derived from pantothenic acid

  and alcohol, 263

  and biosynthesis, 240-43, 244-45

  and energy, 221, 227-29, 234, 236-37

  and ketogenesis, 242-43

  and lipoic acid, 395

  and pantothenic acid, 377

Acetylcholine, 149, 151, 393

Acid-base balance, 112, 188-89

Acidity, of food, 691, 703

Acidosis An abnormally low blood pH (below about 7.35), 188-89

Acne An inflammatory skin eruption that usually occurs in or near the sebacious glands of the face, neck, shoulders, and upper back, 340, 607

Acrodermatitis enteropathica A rare genetic disorder that impairs zinc absorption, 458

Acrolein A pungent decomposition product of fats, generated from dehydrating glycerol component of fats; responsible for the coughing attacks caused by the fumes released by burning fat. This toxic water-soluble liquid vaporizes easily and is highly flammable, 86

Active transport The movement of substances into or out of cells against a concentration gradient. Active transport requires energy (ATP) and involves carrier (transport) proteins in the cell membrane, 71-72, 110, 213

Activities of Daily Living (ADLs) Activities one needs to perform daily, including personal grooming, eating, getting in and out of bed, walking, taking a bath or shower, using the toilet, and dressing, 639

Additives Substances added to food to perform various functions such as adding color or flavor, replacing sugar or fat, improving nutritional content, or improving texture or shelf life, 172, 204, 691-94, 703

Addresses, Appendix K

Adequate Intake (AI) The nutrient intake that appears to sustain a defined nutritional state or some other indicator of health (e.g., growth rate or normal circulating nutrient values) in a specific population or subgroup. AI is used when there is insuf-ficient scientific evidence to establish an EAR, 44-45

Adipocyte A fat cell, 144

Adipose tissue Body fat tissue, 144, 240, 246

  brown, 291

  metabolic profile, 250-51

  and starvation, 249

  and toxins, 247

Adolescence The period between onset of puberty and childhood, 604-9

  and acne, 340

  and body mass index, 298

  and calcium, 422

  pregnancy during, 564

  protein requirement, 197

  and resting metabolism, 290

  and weight, 305

  See also Eating disorders

ADP (adenosine diphosphate) The compound produced upon hydrolysis of ATP, and used to synthesize ATP. Composed of adenosine and two phosphate groups, 224

Advertising, 7, 537, 599, 650

Aerobic air-ROW-bic Referring to the presence or need of oxygen. The complete breakdown of glucose, fatty acids, and amino acids to carbon dioxide and water occurs only via aerobic metabolism. The citric acid cycle and electron transport chain are aerobic pathways, 227, 311

  See also Oxygen energy system

Aerobic endurance The ability of skeletal muscle to obtain a sufficient supply of oxygen from the heart and lungs to maintain muscular activity for a prolonged time, 485, 500

Aflatoxins Carcinogenic and toxic factors produced by food molds, 683

African Americans

  aging, 624

  children, 601

  and diabetes, 117

  and food security, 712

  and hypertension, 431

  and lactose intolerance, 79

  and pregnancy, 558, 561

Africans, 452-53, 720, 721, 727

  diet, 89, 208, 376, 724

Age factor

  and alcohol, 267, 270

  and athletics, 506

  and body mass index, 298-99

  and calcium, 422, 424

  and caloric density, 143-44

ATP (adenosine triphosphate) ah-DEN-oh-seen try-FOS-fate A high-energy compound that is the main direct fuel that cells use to synthesize molecules, contract muscles, transport substances, and perform other tasks, 224, 228, 229-32, 234, 236-37
chemical structure, F-1
and magnesium, 428
and phosphorous, 426
See also ATP-CP energy system; Lactic acid energy system; Oxygen energy system

ATP-CP energy system A simple and immediate anaerobic energy system that maintains ATP levels. Creatine phosphate is broken down, releasing energy and Pi, which is used to form ATP from ADP, 487

Atrophic gastritis An age-related condition in which the stomach loses its ability to secrete acid. In severe cases, ability to make intrinsic factor is also impaired, 388, 620

Autonomic nervous system The part of the central nervous system that regulates the automatic responses of the body; comprised of the sympathetic and parasympathetic systems, 83, 86

Aversion therapy, 263

Avidin A protein in raw egg whites that binds biotin, preventing its absorption. Avidin is destroyed by heat, 379

Bacteria
and citric acid, 703
exercise, 705
and food safety, 674-79
growth temperature, 685, 688
intestinal, 81-82, 87, 127, 358
in stomach, 86
and teeth, 126
and ulcers, 93
See also Immune response; *Salmonella*

Baking soda, 368

Balance, 33-34

Bananas, 417

Barbiturates, 386

Baryophobia barry-oh-FO-bee-ah An uncommon eating disorder that stunts growth in children and young adults as a result of underfeeding, 540

Basal metabolic rate (BMR) A clinical measure of resting energy expenditure that is performed upon awakening, 10 to 12 hours after eating, and 12 to 18 hours after significant physical activity. Often used interchangeably with RMR, 288-90

Base pairs, 553

Basic Four, 35-36

Beans, 105

Beer, 260, 261, 277, 279, 471

Behavior, eating, 4-11, 285-88, 308, 310, 312-14

Behavior modification, 310, 312-14

Beriberi The thiamin-deficiency disease. Symptoms include muscle weakness, loss of appetite, nerve degeneration, and edema in some cases, 20, 369, 372, 727

Beta (β) bond A chemical bond linking two monosaccharides (glycosidic bond), such as in lactose. Cellulose contains beta bonds that cannot be broken by human intestinal enzymes, 109

Beta-carotene, 19, 337-38, 340-42, F-7

Beta-endorphin A type of opiate that produces a sensation of pleasure, 7

Beta-hydroxybutyrate, 242

Beta-oxidation The breakdown of a fatty acid into numerous molecules of the two-carbon compound acetyl coenzyme A (acetyl CoA), 234, 235
and riboflavin, 372

Beverages
diet soda, 692-93
diuretic effect, 402, 406
fruit juices, 594, 633, 635, 689
and iron, 448
meal-replacement, 309
and phosphorous, 426
smart drinks, 394
See also Caffeine; Sports drinks; Tea

Bicarbonate loading. *See* Soda loading

Bicycling, 292

Bifidobacteria, 87

Bifidus factor A compound in human milk that stimulates the growth of *lactobacillus bifidus* bacteria in the infant's intestinal tract, 571

Bile acids, 391, 394

Bile An alkaline, yellow-green fluid that is produced in the liver and stored in the gallbladder. The primary constituents of bile are bile acids, phospholipids, cholesterol, and bicarbonate. Bile emulsifies dietary fats, aiding fat digestion and absorption, 73, 79, 152, 154

Bile duct, E-2

Bile salts, 154, 155

Binge Consumption of a very large amount of food in a brief time (e.g., 2 hr) accompanied by a loss of control over how much and what is eaten, 533

Binge drinking Consuming excessive amounts of alcohol in short periods of time, 270

Binge eating Consumption of a very large amount of food in a brief period of time (e.g., 2 hr) accompanied by a loss of control over how much and what is eaten, 308

Binge-eating disorder An eating disorder marked by repeated episodes of binge eating and a feeling of loss of control of eating. The diagnosis is based on a person's having an average of at least two binge-eating episodes per week for 6 months, 525, 535-37

Bioavailability A measure of the degree to which a nutrient becomes available to the body after ingestion and thus is available to the tissues, 145
of calcium, 423
of iron, 446-47
of minerals, 413, 444
of riboflavin, 373
of thiamin, 371
of zinc, 456

Biochemical assessment Assessment by measuring a nutrient or its metabolite in one or more body fluids such as blood and urine, and in feces. Also called laboratory assessment, 59

Biochemistry, Appendix F

Biocytin A biotin-lysine complex released from digested protein, 378

Biodiversity The countless species of plants, animals and insects that exist on the earth. An undisturbed tropical forest is an example of the biodiversity of a healthy ecosystem, 701

Bioelectrical impedance analysis (BIA) im-PEE-dance The resistance of tissue to the flow of an alternating electric current, which is used to estimate amounts of total body water, lean tissue mass, and total body fat, 301

Biological value (BV) The extent to which protein in a food can be incorporated into body proteins, BV is expressed as the percentage of the absorbed dietary nitrogen retained in the body, 202-3

Biosynthesis Chemical reactions that form simple molecules into complex biomolecules, especially carbohydrates, lipids, protein, nucleotides, and nucleic acids, 224, 230, 234, 237-44

Biotechnology The set of laboratory techniques and processes used to modify the genome of plants or animals, and thus create desirable new characteristics. Genetic engineering in the broad sense, 697, 722-23

Biotin, 81, 378-79, F-12, F-14

Biotinidase An enzyme in the small intestine that releases biotin from biocytin, 379

Birth defects, 17, 273, 340, 384

Black currant seed oil, 150

Bladder, 635

Osteoporosis A bone disease characterized by a decrease in bone mineral density and the appearance of small holes in bones due to loss of minerals, 51, 53, 348, 432-35
and adolescence, 606
Osteoporosis—cont'd
and alcohol, 265
and calcium, 422, 425
in elderly, 638
and exercise, 502
and female athletes, 514
and fluoride, 469
and sodium, 416
Overeaters Anonymous, 309
Overnutrition The long-term consumption of an excess of nutrients. The most common type of overnutrition in the United States is due to the regular consumption of excess kilocalories, fats, saturated fats, and cholesterol, 32, 56
Overweight Body weight in relation to height that is greater than some accepted standard but less than that defined as obesity, 302-5
See also Obesity; Weight; Weight management
Oxalate (oxalic acid) An organic acid in some leafy green vegetables, such as spinach, that binds to calcium to form calcium oxalate, an insoluble compound the body cannot absorb, 413, 434
and iron, 448
Oxaloacetate (acid) A four-carbon intermediate compound in the citric acid cycle. Acetyl CoA combines with free oxaloacetate in the mitochondria to form citrate and enter the cycle, 229, 234-35, 236, 244-45, 491
Oxidation Oxygen attaches to the double bonds of unsaturated fatty acids. Rancid fats are oxidized fats, 147
of amino acids, 237
of glucose, 227-32
Oxidative phosphorylation Formation of ATP from ADP and P_i coupled to the flow of electrons along the electron transport chain, 231
Oxygen energy system A complex energy system that requires oxygen. To release ATP, it completes the breakdown of carbohydrate and fatty acids via the citric acid cycle and electron transport chain, 489-90
Oxygen transport, 444
Oxytocin A pituitary hormone that stimulates the release of milk from the breast, 567
Oysters, 272

Pagophagia, 454
Palatable Pleasant or acceptable to the palate or taste, 504

Palmar grasp Infant's use of entire palm to pick up items; an early gross motor skill, 590
Pancreas The pancreas secretes enzymes that affect the digestion and absorption of nutrients and releases hormones, such as insulin, which regulate metabolism as well as the disposition of the end products of food in the body, 74, 113, 191, E2-E3
and alcohol intake, 265
and Vitamin A, 338
and zinc, 455
See also Glucagon; Insulin
Pancreatic amylase Starch-digesting enzyme secreted by the pancreas, 108
Pancreatic cancer, 211
Pancreatic duct, E-3
Pancreatic lipase, 154
Pangamic acid, 395
Pantothenic acid, 377-78, F-12, F-14
Para-aminobenzoic acid (PABA), 395
Parasites, 726
Parathyroid hormone A hormone secreted by the parathyroid glands in response to low blood calcium. It stimulates calcium release from bone and calcium absorption by the intestines, while decreasing calcium excretion by the kidneys. It acts in conjunction with calcitriol to raise blood calcium. Also called parathormone, 346, 422, 425, 427
Parkinson's disease, 151
Passive diffusion The movement of substances into or out of cells without the expenditure of energy or the involvement of transport proteins in the cell membrane. Also called simple diffusion, 71, 72
Pasta, 100
Pasteurization A process for destroying pathogenic bacteria by heating liquid foods to a prescribed temperature for a specified time, 694, 695
Pathogenic Capable of causing disease, 513
Pathogens, 674-79, 685, 688, 703
Pectin A type of soluble fiber found in fruits, 89, 107
Peer review An appraisal of research against accepted standards by professionals in the field, 23
Pellagra, 20, 376, 727
Pentose A sugar molecule containing five carbon atoms, 102-3
Pentose phosphate pathway, 370
Pepsin A protein-digesting enzyme produced by the stomach, 75, 191
Pepsinogen The inactive form of the enzyme pepsin, 75, 191
Peptidases Enzymes that act on small peptide units by breaking peptide bonds, 191
Peptide, 182, F-1

Peptide bond The bond between two amino acids formed when a carboxyl (−COOH) group of one amino acid joins an amino (−NH$_2$) group of another amino acid, releasing water in the process, 182
Perceived exertion The subjective experience of how difficult an effort is
Percent fat free, 53
Peripheral nervous system
alcohol effect, 265, 268
Peristalsis Per-ih-STAHL-sis The wavelike, rhythmic muscular contractions of the GI tract that propel its contents down the tract, 69-70, 81
Pernicious anemia Result of the inability to absorb vitamin B$_{12}$. Hallmarks of the condition are excess megaloblasts and nerve degeneration that can result in paralysis and death, 389
Personal Responsibility and Work Opportunity Reconciliation Act A 1996 federal welfare reform plan that dramatically changed the nation's welfare system into one that requires work in exchange for time-limited assistance. Also called the Welfare Reform Act, 712
Pesticides Chemicals used to control insects, diseases, weeds, fungi, and other pests on plants, vegetables, fruits, and animals, 679-81, 682, 694
See also Bt gene
Petechiae, 59
pH A measurement of the hydrogen ion concentration, or acidity, of a solution. The pH scale ranges from 0 to 14, with a value of 7 representing neutral pH at which the concentrations of H+ and hydroxyl ions (OH−) are equal. A pH lower than 7 is acidic; a pH higher than 7 is alkaline, 75, 188-89
and chloride, 419
and ketogenesis, 243
and water, 403
Phagocytosis The process by which cells engulf large particles and small microorganisms. Receptors on the surface of cells bind these particles and organisms to bring them into large vesicles in the cytoplasm. From *phago*, "eating," and *cyto*, "cell," 72
Phenobarbital, 373
Phentermine, 315
Phenylalanine, 124-25, 181, 204, F-4
for PKU infants, 595
Phenylketonuria (PKU) An inherited disorder caused by a lack or deficiency of the enzyme that converts phenylalanine to tyrosine, 125, 181-82, 467, 564, 595
Phosphate group A chemical group (−PO$_4$) on a larger molecule, where the phosphorus is single bonded to each of the 4 oxygens,

Photo Credits

Chapter openers created by Studio Montage

All incidental and background photos and art © PhotoDisc, Corbis Digital Images, Hemera Photo Objects

4 (T) © PhotoDisc, (B) © Mickey Pfleger/PictureQuest; 5 Photos courtesy of J.E. Steiner; 6(T1) © Karl Weatherly/PhotoDisc, (T2) © Owen Franken/CORBIS, (T3) © Suza Scalora/PhotoDisc, (T4) © Jules Frazier/PhotoDisc; 6(B) © PhotoDisc; 7 (T) © PhotoDisc, (B) Courtesy of The National Dairy Council; 8 (T) © Bruce Ayers/Tony Stone, (B) © PhotoDisc; 9 (T) © Corbis Digital Images, (M) © PhotoDisc, (B) © Peter Menzel/Stock, Boston Inc./PictureQuest; 10(B) © Corbis Digital Images; 11 © PhotoDisc; 14 (T) © PhotoDisc, (M) © PhotoDisc, (B) © PhotoDisc; 15 (T) © PhotoDisc, (M) © Mitch Hrdlicka/PhotoDisc, (B) © PhotoDisc; 18 (L) © Digital Vision, (R) © Corbis Digital Images; 19 © Corbis Digital Images; 26 Courtesy of the FDA; 32 © NovaStock/Photo Researchers, Inc.; 33(T) © Adobe Image Library; 37 (T) © PhotoDisc, (B) © PhotoDisc; 43 © Hisham F. Ibrahim/PhotoDisc; 44 © Hisham F. Ibrahim/PhotoDisc; 46 all © Jones and Bartlett Publishers; 47 all © Jones and Bartlett Publishers; 49 © Jones and Bartlett Publishers; 54 © Jones and Bartlett Publishers; 64 Photomicrograph of villi © Prof P. Motta/Dept. of Anatomy/University La Sapienza, Rome/Science Photo Library; 66 © PhotoDisc; 86 (a) © EyeWire, (b) © Chris Shorten/Cole Group/PhotoDisc, (c) © PhotoLink/PhotoDisc, (d) © USDA/Science Source/Photo Researchers, Inc., (B) © Dr. E. Walker/Science Photo Library; 94 © PhotoDisc; 100 (TL) © Sylvan Wittwer/Visuals Unlimited, (TR) © David Nance/ARS Photo Library/USDA, (BL) © ARS Photo Library/USDA, (BR) USDA; 105 © Owen Schwartz and B Gunning, from their CDROM on Plant Cell Biology (unpublished); 107(T) © Eyewire, (B) © J. D. Litvay/Visuals Unlimited; 114(T) © Digital Vision, (B) © PhotoDisc; 117 © Barros & Barros/ImageBank; 118 © Don Tremain/PhotoDisc; p.119 © Hemera Photo Objects; 126 © Corbis Digital Images; 127 © Corbis Digital Images; 143 © Steve Mason/PhotoDisc; 144 © Veronica Burmeister/Visuals Unlimited; 145 © PhotoDisc; 150 © Jones and Bartlett Publishers; 159 © W. Ober/Visuals Unlimited; 161 © PhotoDisc; 162 © Hemera Photo Objects; 169 © PhotoDisc; 170 © PhotoDisc; 171 © Hemera Photo Objects; 180 (T) © Digital Vision, (B) © PhotoDisc; 195 (L) © EyeWire, (M) © Keith Brofsky/PhotoDisc, (R) © EyeWire; 196 (T) © Jess Alford/PhotoDisc, (M) © Jules Frazier/PhotoDisc, (B) © PhotoLink/PhotoDisc; 197 © Don Smetzer/Tony Stone; 198 © PhotoDisc; 199 © PhotoDisc; 200 all © PhotoDisc; 201 © PhotoDisc; 204 © Jones and Bartlett Publishers; 206 © Photodisc; 209 (T) © Charles Cecil/Visuals Unlimited, (B) © Seamus Murphy/SABA; 218 Photomicrograph of skeletal muscle © Quest/Science Photo Library; 238 © Adobe Image Library; 246 © Bob Montesclaros/Cole Group/PhotoDisc; 258 (R) © Ryan McVay/PhotoDisc, (L) © Hemera Photo Objects; 259 (TL) © Jack Star/PhotoLink/PhotoDisc, (TR) © Mitch Hrdlicka/PhotoDisc, (B) © Yoav Levy/PictureQuest; 261 © David M. Phillips/Visuals Unlimited; 262(T) © Hemera Photo Objects; 266 (T) © PhotoDisc, (B) © Hemera Photo Objects; 267 © PhotoDisc; 268 © Tomi/PhotoLink/PhotoDisc; 272 (T) © OJ Staats/Custom Medical Stock Photography, (B) © Hemera Photo Objects; 274(L) © Hemera Photo Objects; 276 © Hemera Photo Objects; 279(T) © Hemera Photo Objects; 284 (TL) © Hemera Photo Objects, (TR) © PhotoDisc; 284 illustrations © Font Haus; 285 © PhotoDisc; 287 © AP Photo/John Sholtis; 288 © PhotoDisc; 289 © PhotoDisc; 293 © Jones and Bartlett Publishers Publishers; 299(T) © Jones and Bartlett Publishers, (B) Courtesy of Life Measurement Instruments; 300 © PhotoDisc; 301(T) © Jones and Bartlett Publishers, (B) © Simon Fraser/Newcastle General Hospital/Photo Researchers, Inc.; 302 (L) © SPL/Custom Medical Stock Photo, (R) © SPL/Custom Medical Stock Photo; 308 © Hemera Photo Objects; 309(T) © Hemera Photo Objects; 310 (T) Rubens: The Three Graces, 1640 (oil on canvas), Prado, Madrid, © The Bridgeman Art Library, (M)

Edgar Dega, After the Bath. Mus. D'Orsay, Paris, © Pix/FPG, (B) © AP Photo/Mark J. Terrill; 312 © Karl Weatherly/PhotoDisc; 315 © Michael Philip Manheim/Photo Network/ PictureQuest; 316 © Jones and Bartlett Publishers; 328 (T) © Logical Images/Custom Medical Stock Photography, (B) © EyeWire; 334 © Joe Valbuena/ USDA; 338 © Corbis Digital Images; 339 (T) © Hemera Photo Objects, (B) © Corbis Digital Images; 340 © C Squared Studios/PhotoDisc; 342 © Hemera Photo Objects; 344 © Hemera Photo Objects; 348(T) © Greg Kuchik/PhotoDisc, (B) © Dr. Michael Klein/Peter Arnold, Inc.; 354 (T) © Corbis Digital Images, (B) © Siede Preis/PhotoDisc; 355 © Corbis Digital Images; 356 © CNRI/Science Photo Library/Photo Researcher, Inc.; 358 © CNRI/Science Photo Library/Photo Researchers, Inc.; 359 (T) © Corbis Digital Images, (BL) © PhotoLink/PhotoDisc; 360 © Hemera Photo Objects; 368 (T) © Jones and Bartlett Publishers, (B) © Hemera Photo Objects; 369 © Hemera Photo Objects; 371 © John a. Rizzo/PhotoDisc; 372 © L. V. Bergman/The Bergman Collection; 373 © Richard Pasley/Stock, Boston/PictureQuest; 375 (L) © Digital Vision, (R) © Hemera Photo Objects; 376 © Peter Essick/PictureQuest; 379 © Geostock/ PhotoDisc; 381 © John A. Rizzo/PhotoDisc; 383(L) © Hemera Photo Objects; 385 © PhotoLink/ PhotoDisc; 389 © PhotoLink/PhotoDisc; 391 © Digital Vision; 392 © Hemera Photo Objects ; 393 © Corbis Digital Images; 403 © Hermann Eisenheiss/Photo Researchers, Inc.; 409 © Hemera Photo Objects; 410 © Hemera Photo Objects; 414 © Hemera Photo Objects; 417 © Corbis Digital Images; 419 © CNRI/ Science Photo Library/Photo Researchers, Inc.; 420 © Hemera Photo Objects; 423 © Hemera Photo Objects; 428 © Corbis Digital Images; 429 © Santokh Kochar/PhotoDisc; 434 Photos reprinted with permission from Calcified Tissue Research, 1967; 442(B) © Scott Bauer/ARS Photo Library/USDA; 450 © Cole Group/PhotoDisc; 451 © Hemera Photo Objects; 460 © John A. Rizzo/PhotoDisc; 462 © Martin Rotker/Phototake; 464 © Hemera Photo Objects; 468 © Hemera Photo Objects; 469 © NIH/Custom Medical Stock Photograpy; 470 © Hemera Photo Objects; 472 © Corbis Digital Images; 473 © Hemera Photo Objects; 492 © Hemera Photo Objects; 494 © AP Photo/Nils Meilvang; 496 © Corbis Digital Images; 505 © Hemera Photo Objects; 507 © Jones and Bartlett Publishers; 511 © PhotoDisc; 512 © Hemera Photo Objects; 514 © AP Photo/Kamran Jebrili; 515 © Hemera Photo Objects; 524(R) © PhotoDisc, (L) © PhotoDisc; 526(T) © Hulton-Deutch Collection/CORBIS, (B) © Linda DeBruyn; 529 © Tony Latham/Tony Stone; 531 © RubberBall Productions/EyeWire; 532 © Jack Star/PhotoLink/PhotoDisc; 534 © Jack Star/PhotoLink/PhotoDisc; 535 © RubberBall Productions/EyeWire; 536 illustration © Font Haus; 537 © Jack Star/PhotoLink/PhotoDisc; 539 © AP Photo/AP World Wide; 540 © Gerard Loucel; 548 (T) © Hemera Photo Objects, (B) © PhotoDisc; 551 © Mel Curtis/PhotoDisc; 552 © Lennart Nilsson/ A Child Is Born; 557 © Ian O'Leary/Tony Stone Images; 561 © David H. Wells/CORBIS; 580(TL)© David R. Austen/Stock, Boston/PictureQuest; 580(M) © Lynne Siler/Focus Group/PictureQuest; 580(B) © Michael Newman/PhotoEdit/PictureQuest; 580(TR) © PhotoDisc; 584 © PhotoDisc; 585 © Jones and Bartlett Publishers; 587 © Myrleen Ferguson Cate/Photo Network/PictureQuest; 593 © Gill/Custom Medical Stock Photography; 605 © SW Productions/PhotoDisc; 606 © PhotoDisc; 608 © Rubber Ball Productions/EyeWire; 609 © SW Productions/PhotoDisc; 620(T) © PhotoLink/PhotoDisc, (B) © PhotoLink/PhotoDisc; 634 © Susan Lerner/Design Conceptions/Joel Gordon; 638 © Bill Aron/PhotoEdit; 657 © PhotoDisc; 680 © PhotoDisc; 681 © Scott Camazine/Photo Researchers Inc.; 685(TL) © PhotoDisc, (BL) © PhotoLink/PhotoDisc, (TR) © C Squared Studios/PhotoDisc, (BR) © Siede Preis/PhotoDisc; 689 Illustration courtesy of Partnership for Food Safety Education; 693 Photos © Corbis Digital Images; 695 (T, M) © Corbis Digital Images, (B) © Hemera Photo Objects; 713 (T) © PhotoDisc, (M1) © Skip Nall/PhotoDisc, (M2) © Jack Star/PhotoLink/PhotoDisc, (B) © PhotoDisc; 716 (T) © AP Photo/Danny Johnston, (B) © Bob Daemmrich/Stock, Boston/PictureQuest

Tolerable Upper Intake Levels (UL[1])

Life stage group	Vitamin A[2] (µg/d)	Vitamin D (µg/d)	Vitamin E[3,4] (mg/d)	Niacin[4] (mg/d)	Vitamin B$_6$ (mg/d)	Folate[4] (µg/d)	Vitamin C (mg/d)	Choline (g/d)	Calcium (g/d)	Phosphorus (g/d)	Magnesium[5] (mg/d)
Infants											
0-6 mo	600	25	ND[7]	ND	ND	ND	ND	ND	ND	ND	ND
7-12 mo	600	25	ND	ND	ND	ND	ND	ND	ND	ND	ND
Children											
1-3 y	600	50	200	10	30	300	400	1.0	2.5	3	65
4-8 y	900	50	300	15	40	400	650	1.0	2.5	3	110
Males, females											
9-13 y	1,700	50	600	20	60	600	1,200	2.0	2.5	4	350
14-18 y	2,800	50	800	30	80	800	1,800	3.0	2.5	4	350
19-70 y	3,000	50	1,000	35	100	1,000	2,000	3.5	2.5	4	350
>70 y	3,000	50	1,000	35	100	1,000	2,000	3.5	2.5	3	350
Pregnancy											
≤18 y	2,800	50	800	30	80	800	1,800	3.0	2.5	3.5	350
19-50 y	3,000	50	1,000	35	100	1,000	2,000	3.5	2.5	3.5	350
Lactation											
≤18 y	2,800	50	800	30	80	800	1,800	3.0	2.5	4	350
19-50 y	3,000	50	1,000	35	100	1,000	2,000	3.5	2.5	4	350

Life stage group	Iron (mg/d)	Zinc (mg/d)	Selenium (µg/d)	Iodine (µg/d)	Copper (µg/d)	Manganese (mg/d)	Fluoride (mg/d)	Molybdenum (µg/d)	Boron (mg/d)	Nickel (mg/d)	Vanadium[6] (mg/d)
Infants											
0-6 mo	40	4	45	ND	ND	ND	0.7	ND	ND	ND	ND
7-12 mo	40	5	60	ND	ND	ND	0.9	ND	ND	ND	ND
Children											
1-3 y	40	7	90	200	1,000	2	1.3	300	3	0.2	ND
4-8 y	40	12	150	300	3,000	3	2.2	600	6	0.3	ND
Males, females											
9-13 y	40	23	280	600	5,000	6	10	1,100	11	0.6	ND
14-18 y	45	34	400	900	8,000	9	10	1,700	17	1.0	ND
19-70 y	45	40	400	1,100	10,000	11	10	2,000	20	1.0	1.8
>70 y	45	40	400	1,100	10,000	11	10	2,000	20	1.0	1.8
Pregnancy											
≤18 y	45	34	400	900	8,000	9	10	1,700	17	1.0	ND
19-50 y	45	40	400	1,100	10,000	11	10	2,000	20	1.0	ND
Lactation											
≤18 y	45	34	400	900	8,000	9	10	1,700	17	1.0	ND
19-50 y	45	40	400	1,100	10,000	11	10	2,000	20	1.0	ND

[1]UL = The maximum level of daily nutrient intake that is likely to pose no risk of adverse effects. Unless otherwise specified, the UL represents total intake from food, water, and supplements. Due to lack of suitable data, ULs could not be established for vitamin K, thiamin, riboflavin, vitamin B$_{12}$, pantothenic acid, biotin, carotenoids, arsenic, chromium, or silicon. In the absence of ULs, extra caution may be warranted in consuming levels above recommended intakes.

[2]As preformed vitamin A (retinol) only.

[3]As α-tocopherol; applies to any form of supplemental α-tocopherol.

[4]The ULs for vitamin E, niacin, and folate apply to synthetic forms obtained from supplements, fortified foods, or a combination of the two.

[5]The ULs for magnesium represent intake from a pharmacological agent only and do not include intake from food and water.

[6]Although vanadium in food has not been shown to cause adverse effects in humans, there is no justification for adding vanadium to food and vanadium supplements should be used with caution. The UL is based on adverse effects in laboratory animals and these data could be used to set a UL for adults but not children or adolescents.

[7]ND = Not determinable due to lack of data on adverse effects in this age group and concern with regard to lack of ability to handle excess amounts. Source of intake should be from food only to prevent high levels of intake.

Sources: Data compiled from *Dietary Reference Intakes for Calcium, Phosphorus, Magnesium, Vitamin D, and Fluoride*. Washington, DC: National Academy Press; 1997. *Dietary Reference Intakes for Thiamin, Riboflavin, Niacin, Vitamin B$_6$, Folate, Vitamin B$_{12}$, Pantothenic Acid, and Choline*. Washington, DC: National Academy Press; 1998. *Dietary Reference Intakes for Vitamin C, Vitamin E, Selenium, and Carotenoids*. Washington, DC: National Academy Press; 2000. *Dietary Reference Intakes for Vitamin A, Vitamin K, Arsenic, Boron, Chromium, Copper, Iodine, Iron, Manganese, Molybdenum, Nickel, Silicon, Vanadium, and Zinc*. Washington, DC: National Academy Press; 2001. These reports may be accessed via http://nap.edu.